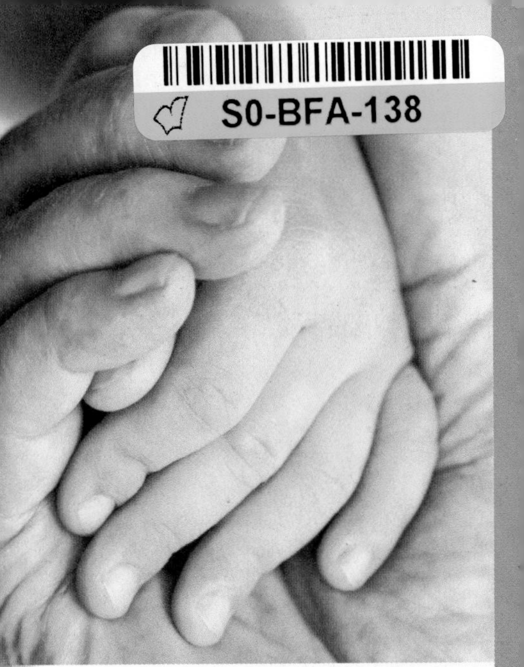

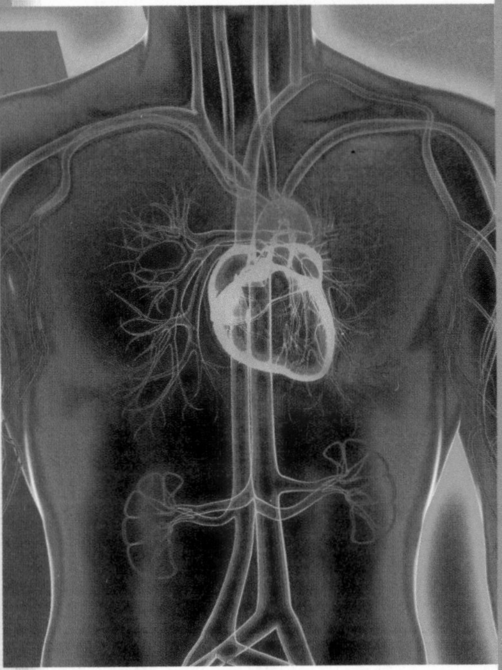

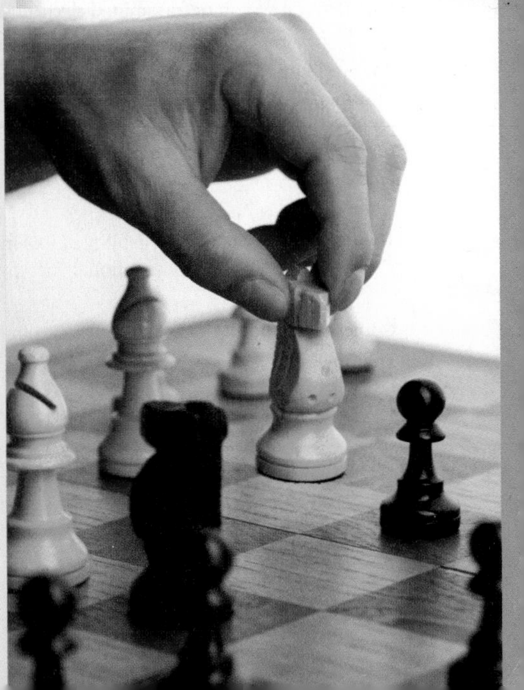

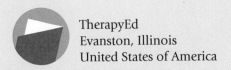

THERAPYED'S

National Occupational Therapy Certification Exam Review & Study Guide

7th EDITION

RITA P. FLEMING-CASTALDY, PHD, OTL, FAOTA
Associate Professor of Occupational Therapy
University of Scranton
Scranton, PA

TherapyEd
Evanston, Illinois
United States of America

Library of Congress Control Number: 00-134576

ISBN: 978-0-9843393-9-6

Copies of this book and software may be obtained from:
TherapyEd
500 Davis Street, Suite 512
Evanston, IL 60201
Telephone (847) 328-5361
Fax (847) 328-5049
www.TherapyEd.com

Preface

The *National Occupational Therapy Certification Exam Review & Study Guide* is designed to assist United States and internationally educated candidates in their preparation for the National Board for Certification in Occupational Therapy (NBCOT®) examination for registered occupational therapists (OTRs®). This *Review and Study Guide* provides a comprehensive overview of the depth and breadth of current occupational therapy practice according to the field's seminal textbooks, the American Occupational Therapy Association's (AOTA's) *Guide to Occupational Therapy Practice*, AOTA's *Standards of Practice*, and AOTA's *Practice Framework*. Since this text's first edition in 2000, many have reported that it has served as an invaluable resource during their professional coursework and clinical affiliations. This text can also be helpful to practitioners who are new to the field, changing practice areas, and/or initiating a new role (e.g., fieldwork supervisor).

The text chapters cover all of the practice domains established by the NBCOT® most current examination blueprint. While the text contributors did not have access to an actual examination or to specific examination items, all chapter content and the computer-based examinations are based on the authors' critical review of the NBCOT®'s most recent publications and the textbooks the NBCOT® identifies as foundational to the examination. Because the NBCOT® examination items cover the entirety of the OT profession, information that is foundational to entry-level OT practice (i.e., anatomy, physiology, kinesiology, theoretical models, OT tools of practice, clinical conditions, and practice standards) is provided. This solid foundation is required to clinically reason through examination items and ensure that the exam candidate acquires the "knowledge essential for effective practice in occupational therapy" (NBCOT®, 2012, p. 5).

Specific methods of evaluation and intervention are provided in chapters organized according to clinical approaches, rather than according to diagnosis. This holistic, integrative approach allows for in-depth coverage while eliminating redundancy and reductionism. It also makes this text compatible with a multitude of OT professional curriculum designs. For example, the chapter on cognitive-perceptual approaches includes evaluation and intervention methods for cognitive-perceptual dysfunction that are relevant to many psychiatric and neurological disorders. References for sources which served as the foundation for text content are provided at the end of each chapter.

Each chapter in this *Review and Study Guide* is presented in an outline format that is easy to read and provides a helpful guide for organizing a study plan. Upon reviewing each chapter's outline, the exam candidate will be able to assess his/her level of comfort with, and mastery of, each content area. Identification of areas of strength and weakness can bolster confidence and help focus studying in an efficient and effective manner. This text is not a substitute for primary resources such as classroom lectures and course textbooks. However, by first using this text, the exam candidate will not spend time extensively studying information already known. Rather, specific areas in which further knowledge is required will be identified, and appropriate study time can be planned. Strategies for effective examination preparation and successful test-taking and opportunities to practice their use via three computer-based examinations are provided.

Completion of this text's simulated examinations will help exam candidates evaluate their preparedness for the certification examination. Consistent with the NBCOT® examination format, this text's examination items are designed to test mastery of professional knowledge by asking the candidate to apply this knowledge to practice situations. Detailed explanations are provided to help exam candidates understand why one answer is considered the best response and the others are incorrect. The critical analysis of this information can be used to identify content areas requiring further study. The critical reasoning skills used to determine the correct responses to the examination items are also analyzed to provide additional information that can guide successful examination preparation.

Table of Contents

Computer Simulated Examinations

Contributors

Marge E. Moffett Boyd, MPH, OTR/L
Coordinator of Academic Studies and Fieldwork
Clinical Instructor, Program of Occupational Therapy
Dominican College
Orangeburg, NY

Ann Burkhardt, OTD, OTR/L, FAOTA
Occupational Therapist
Therapy Resources Management
Fall River, MA

Donna M. Costa, DHS, OTR/L, FAOTA
Associate Professor School of Occupational Therapy
Touro University Nevada
Henderson, NV

Josephine Dolera, PT
Director of Rehabilitation
Union Community Health Center
Bronx, NY

Jan G. Garbarini, MA, OTR/L
Research Coordinator
Occupational Therapy Department
Dominican College
Orangeburg, NY

Glen Gillen, EdD, OTR, FAOTA
Associate Professor
Regenerative and Rehabilitation Medicine
(Occupational Therapy)
Columbia University Medical Center
Programs in Occupational Therapy
Columbia University
New York, NY

Kari Inda, PhD, OTR
Chairperson, Associate Professor
Occupational Therapy Department
Mount Mary University
Milwaukee, WI

Linda Kahn-D'Angelo, ScD, PT
Professor
Department of Physical Therapy
College of Health Professions
University of Massachusetts Lowell
Lowell, MA

William Lambert, MS, OTR/L
Faculty Specialist
Department of Occupational and Physical Therapy
The University of Scranton
Scranton, PA

Regina Lehman, MS, OTR/L
Assistant Professor & Program Director
Occupational Therapy Assistant Program
LaGuardia Community College
Long Island City, NY

Colleen Maher, MS, OTR, CHT
Assistant Professor of Occupational Therapy
University of Sciences
Samson College of Health Sciences
Philadelphia, PA

Colleen De Riitis, MA, OTR/L
Senior Occupational Therapist
Meridian Nursing and Rehabilitation
Brick, NJ

Susan B.O'Sullivan, PT, EdD
Professor Emerita
Department of Physical Therapy
School of Health and Environment
University of Massachusetts Lowell
Lowell, MA

Susan C. Robertson, PhD, OTR/L, FAOTA
Health and Education Resources
Bethesda, MD

Janice Romeo, MA, OTR/L
Retired, Seattle, WA
Formerly Student Coordinator
Rehabilitation Department
Hagedorn Psychiatric Hospital
Glen Gardner, NJ

Julie Ann Starr, PT, MS, CCS
Clinical Associate Professor
Physical Therapy Program
Department of Rehabilitation Sciences
Sargent College of Health and Rehabilitation Sciences
Boston University
Boston, MA

Toni Thompson, MA, OTR/L, C/NDT
Senior Instructor, TherapyEd
Consultant, Shriners Hospitals for Children
Tampa, FL

Patricia Wisniewski, MS, OTR/L, CPRP
Faculty Specialist
Department of Occupational and Physical Therapy
The University of Scranton
Scranton, PA

Acknowledgments

Organizing the depth and breadth of occupational therapy education and practice into a comprehensive review book and study guide can be a daunting task. It can easily become overwhelming if it were not for the capable assistance of others. Kristin Leccese (former University of Scranton graduate assistant), Katherine Regimbal (former University of Scranton work-study employee), and Samantha Zarro and Stephanie Freije (University of Scranton work-study employees) provided essential research and editorial support. Judy Noe of TherapyEd helped obtain and track the copyright permissions which were needed to make sure that this text contained relevant tables and figures to support its content. Past editions of this text benefited from the excellent production and editorial assistance of Jenna Osborn and John Patro (former University of Scranton graduate assistants), Sue Ward (former secretary for TherapyEd), Kathleen Smyth (former personal administrative assistant), and Raymond Siegelman, President of TherapyEd.

1

Certification of the Occupational Therapist, Registered (OTR)

RITA P. FLEMING-CASTALDY

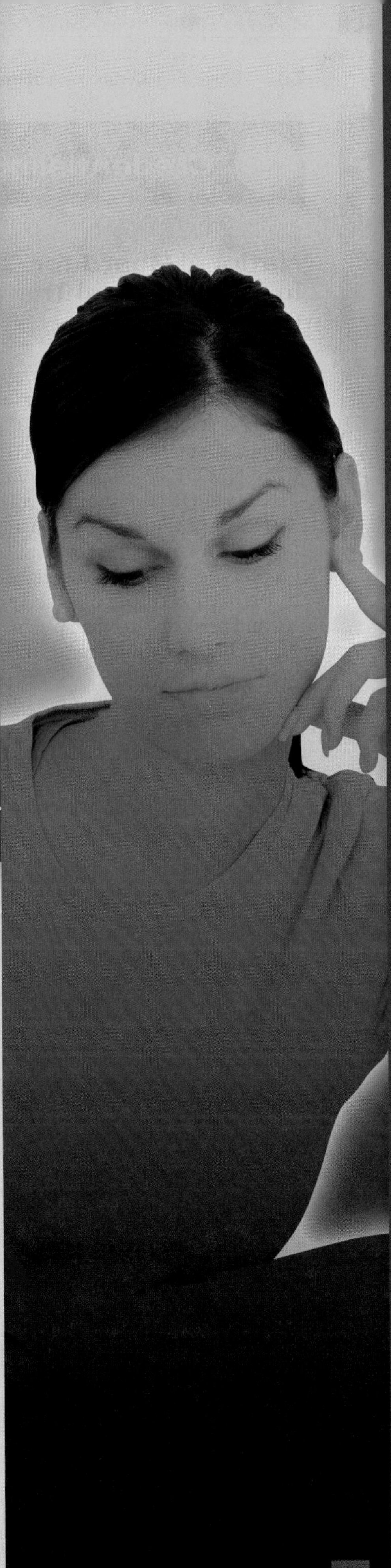

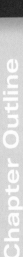

Chapter Outline

Chapter 1

Credentialing Agencies

National Board for Certification in Occupational Therapy (NBCOT)

1. The NBCOT is currently the only national independent credentialing agency for occupational therapy (OT) practitioners, including therapists and occupational therapy assistants (OTAs).
2. The NBCOT develops and implements all policies related to OT professional certification, including the national certification examinations and the NBCOT certification renewal program.
   a. NBCOT holds the copyright to the designations certified occupational therapy assistant (COTA®) and occupational therapist, registered (OTR®).
      (1) Individuals not certified by NBCOT cannot use these credentials.
   b. NBCOT certification is not equivalent to state certification, licensure, or registration.
   c. NBCOT certification is initially granted for three years. Certification must be renewed every three years according to the procedures of the NBCOT Certification Renewal Program.
3. NBCOT's official website (www.nbcot.org) contains all current information about the NBCOT certification process.
   a. As an independent organization, NBCOT can change their certification requirements and procedures at any time; therefore, this website should be consulted on a regular basis by exam candidates.

State Regulatory Boards (SRBs)

1. SRBs are public bodies created by legislation to define and regulate the qualifications a professional must have to practice within his or her state.
2. State regulation may take the form of certification, registration, or licensure.
   a. The terms "registration," "licensure," and "certification" are often used interchangeably even though they are different types of regulations.
   b. Definitions of, and requirements for, state certification, registration or licensure vary from state to state. Therefore, each state regulation should be carefully reviewed to ensure understanding of its requirements and provisions.
      (1) See text's Appendix 3 for contact information for each state.
3. It is against the law to practice OT without meeting state requirements for certification, registration, or licensure.
4. Some states grant temporary practice licenses to individuals eligible to become licensed in the state.
5. SRBs should be contacted directly to obtain their regulations and an application. Most states do not have reciprocal agreements, so you must meet the requirements of every state in which you intend to practice.
6. Most states accept a passing grade on the NBCOT certification exams as one qualifying criterion for initial state licensure, registration, and/or certification.
   a. If you want your NBCOT certification exam score to be sent to an SRB you must indicate this on your application and pay a fee in accordance with NBCOT's Certification Examination Handbook guidelines.
   b. Most states do not require ongoing NBCOT certification to maintain licensure, registration and/or certification.
7. States vary in the additional criteria they require to attain and/or maintain licensure, registration, and/or certification. A passing NBCOT score does not ensure attainment of state licensure registration, or certification.
   a. Occupational therapists who allow their state licensure, registration, or certification to lapse for several years are required by some states to re-take and pass the NBCOT exam in order to renew their state credentials.

Certification Examination Content and Format

Background Information

1. Practice analysis.
   a. NBCOT conducts periodic surveys (typically every five years) of occupational therapy practitioners to validate the domains, tasks, and knowledge statements "appropriate for inclusion on a certification examination for entry-level occupational therapists" (NBCOT, 2012, p. 19).
   b. The analysis of these survey results is used to construct the blueprint of the exam, create exam specifications, and guide the writing of exam items.

c. The exam blueprint implemented in January 2014 was derived from the outcomes of a practice analysis study completed in 2012 (NBCOT, 2012).
   (1) This *Review and Study Guide* presents the most current information available at the time of its publication about the NBCOT exams content, format, administration, and scoring.

2. Certification Examination Development Committee (CEDC).
   a. The CEDC is composed of experts in the exam content areas who represent a diversity of practice settings, geographic regions, and demographics and have completed an item writing training program.
   b. The CEDC uses the exam specifications developed from the practice analysis to guide their item development.
3. Item development.
   a. Exam items are developed to differentiate the presence of inadequate from adequate entry-level practice knowledge and skills.
   b. All exam items are reviewed for appropriateness in measuring the knowledge and skills needed for entry-level OT practice.
   c. All exam items are also reviewed to ensure that the language, context, terminology, descriptions, and content are unbiased, inoffensive, and appropriate to all population groups.

Examination Content

1. The NBCOT exam tests four domains of OT practice with each domain comprising a set percentage of the exam.[1] As of January 2014, these domains and percentages are:
   a. Domain 01: Acquire information regarding factors that influence occupational performance throughout the occupational therapy process: 17%.
   b. Domain 02: Formulate conclusions regarding client's needs and priorities to develop and monitor an intervention plan throughout the occupational therapy process: 28%.
   c. Domain 03: Select interventions for managing a client-centered plan throughout the occupational therapy process: 45%.
   d. Domain 04: Manage and direct occupational therapy services to promote quality throughout the occupational therapy process: 10% (NBCOT, 2012, p. 19).
2. Specific task and knowledge statements for each domain are provided in the ***2012 Practice Analysis of the Occupational Therapist Executive Summary*** which is available on the NBCOT's website.
3. Exam content reflects language typically used in practice and is not based on any one practice framework model.
   a. Certain aspects of a given practice framework (e.g., American Occupational Therapy Association [AOTA]'s) may be integrated into the exam's content if they represent exam specifications as determined by an NBCOT practice analysis.
4. A large item bank is maintained so that each exam will be composed of a unique combination of items drawn from this bank.
   a. Different versions of the exam are offered simultaneously.
   b. Items are selected according to the weightings of exam domains and content areas to ensure each exam contains consistent percentages of each domain and content area.

Examination Format

1. The NBCOT exam is comprised of 170 multiple-choice (MC) items and three simulation test (ST) items.
   a. Each administered exam contains items that NBCOT is pre-testing for future exams.
      (1) The pre-test items are not considered operational and they are not scored.
      (2) The pre-test items are intermixed with the items that are scored. These items have been pre-equated by NBCOT and deemed operational.
      (3) Pre-test items that perform well statistically will become part of the operational pre-equated item bank used for future exams.
      (4) There are no identifying characteristics to distinguish unscored pre-test items from the scored operational items; therefore, you must answer each item as if it counts.
2. Multiple choice (MC) items: Traditional format.
   a. Comprised of an item stem that contains basic information (e.g., a diagnosis and practice setting) followed by a question or statement that addresses a specific aspect of OT practice (e.g., the best evaluation to use).
   b. There are four answer options with only one correct response for each item.

[1] NBCOT examinations taken prior to January 2014 tested the following domains according to their respective percentages: Domain 01 - Gathered information regarding factors that influence occupational performance (13%); Domain 02 - Formulated conclusions regarding client's needs and priorities to develop a client-centered intervention plan (28%); Domain 03 - Selected and implemented evidence-based interventions to support participation in areas of occupation (e.g., ADL, education, work, play, leisure, social participation) throughout the continuum of care (39%); Domain 04 - Upheld professional standards and responsibilities to promote quality in practice (20%) (NBCOT, 2008a).

c. No answers are provided in a combination format (e.g., "b and d," "all," or "none of the above").
d. MC items are non-sequential.
(1) Each item contains a "stand alone" question that does not relate to the ones preceding or following it.

3. Multiple choice (MC) items: Scenario format.
a. Some of the MC items are grouped into a scenario that includes case information or a practice situation.
b. This introduction is then followed by several questions that are related to this information (e.g., the most effective intervention goal, the best treatment method, the recommended discharge plan).
c. Each of the questions in the MC scenario items is presented in the same format as the traditional MC item questions.
(1) Your response to one question does not influence the next question.

4. Simulation test (ST) items.
a. A practice-based case provides the foundation for three to six sections with questions about different aspects of the OT process across a continuum of care.
b. An "opening scene" composed of several sentences will present a practice situation.
(1) This background information may identify a practice setting, a client's diagnosis, some presenting problems, and major occupational roles.
c. Three to six sections sequentially present a question with multiple potential decisions/actions to choose from which measure knowledge, clinical judgment, and critical reasoning.
(1) Each section will have a heading and provide additional information that build on the opening scene.
(2) Each section's question requires the selection of all decisions/actions that are relevant to the section's focus (e.g., screening methods, formulating conclusions regarding treatment needs and priorities, implementing interventions, assessing outcomes).
d. There is more than one correct answer for each section's question.
(1) Once a decision/action is selected, a feedback box appears which describes the consequences of the chosen decision/action.
(a) These outcomes may be positive, negative, or neutral, but they will not be labeled as such.
(b) The use of critical thinking and clinical reasoning is needed to determine the impact of each selection.
(c) This information may be used to make subsequent decision/action selections from the provided decisions/actions, but it cannot be used to reverse a selection.
e. The ST items are designed to replicate real practice situations in which decisions and actions cannot be reversed once they are implemented.

Certification Examination Procedures

Eligibility Requirements for the NBCOT Certification Examination

1. General requirements.
a. Information submitted on the application must be accurate and truthful.
b. Candidates submitting misleading or inaccurate information will be prohibited from taking the certification exam.
c. Information related to felonies must be provided by all candidates.
d. If, after taking the exam, it is determined that a candidate was ineligible to take the exam (or that eligibility was questionable), NBCOT will either hold or void the exam.
e. If a candidate was certified and later found to be ineligible for the exam, certification will be revoked.
(1) NBCOT's Disciplinary Action Committee will review the case to determine if any disciplinary action is warranted and if the candidate will or will not be permitted to take the exam at a future date.

2. Specific requirements.
a. NBCOT clearly delineates exam eligibility requirements for graduates of entry-level post-baccalaureate OT programs within the United States that are accredited by the Accreditation Council for Occupational Therapy Education (ACOTE) of the AOTA and graduates of post-baccalaureate international OT education programs.
(1) Eligibility requirements and application procedures for candidates who are graduates of a NBCOT recognized entry-level post-baccalaureate degree are described in detail in the NBCOT Certification Examination Handbooks.
(2) Eligibility requirements and application procedures for candidates who are NOT

graduates of a NBCOT recognized entry-level post-baccalaureate degree are described in detail in the Occupational Therapist Eligibility Determination (OTED) Handbook.

b. Candidates not seeking NBCOT certification may take the exam to meet state regulatory requirements.
   (1) NBCOT should be contacted directly to obtain information about licensure only application procedures.
   (2) Applications for state credentialing must be submitted to the SRB, not NBCOT.

3. Examination eligibility limit.
   a. There is no limit to the number of times a candidate is eligible to take the exam.
   b. A candidate can continue to take the exam until he/she successfully passes.
   c. All exam candidates should consult the SRB of the state in which they seek to obtain a license to determine the state's standards regarding limits on the number of times the exam can be taken to obtain licensure.

Examination Application Process

1. The NBCOT Certification Examination Handbooks contain all required forms for the exam application and provides specific instructions for completion of the application.
   a. There is a handbook for exam candidates who are graduates of US OT education programs and one for graduates of international OT education programs.
   b. The Certification Examination Handbooks and their corresponding forms are available at http://www.nbcot.org.
      (1) All information from this website can be printed out.
      (2) The exam application can be completed, submitted, and processed on-line or via post-mail.
         (a) NBCOT encourages on-line applications for this process.
         (b) When completing an on-line application, be certain to set up only one account, since NBCOT will charge a fee if a duplicate account is created.
         (c) It is faster and more efficient to check application status on-line.
2. Application directions and procedures must be adhered to strictly.
   a. Applications that are incomplete, inaccurate, and/or do not follow instructions will be rejected and returned to the applicant.
   b. Applications are also returned if there are any problems with the fee payment.
   c. Applications returned to candidates can be resubmitted with the fee payment but this reapplication will delay exam administration.
   d. Review and proof your application carefully before submitting it.
      (1) NBCOT will charge a fee to process any changes or corrections you make to the application after your initial submission.
3. Only one application is required. Do not complete an on-line and a paper post-mailed application.
4. When completing the application, be sure to use your first and last names as they appear on the two forms of identification that you will bring to the testing center.
   a. The names you provide on your application will be those that will be printed on the letter which will authorize you to take the NBCOT exam, so they must match the forms of identification that you will present at the exam administration site.
      (1) If your name changes after your application has been submitted to NBCOT and/or your ATT letter has been generated, you must follow NBCOT guidelines for processing a name change.
5. The NBCOT application process takes approximately 10 to 15 business days to complete.
6. When the application process is completed, candidates will receive an Authorization to Test (ATT) letter from NBCOT.
   a. This ATT letter gives the candidate permission to contact Prometric to schedule an exam administration date.
   b. The ATT letter is valid for 90 days.
      (1) If the given time period expires, the candidate can reactivate the ATT by completing a reactivation form and paying a reactivation fee at any time within one year of the application submission.
      (2) If a candidate does not take an exam within one year of the application submission, the ATT cannot be reactivated. A complete new application is required.
   c. Carefully review your name as it appears on this admission notice to be sure that it matches exactly with the identification that you will present on the exam day.
      (1) To correct any errors on this admissions form, follow NBCOT published guidelines.
   d. This admission notice is required for entry into the exam administration area.
7. Applications do not "roll-over" from year to year.

Special Accommodations

1. Candidates with disabilities can receive accommodations which can support their success on the NBCOT exam; thus, we strongly urge all eligible students to apply for *any and all* accommodations for which they are eligible.
2. Exam candidates seeking accommodations should download the Special Testing Accommodations Handbook and Request Form from the NBCOT website.
   a. All of the steps outlined for requesting STA in this handbook should be strictly followed.
3. The exam application for special testing accommodations (STA) must be filled out accurately with all documentation received by the published deadlines and completed according to the instructions.
   a. Incomplete applications, applications with insufficient documentation, or late applications will not be considered by NBCOT and special accommodations will not be made for a candidate.
   b. All documentation must establish a *current* need for accommodation based on candidate's *current* status.
      (1) The receipt of accommodations during an OT education program does not guarantee that accommodations will be provided for the NBCOT exam.
4. NBCOT uses the definition of disability set forth in the Americans with Disabilities Act (ADA) to determine eligibility for special accommodations.
   a. Candidates must have a documented disability, which can include a mental or physical impairment (e.g., learning, cognitive, or psychological disability; hearing, visual, speech or orthopedic impairment) that substantially limits a major life activity.
5. Candidates who use medical devices which may emit noise (e.g., an insulin pump) must request STA.
6. Candidates who have medical or health conditions (e.g. diabetes) that may require them to have a snack or water and/or take medicine or restroom breaks should contact NBCOT for information about how to obtain special accommodations based on medical necessity.
   a. If a pregnancy results in a medical complication, special accommodations may be considered due to medical necessity; however, these are not automatically granted since pregnancy is not defined as a disability in the ADA.
7. Candidates with temporary conditions that do not meet the ADA definition of disability (e.g., fractures) but who may need accommodations (e.g., wheelchair access) should contact NBCOT for information about how to obtain special testing arrangements.
8. English as a second language is not considered a disability; therefore, the use of a dictionary and/or extra time to complete the exam due to language difficulty are not permitted for individuals for whom English is not the primary language.
9. Text anxiety and technophobia are not defined as disabilities in the ADA; consequently, STA will not be considered for these conditions.
10. Accommodation recommendations made by professionals are considered and reviewed by NBCOT but are not automatically granted.
    a. Denials of requests for accommodations can be appealed according to procedures provided in the Special Accommodations Handbook.
11. NBCOT adheres to ADA's guidelines for accommodations. Accommodations may include:
    a. Architecturally accessible test centers or alternative site arrangements.
    b. Auxiliary aids and services.
    c. Extra exam administration time.
    d. A quiet private room.
    e. Other special accommodations based on documented need.
12. All information about a candidate's disability and request for accommodations is confidential.
    a. NBCOT and its testing agency only communicate with the candidate, the candidate's authorized, verified representative, and/or a professional knowledgeable about the candidate's disability with the candidate's permission.
    b. No information about the candidate's application or request for accommodations is released by NBCOT or its testing agency without the written authorization of the candidate.
13. All accommodations must be approved by NBCOT prior to the exam date.
    a. No requests for accommodations will be approved at the test site.
    b. After taking the exam, a candidate cannot retroactively declare a disability.
14. There are no additional fees required to request or receive accommodations.
15. NBCOT will not issue an ATT letter until after accommodation decisions have been made.

Examination Administration and Scheduling

1. Test centers.
   a. Prometric Test Centers are the only locations in which the NBCOT exam can be administered.
      (1) There are over 10,000 Prometric Test Centers located in over 160 countries throughout the world.

b. Test center and scheduling information is located at www.prometric.com.
c. Exam scheduling should be completed on-line by candidates who are not receiving STA.
(1) Candidates with approved STA must schedule their exam by calling Prometric's Special Condition's Team at 1-800-967-1139.
(a) Not all Prometric sites are able to provide approved STA.
d. Any desired change in an exam administration location after an exam is scheduled must be handled directly by the candidate and Prometric staff.
2. Administration schedule.
a. Exams are offered on a continuous, on demand basis and can be scheduled by a candidate throughout the year.
b. Exams can be scheduled Monday through Saturday for a morning or afternoon administration.
(1) If you are able, try to schedule your exam for the time of day that you are at your best. Do not schedule a morning exam if you are still bleary eyed at 11am or an afternoon exam if you fade after lunch.
(a) Respect your natural rhythms.
(2) Some Prometric centers only schedule afternoon sessions after all morning appointments are filled.
(a) If afternoons are your peak performance time of day, take the time and make the effort to obtain an afternoon exam administration.
(b) Your NBCOT exam administration is *not* the time to ignore your internal clock.
c. Candidates are strongly urged to schedule their exam administration immediately after receipt of the confirmation of eligibility.
(1) NBCOT candidates are competing with all other test-takers who use Prometric services for desired appointment dates and times.
(2) A delay in scheduling an exam administration can result in the need to take the exam at a less preferred time and/or site.
(3) Prometric staff advises that Saturday exams be scheduled a minimum of 6 weeks in advance; weekday exams can be scheduled 2–4 weeks in advance.
d. Candidates who experience a personal or medical emergency that will prevent them from taking a scheduled exam must notify the NBCOT and request a rescheduled exam in writing.
(1) Supporting documentation and payment of a fee must accompany this notification and request.

The Examination Day

Pre-Preparation Plans

1. Be prepared physically.
a. Get a good night's sleep.
b. Eat a well-balanced meal to sustain you.
c. Avoid too much caffeine.
d. Wear clothing that can be comfortable in a warm or cold room and adjusted if the room temperature changes (e.g., a long sleeved cotton knit shirt that you can roll the sleeves up and down); do not wear clothing which can raise unnecessary security concerns (e.g., avoid "hoodies," jackets with pockets, and "cargo" shorts or pants with deep pockets).
(1) It is not advisable to wear a jacket or sweater into the testing area because the doffing of any clothing is not allowed in the testing area. If you want to take the jacket or sweater off during the exam, you will be required to do so in the waiting area.
(2) Head coverings worn for religious reasons (e.g., turbans, yarmulkes, scarves) can be worn into the testing area; they must remain in place during the exam.
(a) Head coverings will be visually inspected before you enter the testing area; any adjustments to a head covering must be made in the waiting area.
(b) The donning of a jacket or sweater hood to cover one's head is not allowed in the testing area.
(c) If you must wear a head covering due to a health reason, you must have received pre-approval from NBCOT for this accommodation.
(3) Your exam administration time will *not* be extended to accommodate for any clothing adjustments made in the waiting area (e.g., doffing a sweater, adjusting a head scarf) nor for the time needed to check out of and then recheck back into the testing area.
(a) It is best to simplify your exam day wardrobe to the greatest extent possible.
e. Go to the rest room before checking in.

Chapter 1

2. Be prepared emotionally.
   a. Remind yourself of past achievements (e.g., completing a rigorous graduate program in occupational therapy) and adopt the attitude that passing the NBCOT exam is one more accomplishment to be added to this list.
   b. Plan to arrive earlier than required to eliminate the anxiety of being late.
   c. If you have never traveled to the test site, do a trial run before your exam date on the same day of the week that you are planning to take the exam.
      (1) Exam day is not the time to discover that mass transportation or traffic patterns are different from those with which you are familiar.
3. If you are late for your exam or need to cancel or reschedule it, you must follow the procedures and pay the fees that are outlined in the Certification Examination Handbook.

Test Center Procedures

1. You ***must*** arrive 30 minutes before your scheduled exam.
   a. It is best to arrive earlier to allow sufficient time to *calmly* check in.
2. No one is admitted without an ATT letter.
3. Two forms of identification, including one primary, non-expired government-issued identification with a photo and signature (e.g., a driver's license, passport, state identification card, green card/permanent resident card, military identification card) and an additional non-expired form of identification (e.g., credit card, ATM card, employee identification card, voter registration card or letter, student identification, or a second form of a primary identification) must be presented at the test center.
   a. Social security cards are not accepted.
   b. Copies of identification are not accepted.
   c. The first and last names on the identifications you present must match the names on your ATT letter exactly.
   d. Both forms of identification must have signatures that match exactly.
   e. No one is admitted without required identification.
   f. If the identifications you present do not match the name on your ATT letter, you will not be allowed to take the exam and your ATT letter will be voided.
      (1) You will be required to request a new ATT letter and pay a reactivation fee.
   g. No name changes can be made on-site at a Prometric center; however, on-site address changes can be made.
4. All candidates are required to complete a biometric-enabled check-in which includes making an electronic record of your identifications, photo imaging, and a digital fingertip record.
   a. A video describing the checkin process can be accessed at http://www.youtube.com/watch?v=g5RHoCOfgpc.
5. Upon check in, if you applied for and obtained STA verify that these special accommodations are available for you.
6. Only a wet marker board, earplugs, eyeglasses/contacts, medications, and/or medical devices (e.g., hearing aids, insulin pumps) are allowed into the test administration area.
   a. All personal items will be visually inspected by Prometric staff.
   b. Adjustments to medical devices must be made in the waiting area.
   c. Headphones and the wet marker board must be obtained from Prometric personnel.
7. Electronic devices (i.e., cell phones, personal digital assistants [PDAs], digital watches, and cameras) are not allowed in ***any*** part of the testing facility.
8. Water and snacks can be stored and accessed in the waiting area.
   a. Some Prometric centers allow small "comfort" items (e.g., tissues, cough drops) to be brought into the test area. Others do not.
   b. All items are carefully checked.
9. A locker is provided to store all personal possessions (e.g., jacket, wallet, purse, watches).
   a. This locker is not accessible until the conclusion of the exam.
10. Food and/or drink are not allowed in the testing area.
    a. Food and/or drink can be consumed in the waiting area.
       (1) Be judicious about your food and drink consumption prior to the exam and during the exam to decrease the need for bathroom breaks.
11. A 10–15 minute tutorial on how to use the computer and complete the ST exam items is available prior to commencement of the exam. After you exit the ST section of the exam, a second 10–15 minute tutorial is provided which provides information on how to complete the MC exam items.
    a. Candidates are strongly advised to take each of these tutorials.
    b. The completion of these tutorials do not count toward the four hour administration time so you can use this time to get physically comfortable (e.g., move the computer screen to decrease glare, adjust the chair, take a bathroom break).
12. Prometric personnel can also provide an orientation to the exam.
    a. They are available prior to the exam's start to answer questions and clarify the exam procedures.
13. If you are assigned an exam location that is dissatisfying for any reason (i.e., poor lighting, computer

screen glare), request a change to another computer cubicle before the exam begins.
   a. You cannot change locations once you have begun the exam.
14. Prometric centers do not dedicate times just for NBCOT test takers. Many individuals taking a variety of exams may be coming, going, or receiving orientation during your exam.
   a. Some individuals find the use of earplugs or headphones helpful in decreasing these auditory distractions.
15. There are no scheduled breaks during the exam unless pre-arranged as an accommodation for a disability or medical necessity.
   a. Restroom breaks are allowed during the exam; however, the exam clock does keep running.
      (1) At the beginning of a break you will need to check out with Prometric staff and after the break you will need to re-check in with Prometric staff.
      (2) This may require waiting while other people check in for their exams or check out and in for their breaks.
16. All areas that are accessible to candidates are videotaped and these tapes are reviewed by Prometric personnel.
17. You are not allowed to talk or read aloud during the exam.
18. If you take a break and are observed using a banned electronic device (e.g., a cell phone, iPad, or personal digital assistant), your exam will be terminated.
   a. The Prometric testing center administrator (TCA) will file a Candidate Proctor Report (CPR) with NBCOT which will detail your infraction.
   b. Your eligibility to take a future NBCOT exam will be determined by NBCOT after a review of the CPR.

Examination Time and Time Keeping

1. There are four hours allowed to complete the exam.
   a. This administration time is *not* divided separately into time to complete the three ST items and the time to complete the 170 MC items.
      (1) You must personally monitor your time to ensure that you complete the exam within the allotted four hours.
      (2) The ST section will be the first one presented during the exam.
         (a) It is recommended that you spend 10–12 minutes to complete each of the three ST items for a total of 30–36 minutes for this exam section. This will allow you to have approximately 3½ hours to complete, the 170 MC items.
         (b) Once the ST item section is completed and the MC section is begun, the ST section cannot be returned to for further review.
2. Additional time is not provided for any reason other than as a pre-approved special accommodation for a disability.
3. There are no scheduled breaks during the exam.
   a. Restroom breaks are allowed during the exam; however, the exam's clock does keep running unless you received breaks as an accommodation.
4. A running clock on the computer will indicate the total exam time remaining and a counter will indicate the number of MC items left to answer so you can readily see if you are progressing at the needed pace.
   a. Periodically check the clock and/or counter to be sure that you are on track with your timing.
      (1) Avoid spending too much time checking this clock and counter.
5. You should allot an average of one minute to complete each MC item.
   a. This pace will enable you to complete 50 MC items in less than an hour, providing you with a 'bank' of approximately 30 minutes that you can use to review and answer more challenging MC items in this exam section.
6. If you are behind schedule, your pace is too slow and you will need to speed up to complete the exam.
   a. Do not belabor difficult questions. Move on to other exam items.
7. If you are ahead of schedule, take a brief breather and congratulate yourself; then maintain this pace, for you can use this additional time later during the exam to take a short break during the MC section.
   a. Some students report feeling listless as the exam progresses and they have found a brief breather re-energized them and enabled them to resume the exam with a positive outlook.

Test Taking Strategies

1. Decrease your anxiety level before you begin by taking the tutorial and asking any and all questions.
2. Don't panic. OT programs are challenging, but you passed your coursework and fieldwork to get to this point so you must have done something right! Remember this and give yourself credit.
3. Pace yourself using the timing advice provided above.
4. Select the best answer(s).
   a. Think logically and eliminate obviously wrong answers.
   b. Jot down notes on the wet marker board. Often visualizing the remaining options of a familiar list (e.g., Allen's Cognitive Levels) will jog one's memory and make it easier to arrive at a correct answer.

c. Narrow your choices to the best possible answers and use your knowledge of the clinical condition and OT standards of practice to clinically reason and determine the best answer.
d. Do not read extra information into the question; just consider what is stated in the question.
   (1) Decide what the question is basically about by looking for key words (e.g., initial intervention, discharge).
e. Avoid thinking "but" and "what if." Often your first instincts are accurate, so decrease second guessing.
f. Do not think about people you know with this condition or practice you've seen in the clinic; think of and apply basic OT principles (i.e., what the book says, not what you saw on fieldwork).
g. It may help to read the answer choices before you read the question scenario. Then you will be able to focus your reading of the scenario on issues directly related to the answer choices.
   (1) It may also help to try to answer the question without reading the answer choices. However, be certain to read all answer choices before making your final choice.
h. The answer should be grammatically consistent with the exam item's question.
   (1) After you have selected your answer, read the question, then your answer. Does it flow? If not, review other options.
      (a) Save this hint for ones you're not sure of. (Who said APA wouldn't come in handy?!)
   (2) If English is your second language, you must remember to "think" in English when reading and answering questions.
      (a) Noting past versus present tense in an item is particularly important.

5. Table 1-1 provides an outline of general test-taking strategies for answering all NBCOT exam items.
6. Table 1-2 provides an outline of specific test-taking strategies for answering MC exam items.
7. Table 1-3 provides an outline of specific test-taking strategies for answering ST exam items.

Completion of the Examination

1. Answers can be recorded by using keystrokes or the mouse.
2. Do not skip exam items.
   a. Although not all of the exam items are scored, there is no way to know which items are operational or not, therefore, you must answer all items to the best of your ability.
3. To answer the ST items, select the decisions/actions that are appropriate to the practice situation provided using the strategies provided in Tables 1-1 and 1-3.

Table 1-1

General Strategies for Answering All NBCOT Exam Items

• Read the exam item carefully before selecting a response to the question posed.
• Employ relevant clinical experience.
  – Remember trends and consistent cases in your experience.
  – Do not call on unusual cases or atypical presentations.
• Read the exam item for key words that set a priority (e.g., pain, acute care).
• Apply clinical reasoning skills to determine the relevance of item info. (i.e., diagnosis, setting, intervention, and theoretical principles).
• Use your knowledge of medical terminology to decipher unknown terms by applying the meanings of known prefixes, suffixes, and root words.
• Select responses that most closely reflect the fundamental tenets of OT (e.g., ethical actions, the use of meaningful occupation).
• Choose client-centered, person-directed actions.
• Identify choices that focus on the emotional well-being of the person.
• Use your clinical judgment to support the best answer.
• Check your answer to see if it is:
  – theoretically consistent with exam scenario.
  – diagnostically consistent with the exam scenario.
  – developmentally consistent with the exam scenario.
• Eliminate choices that contain contraindications as these must be incorrect.
• Consider eliminating options that state "always," "never," "all," or "only" as there are few absolutes in OT practice.
• Eliminate unsafe options.
• Choose answers that reflect entry-level OT practice.
• Remember the NBCOT exam is not a specialty certification exam.

Table 1-2

Specific Strategies for Answering Multiple Choice (MC) Items

• Identify the theme of the MC item. Ask yourself, "What is the question posed REALLY asking?"
• Avoid "reading into" the MC item. Read the question asked and nothing but the question.
• Identify choices that seem similar or equally plausible.
  – If two choices basically say the same thing or use synonyms in their answers both cannot be right; therefore, both can be eliminated.
• Carefully consider choices that are opposites of one another. If you cannot eliminate both opposites right away, one may be the correct answer.
• Determine the best answer using strategies identified in Table 1-1.
  – More than one answer may be "correct." Choose the one that is MOST correct.
• Select positive, active choices rather than passive, negative ones.
• Before changing an answer make sure that you have a good reason to eliminate your original choice and a good reason to make your new choice.
  – Good reasons include realizing that you missed the theme or a key word (e.g., screening) of the exam item or you gained a clue from a subsequent exam item (e.g., SCI levels).
• Do not let second-guessing talk you out of the correct answer.

Table 1-3

Specific Strategies for Answering Simulation Test (ST) Items
• Carefully read the opening scene. Take notes on key information (e.g., dx, age, setting, stage of the OT process). • Do not panic when faced with 6–10 options for you to consider. – You do not have to select only one option. – There will likely be more than one appropriate response to the questions posed by each ST item section. • Eliminate *obviously inappropriate* decisions/actions. *DO NOT* mark these options. Once you make a selection, you *cannot* deselect it. • *Prior to* selecting your first appropriate decision/action, carefully consider the info. provided in the item's "opening scene" and the additional info. provided in each ST item section. • For your *first* decision/action selection, pick the choice that seems *BEST* to you, using all of the general test-taking strategies provided in Table 1-1. • Use the feedback provided about selected decisions/actions to progress through the ST item and guide your subsequent selections. • If the feedback informs you that your choice had less than a desired outcome, use this input constructively to guide your next selection. • Jot down key phrases and brief notes to keep track of your thoughts about the opening scene info., the subsequent section info., and the decision/action feedback. • When considering the options provided, think "What is the outcome?" of each decision/action. If the outcome of the decision/action is consistent with the OT process and standards of practice, moves the client toward goal attainment, and/or solves a given problem, select this option. • If the option is *not* consistent with the OT process and standards of practice, does *not* move the client toward goal attainment, and/or does *not* solve the given problem, do *not* select this option. • If you are uncertain of the appropriateness of an option, scroll back to review the opening scene, and additional section information, the items that you selected, and the provided feedback. You *cannot* deselect a selected response, but this review can help you select your best next step. • *Do not* select an action/decision if you uncertain if it may lead to a negative outcome; points are deducted for these.

a. Once you make a selection, for a ST item question, you cannot deselect it.
b. You can scroll back through the ST item to review its opening scene, section headings, additional section information, the items that you selected, and the provided feedback to guide your subsequent selections.
c. Once you complete a ST item, you cannot return to it.
d. Once you have exited the ST item section you cannot return to it.

4. To answer the MC items use the strategies provided in Tables 1-1 and 1-2.
5. If you are uncertain of an answer to a MC item, mark the item by using the mark/unmark button.
   a. You can return to a marked MC item to review and change the answer (if desired), at any time BEFORE you exit the MC section.
6. Only change the answer to a MC item if you have a good reason to reject your first choice.
   a. Solid reasons for changing an answer include:
      (1) You missed an important key word like "pain," "disorientation," "initial," "best."
      (2) Your original answer was not consistent with the stage of the OT process (e.g., screening, evaluation, intervention, discharge).
      (3) You obtained a solid hint from a subsequent exam item (e.g., SCI levels).
   b. Basically, before you change your answer, you should feel as if a brilliant "light bulb" has been turned on in your brain to illuminate the correct answer.
      (1) If you do not experience a "light bulb" moment, do not change your answer.
7. If you remain unsure of an answer to a MC item make a logical guess. There is no penalty for guessing on MC items, but there is for leaving a question unanswered.
8. Do not communicate with anyone other than Prometric personnel while completing the exam.
   a. An innocent passing remark to another person can be mistaken for an attempt to cheat.
9. Keep your eyes on your own computer screen and do not look at other screens if you take a break.
   a. A fleeting glance at another computer screen can be interpreted as an attempt to cheat.
10. Don't panic if you are stumped by a number of exam item questions.
    a. Focus on what you know, because it is likely you know a lot.
    b. We often tend to remember our "failures" and not our "successes." Be kind to yourself.
11. Congratulate yourself for what you know and make educated guesses on what you don't know. You do not need to answer 100%, 90%, or even 80% of the MC items correctly in order to pass the exam.
12. If you are running out of time on the exam and have not completed the MC item section, pick a letter and mark all remaining answers using that choice.
    a. Laws of probability will result in some of these item answers being correct.
    b. After clicking on your chosen letter for all remaining items use the time you have left to calmly and thoughtfully revisit your answers to determine if your selected answer was correct or not.
       (1) If you determine that your answer was incorrect, use all of the strategies identified in this chapter to determine the best answer and change your response.
       (2) If you determine that your answer was correct, say a silent "YES!" to your self and continue your review of these items until your exam administration time runs out.
    c. Remember there is no penalty in the MC item section for incorrect answers so it does not make sense to leave any answer blank.

After the Examination

Examination Administration Complaints

1. Only complaints regarding an administrative or technical problem with the exam are accepted (e.g., the computer screen freezes).
   a. Prometric centers are in the business of providing optimal environments for test-taking, so administrative and technical problems are rare.
2. If you do experience a problem, *immediately* after you complete your exam, file an on-site administration complaint.
   a. Be very specific about the nature of your complaint, the rationale for the complaint, and any actions that were taken to try to deal with the complaint on-site.
   b. Request a "ticket number" for your complaint from Prometric staff
   c. You must email NBCOT within 24 hours to provide them with a summary of your complaint and its assigned number.
   d. Be certain to adhere to the complaint guidelines in the NBCOT Certification Examination Handbook.
      (1) There are *no* exceptions.
   e. Complaints are investigated by NBCOT and the testing agency and written responses are sent to the candidate.

Examination Scoring and Reporting

1. Item analysis.
   a. All exams use items that NBCOT has analyzed as performing well on previous exams.
   b. All items are pre-equated and determined to have sound statistical attributes.
2. Equating.
   a. The passing score for each exam is statistically adjusted to compensate for differences in the difficulty level of each exam.
   b. This equating aims to ensure that candidates with equivalent abilities will be equally likely to pass the exam.
   c. From NBCOT's and their testing agency's points of view, all exam candidates have a fair and equal chance to pass the exam, regardless of the administration date.
3. Scoring processes.
   a. Only pre-equated operational items are scored; the pre-test items are not scored.
   b. The pre-equated operational MC items are scored by giving points for the one correct answer.
      (1) NO points are deducted if one of other three incorrect answers is chosen or if the answer is left blank.
   c. The pre-equated operational ST items are comprised of three to six sections with multiple decision/action options.
      (1) Points are given for positive decisions/actions that result in optimal outcomes.
      (2) Points are neither given nor deducted if a positive decision/action is not selected.
      (3) Points are deducted for poor decisions/actions that result in negative outcomes.
      (4) Points are neither given nor deducted for decisions/actions that are considered to be neutral.
   d. Statistical procedures convert candidates' raw scores into "scaled scores" which are then comparable for all exams based upon the equating process.
   e. The exam results are reported on a scale from 300 to 600 points.
   f. A scaled score of at least 450 is needed to pass the exam.
   g. This passing score of 450 remains the same for all exam administration dates. There are no adjustments made after the score is determined by the equating process.
4. Scoring schedule and score reporting.
   a. Exam scoring can take up to four weeks.
      (1) Several steps are followed by the testing agency to produce accurate exam reports in as timely a manner as possible.
      (2) Early score results are not given.
   b. Exams are scored weekly.
      (1) The exam scoring schedule is posted on NBCOT's website at www.nbcot.org.
      (2) Exam candidates can access their score report online by logging into their NBCOT account.
      (3) Candidates can typically obtain an unofficial pass/fail score on the next business day after their exam was scored.
         (a) Candidates must use their user name and password to access this score information.
   c. Official score reports are mailed within four to six weeks of the exam administrative date.
      (1) If a report is not received after four weeks of taking the exam, a candidate can submit a Duplicate Score Request form to NBCOT.
   d. Candidates who pass the exam receive a letter of congratulations, a report with their total score, and a wallet card designating their certification status.

e. Candidates who fail the exam receive a report of their total score and information on their performance on each domain of the exam.
   (1) This score report also identifies the regulatory agencies NBCOT has informed about the failing score.

f. Score reports are only provided to exam candidates or their legally verified representative.

g. Score reports can be provided to SRBs and other regulatory agencies upon the written authorization of the exam candidate.

h. Aggregate score reports are provided to the Program Directors of OT Education Programs for candidates who are graduates of their programs.

Waiting For and Receiving Examination Results

1. Accept that the exam is done and over with, and move on to other enjoyable activities.
2. Focus on your successes. Congratulate yourself on items you answered confidently.
3. Avoid focusing on exam difficulties. For example, the exam was not solely about the two obscure diagnoses that you could not recall. Remember, there were many other items about content that you knew well that were scored.
4. Surround yourself with your "fan club," people who assure you of your competencies.
5. Avoid and ignore individuals who continually question the exam's fairness and perseverate about their ability to pass.
6. Ignore rumors about the exam's pass rate.
   a. No one knows this information until it is received in the mail by the exam takers.
   b. OT educational programs do not receive this information prior to the students.
   c. OT educational programs do not receive information identifying the names of students who do not pass the exam.
7. If you passed, congratulate yourself and begin your lifelong pursuit of a rewarding career in occupational therapy.
8. If you did not pass, do not denigrate yourself; rather, make a plan to retake the exam and succeed.

Implications of Not Passing the Examination

1. The implications of not passing the NBCOT exam vary from state to state. You must follow your state regulatory board's (SRB's) procedures for notification of exam failure.
2. If you are currently employed as an occupational therapist or you have specific plans to begin employment, you must notify your employer immediately.
3. Depending on the state, you may be able to continue employment under an extension of a temporary license or have your position reconfigured to be a COTA or a rehabilitation aide/associate, with a corresponding decrease in responsibility and salary.

Retaking the Examination

1. A new and complete application must be submitted to retake the NBCOT exam.
2. NBCOT requires a waiting period after a failed exam administration date before you can take the exam again.[2] Use this time to:
   a. Obtain support to handle your legitimate disappointment.
   b. Review exam results to identify and analyze overall areas of strength and weakness; do not agonize over exact percentages in your score report.
   c. Reflect on your exam experience to identify behaviors that may have hindered success. Common mistakes include:
      (1) Taking too much time to answer difficult questions.
      (2) Becoming anxious or upset over a question that seemed to have no good answer (or two good answers).
      (3) Becoming distracted by the progress of the other test-takers.
      (4) Arriving in a rushed, harried manner.
      (5) Not seeking and obtaining STA when qualified to receive these as a candidate with a disability.
3. Be realistic about the obstacles you can change and those you cannot. For example, if you were stressed due to a traffic jam, you can leave earlier or stay overnight in a nearby hotel. On the other hand, you cannot change the fact that the exam is on a computer even though you have technophobic tendencies.
4. Increase your comfort level with taking a computerized exam by taking the computer-based exams provided on this text's disc.
   a. The disc does not self-destruct after a set number of exam trials; it can be interrupted, returned to, and used repeatedly.
5. If you had received STA for your previous exam, you need to notify NBCOT via accommodations@nbcot.org that you are requesting these accommodations again for your next exam.

[2] As of January 1, 2014, the waiting period is 30 days. Prior to this date, the waiting period was 45 days.

6. If you are eligible for reasonable accommodations but did not previously request them, follow NBCOT's guidelines and adhere to the deadline dates to attain needed STA.
   a. Since the NBCOT exam requires four hours of computer work to complete, carefully and realistically assess your cognitive, physical, and psychosocial abilities for this task.
7. Develop a plan of action to ensure success.
   a. Review this text's Chapter 2 on effective exam preparation and critically evaluate what you did to prepare for your first exam.
   b. Take (or re-take) an exam preparatory course; your first-hand exam experience can make this course even more relevant.
   c. Do not rush to take the next scheduled exam, for that may not allow you sufficient time to adequately prepare for the exam.
      (1) It is better to delay the exam than rush your preparation and risk being under-prepared.
8. Adopt the perspective that your first experience with the exam can be viewed positively, in that you can re-take the exam with a clear idea of what the experience is like.
   a. You are aware of your strong and weak points; therefore, your chances of passing the re-take are greater.
9. Recognize that there are many skilled and competent OT practitioners who did not pass the certification exam on their first (or even their second) attempt.
   a. You can join their ranks by honestly self-assessing your exam preparedness and taking concrete steps to remediate your difficulties and build upon your strengths.
   b. Being able to practice occupational therapy is well worth the effort.

Chapter 1

References

Fleming-Castaldy, R. (2012). *Occupational therapy course manual, 4th edition.* Evanston, IL: TherapyEd.

National Board for Certification in Occupational Therapy (NBCOT). (2013a). *The certification examination handbook for U.S. educated candidates.* Gaithersburg, MD: NBCOT.

National Board for Certification in Occupational Therapy (NBCOT). (2013b). *The certification examination handbook for internationally-educated candidates.* Gaithersburg, MD: NBCOT.

National Board for Certification in Occupational Therapy (NBCOT). (2013c). *Occupational therapist eligibility determination (OTED).* Retrieved August 8, 2013 from http://www.nbcot.org/index.php?option=com_content&view=article&id=294&Itemid=218.

National Board for Certification in Occupational Therapy (NBCOT). (2013d). *National Special Testing Accommodations Handbook and Request Form.* Retrieved August 20, 2013 from http://www.nbcot.org/pdf/spec_accoms/Special-Testing-Accoms-Handbook.pdf.

National Board for Certification in Occupational Therapy (NBCOT). (2012). *2012 executive summary of the practice analysis of the Occupational Therapist Registered* Retrieved August 8, 2012 from http://www.nbcot.org/pdf/OTR_ExecSumm_PA_2012.pdf.

National Board for Certification in Occupational Therapy (NBCOT). (2008a). *2008 executive summary of the practice analysis of the Occupational Therapist Registered.* Retrieved July 2, 2008 from www. nbcot.org.

National Board for Certification in Occupational Therapy (NBCOT). (2008b, March). *Clinical simulation testing webinar for program directors.* Gaithersburg, MD: NBCOT.

National Board for Certification in Occupational Therapy. (2008c). *The NBCOT official OTR study guide: Occupational therapist registered (OTR) certification examination.* Gaithersburg, MD: Author.

Sides, M. & Korcheck, N. (Eds.). (1998). *Successful test-taking: Learning strategies for nurses.* Philadelphia: Lippincott.

2

Principles of Effective Examination Preparation

RITA P. FLEMING-CASTALDY AND KARI INDA

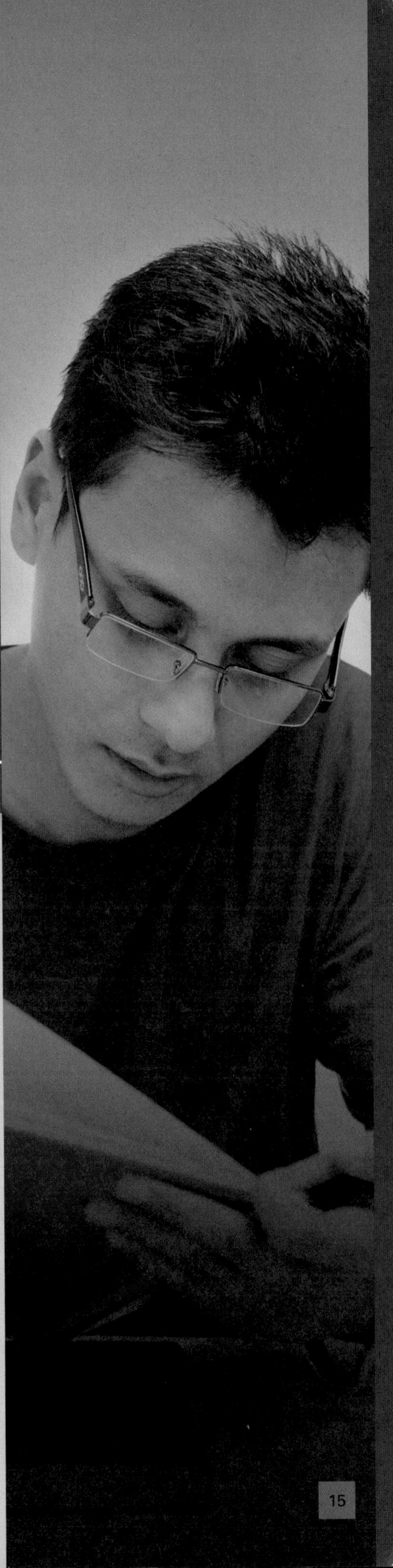

Chapter Outline

Chapter 2

Effective Examination Preparation

Overview and General Guidelines

1. The NBCOT exam tests general knowledge and fundamentals of occupational therapy (OT) in an integrated manner.
   a. There are four main levels of objective exam questions.
      (1) Table 2-1 describes each question level and its relevance to the NBCOT exam and provides related exam preparation strategies.
2. Your clinical and critical reasoning skills will be vital to use to ensure exam success.
   a. Table 2-2 describes the major types of clinical reasoning and how the reflective application of clinical reasoning skills can facilitate exam success.
   b. This chapter provides an extensive discussion about the relationship between critical reasoning and NBCOT exam performance.

Psychological Outlook

1. When preparing for a professional certification exam, your psychological outlook is a critical aspect of effective exam preparation. See Table 2-3.
   a. Fears, doubts, and negative attitudes must be replaced with a positive "I can" outlook.
      (1) Remember that to be eligible for the NBCOT exam, you had to pass a rigorous graduation education program and challenging fieldworks;

Table 2-1

Levels of Exam Questions

QUESTION LEVEL AND DESCRIPTION	RELEVANCE TO NBCOT EXAM	NBCOT EXAM PREPARATION STRATEGY
1. Knowledge Recall of basic information. For example, DSM diagnoses, spinal cord levels, wheelchair measurements.	A solid knowledge foundation of all information related to entry-level OT practice is required to answer practice scenario items. It is highly likely that NO items on the NBCOT exam are solely at this level.	A strong commitment to studying is needed to remember all the information acquired during your OT education. Fortunately, this text provides extensive information in an outline format to ease your review. Memorization of this information is required to be able to readily recall it during the 170 MC and the 3 ST items on the NBCOT exam.
2. Comprehension Understanding of information to determine significance, consequences, or implications. For example, the impact of a tenodesis grasp on function.	The NBCOT exam is not a matching column type of test; therefore, you cannot just recall information to be able to succeed on this exam. You must fully understand the content area to be able to understand the nuances of an exam item. A few items on the NBCOT exam may be at this level.	When studying the text to review basic content and acquire your foundational knowledge, ask yourself how and why this fundamental information is important. Studying with a peer or a study group can provide you with additional insights about the relevance, significance, consequences, and implications of the info. Do not enter the exam without strong comprehension of all major areas of OT practice.
3. Application Use of information and application of rules, procedures, or theories to new situations. For example, the classroom modifications that a therapist would make for a child with autism.	The NBCOT exam requires you to use your knowledge and comprehension as described above, along with the competencies you developed during your clinical fieldworks, in a manner that best fits the specific practice scenario in an exam item. Many NBCOT exam items are at this level for a main goal of the exam is to assess your ability to respond competently to different situations.	Once you have acquired a solid knowledge base and good comprehension skills in all domains of OT as put forth in this text, you should take the computer-based NBCOT simulated practice exams that accompany this text. These exams require you to apply your knowledge in a manner similar to the NBCOT exam. Upon completion of these exams, you receive an analysis of your performance so that you can determine how well you are applying your knowledge.
4. Analysis Recognition of interrelationships between principles & interpretation or evaluation of data presented. For example, the most appropriate focus for discharge planning sessions for a parent with a traumatic brain injury.	The NBCOT exam assumes that you have mastered and comprehend entry-level knowledge and that you can competently apply this information to diverse situations; therefore it will ask you to analyze and respond to ambiguous, not "straight from the book" situations. Most NBCOT exam items are at this level for the main objective of the exam is to determine your ability to be competent in complex practice situations.	Use the analyses of text practice exams described above to reflect on your reasoning mistakes. Critically review the extensive rationales provided in the text for the correct exam answers. Reflecting with a peer or study group can be helpful in determining your gaps in analysis of exam items. Review the text's section on critical reasoning skills and reflect on the questions provided in Table 2-5 to ascertain the actions you need to take to adequately prepare for the complexities of the NBCOT exam.

Table 2-2

Clinical Reasoning Applied to NBCOT Exam Items

TYPE OF REASONING	QUESTIONS TO CONSIDER	RELATIONSHIP TO EXAM SUCCESS
Procedural Reasoning Requires the systematic gathering and interpreting of data to identify problems, set goals, plan intervention, and implement treatment strategies. It is the "doing" of practice.	What does the exam item tell/ask you about: Diagnosis? Symptoms? Prognosis? Assessment methods? Treatment protocols? Theories/practice frameworks to support procedures?	Correct answers on the NBCOT exam will be consistent with the published evaluation standards and intervention protocols for a given clinical condition and congruent with established theories and relevant practice frameworks.
Interactive Reasoning Focuses on the client as a person and involves the therapeutic relationship between the practitioner, the individual, caregivers, and significant others.	What does the exam item tell/ask you about: Rapport building? Family/caregiver involvement? Therapeutic use of self? Teaching/learning styles? Successful collaboration?	Correct answers on the NBCOT exam will have the therapist engaging with the person, family, caregivers, and others in an empathetic, caring, respectful, collaborative, and empowering manner.
Pragmatic Reasoning Considers the context(s) of service delivery including the person's situation and the practice environment to identify the real possibilities for a person in a given setting.	What does the exam item tell/ask you about: Person's client factors? Practice setting characteristics? Reimbursement issues? Legal parameters? Referral options?	Correct answers on the NBCOT exam will be realistic given the person's assets and limitations, his/her environmental supports and barriers, and the practice setting's inherent opportunities and constraints.
Conditional Reasoning Represents an integration of procedural, interactive, and pragmatic reasoning in the context of the client's narrative.[1] Focuses on past, current and possible future social contexts.	What does the exam item tell/ask you about: The individual's unique roles, values, goals? Impact of illness on this person's function? How will the condition's course influence the person's future? Where the person will be able to live after discharge?	Correct answers on the NBCOT exam will take into account all case information that is provided in the item scenario. NBCOT exam items do not include extraneous details so carefully reflect on the relevance of the information provided in each item scenario to determine the best answer.

Reference: Fleming-Castaldy, R. (2010, November 8). The NBCOT examination: Strategies for success. *OT Practice.* 7–10.

Note: [1]The application of narrative reasoning is not likely required during the NBCOT exam since this type of reasoning deals with the individual's occupational story and uses critical imagination to help the person reach an imagined future. This important process is not readily measured by objective exam questions.

thus, your academic and clinical educators have asserted that you possess the knowledge and skills needed for entry-level OT practice by passing you.

b. Because developing a positive attitude can be difficult to do alone, surround yourself with your "fan club," people who know that you will be a terrific occupational therapist.

c. Practice techniques to reduce anxiety during the exam while preparing for the exam.

(1) Techniques of visual imagery, muscle relaxation, controlled diaphragmatic breathing, cognitive-behavioral strategies, meditation, positive self-talk, and/or exercise, can be just as beneficial for you as the individuals with whom you will be working.

2. Keep your "eye on the prize."

a. Write down two reasons why you want to be an occupational therapist.

(1) Keep these statements where you will read them every day so that they help you to stay motivated.

b. Write down two reasons why you *WILL* pass the exam. For instance, "I will pass the certification exam because I have developed a clear study plan and will implement it." "I passed the hardest class in the world with the most difficult teacher ever."

3. If you have previously failed the exam, honestly critique what did not work for you in preparing for and taking your prior exam (e.g., did you not practice taking a complete exam during an uninterrupted four hour period; did you ignore studying professional standards and responsibilities because you found your management class boring?).

a. Develop and implement remediation strategies to effectively deal with these difficulties.

b. Maintain a positive attitude, but be careful and do not accept false reassurance from others.

Structuring a Review of Professional Education

1. Establish your knowledge and skill level.

a. The exam tests general knowledge and fundamentals of occupational therapy in an integrated manner. See Chapter 3 for a review of the profession's tools of practice.

Chapter 2

Table 2-3

Psychology of Successful Test-Taking

CONCEPT	PRINCIPLE	ACTIONS
Control	Only you can determine your future.	• Take charge; determine exactly what is needed to succeed. • Set goals to meet these needs. • Develop and implement concrete plans to succeed.
Self-Awareness	Knowing one's innate capabilities enables one to build on strengths and effectively deal with limitations.	• Critically analyze test-taking errors and content knowledge gaps. • Be honest about your test-taking and content knowledge, strengths and limitations. • Avoid self-defeatist behaviors.
Self-Confidence	Your past accomplishments provide a solid foundation for future success.	• Review exam content prior to completing practice exams. • Use a diversity of learning methods to achieve mastery. • Recognize and celebrate your successes and achievements.
Self-fulfilling Prophecy	Your self-expectancy will influence the outcomes of your efforts.	• Expect success. • Use positive self-talk throughout exam preparation. • Continue to think positively during the exam administration.
Self-esteem	You are a person capable of excellence.	• Remember your personal and academic achievements. • OT academic course work and fieldwork are demanding; give yourself well-earned credit for your success.
Motivation	Your desire to succeed and a fear of failure can be channeled for success.	• Understand that the early stages of studying will have uncertain results. • Remind yourself of what initially motivated you to enter OT school. • Harness fear and establish a do-able study plan.
Courage	Taking responsibility for one's failures is key to success.	• Honestly critique precipitators/reasons for an exam failure. • Do not make excuses. • Do not strive for perfection.
Perseverance	You can only succeed if you persevere.	• Re-establish goals. • Seek support for goal attainment. • Utilize multiple resources to stay on track.
Freedom	You can freely choose your attitude.	• View test-taking as an opportunity. • Keep your "eye on the prize." • Exam success equates to achievement of your goal to become an OT practitioner.

Reference: Sides, M. (1998). Forming the psychology of test-taking success. In M. Sides and N. Korcheck. (Eds). *Successful test-taking: Learning strategies for nurses* (pp. 49–61). Philadelphia: Lippincott.

(1) Your clinical reasoning skills will be vital to use because the NBCOT exam emphasizes the application of knowledge.
(a) Table 2-2 outlines the application of clinical reasoning to multiple choice questions.

b. Critique your knowledge of the four domains that are covered in the NBCOT exam to identify your areas of strength and weakness in order to create a personal study plan. These domains are listed in Chapter 1.

c. Review your academic history to help clarify strengths and weaknesses. Honestly appraise which course topics you mastered and the ones with which you struggled.

d. As you proceed through the chapters in this text rate your knowledge of key content according to a scale of know very well, know adequately, know very little, know nothing.
(1) Based on this critical self assessment, make a personal "OT Knowledge Continuum" for yourself, listing topics from strongest to weakest.
(a) Your aim is to enter the exam with solid knowledge in all critical content areas.

2. Develop and implement an individualized study plan.
a. Content areas that are rated as "know nothing" or "know very little" will become your "Must Study" list.
b. Content areas that are rated as "know very well" or "know adequately" will become your "Review" list.
c. Organize both your "Must Study" list and "Review" list into a logical schedule.
(1) For example, if you are weak in your knowledge about biomechanical evaluation and intervention approaches but have a good recall

of clinical conditions, review the chapter on musculoskeletal conditions and then study the biomechanical chapter.

(a) Studying these two chapters together will provide an integrative learning experience since diagnoses will be included in exam items which test your knowledge about evaluation and intervention approaches.

d. Allocate study time according to your "OT Knowledge Continuum," "Must Study" list, and "Review" list; beginning with your weakest area first.
   (1) After you master a weak content area, reward yourself by reviewing a content area of strength.
   (2) Continue studying to progress along your knowledge continuum, alternating between your "Must Study" list and "Review" list. This will help prevent exam preparation fatigue and burnout.
e. Plan to spend more time studying areas that compose a greater percent of the exam content, especially if these areas are on the low end of your "OT Knowledge Continuum" and on your "Must Study" list.
f. Allow yourself sufficient time to study over a period of time, and set aside enough time to master your weakest areas and to review all areas in general.
   (1) Be realistic about your inherent capabilities (e.g., being a poor memorizer) and your external constraints (e.g., being a single parent who must rely on childcare) when planning the amount of study time needed to ensure success.
   (2) Studying in cram sessions can increase anxiety and result in burnout.
g. Critically assess the study habits you used in OT school to identify routines that worked most effectively for you.
h. Establish a study schedule and routine and adhere to it strictly.
   (1) Study one major content area per study session.
   (2) Limit interruptions.
      (a) Turn off your cell phone so that you are not distracted by phone calls, text messages, emails, tweets, etc. (if needed, lock your cell phone in your car's glove compartment).
      (b) If you are a parent and/or caregiver, arrange for child, elder, and/or respite care.
      (c) DO NOT study by a computer; the latest TravelZoo ad and/or Pininterest post will be far more interesting than supervisory guidelines.
   (3) If an unexpected event results in a loss of planned study time, immediately schedule time to make up for this loss.

3. *DO NOT* take the practice exams in this text until after you have implemented your study plan and gained mastery of your "Must Study" list.
   a. Completing a practice exam before you have attained mastery of essential content will only reinforce that you have key gaps in your foundational knowledge.
      (1) This can diminish confidence, lower self-esteem, and make the prospect of studying more overwhelming.
   b. Completing a practice exam after the full implementation of your study plan will provide you the opportunity to demonstrate your acquired knowledge.
      (1) This can increase confidence, boost self-esteem, and enable your subsequent studying to be more targeted on areas that you had initially not focused on in depth or had not sufficiently mastered.
4. Complete the first practice exam on this text's CD using the test taking strategies provided in Chapter 1.
   a. Reflect on the analysis of your exam performance that will be provided after you complete the exam.
      (1) This analysis will provide information about your content knowledge strengths and gaps and your critical reasoning abilities. Both are important for exam success.
      (2) You can print this analysis out for ongoing review.
   b. Revise your study plan based on this analysis of your exam performance.
      (1) Implement this revised study plan to address identified knowledge gaps.
   c. This chapter provides in-depth information about the relevance of critical reasoning to exam success.
5. Complete the second practice exam on this text's CD using the test taking strategies provided in Chapter 1 that can most effectively address the errors you made on your first practice exam.
   a. Reflect on the analysis of your second exam performance that will be provided after you complete the exam and update your study plan to address remaining content knowledge gaps.
6. Repeat this process for the third exam on the CD.
7. Answering exam items can also assist in identifying your test-taking personality. Acquiring knowledge about your test-taking personality is as important as identifying your content areas of strength and weakness.
   a. Table 2-4 outlines typical test-taking personalities, their corresponding characteristics, and effective behavior management strategies.
8. If you have trouble with any particular content area, use the "Create Your Own Exam" feature on the CD to design individual exams which allow you to focus and practice on your weak area (e.g., neurological disorders and neurophysiological approaches).

Chapter 2

Table 2-4

Personalities of Test-Takers

PERSONALITY TYPE	CHARACTERISTICS	STRATEGIES
The Rusher	• Impatient. • Jumps to conclusions. • Skips key words. • Inadequate consideration of exam items.	• Take practice exams in a timed manner to establish a non-desperate pace and help realize that the time allotted for the exam is sufficient. • Use positive self-talk and relaxation techniques during exam. • Employ the strategies provided in Tables 1-1 to 1-3 to slow your pace and not make the errors that are endemic to rushing.
The Turtle	• Overly slow and methodical. • Over attention to extraneous detail. • Reads and re-reads exam item's details. • Misses theme of exam items.	• Take practice exams in a timed manner to establish a pace of completing each ST item in 10–12 minutes and 50 MC exam items in an hour. • Study in bullet format. • Use the strategies provided in Tables 1-1 to 1-3 to identify each item's focus and select the best answer, and then move on to the next item.
Squisher/Procrastinator	• Puts things off. • Does not reschedule missed study time. • Mastery of exam content is not attained and major knowledge gaps remain.	• Focus on developing a step-by step study plan. • Dig in and get started. • Adopt a "no excuses" attitude. • Join a study group or work with a study partner to stay on track.
Philosopher	• Is a thoughtful, talented, intelligent, and disciplined student. • Excels in essay questions. • Over-analyzes and reads into exam items. • Wants to know everything and answer everything about the topic. • Over-applies clinical knowledge.	• Study in bullet, not paragraph form. • Focus only on the exam item. • Look for simple, straightforward answers. • Remind yourself that your "job" on the exam is to select the best answer for the question posed, not to address all possible aspects of an item's scenario • Apply the strategies provided in Tables 1-1 to 1-3 to stay focused on answering each item as it is presented.
Lawyer	• Is a thoughtful, talented, intelligent and disciplined student. • Picks out some bit of information and builds a case on that. • Reads into a exam item to make a case for a preferred answer instead of determining what the question is asking.	• Focus on what the exam item is asking and only what the exam item is asking. • Remind youself that your "job" is to pass the NBCOT exam, not prove a point. • Remember you can train to be an NBCOT exam item writer and write "better" exam items after you pass the exam.
Second-Guesser	• Often a philosopher who reads into an item. • Frequently looks at the exam item from every angle. • Keeps changing answers, increasing anxiety, thinking less clearly and then changing answers more rapidly.	• Apply the "light bulb" strategy described in Chapter 1. – Identify a good reason to reject your first answer (i.e, missing a key word). – Identify a good reason to select a new answer (i.e., obtaining a solid hint from a subsequent exam item). • If you do not experience a "light bulb" moment, do not change your answer.

Reference: Korchek, N. (1998). Personalities of test-takers. In M. Sides and N. Korcheck. (Eds). *Successful test-taking: Learning strategies for nurses* (77–89). Philadelphia: Lippincott.

9. Be certain to complete computer-based exams in their entirety during a continuous four-hour period to increase comfort with the cognitive, visual, and ergonomic demands of the actual testing situation and help habituate effective test-taking skills.
   a. Simulating the exam in its timed format can increase comfort with the exam format and pace.
   b. Practicing use of the test taking strategies provided in Chapter 1 and the test-taking personality behavior management strategies provided in Table 2-4 during simulated exams will facilitate the habituation of these effective techniques.

10. Do not memorize sample exam items.
   a. Similar items may be on the NBCOT exam and answer choices may even be the same, but a change of only one word (e.g., "initially") can significantly alter the focus of an exam item.
   b. Understanding the rationales for the correct/incorrect answers is most relevant for exam preparation.
      (1) This *Review and Study Guide* contains extensive rationales for the text's three simulated exams.

11. Take a preparatory course.
    a. The style, format, quality, and price of courses will vary, so you will want to assess your learning style, your exam preparation needs, and past participant reviews to select the best course for you.

Key Exam Preparation Resources

1. Effective preparation for the NBCOT exam requires the recognition that there are two components to exam success. They are adequate content knowledge *and* solid objective exam test-taking skills.
2. This *Review & Study Guide* has been designed to be a *primary* content knowledge resource for studying for the exam.
    a. Our chapter authors have used the major OT textbooks identified by NBCOT as providing the foundation for exam items as their chapter references.
    b. If you are particularly weak in a certain area, additional OT textbooks, course notes and handouts can be helpful to supplement your study from this text.
3. Knowledge of exam content does not ensure success on the NBCOT exam.
    a. Competent students with good histories of academic success and satisfactory fieldwork experiences have reported failing the NBCOT exam because they have poor objective exam test-taking skills.
        (1) Entrenched test-taking personalities as described in Table 2-4 must also be effectively managed for exam success.
4. Exam preparatory courses can develop your ability to apply clinical reasoning and critical thinking skills to correctly answer simulation test (ST) items and multiple choice (MC) items.
    a. TherapyEd offers an intensive two-day course that focuses on the self assessment of test-taking abilities and exam content knowledge through the answering and discussion of practice exam items and their answer rationales.
        (1) The effective management of test-taking personalities and the development of an efficient exam preparation plan are emphasized.
        (2) Extensive participant feedback has indicated that this preparatory course when used in combination with this text is highly effective for achieving NBCOT exam success.
        (3) See www.therapyed.com for further information and participant reviews.
5. Fellow exam candidates are a valuable resource and many report studying and/or taking a review course together as a group to be very effective.

Chapter 2

Critical Reasoning and NBCOT Exam Performance

Overview of Critical Reasoning

1. Critical reasoning is a decision-making process which utilizes a person's knowledge, skills, experience, and logic to draw conclusions about everyday situations.
    a. Critical reasoning skills are the foundation for how we reason through the situations we encounter in daily life.
    b. They are the base from which people draw conclusions about their world and what they determine to be true.
    c. When used judiciously, critical reasoning is undertaken with purpose, clarity, accuracy, and thoroughness.

Relationship to the NBCOT Exam

1. Critical reasoning is vitally important for NBCOT exam success.
    a. The NBCOT exam does not merely test the ability to recall facts that are readily found in books.
        (1) Knowledge of facts is a vital foundation for your exam success, but accurately answering the NBCOT exam items requires more than the simple recall of knowledge.
        (2) The NBCOT exam integrates the different levels of objective questions to measure the knowledge, skills, and behaviors needed for competent entry-level practice.
        (3) See Table 2-1 for an outline of the main levels of objective exam questions and their relevance to the NBCOT exam.
    b. Most NBCOT MC items and *ALL* ST exam items focus on contextualized practice situations which test your ability to correctly reason and make prudent decisions about challenging clinical circumstances and/or complex practice situations.
    c. Factual information (e.g., a person's symptoms, diagnosis) must be applied to practice scenarios in which you will need to draw conclusions (e.g., most appropriate intervention, expected outcome).
2. Due to its daily use and intuitive nature, the relationship between critical reasoning and professional

exam success is often not acknowledged. Therefore, the conscious and proactive use of critical reasoning skills is an important part of your NBCOT exam preparation.

a. The three simulated exams in this *Review and Study Guide* provide multiple opportunities for you to demonstrate how well you can reason out challenging practice scenarios as you answer their 510 MC items and nine ST items.
   (1) Each exam item will require you to draw upon your knowledge, skills, and experiences to arrive at a correct conclusion.
      (a) This accurate determination is made through critical reasoning.

3. The development of critical reasoning skills is fostered during OT academic coursework and fieldwork, so at this point you will have developed a solid repertoire of critical reasoning skills.
   a. Your achievement of this level of critical reasoning skills has enabled you to succeed in your pursuit of an OT graduate degree.
   b. These capabilities will serve you well in your preparation for the NBCOT exam.
      (1) Increasing your awareness about how these critical reasoning skills are reflected in NBCOT's MC items and ST items will further enhance your exam success.
4. The following sections will make explicit important facets of critical reasoning skills and help you prepare to successfully complete the NBCOT exam.

Five Subskills of Critical Reasoning

1. There are five subskills of critical reasoning which provide the foundation for good critical reasoning.
   a. They are described by Facione and Facione (1990a, 1990b, 2006) and are based on a consensus of many critical thinking experts about the skills used in reasoning out challenging circumstances.
   b. They include inductive, deductive, analytical, inferential, and evaluative reasoning.
2. These subskills and their relevance to the NBCOT exam are described in the following sections.

Inductive Reasoning

1. The process of reasoning in which the assumptions of an argument are believed to endorse the conclusion, but do not guarantee it.
2. Starts with reasoning in specific situations and then moves to more generalized situations.
3. An important skill clinically because it helps us to look at all our possible options in a circumstance and determine which seems most reasonable.
4. Used in diagnostic thinking to form assumptions about what to expect from a diagnosis as it evolves and changes over time.
5. May start with observations in a specific situation and then lead to drawing conclusions about larger circumstances.
   a. This generalization process can lead to flawed reasoning.
      (1) For example, upon observing a person post-cerebral vascular accident (CVA) with dysarthria, a therapist concludes that all individuals post-CVA have dysarthria, which is untrue.
         (a) This false conclusion is reflective of a faulty reasoning process which applied an observation from a specific situation to a larger, more global assumption.
6. Inductive reasoning must be used cautiously when answering NBCOT exam items because situation-specific knowledge is not an adequate foundation for making universal assumptions.
   a. Be sure you are not erroneous in your reasoning by making hasty generalizations about an exam item practice scenario.
      (1) Generalizations are needed in life and even during the NBCOT exam, but you must be prudent in making such generalizations and not jump to conclusions when answering exam items.
   b. Recognizing the limitations of inductive reasoning is an important part of successful exam performance; additional critical reasoning skills are required to adequately analyze exam items.
7. To help you identify NBCOT exam items that require the formation of assumptions, the analysis of your performance on this text's three practice exams will have a picture of binoculars next to inductive reasoning MC items.

Deductive Reasoning

1. The process of reasoning in which conclusions are drawn based on facts, laws, rules, or accepted principles.
2. The reverse thinking process of inductive reasoning.
3. Starts with information about larger circumstances, broader principles, and general theories and applies this knowledge to specific situations.
   a. For example, a therapist applies the OT ethical principle of veracity to conclude that a fellow therapist who falsely documents a treatment procedure to fraudulently bill Medicare is behaving in an unethical manner.

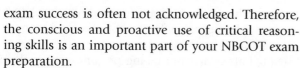

4. Provides important guidelines for OT practice by putting forth protocols (e.g., diagnostic-specific clinical pathways), procedures (e.g., correlation data analysis), rules (e.g., AOTA code of ethics), and laws (e.g., IDEA, ADA) that can be applied to a specific practice scenario without necessitating independent judgment for the situation.
5. Deductive reasoning must be used cautiously when answering NBCOT exam items because erroneous assumptions about the premises of a theory can be made and then mistakenly applied to a specific circumstance.
   a. For example, a therapist who staunchly adheres to the belief that all persons with disabilities want to be independent in all ADL would be wrong to apply this viewpoint to a person from a cultural background that views family-provided assistance as a sign of loving care. This therapist would be deducing from a flawed premise which would lead to a faulty conclusion.
   b. Recognizing the limitations of deductive reasoning is an important part of successful exam performance; the soundness and trustworthiness of the applied procedures, theories, principles, and concepts must be thoughtfully critiqued before they are applied to a specific situation.
6. To help you identify NBCOT exam items that require their correct answer to be based on facts, laws, rules, or accepted principles, the analysis of your performance on this text's three practice exams will have a picture of a microscope next to deductive reasoning MC items.

Analytical Reasoning or Analysis

1. The process of interpreting the meaning of information, determining relationships within the information presented, and then making assumptions or judgments about that information.
   a. Helps to examine ideas and concepts and the relationships between them.
2. Information presented in the form of graphs, charts, tables, and pictures encourage analytical reasoning skills because one must interpret the information that is depicted and determine what it precisely means.
   a. Information can also be presented in a narrative manner that requires one to make a "mental chart" of the information presented.
3. Used in OT practice to interpret exam results (e.g., FIM), categorize information (e.g., define a symptom based on a behavioral description, or determine a diagnosis based on a cluster of reported symptoms).
   a. Important in OT practice, because it helps the therapist determine the potential impact of a clinical condition on occupational performance.
4. Analysis is required to correctly answer many NBCOT exam items.
   a. Analytical reasoning is used when some descriptors are included in an exam item stem (e.g., member characteristics of a mature-level group), but some key descriptors needed to answer the item's question are not provided (e.g., the leader's role in a mature group) leaving the test taker to make assumptions about what the best answer would be (e.g., type of activity used in the group) based on the partial information provided.
5. Analysis exam items are often frustrating since limited information upon which an answer must be selected is provided; however, they accurately reflect the practice reality that OT practitioners rarely have complete information about a person or group.
6. To help you identify NBCOT exam items that require the exam of ideas and concepts and the relationships between them, the analysis of your performance on this text's three practice exams will have a picture of a beaker next to analytical reasoning MC items.

Inferential Reasoning or Inference

1. The process of drawing conclusions or making logical judgments based on facts, concepts, and evidence rather than direct observations.
2. Used in practice situations when a therapist infers the symptoms to expect based on a diagnosis (e.g., a person with a left CVA will exhibit right hemiplegia and aphasia) or the likely progression of a disease or disorder (e.g., amyotrophic lateral sclerosis [ALS] will steadily progress until death while the course of multiple sclerosis [MS] is characterized by exacerbations and remissions).
   a. Inferences about the nature of a disease, all of its possible symptoms and its sequelae are not guaranteed to be 100% accurate; therefore, skilled inference must be based on the therapist's knowledge and experience.
3. Inferential reasoning is also utilized in practice situations when therapists have to decide on a best course of action.
   a. Inferences about clinical courses of action are not guaranteed to be 100% accurate. For example,

when treating an individual with a rotator cuff tear, a therapist cannot be 100% certain that the chosen intervention will result in the successful therapeutic outcome of improved occupational performance. Therefore, skilled inference must be based on the therapist's knowledge and experience.

4. Inferential reasoning is regularly used by therapists in their decision-making process and this reality is precisely why the skill is important for successful NBCOT exam performance.
5. Inference is required to correctly answer many NBCOT exam item questions.
   a. Questions that ask the test taker to determine what is best, most important, or most likely to occur often require inferential reasoning.
   b. Exam items of this nature can be difficult because they ask the test-taker to determine what is believed to be true even though there is no 100% assurance that the selected answer is correct; however, they accurately reflect the realistic uncertainties of OT practice.
6. Inferential reasoning must be used cautiously when answering NBCOT exam items because inadequate consideration of the information presented in an exam item or the use of faulty or hasty logic to determine what may occur in certain situations can lead to the selection of an incorrect answer.
   a. For example, a therapist determines that it is most appropriate for a person with T12 paraplegia to focus on the upper trapezius and levator scapulae muscles in preparation for functional mobility with crutches, rather than the triceps and lower trapezius muscles. This decision is erroneous because it does not consider the nature of the task at hand (i.e., ambulation with crutches).
7. Since quick decisions can lead to suboptimal intervention, the NBCOT exam requires judicious use of inferential reasoning.
8. To help you identify NBCOT exam items that require you to draw conclusions or make logical judgments based on facts, concepts, and evidence rather than direct observations, the analysis of your performance on this text's three practice exams will have a picture of a light bulb next to inferential reasoning MC items.

Evaluative Reasoning or Evaluation

1. The process by which the merits of an argument are weighed for their validity and the inherent value of the argument itself is critiqued.
   a. The determination that an argument "holds any water" or not.
   b. If there is value found in the argument itself, the assignment of a value to it.
2. People make judgments about the merits and value of the information they receive all the time and are often unconscious of the thought process that is involved.
3. In OT practice, evaluative reasoning must be conscious.
   a. A good evaluative thinker listens with a skeptical ear to determine the trustworthiness of information before assigning a value to it.
   b. Accepting information at face value can be a reasoning pitfall since there can be additional information needed to complete an accurate assessment of a situation.
4. Evaluative reasoning helps guide thinking about a correct course of action.
5. Evaluation is often used in OT practice when difficult decisions must be made in areas that have no clear cut answers.
   a. Practice situations can be ambiguous and require the therapist to evaluate the situation, weigh the information presented, and determine a correct course of action, given his/her knowledge and experience.
   b. These dilemmas pose a challenge to practitioners since the correct course of action must be determined.
   c. For example, during an intervention session, a therapist observes bruises on an elder resident in a skilled nursing facility and must determine if the correct course of action is immediately notifying the charge nurse, the physician, adult protective services, and/or the family; or asking the resident to explain the source of the bruises; or documenting the observation and continuing with the session as planned.
6. Pitfalls in evaluative reasoning lie in assigning great value to information that has little value to the situation, not assigning enough value to highly valuable information, and finally not utilizing principles and guidelines that are put into place to help guide one's thinking (e.g., AOTA Code of Ethics, treatment protocols).
   a. For example, a therapist working in home care with a patient who becomes short of breath must determine if he/she should immediately call 911, notify the physician, or continue with the treatment session.
      (1) It would help the therapist to know if the shortness of breath is an expected symptom given the patient's diagnosis, medical history, and past response to treatment. This information would guide the therapist's thinking about a correct course of action.

(2) Evaluative reasoning is important in this clinical situation because the therapist could over-react to the situation and call 911 for expected shortness of breath that often accompanies chronic obstructive pulmonary disease or under-react and fail to call 911 when a person is also complaining of co-occurring severe unremitting substernal pain which can be indicative of a myocardial infarction.

7. Evaluative reasoning is often required during the NBCOT exam to correctly answer exam items about ethical dilemmas.
8. To help you identify exam items that pose challenging practice situations and ethical dilemmas, the analysis of your performance on this text's three practice exams will have a picture of a cogwheel next to evaluative reasoning MC items.

Developing Critical Reasoning Skills for NBCOT Exam Success

1. Since critical reasoning is not learned during a quick lesson or improved upon by simply reading the above basic descriptions of them, it is essential to practice with items that test reasoning skills and provide feedback on your performance.
   a. The good news is that this *Review and Study Guide* provides hundreds of opportunities to develop your reasoning skills.
      (1) Each MC and ST item in this text's three simulated practice exams has an accompanying rationale for the correct and incorrect answer choices.
         (a) The rationale for each of the 510 MC items also include an explanation of its corresponding critical reasoning sub-skill and the knowledge or skill required to select the correct answer.
2. When reviewing the analysis of your exam performance on this text's three simulated practice exams, pay particular attention to the five types of critical reasoning that are listed with each MC item.
   a. The five symbols assigned to designate the different types of critical reasoning are:

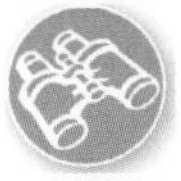 = Inductive Reasoning.

 = Deductive Reasoning.

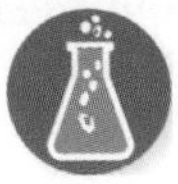 = Analysis Reasoning.

 = Inferential Reasoning.

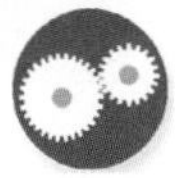 = Evaluative Reasoning.

3. Carefully review this feedback to identify any performance patterns that emerge.
   a. Is your exam performance weaker in a certain area of reasoning?
      (1) Since critical reasoning skills are based on knowledge and day to day experiences, it is not uncommon to be stronger in certain areas of reasoning than others.
4. If you have a weakness in a certain area(s) of reasoning, do not despair.
   a. Being aware of your gaps in reasoning is the first essential step in the development of a corrective plan of action.
5. As you review the rationales provided for the MC items and ST items in this *Review and Study Guide,* refer back to your incorrect responses and see if there is a pattern to the types of items you are answering incorrectly related to a sub-skill of critical reasoning.
   a. Do you notice that you have difficulty with certain types of questions?
6. Once you have identified a weakness in critical reasoning, take some time to reflect on why this is so.
   a. Ask yourself the questions identified in Table 2-5 and determine if they are reflective of your exam performance.
      (1) Questions answered affirmatively can help you identify critical reasoning skills that can be improved.
      (2) Implement the corresponding suggested exam preparation strategies to develop needed critical reasoning skills.
         (a) You can practice applying these critical reasoning strategies by using the "Create Your Own Exam" feature of the accompanying CD. Design practice exams to specifically target areas for improvement and focus on your individual needs
7. An honest appraisal of your performance patterns and the thoughtful application of relevant exam preparation strategies will help build your knowledge of, and acquire experience with, the effective application of critical reasoning skills.
   a. This preparation will help you successfully meet the challenges of the NBCOT exam.

Chapter 2

Table 2-5

Critical Reasoning Self-Assessment Questions

OBSERVED EXAM DIFFICULTY	REASONING CHALLENGE	NBCOT EXAM PREPARATION STRATEGY
Do you: – have difficulty with taking specific information and applying it to larger populations? – select incorrect answers because you can not generalize your knowledge?	Inductive	When studying a specific content area, think about how the discrete information that you are reviewing can be applied to a diversity of situations. Use a reflective "what if" stance to think how this information may be generalized to a broader context. This can be a fun and effective study group activity.
Do you: – prefer to follow your instincts rather than the guidelines that a protocol may provide? – select incorrect answers because you are unfamiliar with established practice standards or major theoretical approaches?	Deductive	Be sure when you study that you master all major facts, laws, rules, and accepted principles that guide OT practice. Carefully review all of the frames of reference, practice models, and intervention protocols and procedures provided in Chapters 11–16 and the AOTA Code of Ethics and legislation information provided in Chapter 4.
Do you: – tend to misinterpret information provided and make poor judgments and apply inadequately conceived assumptions about it? – select incorrect answers because you misjudged the effects of a clinical condition on occupational performance?	Analytical	Be sure to obtain a solid knowledge of all major clinical conditions, their symptoms, diagnostic testing and criteria, anticipated sequelae, and expected outcomes. This information is extensively reviewed in Chapters 6–10 to help you make accurate judgments and correct assumptions about the potential impact of a clinical condition on occupational performance.
Do you: – have difficulty with thinking about how clinical conditions and practice situations may evolve over time? – assume information is valid when in fact it is not true? – select incorrect answers because you have difficulty deciding the best course of action in a practice scenario?	Inferential	When studying the clinical conditions in the chapters identified above, be sure to think about how the presentation of these conditions may sometimes vary from textbook descriptions. Use the knowledge and experience you acquired during your clinical fieldworks to assess the trustworthiness of your assumptions. Study the frames of reference and practice models presented in Chapters 11–14 to develop a solid foundation on how to decide the best course of action based on facts, concepts, and evidence.
Do you: – feel anxious when you have exam items that are ambiguous and you cannot find answers to them in a textbook? – rely on protocols and guidelines more than gut instinct? – select incorrect answers because you become overwhelmed by questions that present ethical dilemmas?	Evaluative	When reviewing specific content, think about the practice ambiguities and ethical dilemmas you observed during your fieldworks related to these areas. Be sure to study the guidelines for ethical decision making that are provided in Chapter 4 to help you evaluate NBCOT question scenarios, weigh the information presented, and determine a correct course action.

This table was adapted with permission from Kari Inda's research on critical reasoning and the OT certification exam.

References

Facione, P. (2006). *Critical thinking: What it is and why it counts.* Millbrae, CA: California Academic Press.

Facione, P. (1990a). *Critical thinking: A statement of expert consensus for purposes of educational assessment and instruction. Research findings and recommendations.* Newark, DE: American Psychological Association.

Facione, P. (1990b). *Critical thinking: A statement of expert consensus for purposes of educational assessment and instruction ("Executive summary: The Delphi report").* Millbrae, CA: California Academic Press.

Facione, N. C., & Facione, P. A. (2006). *The health sciences reasoning test HSRT: Test manual 2006 edition.* Millbrae, CA: California Academic Press.

Fleming-Castaldy, R. (2012). *Occupational therapy course manual,* 4th ed. Evanston, IL: TherapyEd.

Sides, M. & Korcheck, N. (Eds.). (1998). *Successful testtaking: Learning strategies for nurses.* Philadelphia: Lippincott.

Sladyk, K., Gilmore, S., & Tufano, R. (2005). *OT exam review manual,* 4th ed. Thorofare, NJ: Slack.

3

The Process of Occupational Therapy

RITA P. FLEMING-CASTALDY

Chapter Outline

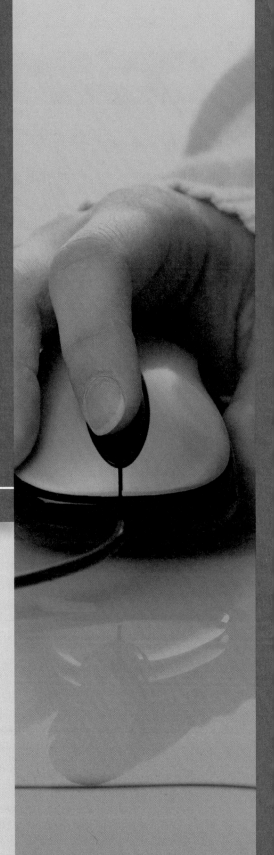

The Process of Occupational Therapy

Overview

1. The occupational therapy (OT) process is comprised of three main aspects of service delivery: evaluation, intervention, and outcomes.
2. This process is client-centered, interactive, and dynamic.
3. The NBCOT exam places a heavy emphasis on the OT process with 90% of the exam focused on direct service delivery to clients; the remaining 10% is focused on the management and direction of OT services throughout the OT process.

Referral, Screening, and Evaluation

Referral

1. The basic request for occupational therapy services. This may also be termed an order or a consultation.
2. Sources include the individual, family or caregivers, physicians, social workers, physical therapists, nurse practitioners, allied health professionals, teachers, administrators, insurance companies, employers, state and local/public and private agencies.
3. The content and form of a referral/order varies among program types and practice areas and can range from the highly specific (e.g., a resting hand splint) to the very general (e.g., evaluate for developmental delay).
4. While anyone can refer themselves or others to OT services, the ability of the occupational therapist to act upon the referral is determined by state licensure laws and/or third party reimbursers.

Screening

1. The acquisition of information to determine the need for an in depth evaluation and to obtain a preliminary understanding of the individual's needs, limitations, assets, and resources.
2. Screening procedures are usually brief and easy to administer since they must be applied to a large number of individuals (i.e., all persons who receive an OT referral need to be screened to determine the appropriateness of the referral).
3. Screening tools measure broad performance abilities and include chart/medical record review, checklists, structured observations, and/or brief interviews with the individual, family, and/or caregivers.
4. The outcome of the screening will determine the client factors, areas of occupation, performance skills, patterns, and/or contexts that require further evaluation.

Evaluation

1. "The comprehensive process of obtaining and interpreting the data necessary to understand the individual, system, or situation" (Hinojosa, Kramer, & Crist, 2005, p. 2).
2. If the individual and the occupational therapist do not share a common language, an interpreter must be used to ensure the validity of the information obtained and that no cultural or religious norms are violated that may compromise the therapeutic process.
3. Obtain a history of the individual's past level of functional performance.
4. Select an appropriate standardized or nonstandardized evaluation tool.
   a. Determine which assessment will attain information essential for setting goals and planning intervention.
   b. Considerations in determining appropriate assessments.
      (1) Individual's baseline functional level, major concerns, and pressing needs as determined through the screening process.
      (2) The environmental context in which the assessment will be conducted.
         (a) The length of stay of the setting influences comprehensiveness of evaluation.
         (b) The primary focus of the setting, (e.g., prevocational versus self management).

(c) Legislative guidelines and restrictions (e.g., in a school setting, assessments must focus on areas related to the child's educational needs).
(d) The facility's resources of space, equipment, and supplies.
(3) The environmental context of the individual's current and expected environment.
(a) Sociocultural aspects including roles, values, norms, supports. (For example, in some cultures home management is only considered a valued role for females, so there is no need to do a home management evaluation for a male of this cultural background.)
(b) Physical environment characteristics. (For example, it would be essential to measure functional mobility endurance for a person who lives in a third floor walk-up apartment.)
(4) The temporal context of the individual and his/her disability.
(a) Person's chronological and developmental age.
(b) Anticipated duration of disability (e.g., short-term, long-term, permanent).
(c) Recent occurrence of illness or exacerbation of a long-standing, chronic condition.
(d) Stage of illness (e.g., acute stage versus terminal stage).
(5) The evaluation tool's compatibility with frame of reference selected to guide intervention planning.
(6) Consider ethical concerns and potential ethical conflicts (Table 3-1).

5. Administer the assessment according to recommended guidelines, administration protocols, and/or standardized procedures.
   a. Observe standard precautions (Tables 3-2 and 3-3).
6. Score or rate assessment results according to published guidelines or standardized procedures.
7. Interpret the assessment results in relation to uniform terminology, the practice framework, and/or a specific frame of reference.
   a. Integrate referral, screening, and diagnostic information and data gathered from assessment.
   b. Relate all information to functional abilities and disabilities relevant to person's roles and environmental contexts.
   c. Use caution when interpreting information based on self report or a highly structured assessment as results may not reflect performance in natural contexts.
   d. Identify functional deficits in occupational performance areas relevant to the individual.
   e. In school/educational settings, assessment information must be related to the multiple aspects of educational performance.
      (1) Academic.
      (2) Mobility.
      (3) Psychosocial.
      (4) Behavioral.
      (5) Self care.
8. Collaborate with the individual, family, caregivers, and other team members to obtain a broader picture of the person's situation and to put the OT assessment results into a larger context.
   a. In school/educational settings, medically necessary OT must be separated from educationally relevant OT.
   b. Referrals to after school, home care, and/or community based OT services are indicated for non-educational OT.
9. Prioritize identified problems in collaboration with the individual to develop intervention plan.
10. Document and communicate the evaluation findings to relevant parties (i.e., consumer, team members, and third party payers).
11. Refer to other professionals or specialists within the profession, as needed, for further evaluation.

Psychometric Properties of Assessments

1. Standardization.
   a. A standardized evaluation is one that is uniform and well-established.
   b. It is always the same in content, administration, and scoring.
   c. Characteristics of a standardized instrument.
      (1) A description of its purpose.
      (2) An administration and scoring protocol.
      (3) Established norms and validity.
2. The administration protocol.
   a. Provides instructions on what to do, ensuring all administrations of the assessment are consistent.
   b. Identifies materials needed for the assessment.
   c. Provides exact wording of directions to give to the individual.
3. The scoring protocol.
   a. Provides ratings and criteria for determining ratings.
   b. Provides norms for the range of ratings for a specific population.
   c. Types of normative data.
      (1) Age.
      (2) Gender.
      (3) Diagnostic groupings.

Table 3-1

Questionnaire for Identifying Potential Conflicts in Assessment

OCCUPATIONAL THERAPIST
• Am I competent to do this assessment? Do I have the necessary knowledge, skills, and attitudes to select, administer, and interpret the results of each evaluation?
• Am I competent to supervise other occupational therapy personnel in the collection of data for this assessment? Am I sure that all delegated tasks are being carried out properly by competent individuals?
• Have I accurately documented the services provided? Is the summary assessment an accurate reflection of the separate evaluations?
OCCUPATIONAL THERAPY ASSISTANT
• Am I competent to carry out the data collection that I am responsible to perform?
• Am I receiving adequate training and supervision to carry out the assigned portions of the assessment process?
• Have I accurately reported the data and contributed to the overall assessment process?
INDIVIDUAL WHO IS BEING ASSESSED (FAMILY, SIGNIFICANT OTHERS, GUARDIAN)
• Has the consumer been informed about the purpose of the assessment, how will it be administered, and by whom? Does this person understand how the results of the assessment will be used?
• Has the individual been informed about how this service will be billed?
• Has the person been given the opportunity to decide if the assessment should be done?
• Are the individual's goals the basis for developing and carrying out the assessment process?
EMPLOYER (FACILITY, AGENCY, COMPANY)
• Is the assessment consistent with the mission of the facility?
• Will there be an accurate billing for services?
• How will the interpretation and recommendations of the therapist be used?
PAYER
• Is the assessment a necessary and billable service?
• If there is not coverage by third-party reimbursement, does the client know this? Has this individual given consent before the initiation of the evaluations?
• Will the therapist and the billing office request fair compensation for the services and request payment only for the services provided?
PROFESSIONAL COLLEAGUES
• Is the referral consistent with the client's goals and needs?
• Is this assessment necessary?
• Are you communicating the results of the assessment clearly so that other members of the service delivery team have useful information?
• Have copyrighted evaluation materials been used according to the laws regulating their use?
• Is it necessary to pay fees to use the evaluation tool? Have they been paid?
• Must the practitioner obtain permission to use the materials?
• Is there specific training and supervision required to conduct the evaluation?
• Does the person carrying out the evaluation hold the appropriate credentials to do so?
• Have you used the correct forms and procedures in conducting the evaluation and reporting the results?
• If it is a standardized evaluation, have you followed the procedures exactly?
COMMUNITY AND SOCIETY
• Is this assessment consistent with the concepts of due process, reparation for wrongs that have been done (physical or emotional), and the fair and equitable distribution of occupational therapy services to individuals needing those services?

From Lesson 10: Ethical considerations. In C.B. Royeen (ed.), *AOTA self-study series: Assessing functions*, (p. 9) by Hansen, R.A. Copyright 1990 by the American Occupational Therapy Association. Reprinted with permission.

Table 3-2

Standard Precautions
OVERVIEW
Standard Precautions combine the major features of Universal Precautions (UP) and Body Substance Isolation (BSI) and are based on the principle that all blood, body fluids, secretions, excretions except sweat, nonintact skin, and mucous membranes may contain transmissible infectious agents. Standard Precautions include a group of infection prevention practices that apply to all patients, regardless of suspected or confirmed infection status, in any setting in which health care is delivered. These include hand hygiene; use of gloves, gown, mask, eye protection, or face shield, depending on the anticipated exposure; and safe injection practices. Also, equipment or items in the patient environment likely to have been contaminated with infectious body fluids must be handled in a manner to prevent transmission of infectious agents (e.g., wear gloves for direct contact, contain heavily soiled equipment, properly clean and disinfect or sterilize reusable equipment before use on another patient). The application of Standard Precautions during patient care is determined by the nature of the health care worker (HCW)–patient interaction and the extent of anticipated blood, body fluid, or pathogen exposure. Standard Precautions are also intended to protect patients by ensuring that health-care personnel do not carry infectious agents to patients on their hands or via equipment used during patient care.
Assume that every person is potentially infected or colonized with an organism that could be transmitted in the health-care setting and apply the following infection control practices during the delivery of health care.
HAND HYGIENE
1. During the delivery of health care, avoid unnecessary touching of surfaces in close proximity to the patient to prevent both contamination of clean hand from environmental surfaces and transmission of pathogens from contaminated hands to surfaces.
2. When hands are visibly dirty, contaminated with proteinaceous material, or visibly soiled with blood or body fluids, wash hands with either a nonantimicrobial soap and water or an antimicrobial soap and water.
3. If hands are not visibly soiled, or after removing visible material with nonantimicrobial soap and water decontaminate hands in the clinical situations described in a–f below. The preferred method of hand decontamination is with an alcohol-based hand rub. Alternatively, hands may be washed with an antimicrobial soap and water. Frequent use of an alcohol-based hand rub immediately following hand washing with nonantimicrobial soap may increase the frequency of dermatitis. Perform hand hygiene:
a. Before having direct contact with patients.
b. After contact with blood, body fluids or excretions, mucous membranes, nonintact skin, or wound dressings.
c. After contact with a patient's intact skin (e.g., when taking a pulse or blood pressure or lifting a patient).
d. If hands will be moving from a contaminated body site to a clean body site during patient care.
e. After contact with inanimate objects (including medical equipment) in the immediate vicinity of the patient.
f. After removing gloves.
4. Wash hands with nonantimicrobial soap and water or with antimicrobial soap and water if in contact with spores (e.g., Clostridium difficile or Bacillus anthracis) is likely to have occurred. The physical action of washing and rinsing hands under such circumstances is recommended because alcohols, chlorhexidine, iodophors, and other antiseptic agents have poor activity against spores.
5. Do not wear artificial fingernails or extenders if duties include direct contact with patients at high risk for infection and associated adverse outcomes (e.g., those in intensive care units [ICUs] or operating rooms).
a. Develop an organizational policy on the wearing of non-natural nails by health-care personnel who have direct contact with patients outside of the groups specified above.
PERSONAL PROTECTIVE EQUIPMENT (PPE)
1. Observe the following principles of use:
a. Wear PPE, as described in 2–4 below, when the nature of the anticipated patient interaction indicates that contact with blood or body fluids may occur.
b. Prevent contamination of clothing and skin during the process of removing PPE.
c. Before leaving the patient's room or cubicle, remove and discard PPE.
2. Gloves
a. Wear gloves when it can be reasonably anticipated that contact with blood or other potentially infectious materials, mucous membranes, nonintact skin, or potentially contaminated intact skin (e.g., of a patient incontinent of stool or urine) could occur.
b. Wear gloves with fit and durability appropriate to the task.
(1) Wear disposable medical examination gloves for providing direct patient care.
(2) Wear disposable medical examination gloves or reusable utility gloves for cleaning the environment or medical equipment.
c. Remove gloves after contact with a patient and/or the surrounding environment (including medical equipment) using proper technique to prevent hand contamination.

(Continued)

Table 3-2

Standard Precautions (*Continued*)

(1) Do not wear the same pair of gloves for the care of more than one patient. Do not wash gloves for the purpose of reuse since this practice has been associated with transmission of pathogens.

d. Change gloves during patient care if the hands will move from a contaminated body site (e.g., perineal area) to a clean body site (e.g., face).

3. Gowns

a. Wear a gown that is appropriate to the task to protect skin and prevent soiling or contamination of clothing during procedures and patient-care activities when contact with blood, body fluids, secretions, or excretions is anticipated.

(1) Wear a gown for direct patient contact if the patient has un contained secretions or excretions.

(2) Remove gown and perform hand hygiene before leaving the patient's environment.

b. Do not reuse gowns, even for repeated contacts with the same patient.

c. Routine donning of gowns upon entrance into a high-risk unit (e.g., ICU, neonatal intensive care unit [NICU], hematopoietic stem cell transplantation [HSCT] unit) is not indicated.

4. Mouth, nose, eye protection.

a. Use PPE to protect the mucous membranes of the eyes, nose, and mouth during procedures and patient-care activities that are likely to generate splashes or sprays of blood, body fluids, secretions, and excretions. Select masks, goggles, face shields, and combinations of each according to the need anticipated by the task performed.

5. During aerosol-generating procedures (e.g., bronchoscopy, suctioning of the respiratory tract [if not using in-line suction catheters], endotracheal intubation) in patients who are not suspected of being infected with an agent for which respiratory protection is otherwise recommended (e.g., M. tuberculosis, SARS, orhemorrhagic fever viruses), wear one of the following: a face shield that fully covers the front and sides of the face, a mask with attached shield, or a mask and goggles (in addition to gloves and gown).

RESPIRATORY HYGIENE/COUGH ETIQUETTE

1. Educate healthcare personnel on the importance of source control measures to contain respiratory secretions to prevent droplet and fomite transmission of respiratory pathogens, especially during seasonal outbreaks of viral respiratory tract infections (e.g., influenza, respiratory syncytial virus [RSV], adenovirus, parainfluenza virus) in communities.

2. Implement the following measures to contain respiratory secretions in patients and accompanying individuals who have signs and symptoms of a respiratory infection, beginning at the point of initial encounter in a health-care setting (e.g., triage, reception and waiting areas in emergency departments, outpatient clinics, and physician offices).

a. Post signs at entrances and in strategic places (e.g., elevators, cafeterias) within ambulatory and inpatient settings with instructions to patients and other persons with symptoms of a respiratory infection to cover their mouths/noses when coughing or sneezing, use and dispose of tissues, and perform hand hygiene after hands have been in contact with respiratory secretions.

b. Provide tissues and no-touch receptacles (e.g., foot pedal–operated lid or open, plastic-lined waste basket) for disposal of tissues.

c. Provide resources and instructions for performing hand hygiene in or near waiting areas in ambulatory and inpatient settings; provide conveniently located dispensers of alcohol-based hand rubs and, where sinks are available, supplies for hand washing.

d. During periods of increased prevalence of respiratory infections in the community (e.g., as indicated by increased school absenteeism, increased number of patients seeking care for a respiratory infection), offer masks to coughing patients and other symptomatic persons (e.g., persons who accompany ill patients) upon entry into the facility or medical office and encourage them to maintain special separation, ideally a distance of at least 3 feet, from others in common waiting areas.

(1) Some facilities may find it logistically easier to institute this recommendation year-round as a standard of practice.

PATIENT PLACEMENT

1. Include the potential for transmission of infectious agents in patient placement decisions.

a. Place patients who pose a risk for transmission to others (e.g., uncontained secretions, excretions or wound drainage, infants with suspected viral respiratory or gasrointestinal infections) in a single-patient room when available.

2. Determine patient placement based on the following principles:

a. Route(s) of transmission of the known or suspected infectious agent.

b. Risk factors for transmission in the infected patient.

c. Risk factors for adverse outcomes resulting from a hospital-acquired infection (HAI) in other patients in the area or room being considered for patient placement.

d. Availability of single-patient rooms.

e. Patient options for room sharing (e.g., cohorting patients with the same infection).

Table 3-2

Standard Precautions (*Continued*)
PATIENT-CARE EQUIPMENT AND INSTRUMENTS/DEVICES
1. Establish policies and procedures for containing, transporting, and handling patient-care equipment and instruments/devices that may be contaminated with blood or body fluids.
2. Remove organic material from critical and semicritical instrument/devices, using recommended cleaning agents before high-level disinfection and sterilization to enable effective disinfection and sterilization processes.
3. Wear PPE (e.g., gloves, gown), according to the level of anticipated contamination, when handling patient-care equipment and instruments/devices that are visibly soiled or may have been in contact with blood or body fluids.
CARE OF THE ENVIRONMENT
1. Establish policies and procedures for routine and targeted cleaning of environmental surfaces as indicated by the level of patient contact and degree of soiling.
2. Clean and disinfect surfaces that are likely to be contaminated with pathogens, including those that are in close proximity to the patient (e.g., bed rails, over bed tables) and frequently touched surfaces in the patient-care environment (e.g., door knobs, surfaces in and surrounding toilets in patients' rooms) on a more frequent schedule compared to that for other surfaces (e.g., horizontal surfaces in waiting rooms).
3. Use Environmental Protection Agency (EPA)–registered disinfectants that have microbiocidal (i.e., killing) activity against the pathogens most likely to contaminate the patient-care environment. Use in accordance with manufacturer's instructions.
a. Review the efficacy of in-use disinfectants when evidence of continuing transmission of an infectious agent (e.g., rotavirus, C. difficile, norovirus) may indicate resistance to the in-use product and change to a more effective disinfectant as indicated.
4. In facilities that provide health care to pediatric patients or have waiting areas with child play toys (e.g., obstetric/gynecology offices and clinics), establish policies and procedures for cleaning and disinfecting toys at regular intervals.
a. Use the following principles in developing this policy and procedures:
(1) Select play toys that can be easily cleaned and disinfected.
(2) Do not permit use of stuffed furry toys if they will be shared.
(3) Clean and disinfect large stationary toys (e.g., climbing equipment) at least weekly and whenever visibly soiled.
(4) If toys are likely to be mouthed, rinse with water after disinfection; alternatively wash in a dishwasher.
(5) When a toy requires cleaning and disinfection, do so immediately or store in a designated labeled container separate from toys that are clean and ready for use.
5. Include multiuse electronic equipment in policies and procedures for preventing contamination and for cleaning and disinfection, especially those items that are used by patients, those used during delivery of patient care, and mobile devices that are moved in and out of patient rooms frequently (e.g., daily).
a. No recommendations are provided for use of removable protective covers or washable keyboards. This is an unresolved issue.
TEXTILES AND LAUNDRY
1. Handle used textiles and fabrics with minimum agitation to avoid contamination of air, surfaces, and persons.
2. If laundry are used, ensure that they are properly designed, maintained, and used in a manner to minimize dispersion of aerosols from contaminated laundry.
SAFE INJECTION PRACTICES
These are not included here since OT practitioners do not give injections. See CDC website.
WORKER SAFETY
Adhere to federal and state requirements for protection of health-care personnel from exposure to bloodborne pathogens.
Reference: Centers for Disease Control and Prevention. (2007). *Guideline for isolation precautions: Preventing transmission of infectious agents in healthcare settings.* Retrieved March 9, 2010 from http://www.cdc.gov/ncidod/dhqp/gl_isolation_standard.html

d. Norms are used for a comparative analysis of an individual's score.
  (1) An individual's characteristics must match the characteristics of the population used to establish the norms (e.g., you cannot compare a 25-year-old's score with norms based on a 10 year-old or a 65-year-old).
  (2) If the client is dissimilar from the "normed" population, interpretations based on these norms would be inaccurate.

Table 3-3

Transmission-based Precautions
There are three categories of Transmission-Based Precautions: Contact Precautions, Droplet Precautions, and Airborne Precautions. Transmission-Based Precautions are used when the route(s) of transmission is (are) not completely interrupted using Standard Precautions alone. For some diseases that have multiple routes of transmission (e.g., SARS), more than one Transmission-Based Precautions category may be used. When used either singly or in combination, they are always used in addition to Standard Precautions. When Transmission-Based Precautions are indicated, efforts must be made to counteract possible adverse effects on patients (i.e., anxiety, depression and other mood disturbances, perceptions of stigma, reduced contact with clinical staff, and increases in preventable adverse events in order to improve acceptance by the patients and adherence by health care workers.
AIRBORNE PRECAUTIONS
In addition to Standard Precautions, use Airborne Precautions, or the equivalent, for patients known or suspected to be infected with serious illness transmitted by airborne droplet nuclei (small-particle residue) that remain suspended in the air and that can be dispersed widely by air currents within a room or over a long distance (for example, Mycobacterium tuberculosis, measles virus, chickenpox virus).
1. Respiratory isolation room.
2. Wear respiratory protection (mask) when entering room.
3. Limit movement and transport of patient to essential purposes only. Mask patient when transporting out of area.
DROPLET PRECAUTIONS
In addition to Standard Precautions, use Droplet Precautions, or the equivalent, for patients known or suspected to be infected with serious illness microorganisms transmitted by large particle droplets that can be generated by the patient during coughing, sneezing, talking, or the performance of procedures (for example, mumps, rubella, pertussis, influenza).
1. Isolation room.
2. Wear respiratory protection (mask) when entering room.
3. Limit movement and transport of patient to essential purposes only. Mask patient when transporting out of area.
CONTACT PRECAUTIONS
In addition to Standard Precautions, use Contact Precautions, or the equivalent, for specified patients known or suspected to be infected or colonized with serious illness transmitted by direct patient contact (hand or skin-to-skin contact) or contact with items in patient environment.
1. Isolation room.
2. Wear gloves when entering room; change gloves after having contact with infective material; remove gloves before leaving patient's room; wash hands immediately with an antimicrobial agent or waterless antiseptic agent. After glove removal and handwashing, ensure that hands do not touch contaminated environmental items.
3. Wear a gown when entering room if you anticipate your clothing will have substantial contact with the patient, environmental surfaces, or items in the patient's room, or if the patient is incontinent or has diarrhea, ileostomy, colostomy, or wound drainage not contained by dressing. Remove gown before leaving patient's room; after gown removal, ensure that clothing does not contact potentially contaminated environmental surfaces.
4. Single-patient-use equipment.
5. Limit movement and transport of patient to essential purposes only. Use precautions when transporting patient to minimize risk of transmission of microorganisms to other patients and contamination of environmental surfaces or equipment.
Reference: Centers for Disease Control and Prevention. (2007). *Guideline for isolation precautions: Preventing transmission of infectious agents in healthcare settings.* Retrieved March 9, 2010 from http://www.cdc.gov/ncidod/dhqp/gl_isolation_standard.html

4. Validity measures the assessment's accuracy to determine if the tool measures what it was intended to measure.
   a. Face validity establishes how well the assessment instrument appears "on the face of it" to meet its stated purpose (e.g., an activity configuration looks like it measures time use).
   b. Content validity establishes that the content included in the evaluation is representative of the content that could be measured (e.g., does the content of a role checklist provide an adequate listing of roles?).
   c. Criterion validity compares the assessment tool to another one with already established validity.
   d. Types of criterion validity.
      (1) Concurrent validity compares the results of two instruments given at about the same time.
      (2) Predictive validity compares the degree to which an instrument can predict performance on a future criterion.
   e. Criterion validity is reported as a correlation. The higher the correlation, the better the criterion validity.
5. Reliability establishes the consistency and stability of the evaluation.

a. If reliable, the evaluation measurements/scores are the same from time to time, place to place, and evaluation to evaluation.
b. Inter-rater reliability or inter-observer reliability establishes that different raters using the same assessment tool will achieve the same results.
c. Test-retest reliability establishes that the same results will be obtained when the evaluation is administrated twice by the same administrator.
d. Reliability is scored as either a correlation or a percentage to identify the degree to which the two items agree/relate.

Assessment Tools

1. Observation involves visual assessment of an individual, his/her behavior, and environmental contexts. An overview of the skills needed for accurate observations is provided in the following section.
2. Interviews involve the therapist asking the individual specific questions. An overview of interviewing techniques is provided in a subsequent section.
3. Self report requires the individual to disclose personal information in an organized manner, e.g., through the completion of a questionnaire.
4. Checklists require the use of a predetermined listing of items against which a person's performance is checked to determine the presence or absence of these items.
5. Rating scales require the individual or therapist to rate reactions, performance, or a set criterion according to an established scale.
6. Goal Attainment Scaling (GAS) uses interviews and rating scales during initial sessions to facilitate clients' participation in the goal-setting process by identifying intervention outcomes that are personally relevant to them; used during post-treatment sessions to assess client progress toward desired goals.
7. Performance tests involve structured guidelines and/or standardized procedures for engaging the individual in performing an activity and for scoring this activity performance.
8. Norm-referenced assessments produce scores that compare the individual's performance to a set population's performance.
9. Criterion-referenced assessments provide scores that compare the individual's performance to a pre-established criterion.
10. Specific assessment tools for client factors, areas of occupation, and performance skills, patterns, and contexts will be reviewed in subsequent chapters.

Observation Skills

1. Observation of a person during actual occupational performance is critical.
2. Observation of performance must be done in different contexts and in structured and unstructured situations.
3. Observation of environmental contexts is also important to assess physical and sociocultural supports or barriers.
4. Use of a structured tool (e.g., COTE) to note observations can increase reliability.
5. Observations must be ongoing to assess the nuances of performance and subtle changes in function.
6. The therapist must be aware of his/her own sociocultural background, as this is the lens through which he/she observes and it can influence the interpretation of observations (e.g., appropriateness of the individual's nonverbal behavior).
7. The therapist's interpretation of his/her observations must be validated by the individual and/or caregiver.

Interviewing Guidelines

1. Establish the purpose of the interview.
   a. Questions asked and information sought should be consistent with stated purpose.
   b. Interviewee should feel each question is relevant and significant.
   c. Irrelevant, spurious, and/or extraneous questions should not be asked.
2. Establish rapport with interviewee.
   a. Initial interview is often the beginning of a long-term therapeutic relationship.
   b. Set an atmosphere of trust by maintaining confidentiality.
   c. Set an atmosphere of respect by being on time, asking pertinent questions, and actively listening.
3. Ask questions in an organized, formalized manner.
   a. Interviews are not casual conversations.
   b. A haphazard approach will not obtain information needed to achieve the purpose of the interview.
   c. Numerous assessment tools are available to guide the interview (e.g., COPM, OPHI). (See Chapter 14.)
4. Observe interviewee's nonverbal communications during the interview.
   a. What is not said during an interview can be as important as what is said.
      (1) Gaps in information presented.
      (2) Affect and mood.
      (3) Physical mannerisms.
      (4) Speech patterns and inflections.
   b. Interpret the congruence or incongruence of nonverbal behaviors with actual verbalizations.

5. Listen before talking.
   a. Counteracts preconceived views of interviewer.
   b. Prevents premature recommendations.
6. Question and re-question, as needed, to obtain essential information.
   a. Follow up questions should be specific.
   b. Open-ended, leading questions facilitate discussion.
   c. Questions that can be answered by yes or no should be avoided.
7. Comment in a limited manner and only when directly related to the stated purpose of the interview.
   a. Reassuring comments are used to facilitate interviewee's participation.
   b. Specific suggestions or advice should only be given if intervention is part of interview's purpose.
8. Answer personal questions directed to interviewer by interviewee in a direct and honest manner.
   a. Purposes of personal questions asked by interviewee.
      (1) To show a general polite interest in interviewer.
      (2) To move the therapeutic relationship to a closer level.
      (3) To indirectly introduce a personal concern of his/her own.
   b. Interviewer should immediately re-direct interviewee to purpose of interview and to him/herself after providing a brief, truthful answer.
9. Lead and direct interview to achieve stated purpose.
10. Interpret verbalizations and nonverbal communications to formulate hypotheses about interviewee's situation.
11. Develop a plan based on the information obtained from the interview and the hypotheses formulated about the person's situation.
    a. Plan can include the need for further evaluation and more information.
    b. The use of an interview to formulate a plan can prevent interviewing just for the sake of interviewing.
    c. Plans for intervention should be developed collaboratively with the individual using a client-centered approach.
12. Maintain confidentiality at all times.

Developmental Considerations in Evaluation

1. Conduct family/teacher interviews and home/classroom observations.
   a. To explore environmental characteristics related to the child's development.
   b. To identify family supports and community resources.
   c. To identify cultural values.
   d. To establish family-centered priorities.
2. Consider appropriate developmental levels in selecting assessments, toys, and other evaluation media.
3. Observe symmetries/asymmetries, stability of trunk, pelvis, hips, and shoulders, at rest and during movement.
4. Observe transitional movement in and out of prone, supine, side-lying, quadruped, sitting, standing, kneeling, half-kneel, and in various sitting positions such as tailor, long, heel, or side-sitting.
5. Assess the quality of movement in and out of the above positions.
6. Assess fine motor coordination.
7. Consider proper positioning and adaptive equipment, seating, and technology needs.
8. Assess cognition in the context of play and other occupations.
9. Assess psychosocial skills such as the child's coping style, frustration tolerance, and social interaction.
10. Consider visual and auditory status and aides.
11. Refer to Chapter 5 for specific pediatric and developmental assessments.

Intervention

Types of Intervention

1. Prevention: interventions designed to promote wellness, prevent disabilities and illnesses, and maintain health.
   a. Primary prevention: the reduction of the incidence or occurrence of a disease or disorder within a population that is currently well or considered to be potentially at risk (e.g., parenting skills classes for teen parents to prevent child neglect or abuse).
      (1) In the AOTA practice framework, primary prevention is termed "create/promote" and "health promotion."
         (a) Interventions focus on providing enrichment experiences to enhance person's occupational performance in their natural contexts.

b. Secondary prevention: the early detection of problems in a population at risk to reduce the duration of a disorder/disease and/or minimize its effects through early detection/diagnosis, early appropriate referral and early/effective intervention (e.g., the screening of infants born prematurely for developmental delays and the immediate implementation of intervention for identified delays).
c. Tertiary prevention: the elimination or reduction of the impact of dysfunction on an individual (e.g., the provision of rehabilitation services to maximize community participation).
d. In the AOTA practice framework, the term "disability prevention" is used to designate interventions that address the needs of persons with or without disabilities who are considered at risk for problems with their occupational performance.
    (1) Interventions focus on preventing the occurrence or minimizing the effects of barriers to occupational performance.

2. Meeting health needs: interventions designed to satisfy inherent, universal human needs. These needs are not automatically met and they include:
    a. Psychophysical: the need for adequate shelter, food, material goods, sensory stimulation, physical activity and rest (e.g., institutionalized orphans confined to cribs require sensorimotor interventions to counter environmental deprivation).
    b. Temporal balance and regularity: the need for a satisfying balance between work/productive activities, leisure/play, and rest (e.g., forced leisure due to involuntary unemployment requires intervention to achieve temporal balance).
    c. Safety: the need to be in an environment free from hazards or threats (e.g., living in a chaotic, abusive home does not meet this need and interventions are needed to ensure safety).
    d. Love and acceptance: the need to be accepted and loved for one's personal attributes and uniqueness, not for one's accomplishments (e.g., the barriers caused by aphasia and ataxia can hinder meeting this need; therefore, supportive interventions are indicated).
    e. Group association: the need to feel a connection to others who share similar interests and goals (e.g., the stigma and symptoms of mental illness can prevent regular interactions with a group; therefore, interventions to develop social interaction skills and provide community supports are indicated).
    f. Mastery: the need to successfully complete an activity or meet a goal because it is interesting and challenging (e.g., deficits in performance components can hinder successful performance and block mastery, therefore interventions to develop performance skills and/or adapt activities are needed).
    g. Esteem: the need to be recognized for one's accomplishments (e.g., a lack of opportunity to do activities perceived as worthwhile by others requires interventions to facilitate recognized contributions).
    h. Sexual: the need for recognition of one's sexuality and the satisfaction of sexual drives (e.g., institutional rules against adult consensual sex prohibit meeting this need and require review and revision). Also, physical impediments to sexuality may require activity adaptations and environmental modifications.
    i. Pleasure: the need to do things just for fun (e.g., the child on an intensive school and home physical rehabilitation program needs an intervention plan supportive of spontaneous play).
    j. Self actualization: the need to engage in activities just for one's self and for personal satisfaction (e.g., the person who writes poetry through an augmentative communication device for the joy of free expression).

3. The change process: interventions designed to achieve behavioral changes and functional outcomes.
    a. This type of intervention is the most commonly used in OT practice and is the most reimbursable.
    b. This process is often the only form of intervention discussed or documented.
    c. Most guidelines for intervention planning and intervention implementation relate directly to this process.
    d. In the AOTA practice framework, the terms "establish/restore/remediation/restoration" are used to distinguish interventions that change a person in some manner.
        (1) Interventions focus on establishing a skill or ability that a person had never developed and/or restoring a skill or ability that the person had lost due to impairment.

4. Management: interventions designed to reduce or minimize disruptive or undesirable behavior that interfere with therapeutic activities or procedures needed to change areas of dysfunction that are the main focus of intervention (e.g., an individual becomes excessively anxious during his/her first use of a wheelchair in an environment outside of the hospital. Supportive interventions are needed to decrease anxiety, thereby enabling the person to work on essential community mobility skills).
    a. In the AOTA practice framework, the terms "modify/compensation/adaptation" are used to distinguish interventions that alter the context or demands of an activity to reduce distracting features.
        (1) Compensation and adaptation techniques are also used to alter the context or demands of an activity to support the person's ability to engage in areas of occupation (e.g., the provision of cues).

5. Maintenance: interventions designed to support and preserve the individual's current functional level (e.g., a reminiscence group to maintain the cognitive and social skills of individuals with early to mid-stage Alzheimer's disease).
   a. No improvement in function is planned due to the chronicity of the disorder or the progression of the disease.
   b. A decline in function is prevented, as much and for as long as possible.
   c. Maintenance programs include familial, environmental, and social supports and consistent and regularly scheduled follow-ups.
   d. While maintenance is not often reimbursed by third-party payers, it is a major type of OT intervention due to the chronic and progressive nature of many disorders with which we work.
   e. In the AOTA practice framework, the term "maintain" is used to designate these interventions.

Intervention Planning

1. The formulation of the plan for intervention based upon an analysis of evaluation results according to selected frame(s) of reference.
2. Collaboration with the individual, family, significant others, and/or caregivers is essential to establish a relevant, meaningful plan that will be followed.
3. Prioritization of problem areas to be addressed in intervention.
   a. Values, interests, and needs of the individual, family, significant others, and caregivers.
   b. Individual's current and expected roles and environmental contexts.
   c. The treatment setting's characteristics, resources, and limitations (e.g., length of stay).
   d. The likelihood that the problem will respond to intervention within the given setting.
      (1) Concrete and specific problems are more likely to be effectively resolved than abstract global ones.
      (2) Services must be available within the setting to effectively address the problem; otherwise a referral is indicated.
4. Formats of written intervention plans can vary from setting to setting.
5. Intervention plan content.
   a. Long-term goals (LTGs): the change in activity limitations and participation restriction that will occur, prior to the termination of intervention, in order to achieve the desired functional occupational performance outcome.
   b. Short-term goals (STGs) or objectives: the component subskills which are to be achieved over shorter time frames, leading to the attainment of the long-term goal.
      (1) STGs must be directly related to the LTG.
      (2) Due to the reality of very brief lengths of stay (LOS) in some settings, only STGs may be accomplished prior to the termination of intervention.
      (3) Referrals to other settings with longer LOS or home care services may be required for intervention to attain LTGs.
   c. Intervention methods.
      (1) The meaningful occupations and purposeful activities and their associated tasks, techniques, procedures, and modalities that are used to achieve goals.
      (2) Methods of intervention must be clearly related to, and theoretically consistent with, the established goals.
      (3) Home programs and/or family caregiver training may be included.
      (4) Adaptive/assistive equipment, orthotics, prosthetics, and/or environmental modifications to meet individual's needs are specified.
   d. Duration, frequency, and number and type of intervention sessions planned to attain goals are specified (e.g., 10 community mobility groups, meeting for 1 hour, 3 times per week).
   e. Recommendations for additional OT services and referrals, if needed, to other professionals are provided.
   f. The design of all intervention plans must actively use clinical reasoning to ensure that each plan's primary focus is on the individual's engagement in occupation and participation in his/her chosen contexts. See this chapter's section on clinical reasoning.
   g. The existing evidence to support potential interventions must be reviewed and used to guide the intervention plan.

Intervention Implementation

1. Fundamental OT principles are used to guide OT interventions. Refer to Table 3-4, "Principles of Occupations."
2. Clinical reasoning is used to ensure that the implementation of intervention is relevant to the individual and the uniqueness of his/her situation. See this chapter's section on clinical reasoning.
3. Overview of OT intervention methods.
   a. Purposeful activities and meaningful occupations are used therapeutically.
   b. Environmental modifications and adaptations are provided to enhance function.

Table 3-4

Principles of Occupations That Support Their Value and Use in Intervention		
PRINCIPLE	**EXPLANATION**	**EXAMPLE**
Occupations and activities act as a therapeutic change agent to *remediate* or *restore*.	People have the potential to improve performance skills, patterns (habits, routines, and rituals), and body functions.	A homemaker who has impairments and problems in motor skills resulting from a stroke benefits more from working in the actual occupation of preparing meals in conjunction with exercises to increase her ROM, muscle strength, and coordination as opposed to solely using exercise equipment and objects stimulating the motor actions of the activity (Gasser-Wieland & Rice, 2002).
The use of new occupations as interventions provides the means for *establishing* performance skills and for developing habits.	The features of the context and environment may have changed and thus may demand the use of new performance skills and habits for the client to perform successfully.	Women with developmental delays and psychiatric conditions had a reduced rate of inappropriate behaviors and increased rate of socially appropriate behaviors in a new community living arrangement when given positive reinforcement in perusing everyday occupations (Holm, Santangelo, Fromuth, Brown, & Walter, 2000).
Valued occupations are *inherently motivating*.	Chosen occupations often are a reflection of what people value and enjoy and thus are more likely to be satisfying.	Older adults were motivated to resume engagement in occupations because of opportunities to reestablish relationships with others during engagement in valued occupations (Chan & Spencer, 2004).
Occupations promote the identification of *values and interests*.	Values influence occupational choice. When active in occupations, one experiences pleasure and satisfaction, thus generating interests (Kielhofner, 2002).	Older adults living within their communities related the three most important activities required for them to remain in their communities as using the telephone, using transportation, and reading; health professionals' list consisted of using the telephone, managing medications and preparing snacks (Fricke & Unsworth, 2001).
Occupations create opportunities to *practice* performance skills and to *reinforce* performance.	The client must have the opportunity to develop patterns that include the remediated skill in routine daily tasks (Holm, Rogers, & Stone, 2003, p. 477).	Elementary students with learning disabilities and handwriting problems who practiced keyboarding in a training program improved written communication skills for performance at school (Handley-More, Deitz, Billingsley, & Coggins, 2003).
Active engagement in occupations produces *feedback*.	Corrective feedback regarding performance helps the client modify behavior.	A computer system was modified for a person with a head injury to provide an auditory prompt to mark the commencement of each planned activity. "I was just sitting there on the sofa doing something like reading a newspaper, and had completely forgotten the swimming bath, the computer started to bleep; oh, what had I forgotten now?" (Erikson, Karlsson, Soderstrom, & Tham, 2004, p. 267).
Engagement in occupations facilitates *mastery* or *competence* in performing daily activities.	Successes motivate further change and continued use and practice of newly learned performance skills during engagement in occupations.	People with severe mental illness developed skills and competence in work and social activities while participating in a supported work setting (Gahnstrom-Strandqvist, Liukko, & Tham, 2003).
Selected occupations promote *participation* with individuals or groups.	Interventions designed to eliminate physical and social barriers increase opportunities for social interaction, leading to increased interaction and sense of control in context and environment.	Children with impaired performance skills used an adapted powered-mobility riding toy, which increased opportunities for participation with other children and adults during the occupation of play (Deitz, Swinth, & White, 2002).
Through engagement in occupations, people learn to *assume responsibility for their own health and wellness*.	Interventions that focus on improving a client's ability to self-direct change in lifestyle choices can lead to a sense of control.	People with chronic disorders who participated in community-based group services developed responsibility for their own health by empowerment of the group members (Taylor, Braveman, & Hammel, 2004).
Occupations exert a positive influence on *health* and *well-being* (Law, 2002b).	Regardless of the presence of impairments, a person may remain active and engaged in healthy occupations.	People with fibromyalgia who successfully used activity modification strategies to complete daily activities reported positive quality of life and health (Lindberg & Schkade, 2001).

(*Continued*)

Chapter 3

Table 3-4

Principles of Occupations That Support Their Value and Use in Intervention (*Continued*)

PRINCIPLE	EXPLANATION	EXAMPLE
Occupations provide the means for people to *adapt* to changing needs and conditions.	A person's capacity for performance is affected by the status of body structures and functions. Permanent loss of capacity necessitates modification of the context and environment and of activity demands.	Patients who had hip fractures demonstrated more efficiency and greater satisfaction in recovering performance skills in daily occupations when modified activity procedures were emphasized (Jackson & Schkade, 2001).
Occupations contribute to the creation and maintenance *of identity* (AOTA, 2002; Christainsen, 1999).	Discovering identity is related to what a person does and to those people with whom they come in contact during daily occupations and activities.	People with injuries to the hand resumed occupations that facilitated resumption of their identity (Chan & Spencer, 2004).
Successful performance in occupation can positively affect *psychological* functioning.	A person's evaluation of performance in occupations and activities influences perceptions about himself or herself.	People recovering from a stroke demonstrated positive views and acceptance of the need for a wheelchair, described opportunities for continuity of previous life activities, maintenance of mobility, and decreased burden on the caregiver (Barker, Reid, & Cott, 2004).
Occupations have unique *meaning* and *purpose* for each person, which influences the quality of performance (AOTA, 2002).	The meaning of occupations refers to the subjective experience one has when engaging in activities.	People recovering from a stroke stood longer when performing personally meaningful tasks (Dolecheck & Schkade, 1999).
Engagement in occupations gives a sense of *satisfaction* and *fulfillment* (AOTA, 2002).	Performance of valued occupations provides for achievement of personal goals in a variety of roles.	Satisfaction through occupations was found when older adults maintained daily routines and engaged in fulfilling occupations (Bontje, Kinebanian, Josephsson, & Tamura, 2004). Goldberg, Brintell, and Golberg (2002) found a correlation between engagement in meaningful activities and life satisfaction.
Occupations influence how people spend time and *make decisions* (AOTA, 2002).	People occupy time through engagement in activity.	In a study of time use, older people spent most of their time completing activities that were meaningful for them and not necessarily the activities that were necessary for them to remain in the community (Fricke & Unsworth, 2001).

From: Moyers, P.A. & Dale, L. (2007). *The guide to occupational therapy practice,* 2nd ed. p. 45–46. Copyright 2007 by the American Occupational Therapy Association. Reprinted with permission.

c. Promotion of engagement in valued occupations is used to foster health and wellness.
d. Adaptive equipment, assistive technology, and orthotic devices are designed, fabricated, and applied to facilitate function.
e. Adaptive equipment, assistive technology, orthotics, and prosthetic use training are provided to promote independence.
f. Physical agent modalities are used to prepare for, or as an adjunct to, engagement in therapeutic functional activities.
g. Ergonomic principles are applied to the performance of meaningful occupations.
h. Standard precautions are observed.
  (1) Standard precautions are the primary strategy for control of nosocomial infection and are used in the care of all persons (Table 3-2).
i. Transmission-based precautions are used for persons with known or suspected infections of highly transmissible or epidemiologically important pathogens.
  (1) Includes airborne precautions, droplet precautions, and contact precautions (Table 3-3).

4. Individual or group interventions may be used. Refer to Table 3-5 for a comparison of indications for "Individual vs. Group Intervention."

Developmental Considerations in Intervention

1. All activities, toys, and other intervention media must be appropriate to the child's developmental level.
2. Play activities should be the primary occupation intervention.

Table 3-5

Individual vs. Group Intervention	
Individual	Learning capacity of the person Amount of attention and skill required from the occupational therapy practitioner owing to body structure and function impairments Need for privacy Need for greater control over the context and environment Difficulty or complexity of occupation and activity demands, performance skills and performance patterns Inappropriate or dangerous behavior of the person
Group	Developing interpersonal skills Engaging in socialization Receiving feedback from people experiencing similar conditions Being motivated by peer role models Learning from other people Placing one's own condition into perspective Developing group normative behavior for successful performance in shared occupations (e.g., work, study, and leisure groups

From: Moyers, P.A. & Dale, L. (2007). *The guide to occupational therapy practice*, 2nd ed. p. 47. Copyright 2007 by the American Occupational Therapy Association. Reprinted with permission.

3. Family education is essential.
   a. Identify environmental characteristics that facilitate the child's development.
   b. Provide advocacy training to link families to community.
   c. Identify psychosocial factors that promote the child's development.
   d. Teach avoidance of behaviors that may interfere with learning.
   e. Consider and respect the family's cultural background.
4. Provide consultation or direct treatment to facilitate school performance and achieve educational goals.
5. Provide treatment to facilitate sensorimotor, cognitive, and psychosocial development.
6. Fabricate or requisition positioning equipment and technological aides for home and/or school.
7. Ensure the proper visual and auditory aides are used during treatment sessions.
8. Review the pediatric and developmental clinical condition information provided in the Clinical Conditions chapters (6–10) for diagnostic-specific interventions.

Reevaluation/Intervention Review

Overview

1. The process of determining whether the individual's occupational performance has improved, declined, or remained the same after intervention.
2. Frequent monitoring of an individual's response to intervention is an integral part of all OT interventions.
3. Effective interventions resulting in the individual's progress require intervention plan modification and an upgrading of goals, as long as there is a reasonable expectation that the individual can improve functional performance.
4. If the individual is not progressing according to plan, different intervention methods, referral(s) to experts in the field or other professions or to another level of care, and/or discharge from intervention may be indicated.

Discharge Planning

1. The process for planning for discontinuation of services.
2. Reasons for discharge.
   a. The individual's goals have been met.
   b. The individual has reached a functional plateau.
   c. The individual does not require skilled services, for maximum benefit has been achieved.
   d. An exacerbation of an illness or a medical crisis requires discharge to a higher level of care.
   e. The person's allotted length of stay in the setting has expired and extension of LOS is not possible.
3. General principles.
   a. Discharge planning begins with the initial evaluation and is an inherent part of the intervention planning process. All interventions should be planned with consideration of the expected, planned discharge environment.
   b. Collaboration with the individual, family, significant others, caregivers, other professionals on the team, employers, and reimbursers is required for an effective and realistic discharge plan.
   c. Discharge may include transfer to a long-term care setting (e.g., a skilled nursing or assistive living facility), to an intermediate care facility (e.g., a halfway house), or to a home setting.
      (1) A pre-discharge home evaluation must be completed to ensure the individual will be safe and to identify needed home adaptations or

supports (e.g., bathroom modifications, home health aide).

d. A well-planned discharge facilitates community integration and maintenance of functional gains.

4. Follow-up referrals for further OT intervention and/or other supportive services must be made.
   a. Home programs.
      (1) Recommendations to the individual, family, significant others, and caregivers on techniques and procedures to maintain and/or improve functional status.
      (2) Training should be provided prior to discharge.
      (3) Information on additional supports should be provided.
   b. Community resources.
      (1) Recommendations and referrals to specific services in the community that can support function (e.g., Alcoholics Anonymous, day treatment).

OT Tools of Practice

Definition

1. The established, legitimate means by which the practitioners of a profession achieve the profession's goals and meet society's needs.

Relevance to Examination

1. While it is unlikely that the NBCOT exam will ask direct questions about the following tools of practice, the use and application of these tools of practice will be needed to decide the best possible answer to exam item questions.

Occupation

1. Definition: goal-directed pursuits which typically extend over time.
   a. They have purpose, value, and meaning to the performer and involve multiple tasks.
   b. They are the ordinary and familiar things that people do every day.
2. Basic concepts of occupation.
   a. Every individual has multiple occupations that are meaningful (e.g., self-care, home management, work and leisure) and needed to function in roles (e.g., parent, worker, student, hobbyist).
   b. Humans are innately occupational beings and are driven by an inherent need for mastery, self-actualization, self-identity, competence, and social acceptance.
   c. Occupations have social, cultural, physical, and temporal contextual dimensions because they involve activities within specific settings and extend over time.
   d. Occupations have symbolic and spiritual dimensions, as individuals infuse individualized meanings into occupations.
   e. Occupations are interdependent (e.g., one must work to pay for leisure; one must have leisure to sustain and renew oneself for work).
   f. Health is attained when the dynamic balance between occupations and rest is appropriate and meets the needs of the individual.
   g. Occupation can be viewed and used as a "means" or a method to change an individual's performance (e.g., playing a board game to increase motor skills).
   h. Occupation can also be viewed and used as an "end" or desired outcome (e.g., playing a board game to improve the ability to engage in age-appropriate social play).
   i. Engagement in occupation to support the individual's participation in environment(s) of choice is the overriding desired outcome of OT.
3. Areas of occupation.
   a. Activities of daily living: activities that involve care of self; often called personal activities of daily living (PADL) or basic activities of daily living (BADL).
   b. Instrumental activities of daily living: activities that involve environmental interaction; they are more complex than self-care and can be optional (e.g., home maintenance, care of others and community mobility activities).
   c. Work: all productive activities that contribute services, goods, or commodities to society, whether financially compensated or not (i.e., a volunteer is working).
   d. Education: activities that involve the student role and participation in an educational environment.
   e. Play/leisure: all activities engaged in for pleasure, relaxation, amusement, and/or self-fulfillment.
   f. Social participation: activities involving interaction with community, family, and peers/friends.

Purposeful Activities

1. Definition.
   a. Doing processes that are directed toward a desired and intended outcome and require energy and thought to engage in and complete.
   b. The goal-directed tasks and/or behaviors that make up occupations.
2. Characteristics of purposeful activities.
   a. Universally, people participate in purposeful activities, although there are personal and sociocultural differences in the manner in which activities are performed (e.g., dressing).
   b. Fundamental to the development and acquisition of performance skills is active participation in purposeful activities (e.g., the development of eye-hand coordination through play).
   c. Fundamental to performance in areas of occupation is engagement in purposeful activities (e.g., to work involves completion of multiple tasks).
   d. Purposeful activities are composed of identifiable parts that can be analyzed.
   e. Purposeful activities are holistic.
   f. Purposeful activities can be manipulated and adapted to be appropriate to, and/or therapeutic for, the individual.
   g. Purposeful activities can be graded along many dimensions to meet the needs of an individual.
   h. Determination of the individual's differential responses to purposeful activities can provide information for the selection of appropriate activities for use in evaluation and intervention.
   i. Verbal and nonverbal communication is facilitated through engagement in purposeful activities.
   j. Organization and ability to focus are enhanced, because purposeful activities provide concrete structure.
   k. Doing is emphasized.
   l. Involvement in, and with, the nonhuman environment is enhanced.
   m. Purposeful activities can vary on a continuum from conscious to not conscious/unconscious.
   n. Purposeful activities vary on a continuum from real to symbolic.
   o. Purposeful activities vary on a continuum from simulated in a clinical setting to real in the individual's natural environment.

Activity/Task Analysis and Synthesis

1. Activity/task analysis.
   a. The breaking down and identification of the component parts of an activity/task.
   b. Determination of the abilities needed to effectively perform and successfully complete the activity/task.
   c. Determination if the activity/task has therapeutic value.
   d. Methods of activity/task analysis.
      (1) Specify the exact activity/task to be analyzed (i.e., not just "dressing" but "donning a sweatshirt").
      (2) Identify and know the procedures, materials, and tools needed to complete the specific activity/task.
      (3) Analyze the activity/task as it is typically performed under ordinary circumstances.
      (4) Analyze the activity/task to be certain that all client factors, performance skills and patterns, and activity/task performance components and contexts are considered.
      (5) Select a frame of reference to determine which aspects of the activity/task are to be emphasized in the analysis.
2. Activity synthesis.
   a. The process of designing an activity for OT evaluation or intervention.
   b. Combines information obtained from the activity analysis with assessment information about the individual to ensure that a suitable match is made between the activity requirements and the person's needs and abilities.
   c. Effective activity synthesis often requires the adaptation and/or gradation of the selected activity.
3. Purposes and methods of activity analysis and synthesis.
   a. Teaching an activity.
      (1) Analyze the nature and sequence of the subtasks within the activity.
      (2) Synthesize to determine the best way to present the activity as a learning experience.
   b. Determining whether an individual can perform an activity.
      (1) Analyze the performance skill requirements of the activity.
      (2) Synthesize by comparing the activity requirements with the individual's functional level.
   c. Adapting an activity.
      (1) Evaluate the individual's functional capabilities.
      (2) Analyze what parts of the activity can be changed.
      (3) Identify what functional aids can be used to allow the individual to successfully perform the activity.
   d. Grading an activity.
      (1) Determine what aspects can be changed along a continuum of performance.
      (2) Identify the individual's performance skill deficit(s) and/or client factors requiring intervention.
      (3) Synthesize to upgrade or downgrade complexity or difficulty level of the activity to meet the needs of the individual.

The Teaching-Learning Process

1. Definition: the process by which the OT practitioner designs experiences to facilitate the individual's acquisition of the knowledge and skills needed for living.
2. Principles of learning.
   a. Learning is influenced by the individual's interests, age, sex, sociocultural factors, and current assets and limitations.
   b. Attention to the learning experience and perception of the situation influence learning.
   c. The learner's sources of motivation must be identified and used for engagement in learning experiences.
   d. Learning goals made by the individual are more likely to be met than goals determined by others.
   e. Learning is enhanced when the individual understands the reason for and purpose of the learning activity.
   f. Learning is increased when it recognizes the individual's current functional level, and is initiated within the person's capabilities (i.e., not too high or too low).
   g. Learning is enhanced when activities and experiences proceed at a rate that is comfortable for the individual.
   h. Individuals who actively participate in the learning process learn more because experiential learning is more effective than didactic learning.
   i. Reinforcement and feedback on the individual's behavior and/or task performance are important parts of the learning experience and can be used to support desired behaviors and extinguish undesirable behaviors.
   j. Learning can be enhanced through trial and error, shaping, and imitation of models.
   k. Frequent repetition and practice in different situations facilitates learning and encourages generalization.
   l. Planned movement from simplified wholes to more complex wholes facilitates integration of what is to be learned.
   m. Inventive solutions to problems (as well as more useful or typical solutions) should be encouraged.
   n. The environment of the learning experience can strongly influence the success of that experience.
   o. Individual differences in the way anxiety affects the individual's learning must be considered.
   p. Conflicts and frustrations, inevitably present in the learning situation, must be recognized and provisions made for their resolution or accommodation.
   q. Continuity between the planned therapeutic learning experiences and the real-life situations for which the individual needs to be prepared facilitates the effective transfer of learning and the generalization of knowledge and skills.
3. Teaching methods.
   a. Definition: ways to present information and/or a task to an individual on a one-to-one basis or in a group.
   b. Demonstration and performance.
      (1) The therapist performs the task and the individual imitates the therapist's performance.
      (2) For example, the therapist demonstrates one-handed cooking techniques, and the use of adaptive equipment, and the individual with a unilateral upper extremity amputation imitates therapist's task performance.
   c. Exploration and discovery.
      (1) A diversity of activities is made available and the individual is permitted to choose any activity and try it without specific instructions or directions.
      (2) For example, in an expressive arts group, members can select from a diversity of media and create individual works.
   d. Explanation and discussion.
      (1) A verbal explanation of the task and a discussion of the activity components to either plan an activity or to review what occurred during the activity are provided by the therapist.
      (2) For example, in a vocational group, the steps for applying for a job are explained and what happened during a job interview is reviewed.
   e. Role play.
      (1) The OT practitioner and/or individual(s) assume roles and act out scenarios to practice behaviors prior to doing the behavior in a real situation.
      (2) For example, the OT practitioner plays the interviewer and the individual plays the job applicant.
   f. Simulation.
      (1) The individual acts out an activity performance using simulated tasks and/or objects.
      (2) For example, using a driving simulator prior to driving in a car on a roadway.
   g. Problem solving.
      (1) The process of teaching a person to analyze a situation, define the problem, outline potential solutions, select the solution that appears to be most viable, implement the solution, evaluate the outcome to determine if problem is resolved, and re-try a new solution, if needed.
      (2) For example, an individual living in a supportive apartment is having a problem getting his/her roommate to share household tasks.
   h. Audiovisual aids.
      (1) The use of slides, videos, and/or audio cassettes to teach material with or without the presence of a therapist.
      (2) For example, an individual with anxiety is provided with relaxation tapes to use at home.

i. Repetition and practice.
   (1) The repetitious engagement in a task to increase accuracy and speed.
   (2) For example, repeatedly closing the fasteners on clothing to decrease the time needed to get ready for work in the morning.

j. Behavioral management.
   (1) The identification of behaviors that require development (e.g., appropriate social skills) and/or require extinction (e.g., hitting people).
   (2) The implementation of a structured program to facilitate the desired behavioral change.
   (3) For example, appropriate social skills are rewarded with praise, whereas aggressive acts lead to a solitary "time out" period.

k. Consumer/family/caregiver education.
   (1) An organized, systematic approach to formally present information to increase knowledge.
   (2) The nature of the illness or disease, including etiology, signs and symptoms, functional implications, prognosis, and interventions are explained.
   (3) The maintenance of roles and occupational performance is emphasized.
   (4) Methods for the prevention of secondary problems (e.g., decubiti), are provided.
   (5) Community resources and supportive services are explored with appropriate referrals made.

Clinical Reasoning

1. Definition: the complex mental processes the therapist uses when thinking about the individual, the disability, and the personal, social, and cultural meanings the individual gives to the disability, the uniqueness of the situation, and him/herself.
2. Value for occupational therapists in practice.
   a. Improves clinical decision making by giving therapists tools for self-conscious reflection on their decisions.
   b. Improves ability to explain the rationales behind therapists' decisions to consumers, family members, team members, and medical finance agencies (e.g., insurers).
   c. Improves job satisfaction by making therapists more aware of the complexity of their work, the value of their practice.
3. Types of clinical reasoning.
   a. Procedural reasoning/scientific reasoning.
      (1) Involves identifying OT problems, goal setting, and treatment planning.
      (2) Involves implementing treatment strategies via systematic gathering and interpreting of client data.
      (3) The actual technical "doing" of practice.
      (4) The reasoning that is documented the most for reimbursement purposes.
   b. Interactive reasoning.
      (1) Deals with how the disability or disease affects the person; focuses on the client as a person.
      (2) Involves the therapeutic relationship between the therapist, the individual, and caregivers.
      (3) Facilitates effective treatment, as it focuses on the personal meaning of illness and disability which can influence how a person engages in treatment (i.e., how motivational issues affect client's performance).
      (4) Congruent with the profession's philosophy and heritage of caring.
   c. Narrative reasoning.
      (1) Deals with the individual's occupational story and focuses on the process of change needed to reach an imagined future.
      (2) Identifies what activities and roles were important to the person prior to illness/injury.
      (3) Analyzes what valued activities and roles the individual can perform now.
      (4) Explores what valued activities and roles are possible in the future, given the person's disability.
      (5) Asks what valued activities and roles the individual would choose as priorities for the future.
      (6) Neglects larger practice area issues in which the client/practitioner interaction is occurring (e.g., pragmatic constraints imposed by reimbursement, equipment, and/or organizational culture).
   d. Pragmatic reasoning.
      (1) Considers the context in which the OT practitioner's thinking occurs.
      (2) States that mental activities are shaped by the situation (i.e., is setting long term or acute?).
      (3) Considers the treatment environment and OT practitioner's values, knowledge, abilities, and experiences.
      (4) Focuses on the treatment possibilities within a given treatment setting.
      (5) Reframes understanding of the influence of personal and practical constraints on OT practice.
      (6) The most effective OT practitioners are able to negotiate pragmatic contextual issues in favor of quality care.
   e. Conditional reasoning.
      (1) Involves an ongoing revision of treatment.
      (2) Focuses on current and possible future social contexts.
      (3) Represents an integration of interactive, procedural, and pragmatic reasoning in the context of the client's narrative.
      (4) Requires multidimensional thinking.

Therapeutic Use of Self

1. Definition: the practitioner's conscious, planned interaction with the individual, family members, significant others, and/or caregivers.
   a. The conscious, planned use of one's personality, unique characteristics, perceptions and insights during the therapeutic process.
2. Purposes of therapeutic use of self.
   a. Provide reassurance and/or information.
   b. Give advice.
   c. Alleviate anxiety and/or fear.
   d. Obtain needed information.
   e. Improve and maintain function.
   f. Promote growth and development.
   g. Increase coping skills.
3. Essential characteristics of therapeutic use of self.
   a. Perception of the individuality and uniqueness of each person.
   b. Respect for the dignity and rights of each individual regardless of past or present situation or possible future potential.
   c. Empathy to enter and share the experiences of an individual while maintaining one's own sense of self.
   d. Compassion to be kind and want to alleviate pain and suffering.
   e. Humility to recognize one's own limitations.
   f. Unconditional positive regard to be non-judgmental and accept, respect, and show concern and liking for each individual as a human being, regardless of presenting behaviors.
   g. Honesty to be truthful and straightforward.
   h. A relaxed manner to leave other concerns aside and schedule sufficient time to be with the person so that external issues do not impede on the relationship.
   i. Flexibility to modify behavior to meet the needs of each individual and deal with circumstances as they arise or change.
   j. Self-awareness to accurately know one's assets and limitations and to be able to make changes as needed to interact more effectively in therapeutic relationships.
   k. Humor to appropriately recognize and/or use what is amusing and comical.
4. Common issues and responses that can affect therapeutic relationships.
   a. Negative attitudes, fear or hostility toward individuals who are different and/or toward the unknown.
   b. Resistance to establishing a rapport due to past rejections and/or fear of future rejection.
   c. Communication difficulties.
      (1) Incongruence between verbal and non verbal communications, (when spoken words do not match a person's facial expression, tone of voice, gestures, or postures), resulting in confusion.
      (2) Language difficulties.
         (a) Psychiatric symptoms such as blocking, circumstantiality, flight of ideas, confabulation, grandiosity, articulated delusions, loosening of association, and/or poverty of content can hinder effective communication.
         (b) Cultural, class, educational, and/or regional differences can result in misunderstandings or lack of comprehension between individuals.
         (c) Misinterpretations can occur due to differences in primary language.
   d. Dependency that is excessive, and hinders the individual's growth toward interdependence and/or independence.
   e. Transference and countertransference.
      (1) Transference is an unconscious response to an individual that is similar to the way one has responded to a significant person (e.g., the therapist is responded to as a parent).
      (2) Countertransference is an unconscious response to transference in which the individual responds in a manner that is expected and desired by the person who has transference toward him/her (e.g., the therapist assumes a parental role toward a client).
   f. Difficulty in expressing feelings due to personal reticence or cultural background.
   g. Over involvement that results in a loss of objectivity or a fear of involvement that leads to detachment.
   h. Difficulty with developing an individual therapeutic style that is a comfortable "fit" so that being a therapist becomes a natural part of one's self.
5. Supervision and support.
   a. Develops the ability to use oneself therapeutically.
   b. Assists with the common issues and responses noted in Section 4 above.
   c. Increases effectiveness in applying therapeutic principles in daily practice.

Group Process, Therapeutic Groups, and Activity Groups

1. Overview of group dynamics.
   a. Group dynamics are the forces which influence the nature of small groups, the interrelationships of their members, the events that typically occur in small groups and ultimately, the outcome(s) of these groups.
   b. Group dynamics can be examined according to the group's structure, content, and process.

2. Group development: the stages groups typically go through from their initial beginnings to their termination.
   a. Origin phase involves the leader composing the group protocol and planning for the group (e.g., size of the group, member characteristics, location of meetings).
   b. Orientation phase involves members learning what the group is about, making a preliminary commitment to the group, and developing initial connections with other members.
   c. Intermediate phase involves members developing interpersonal bonds, group norms, and specialized member roles through involvement in goal-directed activities and clarification of group's purpose.
   d. Conflict phase involves members challenging the group's structure, purposes, and/or processes, and is characterized by dissension and disagreements among members.
      (1) Unsuccessful resolution of this phase results in dissolution of the group.
      (2) Successful resolution of this phase results in modifications to the group that are acceptable to members, enabling the group to proceed to the next phase of development.
   e. Cohesion phase involves members regrouping after the conflict with a clearer sense of purpose and a reaffirmation of group norms and values, leading to group stability.
   f. Maturation phase involves members using their energies and skills to be productive and to achieve group's goals.
   g. Termination phase involves dissolution of the group due to lack of engagement of members, inability to resolve conflict, administrative constraints (e.g., only four sessions allotted for a discharge planning group), goal attainment, or task accomplishment.
3. Group roles: describe the patterns of behavior that are typical within groups.
   a. Instrumental roles are functional and assumed to help the group select, plan, and complete the group's task (e.g., initiator, organizer).
   b. Expressive roles are functional and are assumed to support and maintain the overall group and to meet members' needs (e.g., encourager, compromiser).
   c. Individual roles are dysfunctional and contrary to group roles, for they serve an individual purpose and interfere with successful group functioning (e.g., aggressor, blocker).
4. Group norms: the standards of behavior and attitudes that are considered appropriate and acceptable to the group.
   a. Behavior that falls outside of the group's range of acceptable behavior is considered deviant and is often negatively sanctioned.
   b. Norms can be explicit and clearly verbalized (e.g., confidentiality is maintained by all group members, aggression is not tolerated).
   c. Norms can be non-explicit and not verbalized (e.g., discussion topics that are taboo).
   d. Norms can vary in different groups and can change as a group develops and/or membership changes.
   e. Therapeutic norms.
      (1) Encourage self-reflection, self-disclosure, and interaction among members.
      (2) Reinforce the value and importance of the group by being on time and well-prepared.
      (3) Establish an atmosphere of support and safety.
      (4) Maintain confidentiality and respect.
      (5) Regard group members as effective agents of change by not placing the group leader in the expert role.
5. Group goals: the desired outcomes of the group that are shared by a sufficient number of the group's members.
   a. The group's effort is mostly aimed at attaining these goals.
   b. Group goals provide focus for the group and guidelines for group activities and interactions.
   c. Group goals are not a compilation of individual member goals. Members may have diverse goals but attainment of the group goal will facilitate personal goal achievement.
   d. Benefits of member participation in group goal setting.
      (1) A match between members' goals and group's goal(s).
      (2) Increased understanding of the requirements for achievement of the goal(s).
      (3) Increased appreciation of each member's contribution to achieving group's desired outcomes.
6. Group communication: the process of giving, receiving, and interpreting information through verbal and nonverbal expression.
   a. Effective group communication is a prerequisite to, and a requirement for, all group functioning.
   b. Effective communication occurs in a group when a member sends a message and the message is interpreted by the other group members receiving the message in the manner that the sender intended.
   c. Sending and receiving messages often takes place simultaneously due to the dynamic process of verbal and non-verbal communication.
   d. Communication can take many forms, including monologue, criticism, orders, questions and answers, and open give-and-take.
   e. Group communication that is adaptive may include clarifying goals and the sharing of ideas, experiences, and feelings.
   f. Group communication that is maladaptive may include seeking to control the group by controlling

the channels of communication, and avoidance of specific issues or persons.
7. Group cohesiveness: the degree to which members are committed to a group and the extent of members' liking for the group (i.e., the sense of "we-ness").
   a. Factors that contribute to cohesiveness.
      (1) Extensive interaction between members.
      (2) Similarity or complementariness in member characteristics.
      (3) Perception of relevance of group to individual needs.
      (4) Members' expectation of goal attainment and successful group outcome.
      (5) Democratic leadership and member cooperation.
8. Group decision making: The process of agreeing on a resolution to a problem. The solution may be obtained through different processes.
   a. Unanimous decision in which all group members agree.
   b. Consensus in which members agree to the majority's decision but retain the right to reconsider their decision.
   c. Majority rule in which the majority's decision is accepted with no reevaluation of the decision by members.
   d. Compromise in which a combination of different points of view results in a decision that is different from each distinct point of view.
9. Group leadership styles and membership roles.
   a. Directive leadership takes place when the therapist is responsible for the planning and structuring of much of what takes place in the group.
      (1) This is style needed when the members' cognitive, social, and verbal skills, as well as engagement, are limited (e.g., parallel or project level groups).
      (2) Directive leaders select the activities to be used in the group.
      (3) They provide clear verbal and demonstrated instruction to complete tasks.
      (4) Group maintenance roles and feedback is predominately provided by the directive leader.
      (5) The directive leader's goal is task accomplishment.
   b. Facilitative leadership occurs when the therapist shares responsibility for the group and for group process with the members.
      (1) This style is advised when members' skill levels and engagement are moderate (e.g., egocentric-cooperative, or cooperative).
      (2) Facilitative leaders collaborate with group members to select the activities to be used in a group.
      (3) Members and leaders share instruction throughout the group's process.
      (4) Group maintenance roles and feedback are provided by members with the leader facilitating the process.
      (5) The facilitative leader's goal is to have members acquire skills through experience.
   c. Advisory leadership takes place when the therapist functions as a resource to the members, who set the agenda and structure the group's functioning.
      (1) This style is assumed when members' skills and engagement are high (e.g., cooperative and mature groups).
      (2) Members select and complete the group's activity with leader's advice, if needed.
      (3) Group maintenance roles are independently assumed by group members.
      (4) Feedback occurs as a natural part of the group's self-directed process.
      (5) The advisory leader's goal is to have members understand and self-direct the process.
   d. Refer to Table 3-6 for Medicare guidelines for group therapy member selection and Table 3-7 for Medicare guidelines for group leadership responsibility.
      (1) These guidelines are relevant and helpful standards to apply to all settings that use group interventions.

Table 3-6

Medicare Indicators for Group Membership
THE INDIVIDUAL IS ABLE TO:
• engage willingly in group
• attend to group guidelines/procedures
• actively participate in group process
• benefit from group leadership input
• benefit from group membership/peer input
• respond appropriately throughout group process
• incorporate feedback
• complete activities toward goal attainment
• attain greater benefit from the group intervention than from 1:1 intervention
Reference: *Adapted from United States Government Printing Office Code of Federal Regulations*, Title 42, Volume 3. Retrieved from http://www.cms.gov. December 21, 2003.

Table 3-7

Medicare Criteria for Group Leadership
THE LEADER:
• provides active leadership
• instructs members as a group
• monitors and documents individual's participation and response to intervention
• provides individualized guidance and feedback
• documents person's progress toward goals defined in the individual intervention plan in objective, measurable, functional terms
Reference: *Adapted from United States Government Printing Office Code of Federal Regulations*, Title 42, Volume 3. Retrieved from http://www.cms.gov. December 21, 2003.

10. Co-leadership: occurs when there is sharing of group leadership between two or more therapists.
    a. Advantages.
        (1) Each leader can assume different leadership roles, tasks and styles.
        (2) Both leaders can provide and obtain mutual support.
        (3) Observations and objectivity can increase.
        (4) Co-leaders can share knowledge and skills.
        (5) Co-leaders can model effective behaviors.
    b. Disadvantages may arise and must be dealt with for effective co-leadership.
        (1) Splitting by group member(s) of one leader against the other.
        (2) Excessive competition among co-leaders.
        (3) Unequal responsibilities resulting in an unbalanced work load among co-leaders.
11. Curative factors of groups as defined by Yalom.
    a. Altruism is the giving of oneself to help others.
    b. Catharsis is the relieving of emotions by expressing one's feelings.
    c. Universality comes from recognizing shared feelings and that one's problems are not unique.
    d. Existential factors address accepting the fact that the responsibility for change comes from within oneself.
    e. Self-understanding (insight) involves discovering and accepting the unknown parts of oneself.
    f. Family reenactment leads to understanding what it was like growing up in one's family through the group experience.
    g. Guidance comes from accepting advice from other group members.
    h. Identification involves benefiting from imitation of the positive behaviors of other group members.
    i. Instillation of hope is experiencing optimism through observing the improvement of others in the group.
    j. Interpersonal learning occurs when receiving feedback from group members regarding one's behavior (input).
    k. Interpersonal learning also occurs by learning successful ways of relating to group members (output).
    l. The conscious understanding and facilitation of these curative factors enhances the therapeutic value of a group.
12. Taxonomy of activity groups:
    a. Mosey (1996) provided a standard classification to identify major types of activity groups.
    b. Evaluation group.
        (1) Purpose/focus: to enable client and the therapist to assess client's skills, assets, and limitations regarding group interaction.
        (2) Assumption: to accurately evaluate an individual's functional abilities, one must observe the person in a setting where the skills can be demonstrated.
        (3) Type of client: all individuals who will be involved in groups or who lack group interaction skills.
        (4) Role of the therapist.
            (a) Selects and orients clients to group's purpose.
            (b) Selects activities that require collaboration and interaction and provides needed supplies.
            (c) Does not participate or intervene in group (except to maintain safety, if needed), but observes and reports members' interaction and functional skill level to the treatment team.
            (d) Asks for clients' input.
            (e) Validates assessment and establishes treatment goals with each individual client.
        (5) Suitable activities: tasks that can be completed in one session and require interaction to complete.
    c. Thematic group.
        (1) Purpose/focus: to assist members in acquiring the knowledge, skills, and/or attitudes needed to perform a specific activity.
        (2) Assumptions.
            (a) Improvement of ability to engage in activities outside of group can result from teaching of these activities within group.
            (b) Learning is facilitated by practicing and experiencing needed behaviors, with reinforcement of appropriate behaviors given.
        (3) Type of client.
            (a) Determined by the specific goals of the group.
            (b) Members' needs, concerns, and goals must match the objectives of the group.
            (c) Members must have a minimal group interaction skill level equal to a parallel group skill level.
        (4) Role of the therapist.
            (a) Selects, structures, and grades suitable activities to teach needed skills.
            (b) Interventions vary according to group's level, needs, and goals.
            (c) May range on a continuum from a highly structured, supportive director to a resource advisor.
            (d) Reinforces skill development.
            (e) Attention is not paid to intra- and interpersonal conflicts unless they interfere with or are directly related to the activity.
        (5) Suitable activities.
            (a) Simulated, clearly defined, structured activities which enable members to practice and learn needed skills, attitudes, and knowledge within the group.

(b) Activities selected are directly related to the skills needed to perform the activity outside of the group (e.g., a cooking group to learn how to cook).

d. Topical group.
  (1) Purpose/focus: to discuss specific activities that members are engaged in outside of group to enable them to engage in the activities in a more effective, need-satisfying manner.
    (a) Concurrent topical groups are concerned with activities already engaged in outside of group (e.g., a parenting skills group for parents of children with developmental disabilities).
    (b) Anticipatory topical groups are concerned with activities that are expected to be done in the future (e.g., a discharge planning group for persons completing short-term rehabilitation).
  (2) Assumptions.
    (a) Improvement of ability to engage in specific activities outside of group results from discussion of these activities.
    (b) Discussion of problem areas and potential solutions, reinforcement of appropriate behaviors, and experiential learning facilitate skill acquisition.
  (3) Type of client.
    (a) Individuals who share similar current or anticipatory problems in functioning.
    (b) Members must be at an egocentric-cooperative group skill level.
    (c) Sufficient verbal and cognitive skills to engage in discussion and to problem-solve are present.
  (4) Role of the therapist.
    (a) Facilitate group discussion while maintaining focus on the circumscribed activity.
    (b) Help members problem-solve, give feedback and support, reinforce skill acquisition.
    (c) Share leadership with members; act as a role model.
  (5) Suitable activities.
    (a) Group activity is a verbal discussion on a circumscribed activity that members are engaged in (concurrent) or will be engaged in (anticipatory) outside of group (e.g., parenting, home maintenance, discharge from hospital, work, and leisure).
    (b) Discussion may include members' current or anticipated fears and problems, potential solutions, and coping mechanisms.
    (c) Role play and "homework" may be utilized.

e. Task-oriented group.
  (1) Purpose/focus.
    (a) To increase clients' awareness of their needs, values, ideas, feelings, and behaviors as they engage in a group task.
    (b) To improve intra- and interpsychic functioning by focusing on problems which emerge in the process of choosing, planning and implementing a group activity.
  (2) Assumptions.
    (a) Activities elicit feelings, thoughts, and behaviors.
    (b) Activities are the means by which members can explore and experience these thoughts, feelings, and actions.
    (c) Through activities members can increase their self-awareness and practice new behaviors.
  (3) Type of client.
    (a) Individuals whose primary dysfunction is in the cognitive and socioemotional areas due to psychological or physical trauma.
    (b) Clients with fair verbal skills who can interact with others.
  (4) Role of the therapist.
    (a) Initially, very active, defines group goals and structure.
    (b) Assists with activity selection, offers guidelines and suggestions.
    (c) Facilitates discussion among members.
    (d) Gives feedback and support.
    (e) Assists members in exploring relationships between thoughts, feelings, and actions.
    (f) Encourages members to experiment with new behavior patterns.
    (g) As group develops, the leader is less active, helps members give more feedback and input; however, the therapist remains the leader and ensures that the task is a means to the end, not the end itself.
  (5) Suitable activities.
    (a) Activities that are chosen by members and will create an end product or demonstrable service for the group itself or for persons outside the group.
    (b) Activities are selected, planned, and carried out by members with the understanding that the task is a means to study, understand, and practice behavior.

f. Developmental group.
  (1) A continuum of groups consisting of parallel, project, egocentric-cooperative, cooperative, and mature groups.
  (2) Purpose/focus is to teach and develop members' group interaction skills.
    (a) Parallel.

- To enable members to perform individual tasks in the presence of others.
- To minimally interact verbally and nonverbally with others even though task does not require interaction for successful completion.
- To develop a basic level of awareness, trust, and comfort with others in group.

(b) Project.

- To develop the ability to perform a shared, short-term activity with another member in a comfortable, cooperative manner.
- To develop interactions beyond those that the activity requires.
- To enable members to give and seek assistance.

(c) Egocentric-cooperative.

- To enable members to select and implement a long-range activity which requires group interaction to complete.
- To enable members to identify and meet the needs of themselves and others (e.g., safety, esteem).

(d) Cooperative.

- To enable members to engage in a group activity which facilitates the free expression of ideas and feelings.
- To develop sense of trust, love and belonging, and cohesion.
- To enable members to identify and meet socio-emotional needs.

(e) Mature group.

- To enable members to assume all functional socio-emotional and task roles within a group.
- To enable members to reinforce behaviors which result in need satisfaction and task completion.

(3) Assumptions.

(a) Learning principles are the basis. They are utilized throughout the five developmental levels.

(b) Members are made aware of and helped to engage in appropriate group behavior.

(c) Feedback and reinforcement are utilized. Learning of needed behaviors occurs when adaptive behaviors are reinforced and when maladaptive behaviors are not.

(d) Maladaptive behaviors result from deviations, lags, or insufficiencies in development. These developmental deficiencies can be treated by participating in groups that are similar to the ones in which the skills would have been developed.

(e) Subskills fundamental to mature group function must be acquired in a sequential manner.

(4) Type of clients: individuals with decreased group interaction skills.

(5) Overall role of the therapist.

(a) For all group levels, the therapist assesses the individuals' level and places them in the appropriate group.

(b) Orients all members to group's goals, structure, and norms.

(c) Lower level groups require more active, direct leadership.

(d) As group matures and attains a higher level of group interaction, leadership is shared among members.

(6) Parallel group leadership role.

(a) Provide unconditional positive regard to develop trust.

(b) Actively fill all leadership functions and meets all members' needs.

(c) Reinforce all behaviors appropriate to group, no matter how small.

(d) Provide structure.

(e) Facilitate interaction.

(7) Project group leadership role.

(a) Select and structure activities that can be shared by two or more members.

(b) Fulfill all of members' needs while encouraging members to give and seek assistance and interact beyond activity requirements.

(c) Reinforce cooperation, mild competition, sharing, and interactions.

(8) Egocentric-cooperative group leadership role.

(a) Less of an active, direct leader.

(b) Facilitate and allow members to fulfill functional leadership roles to function independently.

(c) Provide guidelines and assistance as needed.

(d) Reinforce members' meeting needs of self and others.

(e) Serve as a role model.

(9) Cooperative group leadership role.

(a) Act as an advisor, not as a direct leader.

(b) Leader and members are mutually responsible for giving feedback, identifying and meeting needs, and reinforcing behavior.

(10) Mature group leadership role.

(a) Acts as a peer, an equal, a group member.

(b) Members assume all roles with the therapist filling in only if and when needed to maintain group.

(c) All members satisfy needs and reinforce behavior while maintaining a balance between need satisfaction and task completion.

(11) Suitable activities.

(a) Parallel.

- Members perform activities independently of others but in the presence of others.
- Interactions are not required to successfully complete activity.
- Activities should be similar or utilize common tools or materials to facilitate interaction and sharing.
- Activities should be relevant to a person's ability, age, gender, and interest so he/she is more able to interact with and about it.

(b) Project.

- Task is short-term and requires the participation of two or more people.
- Task is shareable and requires interaction to successfully complete.
- Group interaction, not project completion, is emphasized.

(c) Egocentric-cooperative.

- Activity allows 5–10 people to work together.
- It is selected and implemented by members.
- It is longer-term, requiring more than two meetings to complete.

(d) Cooperative.

- Activities facilitate and allow for free expression of ideas and feelings.
- Activity is secondary to need fulfillment and may not produce an end product.

(e) Mature.

- Activity requires a number of people to work together.
- It requires an end product or has an inherent time limit for completion.
- During group, activity may be stopped for members to explore what is going on within the group.

g. Instrumental group.

(1) Purpose/focus.

(a) To help members function at their highest possible level for as long as possible.

(b) To meet mental health needs.

(2) Assumption.

(a) Individuals are functioning at their highest possible level and cannot change or progress.

(b) A supportive, structured environment which provides appropriate activities can prevent regression, maintain function, and meet mental health needs.

(3) Type of client.

(a) Individuals who have demonstrated in treatment an inability to change or progress.

(b) Individuals who can't independently meet their mental health needs and/or need assistance to maintain function due to cognitive, psychological, perceptual-motor, and/or social deficits.

(4) Role of the therapist

(a) Provide unconditional positive regard, support, and structure to create a comfortable, safe environment for patients.

(b) Select and design activities that will meet member's health needs and maintain highest possible level of function.

(c) Assist members with activity as needed.

(d) Make no attempt to changè client.

(5) Suitable activities.

(a) Members can successfully complete activities with structure and assistance of therapist as needed.

(b) Non-threatening and non-demanding.

(c) Interesting, enjoyable and attractive to members.

(d) Meet mental health needs of the person by enabling him/her to experience pleasure, have fun, socialize with others, etc.

(e) Maintain function by providing sensory, cognitive, perceptual-motor, and social input.

h. Role of the OTA in group work.

(1) The OTA is active in all aspects of group work.

(2) Refer to Chapter 14 for additional group information

References

American Occupational Therapy Association. (2010). Standards of practice for occupational therapy. *American Journal of Occupational Therapy, 64* (6, Supplement), S106–S110.

American Occupational Therapy Association. (2006). *Reference manual of the official documents of the American Occupational Therapy Association* (11th ed.). Bethesda, MD: Author.

Asher, I. E. (2007). *An annotated index of occupational therapy evaluation tools,* 3rd ed. Bethesda, MD: AOTA Press.

Case-Smith, J. (Ed.). (2005). *Occupational therapy for children,* 5th ed. St. Louis, MO: Elsevier Mosby.

Hansen, R. A. (1990). Lesson 10: Ethical considerations. In C.B. Royeen (Ed.), *AOTA self study series. Assessing function.* Bethesda, MD: American Occupational Therapy Association.

Hemphill-Pearson, B. J. (1999). *Assessments in occupational therapy mental health: An integrative approach.* Thorofare, NJ: Slack.

Hinojosa, J., & Kramer, P., & Crist, P. (Eds.) (2005). *Evaluation: Obtaining and interpreting data,* 2nd ed. Bethesda, MD: AOTA Press.

Hopkins, H., & Smith, H. (Eds.). (2003). *Willard and Spackman's occupational therapy,* 10th ed. Philadelphia: J.B. Lippincott.

Mailloux, Z., May-Benson, T. A., Summers, C. A., Miller, L. J., Brett-Green, B., Burke, J. P., et al. (2007). The Issue Is - Goal attainment scaling as a measure of meaningful outcomes for children with sensory integration disorders. *American Journal of Occupational Therapy, 61,* 254–259.

McCormack, G., Jaffe, E., Goodman-Lavey, M. (Eds.). (2003). *The occupational therapy manager,* 4th ed. Bethesda, MD: AOTA Press.

Mosey, A. C. (1996). *Psychosocial components of occupational therapy.* New York: Raven Press.

Moyers, P., & Dale, L. (2007). *The guide to occupational therapy practice.* Bethesda, MD: AOTA Press.

Ottenbacher, K. J., & Cusick, A. (1990). Goal attainment scaling as a method of clinical service evaluation. *American Journal of Occupational Therapy, 44,* 519–525.

Trombly, C. (1995). Eleanor Clarke Slagle Lecture Occupation: Purposefulness and meaningfulness as therapeutic mechanisms. *American Journal of Occupational Therapy, 49,* 960–972.

United States Government Printing Office. (2003). *Code of Federal Regulations, Title 42, Volume 3.* Retrieved from http://www. cms.gov. December 21, 2003.

Review Questions

The Process of Occupational Therapy

Below are five questions about key content covered in this chapter. These questions are not inclusive of the entirety of content about the occupational therapy process that you must know for success on the NBCOT exam. These questions are provided to help you "jump start" the thought processes you will need to apply your studying of content to the answering of exam questions; hence they are not in the NBCOT exam format. Exam items in the NBCOT format which cover the depth and breadth of content you will need to know to pass the NBCOT exam are provided on this text's disc. The answers to the below questions are provided in Appendix 4.

1. An occupational therapist is preparing to evaluate a client. What contextual considerations should the therapist take into account when determining the assessments that will be appropriate to use with the client?

2. An occupational therapist owns and operates a pre-school facility for children with developmental, intellectual, and physical disabilities. When should the therapist instruct the facility staff members to use standard precautions? What policies and procedures should the therapist implement for the use of standard precautions in this practice setting?

3. An occupational therapist provides services in a community-based setting which offers individual and group interventions. What factors should the therapist consider when determining if it is best to use an individual intervention versus a group intervention with a client?

4. An occupational therapist working in a long-term care facility co-leads a discharge planning group with a social worker. What are the advantages to this co-leadership? What issues may arise to impede effective co-leadership that the therapist should be prepared to address?

5. An occupational therapist provides services to a group of parents of infants and toddlers who each recently incurred a disability. The therapist plans to use a thematic and a topical group with the clients to address goals related to their parental role. What would be appropriate foci and relevant activities for these groups?

4

Professional Standards and Responsibilities

RITA P. FLEMING-CASTALDY

Chapter Outline

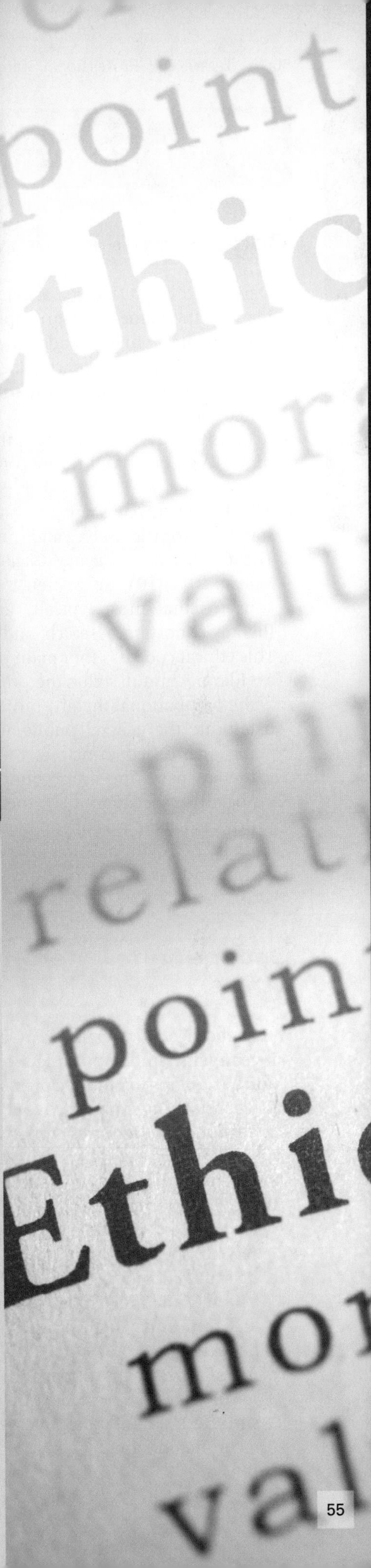

Professional Ethics

Code of Ethics Overview

1. Developed by AOTA as a statement to the public to identify the values and principles used to promote and maintain high standards for the behavior of occupational therapy practitioners.
2. A set of principles that apply to all levels of occupational therapy personnel.
3. Actions that are in violation of the purpose and spirit of AOTA's Code of Ethics are considered unethical by AOTA.
4. All OT practitioners are obligated to uphold these standards for themselves and their colleagues.
5. The *Occupational Therapy Code of Ethics and Ethics Standards* (2010) are written to address the ethical concerns that most typically arise in occupational therapy education, research, and practice.
6. This ethical code has four main purposes. These are:
   a. "Identify and describe the principles supported by the occupational therapy profession.
   b. Educate the general public and members regarding established principles to which occupational therapy personnel are accountable.
   c. Socialize occupational therapy personnel to expected standards of conduct.
   d. Assist occupational therapy personnel in recognition and resolution of ethical dilemmas" (AOTA, 2010, p. 2).

Occupational Therapy Code of Ethics

1. "Beneficence. Principle 1. Occupational therapy personnel shall demonstrate a concern for the safety and well-being of the recipients of their services.... Occupational therapy personnel shall:
   a. Respond to requests for occupational therapy services (e.g., a referral) in a timely manner as determined by law, regulation, or policy.
   b. Provide appropriate evaluation and a plan of intervention for all recipients of occupational therapy services specific to their needs.
   c. Reevaluate and reassess recipients of service in a timely manner to determine if goals are being achieved and whether intervention plans should be revised.
   d. Avoid the inappropriate use of outdated or obsolete tests/assessments or data obtained from such tests in making intervention decisions or recommendations.
   e. Provide occupational therapy services that are within each practitioner's level of competence and scope of practice (e.g., qualifications, experience, and the law).
   f. Use, to the extent possible, evaluation, planning, intervention techniques, and therapeutic equipment that are evidence-based and within the recognized scope of occupational therapy practice.
   g. Take responsible steps (e.g., continuing education, research, supervision, training) and use careful judgment to ensure their own competence and weigh potential for client harm when generally recognized standards do not exist in emerging technology or areas of practice.
   h. Terminate occupational therapy services in collaboration with the service recipient or responsible party when the needs and goals of the recipient have been met or when services no longer produce a measurable change or outcome.
   i. Refer to other health care specialists solely on the basis of the needs of the client.
   j. Provide occupational therapy education, continuing education, instruction, and training that are within the instructor's subject area of expertise and level of competence.
   k. Provide students and employees with information about the Code and Ethics Standards, opportunities to discuss ethical conflicts, and procedures for reporting unresolved ethical conflicts.
   l. Ensure that occupational therapy research is conducted in accordance with currently accepted ethical guidelines and standards for the protection of research participants and the dissemination of results.
   m. Report to appropriate authorities any acts in practice, education, and research that appear unethical or illegal.
   n. Take responsibility for promoting and practicing occupational therapy on the basis of current knowledge and research and for further developing the profession's body of knowledge.
2. Nonmaleficence, Principle 2. Occupational therapy personnel shall intentionally refrain from actions that cause harm.... Occupational therapy personnel shall:
   a. Avoid inflicting harm or injury to recipients of occupational therapy services, students, research participants, or employees.
   b. Make every effort to ensure continuity of services or options for transition to appropriate services

to avoid abandoning the service recipient if the current provider is unavailable due to medical or other absence or loss of employment.

c. Avoid relationships that exploit the recipient of services, students, research participants, or employees physically, emotionally, psychologically, financially, socially, or in any other manner that conflicts or interferes with professional judgment and objectivity.

d. Avoid engaging in any sexual relationship or activity, whether consensual or nonconsensual, with any recipient of service, including family or significant other, student, research participant, or employee, while a relationship exists as an occupational therapy practitioner, educator, researcher, supervisor, or employer.

e. Recognize and take appropriate action to remedy personal problems and limitations that might cause harm to recipients of service, colleagues, students, research participants, or others.

f. Avoid any undue influences, such as alcohol or drugs, that may compromise the provision of occupational therapy services, education, or research.

g. Avoid situations in which a practitioner, educator, researcher, or employer is unable to maintain clear professional boundaries or objectivity to ensure the safety and well-being of recipients of service, students, research participants, and employees.

h. Maintain awareness of and adherence to the Code and Ethics Standards when participating in volunteer roles.

i. Avoid compromising client rights or well-being based on arbitrary administrative directives by exercising professional judgment and critical analysis.

j. Avoid exploiting any relationship established as an occupational therapist or occupational therapy assistant to further one's own physical, emotional, financial, political, or business interests at the expense of the best interests of recipients of services, students, research participants, employees, or colleagues.

k. Avoid participating in bartering for services because of the potential for exploitation and conflict of interest unless there are clearly no contraindications or bartering is a culturally appropriate custom.

l. Determine the proportion of risk to benefit for participants in research prior to implementing a study.

3. Autonomy and confidentiality. Principle 3. Occupational therapy personnel shall respect the right of the individual to self-determination....Occupational therapy personnel shall:

a. Establish a collaborative relationship with recipients of service including families, significant others, and caregivers in setting goals and priorities throughout the intervention process. This includes full disclosure of the benefits, risks, and potential outcomes of any intervention; the personnel who will be providing the intervention(s); and/or any reasonable alternatives to the proposed intervention.

b. Obtain consent before administering any occupational therapy service, including evaluation, and ensure that recipients of service (or their legal representatives) are kept informed of the progress in meeting goals specified in the plan of intervention/care. If the service recipient cannot give consent, the practitioner must be sure that consent has been obtained from the person who is legally responsible for that recipient.

c. Respect the recipient of service's right to refuse occupational therapy services temporarily or permanently without negative consequences.

d. Provide students with access to accurate information regarding educational requirements and academic policies and procedures relative to the occupational therapy program/educational institution.

e. Obtain informed consent from participants involved in research activities, and ensure that they understand the benefits, risks, and potential outcomes as a result of their participation as research subjects.

f. Respect research participant's right to withdraw from a research study without consequences.

g. Ensure that confidentiality and the right to privacy are respected and maintained regarding all information obtained about recipients of service, students, research participants, colleagues, or employees. The only exceptions are when a practitioner or staff member believes that an individual is in serious foreseeable or imminent harm. Laws and regulations may require disclosure to appropriate authorities without consent.

h. Maintain the confidentiality of all verbal, written, electronic, augmentative, and non-verbal communications, including compliance with HIPAA regulations.

i. Take appropriate steps to facilitate meaningful communication and comprehension in cases in which the recipient of service, student, or research participant has limited ability to communicate (e.g., aphasia or differences in language, literacy, culture).

j. Make every effort to facilitate open and collaborative dialogue with clients and/or responsible parties to facilitate comprehension of services and their potential risks/benefits.

4. Social justice Principle 4. Occupational therapy personnel shall provide services in a fair and equitable manner....Occupational therapy personnel shall:

a. Uphold the profession's altruistic responsibilities to help ensure the common good.

b. Take responsibility for educating the public and society about the value of occupational therapy services in promoting health and wellness and reducing the impact of disease and disability.
c. Make every effort to promote activities that benefit the health status of the community.
d. Advocate for just and fair treatment for all patients, clients, employees, and colleagues, and encourage employers and colleagues to abide by the highest standards of social justice and the ethical standards set forth by the occupational therapy profession.
e. Make efforts to advocate for recipients of occupational therapy services to obtain needed services through available means.
f. Provide services that reflect an understanding of how occupational therapy service delivery can be affected by factors such as economic status, age, ethnicity, race, geography, disability, marital status, sexual orientation, gender, gender identity, religion, culture, and political affiliation.
g. Consider offering pro bono ("for the good") or reduced-fee occupational therapy services for selected individuals when consistent with guidelines of the employer, third party payer, and/or government agency.

5. Procedural justice Principle 5. Occupational therapy personnel shall comply with institutional rules, local, state, federal, and international laws and AOTA documents applicable to the profession of occupational therapy....Occupational therapy personnel shall:
a. Be familiar with and apply the Code and Ethics Standards to the work setting, and share them with employers, other employees, colleagues, students, and researchers.
b. Be familiar with and seek to understand and abide by institutional rules, and when those rules conflict with ethical practice, take steps to resolve the conflict.
c. Be familiar with revisions in those laws and AOTA policies that apply to the profession of occupational therapy and inform employers, employees, colleagues, students, and researchers of those changes.
d. Be familiar with established policies and procedures for handling concerns about the Code and Ethics Standards, including familiarity with national, state, local, district, and territorial procedures for handling ethics complaints as well as policies and procedures created by AOTA and certification, licensing, and regulatory agencies.
e. Hold appropriate national, state, or other requisite credentials for the occupational therapy services they provide.
f. Take responsibility for maintaining high standards and continuing competence in practice, education, and research by participating in professional development and educational activities to improve and update knowledge and skills.
g. Ensure that all duties assumed by or assigned to other occupational therapy personnel match credentials, qualifications, experience, and scope of practice.
h. Provide appropriate supervision to individuals for whom they have supervisory responsibility in accordance with AOTA official documents and local, state, and federal or national laws, rules, regulations, policies, procedures, standards and guidelines.
i. Obtain all necessary approvals prior to initiating research activities.
j. Report all gifts and remuneration from individuals, agencies, or companies in accordance with employer policies as well as state and federal guidelines.
k. Use funds for intended purposes, and avoid misappropriation of funds.
l. Take reasonable steps to ensure that employers are aware of occupational therapy's ethical obligations as set forth in this Code and Ethics Standards and of the implications of those obligations for occupational therapy practice, education, and research.
m. Actively work with employers to prevent discrimination and unfair labor practices, and advocate for employees with disabilities to ensure the provision of reasonable accommodations.
n. Actively participate with employers in the formulation of policies and procedures to ensure legal, regulatory, and ethical compliance.
o. Collect fees legally. Fees shall be fair, reasonable, and commensurate with services delivered. Fee schedules must be available and equitable regardless of actual payer reimbursements/contracts.
p. Maintain the ethical principles and standards of the profession when participating in a business arrangement as owner, stockholder, partner, or employee, and refrain from working for or doing business with organizations that engage in illegal or unethical business practices (e.g., fraudulent billing, providing occupational therapy services beyond the scope of occupational therapy practice).

6. Veracity. Principle 6. Occupational therapy personnel shall provide comprehensive, accurate, and objective information when representing the profession.... Occupational therapy personnel shall:
a. Represent the credentials, qualifications, education, experience, training, roles, duties, competence, views, contributions, and findings accurately in all forms of communication about recipients of service, students, employees, research participants, and colleagues.

b. Refrain from using or participating in the use of any form of communication that contains false, fraudulent, deceptive, misleading, or unfair statements or claims.
c. Record and report in an accurate and timely manner, and in accordance with applicable regulations, all information related to professional activities.
d. Ensure that documentation for reimbursement purposes is done in accordance with applicable laws, guidelines, and regulations.
e. Accept responsibility for any action that reduces the public's trust in occupational therapy.
f. Ensure that all marketing and advertising are truthful, accurate, and carefully presented to avoid misleading recipients of service, students, research participants, or the public.
g. Describe the type and duration of occupational therapy services accurately in professional contracts, including the duties and responsibilities of all involved parties.
h. Be honest, fair, accurate, respectful, and timely in gathering and reporting fact-based information regarding employee job performance and student performance.
i. Give credit and recognition when using the work of others in written, oral, or electronic media.
j. Not plagiarize the work of others.

7. Fidelity. Principle 7. Occupational therapy personnel shall treat colleagues and other professionals with respect, fairness, discretion, and integrity.... Occupational therapy personnel shall:
   a. Respect the traditions, practices, competencies, and responsibilities of their own and other professions, as well as those of the institutions and agencies that constitute the working environment.
   b. Preserve, respect, and safeguard private information about employees, colleagues, and students unless otherwise mandated by national, state, or local laws or permission to disclose is given by the individual.
   c. Take adequate measures to discourage, prevent, expose, and correct any breaches of the Code and Ethics Standards and report any breaches of the former to the appropriate authorities.
   d. Attempt to resolve perceived institutional violations of the Code and Ethics Standards by utilizing internal resources first.
   e. Avoid conflicts of interest or conflicts of commitment in employment, volunteer roles, or research.
   f. Avoid using one's position (employee or volunteer) or knowledge gained from that position in such a manner that gives rise to real or perceived conflict of interest among the person, the employer, other Association members, and/or other organizations.
   g. Use conflict resolution and/or alternative dispute resolution resources to resolve organizational and interpersonal conflicts.
   h. Be diligent stewards of human, financial, and material resources of their employers, and refrain from exploiting these resources for personal gain." (AOTA, 2010, pp. 3–10).

Ethics in Practice

1. Ethics guide the behavior and decision making of occupational therapy practitioners to help them determine the morally right course of action.
2. Occupational therapists are often faced with issues and events that challenge their personal values and beliefs and professional ethics.
3. NBCOT examination items may include practice scenarios that reflect ethical distress or ethical dilemmas.
   a. Ethical distress.
      (1) When a therapist knows the correct action to take but an existing barrier prevents the therapist from taking this course of action.
         (a) For example, when an admissions policy to a day treatment program excludes persons with substance abuse histories, yet this program would provide appropriate intervention for a client who is mentally ill and chemically addicted (MICA).
   b. Ethical dilemmas.
      (1) When there are two or more potentially morally correct ways to solve a problem. However, these solutions are exclusive; therefore, choosing one course of action prohibits acting on the other choices.
         (a) For example, a group of occupational therapy private practitioners has the opportunity to bid on a lucrative contract for the provision of services in a school system. However, none of the occupational therapists has pediatric experience. Their options may include not bidding on the contract or bidding on the contract and if the contract is won, incurring the expense of hiring pediatric-trained therapists.
4. Decisions about what are the right or wrong courses of action are based on our profession's Code of Ethics.
   a. NBCOT examination items require the application of the AOTA Code of Ethics.

Patient/Client Abuse

1. It is an ethical responsibility of all occupational therapy practitioners to report any observed or suspected incidents of patient/client abuse or neglect.
   a. This responsibility is in accordance with Principle 1 of the AOTA Code of Ethics which states that occupational therapy personnel must act to ensure "the well-being and safety of the recipients of their services" (AOTA, 2010, p. 3).
   b. The party to whom reporting is required varies from state to state, as do the penalties for not reporting.
      (1) Minimum reporting standards require reporting to one's immediate supervisor.
   c. Occupational therapy practitioners should also provide interventions to victims of abuse and/or neglect. These can include:
      (1) Treatment for physical and emotional injuries.
      (2) Development of a trusting relationship.
      (3) Provision of support to family and loved ones.
      (4) Referral to appropriate disciplines and agencies.
      (5) Contributor to staff training programs to prevent abuse.
2. Facts and figures.
   a. All ages are at risk for abuse.
      (1) Refer to Chapter 5 for specific information on child and elder abuse.
   b. Facts and figures for patient/client abuse are subsumed into institutional elder abuse and abuse of the mentally ill.
3. Definition of abuse.
   a. Abuse is defined as deliberately hurting a patient physically, mentally or emotionally.
   b. Neglect is defined as deliberately withholding services that are necessary to maintain an individual's physical, mental, and emotional health.
   c. Definitions may vary from state to state.
4. Signs of patient/client abuse.
   a. Individual's report of abuse and/or neglect.
   b. Frequent unexplained injuries or complaints of pain without obvious injury.
   c. Burns or bruises suggesting the use of instruments, cigarettes, etc.
   d. Passive, withdrawn, and emotionless behavior.
   e. Lack of reaction to pain.
   f. Sexually transmitted diseases or injury to the genital area.
   g. Unexplained difficulty in sitting or walking.
   h. Fear of being alone with caretakers.
   i. Obvious malnutrition.
   j. Lack of personal cleanliness.
   k. Habitually dressed in torn or dirty clothes.
   l. Obvious fatigue and listlessness.
   m. Begs for food, water, or assistance (especially in regard to toileting).
   n. In need of medical or dental care.
   o. Left unattended for long periods.
   p. Bedsores and skin lesions.

Ethical Decision Making

1. Identify the ethical issues and potential dilemmas.
2. Gather relevant information.
   a. Identify all individuals affected by the issue.
   b. Determine prior history of the issue.
   c. Analyze the dynamics and culture of the setting(s).
   d. Ask open ended questions to obtain descriptive data.
3. Determine conflicting values and areas of agreement.
   a. A commitment to patient autonomy versus the principles of beneficence and nonmaleficence may need to be considered.
4. Identify as many relevant alternative courses of action as possible.
   a. Consider who would take these actions and when these actions would need to occur.
5. Determine all possible positive and negative outcomes for each possible action.
   a. Include outcomes for all participants in the dilemma. An ethical dilemma never involves just one person.
   b. It can take time and thought to identify all those who may possibly have a "stake" or will be touched by a specific decision.
6. Weigh, with care, the consequences of each outcome.
   a. This step includes the process of reordering or rearranging parts of different decisions to arrive at a new alternative which may be the best possible course of action.
7. Seek input from others (i.e., supervisors).
   a. Provide information in an anonymous fashion which enables the individual to give advice in a more objective manner and to provide recommendations that cannot be construed to be biased or prejudicial.
8. Apply best professional judgment to choose the action(s) to recommend.
9. Contact any and all agencies that have jurisdiction over a practitioner if there are questions about potential ethical violations that could cause harm or have the potential to cause harm to a person.
10. Determine desired and/or potential outcome of filing an ethical complaint.

Ethical Jurisdiction of Occupational Therapy

American Occupational Therapy Association (AOTA)

1. The profession's official membership organization which develops, publishes, and disseminates the field's ethical code.
2. AOTA's Code of Ethics is a statement to the public that identifies the values and principles used to develop, endorse, and sustain high standards of behavior for OT practitioners.
   a. A set of principles that apply to all levels of OT personnel.
   b. All occupational therapy practitioners are obligated to uphold these standards for themselves and their colleagues.
3. Actions that are in violation of the purpose and spirit of AOTA's Code of Ethics are considered unethical by AOTA.
4. These ethical standards are often the guide by which other bodies judge professional behaviors to determine if malpractice has occurred.
5. As a voluntary membership organization, AOTA has no direct authority over practitioners (occupational therapists and OTAs) who are not members, and no direct legal mechanism for preventing nonmembers who are incompetent, unethical, or unqualified from practicing.
6. Ethics Commission.
   a. The component of AOTA that is responsible for the Code of Ethics and the Standards of Practice of the profession.
   b. The Ethics Commission is responsible for informing and educating members about current ethical issues, upholding the practice and education standards of the profession, monitoring the behavior of members, and reviewing allegations of unethical conduct.
      (1) Ethical complaints filed with the Ethics Commission initiate an extensive, confidential review process according to AOTA's established enforcement procedures for occupational therapy Code of Ethics.

National Board for Certification in Occupational Therapy (NBCOT)

1. The national credentialing agency for occupational therapy practitioners.
   a. Certifies qualified persons as OTR®s and COTA®s initially through a written examination for entry-level practitioners.
   b. NBCOT also maintains OTR® and COTA® certification through a voluntary certification renewal program.
   c. Jurisdiction is over all NBCOT certified occupational therapy practitioners as well as those eligible for NBCOT certification.
2. As a voluntary credentialing agency, NBCOT has no direct authority over OT practitioners who are not certified by NBCOT, and no direct legal mechanism for preventing uncertified practitioners who are incompetent, unethical, or unqualified from practicing.
3. NBCOT has developed investigatory and disciplinary action procedures for NBCOT certified practitioners whose practices raise concern due to incompetence, unethical behavior, and/or impairment.

State Regulatory Boards (SRBs)

1. Public bodies created by state legislatures to assure the health and safety of the citizens of that state.
   a. Their specific responsibility is to protect the public from potential harm that might be caused by incompetent or unqualified practitioners.
   b. State regulation may be in the form of licensure, registration or certification. (See text's Appendix 2.)
   c. Each state has legal guidelines that usually specify the scope of practice of the profession, and the qualifications that must be met to practice in that state.
2. Ethical jurisdiction.
   a. SRBs usually provide a description of ethical behavior. In many instances, SRBs have adopted AOTA's Code of Ethics for this purpose.
   b. By the very nature of their limited jurisdiction (i.e., only over practitioners practicing in their state), SRBs can monitor a profession closely.
   c. SRBs have the authority by law to discipline members of a profession if the public is determined to be at risk due to malpractice.
   d. SRBs also intervene in situations where the individual has been convicted of an illegal act that is directly connected with professional practice (i.e., fraud or misappropriation of funds through false billing practices).
   e. Since SRBs are primarily concerned with the protection of the public from harm, they will typically limit their review of complaints to those involving such a threat.

Disciplinary Actions for Ethical Violations & Professional Misconduct

1. When the AOTA, NBCOT, and/or a SRB determine that a person has violated their standards for ethical practice, different actions can be used as a disciplinary measure.
   a. These actions are based on agency internal investigations to determine the severity of an infraction and can include:
      (1) Reprimand: the private communication of the respective agency's disapproval of a practitioner's conduct.
      (2) Censure: a public statement of the respective agency's disapproval of a practitioner's conduct.
      (3) Ineligibility: the removal of eligibility for membership, certification, or licensure by the respective agency for an indefinite or specific time period.
      (4) Probation: the requirement that a practitioner meet certain conditions (e.g., further education, extensive supervision, individual counseling, participation in a substance abuse rehabilitation program) to retain membership, certification, or licensure by the respective agency.
      (5) Suspension: the loss of membership, certification, or licensure for a specific time period.
      (6) Revocation: the permanent loss of membership, certification, or licensure.
2. All of the above actions (except for reprimand) are made public by the respective agencies.
   a. Disciplinary actions that are made public by one agency (e.g., NBCOT) can trigger an investigation into a practitioner's professional conduct by other practice jurisdictions (e.g., SRBs).

Common Law Related to Professional Misconduct & Malpractice

1. Common law evolves from legal decisions and can impact occupational therapists.
   a. Malpractice suits can be filed by individuals and/or their caregivers if the occupational therapist is viewed to be personally responsible for negligence or other acts that resulted in harm to a client.
      (1) Negligence.
         (a) Failure to do what other reasonable practitioners would have done under similar circumstances.
         (b) Doing what other reasonable practitioners would not have done under similar circumstances.
         (c) The end result was harm to the individual.
         (d) Every individual (occupational therapist, student occupational therapist, OTA or student OTA) is liable for their own negligence.
   b. Supervisors or superiors may also assume the liability of their workers if they provided faulty supervision or inappropriately delegated responsibilities.
   c. The institution usually assumes liability if an individual was harmed as a result of an environmental problem.
      (1) Falls resulting from slippery floors, poorly lit areas, lack of grab bars.
   d. The institution is also liable if an employee was incompetent or not properly licensed.
   e. Personal malpractice insurance is advisable for all levels of OT practitioners.

OT Practitioner Roles

General Information

1. OT practitioners include occupational therapists and occupational therapy assistants (OTAs).
2. Due to the implementation of the voluntary NBCOT certification renewal program, all occupational therapists may not be OTR®s and all OTAs may not be COTA®s.
3. OT aides have an important role but are not considered OT practitioners.
4. OT practitioners can assume a variety of roles including entry to advanced level practitioner, peer and/or consumer educator, fieldwork educator, supervisor, administrator, consultant, fieldwork coordinator, faculty member, academic program director, researcher/scholar, and/or entrepreneur.
5. Role development and advancement depends on practitioner's experience, education, practice skills, and professional development activities (i.e., self study, continuing education, advanced degrees).

OT Assistant (OTA) Information

1. OTAs are graduates of ACOTE accredited technical educational programs which are generally two years in duration, resulting in an Associate's degree or a Certificate.

2. An OTA can expand their role by establishing service competency.
   a. Service competency is the ability to use the specified intervention in a safe, effective, and reliable manner, (i.e., the OTA and occupational therapist can perform the same or equivalent procedure and obtain the same results).
   b. OTAs who establish service competency do not become independent; they continue to work under the occupational therapist's supervision.
3. OTA's primary role is to implement treatment.
   a. OTAs can contribute to the evaluation process but they cannot independently evaluate or initiate treatment prior to the occupational therapist's evaluation.
   b. OTAs can contribute to development and implementation of the intervention plan and the monitoring and documenting of the individual's response to intervention under the occupational therapist's supervision.
4. OTAs can be activities directors in skilled nursing facilities (SNFs) and can supervise OT aides.
5. AOTA supports the independent practice of OTAs with advanced level skills who work for independent living centers.
   a. State licensure laws and scope of practice legislation may supersede this recommendation.

OT Aide Roles

1. Although OT aides are not considered OT practitioners, the use of OT aides has increased in response to changes in the health care system (i.e., pressures to control costs have resulted in the delegation of non-skilled tasks to aides).
2. OT aides can be trained by OTAs or occupational therapists to perform specific non-skilled tasks.
3. The occupational therapist is responsible for the determination and delegation of the client and non-client tasks an aide performs and the outcome of these activities.
   a. Non-skilled non-client tasks aides may perform include routine maintenance and clerical activities (e.g., preparation of clinic area for intervention, organizing supplies).
   b. Non-skilled client tasks (e.g., contact guarding a client during transfers) can only be delegated to an OT aide after the occupational therapist has determined that the following conditions have been met.
      (1) The anticipated result of the delegated task is known.
      (2) The performance of the delegated task is clearly established and predictable and does not require any adaptation, judgment, and/or interpretations by the aide.
      (3) The patient's situation and the practice environment are stable and will not require any adaptation, judgment, and/or interpretations by the aide.
      (4) The patient has previously demonstrated some capabilities in performing the task.
      (5) The aide has been appropriately trained in the competent performance of the task and is able to demonstrate service competency in task performance.
      (6) The aide has received specific instructions on task implementation relevant to the specific client with whom the aide will be performing the delegated task.
      (7) The aide knows the precautions of the designated task and patient signs and symptoms that could indicate the need to seek assistance from the OTA or occupational therapist.
4. The performance of tasks performed by OT aides must be supervised by an OTA or occupational therapist and this supervision must be documented.

Supervisory Guidelines for OT Personnel

General Supervision Information

1. Supervision is the process in which two or more individuals collaborate to establish, maintain, promote, or enhance a level of performance and quality of service.
2. It is a mutually respectful joint effort between supervisor and supervisee.
3. It promotes professional growth and development and facilitates mentoring.
4. It ensures appropriate training, education, and use of resources for safe and effective service provision.
5. Supervision facilitates innovation, supports creativity, and provides encouragement, guidance, and support while working toward attainment of a shared goal.
6. Only OT practitioners can supervise OT practice, OT aides cannot supervise OT practice.
7. Occupational therapists can practice autonomously and do not require any supervision to provide OT services.

a. Occupational therapists are responsible and accountable for all aspects of OT service delivery.
b. To develop best practice competencies and foster professional growth, occupational therapists should use supervision and mentorship.

8. OT assistants must be supervised by occupational therapists for any and all aspects of the OT service delivery process.

Methods of Supervision

1. Direct: face-to-face contact between supervisor and supervisee.
   a. Includes co-treatment, observation, instruction, modeling, and discussion.
2. Indirect: non face-to-face contact between supervisor and supervisee.
   a. Includes electronic, written and telephone communications.

The Supervision Continuum

1. Supervision occurs along a continuum that includes close, routine, general, and minimum.
   a. Close: daily, direct contact at the site of work.
   b. Routine: direct contact at least every two weeks at the site of work, with interim supervision occurring by other methods such as telephone or written communication.
   c. General: at least monthly direct contact with supervision available as needed by other methods.
   d. Minimal: provided only on a needed basis, and may be less than monthly.
2. Formal supervision can be supplemented by functional supervision, which is the provision of information and feedback to coworkers (a sharing of expertise).
3. The degree, amount, and pattern of supervision required can vary depending on the:
   a. Practitioner's knowledge and skills.
   b. Complexities of client needs and caseload characteristics and demands.
   c. State laws, licensure requirements, and other regulatory mandates.
   d. Practice setting type and facility procedures.
4. An OT assistant providing services to an acutely ill person with rapidly changing status on an inpatient unit will require a closer occupational therapist/OTA partnership than an OT assistant providing services to a more stable client in a long-term care residential facility.
5. The supervising occupational therapist determines the type of supervision that is most appropriate.
6. Ethically, the OT supervisor must ensure that the type, amount, and pattern of supervision match the supervisee's level of role performance. See Table 4-1.
7. OT aide supervision may be intermittent or continuous depending on the task being performed.
   a. Intermittent supervision is sufficient for non-patient related tasks. It requires periodic discussion, demonstration, or contact between the supervisor and aide on at least a monthly basis.
   b. Continuous supervision is required for client-related tasks. A supervisory OTA or occupational therapist must be within auditory and/or visual contact in the immediate area of the aide during the aide's task performance.

Specific OT Roles and Supervisory Guidelines

1. Occupational therapist.
   a. Functions to provide quality OT services (assessment, intervention, program planning and implementation, discharge planning, related documentation and communication).
   b. Can be direct, indirect, or consultative in nature, and can range from entry level to advanced level depending on experience, education, and practice skills.
   c. The occupational therapist has ultimate responsibility for service provision.
   d. Occupational therapists who do not have access to formal supervision are advised to seek mentoring to facilitate professional growth and develop best practice skills.
2. Occupational therapy assistant (OTA).
   a. Functions to provide quality OT services to assigned individuals under supervision of an occupational therapist.
   b. Can range from entry level to advanced level depending on experience, education, and practice skills.
   c. Development from entry level to advanced level is dependent upon development of service competency.
3. Educator (consumer, peer).
   a. Functions to develop and provide training or educational offerings related to OT's domain of concern to consumer, peer, and community groups or individuals.
   b. Can be an occupational therapist or an OTA with appropriate supervision.
4. Fieldwork educator.
   a. Functions as the manager of Level I and/or II fieldwork in a practice setting, providing students with

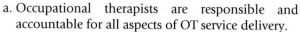

Table 4-1

Guide for Supervision of Occupational Therapy Personnel

OCCUPATIONAL THERAPY PERSONNEL	SUPERVISION	SUPERVISES
Entry-level OT* (working on initial skill development or entering new practice) (AOTA, 1993a, p. 1088)	Not required. Close supervision by an intermediate-level or an advanced-level OT recommended.	Aides, technicians, all levels of OTAs, volunteers, Level I fieldwork students.
Intermediate-level OT* (working on increased skill development and mastery of basic role functions, and demonstrates ability to respond to situations based on previous experience) (AOTA,1993a, p. 1088)	Not required. Routine or general supervision by an advanced-level OT recommended.	Aides, technicians, all levels of OTAs, Level I and Level II fieldwork students, entry-level OTs.
Advanced-level OT* (refining specialized skills with the ability to understand complex issues affecting role functions) (AOTA, 1993a, p. 1088)	Not required. Minimal supervision by an advanced-level OT is recommended.	Aides, technicians, all levels of OTAs, Level I and Level II fieldwork students entry-level and intermediate-level OTs.
Entry-level OTA* (working on initial skill development or entering new practice) (AOTA, 1993a, p. 1088)	Close supervision by all levels of OTs, or an intermediate or an advanced-level OTA who is under the supervision of an OT.	Aides, technicians, volunteers.
Intermediate-level OTA* (working on increased skill development and mastery of basic role functions, and demonstrates ability to respond to situations based on previous experience) (AOTA, 1993a, p. 1088)	Routine or general supervision by all levels of OTs, or an advanced-level OTA, who is under the supervision of an OT.	Aides, technicians, entry-level OTAs, volunteers, Level I OT fieldwork students, Level I and II OTA fieldwork students.
Advanced-level OTA** (refining specialized skills with the ability to understand complex issues affecting role functions) (AOTA, 1993a, p. 1088)	General supervision by all levels of OTs, or an advanced-level OTA, who is under the supervision of an OT.	Aides, technicians, entry-level and intermediate-level OTAs, volunteers, Level I OT fieldwork students, Level I and Level II OTA fieldwork students.
Personnel other than occupational therapy practitioners assisting in occupational therapy service (aides, paraprofessionals, technicians, volunteers)*** (AOTA, 1993a, p. 1088)	For non-client related tasks, supervision is determined by the supervising practitioner. For client-related tasks, continuous supervision is provided by all levels of practitioners.	No supervisory capacity.

*Refer to the *Occupational Therapy Roles* document for descriptions of entry-level, intermediate-level, and advanced-level OTs and OTAs (AOTA, 1993a).

**Although specific state regulations may dictate the parameters of certified occupational therapy assistant practice, the American Occupational Therapy Association supports the autonomous practice of the certified occupational therapy assistant practitioner in the independent living setting (AOTA, 1993b, p. 1079). (*Note.* Removed from active files and placed in archives April 1999).

***Students are not addressed in this category. The student role as a supervisor is addressed in the Essentials and Guidelines for an Accredited Educational Program for the Occupational Therapist (AOTA, 1991a) and Essentials and Guidelines for an Accredited Educational Program for the Occupational Therapy Assistant (AOTA, 1991b).

From: Guide for supervision of occupational therapy. *American Journal of Occupational Therapy, 53* (p. 594) by the American Occupational Therapy Association Commission on Practice. Copyright 1999 by the American Occupational Therapy Association. Reprinted with permission.

opportunities to practice and implement practitioner competence.

(1) Entry level occupational therapists and OTAs may supervise Level I fieldwork students.[1]

(2) Occupational therapists with one year practice-based experience may supervise OT Level II students.

(3) OTAs with 1 year of practice experience may supervise OTA Level II fieldwork students.

(4) Three years of experience are recommended for individuals supervising programs with multiple students and multiple supervisors.

5. Supervisor.
   a. Functions as the manager of the overall daily operation of OT services in a defined practice area(s).
   b. Can be an occupational therapist or an OTA.
   c. Experienced OTAs may supervise other OTAs administratively as long as service protocols and documentation are supervised by an occupational therapist.

[1]According to ACOTE standards, currently licensed and professionally credentialed personnel may supervise Level I fieldwork students. This standard includes occupational therapists and occupational therapy assistants and non-OT personnel such as nurses, nurse practitioners, psychologists, vocational counselors, physician assistants, recreation therapists, teachers, speech therapists, social workers, and physical therapists.

6. Administrator.
   a. Functions to manage department, program, services, or agency providing OT services.
   b. Can be an occupational therapist with a graduate degree or continuing education relevant to management and experience appropriate to the size and scope of department and program(s), (i.e., a minimum of 3–5 years of experience).
7. Consultant.
   a. Functions to provide OT consultation to individuals, groups, or organizations.
   b. Can be an occupational therapist or an OTA at the intermediate or advanced practice level.
   c. The occupational therapist and OTA are responsible for obtaining the appropriate level of supervision to meet regulatory and professional standards.
8. Academic setting fieldwork coordinator.
   a. Functions to manage fieldwork within the OT academic setting.
   b. Can be an occupational therapist or an OTA with a recommended three years of practice experience and experience in supervising fieldwork students.
   c. General supervision by the OT academic program director is recommended.
   d. Close to routine supervision is recommended for new faculty.
9. Faculty.
   a. Functions to provide formal academic education to occupational therapist or OTA students.
   b. Can be an occupational therapist or an OTA with an appropriate advanced professional degree and intermediate to advanced skills in teaching.
   c. General supervision is recommended by academic program director.
   d. Close to routine supervision for new, adjunct, and part-time faculty by program director.
10. Program director (academic setting).
   a. Functions to manage the occupational therapist or OTA education program with an appropriate advanced professional degree, experience as a faculty member, and experience or continuing education in academic management.
   b. General to minimal administrative supervision from designated administrative officer (e.g., Academic Dean).
11. Researcher/scholar.
   a. Functions to perform scholarly work of the profession, i.e., examining, developing, refining, and/or evaluating the profession's theoretical base, philosophical foundations, and body of knowledge.
   b. Can be an occupational therapist or an OTA with additional self study, continuing education, experience, and formal education related to research and scholarly activities.
   c. OTAs can contribute to research process.
   d. Additional academic qualifications are needed for OTAs to be principal investigators.
   e. Supervision needs range from close to minimal depending on skills of researcher/scholar and scope of the project.
12. Entrepreneur.
   a. Functions as a partially or fully self-employed individual who provides OT services.
   b. Can be an occupational therapist or an OTA who meets state regulatory requirements.
   c. OTAs who provide direct service have the responsibility to obtain appropriate supervision from an occupational therapist.

Team Roles and Principles of Collaboration

Overview

1. A team is a group of equally important individuals with common interests collaborating to develop shared goals and build trusting relationships to achieve these shared goals.
2. Members of the team include the patient/client/consumer; his/her family, significant others, and/or caregivers; healthcare professionals; and the reimburser's gatekeepers.
3. Professional members on team will vary according to practice setting.
4. The consumer, family, significant other, and/or caregiver role on the team has become increasingly important. Collaboration with these individuals is even mandated by law (e.g., OBRA, IDEA; see this chapter's section on legislation).

Principles of Collaboration

1. Factors that influence effective team functioning.
   a. Member skill and knowledge.
   b. Membership stability.
   c. Commitment to team goals.
   d. Good communication.
   e. Membership composition.
   f. A common language.
   g. Effective leadership.
2. Recognize that all members of the team are equally important.
   a. No one's opinion or area of competence takes precedence over the other.
      (1) Facility chain of command guidelines will determine who is ultimately responsible for the team's decision.

3. Understand principles of team collaboration and that correct exam answers will adhere to these principles.
4. Know the different types of teams and their respective limits and benefits for team efficacy.
5. Know all potential team members and their respective role responsibilities. NBCOT exam items can ask questions that require an answer that includes a referral to another team member.
6. Recognize that OT practitioners are competent in many domains of concern but our scope of practice does have its limits.
   a. Be prepared to recognize these limits. For example, a parent distraught over his/her child's traumatic brain injury angrily questions the meaning of life and the relevance of his/her faith. A correct answer would include active listening and a referral to pastoral care.

Types of Teams

1. Intradisciplinary.
   a. One or more members of one discipline evaluate, plan, and implement treatment of the individual.
   b. Other disciplines are not involved; communication is limited, thereby limiting perspectives on the case.
   c. This "team" is at risk due to potential narrowness of perspective.
   d. Comprehensive, holistic care can be questionable.
2. Multidisciplinary.
   a. A number of professionals from different disciplines conduct assessments and interventions independent from one another.
   b. Members' primary allegiance is to his/her discipline. Some formal communications occur between team members.
   c. Limited communication may result in lack of understanding of different perspectives.
   d. Resources and responsibilities are individually allocated between disciplines; therefore, competition among team members may develop.
3. Interdisciplinary.
   a. All disciplines relevant to the case at hand agree to collaborate for decision making.
   b. Evaluation and intervention is still conducted independently within defined areas of each profession's expertise. However, there is a greater understanding of each discipline's perspective.
   c. Members are directed toward a common goal and not bound by discipline line-specific roles and functions.
   d. Members tend to use group process skills effectively (e.g., during team treatment planning meetings).
   e. The exchange of information, prioritization of needs and allocation of resources and responsibilities are based on members' expertise and skills, not on "turf" issues.
4. Transdisciplinary.
   a. Characteristics of interdisciplinary teams are maintained and expanded upon.
   b. Members support and enhance the activities and programs of other disciplines to provide quality, efficient, cost-effective service.
   c. Members are committed to ongoing communication, collaboration, and shared decision making for the patient/client's benefit.
   d. Evaluations and interventions are planned cooperatively, yet one member may take on multiple responsibilities. Role blurring is accepted.
   e. Ongoing training, support, supervision, cooperation, and consultation among disciplines are important to this model, ensuring that professional integrity and quality of care is maintained.
5. Team efficacy.
   a. Interdisciplinary and transdisciplinary teams are the most common and considered the most effective in today's health care system.

Lay Team Members and Role Responsibilities

1. Consumer.
   a. The most important and primary member of the treatment team.
   b. The consumer's occupations, values, interests, and goals must be determined and used in all treatment planning.
      (1) If the consumer and the therapist do not share a common language, an interpreter must be used.
2. Family/primary caregiver.
   a. Family's sociocultural background, socioeconomic status, and caregiving tasks, needs, and skills must be considered as they can impact on the outcome of intervention.
      (1) If the family and the therapist do not share a common language, an interpreter must be used.

Para-professional Team Members and Role Responsibilities

1. Personal Care Assistants (PCAs)/Home Health Aides (HHAs).
   a. Individuals who provide primary care to enable a person with a disability to remain in his or her own home.
   b. Most states require some minimum training and certification as a HHA/PCA. Standards and educational requirements can vary greatly from state to state.

c. Responsibilities.
   (1) Personal care such as bathing, grooming, dressing, and feeding.
   (2) Home management such as shopping, cleaning, and cooking.
   (3) Supervision of home programs as directed by a therapist.
d. Due to the tremendous importance this role has in maintaining a person with a disability in his or her own home, OT collaboration with HHAs/PCAs is critical.
e. Occupational therapists can also educate and train consumers on the hiring, training, and supervision of HHAs/PCAs.

Professional Team Members and Role Responsibilities

1. Alternative practitioners.
   a. May include massage therapists, acupuncturists, Reiki practitioners, and others.
   b. Training and licensure requirements vary greatly.
   c. The roles and tasks of alternative practitioners will be determined by state practice regulations and reimburser's guidelines.
2. Athletic trainer.
   a. An allied health professional.
   b. Assesses athletes' risk for injury, conducts injury prevention programs, and provides treatment and rehabilitation under the supervision of a physician when athletic trauma occurs.
3. Audiologist.
   a. A professional who is a graduate of an educational program in audiology.
   b. Administers assessments to determine an individual's auditory acuity, level of hearing impairment, and damage site(s) in the auditory system.
   c. Provides recommendations for assistive devices (e.g., hearing aids) and/or special training to enhance residual hearing and/or adapt to hearing loss.
4. Biomedical engineer.
   a. A graduate of an engineering program who specializes in the biomedical application of engineering theory and technology.
   b. Serves as a technical expert to recommend commercial products, adapt available devices, and/or modify existing environments.
   c. Develops, designs, and fabricates customized equipment, devices, and techniques.
5. Certified orthotist (CO).
   a. Evaluates the need for orthotic equipment (splints, braces).
   b. Designs, fabricates, and fits orthoses for individuals to prevent or correct deformities and/or support body parts weakened by injury, disease, or congenital deformity.
   c. Educates the client on purpose of orthoses, recommended care, and wearing schedule.
   d. May be an occupational therapist, a physical therapist, or an individual with specialized training.
6. Certified prosthetist (CP).
   a. Evaluates the need for a prosthesis.
   b. Designs, fabricates, and fits prosthesis for an individual to ensure proper fit and to promote functional abilities.
   c. Educates client and/or caregiver(s) about the use and care of the prosthesis.
   d. Works directly with occupational therapists, physical therapists, and physicians.
7. Chiropractor (DC).
   a. A professional who is a graduate of an educational program in chiropractic who is usually licensed by state boards.
   b. Assesses the individual's spinal column and intervenes to restore and maintain health and decrease and eliminate pain.
8. Dietician/clinical nutritionist.
   a. A licensed professional who is a graduate of an accredited educational program and who passed a national registration examination.
      (1) Practitioners who pass this registration examination are credentialed as Registered Dietician (RD) or Dietician Technician, Registered (DTR), depending on level of education.
   b. Evaluates individuals' nutritional status and dietary needs.
   c. Provides nutrition therapy for diseases such as diabetes and preventive counseling for issues such as obesity.
9. Expressive/creative arts therapist.
   a. Professionals who are graduates of specialized education programs.
   b. Depending on the state, they may or may not be licensed or registered.
   c. Includes art, dance/movement, music, horticulture, and poetry therapists.
   d. Conducts individual and/or group interventions which use select expressive modalities to facilitate self-expression, self-awareness, social skills, symptom reduction and management.
10. Job coach.
   a. Provides on-site, one-on-one training to employees with disabilities to help them learn to perform their jobs accurately, efficiently, and safely; and acclimate to the work environment.
   b. Performs job analyses at work sites to match people with optimal positions.
   c. Conducts assessments, develops jobs, and provides counseling, travel and mobility training, and other services required to retain employment.
   d. The job coach's degree of involvement with the employee decreases over time as the employee

masters the job with follow-up services provided as needed.

11. Nurse practitioner (NP).
    a. An advanced practice nurse who has completed post-professional graduate education to obtain a Master's or a Doctoral degree in nursing.
    b. NPs are nationally certified in specific areas of specialty (e.g., pediatrics, geriatrics, family practice, acute care).
    c. Depending on a state's scope of practice act, NPs can serve as primary care providers, prescribe medications, and complete referrals for occupational therapy and other rehabilitative services.
    d. Diagnoses, treats, and manages acute and chronic medical conditions.
12. Nurse, registered (RN).
    a. A licensed professional who is a graduate of an accredited nursing education program.
    b. Serves as the primary liaison between the individual and physician.
        (1) Often serves as the primary case manager.
    c. Monitors vital signs, symptoms, and behaviors.
    d. Dispenses medications and assists the physician with the titration of medications.
    e. Performs or supervises bedside care and assists with ADL in collaboration with the occupational therapist.
    f. Conducts group and individual interventions related to wellness and prevention and disease and symptom management (e.g., medication education).
    g. Performs patient, family, and caregiver education to facilitate recovery and maximize quality of life.
    h. Supervises and is assisted by licensed practical nurses (LPNs), certified nursing assistants (CNAs), and aides.
        (1) Due to the major role LPNs, CNAs, and aides have in providing direct care to individuals. OT collaboration with these team members is essential.
13. Optometrist/vision specialist.
    a. A professional who is a graduate of an educational program in optometry.
    b. Examines the eye to determine visual acuity, level of visual impairments, and damage to or disease in the visual system.
    c. Prescribes assistive devices (e.g., corrective lenses) and recommends other appropriate treatment (e.g., visual-motor training).
    d. Optometrists can refer individuals to outpatient OT.
14. Pastoral care.
    a. Serves as the spiritual advisor to the individual, his/her family, caregivers, and the team.
    b. Provides individual, couple, and family counseling in a non-denominational manner.
15. Physiatrist.
    a. A physician who specializes in physical medicine and rehabilitation and is certified by the American Board of Physical Medicine and Rehabilitation.
    b. Leads the rehabilitation team and works directly with occupational, speech, and physical therapists and others to maximize rehabilitation outcome for persons with physical disorders.
    c. Diagnoses and medically treats individuals with musculoskeletal, neurological, cardiovascular, pulmonary, and/or other body systems disorders.
16. Physical therapist (PT).
    a. A licensed professional who is a graduate of an accredited physical therapy education program at a baccalaureate or graduate level.
    b. Evaluates clients' physical motor skills.
    c. Develops plan of care, and administers or supervises treatment to develop, improve and/or maintain client's physical motor skills, to alleviate pain, and to correct or minimize physical deformity.
    d. Delegates portions of treatment program to supportive personnel, e.g., physical therapist assistant (PTA).
    e. Supervises and directs supportive staff (PTA, PT aide) in designated tasks.
    f. Re-evaluates and adjusts plan of care as appropriate.
    g. Performs and documents final evaluation and establishes discharge and follow-up plans.
17. Physical therapist assistant (PTA).
    a. A skilled allied health care technologist, usually with a two year associate's degree.
    b. Must work under the supervision of a physical therapist.
        (1) If the supervisor is off-site, delegated responsibilities must be safe and legal practice with ready access to the supervisor.
        (2) In home health, required periodic joint on-site visits or treatments with physical therapist.
    c. Able to adjust treatment procedure in accordance with the patient's status.
    d. May not evaluate, develop, or change plan of care, or write discharge plan or summary.
18. Physician's assistant (PA).
    a. A professional who is a graduate of an accredited physician's assistant educational program and who has passed a national certification examination.
    b. Performs routine diagnostic, therapeutic, preventative, and health maintenance services.
    c. Specializations can include family medicine, geriatrics, pediatrics, obstetrics, orthopedics, psychiatry, and emergency care.
    d. Must work under the direction of and be supervised by a physician.
19. Primary care physician (PCP).
    a. A physician who serves as the "gatekeeper" of services for consumers in managed health care systems.

b. Provides primary health care services and manages routine medical care.
c. Makes referrals, as needed, to other health care providers and services including specialty tests and examinations, rehabilitation services, and occupational therapy.
d. PCPs can be a doctor of medicine (MD) or a doctor of osteopathy (DO).
(1) DOs undergo a similar education as MDs with the addition of specific training in osteopathic medicine techniques.

20. Psychiatrist.
a. A physician who specializes in mental health and psychiatric rehabilitation.
b. Leads the rehabilitation team and works directly with occupational therapists, psychologists, social workers, and others to maximize rehabilitation outcomes for persons with psychiatric disorders.
c. Diagnoses and medically treats individuals with psychiatric disorders.
d. Responsible for ordering transfers to long term care settings and for determining competence and the need for involuntary treatment.

21. Psychologist.
a. A professional with a Ph.D. in psychology.
b. Evaluates psychological and cognitive status with standardized and non-standardized assessments including intelligence/IQ (Stanford-Binet, Wechsler), Projective (Rorschach), Personality (Minnesota Multiphasic Personality Inventory), Neuropsychological and Interest Inventories (Strong-Campbell).
c. Provides individual, couple, family, and group supportive therapy, cognitive retraining, and behavior modification.

22. Recreational therapist/therapeutic recreation specialist.
a. A professional who is a graduate of a baccalaureate or graduate level recreation therapy education program.
b. Conducts individual and/or group interventions to develop leisure interests and skills; to facilitate community, social, and recreational integration; to manage stress and symptoms; and to adjust to disability.
c. May be called an activities therapist but the two positions are not synonymous. activities therapists may only have on-the-job training.

23. Respiratory therapy technician certified (CRT).
a. A technically trained professional with an Associate's Degree who has passed a national certification examination.
b. Administers respiratory therapy as prescribed and supervised by a physician.
c. Performs pulmonary function tests and intervenes through oxygen delivery, aerosols, and nebulizers.

24. Social worker.
a. A licensed/registered professional who is a graduate of an accredited educational social work program at a baccalaureate level (BSW) or at a graduate level (MSW).
b. Upon passing a national certification examination, a social worker is eligible to use the credentials Certified Social Worker (CSW).
(1) In states with licensure requirements, a social worker may have the credential of licensed clinical social worker (LCSW).
c. Assesses client's social history and psychosocial functioning via clinical interviews and structured assessments.
d. Assists clients, families and caregivers with accessing social support services (e.g., home care, support groups) and obtaining needed reimbursement/funding (e.g., Medicaid, food stamps) through the completion of required application processes and through active advocacy.
e. Provides individual, couple, and family counseling.
f. Serves as a primary care manager, enabling individual to function optimally and maintain quality of life.
g. Provides crisis intervention and recommendations for additional services.
h. Contributes to discharge plan and completes tasks needed for implementation of discharge orders (e.g., application to a SNF).
i. Supervises and is assisted by social work assistants.

25. Special educator/teacher.
a. A professional teacher certified to provide education to children with special needs.
(1) Visual and/or hearing impairments.
(2) Emotional and psychosocial disabilities.
(3) Physical and sensorimotor disabilities.
(4) Developmental disabilities.
(5) Learning and cognitive disabilities.
b. Assesses and monitors student learning, plans and implements instructional activities, and addresses the special developmental and educational needs of each student.
c. Advanced training in instructional methods for teaching children with special needs to develop to their fullest educational potential is required.
d. Additional training in teaching children with multiple disabilities is often needed.
e. May be assisted by teacher aides who provide direct care and "hands-on" support to students in the classroom.
(1) Collaboration with aides is required for effective follow-through of OT programming in school settings.

26. Speech-language pathologist (SLP), or speech therapist (ST).
    a. A professional who is a graduate of an accredited educational program in speech-language pathology.
    b. Assesses language and speech abilities and impairments.
    c. Develops and conducts intervention programs to restore, improve, or augment the communication of persons with speech and/or language impairments.
    d. May receive advanced training and specialize in oral-motor functioning (e.g., the evaluation and treatment of dysphagia).
27. Substance abuse counselor.
    a. A professional who may come from a diversity of educational backgrounds (psychology, social work, occupational therapy) who has completed a specialized training program.
    b. Provides individual and/or group intervention.
    c. Certified Alcohol Counselor (CAC) and Certified Alcohol and Drug Counselor (CADC) are the two main credentials designating this specialized role.
28. Vocational rehabilitation counselor.
    a. A professional who is a graduate of an educational program in vocational rehabilitation.
    b. If certified, the counselor is able to use the credential of Certified Rehabilitation Counselor (CRC).
    c. Evaluates prevocational skills and vocational interests and abilities via standardized and nonstandardized assessments to determine an individual's employability.
    d. Provides counseling to maximize the individual's vocational potential.
    e. Refers individual to appropriate vocational programming and/or job placement.
    f. Serves as liaison between the individual and state educational and vocational departments for persons with disabilities to obtain funding for needed services.

The United States Health Care System

Overview

1. A group of decentralized subsystems serving different populations.
2. Health care in the United States is overwhelmingly insured and delivered by privately owned companies.
3. The Patient Protection and Affordable Care Act (ACA), signed into law in 2010 with implementation to continue into 2016, seeks to expand access to health insurance for all Americans and improve the quality of health care provided in the United States. Key components of the ACA are:
    a. Accountable Care Organizations (ACOs) provide financial incentives for health care providers who develop an integrated network to collaborate when treating patients across care settings and care episodes.
        (1) The aim is to lower health care costs while meeting quality performance standards.
    b. Patient-Centered Medical Homes (PCMHs or medical homes) are places of care designed to meet patients' complete needs for mental and physical health via preventative, acute care, and disability/chronic illness management services.
4. Relatively small federal and state governmental programs work in conjunction with a large private sector; however, the government pays for a large portion of these private sector services through Medicare and Medicaid reimbursement.
    a. ACA has provided states with the ability to expand Medicaid services; however, several states have opted out.
5. Decentralization results in overlap in some areas and competition in others; therefore, health care is primarily a business that is market-driven.
    a. Patients and clients are viewed as consumers due to this economic focus.
    b. Cost containment while maintaining quality of service is a delicate balancing act that is not always achieved.

Health Care Regulations

1. Health care is a highly regulated industry with most established practices mandated by federal and state laws.
    a. Due to the great variance in state laws, the NBCOT exam will only test knowledge of federal regulations.
2. The Center for Medicare and Medicaid Services (CMS), a division of U.S. Department of Health and Human Services (HHS) is the federal agency which develops rules and regulations pertaining to federal laws governing the Medicare and Medicaid programs.
    a. Facilities that participate in Medicare and/or Medicaid programs are monitored regularly for compliance with CMS guidelines by federal and state surveyors.

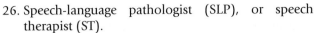

b. Facilities that repeatedly fail to meet CMS guidelines lose their Medicare and/or Medicaid certification(s).
c. Long-term settings, i.e., skilled nursing facilities (SNFs), are strongly influenced by CMS regulations since Medicare and/or Medicaid pays for all or most of the expense of long-term care.
d. CMS is divided into several centers.
   (1) The Center for Beneficiary Choices: focuses on Medicare Choice and Medigap.
   (2) The Center for Medicare Management: focuses on traditional fee-for-service Medicare.
   (3) The Center for Medicaid and State Operations: focuses on state administered programs like Medicaid and State Children's Health Insurance Program (SCHIP).
   (4) Center for Program Integrity: provides oversight of Medicare and Medicaid programs to ensure their integrity and coordinate resources and best practices to improve programs.
   (5) Center for Medicare and Medicaid Innovation: established by the ACA, this center develops and tests new service delivery and payment models for maintaining or improving the quality of care in CMS managed programs (i.e., Medicare, Medicaid and CHIP), while controlling program costs.

3. Standards related to safety are set forth and enforced by the Occupational Safety and Health Administration (OSHA), a division of the U.S. Department of Labor.
   a. Structural standards and building codes are established and enforced by OSHA to ensure the safety of structures.
   b. The safety of employees and consumers is regulated by OSHA standards for handling infectious materials and blood products, controlling blood borne pathogens, operating machinery, and handling hazardous substances.
4. State accreditation to obtain licensure for a health care facility is mandatory. Individual states develop their own requirements, with state agencies enforcing these regulations.
5. Local or county entities also develop regulations pertaining to health care institutions (e.g., physical plant safety features such as fire, elevator, and boiler regulations).

Voluntary Accreditation

1. Voluntary accreditation and self-imposed compliance with established standards is sought by most health care organizations, e.g., hospitals, skilled nursing facilities (SNFs), home health agencies, preferred provider organizations (PPOs), rehabilitation centers, health maintenance organizations (HMOs), behavioral health (including mental health and chemical dependency) facilities, physicians' networks, hospice care, long term care facilities, and others.
2. Accreditation is a status awarded for compliance with established standards.
3. Accreditation ensures the public that a health care facility is adequately equipped and meets high standards for patient care, and employs qualified professionals and competent staff.
4. Accreditation affirms the competence of practitioners and the quality of health care facilities and organizations.
5. Accreditation through an accrediting agency is voluntary; however, it is mandatory to receive third party reimbursement and to be eligible for federal government grants and contracts.
6. CMS and many states accept certain national accreditations as meeting their respective requirements for participation in the Medicare and Medicaid programs and for a license to operate.
7. Voluntary accrediting agencies include the Joint Commission (JCAHO), Commission on Accreditation of Rehabilitation Facilities (CARF), and the Accreditation Council for Services for Mentally Retarded and Other Developmentally Disabled Persons (AC-MRDD) and others.

The Accreditation Process

1. Accreditation is initiated by the organization submitting an application for review or survey by the accrediting agency.
2. A self-study or self-assessment is conducted to examine the organization based on the accrediting agency's standards.
3. An on-site review is conducted by an individual reviewer or surveyor or a team visiting the organization.
4. The accreditation and the re-accreditation process involve all staff. Tasks include document preparation, hosting the site visit team, and interviews with accreditors.
5. Once accredited, the organization undergoes periodic review, typically every three years.

Value of Accreditation to Occupational Therapy

1. Self-study and self-assessment can be an opportunity to identify areas of strength, validate competence, and promote excellence.

2. Areas needing improvement can be identified (i.e., procedures can be streamlined and additional resources can be obtained, team communication can be enhanced).
3. Program goals are clarified.
4. Practice is defined and documented.
5. Accreditors can share information regarding best practices.
6. An increased recognition of OT's contributions to the agency and identification of functional outcomes can result in increased visibility for OT and increased referrals.

Payment for Occupational Therapy Services

Key Terms

1. Beneficiary: a person receiving services. In skilled nursing facilities (SNFs), the term "resident" is used.
2. Capitation.
   a. Payment system under which the provider is paid prospectively (i.e., on a monthly basis) a set fee for each member of a specific population (i.e., health plan members) regardless if no covered health care is delivered or if extensive care is delivered.
   b. Payment is typically determined in terms of "per member per month" (PMPM).
   c. The healthier the enrollees (and the fewer services used), the more the provider retains of the total PMPM payment.
3. Co-insurance: the monetary amount to be paid by a patient, usually expressed as a percentage of total charge.
4. Clinical/critical pathway: a standardized recommended intervention protocol for a specific diagnosis.
5. Deductible: the amount a patient must pay to a provider before the insurance benefits will pay; usually expressed as an annual dollar amount.
6. Denial: the refusal by a payer to reimburse a provider for services rendered. Reasons for denial include benefits exhausted, duplication of services, and services not indicated.
7. Diagnosis code: a code that describes a patient's medical reason or condition that requires health service.
8. Diagnostic related groups (DRGs): the descriptive categories established by CMS that determine the level of payment at a per case rate.
9. Fee for service: the payment system under which the provider is paid the same type of rate per unit of service. Traditionally, payer pays 80% and patient or provider is responsible for the remaining 20%.
10. Health insurance marketplace: established by the ACA to allow consumers to compare the cost of insurance plans in their area.
    a. Also know as health care exchanges.
11. Health maintenance organization (HMO): the most common form of managed care. Maintains control over services by requiring enrollees to see only doctors within the HMO network and to obtain referrals before seeking specialty or ancillary care.
12. Managed care: a method of maintaining some control over costs and utilization of services while providing quality health care. Managed care organizations (MCOs) include HMOs and PPOs.
13. Per diem: a negotiated, per day fee for service. Typically used for inpatient hospital stays and skilled nursing facilities.
14. Preferred provider organization (PPO): a form of managed care that is similar to an HMO but usually offers a greater choice of providers. However, as choices increase, percentage of payment decreases.
15. Private payment: the individual receiving services is responsible for payment.
16. Procedure codes: codes that describe specific services performed by health professionals.
17. Prospective payment system (PPS): the nationwide payment schedule that determines the Medicare payment for each inpatient stay of a Medicare beneficiary based on DRGs.
18. Provider: the entity responsible for the delivery and quality of services. Providers bill Medicare, HMOs and PPOs for services rendered.
19. Third party payers: agencies and companies who are the primary reimbursers for health care in the U.S. (e.g. Blue Cross). HMOs and PPOs are also third party payers.
20. Treatment authorization request (TAR): The Medicaid form a primary care provider must complete to document the need for requested medically necessary covered services and their supporting rationale.
21. Usual and customary rate (UCR): the average cost of specific health care procedures in a geographic area. This is the maximum amount the insurer will pay for a service and covered expense.
22. Vendor/supplier: the entity which supplies services.

Private Insurance and Managed Care Plans

1. Largest source of insurance payment in the United States.
   a. These plans can be managed by for profit or not for profit companies, organizations, and/or networks.
   b. There are broad variations among plans and plan options.
      (1) The ACA has mandated the establishment of insurance "exchanges" (also called a marketplace) to allow people to comparision shop on line for health insurance plans offered by different companies.
2. Many private insurers contract with Medicare to handle the day to day operations of Medicare. They are called intermediaries.
3. Insurers (e.g., Blue Cross/Blue Shield, Aetna, MetLife, and Prudential), offer many insurance products including PPOs, HMOs, and MCOs.
4. Coverage cannot be assumed based on the name of plan alone.
   a. Co-insurance, deductibles, and co-payments are common.
   b. Most plans cover for OT in hospitals.
   c. Outpatient coverage varies greatly.
   d. Total number of visits and/or type and amount of services per diagnosis are limited.
5. Historically, private insurers have not been federally regulated.
6. Under the ACA, federal regulations have been established for private insurance coverage. Key ones include:
   a. Insurers must provide essential benefits to participants in their plans; these include mental health, substance abuse, and behavioral health treatment; rehabilitative, habilitative, and chronic disease management services and devices; and preventative and wellness services.
   b. Insurers can no longer refuse coverage to persons with pre-existing conditions.
   c. Insurers cannot raise insurance premiums based on a person's occupation, gender, pre-existing condition, health status, or claim history,
   d. Insurers must allow young adults until their 26th birthday to be covered under their parents' plans, if these plans cover dependents.
   e. Insurers cannot set caps on annual and lifetime coverage.
7. States can set their own requirements and regulations for insurers who operate within their borders.
   a. As a national examination, the NBCOT examination will not test state-specific requirements or regulations.
8. Cost controlling payment strategies such as case management, precertification or preauthorization, mandatory second opinions, and preferred provider networks are often implemented.
9. Occupational therapists can join health care provider panels and/or a preferred provider network.
10. Due to the great variability in private insurance coverage, the NBCOT examination will not ask specific questions about private insurance.
    a. However, knowledge of industry trends such as those identified above will be helpful in answering management questions.

Medicare

1. General information.
   a. Largest single payer for OT services.
   b. Administered by CMS.
   c. Intermediaries determine if services provided are within Medicare guidelines.
   d. Persons eligible for Medicare medical coverage for health care services.
      (1) Persons 65 years or older.
      (2) Individuals of all ages with end stage renal disease/permanent kidney failure that may require dialysis treatment or a kidney transplant.
      (3) Persons with a long-term disability (e.g., ALS, MS) who have received government-funded disability benefits for 24 months may be eligible.
      (4) Retired railroad workers.
2. Part A: pays for inpatient hospital, skilled nursing facility (SNF), home health, rehabilitation facilities, and hospice care.
   a. Part A is automatically provided to all who are covered by the Social Security System that meet the above coverage criteria.
   b. Services provided in acute care hospitals receive a prospective, predetermined rate based on DRGs (Diagnostic Related Groups).
      (1) The DRG per case rate covers all services including OT.
      (2) It is a fixed dollar amount for patient care for each diagnosis regardless of length of stay (LOS) or number of services provided.
      (3) Treatment supplies (i.e., adaptive equipment, splints) are included in this per case rate.
      (4) Individual hospitals determine the combination of services a patient will receive.
   c. Part A covered services have specific time limits and also require deductible and coinsurance payments by the beneficiary.
      (1) Annual deductible fees must be paid by patient.
      (2) Twenty percent of home health care must be paid by patient.

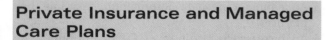

3. Part B: pays for hospital outpatient physician and other professional services including OT services provided by independent practitioners.
   a. Part B is considered a Supplemental Medical Insurance Program and therefore must be purchased by the beneficiary, usually as a monthly premium.
   b. Part B services have no specific time limit and require 20% co-payment.
4. Criteria for coverage of occupational therapy services.
   a. Prescribed by a physician or furnished according to a physician-approved plan of care.
   b. Performed by a qualified occupational therapist or an OTA under the general supervision of an occupational therapist.
   c. Service is reasonable and necessary for treatment of individual's injury or illness.
   d. Diagnosis can be physical, psychiatric, or both. There are no diagnostic restrictions for coverage.
   e. OT must result in a significant, practical improvement in the person's level of functioning within a reasonable period of time.
5. The primary difference between Part A and Part B is the frequency in which the individual receives services. Inpatient Part A coverage requires services for a minimum of 5 days per week services. Part B typically covers 3 days per week outpatient services.
6. Medicare does not cover most chronic illnesses, long term supportive care, or all medical expenses incurred when ill.
7. OT in SNFs is covered if the patient requires skilled nursing or skilled rehabilitation (i.e., OT, PT, ST) on a daily basis (i.e., minimum 5 days/week).
   a. Reimbursement is based upon resource utilization groups (RUGs).
   b. Reimbursement is also provided for the designing of a maintenance plan and for the occasional reevaluation of this plan's effectiveness.
   c. Reimbursement is typically not provided for a therapist to carry out the maintenance plan.
   d. Evaluation and training of caregivers is considered part of the design and reevaluation of a maintenance plan.
   e. The competence of caregivers to carry out the maintenance plan must be documented prior to discharge from OT.
   f. In 2013, existing Medicare policy about reimburseable skilled services was clarified.
      (1) The restorative potential of a person was determined to *not* be the sole payment criteria for skilled services.
      (2) Services to prevent or slow deterioration and maintain a person at the highest functional level possible must be recognized as skilled and covered if these services are reasonable and neccessary.
         (a) If these services can be performed safely and effectively by unskilled personnel, coverage for skilled service is not mandated.
8. OT in home care is covered if the individual is homebound and needed intermittent skilled nursing care, PT, or ST before OT began. OT services can continue after need for skilled nursing, PT, or ST has ended.
   a. Homebound status criteria.
      (1) The person is typically not able to leave the home; i.e., is "confined" to the home.
         (a) "Confinement" may be due to the need for the aid of ambulatory devices, the assistance of others, or special transportation.
         (b) It considers medical, physical, cognitive, and psychiatric conditions.
      (2) If the person leaves the home it requires "considerable and taxing effort" (CMS 2010).
      (3) A person may leave his/her home for medical appointments (e.g., kidney dialysis) and non-medical short-term and infrequent appointments/events (e.g., a trip to a hairdresser, attendance at religious services).
      (4) The need for adult day care does not preclude a person from receiving home health services.
   b. Home health agencies (HHAs) are reimbursed under a prospective payment system (PPS).
      (1) This rate per episode of care reimbursement system applies to all home health services including all forms of therapy and medical supplies.
      (2) Durable medical equipment is excluded from HHA PPS.
      (3) The HHA PPS uses a classification system called Home Health Resource Groups (HHRGs) to determine an episode payment rate.
      (4) An episode is defined as a 60-day period beginning with the first billable visit and ending 60 days after the start of care.
   c. An initial assessment visit and a comprehensive assessment using the Outcome and Assessment Information Set (OASIS) must be completed to verify the person's eligibility for Medicare home health benefits, the continuing need for home care, and to plan for the person's nursing, medical, social, rehabilitative, and discharge needs.
      (1) Occupational therapists can complete the initial OASIS if the need for OT establishes program eligibility.
      (2) The initial assessment must be completed within 48 hours of referral or within 48 hours of the person's return home.
      (3) Occupational therapists can conduct follow-up, transfer, and discharge evaluations.

   d. AOTA is actively working to change federal legislation to have OT identified as an initial qualifying service for home health care, so barriers to OT home health services my be removed in the future.
9. OT in hospice care is provided to persons who are certified as terminally ill (medical prognosis of fewer than 6 months to live).
   a. OT services are provided to enable a patient to maintain functional skills and ADL performance and/or to control symptoms.
10. OT is covered as an outpatient service when provided by or under arrangements with any Medicare Certified provider (i.e., hospital, SNF, home health agency, rehabilitation agency, a clinic) or when provided as part of comprehensive rehabilitation facility services (CORF).
11. OT services can also be covered if provided by a Medicare certified occupational therapist in independent practice (OTIP) when services are provided in the therapist's office or in the patient's home.
   a. Payment is according to the fee schedule entitled the Resource Based Relative Value Scale (RBRVS).
12. Criteria for coverage of OT services rendered in a physician's office or in a physician-directed clinic.
   a. The occupational therapist or OTA is employed by the physician or clinic.
   b. The service is furnished under physician's direct supervision and the services are directly related to the condition for which the physician is treating the patient.
   c. OT service fees are included on the physician's bill to Medicare.
13. Criteria for coverage of partial hospitalization (PHP) services in a hospital-affiliated or community mental health psychiatric day program.
   a. The beneficiary would otherwise have required inpatient psychiatric care.
   b. OT services are covered under general Medicare guidelines (i.e., MD's prescription, reasonable and necessary, function expected to improve).
   c. Active treatment incorporating an individualized multi-disciplinary intervention plan to attain measureable, time-limited, medically necessary, functional goals directly related to the reason for admission must be provided.
      (1) Psychosocial programs that provide structured diversional, social, and or recreational, services or vocational rehabilitation do not meet the criteria for active treatment in a PHP and are not reimbursable under Medicare.
14. All of the above standards can change when and if new federal legislative guidelines are passed for Medicare.

Medicare Coverage of Durable Medical Equipment, Prostheses, and Orthoses

1. Rental or purchase expenses for durable medical equipment (DME) are covered if used in beneficiary's home and if necessary and reasonable to treat an illness or injury or to improve functioning.
2. A physician's prescription is needed and must include diagnosis, prognosis, and reason for DME need.
3. Criteria for durable medical equipment.
   a. Repeated use can be withstood.
   b. Primarily and customarily used for a medical purpose (e.g., a wheelchair or walker).
   c. Generally not useful to a person in the absence of injury or illness.
4. Self-help items, bathtub grab bars, and raised toilet seats are not reimbursable because other people can use them and they are not considered medically necessary.

Medicaid

1. General information.
   a. A state/federal health insurance program for persons who have an income that is below an established threshold and/or have a disability.
   b. States administer the program but receive at least 50% of their funding from the federal government.
      (1) Under the ACA, states are receiving increased federal contributions to expand their Medicaid programs.
   c. Includes federally mandated services and state optional services.
   d. Mandated services must be provided if a state receives federal funds.
   e. Coverage of optional services varies greatly from state to state.
      (1) As a result, questions about state specific Medicaid coverage cannot be on the NBCOT examination.
2. Mandated Medicaid services (pre-ACA).
   a. Inpatient and hospital services.
   b. Outpatient (e.g., laboratory work, x-rays, skilled nursing) and physicians' services.
   c. Home health (level and amount of care can vary).

d. Early periodic screening diagnosis, and treatment services (EPSDT) for persons 21 years old and younger.
e. Services identified as needed to treat a condition during EPSDT (including OT) must be provided.
f. SNFs receiving Medicaid must provide skilled rehabilitation services (including OT) to residents who require them.

3. Optional Medicaid services (pre-ACA).
   a. Occupational therapy, physical therapy, speech language therapy.
   b. Durable medical equipment.
   c. Services provided by independently practicing licensed professionals including psychologists, psychiatric social workers, and other mental health professionals.
   d. Targeted case management.
   e. Prescription medication.
   f. Dental care, eyeglasses.
   g. Crisis response services.
   h. Transportation.
   i. Psychiatric inpatient services for persons aged under 21 or over 65.
   j. Related services (including OT) provided by school systems to children with disabilities. (Note: This provision overlaps IDEA legislation and has led to questioning as to whether services to individual children should be funded as an educational or a health care service).
4. Under the ACA, Medicaid must provide the same minimum essential benefits that are provided in the insurance exchanges established by the ACA.
   a. States are not required to expand their Medicaid programs and they have varied in their response to the ACA; thus, questions about state specific Medicaid coverage cannot be on the NBCOT examination.
   b. See prior information on the ACA.
5. Medicaid reform.
   a. Due to rapidly rising costs there is an increased press for cost containment.
   b. States are examining ways to reformulate Medicaid benefits.
   c. Reform options may include placing caps or other limitations on types and length of therapy, reducing or eliminating optional benefits, and/or developing and implementing managed care approaches.
   d. Individual states can apply to the federal government for a waiver which gives the state flexibility in the types of services and delivery systems they provide under Medicaid.

Workers' Compensation

1. Designed to compensate employees who have job-related illness or injuries.
2. Funded jointly by individual employers or groups of employers and state governments.
3. Each state has a workers' compensation commission board which determines regulations for employer participation, benefit provision, employee coverage, and insurance administration.
4. Administration can be through contract with private insurance companies or through individual employers or groups of employers who administer their own programs. This is known as self-insuring.
5. Coverage varies from state to state, with many states initiating cost-containment measures including limits on choice of providers, use of set fee schedules, utilization review, and managed care.
6. Workers compensation programs include cash benefits and medical benefits. OT services may be included.
7. Rehabilitation and disability management to return the person to gainful employment is a primary focus.

Personal Payment and "Pro Bono" Care

1. Individuals whose health insurance has discontinued coverage of OT services may elect to pay for these services personally, providing that benefit can be derived from continued services.
2. Individuals without health insurance or with no coverage for rehabilitative services may also pay for OT personally.
3. The services of occupational therapists practicing in non-medical settings, (e.g., wellness and prevention programs) are generally not covered by insurers so their clients must private pay.
4. "Pro Bono" or free or reduced rate care may be supported by the individual therapist's personal donation of services or through philanthropic donations.

Documentation for Reimbursement

1. Refer to the following section for guidelines on documenting effectively in order to receive payment for services.

Occupational Therapy Documentation Guidelines

Purpose of Documentation

1. Provides a legal, serial record of client's condition, evaluation, and re-evaluation results, course of therapeutic intervention and response to intervention from referral to discharge.
2. Serves as an information resource for client care, can be used by a covering therapist in absence of primary therapist.
3. Enhances communication among health care or educational team members.
4. Provides data for use in intervention, program evaluation, research, education, and reimbursement.
5. Electronic medical records (EMRs)/electronic health records (EHRs) provide digital versions of paper charts.

General Documentation Standards

1. Legible handwriting must be used for handwritten documentation.
   a. Illegible notes can result in miscommunication.
2. Documentation for an electronic medical record (EMR)/electronic health record (EHR) must adhere to all established documentation standards.
3. Correct grammar and spelling is required.
   a. Errors detract from a professional presentation.
4. Concise but complete information should be recorded.
   a. If it is not recorded, it does not exist and never happened.
   b. Non-important, extraneous details (i.e., color of clothing) should be left out.
5. Objective statements, with clear distinctions between facts and behavioral data and opinions and interpretations, are required.
6. All documentation must be current and accurate.
7. Institution and/or program guidelines, as well as reimbursers'/third party payers' guidelines must be followed.
   a. Non-compliance can result in services and/or payment being denied.
8. Standard, well recognized, abbreviations (i.e., ROM, MMT) should be the only ones used.
   a. Avoid alphabet soup.
   b. Write in functional terms using uniform terminology consistent with AOTA's Standards of Practice and state practice acts.
9. Person first language should be used at all times (e.g., "a parent with schizophrenia," or "the student with an intellectual disability," not "the schizophrenic," "the retarded").
10. Client's name and ID number should be on every page.
11. The blocking out or deletion of information is unacceptable.
    a. In handwritten notes, errors must be crossed out with one line, initialed, and dated. Black or blue ink is used at all times.
12. The complete date (i.e., day, month, and year) must be provided.
13. The type of documentation (i.e., initial note, progress note, discharge plan) should be identified.
14. Compliance with confidentiality standards is mandated (i.e., do not put other clients' names in a note).
15. Informed consent for treatment can only be given by a competent adult.
    a. Minors or adults determined to be incompetent must have written consent provided by a parent, legal guardian, person with power of attorney, or proxy.
16. A full signature (first and last name with professional designations) should directly following documentation content with no space left between the content and signature.
17. Countersignature by an occupational therapist on documentation written by an OTA or a student if required by law or the facility.
18. Occupational therapy notes and records are legal documents; thus, all documentation may be subject to subpoena.
    a. Adherence to documentation standards is a must.

OTA Documentation Guidelines

1. OTAs are qualified to write notes in medical charts and other documentation formats.
2. OTA notes are not required to be cosigned by an occupational therapist by the AOTA, but state and federal governments may mandate cosigning as a tangible way to demonstrate compliance with OTA supervisory laws and regulations.
3. AOTA recommends OTA notes which will be included in medical charts, Individualized Education Plans (IEPs), and other legal documents be cosigned by an occupational therapist.
   a. As official documents, these records may be subject to subpoena.

Content of Documentation

1. Identification and background information.
   a. Name, age, gender, date of admission, treatment diagnosis, and case number if one exists.
   b. Referral source, reason for referral, chief complaint relevant to OT's domain of concern.
   c. Pertinent history that indicates prior levels of function and support systems, including applicable developmental, educational, vocational, socioeconomic, and medical history. This can be brief.
   d. Secondary problems or preexisting conditions that may affect function or treatment outcomes.
   e. Precautions, risk factors and contraindications, medications, surgery dates.
2. Evaluation and reevaluation documentation.
   a. Assessments administered and the results.
   b. Summary and analysis of assessment findings in measurable, functional terms.
      (1) Sufficient baseline objective data.
      (2) In reevaluation, compare findings to initial findings.
      (3) Indicate change, if any.
   c. References to other pertinent reports and information including relevant psychological, social, and environmental data.
   d. Occupational therapy problem list, specific and sufficient to develop intervention plan.
   e. Recommendations for occupational therapy services (can include recommendation that no OT services are indicated).
   f. Client's understanding of current status and problems, his or her subjective complaints.
   g. Client's interest and desire to participate in therapy.
3. Intervention plan documentation.
   a. A prioritized problem list.
   b. Goals related to problem list and indicating potential for function and improvement.
   c. The structure of a goal statement.
      (1) The person who will exhibit the skill, almost always written as "the patient/client will." However, the caregiver, family member, and/or teacher may be the focus of the goal.
      (2) The desired functional behavior that is to be demonstrated or increased as the outcome of intervention.
      (3) The underlying factors (e.g., performance component deficits) that must be remediated to achieve functional outcome.
      (4) The circumstances under which the behavior must be performed or the conditions necessary for the behavior (e.g., independent, with cueing, with assistance).
      (5) The degree at which the behavior is exhibited (e.g., 3 out of 4 times, minimum number of repetitions).
   d. Short and long term goals written in a SMART manner.
      (1) Specific. For example, not "increase self-care skills"; rather, "develop ability to button shirt using non-dominant hand."
      (2) Measurable, as to number of times or a percent.
      (3) Attainable, as to what can be realistically achieved. For example, one hundred percent return is unlikely.
      (4) Relevant, to roles and expected environment.
      (5) Time-limited, anticipated time to achieve goals.
         (a) Time allotted for goal attainment must be relevant to setting's LOS (e.g., in acute care, goals are measured in days whereas in long term care, weekly or monthly goals are acceptable).
      (6) The acronym RUMBA is similarly used to guide documentation (R = realistic/relevant, U = understandable, M = Measureable, B = behavioral, A = attainable/achievable).
   e. Long term goals must indicate the final desired functional outcome before discharge, regardless of LOS.
      (1) A clear reason for skilled therapeutic intervention.
      (2) Statement of potential functional outcome that is clearly related to goal.
   f. Activities and/or treatment procedures and methods related to stated goals and problems.
   g. Type, amount, frequency of treatment needed to accomplish goals (how many times/week/day? how long are sessions?).
   h. Explanation of treatment plan to client and a provision of statement of goals in client's words.
4. Intervention implementation documentation.
   a. Activities, procedures, and modalities used.
   b. Client's response to treatment and the progress toward goal attainment as related to problem list.
   c. Goal modification when indicated by the response to treatment. Rationale for changes in goals needed.
   d. Change in anticipated time to achieve goals with rationale for change and new time frame specified.
   e. Attendance and participation with treatment plan (attendance can be a check format).
   f. Statement of reason for individual missing treatment.
   g. Assistive/adaptive equipment, orthoses, and prostheses if issued or fabricated, and specific instructions for the application and/or use of the item, including wearing schedule and care.
   h. Patient-related conferences and communication with physicians, third party payers, case manager, team members, etc.
   i. Home programs developed and taught to client and/or caregiver(s).
   j. Client's and/or caregiver's compliance with home program.
5. Discharge plan documentation.
   a. Summary of evaluation and intervention.
   b. Compare initial and discharge status.

c. Specify number of sessions, goals achieved, and functional outcome.
d. Reason for discharge.
(1) Goals attained.
(2) Client no longer making functional gains.
(3) Client refuses or is noncompliant with intervention.
(4) Client moves to another location.
(5) Setting not appropriate to individual's needs.
e. Home programs to be followed after discharge.
f. Client and family education.
g. Equipment provided and/or ordered.
h. Follow-up plans/recommendations with rationales.
i. Referral(s) to other health care providers and community agencies.

Specific Documentation Formats

1. Problem Oriented Medical Record (POMR): a system of providing structure for progress note writing that is based on a list of problems based on assessment.
a. SOAP notes.
(1) Subjective: information reported by the client, family, or significant other.
(2) Objective: diagnosis, medical information and history, and measurable, observable data obtained through formal assessments.
(3) Assessment: therapist's interpretation and clinical reasoning based on objective data includes analysis of client's status and goals and a prioritized problem list.
(4) Plan: the therapist's specific plan of intervention to resolve identified problems and meet stated goals.
2. Consultation reports: meetings and/or phone conversations with team members, other professionals, the individual, and his/her caregivers.
3. Critical incident reports: significant, out of the norm events that may occur during OT evaluation or intervention (e.g., the individual slips during a transfer).
4. All of the above must comply with general documentation standards and contain all fundamental components of documentation.

Documentation for Reimbursement

1. Coding and billing for services.
a. To be reimbursed, OT services must be properly coded and billed, as required by reimbursers.
b. Practitioners must represent their services in terms of diagnosis and procedure codes.
c. Diagnosis codes describe person's condition or medical reason for requiring services.
(1) The International Classification of Diseases, 9th Revision, Clinical Modification (ICD-9-CM) is the most frequently used diagnosis-coding system in the United States.
(2) ICD-9-CM is updated annually so all billing documentation must use current version. Due to these annual updates, the NBCOT examination would not include specific codes.
(3) Each service, procedure, supply, or piece of equipment must be related to the ICD-9-CM code.
d. Procedure codes describe the specific services provided by health care professionals.
(1) HCFA Common Procedure Coding System (HCPCS) is most widely used.
(2) HCPCS includes the Physician's Current Procedural Terminology (CPT).
(3) The most current HCPCS and CPT codes must be used as they are updated annually. Due to these annual updates, the NBCOT examination would not include specific codes.
(4) Specific codes that most closely describe the service(s) provided should be used. Each procedure, modality, and/or treatment should be coded.
e. Specific billing forms are used by institutional providers (i.e., hospitals and home health agencies) and by physicians and occupational therapists in independent practice for Medicare, Medicaid, and most states' workers' compensation programs. Form numbers may change, so NBCOT should not ask questions about specific forms.
f. Effective July 1, 2013, outpatient occupational therapy services provided under Medicare Part B must report functional data on their claims in the form of new G-codes.
(1) G-codes identify the primary issue being addressed by therapy; modifiers are used to report the person's impairment/limitation/restriction.
(a) All G-codes are available to be used by all therapy disciplines (i.e., OT practitioners can use the codes for mobility, memory, swallowing, and cognition).
(2) G-codes will be used to track patient outcomes over time.
g. OTAs are generally not eligible for direct payment because they require supervision and do not perform evaluations.
2. Documentation "red flags."
a. The use of certain words, terms, and/or physician's errors can result in delay, denial, and/or discharge from services.

b. Avoid these in all documentation, unless they are true and accurate representations of a client's status.
c. If a client has met his/her goals and/or is no longer making significant functional gains, this must be documented and the client may need to be discharged from services.
   (1) Under Medicare, services can continue to be provided if they are needed to prevent deterioration and enable the person to function at their maximal potential.
d. Words to carefully consider, for they do not reflect progress.
   (1) Chronic.
   (2) Status quo, no change in status.
   (3) Maintaining.
   (4) Little change.
   (5) Plateau.
   (6) Making slow progress.
   (7) Stable or stabilizing.
e. Words to carefully consider, for they do not reflect potential for improvement.
   (1) Same as.
   (2) Uncooperative, noncompliant.
   (3) Dislikes therapy.
   (4) Confused/disoriented.
   (5) Inability to follow directions.
   (6) Patient refused to participate.
   (7) Custodial care needed.
   (8) Treatment repeated.
   (9) Repeated instruction.
   (10) Unmotivated.
   (11) Extreme depression.
   (12) Fair to poor potential.
   (13) Chronic/long-term condition.
   (14) General weakness.
f. Errors in physician's orders, for they can result in denial or delay of payment for OT services.
   (1) Incomplete or non-specific orders.
   (2) Orders with a span of frequency over the duration of intervention (e.g., 2–3 times/week for 4–6 weeks).
   (3) Orders that do not state a specific type of intervention (e.g., activities, splint or equipment, as needed).
   (4) Orders that cover only evaluation but intervention has been initiated.
   (5) Order is specific to a certain type of treatment, but the treatment plan does not include it.
   (6) Order does not include duration of treatment.
   (7) The plan changes mid-month but the order is not updated to meet the new plan change.
   (8) There is no discharge order or there is no order immediately after treatment ends.

Documentation for Medicare Reimbursement

1. Overview.
   a. Many private reimbursers and state Medicaid programs follow federal Medicare guidelines, so if documentation meets Medicare standards it will generally be acceptable to other insurers.
   b. It is advisable to get copies of state and individual insurers' guidelines for OT services, as adherence to these guidelines will be critical for reimbursement.
      (1) Due to the potential wide variance in these guidelines, the NBCOT examination should not test information beyond the established federal Medicare guidelines.
   c. Previously stated standards and guidelines for documentation apply to reimbursement for Medicare.
2. Medicare prescription documentation.
   a. Required from a physician as defined by state practice acts.
   b. The certification could be:
      (1) A signature on the bottom of the note.
      (2) An MD signed 700 or 701 form.
      (3) A sheet stapled to the note with the MD signature and a statement reading "I certify that I approve of the attached treatment plan."
   c. Make sure diagnoses are acute, not chronic.
      (1) Rephrase the diagnosis for the physician if needed.
      (2) Use onset dates of within 60 days of admission to services, if possible. (Example: instead of rheumatoid arthritis (RA) x 10 years, use acute exacerbation of RA as of 1-15-14).
3. Intervention documentation.
   a. Content must indicate that the treatment shows a level of complexity and sophistication, or the condition of the patient must be of a nature that requires the judgment, knowledge, and skills of a qualified therapist. This statement is as per Medicare.
   b. Skilled rehabilitation intervention is mandatory.
      (1) Delineate the specific skilled care rendered. This is the biggest cause for retroactive denial.
      (2) Notes must show therapeutic intervention. Example: dressing does not indicate therapeutic concerns. Decreasing extensor tone to enable dressing meets these criteria.
   c. Skilled care rendered must match the diagnosis and the physician's order.
   d. Services must be unique to OT and not sound like PT or SLP. Medicare does not pay for duplication of services.
   e. In home care, homebound status due to functional limitations must be clearly delineated.

(1) If the diagnosis may not render the individual homebound, explain why this particular person is homebound.
(2) Do not give a reviewer any doubt that this person does not meet Medicare homebound criteria (e.g., do not state client not at home when you arrive. Rather state there was no answer to a locked door.)

f. Document honestly, but not over optimistically. Medicare reviewers are interested in determining the need for continued intervention.
(1) If a person has improved but can benefit from further intervention, document this need, rather than emphasizing the improvement.
(a) Provide behavioral observations that substantiate need for further care.

g. Practical improvement should be noted with functional change.
(1) If improvements are not made, the client should be discharged in a timely fashion.
(2) If there is a reason for the lack of progress, it should be noted.

h. Documentation must also demonstrate that the patient is making significant functional improvement in a reasonable and generally predictable period of time.
(1) Some improvement must be made at least on a weekly basis; otherwise treatment will be considered maintenance.
(a) Documentation to support the provision of services to persons not expected to improve must substantiate the need for skilled services to prevent deterioration and maximize function.
(2) If progress is slower than expected, document extenuating circumstances and/or limiting factors (e.g., a secondary diagnosis).
(3) Medicare does not reimburse for OT practitioners to implement maintenance treatment; this is considered unskilled service.
(4) Payment for designing a maintenance program and making periodic but infrequent evaluations of the program's effectiveness is provided.

i. The service must be reasonable and necessary.
(1) Was the service effective and completed in a timely fashion?
(2) In long term care, if the treatment does not lessen the amount of care needed by staff, what made the service worthwhile?

Federal Legislation Related to Occupational Therapy

Overview

1. Historically, the opportunities available to and the roles afforded to persons with disabilities have been influenced by federal legislation.
2. Federal laws establish numerous standards and provide funding for health benefits, medical services, rehabilitation, early intervention, education, vocational programming, professional training, and research.
3. These laws directly affect the profession of occupational therapy by establishing practice guidelines and reimbursement standards.
4. Major social movements that have precipitated federal legislation and/or have resulted from federal legislation include deinstitutionalization, early intervention, mainstreaming, and full inclusion.
5. State laws also influence OT practice but, due to their variability, would not be included in a national examination.
6. To ensure best practices, occupational therapists have an ethical responsibility to know federal and state laws and regulations; consequently the NBCOT examination may require knowledge about key legislation.

Patient Protection and Affordable Care Act (ACA)

1. Consists of 10 separate legislative titles that seek to improve the accessibility, fairness, quality, efficiency, accountability, and affordability of health insurance coverage in the United States.
2. See prior section on payment for OT services for ACA details.

Health Insurance and Portability Accountability Act (HIPAA)

1. Sets standards and safeguards to assure the individual's right to continuity in health care coverage and to ensure privacy and security of health care records.

2. All persons must be informed of the setting's privacy policies and a good faith effort must be made to obtain written acknowledgement from each person about his/her attainment of this knowledge.
   a. If the person refuses to sign, the provider should document the efforts made; failure to obtain written acknowledgement is not a violation of the rule.
   b. Written consent must be obtained from a person before any personal health information is used or disclosed in the provision of treatment, obtainment of payment, or the carrying out of any healthcare related operations.
      (1) Exemptions to the written notification/acknowledgement are allowed if the attainment of this will prevent or delay timely care (i.e., emergency care). Written acknowledgement must be obtained as soon as possible.
      (2) If language barriers preclude signed acknowledgement, treatment can occur if the physician believes consent is implied.
3. Prior to discussing a person's status with a family member/significant other or other provider, the provider must obtain the person's permission, or give the person the opportunity to object.
   a. Providers can use their clinical judgment to determine whether to discuss the person's case with others if the person cannot give permission or objects.
      (1) Documentation for this decision is essential (e.g., person is at risk of harming self due to lack of judgment; consultation with a specialist is essential to ensure quality of care).
   b. All information used or disclosed about a person's status must be limited to the minimum needed for the immediate purpose.
4. The HIPAA Privacy Rule requires that all providers protect patient confidentiality in all forms (i.e., oral, written, and electronic) and implement appropriate physical, technical, and administrative safeguards to assure this privacy.
   a. Settings must reduce the physical identifiability of patient information; i.e., door tags and white boards can only list last names, no diagnoses or treatment procedures may be listed, sign-in sheets with names only are allowed.
   b. Charts and any documentation with patients' names or other identifiers must be stored out of public view and in secure locations.
   c. Opaque covers should be used for clipboards that contain paperwork with patient information.
   d. All computers that are used to record, document, or transmit patient information should be equipped with monitor privacy screens.
   e. All faxes must contain cover sheets noting confidentiality of accompanying information and be sent only to dedicated fax machines in secure locations.
   f. All e-mails must use password protection and encryption if going over the Internet.
   g. All faxes and computer printouts must be immediately destroyed or placed in the person's chart, as most appropriate.
   h. All conversations regarding a person's health status must be done in private areas, in low tones, and with minimal disclosure.
5. An individual has the right to access all of his/her records.
   a. Providers can charge reasonable copying costs and have 30–60 days to respond.
   b. Individuals have the right to request that information in their record be amended.
      (1) The provider can refuse the request, providing his/her rationale.
      (2) The provider can comply with the request by documenting the request and the reason for compliance. The original documentation should not be removed/excised.
6. HIPAA does not exclude treatment from occurring in group settings or open clinics.
   a. Discussion regarding treatment should be done quietly and, if possible, behind a screen/room divider.
7. HIPAA does not require a guarantee of 100% confidentiality; it does require reasonable and vigilant safeguards.
8. HIPAA guidelines for research are complex but they are congruent with the established guidelines for human subject research and Institutional Review Board (IRB) standards.
   a. A limited data set that does not include any identifiable patient information can be used in research without patient approval (e.g., diagnosis, age, length of stay).
9. The Administrative Simplification rules also provide standardization of codes and formats for medical data.
10. HIPAA does not override state laws that further restrict privacy and it defers to state laws governing minors.

Key Legislation Related to Overall Disability Rights

1. Medicare Title 18-PL 89-97.
   a. Established Medicare and Supplemental Security Income (SSI).
   b. SSI enables persons with disabilities to receive a monthly income enabling them to live in the community.
2. Rehabilitation Act of 1973.

a. Prohibits discrimination on the basis of disability in any program or activity that receives federal assistance.
b. Required all federal agencies to develop action plans for the hiring, placement, and advancement of persons with disabilities.
c. Required contractors who received federal contracts over a pre-set amount to take affirmative action to employ persons with disabilities.

3. Fair Housing Act.
   a. Prohibits discrimination on the bases of disability, religion, sex, color, race, national origin, and familial status.
   b. Required owners of housing to make reasonable exceptions to their standard tenant policies to allow individuals with disabilities equal housing opportunities (e.g., allowing a seeing eye or service dog in a "no-pets" apartment).
   c. Required that tenants with disabilities be allowed to make reasonable modifications to common use areas and to their private living space to enable access.
      (1) The housing owner is not required to fund these modifications.
   d. Required that newly constructed multifamily residences (4 or more apartments) be built to meet established accessibility standards.
4. Omnibus Budget Reconciliation Act (OBRA) of 1981.
   a. Affirmed application of Section 504 of the Rehabilitation Act of 1973, which prohibits discrimination in federally funded programs to a diversity of services (i.e., Head Start programs, block grant programs, community development programs).
   b. Provided Medicaid financing for community-based services for people with developmental disabilities when services were demonstrated to be less expensive than institutional care.
5. Americans with Disabilities Act (ADA).
   a. Prohibits discrimination against qualified persons with disabilities in employment, transportation, accommodations, telecommunications, and public services.
   b. Criteria for classifying an individual as disabled.
      (1) A person with a physical or mental impairment that substantially limits one or more major life activities.
      (2) A person having a record of such an impairment.
      (3) A person regarded as having such an impairment.
   c. Individuals who are actively abusing substances or compulsively gambling or persons who have kleptomania, pyromania, or sexual behavior disorders are not protected by ADA.
   d. Title I—Employment.
      (1) Prohibits employers from discriminating against persons with disabilities in any aspect or phase of employment including recruitment, hiring, working conditions, hours, promotion, training opportunities, termination, social activities, and other privileges of employment.
      (2) Allows questions about one's ability to perform a job but prohibits inquiries as to whether one has a disability.
      (3) Prohibits employment tests that tend to screen out people with disabilities.
      (4) A "qualified individual with a disability" means a person with a disability who is able to perform the "essential functions" of a job (that is, the tasks fundamental to the position) with or without reasonable accommodations.
      (5) "Reasonable accommodations" must be provided by businesses with 15 or more employees to persons with disabilities to enable them to perform essential job functions unless such accommodations would impose an "undue" hardship on the business.
         (a) Types of reasonable accommodations.
            - Acquisition or modification of equipment or devices.
            - Modifications or adjustments to examinations, training materials, or publications.
            - Provision of ancillary aids or services.
            - Modified or part-time work schedules, job restructuring, or reassignment to a vacant position.
            - Improvement of existing facilities used by employee so they are usable by and accessible to persons with disabilities and/or other similar accommodations.
         (b) Types of auxiliary aids and services.
            - Taped texts, qualified readers, or other methods that can effectively make visually delivered materials accessible to persons with visual impairments.
            - Qualified interpreters or other methods that can effectively make aurally delivered materials accessible to persons with hearing impairments.
            - Modification or acquisition of devices or equipment.
            - Similar actions or services that increase accessibility.
         (c) Undue hardship is defined as action that would be significantly difficult or overly expensive given the financial resources of the employer, its size, and major functions.
      (6) The United States Government, Indian Tribes, and/or private tax-exempt membership clubs are exempt from ADA employer guidelines.

e. Title II Public Services.
  (1) Mandates that state and local governments and their departments, agencies, and/or component parts may not discriminate against, exclude, or deny persons with disabilities participation in or benefit from the services, programs, or activities of these public entities.
    (a) This includes transportation, public education, employment, recreation, social services, health care, courts, town meetings, and voting.

f. Title III Public Accommodations and Services operated by Public Entities.
  (1) Mandates that places of public accommodation (i.e., hospitals, health care providers' offices, schools, day care centers, and other places of accommodation, restaurants, theatres) may not discriminate against persons with disabilities with respect to their participation in or ability to benefit from the service, goods, facility, use, or other programming aspects.
  (2) Public places operated by private entities must be designed, constructed, and altered to comply with accessibility standards.
    (a) All new construction of public accommodations must be accessible.
    (b) Physical barriers in existing facilities must be removed if removal is able to be carried out without much difficulty or expense.
    (c) The United States Government, Indian Tribes, religious organizations, and/or private tax-exempt membership clubs are exempt from ADA accessibility standards.
  (3) Private services that serve the public (e.g., restaurants, stores, and theaters) cannot discriminate in the provision of services.
  (4) Public transportation systems must be accessible.
  (5) Private transportation systems must be accessible and non-discriminatory (e.g., livery services, taxis, tour bus companies).

g. Title IV Telecommunications.
  (1) All televisions must include closed captioning.
  (2) Telephone companies must provide telecommunications relay services (TRS) to persons with hearing or speech impairments 24 hours per day, 7 days per week.

6. Ticket to Work and Work Incentives Improvement Act (TWIIA).
  a. Strives to make it more realistic and easier for a person with a disability to work.
  b. Removes a major disincentive to work by allowing individuals with disabilities to maintain their Medicare or Medicaid health care benefits.
    (1) Allows an individual with a disability to keep Medicare benefits for an additional 54 months after starting work.
    (2) Eliminates limits on Medicaid 'buy in' options.
  c. Enables consumers to have a choice in their service provider beyond public assistance programs.
  d. Establishes community-based vocational planning and assistance programs.
  e. Increases consumer choices for accessing employment support services.
  f. All states can design their own program.

7. Work Investment Act (WIA).
  a. Established a federally sponsored national employment and vocational training system.
  b. Established a "One-Stop" delivery system for all adults aged 18 or older seeking access to employment and training services. This means traditionally separate "unemployment" offices and "vocational rehabilitation services" are now available at a "One-Stop Center."
    (1) Availability of all employment and training services at a One-Stop Center is aimed to allow for universal access for person with disabilities, a core principle of WIA.
    (2) Categories of One-Stop services.
      (a) Core services, which include outreach, intake and orientation; initial assessment; eligibility determination for services; assistance with job search and placement; job market information and career counseling.
      (b) Intensive services for individuals who do not attain successful employment after receipt of core services. Services can include comprehensive assessments of service needs and skill level, development of individualized plans for employment, case management, and counseling.
      (c) Training services for individuals who do not attain successful employment after receipt of core and intensive services. These services are typically provided off-site from the One-Stop Center and can include adult education and literacy training, on-the-job training, and individualized vocational training.
    (3) The One-Stop system of services is provided through a network in each state. The names of these systems can vary from state to state.
  c. Persons determined to be eligible for WIA services receive an Individual Training Account (ITA) which is used to obtain services from any approved provider. Specific ITA procedures can vary from state to state.
  d. Services for youth (aged 14–21) with disabilities are also provided for in the WIA to assist in a successful transition from school to work.

Select Legislation Specific to Technology

1. Technology Related Assistance for Individuals with Disabilities Act.
   a. Funded the development of technology and technologic aids for persons with disabilities to improve communication, mobility, self-care, transportation, and education.
2. Title IV Telecommunications of the ADA. See Section on the ADA.
3. Telecommunications Act of 1996.
   a. Required providers of telecommunications systems and manufacturers of telecommunications equipment to make services and equipment useable by and accessible to individuals with disabilities, if at all possible.
   b. Examples of services and equipment covered by this act are cell phones, pagers, call waiting, caller ID, and operator assistance.

Legislation Specific to Pediatric Practice

1. Child Abuse Prevention and Treatment Act
   a. Defines child abuse and neglect as mental or physical injury, negligent treatment, maltreatment, or sexual abuse of a child less than 18 years of age by a person responsible for the child's welfare under circumstances that indicate that a child's welfare or health is being threatened or harmed.
   b. Mandates professionals to report abuse and neglect to law enforcement officials.
   c. Occupational therapists are included in this list of mandated reporters.
   d. OT practitioners can also serve as child welfare advocates.
   e. Direct OT intervention may be needed to remediate the emotional or physical disorders that result from abuse.
      (1) See Chapter 5 for further information about child abuse.
2. Early Intervention and Education Acts.
   a. Multiple acts have provided the foundation for current early intervention and education services. These include:
      (1) Mandates for free and appropriate education (FAPE) for all children regardless of ability or disability, (aged 3–21) in the least restrictive environment.
         (a) Mainstreaming (i.e., integrating children with disabilities into classrooms) was the means to ensure education is provided in the least restrictive environment
      (2) Requirements that public schools provide OT to special education students if OT is needed for the student to benefit from the special education.
      (3) The designation of occupational therapy as a primary early intervention service.
      (4) Funding for family support services. and programs to train professionals in early intervention.
      (5) Recommendations for states to develop infant and toddler programs (birth to 3 years).
         (a) Programs are voluntary and vary from state to state but all states participate to some degree.
         (b) OT is considered a primary developmental service.
3. Reauthorization and Amendment of Individuals with Disabilities Education Act.
   a. Emphasizes that the purpose of the Individualized Education Plan (IEP) is to address the child's unique needs as related to his/her disability and decide how these needs can be served so the child has full access to the general education curriculum and can participate in the general education classroom.
   b. Clarifies that the individual education plan (IEP) can include consideration of assistive technology and behavioral interventions, strategies, and supports (an area in which OT can offer a great deal).
   c. States that IEP planning team is open to related personnel at the request of the parent or school, in addition to the regular education teacher, if the student is in a regular education class.
   d. States that the education the student receives should prepare him/her for independent living and employment in adult life.
      (1) Transitional planning begins at the age of 14 (or younger if indicated) to help the student plan a course of study that will lead to post-school goals.
      (2) Transition services begin at the age of 16 (or younger if indicated) to provide student with a coordinated set of services to attain post-school goals.
         (a) These services can include community experience, specific instruction, and/or ADL and vocational assessment and intervention.
      (3) The student must be invited to attend IEP meetings that discuss his/her transition planning and services to allow for self-advocacy and self determination.
      (4) This transition plan must be updated annually with appropriate service revision provided.
   e. Maintains the established definition of related services (including OT).
   f. Expands orientation and mobility services by broadly interpreting them to include all children with disabilities.

g. Students with disabilities may be punished in the same manner as other students for serious offenses (i.e., carrying illicit drugs or a weapon). However, disciplinary prevention measures are stressed.
h. Educational and related services still must be received by the child even if he/she is removed to an alternative placement.
i. Clarifies early intervention services and systems.
    (1) Mandates an Individual Family Service Plan (IFSP) for children 0–2 years of age.
    (2) OT is identified as a primary early intervention service.

4. Individuals with Disabilities Education Improvement Act (IDEA 2004).
    a. Directly addresses the student's functional performance along with academic performance.
        (1) Requires that evaluations for IDEA eligibility include relevant functional and developmental information, not just academic achievement data.
        (2) Expands the IEP's annual goals to include academic and functional goals.
        (3) Specifies that accommodations must be provided as needed to measure the functional performance and academic achievement of all students with disabilities.
        (4) Enables services to be provided to students as soon as learning needs become apparent via a Response to Intervention (RtI) approach.
            (a) RtI provides evidence-based early intervention services to children who are having difficulty learning to prevent academic failure.
    b. Provides for the piloting of a multi-year (not to exceed 3 years) IEP to allow for long-term planning and to coincide with a child's "natural" transitions (e.g., pre-school to elementary school, middle school to high school).
        (1) Plan is optional for parents.
    c. Provides for increased flexibility in IEP meetings.
        (1) Allows IEP team members to be excused from IEP meetings if their area of concern is not being addressed or modified at the meeting or if a written report is submitted prior to the meeting.
            (a) District and parental approval for a team member's absence is required.
            (b) Parental approval must be in writing.
        (2) Allows IEP revisions and/or amendments to be made by parents and districts after an annual IEP meeting.
            (a) Parents must be provided with a written copy of the revised/amended IEP.
        (3) Allows the use of technological alternatives to face-to-face IEP meetings (i.e., videoconferences conference calls).
    d. Requires that recommendations for early intervention, special education, related, and supplementary services and aids be made based on peer-reviewed research to the extent that this is practical.
        (1) This requirement raises concern that established intervention methods may be questioned due to a real or perceived lack of evidence supporting their efficacy.
        (2) This requirement may spur research on early intervention and school-based OT to support evidence-based practice.
    e. Clarifies that a screening done by a specialist is not equivalent to an evaluation for eligibility for IDEA services.
        (1) OT practitioners can conduct informal classroom-based screenings and provide consultations for classroom modifications and other teaching strategies without completing a formal evaluation according to IDEA procedures.
    f. Requires that all students with disabilities be assessed in compliance with the No Child Left Behind Act.
        (1) The IEP team determines if the student should take an alternative assessment or the standard assessment with or without accommodations.
    g. Provides for early coordinated intervening services for general education students from kindergarten through 12th grade who do not require special education services but who do need additional supports to succeed in school.
    h. Clarifies that the purpose of the IDEA is to prepare children with disabilities for further education, employment, and independent living.
    i. Allows school personnel to individually consider each case of a student with a disability who violates the school's code of conduct.
        (1) Students with disabilities who are disciplined must:
            (a) be provided with services to continue to progress towards achieving their IEP goals.
            (b) receive appropriate functional behavioral assessments and interventions and service modifications as needed to address their conduct violation(s).
    j. Allows each state to define developmental delay criteria to determine if an infant or toddler is eligible for early intervention in that state.
        (1) Typically, states define developmental delays quantitatively (e.g. a percentage of delay according to a standardized developmental assessment).
    k. Requires that an IFSP be completed to include:
        (1) the infant's or toddler's developmental level.
        (2) family priorities, concerns, and resources.
        (3) the infant's or toddler's natural environments.
        (4) measureable outcomes.
        (5) projected, length, frequency and duration of research-based services.
        (6) transition plans to pre-school or other services, as appropriate.

l. Clarifies the role of the parent and IFSP team in determining the site for service provision.
   (1) Requires states to maximize the provision of early intervention services in the infant's or toddler's natural environments, as appropriate.

m. Requires states to establish procedures for the referral of infants and toddlers who are victims of abuse and/or neglect to early intervention services.
   (1) This provision was also included in the Keeping Children and Families Safe Act.

5. No Child Left Behind Act (NCLB).
   a. A general education law which emphasizes standards-based education.
   b. Considers occupational therapists to be pupil services personnel and sets no requirements for OT services.
   c. Requires schools to provide accommodations, if needed by students, for mandated tests.
      (1) OT practitioners can recommend testing alternatives and/or classroom accommodations.

Legislation Specific to Gerontic Practice

1. Age Discrimination in Employment Act.
   a. Prohibits employment practices that discriminate or unfairly affect workers 40 years and older.
   b. Prohibits mandatory retirement of older workers. Employers cannot fix a retirement age.
2. Freedom to Work Act.
   a. Amended the Social Security Act to enable Americans receiving retirement Social Security (SS) benefits (currently 65 years old) to be able to work without affecting their SS income.
      (1) There are no income restrictions in this amendment.
3. Omnibus Budget Reconciliation Act (OBRA) of 1990.
   a. Applied to all nursing homes that receive federal money for Medicare or Medicaid patients.
   b. Emphasized attending to resident rights, autonomy, and self determination; providing quality of care; and enhancing quality of life within nursing homes.
   c. Mandated a comprehensive resident assessment system, the Minimal Data Set (MDS), which is administered upon admission and thereafter on an annual basis, unless there is a significant change in the resident's condition.
      (1) MDS is coordinated by an RN. Occupational therapists can contribute information.
   d. Psychosocial well-being and activity pursuit patterns must be considered along with the resident's physical condition and cognitive abilities.
      (1) This has broadened OT's role in nursing homes.
   e. Mandated that the evaluation and treatment of conditions found during the MDS follow specific guidelines called the Resident Assessment Protocols (RAPS).
      (1) The structured approach to assessment is called the Resident Assessment Instrument (RAI).
      (2) Individualized care plans must be established within specific time frames.
   f. The enhancement of quality of life through restraint reduction and the provision of restraint-free environments are strongly emphasized.
      (1) Nursing homes must show evidence of consultation by an occupational or physical therapist for consideration of interventions that are less restrictive than restraints.
      (2) Occupational therapists are frequently consulted for ADL treatment, seating adaptations, positioning ideas, environmental modifications, psychosocial interventions, and activity programming.
   g. Aims to guarantee that residents have the right to choose how they want to receive care and live their lives.
      (1) Residents should have a choice in determining their ADL, including community activities.
      (2) Residents should be able to function as independently as possible.
   h. Post discharge plans must meet specific criteria including client or caregiver education

Service Delivery Models and Practice Settings

Overview

1. A working knowledge of service delivery models and practice settings ensures that OT practitioners make educated decisions about their employment and competent referrals for their clients.
2. As a result of legislative initiatives and health care system changes, service delivery is evolving from medical-based models and settings to more community and home-based models and settings (e.g., IDEA has solidified schools as a practice setting).

3. Implications for OT practice.
   a. Fewer practitioners will work in hospitals and long term care facilities.
   b. More practitioners will work in community and home-based settings (e.g., day treatment, home care, school settings).

Models of Practice

1. Criteria for determining a model of practice.
   a. The type of setting.
   b. Philosophy and mission of the particular setting and department.
   c. The role the therapist plays as a team member within that particular setting.
2. Medical model.
   a. Views the individual with a disability as a person who has incurred a physiological insult that has resulted in reduced functional capacity.
   b. Focus is placed on identifying the disease or dysfunction.
   c. Treatment addresses the disease or dysfunction (performance components) contributing to decreased functional skills.
   d. OT frames of reference address the pathological process of the disease or dysfunctions (e.g., biomechanical, neurodevelopmental).
3. Education model.
   a. Views the individual with a disability as lacking knowledge or skills.
   b. Focus is placed on learning and making the behavioral changes needed to interact successfully in the environment.
   c. An individual's skill deficits are determined, and related goals are established, to promote learning to adequately perform within a particular environment.
   d. Behaviors are measured in terms of obtaining skills, knowledge, and competency to successfully meet the demands of the environment.
   e. OT frames of reference are based on learning theories to facilitate adaptation in the environment (e.g., role acquisition, cognitive remediation).
4. Community model.
   a. Views the individual with a disability as lacking skills, resources, and supports for community participation.
   b. Focus is placed on identifying and developing the skills needed for one's expected environment.
   c. If skills cannot be developed, community resources and supports are identified and developed to enable functioning within one's chosen environment.
   d. OT frames of reference promote development of performance skills and/or areas of occupation within the individual's performance contexts (e.g., life-style performance, occupation adaptation).
5. Telehealth model.
   a. A service delivery model which can include features of the above models by providing medical, rehabilitative and/or educational services to persons via telecommunications technologies.

Institutional Practice Settings

1. Acute care hospitals.
   a. Admission is for a medical or psychiatric diagnosis that cannot be treated on an outpatient basis.
      (1) Initial onset of a new illness or major health problem.
      (2) Acute exacerbation of a chronic illness.
      (3) In psychiatry, a person may be involuntarily admitted to an acute unit if he/she is considered to be a danger to self or others, or as having a grave disability.
   b. Length of stay (LOS) is determined by diagnosis and presenting symptoms.
      (1) LOS can be limited to 1–7 days.
      (2) Longer LOS requires significant documentation to justify need for further hospitalization.
      (3) Ongoing need for care frequently results in discharge to another setting.
   c. OT evaluation process focuses on quick and accurate screening of major difficulties impeding function (e.g., cognitive status, home safety skills).
   d. OT intervention focus.
      (1) Stabilization of client's status.
      (2) Engagement of the client in the therapeutic relationship and purposeful activities/meaningful occupations so that he/she can see that change is possible, thereby increasing motivation to pursue follow-up.
      (3) Discharge planning and after-care referrals.
      (4) Family, caregiver, and consumer education.
   e. The role of an acute care occupational therapist can be a generalist or a specialist (e.g., neonatology, burns).
      (1) Specialized practice roles require advanced knowledge and skills and therefore would not be evaluated on the NBCOT examination.
2. Sub-acute care/intermediate care facilities (ICFs).
   a. Admission is for a medical or psychiatric diagnosis that has progressed from an acute stage but has not stabilized sufficiently to be treated on an outpatient basis.
   b. Length of stay (LOS) is determined by diagnosis and presenting symptoms.
      (1) LOS can range from 5–30 days.
      (2) Longer LOS requires significant documentation to justify need for further hospitalization.

(3) Ongoing need for intervention or long-term care frequently results in discharge to another setting.

c. OT evaluation can include more in-depth assessments and more thorough observations of client's functional performance.

d. OT intervention focus.

(1) Functional improvements in performance skills and areas of occupation.

(2) Active engagement of the client in the treatment planning, implementation, and re-evaluation process.

(3) Discharge planning to expected environment.

e. Sub-acute care and ICFs can be housed in hospitals or skilled nursing facilities (SNFs).

3. Long-term acute care hospital (LTAC).

a. Admission is for chronic or catastrophic illnesses or disabilities that require extensive medical care and/or dependency on life support or ventilators.

(1) Patients often have multiple diagnoses with major complications.

b. The average length of stay is greater than 25 days to maintain Medicare certification.

c. OT evaluation and intervention is often limited by the population's severe and complex medical needs.

(1) For all clients, evaluation and intervention is concerned with palliative care and the prevention and treatment of complications (e.g., positioning to prevent decubiti and contractures).

(2) For individuals who are cognitively intact, the focus of evaluation and intervention is mastery of the environment and the attainment of client-centered goals.

4. Rehabilitation hospitals.

a. Admission is for a disability that is medically stable but which has residual functional deficits requiring skilled rehabilitation services.

b. Length of stay (LOS) is determined by presenting deficits and rehabilitation potential.

(1) LOS can range from a week to months.

(2) Documentation requirements supporting the need for an extended LOS are dependent upon institutional, state, and third party payer guidelines.

(3) LOS ends when coverage is expended. The client is then discharged to the appropriate environment.

(a) A skilled nursing facility.

(b) A supportive community residence.

(c) Home/independent living.

c. OT evaluation can be extensive and focus on all performance skills and patterns, areas of occupation, and occupational roles that will be required in the expected environment.

(1) Environmental assessments of planned discharge environment must be completed.

d. OT intervention focus.

(1) Functional improvement in performance skills and patterns, areas of occupation, and occupational roles.

(2) Development of compensatory strategies for residual deficits and client factors.

(3) Provision of adaptive equipment and training in use of the equipment to promote independent function.

(4) Modification of the discharge environment, as needed, to enhance function.

(5) Education of the individual, family, and caregivers on abilities, limitations, compensatory techniques, and advocacy skills.

5. Long-term hospitals.

a. Admission is for a medical or psychiatric diagnosis that is chronic with the presence of symptoms that cannot be treated on an outpatient basis.

b. Length of stay (LOS) is determined by diagnosis and presenting symptoms.

(1) LOS can range from a month to years.

(2) Documentation requirements supporting need for increased LOS are dependent upon institutional, third party payer, and/or state guidelines.

(3) LOS in private long-term hospitals is determined by insurance coverage. When coverage is expended, an alternative discharge environment is needed for the client.

(a) A state run long-term hospital.

(b) A skilled nursing facility.

(c) Home or supportive residence.

c. OT evaluation can be extensive due to increased LOS.

d. OT intervention focus.

(1) Functional improvements in performance skills and patterns and areas of occupation.

(2) Development of compensatory strategies for residual deficits and client factors.

(3) Maintenance of quality of life.

(4) Development of skills for discharge to the least restrictive environment.

6. Skilled nursing facilities (SNFs)/Extended care facilities (ECFs).

a. Admission is for a medical or psychiatric diagnosis that is chronic and requires skilled care, but the individual's illness is stable with no acute symptoms.

b. Due to managed care constraints on acute hospital stays, many individuals are being admitted to SNFs for medical care and rehabilitation.

c. Length of stay (LOS) can range from 1 month to the individual's lifetime. Several factors influence LOS.

(1) The progression of the illness.

(2) Availability of family or community supports.

(3) Insurance coverage.

d. OT evaluation and intervention is guided by Medicare standards.
   (1) For individuals with rehabilitation potential, the focus of evaluation and intervention is the same as identified under Rehabilitation Hospitals.
   (2) For individuals without rehabilitation potential, evaluation and intervention is more concerned with palliative care and the maintenance of quality of life.

7. Forensic settings.
   a. Admission is due to engagement in criminal activity by a person. The person can be remanded to a variety of settings depending on the nature of the crime and if he/she has a psychiatric diagnosis.
      (1) Jail: a city or county facility which is the individual's first entry into the criminal justice system and the placement for those convicted of crimes with sentences of less than a year.
      (2) Prison: a state or federal facility for individuals found guilty of crimes with sentences greater than a year.
      (3) Forensic psychiatric hospital or unit: a specialized hospital or unit within a hospital which provides inpatient psychiatric care for individuals convicted of a crime and found guilty but mentally ill or not guilty by reason of insanity.
   b. Length of stay is determined by court-ordered directives and criminal sentences.
   c. The availability and quality of services varies greatly from none in most jails to extensive in some forensic hospitals.
   d. Due to serious gaps in mental health services, the incarceration rate of persons with mental illness has increased significantly (e.g., a homeless person with schizophrenia steals food due to hunger).
   e. OT evaluation and intervention focus.
      (1) Determination of individual's competency to stand trial, in forensic psychiatry settings.
      (2) Areas similar to those described under Rehabilitation Hospitals to develop community living skills needed for successful community reintegration upon release.
      (3) Facilitation of skills and provision of structured programs to enable the person to function at his/her highest level within their current environment since discharge may be delayed or not possible, depending on the nature of the crime.
      (4) Restoration of competency to stand trial in forensic psychiatry settings.

8. Outpatient/ambulatory care.
   a. An individual who does not require hospitalization but has functional deficits requiring evaluation and intervention may receive OT services on an outpatient basis in private clinics, medical offices, and/or hospital satellite centers.
   b. Focus of outpatient care is diagnostic evaluations, interventions to increase functional performance, consumer education, and prevention.

Community-Based Practice Settings

1. Early intervention programs.
   a. Acceptance criteria for an early intervention evaluation are based on "at risk" status of the infant or toddler who is under the age of three.
      (1) Birth complications.
      (2) Suspected delays in development.
      (3) Failure to thrive.
      (4) Maternal substance abuse during pregnancy.
      (5) Birth to an adolescent/teen mother.
      (6) Established disability/diagnosis.
   b. Acceptance criteria for early intervention services are based on the following criteria.
      (1) The extent of the developmental delay (typically a 33% delay in one area of development or a 25% delay in two areas).
      (2) An established diagnosis/disability.
   c. Length of service provision.
      (1) If the infant/child qualifies for services, an infant family service plan is completed by the service coordinator after a review of all assessments and in collaboration with the family and early intervention team.
      (2) Six-month reviews are submitted by all professionals to determine if services should continue.
   d. Occupational therapy evaluation.
      (1) Assessment of five developmental areas.
         (a) Cognitive.
         (b) Physical.
         (c) Communication.
         (d) Social-emotional.
         (e) Adaptive.
      (2) Determination of the effects of current development on the occupational areas of play and activities of daily living.
      (3) Evaluations need to be written in a strength-oriented manner.
      (4) Functional goals must be written in family friendly terms and include levels of functioning, unique needs, and recommended services.
   e. Occupational therapy intervention process.
      (1) Development of cognitive/process, psychosocial/communication/interaction, and sensorimotor skills.
      (2) Development of play and activities of daily living skills.
      (3) Provision of family education.
      (4) Provision of advocacy and advocacy training.

(5) Transition planning from early intervention to preschool is essential.

2. Schools.
   a. Acceptance criteria for OT services as a related service in an educational setting.
      (1) The child requires special education services, and OT will enable the child to benefit from special education.
      (2) OT will facilitate the child's participation in educational activities and enhance the child's functional performance.
      (3) Referrals are received from the previous agency that provided early intervention services, the child's teacher, and/or school's child study team.
      (4) The school reviews the referral and, if indicated, recommends an OT evaluation.
         (a) If an OT evaluation has already been completed, the need for OT intervention services is discussed.
         (b) The frequency, length of sessions, and duration of the intervention are also determined.
   b. Length of services is dependent upon the impact of OT services on the child's abilities and prevention of loss of abilities.
      (1) If OT services can improve the child's ability to participate in education-related activities and allow full access to the general education curriculum, services can be continued.
      (2) A review of services and progress made towards the child's individualized education plan (IEP) is conducted on an annual basis.
   c. OT evaluation.
      (1) Assess client factors, performance skills and patterns and areas of occupation, that impact on the educational and functional performance of the child within the school.
         (a) Findings are used to contribute to the IEP, in which goals and objectives are formulated to address the overall educational needs of the student.
      (2) Assess the child's functional and developmental level to contribute to the Functional Behavioral Analysis.
   d. OT intervention focus.
      (1) Based on an educational model versus a medical model.
      (2) Addresses the student's functional performance along with academic performance.
      (3) Activities are utilized to address the goals and objectives documented in the IEP using both corrective and compensatory methods.
      (4) Assistive technology and transition services, in accordance with the regulations of IDEA, are provided.
      (5) Performance skill deficits and client factors (i.e., sensorimotor, cognitive/process, and psychosocial/communication/interaction) are treated to improve the child's ability to participate in and perform education-related activities within a school setting.
      (6) Skills in the performance areas of ADL, school, and play are developed to improve the child's ability to participate in and perform education-related activities within a school setting.
      (7) Skills for adult life post-school are developed in accordance with the student's transition plan.
   e. The OT practitioner needs to know the school district's and state's funding sources, and regulations and interpretations of the federal laws regarding education (see this chapter's section on legislation).
   f. The role of OT practitioners in school-based practice has expanded beyond education-related services to include programs that address students' psychosocial needs and prevent school violence.
      (1) Behavioral Intervention Plans which include Response to Intervention (RtI), Early Intervening Services (EIS), and Positive Behavioral Supports (PBS) may be a component of school-based OT service provision
         (a) Response to Intervention (RtI) is an evidence-based, structured intervention approach that uses Early Intervening Services (EIS) to address academic difficulties and Positive Behavioral Supports (PBS) to address behavioral problems early in a child's education.

3. Supported education programs.
   a. Participant criteria include adolescents or adults who require intervention to develop skills that are needed to succeed in secondary and/or post-secondary education.
      (1) The person may have never developed these skills or lost them due to a psychiatric disability or mental health problems.
   b. Length of stay is determined by agency's funding and person's attainment of goals.
      (1) Discharge is upon entry into, or completion of, an educational program or the attainment of a graduate equivalency degree (GED).
   c. OT evaluation is focused on the individual's client factors, performance skills and patterns that impact on the occupational role of student.
   d. OT intervention focus.
      (1) Improvement in performance skills and patterns that are needed for the occupational role of student (e.g., time management and task prioritization).

(2) Education and training in compensatory strategies to support academic performance (e.g., studying in a quiet room).

(3) Exploration of participant's educational interests and aptitudes to ensure self-determined engagement in a school, college, technical training program, or community-based adult-education class(es).

4. Prevocational programs.
   a. Participant criteria include adolescents or adults who require intervention to develop skills that are prerequisite to work.
      (1) The person may have never developed these skills due to developmental delays, environmental insufficiencies, illness, or disability.
      (2) The person may have lost these skills due to illness or disability.
   b. Length of stay is determined by agency's funding and person's attainment of goals.
      (1) Discharge is usually to a vocational program.
      (2) Discharge to a work setting can occur if sufficient abilities are developed.
   c. OT evaluation is focused on the individual's task skills, social interaction skills, work habits, interests, and aptitudes.
   d. OT intervention focus.
      (1) Improvement in task skills and social skills that is prerequisite to vocational training or work.
      (2) Development of work habits and abilities.
      (3) Exploration of work interests and aptitudes to ensure discharge to a relevant vocational training program, school, or work setting.
5. Vocational programs.
   a. Acceptance is for the development of specific vocational skills.
      (1) Person has the prerequisite abilities to work (e.g., good task skills and work habits) but requires training for a specific job and/or ongoing structure, support and/or supervision to maintain employment.
      (2) Person has to develop his/her work capacities to a level acceptable for competitive employment (e.g., strength and endurance).
   b. Length of stay is determined by agency's funding and attainment of goals.
      (1) In rehabilitation workshops (formerly called sheltered workshops) and supportive employment programs, discharge is not always a goal.
         (a) Maintenance of the person in these structured work environments can be the desired objective for some individuals while others will be discharged to other programs or to work.
      (2) Transitional employment programs (TEPs) are generally time limited (3–6 months) with discharge to competitive employment, supportive employment, or rehabilitation workshops.
      (3) Employee assistance programs (EAPs) provide ongoing support, intervention, and referrals as needed to a company's employees to enable these individuals to maintain this employment.
   c. OT evaluation is focused on the individual's functional skills and deficits related to work in his/her current and expected vocational environment.
   d. OT intervention focus.
      (1) Remediation of underlying performance skill deficits and compensation for client factors that affect the work performance area.
      (2) Development of general work abilities and specific job skills.
      (3) Consultation to and/or supervision of vocational direct care staff.
      (4) Identification and implementation of reasonable accommodations in accordance with ADA.
      (5) Referral to state offices of vocational and educational services (i.e., "One-Stop Centers") for persons with disabilities for further evaluation, education, and training.
6. Residential programs.
   a. Admission is for a developmental, medical or psychiatric condition that has resulted in functional deficits that impede independent living but are not severe enough to require hospitalization.
      (1) Residential programs are on a continuum from 24-hour supervised quarter way houses, halfway houses, or group homes, to supportive apartments with weekly or biweekly "check-in" supervision.
      (2) The degree of functional impairment determines the residential level of care needed.
   b. Length of stay for transitional living programs (e.g., quarter way and halfway house programs) is determined by agency's funding.
      (1) Long-term and permanent housing options (i.e., group homes and supportive apartments) are available and are funded through the individual's social service benefits.
   c. OT evaluation is focused on assessment of the individual's skills for living in the community and determination of the social and environmental resources and supports needed to maintain the individual in his/her current and expected living environment.
   d. OT intervention focus.
      (1) Consultation to and/or supervision of residential program staff.
      (2) Remediation of underlying performance skill deficits and compensation for client factors that affect independent living skills.

(3) ADL training, activity adaptation, and environmental modifications to facilitate community living skills.
(4) Referral to appropriate residential services along the continuum of care as individual's functional level improves.
(5) Education about ADA, the Fair Housing Act, and Section 8 Housing.

7. Partial hospitalization/day hospital programs.
  a. Admission is for a medical or psychiatric condition that has been sufficiently stabilized to enable an individual to be discharged home or to a community residence (e.g., a halfway house or supported apartment); however, the individual still has symptoms remaining which require active treatment.
  b. Treatment is up to 5 days per week with multiple interventions scheduled each day.
  c. Length of stay (LOS) is determined by diagnosis, presenting symptoms, and response to treatment.
    (1) LOS can vary from 1 week to 6 months.
    (2) Documentation requirements supporting the need for an extended LOS are dependent upon institutional, state, and/or third party payer guidelines.
    (3) Once LOS is expended, discharge is usually to a less intensive community day program.
  d. OT evaluation is focused on the individual's functional skills and deficits in his/her performance areas and the occupational roles that are required in his/her current and expected environment(s).
  e. OT intervention focus.
    (1) Functional improvement in areas of occupation and occupational role functioning.
    (2) Remediation of underlying performance skill deficits and compensation for client factors that affect functional performance.
    (3) Development of skills for community living and identification of community supports for community participation.

8. Clubhouse programs.
  a. Membership is open to adults and elders with a current mental illness or a history of mental illness.
    (1) All members have equal access to all clubhouse functions and opportunities regardless of functional level or diagnosis.
    (2) Individuals who pose a significant and direct threat to the safety of the clubhouse community are the only persons excluded.
  b. Services are provided by staff and members with the responsibilities of operating the clubhouse shared equally by staff and members under the oversight of a director.
    (1) Due to this role equality, it can be difficult to distinguish between members and paid staff.
    (2) Staff's main role is to engage membership, provide needed support and structure, and enable recovery.
  c. Individual schedules will vary to meet each person's unique needs and interests.
    (1) Clubhouses are open at least 5 days per week. Many are open 7 days per week.
    (2) The daily schedule is organized around the "work-ordered" day, which parallels typical working hours to engage members and staff in the running of the clubhouse.
    (3) Evening and weekend schedules are focused on avocational interests and recreational pursuits.
    (4) Additional services that can be provided include literacy and education programs, transitional employment placements, independent employment assistance, community support and outreach services, housing programs, and legal and financial advisement.
  d. Length of stay is indefinite and members can exit and re-enter a clubhouse community at will.
  e. OT evaluation and intervention is not provided in a formalized manner.
    (1) The role of the OT is integrated into the clubhouse model which has staff acting as generalists who contribute to the development and enrichment of members' abilities and the promotion of their recovery.

9. Adult day care.
  a. Admission is for adults and elders with chronic physical and/or psychosocial impairments, and/or for individuals who are frail but semi-independent.
  b. Services are provided in a congregate or group setting.
  c. Individual schedules will vary.
    (1) Flexibility in scheduling is provided to address daily caregiver needs and allow for planned respite.
    (2) Schedules can range from one afternoon per week to 5 full days.
  d. Length of stay is indefinite.
    (1) Ongoing services are provided to individuals with chronic conditions who might otherwise be institutionalized or to individuals who are frail and need ongoing support (e.g., cooked meals, socialization opportunities).
  e. OT evaluation is focused on the individual's functional skills and deficits in the areas of occupation, his/her home environment, and the adult day center's environment.
  f. OT intervention focus.
    (1) Maintenance of the healthy, functional aspects of the individual and facilitation of adaptation to impairments.

(2) Engagement in purposeful activities that provide appropriate stimulation, reflect life-long interests, develop new interests, and foster a sense of community with other participants.
(3) Caregiver education, support groups, home visits, consultations, and referrals to community resources.
(4) Modifications to the day care center's environment and the individual's home environment to maximize the person's comfort in, and mastery and control of, these environments.

10. Outpatient/ambulatory care.
    a. Admission is for a medical or psychiatric condition that is not serious enough to warrant hospitalization or for a condition that has sufficiently stabilized to enable the individual to be discharged from a hospital but remaining symptoms require active treatment.
    b. Treatment is usually provided in short 30–60 minute sessions once a day for up to 5 days a week.
    c. Length of stay is determined by diagnosis, presenting symptoms, response to treatment, and insurance coverage or ability to pay a fee for service.
    d. OT evaluation focused on the individual's client factors and functional assets and deficits in his/her performance skills and patterns, areas of occupation, and his/her home, work and leisure environments.
    e. OT intervention focus.
        (1) Active engagement of the client in the treatment planning, implementation, re-evaluation, and discharge process.
        (2) Remediation of underlying performance skill deficits that affect functional occupational performance.
        (3) Functional improvements in performance areas and occupational roles.
        (4) Compensatory strategies for remaining performance skill deficits and client factors.
        (5) Consumer, family, and caregiver education.
11. Home health care.
    a. Acceptance criteria for home health services.
        (1) Presence of a medical or psychiatric condition that is not serious enough to warrant hospitalization or for a condition that has sufficiently stabilized to enable the individual to be discharged from a hospital but that still has remaining symptoms requiring active treatment.
        (2) Reimbursers can have strict and variable criteria for qualifying for home health care. See earlier section on Medicare and third party reimbursement.
    b. Treatment is usually provided in 60-minute sessions, once a day for up to 5 days a week, as determined by insurance coverage.
    c. Length of stay is determined by diagnosis, presenting symptoms, response to treatment, insurance coverage, or ability to pay a fee for service.
    d. OT evaluation is focused on the individual's client factors and functional skills and deficits in his/her performance skills and patterns, areas of occupation, and the occupational roles that are required in the current and expected environment(s).
    e. OT intervention focus.
        (1) Active engagement of the client, family, and caregivers in the treatment planning, implementation, and re-evaluation process.
        (2) Functional improvement in areas of occupation and occupational role functioning within the home.
        (3) Remediation of underlying performance skill deficits and compensation for client factors that affect functional performance within the home.
        (4) Education of the family, caregivers, and/or home health aides to provide appropriate care and/or assistance as needed.
        (5) Environmental modifications and activity adaptations that maintain optimal functioning and improve quality of life.
        (6) Increasing ability to resume occupational roles outside of the home.
        (7) Prevention of hospitalization and avoidance or delay of residential institutional placement.
12. Hospice.
    a. Acceptance criteria for hospice services.
        (1) Terminal illness that has a life expectancy of 6 months or less.
    b. Services are most often provided in the home with the type and quantity of services determined by the needs of the individual, his/her family, significant others, and caregivers.
        (1) Hospice services may also be provided in an independent facility or in a special unit of a SNF or a hospital.
    c. Length of stay is determined by the person's terminal outcome.
    d. OT evaluation is focused on determining the individual's occupational functioning and his/her physical, psychosocial, spiritual, and environmental needs that are most important to him/her.
    e. OT intervention focus.

(1) Maintenance of the individual's control over his/her life.
(2) Facilitation of engagement in meaningful occupations and purposeful activities that are consistent with the individual's roles, values, choices, interests, aspirations, abilities, and hopes and that contribute to a satisfactory quality of life.
(3) Reduction or removal of distressing symptoms and pain.
(4) Environmental modifications and activity adaptations that maintain optimal functioning and improve quality of life.
(5) Caregiver and family education and support to maintain optimal functioning and improve quality of life for all.

13. Case management programs.
 a. There are two different focuses to case management programs: one is clinical, one is administrative.
  (1) Clinical case management provides individualized support and intervention to a client with a serious illness which significantly limits his/her ability to access and/or engage in existing community services and/or therapeutic programs, ensuring that the person is able to remain in the community and not be re-hospitalized.
  (2) Administrative case management connects a person with a serious illness to the appropriate and needed community services and/or therapeutic programs, overseeing this service provision to ensure that quality of care in a cost-effective manner is achieved.
 b. Services can be provided in an office and/or in the individual's home and community.
 c. Length of stay is determined by the individual's ability to independently access needed services and by funding availability.
 d. OT evaluation is focused on the individual's client factors and functional skills and deficits in his/her performance skills and patterns, areas of occupation, and the occupational roles that are required in his/her current expected environment.
  (1) Assessment of the individual's supports and barriers for community integration is critical.
 e. Case management interventions can be purely referral-based in the administrative model or encompass the full range of interventions in the clinical model, (e.g., one-on-one counseling, family education, ADL training, community re-entry, etc.).
  (1) Both models aim to prevent regression and re-hospitalization and promote optimal functioning and quality of life.
  (2) Both models actively engage the individual and family in treatment planning, implementation, and the reevaluation process.
  (3) Both models plan discharge, if appropriate, to an environment that will best serve an individual's needs.

14. Wellness and prevention programs.
 a. Acceptance is most often by individual's self-referral to meet a personal need or by an institution's provision of a program to its members or employees (e.g., a parenting skills class for pregnant teens in a school).
 b. Programs have been developed to serve populations considered at risk and are held in offices or individual's residences and/or at community sites.
 c. Length of stay is determined by the individual. It is usually influenced by program's planned length (e.g., a six-week joint protection program) or by individual's achievement of a desired outcome (e.g., smoking cessation).
 d. OT evaluation focuses on risk factors for illnesses and disabilities and the individual's functional skills and deficits in the occupational roles that are required in his/her current and expected environment.
 e. OT intervention focus.
  (1) Disease prevention and health promotion.
  (2) Interventions can range from the traditional domain of OT (e.g., home safety and environmental modifications), to contemporary areas of concern (e.g., stress management, life coaching).
  (3) Refer to Chapter 3 for definitions of and specific interventions for primary, secondary, and tertiary prevention.

Private/Independent Practice

1. In any and all of the above community and institutional settings, the OT practitioner can work in an entrepreneurial manner by negotiating a fee for service agreement and/or a long term contract.
2. Private practitioners can also open their own free-standing clinics.
3. A provider number is required for a private practitioner to receive third party payment.
4. Private practitioners must abide by all state and third party payer regulations for evaluation, intervention, and documentation.

Service Management

Management Principles, Functions, and Strategies

1. Managers that have a positive attitude about change and innovation fosters best practice.
2. Successful management supports open communication, team building, decentralization of resources, and the sharing of power.
3. Managers that utilize strategic thinking in a systems model can respond proactively to market demands and changes.
4. The use of different management styles (i.e., the manager's characteristic way of performing management tasks) has a significant impact on productivity, change and growth. See text's section on leadership styles.
5. Managers' understanding and application of theories of motivation and behavior facilitates appropriate and effective responses to situations, fosters program efficacy, and promotes employee satisfaction.
6. Administrative functions of management include program development, fiscal and personnel management, and program evaluation.
   a. Subsequent chapter sections provide specific information about each major function.
7. Management by Objective (MBO): a complete system of management based upon a core set of goals to be accomplished by a program.
   a. Mission and goals are established.
   b. Measurable objectives are quantified.
   c. Specific time frames for accomplishment of objectives are established.
   d. Staff training needs and deterrents to progress are identified.
   e. Program evaluation is instituted.

Program Development

1. Purposes of developing specific programs.
   a. To directly meet the needs of a specific population(s) or group(s).
   b. To clearly focus evaluation and intervention efforts and activities.
   c. To increase visibility and use of available services (e.g., offering an outpatient cardiac rehabilitation program is more visible than individual referrals, resulting in increased recognition and utilization of this service).
   d. To convert an idea into a practice reality.
2. Four basic steps of program development.
   a. Needs assessment.
      (1) Describe the community; its physical, social, cultural and economic factors; and populations at risk.
      (2) Describe the target population's demographics, disorder(s), functional level(s), and presenting problem(s).
      (3) Identify specific needs of target population.
         (a) Perceived needs of the population as reported by others (e.g., family, physicians, other professionals).
         (b) Felt needs as stated by the individual members of the target population.
         (c) Real needs, which are the actual disabilities and functional limitations of the target population.
      (4) Determine discrepancy between real needs and felt needs.
      (5) Establish unmet needs according to priority.
      (6) Identify resources available for program implementation.
         (a) Formal or institutional resources such as staff, supplies, money, space.
         (b) Informal resources such as family, friends, cultural or religious figures, self-help/consumer groups.
      (7) Needs assessment methods.
         (a) Survey, interview, or self report of target population. A representative sample is required.
         (b) Key informant, which involves the surveying of specific individuals who are knowledgeable about the target population needs.
         (c) Community forums to obtain information through public meetings or panels.
         (d) Service utilization review of records and reports.
         (e) Analysis of social indicators to identify social, cultural, environmental, and/or economic factors that can predict problems.
   b. Program planning.
      (1) Define a focus for the program based on the needs assessment results.
         (a) Problem areas, functional limitations, and unmet needs that are relevant to the majority of the target population are the priority focus.
         (b) Program level of difficulty as determined by the range of population's functional levels

and the level required by the current and expected environment.

(2) Adopt a frame or frames of reference that are most likely to successfully address and meet the needs that are program's focus.

(3) Establish objectives and goals of the program specifically related to primary focus.

(a) Individual goals which will be met by the program are set.

(b) Programmatic goals which establish standards for program evaluation are determined.

(4) Describe integration of program into existing system of care.

(a) Establish realistic timetable for program implementation.

(b) Define staff roles, responsibilities, and assignments.

(c) Identify methods for professional collaboration.

(d) Determine the physical setting and space requirements.

(e) Consider potential barriers to program implementation.

(f) Develop methods to effectively deal with identified obstacles before program implementation.

(5) Develop a system of referral for entry into, completion of, and discharge from the program.

(a) Evaluation protocols to standardize information to be obtained from each person referred to the program and to assess the type of program services needed.

(b) Criteria for acceptance into the program and for movement through program levels.

(c) Discharge criteria to determine when an individual has achieved maximum gain from the program, usually defined as the achievement of program goals.

(6) Describe the fiscal implications of program plan.

(a) Determine projected volume or service demand to estimate revenue.

(b) Identify resource utilization and projected expenses to estimate costs.

(c) Directly compare estimated revenue and estimated expenses to determine financial viability of program.

c. Program implementation.

(1) Initiate program according to timetable and steps set forth in the program plan.

(2) Document program activities, procedures, and use.

(3) Communicate and coordinate with other programs within the system.

(4) Promote program to ensure it reaches target population.

d. Program evaluation. See this chapter's section on program evaluation and quality improvement.

Fiscal Management

1. Purposes of fiscal management.

a. To ensure cost-effective services and programs are planned and implemented.

b. To meet the demands of a managed health care system.

c. To remain competitive in a market-driven practice environment.

2. Major fiscal management tasks.

a. Develop revenue and volume projections.

b. Use cost-effective charging procedures and fee structures.

c. Manage payroll and staffing budgets.

d. Schedule staff in a cost-effective manner that meets productivity standards.

e. Plan for short- and long-term program needs including capital expenses.

f. Manage general, administrative, and operating expenses.

g. Meet organization's revenue expectations.

3. Budget terms and concepts.

a. A budget financially projects, for a specified time period, the costs of managing a program and the anticipated revenue from service provision.

b. Budget periods vary from multi-year (5–10 years) for capital expenses to annual for personnel and supply expenses.

c. Budget revisions may be needed as program(s) or service(s) change due to ongoing program evaluation.

d. Capital expense budgets.

(1) Permanent or long term purchases such as an ADL kitchen or for new facilities, such as a new wing for a work hardening program.

(2) Typically any item or action above a fixed amount (e.g., $500.00) is considered a capital expense.

(3) Capital items are separated from other expenses due to depreciation of value and possible tax credits for purchases and investments.

e. Operating expense budgets.

(1) The daily financial activity of a program or service.

(2) Information on revenue, volume, and direct and indirect expenses.

(a) Direct expenses include costs related to OT service provision, such as salaries and benefits (e.g., vacation and sick time), office supplies (e.g., pen, paper), and treatment equipment (e.g., ADL materials).

(b) Indirect expenses include costs shared by the setting as a whole such as utilities, housekeeping, and marketing.
(c) Fixed expenses remain at the same level even when there are changes in the amount of services provided (e.g., rent).
(d) Variable expenses change in direct proportion to the amount of services provided (e.g., splinting materials).

f. Full-time equivalent (FTE).
(1) The amount of time a full-time staff employee works; in the United States, 8 hours/day, 5 days/week.
(2) A budget formula used to determine the number of personnel providing direct care.
(a) Two practitioners who do administrative tasks half of the day and direct care half of the day would equal one FTE.
(b) Three part-time employees would equal 1.5 FTEs.

g. Productivity standards.
(1) Establishes the amount of direct care and reimbursable service(s) each therapist is to provide per day.
(2) Managed care pressures have increased productivity expectations in some practice areas resulting in ethical dilemmas and/or ethical distress.

h. Break-even analysis.
(1) Also called cost-volume-profit analysis.
(2) Determines the volume of services needed to be provided for revenues to equal cost and profits to equal zero.

i. Accounts payable.
(1) The debts within a budget.
(2) Indicates payments that are due for purchases or services rendered (e.g., to an equipment supplier, a landlord).

j. Accounts receivable.
(1) The assets within a budget.
(2) Indicates payments that are owed to the program, setting, or institution (e.g., consultation fees).

Personnel Management

1. The oversight of OT practitioners and support personnel and the services they provide.
2. Purposes of personnel management.
a. To serve as the link between the individuals working for an organization and the larger organizational structure.
b. To attain best practice from personnel.
3. Major personnel management tasks.
a. Design work roles and write job descriptions.
b. Recruit, select, and orient personnel to perform the roles.
c. Supervise and evaluate personnel to ensure adequate role performance and the attainment of organizational goals.
d. Support personnel's ongoing professional development.
e. Deal with difficult personnel issues as they arise.
4. Job description: a statement of the job's expectations, duties, and purpose and its supervisory relationships. It should include:
a. Position's title and department.
b. Skilled and non-skilled requirements of the job including education, special training, experience, physical demands, and licensure requirements.
c. Specific responsibilities, duties, and performance standards in detail.
d. Supervisor(s) and supervisory relationships: decision making authority and degree of autonomy.
5. Recruitment: the process of determining staffing needs, predicting turnover and vacancies, and identifying and recruiting potential replacements to maintain the staffing levels required to meet program objectives.
a. Identify the position available and determine its job description.
b. Attract potential qualified applicants.
(1) Advertise in trade publications, state and national OT association newsletters, and/or on-line.
(2) Network internally within own organization and externally at local, state, and/or national OT meetings and conferences and through established OT contacts.
(3) Conduct open houses, job fairs, and workshop.
(4) Direct mail recruitment information to OT practitioners.
(5) Use placement agencies.
(6) Train and educate fieldwork students.
c. Screen interested applicants for an interview.
(1) Review applications and resumes.
(2) Check references.
d. Interview screened applicants to determine suitability for position.
(1) Obtain information about relevant experience and career goals.
(2) Verify knowledge and skills.
(3) Use open-ended semi-structured questions to facilitate discussion.
(4) Ask the same questions of every candidate.
(5) Take notes of applicants' responses.
(6) Questions to the applicant that violate civil rights legislation or ADA should not be asked.
(a) Age.
(b) Sexual orientation.
(c) Marital status or family composition.
(d) Race or national origin, religion, or political beliefs.
(e) Physical, mental, or cognitive disabilities.

(7) Share information about the position's salary, benefits, work hours, job description, and advantages and limitations of the organization.

e. Make the job offer.

(1) Contact selected applicant to offer position.

(2) Upon applicant's acceptance of position, confirm terms of employment, starting date, salary, and licensure requirements.

6. Orientation of staff.

a. The process of providing specific information to a new employee to increase the ease and effectiveness of his/her transition into his/her new position.

(1) Introduce key coworkers, managers, and department heads.

(2) Provide specific information about the organization's and department's mission, policies, and procedures.

(3) Distribute manuals, checklists, and/or handouts with recommended standards on how to perform required tasks competently.

(4) Tour the facility and department to learn locations of resources, support services, equipment, and materials.

7. Supervision of personnel. See this chapter's section on supervision.

8. Performance evaluation/appraisal.

a. The process of evaluating staff performance according to established performance expectations.

b. Steps in performance appraisal.

(1) Articulate specific and clear expectations for performance.

(2) Document positive performance to substantiate quality care and to support recommendations for merit pay, raises, bonuses, and/or promotions.

(3) Document substandard performance to identify areas requiring quality improvement, further training, increased supervision, and/or disciplinary action.

(4) Meet privately with employee to discuss written performance appraisal, allow employee feedback, and develop a plan for remediation, if needed, and a plan for ongoing professional development.

9. Disciplinary action.

a. The process of informing an employee that his/her job performance is unacceptable, the organization's procedures for an administrative review of disciplinary actions and the organization's employee grievance procedures.

b. Criteria for fair disciplinary action.

(1) Written documentation of problem behaviors and expectations for improvement.

(2) Referral to counseling and/or other services needed to improve performance.

(3) Clear and documented warnings of consequences for unremediated behavior.

(4) Consequences that are impersonal, immediate, and consistent.

(5) Continuous documented monitoring of employee's behavior until the employee achieves satisfactory job performance, resigns voluntarily, or is terminated.

10. Retention and motivation of staff.

a. The process of identifying understanding, and meeting employees' needs, expectations, and desired rewards.

b. Motivating job characteristics.

(1) A fair and competitive salary and benefits package.

(2) Job security, realistic performance expectations, and fair employment policies.

(3) A good working environment with a relaxed, friendly atmosphere, adequate physical space, and sufficient current equipment and supplies.

(4) Challenging, satisfying work and diverse caseloads.

(5) Competent supervision with adequate feedback on job performance.

(6) Active mentorship and support for professional development.

(7) Tuition reimbursement and financial support for conferences, workshops, and/or post-professional education.

(8) Recognition of contributions and achievements.

11. Staff development.

a. The process of continually upgrading employees' knowledge and skills to provide competent, current, and caring OT services in changing and challenging delivery systems.

b. Staff development steps.

(1) Assess employees' development needs and interests.

(2) Assess organization's strategic plan to identify existing and new areas planned for OT service that may require staff training.

(3) Provide mentorship and supervision.

(4) Provide educational in-services, workshops, and practical on-site experiences.

(5) Support self-directed learning, such as journal reviews, self-study courses, on-line networking, teleconferencing, off-site workshops, and/or post-professional education.

Program Evaluation and Quality Improvement

1. The systematic review and analysis of care provided to determine if this care is at an acceptable level of quality.
2. Purposes of program evaluation.

a. To measure the effectiveness of a program; that is, were program goals accomplished.
b. To use information obtained in the evaluation to improve services and assure quality.
c. To meet external accreditation standards (see this chapter's section on voluntary accreditation).
d. To identify program problems/limitations and to resolve them.

3. Major types and terms.
   a. Quality improvement (QI): a system-oriented approach that views limitations and problems proactively as opportunities to increase quality.
      (1) Prevention is emphasized.
      (2) Blame is not attributed to persons; problems are related to organizational improvement needs.
   b. Total quality management (TQM): the creation of an organizational culture that enables all employees to contribute to an environment of continuous improvement to meet or exceed consumer needs.
   c. Performance assessment and improvement (PAI): a systematic method to evaluate the appropriateness and quality of services.
      (1) Utilization of an interdisciplinary systems focus.
      (2) A client-centered approach which focuses on the rights, assessment, care, and education of the person.
      (3) Organizational ethics, improved organizational performance, leadership, and management are emphasized.
   d. Goal attainment scaling (GAS): an evaluation tool that attains clients' goals for intervention and measures goal attainment and intervention outcomes after a specified time period.
      (1) See Chapter 14.
   e. Utilization review: a plan to review the use of resources within a facility.
      (1) Determination of medical necessity and cost efficiency.
      (2) Often a component of a QI or PAI system.
   f. Statistical utilization review: reimbursement claims data are analyzed to determine the most efficient and cost-effective care.
   g. Peer review: a system in which the quality of work of a group of health professionals is reviewed by their peers.
   h. Professional review organization (PRO): groups of peers who evaluate the appropriateness of services and quality of care under reimbursement and/or state licensure requirements.
   i. Prospective review.
      (1) Evaluation of proposed intervention plan that specifies how and why care will be provided.
      (2) Used by third party payers to approve proposed occupational therapy intervention program.
   j. Concurrent review.
      (1) Evaluation of ongoing intervention program during hospitalization, outpatient, or home care treatment.
      (2) Method to ensure appropriate care is being delivered.
      (3) Often a component of a QI or PAI system.
   k. Retrospective review.
      (1) Audits of medical records after intervention were rendered.
      (2) Method to ensure appropriate care was given.
      (3) A UR tool for third party payers that can be time consuming and costly.
   l. Risk management: a process that identifies, evaluates, and takes corrective action against risk and plans, organizes and controls the activities and resources of OT services to decrease actual or potential losses.
      (1) Potential risks are client or employee injury and property loss or damage with resulting liability and financial loss.
      (2) Occupational therapists are responsible to ensure proper maintenance of equipment and a safe treatment environment.
      (3) Staff education and training (e.g., annual certification/recertification in CPR) is required.
      (4) Effective communication with consumers (e.g., informed consent) and with team members is required.
      (5) Risk management is an integral part of program evaluation.
      (6) If risk management fails and an incident occurs, completion of an incident report according to setting's standards is required.

4. Methods of program evaluation.
   a. Describe program objectives and goals to determine program outcome criteria.
   b. Identify measurable indicators based on objectives and goals.
   c. Describe population, staff, services provided, intervention methods, scope of care, and length of treatment.
   d. Design an evaluation study.
   e. Select methods to collect data.
      (1) Direct observation and/or review of client charts.
      (2) Safety checklists, incident reports, and/or client/family complaints.
      (3) Surveys of clients, families and/or staff.
      (4) Review of treatment sessions and missed treatments.
      (5) Initial, discharge, and follow-up assessments.
      (6) Review of statistics on costs and service volume.
   f. Collect and organize data.
   g. Evaluate and analyze results and limitations of the study.

h. Report results, highlighting information to determine program's efficacy.
i. Use results to initiate appropriate program actions.
   (1) Continue and/or expand programs that have demonstrated good efficacy/positive outcomes.
   (2) Change or modify programs that have demonstrated limited efficacy/satisfactory outcomes.
   (3) Discontinue programs that have demonstrated poor efficacy/unsatisfactory outcomes.
j. Evaluate effectiveness of actions.

Marketing/Promotion

1. A managerial process that analyzes consumer need(s), plans and designs a service or product to meet the identified market need(s), and implements strategies and actions to promote consumer use of the service or product.
2. Major marketing tasks.
   a. Analyze market opportunities.
      (1) Conduct a self audit to assess the strengths and weaknesses of oneself and/or one's organization.
      (2) Conduct a consumer analysis to determine consumer need(s) and desire(s) for services or products.
      (3) Identify potential competitors to clarify areas of service overlap/product similarity and to identify areas that are underserved or unserved.
      (4) Assess the environment to determine political, sociocultural, economic, and/or demographic factors that may impact on the product(s) or service(s).
   b. Analyze the market to be targeted for purchase of product(s) or service(s).
      (1) Research selected target market(s) to determine validity of perceived market needs and wants.
      (2) Divide market into segments to identify groups of consumers with similar characteristics, interests, and needs that will influence their purchase of the product(s) or service(s).
   c. Develop marketing strategies to address the 5 Ps (product, price, place, promotion, and position) of a market plan for the OT service.
      (1) Product: the service or thing that is being offered to the market (e.g., a work hardening program, adaptive equipment).
      (2) Price: the financial, physical, and psychological cost of doing business.
      (3) Place: the distribution method for getting a product or service to the target market for providing the target market with access to the product or service.
      (4) Promotion: all efforts to communicate information about the product or service to the target market or market segment that makes the product or service visible and desirable.
      (5) Position: the place the product or service holds in relation to similar products or services available in the marketplace.
   d. Implement and evaluate the marketing plan.
      (1) The implementation and evaluation of marketing efforts must always consider ethics (i.e., truth in advertising).
      (2) Undifferentiated marketing: the use of the same marketing strategies and activities with the complete market (e.g., promoting the OT profession to the general public).
      (3) Differentiated marketing: the design and use of marketing strategies and activities for different market segments (e.g., promoting OT specialties to different consumer self-help groups).
      (4) Concentrated marketing: the design and use of specific marketing strategies and activities to concentrate on one market segment (e.g., the elderly).
      (5) Ongoing assessment and periodic review is needed to determine market plan's effectiveness and to modify, as needed.
3. Methods
   a. Marketing instruments that can be employed to address the 5 Ps include:
      (1) Advertising and publicity releases.
      (2) Sales promotions, discounts, and bonuses.
      (3) Personal contact selling and networking.
      (4) Word of mouth recommendations.

Fieldwork Education

1. A key service management function is to develop, implement, and support clinical fieldwork education for OT and OTA students.
   a. ACOTE guidelines for Level I and Level II fieldwork education are to be followed.
   b. Supervisory qualifications and guidelines for fieldwork educators are provided in this chapter's section on OT practitioner roles and supervision.
2. Fieldwork education managerial tasks.
   a. Collaboration with the academic education program to develop specific fieldwork learning objectives and activities consistent with the facilities' and school's philosophies and missions.
   b. Development of professional development plans and activities for the students' clinical supervisors to ensure adequate fieldwork supervision.

c. Establishment of departmental policies and procedures for a student program and its supervision.
d. Assurance of quality care provided by student(s) according to established program standards and professional ethics.
e. Evaluation and supervision of students' performance and completion of ACOTE's evaluation tool.
f. Completion of cost-benefit analysis to collect data for institutional support of clinical education.

Research

Purposes of Research

1. Critical evaluation and consumption of research literature enhances one's theoretical and philosophical foundations, improves clinical reasoning and critical thinking, increases professional knowledge and skills, and facilitates evidence-based decision-making.
2. Application of research literature ensures practice is current, meaningful, and competent which ultimately improves the quality of life of individuals receiving OT services.
3. Knowledge of research provides opportunities to address questions that arise daily in professional practice.
4. The development and implementation of research projects that test and establish the efficacy of OT evaluation and intervention is essential to the provision of evidence-based practice (EBP).
   a. Establishment of the relevance and efficacy of OT can influence public health, social and educational policy, thereby impacting on the delivery of OT services.
   b. Recent legislation (e.g. IDEA 2004 and No Child Left Behind) place increase emphasis on the provision of EBP.
5. Acquisition of scientific knowledge can provide answers to practice questions and help solve problems encountered in practice.
6. Development of a body of professional research contributes to the science of a profession and provides a body of knowledge to guide practitioners.
7. Participation in research to evaluate program outcomes is a requirement of most practice settings and accrediting bodies.

Quantitative Methodology/ Design Types

1. True-experimental: the classic two-group design which includes random selection and assignment into an experimental group that receives treatment or a control group that receives no treatment. All other experiences are kept similar.
   a. The two levels of treatment (some and none) together constitute the independent variable being manipulated.
   b. The comparison of their status on some variable (i.e., the outcome) that might be influenced by treatment constitutes the dependent variable.
   c. A cause and effect relationship between the independent and dependent variable is examined.
   d. In human subject research, it is often difficult to design pure experimental designs.
2. Quasi-experimental: an independent variable is manipulated to determine its effect on a dependent variable but there is a lesser degree of researcher control and/or no randomization.
   a. Used often in health care research in which it is unethical to control or withhold treatment.
   b. Used to study intact groups created by events or natural processes.
3. Non-experimental/correlational: there is no manipulation of independent variable; randomization and researcher control are not possible.
   a. Used to study the potential relationships between two or more existing variables (e.g., attendance at a day program and social interaction skills).
   b. Describes relationships, predicts relationships among variables without active manipulation of the variables.
   c. Limitations.
      (1) Cannot establish cause and effect relationships; limits interpretation of results.
      (2) May fail to consider all variables that enter into a relationship.
   d. Degree of relationship is expressed as correlational coefficient, ranging from −1.00 and +1.00.
   e. Examples of correlation research.
      (1) Retrospective: investigation of data collected in the past.
      (2) Prospective: recording and investigation of present data.
      (3) Descriptive: investigation of several variables at once; determines existing relationships among variables.
      (4) Predictive: used to develop predictive models.

f. Can be "ex post facto" (after the fact) research because variables may be studied after their occurrence (e.g., post-diagnosis adjustment).

Qualitative Methodology/Design Types

1. A form of descriptive research that studies people, individually or collectively, in their natural social and cultural context.
2. A systematic, subjective approach to describe real-life experiences and give them meaning.
3. It is rich in verbal descriptions of people and phenomena based on direct observation in naturalistic settings.
4. The process of the study is considered as important as the specific outcome data.
5. Types of qualitative research.
   a. Phenomenological: a study of one or more persons and how they make sense of their experience.
      (1) Minimal interpretations by the investigator.
      (2) Meanings can only be ascribed by participants.
   b. Ethnographic: patterns and characteristics of a cultural group, including values, roles, beliefs, and normative practices, are intensely studied.
      (1) Extensive field observations, interviews, participant observation, examination of literature and materials, and cultural immersion are used.
      (2) Used in health care to understand an insider's perspective to develop meaningful services (e.g., a study of a nursing home).
   c. Heuristic: complete involvement of the researcher in the experience of the subject(s) to understand and interpret a phenomenon.
      (1) Aim is to understand human experience and its meaning.
      (2) Meanings can only be understood if personally experienced.
   d. Case study: a single subject or a group of subjects is investigated in an in-depth manner.
      (1) Purpose can be description, interpretation, or evaluation.
      (2) This method is easy to use in most practice settings.
6. To attain rigor in qualitative research, the trustworthiness of a study should be critiqued and are strategies to increase trustworthiness should be employed. Trustworhiness criteria include:
   a. Credibility: the researcher's level of confidence that his/her findings truthfully reflect the reality of a study's participants and the study's context.
      (1) Credibility is attained when the researcher does not have preconceived notions about a study and allows for multiple truths to emerge from the findings, as revealed by the participants.
         (a) Credibility can be enhanced by extended and varied field experience, reflexivity via completion of a field journal, sampling, triangulation of data, interview techniques, and member checks.
   b. Transferability: how well other researchers can fit a study's findings into similar conrexts; the "goodness of fit" between the contexts of two studies.
      (1) Transferability is evident when a researcher provides sufficient descriptive data to allow comparison by other researchers.
         (a) Transferability can be enhanced by use of a nominated sample, comparision of sample characteristics to available demographic data, and dense description of the study's participants and contexts.
   c. Dependability: the inclusion of the full range of data, including outlier or atypical findings.
      (1) Dependability is attained when all participants' experiences/perspectives are considered important and reported.
         (a) Dependability can be enhanced by a dependability audit, triangulation of data, comprehensive description of research methods, peer review, member check, code-recode procedures, and step-wise replication.
   d. Confirmability: the degree to which a study's conclusions are based on the data.
      (1) Confirmability is attained when data is truthful.
      (2) Confirmability can be enhanced by a confirmabillity audit, member check, researcher reflexivity, and triangulation of data.

Essentials of the Research Process

1. Formulation of a philosophical foundation to reflect researcher's view of, and assumptions about, learning, human behavior, and other phenomena related to health and human services.
2. Identification of a broad issue, topic or problem of interest and relevance that warrants scientific investigation.
3. Review and synthesis of research literature related to identified area of interest.
   a. Conduct a comprehensive and systematic literature search.
      (1) Define the parameters and boundaries of the search according to the research question's main concepts and constructs.
      (2) Use databases, indices, and abstracts along with the support of a reference librarian.

(3) Organize literature obtained according to relevance and concepts and take notes to summarize content.
(4) Critically evaluate literature reviewed (see 3b below).
(5) Recognize that the literature may need to be re-visited and/or re-searched as the study progresses and/or when its results are analyzed.

b. Critique of published research.
(1) Analyze the purpose, relevance, and meaningfulness of the study.
(2) Assess the comprehensiveness of the study's literature review.
(3) Examine the congruence between the purpose, literature, methodology, findings, and conclusions.
(4) Assess the adequacy of the research procedures to address the study's question or focus.
(5) Analyze the comprehensiveness of data analyses, interpretation, conclusions, and limitations.

4. Utilization of a theoretical base to frame the research problem or area of concern to ensure that the resulting research contributes to, or builds upon, theory.
5. Development of a specific question or focus for research.
a. In quantitative/experimental research this is very specific, detailing the exact variables to be studied.
b. In qualitative/naturalistic research, this is a broad question called a "query" that will develop specificity over the course of the study.
6. Selection of a research design.
a. In quantitative/experimental research, the design is highly standardized.
b. In qualitative/naturalistic research, the design is more fluid.
7. Formulation of methodology (see section on research design types).
8. Determination of study's length.
9. Identification of study's participants/population sample.
a. Based on a literature review, the study's hypothesis and goals, determine a target population's desired characteristics.
b. Describe criteria for selecting a sample of the population to be study's participants.
c. Determine sampling method.
(1) Random: individuals are selected through the use of a table of random numbers.
(2) Systematic: individuals are selected from a population list by taking individuals at specified intervals (e.g., every 10th name).
(3) Stratified: individuals are selected from a population's identified subgroups based on some pre-determined characteristic (e.g., by diagnosis) that correlates with the study.
(4) Purposive: individuals are purposefully and deliberately selected for a study (e.g., all consumers of a program for a QI study).
(5) Convenience: individuals are selected who meet population criteria based upon availability to the researcher.
(6) Network/snowball: study subjects provide names of other individuals who can meet study criteria.

d. Obtain informed consent from all participants.

10. Collection of data using established principles for collecting research information.
a. Information obtained must be relevant and sufficient to answer the specific research question or query.
b. The method of data collection selected must be realistic given the practical limitations of the researcher, the type of research design, and the nature of the research problem.
c. Use of a combination of data collection methods can be useful and more fully answer a research question or query.
11. Methods of data collection.
a. Methods range along a continuum from unstructured observations to highly structured, fixed choice questionnaires.
b. Most methods are used in both qualitative and quantitative research.
c. Most methods are used in conjunction with other data collection techniques.
d. Observation.
(1) In quantitative research, observations are structured and formalized.
(2) In qualitative research, observations are unstructured and ever-changing according to the contexts and results of the observations.
(3) Observations may be made of nonhuman objects, such as equipment, or human subjects during actual performance or via videotapes.

e. Interview.
(1) Used to gather information in ethnographic and survey research.
(2) In survey research, interviews can be face-to-face or by telephone.
(3) In ethnographic research, interviews are always face-to-face.

f. Written questionnaires.
(1) In quantitative research, questionnaires must be structured.
(2) In qualitative research, questions may be unstructured.

(3) Distribution may be by mail, e-mail, or in-person, with instructions to complete at that moment or at respondent's convenience and with directions to return the completed questionnaire to researcher by a specific date.
(4) Surveys are a major type of questionnaire used in research.

g. Survey instruments.
(1) Surveys are nonexperimental instruments designed to measure specific characteristics.
(2) Survey questions can be open-ended questions or closed-ended questions.
(a) Semantic differential: a point scale with opposing adjectives at two extremes, measuring affective meaning.
(b) Likert scale: respondents indicate their level of agreement, usually on a five point scale.
(c) Guttmann scale rank ordering: the respondent places a number alongside a list of items, indicating their order of importance. Sometimes only 2–3 items are asked for, other times a whole list may be prioritized. It is difficult (and irrelevant) to prioritize more than 10.
(d) Multiple choice: a statement is provided, sometimes in a question format, and the respondent selects the item most reflective of their opinion. Used to elicit opinions or attitudes.
(e) Incomplete sentences: a phrase is provided to indicate a certain domain of concern and the respondent completes the sentence. Used to find out opinions, attitudes, knowledge, styles of behavior, personality traits.
(3) Survey design research typically uses large samples through mail, telephone, or face-to-face contact.
(4) Benefits of survey research.
(a) The ability to obtain a large number of participants at a relatively low cost.
(b) The ability to measure numerous variables with one instrument.
(c) The ability to use the data obtained in multiple ways through statistical manipulation during data analysis.
(5) Disadvantages to survey research.
(a) Limited or poor response rate.
(b) Missing or inaccurately completed data.
(c) Most disadvantages to survey research can be minimized with the development and use of a good survey instrument; therefore, it is advisable for all researchers to carefully critique and pilot their survey before its use in a research study.

h. Artifact and record review.
(1) Used to gather information in all types of research.
(2) May be the sole data collection method in historical research.
(3) A review of written records can include medical records, publications, letters, and/or minutes of meetings and conferences.
(4) A review of artifacts may include physical items such as personal objects in a person's home, adaptive equipment and/or audiovisuals.

i. Hardware instrumentation.
(1) Mechanical or physical instruments with established reliability and validity that measure independent variables (e.g., goniometers).

j. Tests and assessments.
(1) Use to measure independent variables, (e.g., performance components, interests and values).
(2) Published tests with established reliability and validity are preferred.
(3) If there are no existing tests or assessments available to collect information sought by the research, an instrument can be constructed in accordance with established test construction guidelines.
(4) Refer to Chapter 3 for the psychometric characteristics of evaluations and definitions of assessments.

12. Analysis and interpretation of data using descriptive statistics.
a. Measures of central tendency: a determination of average or typical scores.
(1) Mean: the arithmetic average of all scores.
(a) The most frequently used measure of central tendency; appropriate for interval or ratio data.
(2) Median: the midpoint, 50% of scores are above the median and 50% of scores are below; appropriate for ordinal data.
(3) Mode: the most frequently occurring score; appropriate for nominal data.
b. Measures of variability: a determination of the spread of a group of scores.
(1) Range: the difference between the highest score and the lowest score.
(2) Standard deviation (SD): a determination of variability of scores (difference) from the mean.
(a) The most frequently used measure of variability.
(b) Appropriate with interval or ratio data.
(3) Normal distribution: a symmetrical bell-shaped curve indicating the distribution of scores; the mean, median, and mode are similar.

(a) Half the scores are above the mean and half the scores are below the mean.
(b) Most scores are near the mean, approximately 68% of scores fall within +1 or −1 SD of the mean.
(c) Frequency of scores decreases further from the mean.
(d) Distribution may be skewed (not symmetrical) rather than normal: scores are extreme, clustered at one end or the other; the mean, median, and mode are different.

(4) Percentiles and quartiles: describe a score's position within the distribution, relative to all other scores.
(a) Percentiles: data is divided in 100 equal parts; position of score is determined.
(b) Quartiles: data is divided into 4 equal parts and position of score is placed accordingly.

13. Analysis and interpretation of data using inferential statistics.
a. Determines how likely the results of a study of a sample can be generalized to the whole population.
b. Standard error of measurement: an estimate of expected errors in an individual's score; a measure of response stability or reliability.
c. Tests of significance: an estimation of true differences, not due to chance; a rejection of the null hypothesis.
(1) Alpha level: pre-selected level of statistical significance.
(a) Most commonly .05 or .01: indicates that the expected difference is due to chance, e.g., at .05, only 5 times out of every 100 or a 5% chance, often expressed as a value of P.
(b) There are true differences on the measured dependent variable.
(2) Degrees of freedom: based on number of subjects and number of groups; allows determination of level of significance based on consulting appropriate tables for each statistical test.
(3) Errors.
(a) Standard error: expected chance variation among the means, the result of sampling error.
(b) Type I error: the null hypothesis is rejected by the researcher when it is true, e.g., the means of scores are concluded to be truly different when the differences are due to chance.
(c) Type II error: the null hypothesis is not rejected by the researcher when it is false, e.g., the means of scores are concluded to be due to chance when the means are truly different.

d. Parametric statistics: testing is based on population parameters; includes tests of significance based on interval or ratio data.
(1) T test: a parametric test of significance used to compare two group means and identify a difference at a selected probability level (e.g., 0.05).
(2) Analysis of variance (ANOVA): a parametric test used to compare two or more treatment groups or conditions at a selected probability level.
(3) Analysis of covariance (ANCOVA): a parametric test used to compare two or more treatment groups or conditions while also controlling for the effects of intervening variables (covariates), e.g., two groups of subjects are compared on the basis of upper extremity functional reach using two different types of assistive devices; subjects in one group have longer arms than subjects in the second group; arm length then becomes the covariate that must be controlled during statistical analysis.

e. Nonparametric statistics: testing not based on population parameters; includes tests of significance based on ordinal or nominal data.
(1) Used when above parametric assumptions cannot be met; less powerful than parametric tests, more difficult to reject the null hypothesis.
(2) Chi square test: a nonparametric test of significance used to compare data in the form of frequency counts occurring in two or more mutually exclusive categories, e.g., subjects rate treatment preferences.

f. Correlational statistics: used to determine relationships between two variables; e.g., compare progression of radiologically observed joint destruction in rheumatoid arthritis and its relationship to demographic variables (gender, age), disease severity, and exercise frequency.
(1) Pearson product-moment coefficient (r): used to correlate interval or ratio data.
(2) Spearman's rank correlation coefficient (rs): a nonparametric test used to correlate ordinal data.
(3) Intraclass correlation coefficient (ICC): a reliability coefficient based on an analysis of variance.
(4) Strength of relationships: positive correlations range from 0 to +1.0; indicates as variable X increases, so does variable Y.
(a) High correlations: 0.70 to +1.00.
(b) Moderate correlations: 0.35 to 0.69.
(c) Low correlations: 0 to 0.34.

(d) 0 means no relationship between variables.
(e) Negative correlations range from −1.0 to 0: indicates as variable X increases, variable Y decreases; an inverse relationship.

(5) Common variance: a representation of the degree that variation in one variable is attributable to another variable.

14. Report and dissemination of research findings.
   a. Results section.
      (1) In quantitative/experimental research, report all factual data with no interpretation.
      (2) In quantitative/experimental research report all findings with no bias towards reporting only results supportive of the study's hypothesis.
      (3) In qualitative/naturalistic research, results, conclusions, and interpretation are discussed in an integrated manner.
         (a) Descriptions, illustrative quotations, and brief examples are used.
         (b) Writing format used depends on the qualitative/naturalistic design of the study.
   b. Conclusions section.
      (1) Interpretation of the results.
      (2) Comparison of study's findings to those presented in the literature review.
      (3) Analysis of findings supportive and nonsupportive of the hypothesis.
   c. Summary.
      (1) Major contributions, practical or theoretical implications that can be drawn from the study.
      (2) Brief suggestions for improvements to the study's design and procedures.
      (3) Proposals for new research based on study's findings.

Ethical Considerations

1. Participants must be provided with full disclosure of study's purpose, methodology, and the nature and scope of expected participation.
2. Participants must be informed of any potential risk or discomforts and a plan to remediate risk or discomfort must be developed and provided to participants.
3. Participation in the study must be voluntary.
   a. Participants' right to withdraw from a study must be protected.
   b. Participants' refusal to answer certain questions and/or participate in a specific procedure must be respected and honored.
4. Confidentiality of all participants identifying information must be ensured at all times.
5. Institutional Review Board (IRB) approval must be obtained for all human subject research.
   a. IRBs (or Human Subjects Boards) are mandated by the government to be established at all institutions that are involved in research. This includes educational and health care settings.
   b. IRB approval is required to receive federal (and most other) research grants.
   c. Proposals for research must be submitted to, and approved by, an IRB prior to implementation of the research study.
   d. IRBs review research proposals to ensure that all of the above ethical standards for research have been considered by the researcher.

Professional Development

1. All occupational therapy practitioners have an ethical responsibility to engage in professional development activities which maintain and enhance their competence and ability to provide client-centered, occupation-based, and evidence-based practice.
2. Professional development activities are required to develop advanced and specialized knowledge and skills beyond entry-level competencies.
3. Supervisory feedback, peer review, and active self reflection should be used to identify professional development needs and establish professional development goals.
4. Practitioners should seek and participate in professional development activities that are relevant to their practice setting, client population, job responsibilities, and professional goals.
   a. Activities can include (but are not limited to) facility-based training, active professional association membership and conference participation, continuing education workshops and/or on-line courses, independent study, professional presentations and publications, and research.
5. Professional development tools (PDTs) are available to guide the self-assessment of professional development needs and interests and develop a professional development plan.
6. Most state regulatory boards (SRBs) and the NBCOT require evidence of participation in professional development activities to maintain licensure and certification, respectfully.
   a. The amount and nature of these requirements vary between different jursdictions.
      (1) It is the practitioner's responsibility to ensure that all professional development requirements are fulfilled within the required timeframe (e.g., every 2–3 years) and that all documentation (e.g., proof of continuing education units [CEUs] earned) is available for review upon request by a SRB or the NBCOT.
         (a) The use of professional portfolio is an effective means to track and document professional development activities.

References

Alexander, T. C. (October 20, 2003). Capital briefing: Members want to know. *OT Practice*, 7.

American Dietetic Association. (2005). *Scope of dietetics practice framework*. Chicago: American Dietetic Association.

American Occupational Therapy Association. (2010). Occupational therapy code of ethics and ethics Standards (2010), *American Journal of Occupational Therapy, 64*(6, Supplement), S17–S26.

American Occupational Therapy Association. (2010). Enforcement procedures for occupational therapy code of ethics. *American Journal of Occupational Therapy, 64*(6, Supplement), S4–S16.

American Occupational Therapy Association. (2010). Standards of practice for occupational therapy. *American Journal of Occupational Therapy, 64*(6, Supplement), S106–S110.

American Occupational Therapy Association. (2009). Guidelines for supervision, roles, and responsibilities during the delivery of occupational therapy services. *American Journal of Occupational Therapy, 63*, 797–803.

American Occupational Therapy Association. (2006). *The new IDEA: Summary of the Individuals with Disabilities Education Improvement Act of 2004* (P.L. 108–446). Bethesda, MD: Author.

American Occupational Therapy Association. (2006). *Reference manual of the official documents of the American Occupational Therapy Association*, 11th ed. Bethesda, MD: Author.

American Occupational Therapy Association. (2005). *Standards for continuing competence American Journal of Occupational Therapy, 59* 661–662.

American Occupational Therapy Association. (2004a). Guidelines for supervision, roles, and responsibilities during the delivery of occupational therapy services. *American Journal of Occupational Therapy, 58*, 663–667.

American Occupational Therapy Association. (2003). *Professional development tool.* Bethesda, MD: Author. Retrieved August 20, 2013 from http://www.aota.org/pdt.

Braveman, B. (2006). *Leading and managing occupational therapy services.* Bethesda, MD: AOTA Press.

Case-Smith, J. (Ed.). (2005). *Occupational therapy for children*, 5th ed. St. Louis, MO: Elsevier Mosby.

Centers for Medicare and Medicaid Services (CMS). (2010). Medicare and home health care Retrieved September 15, 2013 from http://www.medicare.gov/Pubs/pdf/10969.pdf.

Centers for Medicare and Medicaid Services (CMS). (2009). *Medicaid benefit policy manual.* Washington DC: Author.

Chandler, B. (2008, January 21). School System Special Interest Section. *OT Practice*, 25.

Clark, G. (2008). The infants and toddlers with disabilities program (Part C of IDEA). *OT Practice, 13I*(1), CE-1–CE-8.

Clifton, D. (2004, December). Workers' Comp: A plethora of opportunities. *Rehab Management*, 32, 34–36.

Department of Training, *Training manual* (2001). Department of Health and Human Services, Trenton New Jersey.

DePoy, E., & Gitlin, L. N. (2005). *Introduction to research: Understanding and applying multiple strategies*, 3rd ed. St. Louis, MO: Mosby.

Diffendal, J. (2001, April 30). Coming out of retirement: Do working retirees need your services? *OT Advance*, 33, 36.

Gennerman, M. (2005, May 9). CPT coding: Defining our practice. OT Practice, 19–23.

Grossman, J., & Bortone, J. (2000). Program development. In R.P. Cottrell (Ed.), *Proactive approaches in psychosocial occupational therapy*. (pp 39–45) Thorofare, NJ: Slack.

Hopkins, H. & Smith, H. (Eds.). (2003). *Willard and Spackman's occupational therapy*, 10th ed. Philadelphia: J.B. Lippincott.

Hussey, S., Sabonis-Chafee, B., & O'Brien, J. (2007). *Introduction to occupational therapy*, 3rd ed. St. Louis, MO: Elsevier Mosby.

International Center for Clubhouse Development. (1994). *Standards for clubhouse programs*. New York, Author.

Jacobs, K. (2000). Innovation to action: Marketing occupational therapy. In R. P. Cottrell (Ed.), *Proactive approaches in psychosocial occupational therapy*. (pp 505–507) Thorofare, NJ: Slack.

Jacobs, K., & Logigan, M. K. (1999). *Functions of a manager in occupational therapy*, 3rd ed. Thorofare, NJ: Slack.

Jimmo vs Sebelius settlement agreement fact sheet. (2013). Retrieved September 21, 2013 from http://www.cms.gov/Medicare/Medicare-Fee-for-Service-Payment/SNFPPS/Downloads/Jimmo-FactSheet.pdf

Job Accommodation Network (2009). *Accommodation and compliance series: The ADA Amendments Act of 2008*. Morgantown, WV: Author.

Johnson, K. V. (2000, September). Home health PPS: The new payment system. *OT Practice*. CE1–CE8.

Kielhofner, G. (2006). *Research in occupational therapy: Methods of inquiry for enhancing practice*. Philadelphia: F. A. Davis.

Kornblau, B. & Burkhardt, A. (2012). *Ethics in rehabilitation: A clinical perspective*, 2nd ed. Thorofare, NJ: Slack.

Kreftling L. (1991). Rigor in qualitative research: The assessment of trustworthiness. *American Journal of Occupational Therapy, 45*, 214–222.

Kyler, P. (Ed.). (2005). *Reference guide to the occupational therapy code of ethics*. Bethesda, MD: American Occupational Therapy Association.

Leary, D., & Mardirossian, J. (2000, Sept. 11) Ethical knowledge = collaborative power. *OT Practice*, 19–22.

McCormack, G., Jaffe, E., & Goodman-Lavey, M. (Eds.). (2003). *The occupational therapy manager*, (4th ed.). Bethesda, MD: American Occupational Therapy Association.

Medcom. (2003). HIPAA: *A guide for health care workers*. Cypress, CA: Author.

Moyers, P, & Dale, L. (2007). *The guide to occupational therapy practice*. Bethesda, MD: American Occupational Therapy Association.

Murer. C. (2007, October). Psychiatric partial hospitalization: An overview. *Rehabilitation Management*, 48–49.

National Board for Certification in Occupational Therapy (NBCOT). (2008). *Qualifications and compliance review information*. Gaithersburg, MD: Author.

National Board for Certification in Occupational Therapy. (NBCOT). (2007, Fall/Winter). *Report to the profession*. Gaithersburg, MD: Author.

National Council on Disability and National Urban League. (2000). *A guide to disability rights laws*. Washington, DC: Author.

Opp, A. (2007, September 27). Reauthorizing No Child Left Behind: Opportunities for OT. *OT Practice*, 9–13.

Ottenbacher, K. J., & Cusick, A. (1990). Goal attainment scaling as a method of clinical service evaluation. *American Journal of Occupational Therapy, 44*, 519–525.

Patient and elder abuse (2001). Tennessee Bureau of Investigation, *Tennessee Anytime*, Available: www.tbi.state.tn.us/PATIENTABUSE.

Scaffa, M. (2001). *Occupational therapy in community-based practice settings*. Philadelphia, PA: F.A. Davis.

Schindler, V. P. (2000). Occupational therapy in forensic psychiatry. In R. P. Cottrell (Ed.), *Proactive approaches in psychosocial occupational therapy* (pp 319–325). Thorofare, NJ: Slack.

Shadish, W. Cook, T., & Campbell, D. (2002). *Experimental and quasi-experimental designs for generalized causal inference*. Boston: Houghton Mifflin.

United States Government Printing Office. (2003). *Code of Federal Regulations*, Title 42, Volume 3. Retrieved from http://www.cms.gov. December 21, 2003.

Vance, K., McGuire, M. J., & Nanof, T. (2009). Medicare coverage of occupational therapy in the home and community. *OT Practice, 14*(13), CE-1–CE-8.

Wilmarth, C. (2009, November 9). Using aides to provide therapy. *OT Practice*, 8.

Review Questions

Professional Standards and Responsibilities

Below are five questions about key content covered in this chapter. These questions are not inclusive of the entirety of content on occupational therapy professional standards and responsibilities that you must know for success on the NBCOT exam. These questions are provided to help you "jump start" the thought processes you will need to apply your studying of content to the answering of exam questions; hence they are not in the NBCOT exam format. Exam items in the NBCOT format which cover the depth and breadth of content you will need to know to pass the NBCOT exam are provided on this text's disc. The answers to the below questions are provided in Appendix 4.

1. You are working in a skilled nursing facility. An administrator asks you to actively treat a new resident who is very frail with multiple medical complications. Upon admission, you had evaluated the resident and determined that the resident would not be able to tolerate occupational therapy services. During the evaluation, the resident had stated that chronic pain made all activities very difficult. Pain relief and rest were the only things the resident identified as personally desired. How should you respond to the adminstrator's request? Which principles of the AOTA Code of Ethics should you use to guide your response? Explain how these principles relate to this situation.

2. A large regional health care system provides occupational therapy services across the continuum of care. Settings in which occupational therapy services are provided include an acute care hospital, an outpatient clinic, a subacute rehabilitation unit, a skilled nursing facility (SNF), a palliative care unit, and a home health agency. All settings employ occupational therapists and occupational therapy assistants. What factors should be considered when determining the level of supervision that the occupational therapist should provide to the occupational therapy assistant? What is a key determinant for deciding if an occupational therapy assistant (OTA) can ethically be given more responsibility?

3. An occupational therapist is opening a private practice. What procedures should the therapist implement to ensure full compliance with the Health Insurance and Portability Accountability Act (HIPAA)?

4. You are beginning a new job as an occupational therapist for a Medicare-certified home health agency. Most of your clients will have limited independence or be dependent in basic activities of daily living. What are key Medicare guidelines for home-based occupational therapy you must consider when working with these individuals and their caregivers?

5. You are developing a new driver rehabilitation program. What are important issues for you to consider as you develop your budget and fiscal mangement plan?

5

Human Development Across the Lifespan: Pediatric Through Geriatric Considerations for Occupational Therapy Practice

MARGE E. MOFFETT BOYD, JAN G. GARBARINI, LINDA KAHN D'ANGELO, SUSAN B. O'SULLIVAN, AND RITA P. FLEMING-CASTALDY

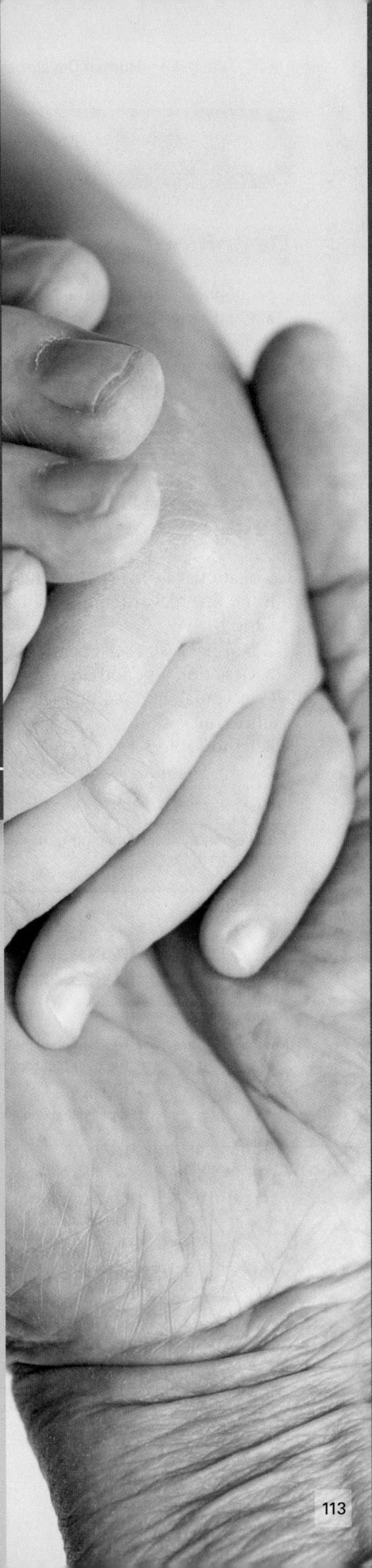

Chapter Outline

Human Development

Definition

1. Sequential changes in the function of the individual.
   a. Qualitative or quantitative.
   b. Influenced by biologic determinants and biopsychosocial environmental experiences.

Sensorimotor Development

Fetal Sensorimotor Development

1. Gestational age: age of the fetus or newborn, in weeks, from first day of mother's last normal menstrual period.
   a. Normal gestational period 38–42 weeks.
   b. Gestational period divided into three trimesters.
2. Conceptual age: age of a fetus or newborn in weeks since conception.
3. Refer to Table 5-1.

Development of Sensorimotor Integration

1. Prenatal period.
   a. Responds first to tactile stimuli.
   b. Reflex development.
   c. Innate tactile, proprioceptive, and vestibular reactions.
2. Neonatal period.
   a. Tactile, proprioceptive and vestibular inputs are critical from birth onward for the eventual development of body scheme.

Table 5-1

Fetal Sensorimotor Development

	FIRST TRIMESTER	SECOND TRIMESTER	THIRD TRIMESTER
Muscle Spindle	• Muscle starts to differentiate • Tissue becomes specialized	• Motor end plate forms • Clonus response to stretch	• Some muscles are mature and functional, others still maturing
Touch and Tactile System	• First sensory system to develop • Response to tactile stimulus	• Receptors differentiate	• Touch functional • Actual temperature discrimination at the end of the third trimester • Most mature sensory system at birth
Vestibular System	• Functioning at the end of the first trimester (not completely developed)		
Vision	• Eyelids fused • Optic nerve and cup being formed	• Startle to light • Visual processing occurs	• Fixation occurs • Able to focus (fixed focal length)
Auditory		• Will turn to auditory sounds	• Debris in middle ear, loss of hearing
Olfactory			• Nasal plugs disappear, some olfactory perception
Taste	• Taste buds develop		• Can respond to different tastes (sweet, sour, bitter, salt)
Movement	• Sucking, hiccuping • Fetal breathing • Quick generalized limb movement • Positional changes • 7½ weeks; bend neck and trunk away from perioral stroke	• Quickening • Sleep states • Grasp reflex • Reciprocal and symmetrical limb movements	• 28 weeks primitive motor reflexes • Rooting, suck, swallow • Palmar grasp • Plantar grasp • MORO • Crossed extension

O'Sullivan, S. B. & Siegelman, R. P. (2000). *National Physical Therapy Examination Review and Study Guide,* (p. 148). Concord, MA: International Educational Resources. Reprinted with permission.

b. Vestibular system, although fully developed at birth, continues to be refined and impacts on the infant's arousal level.
   (1) Helps the infant to feel more organized and content.
c. Visual system develops as infant responds to human faces and items of high contrast placed approximately 10 inches from face.
d. Auditory system is immature at birth and develops as the infant orients to voices and other sounds.

3. First six months.
   a. Vestibular, proprioceptive, and visual systems become more integrated and lay the foundation for postural control, which facilitates a steady visual field.
   b. Tactile and proprioceptive systems continue to be refined, laying the foundation for development of somatosensory skills.
   c. Visual and tactile systems become more integrated as the child reaches out and grasps objects, laying the foundation for eye-hand coordination.
   d. Infant movement patterns progress from reflexive to voluntary and goal-directed.
4. Six to twelve months.
   a. Vestibular, visual, and somatosensory responses increase in quantity and quality as the infant becomes more mobile.
   b. Tactile and proprioceptive perceptions become more refined, allowing for development of fine motor and motor planning skills.
   c. Tactile and proprioceptive responses also lead to midline skills and eventual crossing of midline.
   d. Auditory, tactile, and proprioceptive perceptions are heightened allowing for development of sounds for the purpose of communication.
   e. Tactile, proprioceptive, gustatory, and olfactory perceptions are integrated, allowing for primitive self-feeding.
5. Thirteen to twenty-four months.
   a. Tactile perception becomes more precise allowing for discrimination and localization to further refine fine motor skills.
   b. Further integration of all systems promotes complexity of motor planning as the toddler's repertoire of movement patterns expands.
   c. Symbolic gesturing and vocalization promotes ideation, indicating the ability to conceptualize.
   d. Motor planning abilities contribute to self concept as the toddler begins to master the environment.
6. Two to three years.
   a. This is a period of refinement as the vestibular, proprioceptive, and visual systems further develop, leading to improved balance and postural control.
   b. Further development of tactile discrimination and localization lead to improved fine motor skills.
   c. Motor planning and praxis ideation also progress during this period.
7. Three to seven years.
   a. Child is driven to challenge sensorimotor competencies through roughhouse play, playground activities, games, sports, music, dancing, arts and crafts, household chores, and school tasks.
      (1) These activities also provide opportunities to promote social development and self-esteem.

Reflex Development and Integration

1. Predictable motor response elicited by tactile, proprioceptive, or vestibular stimulation.
2. Primitive reflexes are present at or just after birth and typically integrate throughout the first year.
3. The persistence or reemergence of these primitive reflexes are indicative of central nervous system (CNS) dysfunction that may interfere with motor milestone attainment, patterns of movement, musculoskeletal alignment, and function.
4. Refer to Table 5-2 for reflex time tables, stimuli, responses, and functional and occupational relevance.
5. Refer to Figures 5-1 to 5-10 for pictures of some key reflexes.

Motor Development

1. Performance of occupational roles can be enhanced or inhibited based on the reflex development and integration noted above and in additional areas noted below.
   a. Crossing the midline: as the child becomes more mobile, movement against gravity and weight-shift increase, leading to eventual crossing of the midline, often in an attempt to reach for a toy, while weight bearing on the opposing upper extremity for balance (begins at 9–12 months).
   b. Laterality: hemispheric specialization for specific tasks varies with different individuals (handedness is considered to be stable by age five; however, strong preferences can be seen much earlier).
   c. Bilateral integration: as the child experiments with movement, the nervous system is stimulated, and the resulting sensations help the child to coordinate the two sides of the body (begins at 9–12 months).
   d. Fine motor coordination and dexterity. (See section on development of hand skills.)
   e. Visual-motor integration is dependent upon the lower level skills of visual attention, visual memory, visual discrimination, kinesthesia, position in space, figure ground, form constancy, and spatial relations.
   f. Oral-motor control, which is developed in the area of feeding, provides the foundation for early oral communication and later language development.

Table 5-2

Overview of the Most Important Reflexes

REFLEX	ONSET AGE	INTEGRATION AGE	STIMULUS	RESPONSE	RELEVANCE
Rooting	28 wks gestation	3 months	Stroke the corner of the mouth, upper lip, and lower lip	Movement of the tongue, mouth, and/or head toward the stimulus	Allows searching for and locating feeding source
Suck-swallow	28 wks gestation	2–5 months	Place examiner's index finger inside infant's mouth with head in midline	Strong, rhythmical sucking	Allows ingestion of nourishment
Traction	28 wks gestation	2–5 months	Grasp infant's forearms and pull-to-sit	Complete flexion of upper extremities	Enhances momentary reflexive grasp
Moro	28 wks gestation	4–6 months	Rapidly drop infant's head backward	First phase: arm extension/abduction, hand opening Second phase: arm flexion and adduction	Facilitates ability to depart from dominant flexor posture: protective response
Plantar grasp	28 wks gestation	9 months	Apply pressure with thumb on the infant's ball of the foot	Toe flexion	Increases tactile input to sole of foot
Galant	32 wks gestation	2 months	Hold infant in prone suspension, gently scratch or tap alongside the spine with finger, from shoulders to buttocks	Lateral trunk flexion and wrinkling of the skin on the stimulated side	Facilitates lateral trunk movements necessary for trunk stabilization
Asymmetric tonic neck	37 wks gestation	4–6 months	Fully rotate infant's head and hold for 5 seconds	Extension of extremities on the face side, flexion of extremities on the skull side	Promotes visual hand regard
Palmar grasp	37 wks gestation	4–6 months	Place examiner's finger in infant's palm	Finger flexion; reflexive grasp	Increases tactile input on the palm of the hand
Tonic labyrinthine - Supine	> 37 wks gestation	6 months	Place infant in supine	Increased extensor tone	Facilitates total-body extensor tone
Tonic labyrinthine - Prone	> 37 wks gestation	6 months	Place infant in prone	Increased flexor tone	Facilitates total-body flexor tone
Labyrinthine/optical (head) righting	birth - 2 months	persists	Hold infant suspended vertically and tilt slowly (about 45°) to the side, forward, or backward	Upright positioning of the head	Orients head in space; maintains face vertical
Landau	3–4 months	12–24 months	Hold infant in horizontal prone suspension	Complete extension of head, trunk, and extremities	Breaks up flexor dominance; facilitates prone extension
Symmetric tonic neck	4–6 months	8–12 months	Place infant in the crawling position and extend the head	Flexion of hips and knees	Breaks up total extensor posture; facilitates static quadruped position
Neck righting (NOB)	4–6 months	5 years	Place infant in supine and fully turn head to one side	Log rolling of the entire body to maintain alignment with the head	Maintains head/body alignment; initiates rolling (first ambulation effort)
Body righting (on body) (BOB)	4–6 months	5 years	Place infant in supine, flex one hip and knee toward the chest and hold briefly	Segmental rolling of the upper trunk to maintain alignment	Facilitates trunk/spinal rotation
Downward parachute (protective extension downward)	4 months	Persists	Rapidly lower infant toward supporting surface while suspended vertically	Extension of the lower extremities	Allows accurate placement of lower extremities in

Table 5-2

Overview of the Most Important Reflexes (*Continued*)

REFLEX	ONSET AGE	INTEGRATION AGE	STIMULUS	RESPONSE	RELEVANCE
Forward parachute (protective extension forward)	6–9 months	Persists	Suddenly tip infant forward toward supporting surface while vertically suspended	Sudden extension of the upper extremities, hand opening, and neck extension	Allows accurate placement of upper extremities in anticipation of supporting surface to prevent a fall
Sideward parachute (protective extension sideward)	7 months	Persists	Quickly but firmly tip infant off-balance to the side while in the sitting position	Arm extension and abduction to the side	Protects body to prevent a fall; supports body for unilateral use of opposite arm
Backward parachute (protective extension backward)	9–10 months	Persists	Quickly but firmly tip infant off-balance backward	Backward arm extension or arm extension to one side spinal rotation	Protects body to prevent a fall; unilaterally facilitates
Prone tilting	5 months	Persists	After positioning infant in prone, slowly raise one side of the supporting surface	Curving of the spine toward the raised side (opposite to the pull of gravity); abduction/extension of arms and legs	Maintain equilibrium without arm support; facilitate postural adjustments in all positions
Supine tilting and Sitting tilting	7–8 months	Persists	After positioning infant in supine or sitting, slowly raise one side of the supporting surface	Curving of the spine toward the raised side (opposite to the pull of gravity); abduction/extension of arms and legs	Maintain equilibrium without arm support; facilitate postural adjustments in all positions
Quadruped tilting	9–12 months	Persists	After positioning infant on all fours, slowly raise one side of the supporting surface	Curving of the spine toward the raised side (opposite to the pull of gravity); abduction/extension of arms and legs	Maintain equilibrium without arm support; facilitate postural adjustments in all positions
Standing tilting	12–21 months	Persists	After positioning infant in standing, slowly raise one side of the supporting surface	Curving of the spine toward the raised side (opposite to the pull of gravity); abduction/extension of arms and legs	Maintain equilibrium without arm support; facilitate postural adjustments in all positions

From: *Foundations for practice in the neonatal intensive care unit and early intervention,* (Volume 2, p. 35) by Vergara, E. Copyright 1993 by the American Occupational Therapy Association, Bethesda, MD. Reprinted with permission.

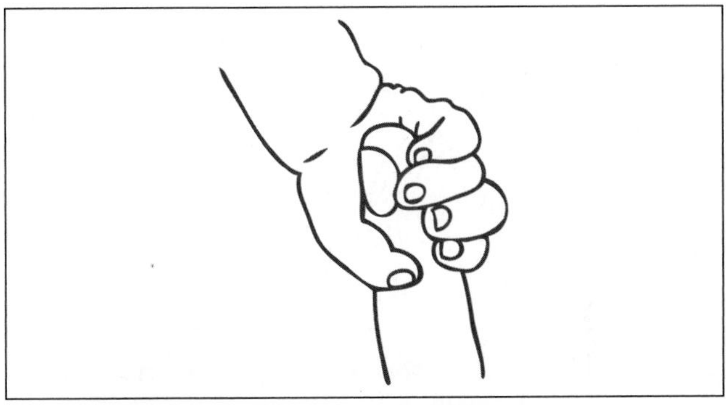

Figure 5-1 Palmar Grasp Reflex

Groenweghe, Marisa with permission.

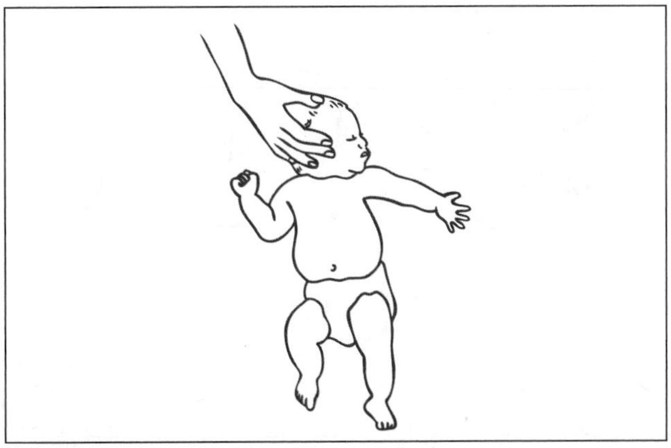

Figure 5-2 Asymmetric Tonic Neck Reflex (ATNR)

Groenweghe, Marisa with permission.

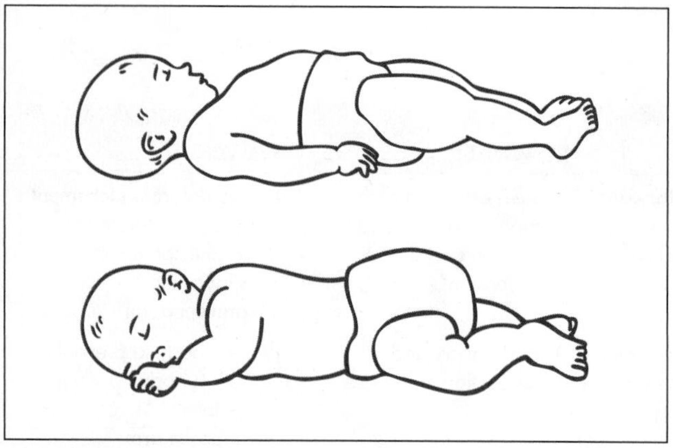

Figure 5-3 Tonic Labyrinthine Reflex (TLR)
Groenweghe, Marisa with permission.

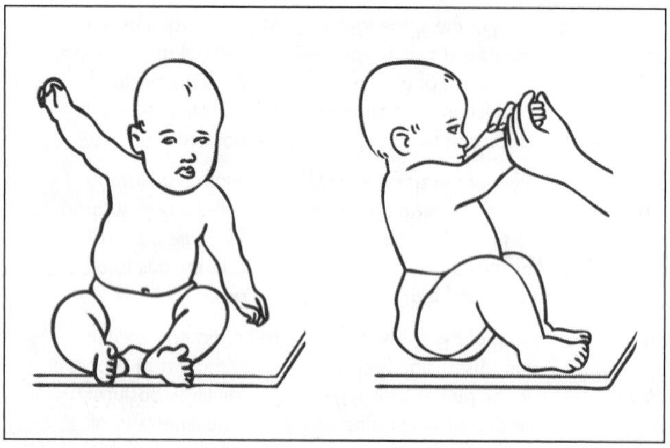

Figure 5-4 Optical Righting Reaction
Groenweghe, Marisa with permission.

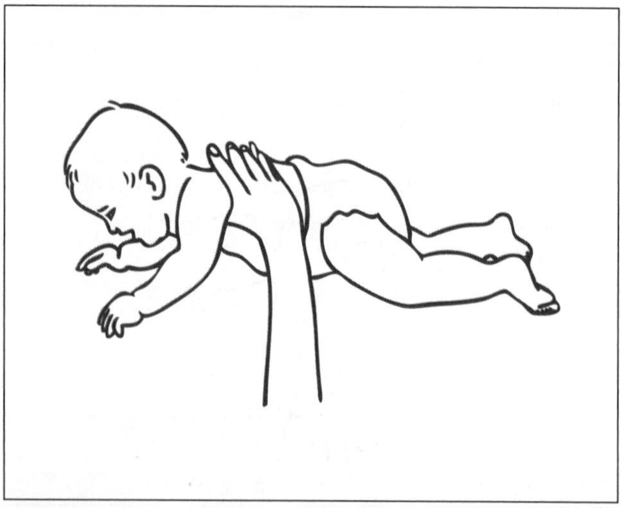

Figure 5-5 Landau Reaction
Groenweghe, Marisa with permission.

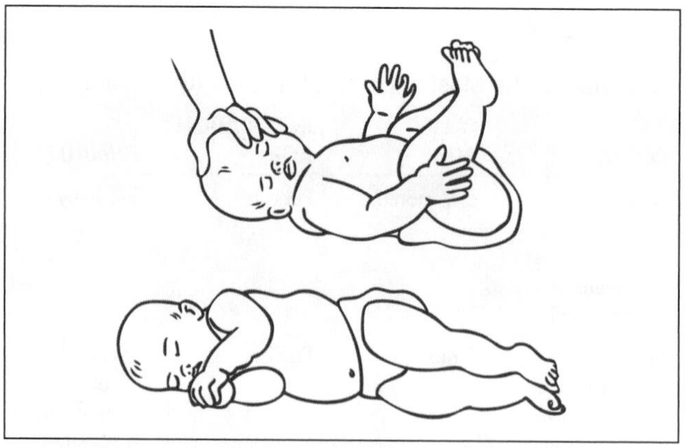

Figure 5-6 Neck on Body (NOB)
Groenweghe, Marisa with permission.

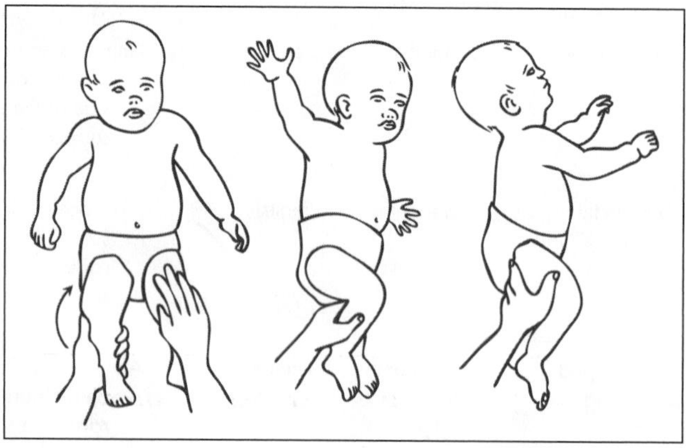

Figure 5-7 Body Righting Reaction on Body (BOB)
Groenweghe, Marisa with permission.

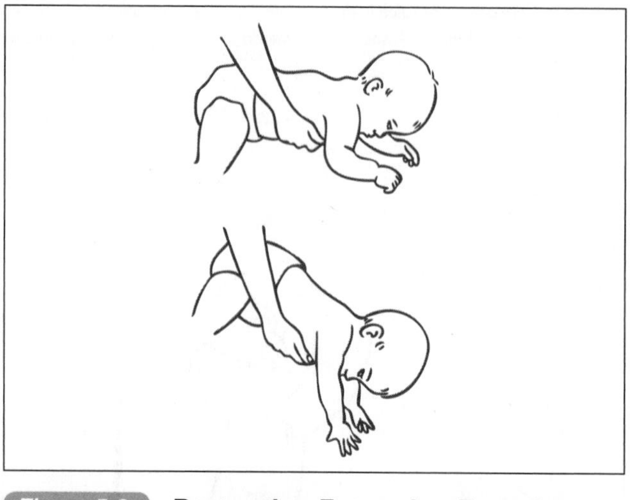

Figure 5-8 Protective Extension Reaction Forward
Groenweghe, Marisa with permission.

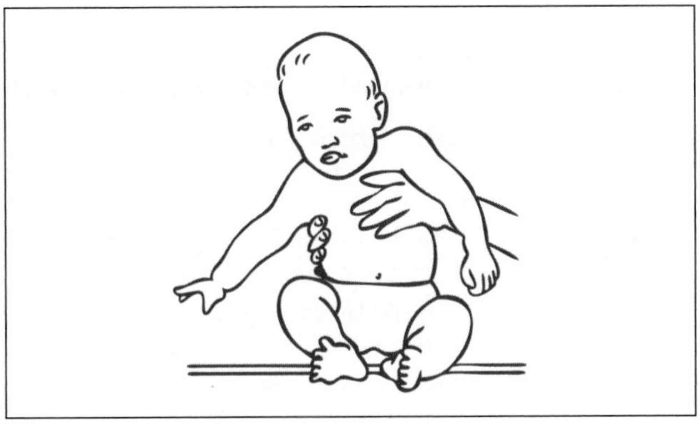

Figure 5-9 **Protective Extension Reaction Sideward**

Groenweghe, Marisa with permission.

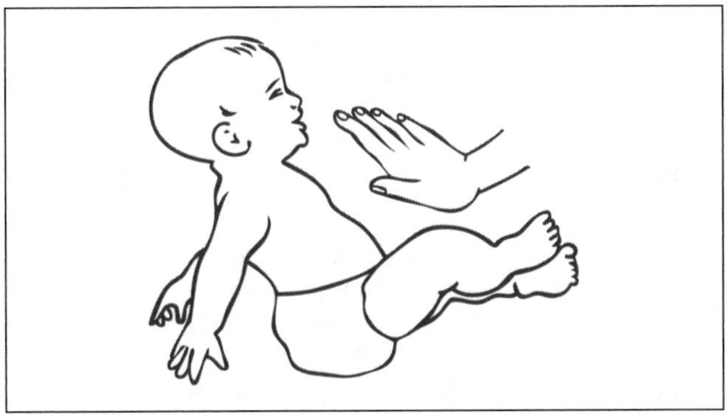

Figure 5-10 **Protective Extension Reaction Backward**

Groenweghe, Marisa with permission.

2. General principles of motor development.
   a. Occurs in a cephalocaudal/proximal to distal direction.
   b. Progresses from gross to fine movement.
   c. Progresses from stability to controlled mobility.
   d. Occurs in a spiraling manner, with periods of equilibrium and disequilibrium.
   e. Sensitive periods occur when the infant/child is affected by environmental input.
3. Normal sensorimotor development in key positions (Tables 5-3 and 5-4).
4. Important aspects in the development of upper extremity function.
   a. Head and trunk control.
   b. Eye/hand interaction, sensory-perceptual interaction.
   c. Shoulder-scapular stability/mobility.
   d. Humeral control.
   e. Elbow control.
   f. Forearm control.
   g. Wrist control.
   h. Thumb opposition and stability.
   i. Palmar arches of hand.
   j. Isolated finger control.

Table 5-3

Sensorimotor Development Mobility and Stability

AGE	GROSS MOTOR SKILL
Prone Position	
0–2 mo	Turns head side to side Lifts head momentarily Bends hips with bottom in air Lifts head and sustains in midline Rotates head freely when up Able to bear weight on forearms Able to tuck chin and gaze at hands in forearm prop Attempts to shift weight on forearms, resulting in shoulder collapse
5–6 mo	Shifts weight on forearms and reaches forward Bears weight and shifts weight on extended arms Legs are closer together and thighs roll inward toward natural alignment Hips are flat on surface Equilibrium reactions are present
5–8 mo	Airplane posturing in prone position; chest and thighs lift off surface
7–8 mo	Pivots in prone position Moves to prone position to sit
9 mo	Begins to dislike prone position
Supine Position	
0–3 mo	Head held to one side Able to turn head side to side
3–4 mo	Holds head in midline Chin is tucked and neck lengthens in back Legs come together Lower back flattens against the floor
4–5 mo	Head lag is gone when pulled to a sitting position Hands are together in space
5–6 mo	Lifts head independently Brings feet to mouth Brings hands to feet Able to reach for toy with one or both hands Hands are predominantly open
7–8 mo	Equilibrium reactions are present
Rolling	
3–4 mo	Rolls from prone position to side accidentally because of poor control of weight shift Rolls from supine position to side
5–6 mo	Rolls from prone to supine position Rolls from supine position to side with right and left leg performing independent movements Rolls from supine to prone position with right and left leg performing independent movements
6–14 mo	Rolls segmentally with roll initiated by the head, shoulder, or hips

(Continued)

Chapter 5

Table 5-3

Sensorimotor Development Mobility and Stability (*Continued*)

AGE	GROSS MOTOR SKILL
Creeping	
7 mo	Crawls forward on belly
7–10 mo	Reciprocal creep
10–11 mo	Creeps on hands and feet
11–12 mo	Creeps well
Sitting	
0–3 mo (held in sitting)	Head bobs in sitting Back is rounded Hips are apart, turned out, and bent Head is steady Chin tucks; able to gaze at floor Sits with less support Hips are bent and shoulders are in front of hips
5–6 mo (supports self in sitting)	Sits alone momentarily Increased extension in back Sits by propping forward on arms Wide base, legs are bent Periodic use of "high guard" position Protective responses present when falling to the front
5–10 mo (sits alone)	Sits alone steadily, initially with wide base of support Able to play with toys in sitting position
6–11 mo	Gets to sitting position from prone position
7–8 mo	Equilibrium reactions are present Able to rotate upper body while lower body remains stationary Protective responses are present when falling to the side
8–10 mo	Sits well without support Legs are closer; full upright position, knees straight Increased variety of sitting positions, including "w" sit and side sit Difficult fine motor tasks may prompt return to wide base of support
9–18 mo	Rises from supine position by first rolling over to stomach then pushing up into four-point position
10–12 mo	Protective extension backwards, first with bent elbows then straight elbows Able to move in and out of sitting position into other positions
11–12 mo	Trunk control and equilibrium responses are fully developed in sitting position Further increase in variety of positions possible
11–24 mo +	Rises from supine by first rolling to side then pushing up into sitting position

Table 5-3

Sensorimotor Development Mobility and Stability (*Continued*)

AGE	GROSS MOTOR SKILL
Standing	
0–3 mo	When held in standing position, takes some weight on legs
2–3 mo	When held in standing position, legs may give way
3–4 mo	Bears some weight on legs, but must be held proximally Head is up in midline, no chin tuck Pelvis and hips are behind shoulders Legs are apart and turned outward
5–10 mo	Stands while holding onto furniture
5–6 mo	Increased capability to bear weight Decreased support needed; may be held by arms or hands Legs are still spread apart and turned outward Bounces in standing position
6–12 mo	Pulls to standing position at furniture
8–9 mo	Rotates the trunk over the lower extremities Lower extremities are more active in pulling to a standing position Pulls to a standing position by kneeling, then half-kneeling
9–13 mo	Pulls to standing position with legs only, no longer needs arms Stands alone momentarily
12 mo	Equilibrium reactions are present in standing
Walking	
8 mo	Cruises sideways
8–18 mo	Walks with two hands held
9–10 mo	Cruises around furniture, turning slightly in intended direction
9–17 mo	Takes independent steps, falls easily
10–14 mo	Walking: stoops and recovers in play
11 mo	Walks with one hand held Reaches for furniture out of reach when cruising Cruises in either direction, no hesitation
15 mo	Able to start and stop in walking
18 mo	Seldom falls Runs stiffly with eyes on ground
Release	
0–1 mo	No release; grasp reflex is strong
1–4 mo	Involuntary release
4 mo	Mutual fingering in midline
4–8 mo	Transfers object from hand to hand
5–6 mo	Two-stage transfer; taking hand grasps before releasing hand lets go

Table 5-3

Sensorimotor Development Mobility and Stability (*Continued*)	
AGE	**GROSS MOTOR SKILL**
Release (cont.)	
6–7 mo	One-stage transfer; taking hand and releasing hand perform actions simultaneously
7–9 mo	Volitional release
7–10 mo	Presses down on surface to release
8 mo	Releases above a surface with wrist flexion
9–10 mo	Releases into a container with wrist straight
10–14 mo	Clumsy release into small container; hand rests on edge of container
12–15 mo	Precise, controlled release into small container with wrist extended

Modified from Bly, L. (1993). *Normal development in the first year of life.* Tucson, AZ: Therapy Skill Builders; Illingworth, R. S. (1991). *The normal child: Some problems of the early years and their treatment,* 10th ed. Edinburgh: Churchill-Livingstone; Knobloch, H., & Pasamanick, B. (1974). *Gesell and Amatruda's developmental diagnosis: The evaluation and management of normal and abnormal neuropsychological development in infancy and early childhood.* Hagerstown, MD: Harper and Row; Gilfoyle, E., Grady, A., & Moore, J. (1990). *Children adapt.* Thorofare, NJ: Slack.

Case-Smith, J., Allen, A. S., & Pratt, P. N. (1996). *Occupational therapy for children,* 3rd ed. (pp. 49–50). St. Louis, MO: Mosby-Year Book. Reprinted with permission.

Table 5-4

Development of Stair Climbing and Jumping/Hopping Skills	
AGE	**SKILL**
Stair Climbing	
15 mo	Creeps up stairs
18–24 mo	Walks up stairs while holding on Walks down stairs while holding on
18–23 mo	Creeps backwards down stairs
2–2½+ yr	Walks up stairs without support, marking time Walks down stairs without support, marking time
2–2½–3 yr	Walks up stairs, alternating feet
3–3½ yr	Walks down stairs, alternating feet
Jumping and Hopping	
2 yr	Jumps down from step
2½+ yr	Hops on one foot, few steps
3 yr	Jumps off floor with both feet
3–5 yr	Jumps over objects
3½–5 yr	Hops on one foot
3–4 yr	Gallops, leading with one foot and transferring weight smoothly and evenly
5 yr	Hops in straight line
5–6 yr	Skips on alternating feet, maintaining balance

Modified from Gesell, A., & Amatruda, C. S. (1947). *Developmental diagnosis.* New York, NY: Harper and Row; Bayley, N. (1993). *Bayley scales of infant development* (rev ed.). New York, NY: Psychological Corporation; Knobloch, H. & Pasamanick, B. (1974). *Gesell and Amatruda's developmental diagnosis: The evaluation and management of normal and abnormal neuropsychological development in infancy and early childhood.* Hagerstown, MD: Harper and Row.

Case-Smith, J., Allen, A. S., & Pratt, P. N. (1996). *Occupational therapy for children,* 3rd ed. (p. 59). St. Louis, MO: Mosby-Year Book. Reprinted with permission.

5. Important components in the development of hand skills.
   a. Reaching skills.
      (1) Visual regard accompanied by swiping/batting, with closed hand and abducted shoulder (newborn).
      (2) Hands come together at midline for bilateral reaching with shoulders abducted with partial internal rotation, forearm pronation, and full finger extension (4 months).
      (3) Increased dissociation of body sides, allows for unilateral reaching with less abduction and internal rotation of the shoulder, and the hand is more open (6 months).
      (4) As trunk stability improves, shoulder flexion with slight external rotation, elbow extension, forearm supination, and slight wrist extension begin to emerge (9 months).
   b. Grasping skills according to Erhardt Prehension Developmental Levels.
      (1) Grasp of the pellet (prone or sitting).
         (a) No voluntary grasp or visual attention to the object (natal).
         (b) No attempt to grasp, but visually attends to the object (3 months).
         (c) Raking and contacting object (6 months).
         (d) Inferior-scissors grasp: raking object into palm with adducted totally flexed thumb and all flexed fingers, or two partially extended fingers (7 months).
         (e) Scissors grasp: between thumb and side of curled index finger, distal thumb joint slightly flexed, proximal thumb joint extended (8 months).
         (f) Inferior pincer grasp: between ventral surfaces of thumb and index finger, distal thumb joint extended, beginning of thumb opposition (9 months).
         (g) Pincer grasp: between distal pads of thumb and index finger, distal thumb joint slightly flexed, thumb opposed (10 months).
         (h) Fine pincer grasp: between fingertips or fingernails, distal thumb joint flexed (12 months).
         (i) Refer to Figure 5-11.

(2) Grasp of the cube.
  (a) Neonate visually attends to object, grasp is reflexive.
  (b) Visually attends to object and may swipe. Sustained voluntary grasp possible only upon contact, ulnar side used, no thumb involvement, wrist flexed (3 months).
  (c) Primitive squeeze grasp: visually attends to object, approaches if within 1 inch, contact results in hand pulling object back to squeeze precariously against the other hand or body, no thumb involvement (4 months).
    (1) Between 4 and 5 months the infant begins to progress toward a palmar grasp, the infant's thumb begins to adduct with fingers pressed against the ulnar side of the palm, progressing in the direction of the center of the palm toward a palmar grasp. This is sometimes referred to as an ulnar-palmar grasp.
  (d) Palmar grasp: fingers on top surface of object press it into center of palm with thumb adducted (5 months).
  (e) Radial-palmar grasp: fingers on far side of object press it against opposed thumb and radial side of palm (6 months), with wrist straight (7 months).
  (f) Radial-digital grasp: object held with the opposed thumb and fingertips, space visible between (eight months) with wrist extended (9 months).
  (g) Refer to Figure 5-12.

c. Releasing skills: initially, involuntary dropping, then object is pulled out of one hand by the other hand. (See Table 5-3).
  (1) Development progresses from no release (0–1 month) to involuntary release (1–4 months) to

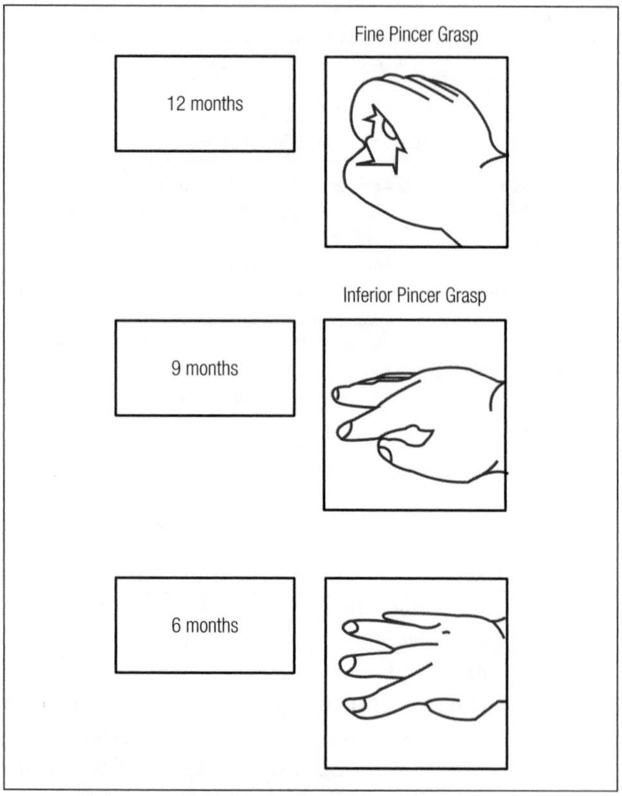

Figure 5-11 Developmental Levels: Grasp of the Pellet

Illustrations from *The Erhardt Developmental Prehension Assessment,* copyright 1994 by Rhoda P. Erhardt. Published by Erhardt Developmental Products, 2379 Snowshoe Court, Maplewood, MN 55119, (651) 730-9004. Reprinted by permission.

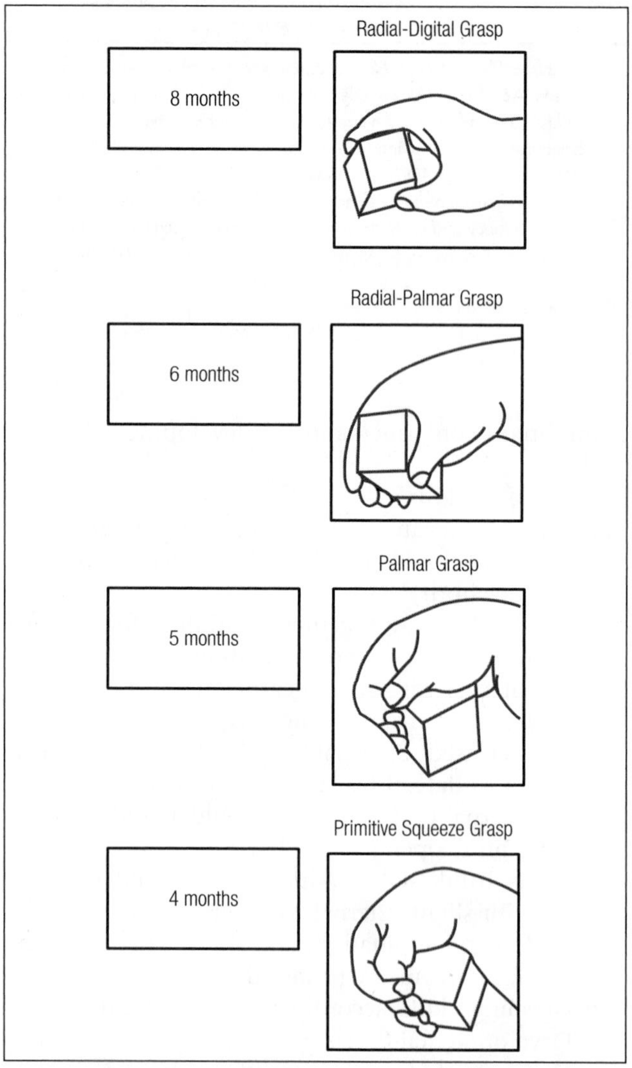

Figure 5-12 Developmental Levels: Grasp of the Cube

Illustrations from *The Erhardt Developmental Prehension Assessment,* copyright 1994 by Rhoda P. Erhardt. Published by Erhardt Developmental Products, 2379 Snowshoe Court, Maplewood, MN 55119, (651) 730-9004. Reprinted by permission.

two-stage transfer (5–6 months) to one-stage transfer (6–7 months) to voluntary release (7–9 months).
(2) By 9 months, release by full arm extension.
(3) Refinement continues up to age four with the attainment of graded release.

d. Carrying skills: involves a combination of movements of the shoulder, body and distal joints of the wrist and hand to hold the item, making appropriate adjustments as necessary to maintain this hold.

e. Bilateral hand use: asymmetric movements prevail until 3 months, and then symmetric movements emerge until 10 months.
(1) By 12 to 18 months, the baby uses both hands for different functions.
(2) At 18 to 24 months, manipulation skills emerge.
(3) The ability to use two different hands for two very different functions emerges at age 2½ years.

f. Manipulating skills according to Exner's Classification System.
(1) Finger-to-palm translation: a linear movement of an object from the fingers to the palm of the hand; e.g., picking up coins (12–15 months).
(2) Palm-to-finger translation: with stabilization, a linear movement of an object from the palm of the hand to the fingers; e.g., placing coins in a slot (2–2½ years).
(3) Shift: a linear movement of an object on the finger surfaces to allow for repositioning of the object relative to the finger pads; e.g., separating 2 pieces of paper (3–5 years), rolling a piece of clay into a ball (3–6+ years), shifting on marker or pencil (5 to 6+ years).
(4) Simple rotation: the turning or rolling of an object held at the finger pads approximately 90 degrees or less; e.g., unscrewing a small bottle cap (2–2½ years).
(5) Complex rotation: the rotation of an object 360 degrees; e.g., turning a pencil over to erase (6–7 years).
(6) In-hand manipulation with stabilization: several objects are held in the hand and manipulation of one object occurs, while simultaneously stabilizing the others; e.g., picking up pennies with thumb and forefinger while storing them in the ulnar side of the same hand (6–7 years).

g. Pre-writing skills.
(1) Palmar-supinate grasp: writing tool held with fisted hand, wrist slightly flexed and slightly supinated away from mid-position; arm moves as a unit (1–1½ years).
(2) Digital-pronate grasp: writing tool held with fingers, wrist neutral with slight ulnar deviation, and forearm pronated; arm moves as a unit (2–3 years).
(3) Static tripod posture: writing tool held with crude approximation of thumb, index, and middle fingers, ring and little fingers only slightly flexed, grasped proximally with continual adjustments by other hand, no fine localized movements of digit components; hand moves as a unit (3½–4 years).
(4) Dynamic tripod posture: writing tool held with precise opposition of distal phalanges of thumb, index, and middle fingers, ring and little fingers flexed to form a stable arch, wrist slightly extended, grasped distally, MCP joints stabilized during fine, localized movements of PIP joints (4½–6 years).
(5) Refer to Figure 5-13.

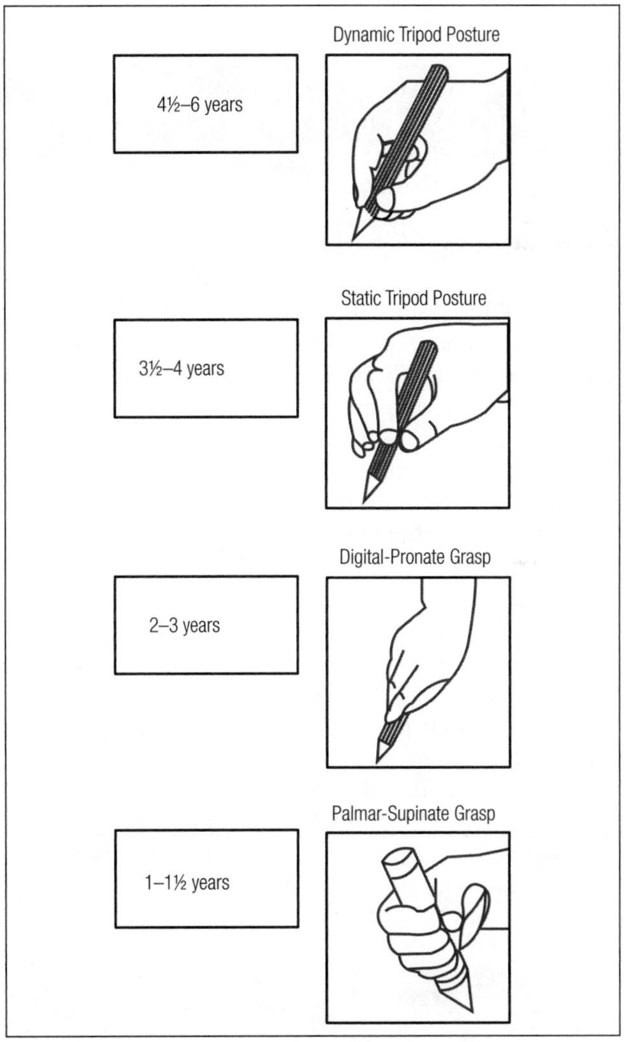

Figure 5-13 Developmental Levels: Pre-Writing Skills

Illustrations from *The Erhardt Developmental Prehension Assessment*, copyright 1994 by Rhoda P. Erhardt. Published by Erhardt Developmental Products, 2379 Snowshoe Court, Maplewood, MN 55119, (651) 730-9004. Reprinted by permission.

Chapter 5

h. Scissor skills.
(1) Prerequisite skills for using scissors include the ability to:
(a) Open and close a hand.
(b) Isolate or combine the movements of the thumb, index, and middle fingers.
(c) Use hands bilaterally; one hand cuts with the scissors, while the other hand stabilizes the item being cut.
(d) Coordinate arm, hand, and eye movements.
(e) Stabilize the wrist, elbow, and shoulder joints so that movement can occur at the distal joints.
(f) Interact with the environment in the constructive developmental play stage.
(2) Stages of development of scissor skills, the child sequentially:
(a) Shows an interest in scissors, 2–3 years.
(b) Holds and snips with scissors, 2–3 years.
(c) Opens and closes scissors in a controlled fashion, 2–3 years.
(d) Manipulates scissors in a forward motion, 3–4 years.
(e) Coordinates the lateral direction of the scissors, 3–4 years.
(f) Cuts a straight forward line, 3–4 years.
(g) Cuts simple geometric shapes, 3–4 years.
(h) Cuts circles, 3½–4½ years.
(i) Cuts simple figure shapes, 4–6 years.
(j) Cuts complex figure shapes, 6–7 years.

Psychosocial Development and Major Theorists

Overview

1. The NBCOT examination will likely not ask specific questions about psychosocial developmental theories, but the application of this knowledge may be needed to correctly answer exam items.
   a. The application of lifespan psychological theories can help determine a developmentally appropriate answer to an exam item question.
2. Occupational therapists need to know and understand the biological processes that are dependent on maturation.
   a. Occupational therapists consider these stages of development to be important in an individual's occupational performance.
3. Developmental psychological theories are not sufficient to understand the complexity involved in human occupational performance.
   a. The Occupational Practice Framework considers psychological theories as partially contributing to occupational performance.

Erik Erikson

1. Ego adaptation is the adaptive response of the ego in the development of the personality.
2. Eight stages of man are identified and include a critical personal-social crisis that when resolved by the individual gives the individual a sense of mastery and results in the acquisition of a personality quality.
   a. Stage 1, Basic trust vs. mistrust: the infant/baby realizes that survival and comfort needs will be met; hope is integrated into the personality (birth to 18 months).
   b. Stage 2, Autonomy vs. doubt and shame: the child realizes that he/she can control bodily functions; self-controlled will is integrated into the personality (2 to 4 years).
   c. Stage 3, Initiative vs. guilt: the child gains social skills and a gender role identity; a sense of purpose is integrated into the personality (preschool age).
   d. Stage 4, Industry vs. inferiority: the child gains a sense of security through peers and gains mastery over activities of his/her age group; a feeling of competency is integrated into the personality (elementary school age).
   e. Stage 5, Self-identity vs. role diffusion: the teenager begins to make choices about adult roles, and with the resolution of this identity crisis a sense of fidelity or membership with society is integrated into the personality (teenage years).
   f. Stage 6, Intimacy and solidarity vs. isolation: the young adult establishes an intimate relationship with a partner and family; the capacity to love is achieved (young adulthood).
   g. Stage 7, Generativity vs. self-absorption: the adult finds security in the contribution of his/her chosen personal/professional roles; the capacity to care is achieved (middle adulthood).

h. Stage 8, Integrity vs. despair: the mature adult reflects on his/her own value, and shares with the younger generation the knowledge gained; wisdom is acquired (maturity).

Lawrence Kohlberg

1. Stages of Moral Development.
   a. Level 1, preconventional morality: occurs up until the age of 8.
      (1) Stage 1, punishment and obedience: the child is obedient in order to avoid punishment.
      (2) Stage 2, instrumental relativism: the child makes moral choices based on the benefit to self and sometimes to others.
   b. Level 2, conventional morality: occurs at about 9 or 10 years of age.
      (1) Stage 1, social conformity: the child desires to gain the approval of others.
      (2) Stage 2, law and order: rules and social norms are internalized.
   c. Level 3, postconventional morality: age range can vary, and not all will achieve this level.
      (1) Social contracts: the young adult has social awareness and an awareness of the legal implications of decisions/actions.

Abraham Maslow

1. Maslow developed a hierarchy of basic human needs, proposing that if the lower-level needs are not met, the individual is unable to work on higher-level pursuits.
   a. Physiological: basic survival needs (i.e., food, water, rest, warmth).
   b. Safety: the need for physical and physiologic security.
   c. Love and belonging: the need for affection, emotional support, and group affiliation.
   d. Self-esteem: the need to believe in one's self as a competent and valuable member of society.
   e. Self-actualization: After attaining all of the psychosocial developmental milestones an individual's development of creativity, morality, spontenaity, lack of predjudice, acceptance of facts and problem-solving becomes integrated at this highest level of individual capability.

Cognitive Development

Jean Piaget

1. Described the process of cognitive development from birth to adolescence.
2. Major constructs.
   a. Adaptation: responding to environmental challenges as they occur.
   b. Mental schemes: organizing experiences into concepts.
   c. Operations: the cognitive methods used by the child to organize schemes and experiences to direct subsequent actions.
   d. Adapted intelligence or cognitive competence.
   e. Equilibrium: the balance between what the child knows and can act on and what the environment provides.
   f. Assimilation: the ability to take a new situation and change it to match an existing scheme or generalization.
   g. Accommodation: the development of a new scheme in response to the reality of a situation, or discrimination.
3. Hierarchical development of cognition.
   a. Sensorimotor period, ages birth to 2 years.
      (1) Reflexive stage: schemes begin in response to reflexes (1 month).
      (2) Primary circular reactions: child learns about cause and effect as a result of reflexive sensorimotor patterns that are repeated for enjoyment (2 to 4 months).
      (3) Secondary circular reactions: voluntary movement patterns emerge due to coordination of vision and hand function, and an early awareness of cause and effect develops (5 to 8 months).
      (4) Coordination of secondary schemata: voluntary movement in response to stimuli that cannot be seen such as in object permanence, and early development of decentered thought (9 to 12 months).
      (5) Tertiary circular reactions: the child seeks out new schemes, with improved gross and fine motor abilities; tool use begins (12 to 18 months).
      (6) Inventions of new means through mental combinations: the child demonstrates insight

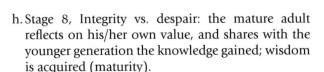

and purposeful tool use, and explores problem solving options. The ability to represent concepts without direct manipulation emerges (18 months to 2 years).

(7) Child progresses from reflexive activity to mental representation, to cognitive functions of combining and manipulating objects in play.

b. Preoperational period, ages 2 to 7 years.

(1) Classification: categorizing objects according to similarities and differences.

(2) Seriation: the relationship of one object or classification of objects to another.

(3) Conservation: the end product of the preoperational period. The child is able to recognize the continuities of an object or class of objects in spite of apparent changes.

(4) The preoperational period is divided into two phases.

(a) Preconceptual: the child expands vocabulary and symbolic representations (2 to 4 years).

(b) Intuitive thought phase: the child imitates, copies or repeats what is seen or heard and bases conclusions on what the child believes to be true rather than on logic. Inductive reasoning denotes a transition to the next stage (4 to 7 years).

(5) Child progresses from dependence on perception, and egocentric orientation to logical thought, for solving problems. Child enjoys symbolic and verbal play.

c. Concrete operations, ages 7 to 11 years.

(1) Reversibility: an expansion of conservation, leads to increased spatial awareness.

(2) Rules: as rules are better understood, they are also applied.

(3) Empirical-inductive thinking: the child solves problems with the information that is obvious and present.

(4) Child uses logical thinking on observed or mentally represented objects, enjoying games with rules which help the child adjust to social demands.

d. Formal operations, ages 11 through the teen years.

(1) Hypothetical-deductive thinking, the ability to analyze and plan.

(2) Child uses logic to hypothesize many ways to solve problems, and can draw from past and present experiences to imagine what can have an effect on future situations.

4. Piaget stated that maturation of cognition is dependent on the following items.

a. Organic growth, especially the maturation of the nervous system and endocrine glands.

b. Experience in the actions performed on objects.

c. Social interaction and transmission.

d. A balance of opportunities for both assimilation and accommodation.

Major Milestones in Cognitive Development

1. Early object use.

a. Child focuses on action performed with objects; e.g., banging, shaking (3–6 months).

b. Child explores characteristics of objects and expands the range of schemes; e.g., pulling, turning, poking, tearing (6–9 months).

c. Child combines objects in relational play, such as objects in containers (8–9 months).

d. Child notices the relation between complex actions and consequences such as opening doors, placing lids on containers, and differential use of schemes based on the toy being played with; e.g., pushing a train or rolling a ball (9–12 months).

e. Child acts on objects with a variety of schemes (12 months +).

f. Child links schemes in simple combinations; e.g., placing a baby in carriage and then pushing the carriage (12–15 months).

g. Child links multi-scheme combinations into a meaningful sequence; e.g., putting food in a bowl, scooping the food using a spoon, and feeding a doll (24–36 months).

h. Child links schemes into a complex script (36–42 months).

2. Problem-solving skills.

a. 6–9 months.

(1) Child finds object after watching it disappear; e.g., toy covered by cloth.

(2) Child uses movement as a means to an end; e.g., rolling to secure toy.

(3) Child anticipates movement of objects in space; e.g., looking toward trajectory of object circling the child's head.

(4) Child attends to consequences of actions; e.g., banging toy and realizing it makes noise.

(5) Child repeats actions to repeat consequences; e.g., banging toy to hear noise.

b. 9–12 months.

(1) Child is able to use a tool after demonstration, e.g., using a stick to secure a toy that is out of reach.

(2) Child's behavior becomes more goal directed.

(3) Child performs an action to produce a response.

c. 12–15 months.

(1) Child recruits the help of an adult to achieve a goal.

(2) Child attempts to activate a simple mechanism.

(3) Child turns and inspects objects.

(4) Child uses a trial and error approach to new challenges.

d. 18–21 months.

(1) Child attends to shapes of things and uses them appropriately.

(2) Child begins to think before acting.

(3) Child uses tool to obtain a favored object.

(4) Child begins to replace trial and error with a thought process in order to attain a goal.

(5) Child can operate a mechanical toy; e.g., an on-off switch.

(6) Child can predict effects or presume causes.

e. 21–24 months.

(1) Child recognizes operations of several mechanisms.

(2) Child matches circles, squares, triangles, and manipulates objects into small openings; e.g., shape sorters.

f. 24–27 months.

(1) Child discriminates sizes.

g. 24–30 months.

(1) Child can build with blocks horizontally and vertically.

h. 27–30 months.

(1) Child begins to relate experiences to one another, based on logic and knowledge of previous experiences.

(2) Child can make a mental plan of action without acting it out.

(3) Child can see relationships between experiences; e.g., if the balloon is popped, it will make a loud noise.

i. 36–48 months.

(1) Child can build a tower of nine cubes, demonstrating balance and coordination.

(2) Child can organize objects by size and build a structure from a mental image.

j. 48–60 months.

(1) Child can build involved structures combining various planes, along with symmetrical designs.

(2) Child is able to utilize spatial awareness, cause-and-effect, and mental images in problem solving.

3. Symbolic play.

a. 12–16 months.

(1) Basic "make believe" play, primarily involving self; e.g., eating, sleeping.

b. 12–18 months.

(1) Child can project "make believe" play on objects and others.

(2) Child uses a variety of schemes in imitating familiar activities.

c. 18–24 months.

(1) Child increases the use of non-realistic objects in pretending; e.g., substituting a block for a train.

(2) Child has inanimate objects perform familiar activities; e.g., a doll washing itself.

d. 24–48 months.

(1) See the following section.

Development of Play

Categories of Play

1. Exploratory play, 0–2 years.

a. Child engages in play experiences through which the child develops a body scheme.

b. Sensory integrative and motor skills are also developed as the child explores the properties and effects of actions on objects and people.

c. Child plays mostly with parents/caregiver(s).

2. Symbolic play, 2–4 years.

a. Child engages in play experiences through which the child formulates, tests, classifies, and refines ideas, feelings, and combined actions.

b. This form of play is associated with language development.

c. Objects that are manageable for the child in terms of symbolization, control, and mastery are preferred by the child.

d. Child is mostly involved in parallel play with peers and begins to become more cooperative over time.

3. Creative play, 4–7 years.

a. Child engages in sensory, motor, cognitive, and social play experiences in which the child refines relevant skills.

b. Child explores combinations of actions on multiple objects.

c. Child begins to master skills that promote performance of school and work related activities.

d. Child participates in cooperative peer groups.

4. Games, 7–12 years.

a. Child participates in play with rules, competition, social interaction, and opportunities for development of skills.

b. Child begins to participate in cooperative peer groups with a growing interest in competition.

c. Friends become important for validation of play items and performance, while parents assist and validate in the absence of peers.

Chapter 5

Self-Care Development

Feeding

1. Oral-motor development.
   a. Prior to 33 weeks of gestation an infant is fed by non-oral means.
   b. 35 weeks of gestation or after: jaw and tongue movements are strong enough to allow for feeding.
   c. 40 weeks of gestation: rooting reflexes, gag and cough reflex are present for up to four months, protecting the airway and decreasing the chances of aspiration.
   d. 4–5 months: munching occurs consisting of a phasic bite and release of a soft cookie.
   e. 6 months: strong up and down movement of the tongue.

Table 5-5

Developmental Continuum in Self-Feeding and Associated Component Areas

AGE (MO)	EATING AND FEEDING PERFORMANCE	CONCURRENT CHANGES IN PERFORMANCE COMPONENTS		
		SENSORIMOTOR	COGNITION	PSYCHOSOCIAL
5–7	Takes cereal or poured baby food from spoon.	Has good head stability and emerging sitting abilities; reaches and grasps toys; explores and tolerates various textures (e.g., fingers, rattles); puts objects in mouth.	Attends to effect produced by actions, such as hitting or shaking.	Plays with caregiver during meals and engages in interactive routines.
6–8	Attempts to hold bottle but may not retrieve it if it falls; needs to be monitored for safety reasons.		Object permanence is emerging and infant anticipates spoon or bottle.	Is easily distracted by stimuli (especially siblings) in the environment.
6–9	Holds and tries to eat cracker but sucks on it more than bites it; consumes soft foods that dissolve in the mouth; grabs at spoon but bangs it or sucks on either end of it.	Good sitting stability emerges; able to use hands to manipulate smaller parts of rattle; guided reach and palmer grasp applied to hand-to-mouth actions with objects.	Uses familiar actions initially with haphazard variations; seeks novelty and is anxious to explore objects (may grab at food on adult's plate).	Recognizes strangers; emerging sense of self.
9–13	Finger-feeds self a portion of meals consisting of soft table foods (e.g., macaroni, peas, dry cereal) and objects if fed by an adult.	Uses various grasps on objects of different sizes; able to isolate radial fingers on smaller objects.	Has increased organization and sequencing of schemes to do desired activity; may have difficulty attending to events outside visual space (e.g., position of spoon close to mouth).	Prefers to act on objects than be passive observer.
12–14	Dips spoon in food, brings spoonful of food to mouth, but spills food by inverting spoon before it goes into mouth.	Begins to place and release objects; likely to use pronated grasp on objects like crayon or spoon.	Recognizes that objects have function and uses tools appropriately; relates objects together, shifting attention among them.	Has interest in watching family routines.
15–18	Scoops food with spoon and brings it to mouth.	Shoulder and wrist stability demonstrate precise movements.	Experiments to learn rules of how objects work; actively solves problems by creating new action solutions.	Internalizes standards imposed by others for how to play with objects.
24–30	Demonstrates interest in using fork; may stab at food such as pieces of canned fruit; proficient at spoon use and eats cereal with milk or rice with gravy with utensil.	Tolerates various food textures in mouth; adjusts movements to be efficient (e.g., forearm supinated to scoop and lift spoon).	Expresses wants verbally; demonstrates imitation of short sequence of occupation (e.g., putting food on plate and eating it).	Has increasing desire to copy peers; looks to adults to see if they appreciate success in an occupation; interested in household routines.

Shepherd, J. (2005). Activities of daily living and adaptations for independent living. In J. Case-Smith, (Ed.), *Occupational therapy for children*, 5th ed. (p. 489). St. Louis, MO: Elsevier Mosby. Reprinted with permission.

f. 7–8 months: beginning of mastication of soft and mashed foods with diagonal jaw movement.
g. 9 months: lateral tongue movements make mastication of soft and mashed food effective, able to drink from a cup; however, jaw is not firm.
h. 12 months: jaw is firm; there is rotary chewing allowing for a good bite on a hard cookie.
i. 24 months: able to chew most meats and raw vegetables.

2. Evaluation of feeding.
   a. Parent interview including parent's concerns, feeding history, behavior during feeding, weight gain or loss.
   b. Medical and developmental history.
   c. Observation of feeding including postural control; oral sensitivity; motor control of the jaw, lip, tongue, and cheek; and coordination and endurance of all.
   d. Recommendation for videofluoroscopy swallow study especially if the child has a high risk of aspiration (refer to Chapter 9).
3. Intervention for oral motor control.
   a. Appropriate positioning to allow for neutral pelvic alignment and trunk stability either in caregiver's lap or chair (infant seat or wheelchair); avoid head extension to prevent asphyxiation as a result of closing of the airway.
   b. Hand positioning of the caregiver: place the index finger longitudinally under the child's lip, middle finger under the jaw, and place the thumb on the lateral end of the mandible.
   c. Facilitate lip closure by applying slight upward pressure of the index finger under the child's lip.
   d. Facilitate jaw closure by firm upper pressure of the middle finger under the jaw.
   e. Hand positioning of the index and middle fingers to assist in inhibiting tongue thrust.
      (1) Press bowl of spoon downward and hold on tongue.
   f. Facilitate swallow by lip closure, and by placement and slight downward pressure of the spoon on the middle aspect of the tongue.
   g. Facilitate chewing by placement of foods, such as long soft cooked vegetables, between the gum and teeth.
   h. Integrate preventive measures to work out of abnormal patterns.
      (1) Provide firm downward pressure, using a spoon, on the middle aspect of the tongue in presence of a tonic bite reflex.
      (2) Prevent tongue retraction to avoid choking.
      (3) Facilitate lip closure for a tongue thrust that can result in loss of liquid and food, drooling, and failure to thrive.
      (4) Decrease tactile sensitivity prior to feeding as well as at other times, by providing firm pressure; encourage sucking/chewing on a cloth; rub gums, palate, and tongue; promote oral exploration of toys; use a NUK toothbrush; and vary texture of foods, gradually introducing mashed potatoes mixed with other vegetables and soft meats.

Table 5-6

Development of Self-Dressing Skills

AGE (YRS)	SELF-DRESSING SKILL
1	Cooperates with dressing (holds out arms and feet) Pulls off shoes, removes socks Pushes arms through sleeves and legs through pants
2	Removes unfastened coat Removes shoes if laces are untied Helps pull down pants Finds armholes in pullover shirt
2½	Removes pull-down pants with elastic waist Assists in pulling on socks Puts on front-button coat or shirt Unbuttons large buttons
3	Puts on pullover shirt with minimal assistance Puts on shoes without fasteners (may be on wrong foot) Puts on socks (may be with heel on top) Independently pulls down pants Zips and unzips jacket once on track Needs assistance to remove pullover shirt Buttons large front buttons
3½	Finds front of clothing Snaps or hooks front fastener Unzips front zipper on jacket, separating zipper Puts on mittens Buttons series of three or four buttons Unbuckles shoe or belt Dresses with supervision (needs help with front and back)
4	Removes pullover garment independently Buckles shoes or belt Zips jacket zipper Puts on socks correctly Puts on shoes with assistance in tying laces Laces shoes Consistently identifies the front and back of garment
4½	Puts belt in loops
5	Ties and unties knots Dresses unsupervised
6	Closes back zipper Ties bows Buttons back buttons Snaps back snaps

Shepherd, J. (2005). Activities of daily living and adaptations for independent living. In J. Case-Smith, (Ed.), *Occupational therapy for children*, 5th ed. (p. 547). St. Louis, MO: Elsevier Mosby. Reprinted with permission.

i. Consider and utilize the appropriate texture of foods as related to the child's feeding problems. Thick foods are easier to swallow and manage, especially if a tongue thrust is present.
j. A major role of the therapist is to assist the caregiver in considering and promoting a pleasant social atmosphere for feeding by utilizing positioning and handling techniques to promote eye contact and bonding in a relaxed environment.
k. Consider the developmental sequence of feeding skills
(1) Refer to Table 5-5.

Development of Dressing Skills

1. Refer to Table 5-6.

Development of Toileting Skills

1. Refer to Table 5-7.

Table 5-7

Typical Developmental Sequence of Toileting

APPROX. AGE (YR)	TOILETING SKILL
1	• Indicates discomfort when wet or soiled • Has regular bowel movements
1½	• Sits on toilet when placed there and supervised (short time)
2	• Urinates regularly
2½	• Achieves regulated toileting with occasional daytime accidents • Rarely has bowel accidents • Tells someone that he or she needs to go to the bathroom • May need reminders to go to the bathroom • May need help with getting on the toilet
3	• Goes to bathroom independently; seats himself or herself on the toilet • May need help with wiping • May need help with fasteners or difficult clothing
4–5	• Is independent in toileting (e.g., tearing toilet paper, flushing, washing hands, managing clothing)

Shepherd, J. (2005). Activities of daily living and adaptations for independent living. In J. Case-Smith, (Ed.), *Occupational therapy for children*, 5th ed. (p. 543). St. Louis, MO: Elsevier Mosby. Reprinted with permission.

Development of Home Management Skills

1. Refer to Table 5-8.

Table 5-8

Developmental Sequence for Household Management Tasks

AGE	TASK
13 months	Imitates housework
2 years	Picks up and puts toys away with parental reminders Copies parents' domestic activities
3 years	Carries things without dropping them Dusts with help Dries dishes with help Gardens with help Puts toys away with reminders Wipes up spills
4 years	Fixes dry cereal and snacks Helps with sorting laundry
5 years	Puts toys away neatly Makes a sandwich Takes out trash Makes bed Puts dirty clothes in hamper Answers telephone correctly
6 years	Does simple errands Does household chores without redoing Cleans sink Washes dishes with help Crosses street safely
7–9 years	Begins to cook simple meals Puts clean clothes away Hangs up clothes Manages small amounts of money Uses telephone correctly
10–12 years	Cooks simple meals with supervision Does simple repairs with appropriate tools Begins doing laundry Sets table Washes dishes Cares for pet with reminders
13–14 years	Does laundry Cooks meals

Shepherd, J. (2005). Activities of daily living and adaptations for independent living. In J. Case-Smith, (Ed.), *Occupational therapy for children*, 5th ed. (p. 558). St. Louis, MO: Elsevier Mosby. Reprinted with permission.

Occupational Therapy Developmental Evaluation

Overall Components

1. Information regarding the mother's pregnancy and specifics of birth history.
   a. Apgar score of the infant's heart rate, respiration, reflex irritability, muscle tone, and color is measured at one, five, and 10 minutes after birth, each item receives a rating of 0, 1 or 2 The highest score possible is 10 points indicating a newborn's well-being.
   b. Number of weeks premature, adjusted age.
   c. Number of days/weeks in incubator, intubated and/or on ventilator, or nasogastric tube.
2. Medical history: admissions and length of hospitalizations for illness, disease, surgery, and medications.
3. Developmental history: important developmental milestones, their time of achievement, and any difficulties or problems surrounding their attainment.
4. Parent interview to address the above, and the parent's perspective on developmental progress and/or concerns, home situation, family history, school history, support systems, and insurance coverage.

Assessment of the Newborn, Infant, and Child

1. Neurobehavioral organization: signs of stress or stability.
   a. Neurobehavioral subsystems: based on synactive theory of development (i.e., subsystems continuously interact with each other and with the environment as evidenced by the infant's levels of stress or stability).
      (1) Autonomic system: physiological instability orstability.
      (2) Motor system: fluctuating tone with uncontrolled activity or consistent tone with controlled activity.
      (3) Emotional state: disorganized, calm, alert.
      (4) Attention-interaction: stress signals upon attempts at attending to stimuli, difficulty shifting attention, focused responsiveness to stimuli, and fluid shifting of attention.
      (5) Self-regulation: ability to self-organize and balance of subsystems
   b. Testing of reflex integration. (Table 5-2).
   c. Muscle tone.
2. Musculoskeletal status.
   a. Skeletal status including extremity and spine deformities.
   b. Range of motion status.
   c. Posture at rest and posture during active movement (see neuromotor assessments).
   d. See Chapter 6 on evaluation and intervention for musculoskeletal dysfunction.
3. Developmental assessments.
   a. There are many published tools that measure neonate, infant, and child development.
   b. Currently the NBCOT examination may include a description of evaluation methods and/or the names of specific published assessment tools; therefore, a review of major developmental assessments is important for examination preparation.
      (1) This can also increase understanding and knowledge of major principles and approaches in the evaluation of normal and abnormal development.
      (2) This can further strengthen the clinical reasoning skills needed to answer questions that address evaluation.
4. As of the publication of this text, NBCOT has not made public the names of all of the specific assessments that may be on the examination.
   a. The assessments included in this chapter are based on the authors' review of NBCOT self-assessment tools, major OT textbooks and feedback obtained from OT practitioners regarding developmental measures used in practice.

Developmental Assessments of Neonates

1. Assessment of Preterm Infants' Behavior (APIB).
   a. Focus: assesses infant's pattern of developing behavioral organization in response to increasing sensory and environmental stimuli.
      (1) An extension and refinement of the Neonatal Behavioral Assessment Scale (NBAS).
   b. Method: a behavior checklist and scale.
   c. Scoring and interpretation.
      (1) Scores are obtained prior to administration for a baseline, during administration and following administration.
      (2) Scores reflect the degree of facilitation provided by the examiner.
      (3) Eye movements and asymmetry of performance are measured.
      (4) Function and integration of the physiological, motor, state, attentional/interactive, and regulatory systems are determined.

(5) Interpretation of scores allows the therapist to plan interventions, measure outcomes, and plan follow-up.

d. Population: pre-term and full-term infants.

2. Neurological Assessment of Pre-term and Full-term New-born Infant (NAPFI).

a. Focus: a rating scale consisting of a brief neurological examination incorporated into routine assessment.

(1) Can be used with newborns in an incubator and/or on a ventilator if handling can be tolerated.

(2) Habituation, movement and tone, reflexes, and neurobehavioral responses including state transition, level of arousal and alertness, auditory and visual orientation, irritability, consolability, and cry are assessed.

b. Method: items are administered in a sequence; first in a quiet or sleep state, followed by items not influenced by state, then during the awake state.

c. Scoring and interpretation.

(1) The infant's state is recorded, based on six gradings of state, for each item.

(2) Interpretation of scores allows the therapist to document a pattern of responses to reflect neurological functions and identify deviations for diagnosis.

(3) A comparison of pre-term with full-term infant behavior is provided.

d. Population: pre-term and full-term newborn infants.

Overall Development Assessments

1. Denver Developmental Screening Test II.

a. Focus: standardized task performance and observation screening tool for early identification of children at risk for developmental delays in four areas including personal-social, fine motor-adaptive, language, and gross motor skills.

b. Method.

(1) Test includes 125 test items.

(2) Test items below the child's chronological age level are administered with sequential progression toward higher level chronological items until the child fails three items.

(3) Behaviors observed during the screening are marked on a checklist.

(4) Questionnaires for home screening of environments and prescreening of development are available to administer to parents/caregivers.

c. Scoring and interpretation.

(1) Each item scored indicates the chronological age at which it is expected to be performed. The child's score on that item is compared to determine whether the child's performance is age appropriate or delayed, and is marked as pass or fail.

(2) The test is discontinued when three items are failed.

(3) The screening allows for interpretation of a child's performance in terms of being normal, abnormal, questionable, or unstable in personal-social, fine motor-adaptive, language, and gross motor abilities.

(4) Interpretation of findings must be considered in the context of other pertinent information and with ongoing observations.

d. Population: 1 month to 6 years.

2. Bayley Scales of Infant Development, 3rd Edition (BSID-III).

a. Focus: standardized rating scales that assess multiple areas of development to attain a baseline for intervention and to monitor progress.

(1) Evaluates five domains: cognitive, language, and motor, which are performance based tasks, and social-emotional and adaptive behavior skills.

b. Method.

(1) Age appropriate items are selected from items on the different domain scales.

(2) Involves parent(s) completing two questionnaires.

c. Scoring and interpretation.

(1) Composite scores yield qualitative descriptors and performance levels for each domain.

(2) Results are used to plan interventions for any delays.

d. Population: 1 to 42 months.

3. First STEP Screening Test for Evaluating Preschoolers.

a. Focus: a checklist and rating scale which identifies preschool students at risk and in need of a more comprehensive evaluation.

b. Method.

(1) It assesses five areas/domains as identified by IDEA which include cognition, communication, physical, social and emotional, and adaptive functioning.

(a) Table-top tasks are administered while sitting across from the child; additional space is needed for gross motor tasks.

(2) An optional Social-Emotional Rating Scale is rated by the examiner based on the child's behavior during testing.

(3) An optional Adaptive Behavior Checklist is rated by the examiner according to the information obtained from a parent or caregiver interview regarding daily functioning.

(4) An optional Parent-Teacher Scale provides additional information not obtained during the testing.

c. Scoring and interpretation.
   (1) Each item has criteria for grading and scores for each domain are totaled.
   (2) Total domain scores are converted to composite scores to determine whether the child's performance is within an acceptable level or if the child is at risk.
   (3) The determination of a child's strengths and areas needing improvement guide treatment planning.
d. Population: 2 years 9 months through 6 years 2 months.

4. Hawaii Early Learning Profile, Revised (HELP).
   a. Focus: non-standardized scale of developmental levels. An educational curriculum-referenced test that assesses six areas of function including cognitive, language, gross motor, fine motor, social-emotional, and self-help.
   b. Methods.
      (1) Administered in the child's natural environment and in the context of the family during typical routines.
      (2) Developmentally appropriate items are administered according to established protocols.
      (3) A protocol using a warm-up period, structured play, and snack time is recommended.
   c. Scoring and interpretation.
      (1) Developmental age range levels of skills in each of the six areas can be approximated.
      (2) Specification of skills noted on a chart can be transferred to a checklist for analysis of expected skills that are absent.
      (3) A description of behavior and possible causes of difficulty, all within the context of the family and environment, can be obtained.
      (4) Developmental structuring of skills is provided in the form of a sequence of conceptual strands, so skills needed as a foundation for more advanced skills are provided.
   d. Population: children, ages birth through 3 years, with developmental delay, disabilities, or at risk. HELP for Preschoolers is available for children ages 3 to 6, with and without delays.

5. Miller Assessment for Preschoolers (MAP).
   a. Focus: standardized task performance screening tool that assesses sensory and motor abilities consisting of foundation and coordination indexes, cognitive abilities including verbal and nonverbal indexes, and combined abilities which include a complex tasks index.
   b. Method.
      (1) Items are administered that relate to the age of the subject.
      (2) Supplemental nonstandardized observations may be administered.
   c. Scoring and interpretation.
      (1) Measures are obtained in sensory and motor abilities, cognitive abilities, and combined abilities.
      (2) The child's performance is compared with norms.
      (3) Percentile equivalents can be obtained for each index and for performance overall.
      (4) Results used for treatment planning.
   d. Populations: 2 years 9 months to 5 years 8 months.

6. Pediatric Evaluation of Disability Inventory (PEDI).
   a. Focus: standardized behavior checklist and rating scale that assesses capabilities and detects functional deficits, to determine developmental level, monitor the child's progress and/or to complete a program evaluation.
      (1) Modifications and Caregiver Assistance Scales determine the level of assistance and adaptations needed to enhance participation.
   b. Method.
      (1) Observation, interview, and scoring of the three domains.
         (a) Self-care, mobility, and social skills and their functional sub-units are assessed.
   c. Scoring and interpretation.
      (1) The score forms include the areas of functional skills, caregiver assistance, and modifications.
         (a) The three sections are scored separately.
      (2) Identifies children with patterns of delay.
      (3) Progress and outcomes can be monitored.
   d. Population: 6 months to 7.5 years.

Motor Assessments

1. Bruininks-Oseretsky Test of Motor Proficiency (2nd ed.) (BOT-2).
   a. Focus: standardized test assesses and provides an index of overall motor proficiency; fine and gross motor composites, including consideration of speed, duration, and accuracy of performance, and hand and/or foot preferences.
   b. Method.
      (1) There is a long and short form with 8 subtests: fine motor precision, fine motor integration, manual dexterity, bilateral coordination, balance, running speed and agility, upper limb coordination and strength.
         (a) Hand and foot preference is initially determined.
   c. Scoring and interpretation.
      (1) A total motor composite score consists of four motor areas: fine manual control, manual coordination, body coordination, and strength and agility.

(2) Age equivalency and descriptive categories, and performance scores indicate motor strengths and weaknesses.
(3) Scores may be used as a basis for suggesting treatment goals and to evaluate change.

d. Population: 4 years to 21 years.

2. Erhardt Developmental Prehension Assessment (EDPA) Revised and Short Screening Form (EDPA-S).
   a. Focus: observation checklist based on performance which assesses three clustered areas including involuntary arm-hand patterns; voluntary movements of approach; and prewriting skills.
      (1) EDPA allows for charting and monitoring of prehensile development.
      (2) EDPA-S identifies developmental gaps in prehensile development and the need for further assessment.
   b. Method.
      (1) Test is administered in sections according to the appropriate age level.
      (2) There are 341 test components in the EDPA categorized according to involuntary arm hand patterns, voluntary movements, and prewriting skills.
      (3) The EDPA-S contains 128 components.
   c. Scoring and interpretation.
      (1) Part One: right and left hand scores are scored as normal or well-integrated, not present or emerging, or abnormal.
      (2) Part Two: scores are placed into a developmental level for each cluster.
      (3) Part Three: function is determined for involuntary arm-hand patterns, voluntary movements, and prewriting skills.
      (4) Gaps in hand skills and developmental levels can be determined.
         (a) Intervention can be planned and provided depending on individual needs.
   d. Population: Children of all ages and cognitive levels with neurodevelopmental disorders.
3. Peabody Developmental Motor Scales (2nd ed.) (PDMS-2).
   a. Focus: standardized rating scales of gross and fine motor development.
   b. Method.
      (1) Gross and fine motor subtests measure reflexes, sustained control, locomotion, object manipulation, grasping, and visual motor integration.
      (2) Test items are administered one level below the child's expected motor age in order to obtain a basal age level.
      (3) Test is discontinued with three consecutive scores of zero.
   c. Scoring and interpretation.
      (1) A developmental profile of gross and fine motor skills is provided.
      (2) Standard scores are provided.
      (3) Strengths and weaknesses are indicated once the percentile ranks are grafted.
      (4) A motor activity program useful for planning and implementing training is provided.
   d. Population: children, ages birth to 6 years, with motor, speech-language, and/or hearing disorders.
4. Toddler and Infant Motor Evaluation (TIME).
   a. Focus: assesses the quality of movement.
   b. Method.
      (1) Five primary subtests assess mobility, stability, motor organization, social/emotional abilities, and functional performance.
      (2) Quality rating, component analysis, and atypical positions can be assessed by clinicians with advanced training.
   c. Scoring and interpretation.
      (1) Cutoff scores are indicative of moderate or significant motor delays.
      (2) Subtests give more specific information.
   d. Population: Birth to 3 years and 6 months.

Visual motor and Visual Perception Assessments

1. Beery-Buktenica Developmental Test of Visual Motor Integration-VMI, 6th edition.
   a. Focus: assesses visual motor integration.
      (1) Can be used as a classroom screening tool.
   b. Method.
      (1) The child copies 24 geometric forms which are sequenced according to level of difficulty.
      (2) Once the child fails to meet grading criteria for three consecutive forms, the test is discontinued.
   c. Scoring and interpretation.
      (1) Raw score can be translated to percentile ranks, standard score, and age equivalency.
      (2) Average scores fall between 80 and 120 and average percentiles fall between 25 and 75.
   d. Population: Two years to 100 years.
      (1) The revised edition provides new norms for ages two through 18 years.
         (a) The adult norms for ages 19 and older have not been updated.
2. Developmental Test of Visual Perception (2nd Edition) (DTVP-2) and Developmental Test of Visual Perception – Adolescent and Adult (DTVP-A).
   a. Focus: assesses visual perceptual skills and visual motor integration for levels of performance and for designing interventions and monitoring progress.

b. Method.
(1) DTVP-2 is comprised of eight subtests including eye-hand coordination, copying, spatial relations, visual-motor speed, position in space, figure-ground, visual-closure, form-constancy.
(2) DTVP-A is comprised of four subtests of visual motor integration, composite index, and motor-reduced visual perception composite index.
c. Scoring and interpretation.
(1) Raw scores, age equivalents, percentiles, subtest standard scores, and composite quotients are provided.
(2) Three indexes provided.
(a) General visual perceptual.
(b) Motor-reduced visual perception.
(c) Visual motor integration.
d. Population: children aged 4 to 10 years for the DTVP-2; adolescents and adults aged 11 to 74 years for the DTVP-A.

3. Erhardt Developmental Vision Assessment (EDVA) and Short Screening Form (EDVA-S).
a. Focus: a behavior rating scale to determine visuomotor development that assesses involuntary visual patterns including eyelid reflexes, pupillary reactions, doll's eye responses, and voluntary patterns including fixation, localization, ocular pursuit, and gaze shift.
b. Method.
(1) There are 271 test items organized developmentally into seven clusters.
(2) The clusters are presented and items are sequenced developmentally.
(3) Upon administration of each item, a response is scored for each eye.
(4) Models for assessment and management, and items required for testing are provided.
c. Scoring and interpretation.
(1) Responses are scored as normal, well-integrated, emerging, or not present.
(2) A developmental level is provided for each cluster and a final developmental level is estimated.
(3) EDVA-S includes 67 components of permanent vision patterns, and is scored in the same manner as EDVA.
(a) If a test item is scored emerging or not present, a full evaluation using EDVA is indicated.
(4) Baseline levels allow for identification of delays, and also determine the sequenced developmental items that have not been attained.
(a) A baseline also allows progress to be tracked and interventions to be established.
(5) Findings will determine indications for an ophthalmic evaluation.
d. Population: birth to 6 months. Since the 6-month level is considered the norm, the EDVA-S can be used for assessing older children.

4. Preschool Visual Motor Integration Assessment (PVMIA).
a. Focus: a standardized norm referenced assessment which evaluates visual motor integration and visual perceptual skills of preschoolers, including perception in space, awareness of spatial relationships, color and space discrimination, matching two attributes simultaneously and the ability to reproduce what is seen and interpreted.
b. Method: two performance subtests and two behavioral observation checklists.
(1) The Drawing subtest requires the child to recognize and reproduce lines and shapes that increase in level of complexity.
(2) The Block Patterns subtest requires the child to recognize color and shape and reproduce block patterns and match block pictures using three-dimensional blocks.
(3) It has a section that first predetermines that the child has the requisite skills to continue with the test items.
(4) The behavioral observation checklists are completed during testing by the administrator to document observed behaviors in an orderly manner to be used in test interpretation.
c. Scoring and interpretation:
(1) The child's fine motor skills and visual perceptual abilities are examined separately, to the extent possible.
(2) Each task has specific criteria listed on the score sheet.
(3) To attain the precision needed to accurately score the child's final products, templates and a ruler are provided to be used when scoring each subtest.
(4) Raw scores are converted to standard scores and percentile ranges for both subtests and for the total test.
(a) Impairments are indicated by standards scores below 80 and percentile scores below 25.
(5) Administrator's recorded behavioral observations of the child during the testing are not included in the score. These observations are used in test interpretation and subsequent intervention planning.
(6) Interpretation of the child's performance and current emerging abilities are made based upon the combination of numerical scores, behavioral observations, and error analysis.
d. Population: preschoolers aged 3½ to 5½ years old.

5. Motor-Free Visual Perception Test (MVPT-3)
   a. Focus: a standardized, quick evaluation to assess visual perception (excludes motor components) in five areas including spatial relationships, visual discrimination, figure-ground, visual closure, and visual memory.
   b. Method.
      (1) The number of items administered depends on the child's age.
         (a) For children aged 4 to 10 years, items 1–40 are administered; for persons aged 10 years or older, items 14–65 are administered.
   c. Scoring and interpretation
      (1) Raw scores are translated into perceptual ages and perceptual quotients.
      (2) Average performance is determined as a standard score of 80–120 and percentile ranks of 25–75.
   d. Population: children and adults aged 4 to 95 years.
6. Motor-Free Visual Perception Test-Vertical (MVPT-V).
   a. Focus: evaluation of individuals with spatial deficits, due to hemi-field visual neglect or abnormal visual saccades.
   b. Method: Thirty-six items vertically placed are used to assess spatial relationships, visual discrimination, figure ground, visual closure, and visual memory (excluding motor components).
   c. Scoring and interpretation.
      (1) Provides perceptual ages and perceptual quotients.
      (2) Inadequate performance is determined as a score of 85 or less.
   d. Population: children and adults with visual field cuts or without visual impairments.
      (1) Appropriate for individuals with brain injury since it reduces confounding variables.
7. Test of Visual-Motor Skills (TVMS) and Test of Visual-Motor Skills: Upper Level (TVMS-UL).
   a. Focus: assesses eye hand coordination skills for copying geometric designs.
   b. Method.
      (1) The individual copies and draws geometric designs which become sequentially more complex.
         (a) There are 23 geometric forms in the TVMS which are scored for 8 possible errors and 16 in the TVMS: UL which are scored for 9–22 possible errors in motor accuracy, motor control, motor coordination, and psychomotor speed.
      (2) Test behavior is also documented.
   c. Scoring and interpretation.
      (1) The resulting score can be translated into a motor age, standard score, and percentile rank.
      (2) Characteristics and errors of the drawings are examined and provide clinical information.
      (3) Information is used to establish a treatment plan.
   d. Population.
      (1) TVMS: Two through 13 years.
      (2) TVMS- UL: Twelve through 40 years.
8. Test of Visual-Perceptual Skills (3rd ed.) (TVPS3).
   a. Focus: assesses visual-perceptual skills and differentiates these from motor dysfunction, as a motor response is not required.
   b. Method.
      (1) Seven visual-perceptual skills including visual discrimination, visual memory, visual-spatial relationships, visual form constancy, visual sequential memory, visual figure-ground and visual closure are assessed.
      (2) Test items are presented in a multiple choice format and are sequenced in complexity.
         (a) If subjects have three consecutive errors, the test is discontinued.
      (3) The individual looks at the test item and then selects the correct choice among all possible responses on the test plate.
      (4) Behavior observed during testing is also recorded.
   c. Scoring and interpretation.
      (1) Indications of visual perceptual problems are determined by standard scores below 80 and percentile ranks below 25.
      (2) Information is used to establish an intervention program to address deficits which impact on learning.
   d. Population: Four through 19 years.

Sensory Processing Assessments

1. Sensory Profile (SP): Infant/Toddler Sensory Profile.
   a. Focus: measures reactions to daily sensory experiences.
   b. Method.
      (1) Obtains caregiver's judgment and observation of a child's sensory processing, modulation, and behavioral and emotional responses in each sensory system via a caregiver questionnaire.
   c. Scoring and interpretation.
      (1) Cutoff scores indicate typical performance and probable, definite, and significant differences.
         (a) Differences indicate which sensory system is hindering performance.
         (b) Can be used for intervention planning.
   d. Population.
      (1) Infants and toddlers from birth to 36 months.
2. Sensory Profile (SP): Adolescent/Adult Sensory Profile.

a. Focus: allows clients to identify their personal behavioral responses and develop strategies for enhanced participation.
b. Method.
(1) A questionnaire measures individual's reactions to daily sensory experiences.
c. Scoring and interpretation.
(1) Cutoff scores indicate typical performance and probable, definite, and significant differences.
(a) Differences indicate which sensory system is hindering performance.
(b) Can be used for intervention planning.
d. Population: Individuals from 11 to 65 years old.

Psychological and Cognitive Assessments

1. Childhood Autism Rating Scale (CARS).
a. Focus: determines the severity of autism (i.e., mild, moderate or severe) and distinguishes children with autism from children with developmental delays who do not have autism.
b. Method.
(1) An observational tool is used to rate behavior.
(a) Fifteen descriptive statements include characteristics, abilities, and behaviors that deviate from the norm.
c. Scoring and interpretation.
(1) Scores below 30 = no autism.
(2) Scores of 31 to 36.5 = mild to moderate autism.
(3) Scores of 37 to 60 = severe autism.
d. Population: children over 2 years of age who have mild, moderate, or severe autism.
2. Coping Inventory and Early Coping Inventory.
a. Focus: assesses coping habits, skills, and behaviors, including effectiveness, style, strengths, and vulnerabilities to develop intervention plans for coping skills.
b. Method.
(1) Coping Inventory: questionnaire assesses coping with self and coping with environment according to three categories of coping styles: productive, active, and flexible.
(2) Early Coping Inventory: questionnaire assesses the effectiveness of behaviors according to sensorimotor organization, reactive behavior, and self-initiated behavior
c. Scoring and interpretation.
(1) Determines the level of adaptive behavior and whether or not intervention is needed.
(2) A coping profile can be grafted for each dimension.
d. Population.
(1) Coping Inventory: 15 years and above.
(2) Early Coping Inventory: 4 to 36 months.

Play Assessments

1. Play History.
a. Focus: assesses play behavior and play opportunities.
b. Method
(1) The primary caregiver provides information about a child in three categories including general information, previous play experience, and actual play that occurs over three days of play.
(a) Previous play experiences and actual play, consisting of nine aspects that address the form and content of behavior, are analyzed according to materials, action, people, and setting.
c. Scoring and interpretation.
(1) A description of play is obtained and play dysfunction is determined.
(2) A treatment plan can be developed based on strengths and deficits.
d. Population: children and adolescents.
2. Revised Knox Preschool Play Scale (RKPPS).
a. Focus: Observations of play skills to differentiate developmental play abilities, strengths and weakness, and interest areas.
b. Method.
(1) Administered in a natural indoor and outdoor environment with peers.
(a) Two 30-minute periods of observations are completed indoors and outdoors.
(2) Observations are organized according to 6-month increments up to age 3.
(3) Four dimensions of play including space management, material management, pretense/symbolic (including imitation), and participation are assessed.
c. Scoring and interpretation.
(1) The four dimensions of play are described.
(a) Each dimension contains behavioral descriptions/factors.
(2) The mean scores of all four dimension scores provide a play age score indicative of the child's play maturity.
(3) The effectiveness of treatment can also be determined.
d. Population: 0 through 6 years.
(1) It is useful with children for whom standardized testing may not be appropriate.
3. Test of Playfulness (ToP) Revised Version 3.5
a. Focus: Assesses a child's playfulness based on observations according to four aspects of play.
b. Method.
(1) Observed behaviors are rated according to intrinsic motivation, internal control, disengagement from constraints of reality, and framing.

(2) The extent, intensity, and skillfulness of play are also observed and rated.

c. Scoring and interpretation.

(1) Scores in the 25 percentile or below indicate the need for intervention.

d. Population: 15 months to 10 years.

4. Transdisciplinary Play-Based Assessment (TPBA).

a. Focus: measures child's development, learning style, interaction patterns, and behaviors to determine need for services.

b. Method.

(1) Non-standardized play assessment employing team observations based on six phases.

(2) Observations are categorized into the developmental domains of cognitive, social-emotional, communication and language, and sensorimotor.

c. Scoring and interpretation.

(1) A program plan is developed and can include developmental levels, family assessment, intervention services and strategies to promote an appropriate activity environment.

(2) A curriculum is available to address particular needs

d. Population: Infancy to 6 years.

5. See Chapter 15 for additional information on the evaluation of play.

Social Participation Assessments

1. Participation Scale (P Scale) (Version 6.0).

a. Focus: a measure of restrictions in social participation related to community mobility, access to work, recreation, and social interaction with family, peers, neighbors, etc.

b. Method.

(1) Eighteen-item questionnaire addressing the nine domains of participation identified in the International Classification of Function, Disability, and Health.

(2) Self-care, mobility, and social function and their functional sub-units are assessed.

(a) The score forms include the areas of functional skills, caregiver assistance and modifications.

c. Scoring and interpretation.

(1) Scores above 12 on the scale (ranging from 0 to 90) indicate the need for intervention.

d. Population: 15 years and older with physical disabilities.

2. School Function Assessment (SFA).

a. Focus: assesses and monitors functional performance in order to promote participation in a school environment.

(1) It does not measure academic performance.

b. Method.

(1) A criterion referenced questionnaire assesses the student's: level of participation, type of support currently required, and performance on school related tasks.

c. Scoring and interpretation.

(1) Two different scoring mechanisms.

(a) Basic level of criterion cutoff scores: scores falling below the cutoff point indicate a performance that does not meet expectations.

(b) Advanced level scores range from 0 to 100, indicating appropriate grade level functioning.

Lifespan and Occupational Therapy Developmental Theorists

Overview

1. The NBCOT examination will likely not ask specific questions about lifespan and OT developmental theories, OT frames of reference, or models of practice, but the application of this knowledge may be needed to correctly answer test questions.
2. Understanding that development occurs in many dimensions throughout the lifespan, with specific tasks being considered typical for each life stage, can be helpful in determining an answer that is developmentally appropriate for an exam item scenario.

Havighurst

1. Proposed that people need to develop certain skills at different ages to meet social standards.
2. Believed that these developmental tasks rely on biological, psychological, and sociological conditions.

a. Proposed that there are certain sensitive periods, when biological, psychological, and sociological conditions are optimal for the accomplishment of a developmental task.
b. Described "teachable moments," referring to the sensitive periods when conditions are optimal for integration of previous knowledge and the accomplishment of new developmental task with assistance.

3. Six stages of development are described along with specific developmental tasks for each stage.
4. In current society, the tasks of some stages may occur later than described by Havighurst.
5. Tasks of infancy and childhood.
   a. Walk.
   b. Take solid food.
   c. Talk.
   d. Control elimination of body wastes.
   e. Develop sex differences and sexual modesty.
   f. Develop physiologic stability.
   g. Understand concepts of social and physical reality.
   h. Develop emotional ties with parents, siblings, and others.
   i. Understand right from wrong, conscience evolves.
6. Tasks of middle childhood.
   a. Develop physical skills needed for games.
   b. Establish healthy self-concept.
   c. Make friends with children of the same age.
   d. Read, write, and calculate.
   e. Acquire a fund of information necessary for everyday life.
   f. Develop morality and values.
   g. Formulate opinions about social groups and institutions.
7. Tasks of adolescence.
   a. Establish relationships with male and female friends of same age, increasing in quantity and quality.
   b. Develop gender social role.
   c. Become comfortable with and respect one's changing body.
   d. Decrease emotional reliance on parents/other adults.
   e. Prepare for marriage and family life.
   f. Prepare for economic career.
   g. Develop a value system to shape behavior or develop one's own philosophy.
   h. Behave in a socially responsible manner.
8. Tasks of early adulthood.
   a. Choose a partner.
   b. Adjust to a partner.
   c. Start a family.
   d. Raise children.
   e. Manage a home.
   f. Pursue an occupation.
   g. Develop civic responsibility.
   h. Join/form a compatible social group.
9. Tasks of middle adulthood.
   a. Guide adolescents toward becoming responsible and well adjusted adults.
   b. Engage in adult civic and social responsibility.
   c. Progress in an occupational career.
   d. Pursue leisure-time activities.
   e. Relate to partner as a person.
   f. Deal with and accept physiologic changes of middle age.
   g. Accept aging parents.
10. Tasks of later adulthood.
   a. Cope with decreasing physical strength and health.
   b. Adjust to retirement and reduced income.
   c. Adjust to death of a spouse/partner.
   d. Affiliate with one's age-group.
   e. Change social roles.
   f. Arrange for the most appropriate and appealing living environment.

Lela Llorens

1. Individual is viewed from two perspectives.
   a. Specific period of time, referred to as horizontal development.
   b. Over the course of time, referred to as longitudinal/chronological development.
2. Both of these perspectives occur simultaneously.
3. The integration of these two aspects is critical to normal development.
4. The role of the occupational therapist is to facilitate development and assist in the mastery of life tasks and the ability to cope with life expectations.
5. Lloren's frame of reference integrated many of the concepts of Gesell, Amatruda, Erikson, Havighurst, and Freud.

Anne Mosey

1. Recapitulation of ontogenesis frame of reference.
   a. The development of adaptive skills, essential learned behaviors, is considered critical for successful participation in occupational performance.
2. Six major adaptive skills along with subskills are delineated.
   a. Sensory integration of vestibular, proprioceptive, and tactile information for functional use.
      (1) Integration of the tactile subsystems (0–3 months).

(2) Integration of primitive postural reflexes (3–9 months).
(3) Maturation of righting and equilibrium reactions (9–12 months).
(4) Integration of two sides of the body, awareness of body parts and their relationship, and motor plan gross movements (1–2 years).
(5) Motor plan fine movements (2–3 years).

b. Cognitive skill: the ability to perceive, represent, and organize sensory information to think and problem solve.
(1) Utilization of inborn behavioral patterns for environmental interaction (0–1 month).
(2) Interrelation of visual, manual, auditory, and oral responses (1–4 months).
(3) Early exploration of the environment and interest in outcomes of actions: remembers action responses, believes that own actions cause responses, and has an awareness of the relation of these actions and events (4–9 months).
(4) Utilization of deliberate actions to achieve a goal: object permanence begins, anticipation of familiar events, imitation, interest in sizes/shapes, and perception of other objects as partially causal (9–12 months).
(5) Utilization of a trial and error approach to problem solving: tool use, begins to realize that alternate routes can be used, remembers the order of a simple sequence, and realizes that others can cause events to happen (12–18 months).
(6) Formulation of mental pictures: pretends, early cause and effect, manipulates objects in space, has a clearer understanding that others can manipulate the environment (18 months–2 years).
(7) Representation of objects in terms of felt experiences: understands that there are consequences to actions; that others cannot read your mind, and recognizes that events have causes (2–5 years).
(8) Representation of objects by name: begins to understand that other people may have differing opinions (6–7 years).
(9) Comprehension that different labels can be used for the same object, use of formal logic and speculation (11–13 years).

c. Dyadic interaction skill: the ability to participate in a variety of dyadic relationships.
(1) Family relationships (8–10 months).
(2) Playmate relationships (3–5 years).
(3) Superior/authority relationship interactions (5–7 years).
(4) Friend relationships (10–14 years).
(5) Peer-superior relationships (15–17 years).
(6) Intimate/sharing/committed relationships (18–25 years).
(7) Caring/unselfish relationships (20–30 years).

d. Group interaction skill: the ability to engage in a variety of primary groups.
(1) Parallel group: minimal awareness of or interaction with others (18 months–2 years).
(2) Project group: limited in duration, cooperation, and sharing (2–4 years).
(3) Egocentric group: cooperation, competition, longer in duration, builds self-esteem (9–12 years).
(4) Cooperative group: compatible group, members concerned with meeting the needs of fellow members (9–12 years).
(5) Mature group: differing roles, concerned with completion of task as well as meeting the needs of fellow members (15–18 years).

e. Self-identity skill: the ability to perceive the self as a relatively autonomous, holistic, and acceptable person who has permanence and continuity over time.
(1) Self as a valued person (9–12 months).
(2) Assets and limitations of the self (11–15 years).
(3) Self as self-directed (20–25 years).
(4) Self as a productive, contributing member of a society (30–35 years).
(5) Self identity as an independent individual (35–50 years).
(6) Understanding the aging process of one's self and eventual death as part of the life cycle (45–60 years).

f. Sexual identity skill: the ability to feel comfortable about one's sexual nature and to engage in continued sexual relationship that takes into account mutual satisfaction of sexual needs.
(1) Act on the basis of one's pregenital sexual nature (4–5 years).
(2) Sexually mature as a positive growth experience (12–16 years).
(3) Give and receive sexual gratification (18–25 years).
(4) Sustain sexual relationship with mutual satisfaction of sexual needs (20–30 years).
(5) Accept sex-related physiological changes that occur as a natural part of the aging process (40–60 years).

Child Abuse

Overview: Facts and Statistics

1. In the United States, child abuse is a major social justice crisis. The below facts are provided to highlight the need for occupational therapists to be vigilant about the potential of child abuse and neglect in all interactions with children and adult survivors. These statistics will not be on the NBCOT examination.
   a. A report of child abuse is made every ten seconds.
   b. In 2007, an estimated 3.2 million child abuse reports and allegations were made involving approximately 5.8 million children.
   c. Almost five children die each day as a result of child abuse.
      (1) More than 75% of these deaths are children under the age of four.
      (2) The death of children as a result of maltreatment is thought to be significantly underreported with the majority (60–85%) of child fatalities caused by maltreatment not recorded as such on death certificates.
2. Child abuse can occur in any family. It is evident at all socio-economic levels, in all ethnicities, cultural groups, and religions and at all levels of education.
3. Females make up 58% of abusers and are more likely to be involved in neglect or physical abuse.
4. Males make up 42% of abusers and are more likely to be involved in sexual abuse.
5. 79% of the cases involved abuse by one or both of the parents.
6. The effects of child abuse and neglect continue into adulthood.
   a. It is estimated that the cycle of abuse is continued by 30% of abused and neglected children who as parents abuse their own children,
   b. Approximately 80% of 21 year olds who survived child abuse have at least one diagnosed psychological disorder.
   c. 31% of women in prison and 14% of men in prison in the United States are survivors of child abuse.
   d. Over 60% of adults in drug rehabilitation centers report being survivors of child abuse or neglect.

Definition of Child Abuse

1. Any behavior directed toward a child by a parent, guardian, caregiver, other family member, or other adult that endangers or impairs a child's physical or emotional health and development.

Types of Child Abuse

1. Physical.
2. Emotional or mental.
3. Sexual.
4. Neglect.

Signs of Abuse

1. General signs of abuse.
   a. Withdrawal.
   b. Nightmares.
   c. Running away.
   d. Anxiety or depression.
   e. Guilt.
   f. Mistrust of adults.
   g. Fear.
   h. Aggressiveness.
2. Signs and symptoms of physical abuse.
   a. The child reports being physically mistreated.
   b. Unexplained injuries.
   c. Repeated injuries.
   d. Abrasions and lacerations.
   e. Small circular burns such as cigarette or cigar burns.
   f. Burns with a "doughnut" shape on the buttocks that may indicate scalding, or any burn that shows the pattern of an object used to inflict injury, such as an iron.
   g. Friction burns such as those from a rope.
   h. Unexplained fractures.
   i. Denial, unlikely explanations, or delays in treatment on the part of the caregiver.
3. Signs and symptoms of emotional or mental abuse.
   a. The child reports being verbally and/or emotionally mistreated.
   b. Aggressive or acting out behavior such as lying or stealing.
   c. Shy, dependent, or defensive appearance.
   d. Verbally abuses others with language that appears to have been directed toward them.
4. Signs and symptoms of sexual abuse.
   a. The child reports being inappropriately approached, touched, and/or assaulted.
   b. Abuse may be physical (e.g., touching), non-physical (e.g., indecent exposure), or violent (e.g., rape), so signs may include emotional and physical indicators.
   c. Precocious sexual behavior or knowledge.
   d. Copying adult sexual behavior.

e. Inappropriate sexual behavior (e.g., putting tongue in other's mouth when kissing).
f. Soreness or injury around the genitals.
g. Reluctance or refusal to let caregivers wash parts of the body.
h. Sexual play.

5. Signs and symptoms of neglect.
a. Poorly nourished appearance or inadequately clothed.
b. Consistently tired or listless behavior.
c. Inconsistent attendance at school.
d. Poor hygiene or obsession with cleanliness.
e. Left alone in dangerous situations, for long periods of time and/or at an inappropriate young age.
f. Unable to relate well to adults or form friendships.

Role of Occupational Therapy

1. Mandatory reporting.
a. The federal Child Abuse Prevention and Treatment Act (CAPTA) defined child abuse and neglect and established mandates for professionals to report abuse and neglect to law enforcement officials.
b. All states must have child abuse and neglect reporting laws to qualify for federal funding under CAPTA.
c. All states require reporting of known or suspected cases of child abuse or neglect by health care providers.
(1) Standards for reporting may vary.
(2) Reporting to the therapist's direct supervisor may/may not be sufficient.
(a) The therapist should immediately report any and all concerns to his/her OT supervisor but he/she must be prepared to follow-up as necessary.
d. Failure to report suspected child abuse may be considered a crime.
e. In most states, good faith reporting is immune from liability.
f. All states require reporting to be made to a law enforcement agency or child protective services.

2. Occupational therapy intervention.
a. Treat physical injuries, emotional injuries, and developmental delays.
b. Develop a trusting relationship with child and non-abusive caregivers.
c. Provide support to non-abusive caregivers.
d. Refer to appropriate disciplines and agencies.

Aging

General Concepts and Definitions

1. Aging: the process of growing old.
a. Describes a wide array of physiological changes in the body systems.
b. A complex and variable process.
c. Common to all members of a given species.
d. Aging is developmental, occurs across the life span.
e. Progressive with time.
f. Evidence of aging.
(1) Decline in homeostatic efficiency.
(2) Decline in reaction time.
(a) Increased probability that reaction to injury will not be successful.
g. Varies among and within individuals.

2. Aging changes.
a. Cellular changes.
(1) Increase in size; fragmentation of Golgi apparatus and mitochondria.
(2) Decrease in cell capacity to divide and reproduce.
(3) Arrest of DNA synthesis and cell division.
b. Tissue changes.
(1) Accumulation of pigmented materials, lipofuscins.
(2) Accumulation of lipids and fats.
(3) Connective tissue changes: decreased elastic content, degradation of collagen; presence of pseudoelastins.
c. Organ changes.
(1) Decrease in functional capacity.
(2) Decrease in homeostatic efficiency.

3. Gerontology: the scientific study of the factors impacting the normal aging process and the effects of aging.

4. Geriatrics: the branch of medicine concerned with the illnesses of old age and their care.

5. Ageism: discrimination and prejudice leveled against individuals on the basis of their age.
a. Isolates elders socially.
b. Permits attitudes and policies that discourage elders from full participation in work, leisure and other meaningful occupations.
c. Perpetuates fears of aging.
d. Diminishes quality of life.

Demographics, Mortality, and Morbidity

1. Life span: maximum survival potential, the inherent natural life of the species; in humans 110–120 years.
2. Senescence: the weakening of the body at a gradual but steady pace during the last stages of adulthood through death.
3. Life expectancy: the number of years of life expectation from year of birth.
   a. 78.8 years; in United States women live 5.1 years longer than men.
   b. Current trends are contributing to increased life expectancy.
      (1) Advances in health care, improved infectious disease control.
      (2) Advances in infant/child care, decreased mortality rates.
      (3) Improvements in nutrition and sanitation.
4. Categories of elderly.
   a. Young elderly: ages 65–74.
   b. Old elderly: ages 75–84.
   c. Oldest elderly: ages > 85.
5. Persons over 65: represents a rapidly growing segment with lengthening of life expectancy; currently 12.5% of US population; by year 2030, expected over 65 population will be 22% of US population.
6. Socioeconomic factors.
   a. Half of all older women are widows; older men twice as likely to be married as older women.
   b. Most live on fixed incomes: social security is the major source of income; poverty rate for persons over 65 is 11.4%; another 8% live near the poverty rate.
   c. About half of older persons have completed high school.
   d. Non-institutionalized elderly: most live in family setting.
   e. Institutionalized elderly: about 5% of persons over 65 reside in nursing homes; percentage increases dramatically with age (22% of persons over 85).
7. Leading causes of death (mortality) in persons over 65, in order of frequency.
   a. Coronary heart disease (CHD), accounts for 31% of deaths.
   b. Cancer, accounts for 20% of deaths.
   c. Cerebrovascular disease (stroke).
   d. Chronic obstructive pulmonary disease (COPD).
   e. Pneumonia/flu.
8. Leading causes of disability/chronic conditions (morbidity) in persons over 65, in order of frequency.
   a. Arthritis, 49%.
   b. Hypertension, 37%.
   c. Hearing impairments, 32%.
   d. Heart impairments, 30%.
   e. Cataracts and chronic sinusitis, 17% each.
   f. Orthopedic impairments, 16%.
   g. Diabetes and visual impairments, 9% each.
   h. Most older persons (60–80%) report having one or more chronic conditions.
9. Health care costs.
   a. Older persons account for 12% of population and 36% of total health care expenditures.
   b. Older persons account for 33% of all hospital stays, 44% of all hospital days of care.

Theories of Aging

1. Biological theories.
   a. Genetic: aging is intrinsic to the organism; genes are programmed to modulate aging changes, overall rate of progression.
      (1) Individuals vary in the expression of aging changes; e.g., graying of hair, wrinkling of skin.
      (2) Polygenic controls exist (multiple genes are involved): no one gene can modulate rate of development in all aspects of aging.
      (3) Premature aging syndromes (progeria) provide evidence of defective genetic programming; individuals exhibit premature aging changes, i.e., atrophy and thinning of tissues, graying of hair, arteriosclerosis, etc.
         (a) Hutchinson-Gilford syndrome: progeria of childhood.
         (b) Werner's syndrome: progeria of young adults.
   b. Doubling/biologic clock (Hayflick limit theory): functional deterioration within cells is due to limited number of genetically programmed cell doublings (cell replication).
   c. Free radical theory: free radicals are highly reactive and toxic forms of oxygen produced by cell mitochondria. The released radicals:
      (1) Cause damage to cell membranes and DNA cell replication.
      (2) Interfere with cell diffusion and transport, resulting in decreased O_2 delivery and tissue death.
      (3) Decrease cellular integrity, enzyme activities.
      (4) Result in cross-linkages: chemical bonding of elements not generally joined together; interferes with normal cell function.
      (5) Result in accumulation of aging pigments, lipofuscins.
      (6) Can trigger pathologic changes: atherosclerosis in blood vessel wall; cell mutations and cancer.
   d. Cell mutation (intrinsic mutagenesis): errors in the synthesis of proteins (DNA, RNA) lead to exponential cascade of abnormal proteins and aging changes.

e. Hormonal theory: functional decrements in neurons and their associated hormones lead to aging changes.
   (1) Hypothalamus, pituitary gland, adrenal gland are the primary regulators, timekeepers of aging.
      (a) Thyroxine is the master hormone of the body; controls rate of protein synthesis and metabolism.
      (b) Secretion of regulatory pituitary hormones influence thyroid.
   (2) Decreases in protective hormones: estrogen, growth hormone, adrenal DHEA (dehydroepiandrosterone).
   (3) Increases in stress hormones (cortisol): can damage brain's memory center, the hippocampus, and destroy immune cells.
f. Immunity theory: thymus size decreases, shrivels by puberty, becomes less functional; bone marrow cell efficiency decreases; results in steady decrease in immune responses during adulthood.
   (1) Immune cells, T-cells, become less able to fight foreign organisms; B-cells become less able to make antibodies.
   (2) Autoimmune diseases increase with age.

2. Environmental theories (stochastic or non-genetic theories).
   a. Aging is caused by an accumulation of insults from the environment.
   b. Environmental toxins include: ultraviolet, crosslinking agents (unsaturated fats), toxic chemicals (metal ions, Mg, Zn), radiation, and viruses.
   c. Can result in errors in protein synthesis and in DNA synthesis/genetic sequences (error theory), cross-linkage of molecules, mutations.
3. Psychological theories.
   a. Stress theory: homeostatic imbalances result in changes in structural and chemical composition.
      (1) General Adaptation Syndrome (Selye): initial alarm reaction, progressing to stage of resistance, progressing to stage of exhaustion.
      (2) Closely linked to hormonal theory.
   b. Erickson's bipolar theory of lifespan development: stages of later adulthood.
      (1) Integrity: individual exhibits full unification of personality; life is viewed with satisfaction (productive life, sense of satisfaction), remains optimistic, continues to grow.
      (2) Despair: individual lacks ego integration: life is viewed with despair (fear of death, feelings of regret and disappointment, missed opportunities).
4. Sociological theories: life experience/lifestyles influence aging process.
   a. Activity theory: older persons who are socially active exhibit improved adjustment to the aging process; allows continued role enactment essential for positive self-image and improved life satisfaction.
   b. Disengagement theory: distancing of an individual or withdrawal from society; reduction in social roles leads to further isolation and life dissatisfaction.
   c. Dependency: increasing reliance on others for meeting physical and emotional needs; focus is increasingly on self.
5. An integrated model of aging assumes aging is a complex, multifactorial phenomenon in which some or all of the above processes may contribute to the overall aging of an individual; aging is not adequately explained by any single theory.

Muscular System Changes and Adaptation in the Older Adult

1. Age-related changes.
   a. Changes may be due more to decreased activity levels (hypokinesis) and disuse than from the aging process.
   b. Loss of muscle strength: peaks at age 30, remains fairly constant until age 50; after which there is an accelerating loss, 20–40% loss by age 65 in the non-exercising adult.
   c. Loss of power (force/unit time): significant declines, due to losses in speed of contraction, changes in nerve conduction and synaptic transmission.
   d. Loss of skeletal muscle mass (atrophy): both size and number of muscle fibers decrease, by age 70 lose 33% of skeletal muscle mass.
   e. Changes in muscle fiber composition: selective loss of Type II, fast twitch fibers, with increase in proportion of Type I fibers.
   f. Changes in muscular endurance: muscles fatigue more readily.
      (1) Decreased muscle tissue oxidative capacity.
      (2) Decreased peripheral blood flow, oxygen delivery to muscles.
      (3) Altered chemical composition of muscle: decreased myosin ATPase activity, glycoproteins and contractile protein.
      (4) Collagen changes: denser, irregular due to cross-linkages, loss of water content and elasticity; affects tendons, bone, cartilage.
2. Clinical implications.
   a. Movements become slower.
   b. Increased complaints of fatigue.
   c. Connective tissue becomes denser and stiffer.
      (1) Increased risk of muscle sprains, strains, tendon tears.
      (2) Loss of range of motion: highly variable by joint and individual's activity level.
      (3) Increased tendency for fibrinous adhesions, contractures.

d. Decreased functional mobility, limitations to movement.
e. Gait may become unsteady due to changes in balance, strength; increased need for assistive devices.
f. Increased risk of falls.

3. Strategies to slow or reverse changes.
   a. Improve health.
      (1) Correct medical problems that may cause weakness: hyperthyroidism, excess adrenocortical steroids (e.g., Cushing's disease, steroids); hyponatremia (low sodium in blood).
      (2) Improve nutrition.
      (3) Address alcoholism/substance abuse.
   b. Increase levels of physical activity, stress functional activities, and activity programs.
      (1) Gradually increase intensity of activity to avoid injury.
      (2) Plan and include adequate warm-ups and cool downs; appropriate pacing and rest periods.
   c. Provide strength training to increase/maintain muscle strength required for functional activity.
      (1) Significant increases in strength are noted in older adults with isometric and progressive resistive exercise regimes.
      (2) High-intensity training programs (70–80% of one-repetition maximum) produce quicker and more predictable results than moderate intensity programs; both have been successfully used with the elderly.
      (3) Age not a limiting factor; significant improvements noted in 80- and 90-year-old elders who were frail and institutionalized.
      (4) Improvements in strength can improve functional abilities and occupational performance.
      (5) Maintain newly gained and existing strength and incorporate into functional activities.
   d. Provide flexibility and range of motion exercises to increase range of motion needed for functional activity.
      (1) Utilize slow, prolonged stretching, maintained for 20–30 seconds.
      (2) Tissues heated prior to stretching are more distensible, e.g., warm pool.
      (3) Maintain newly gained range: incorporate into functional activities.
      (4) Mobility gains are slower with older adults.

Skeletal System Changes and Adaptations in the Older Adult

1. Age-related changes.
   a. Cartilage changes: decreased water content, becomes stiffer, fragments, and erodes; by age 60 more than 60% of adults have degenerative joint changes, cartilage abnormalities.
   b. Loss of bone mass and density: peak bone mass at age 40; between 45 and 70 bone mass decreased (women by about 25%; men 15%); decreases another 5% by age 90.
      (1) Loss of calcium, bone strength: especially trabecular bone.
      (2) Decreased bone marrow red blood cell production.
   c. Intervertebral discs: flatten, less resilient due to loss of water content (30% loss by age 65) and loss of collagen elasticity; trunk length, overall height decreases.
   d. Senile postural changes.
      (1) Forward head.
      (2) Kyphosis of thoracic spine.
      (3) Flattening of lumbar spine.
      (4) With prolonged sitting, tendency to develop hip and knee flexion contractures.
2. Clinical implications.
   a. Maintenance of weight bearing is important for cartilaginous/joint health and mobility.
   b. Increased risk of falls and fractures.
3. Strategies to slow or reverse changes.
   a. Postural exercises: stress components of good posture.
   b. Weight bearing (gravity-loading) exercise can decrease bone loss in older adults, e.g., walking, stair climbing, all activities that are performed in standing.
   c. Nutritional, hormonal and medical therapies.
   d. See Chapter 16 for information on fall prevention.

Neurological System Changes and Adaptations in the Older Adult

1. Age-related changes.
   a. Atrophy of nerve cells in cerebral cortex: over-all loss of cerebral mass/brain weight of 6–11% between ages of 20 and 90; accelerating loss after age 70.
   b. Changes in brain morphology.
      (1) Gyral atrophy: narrowing and flattening of gyri with widening of sulci.
      (2) Ventricular dilation.
      (3) Generalized cell loss in cerebral cortex: especially frontal and temporal lobes, association areas (prefrontal cortex, visual).
      (4) Presence of lipofuscins, senile or neuritic plaques, and neurofibrillary tangles (NFT): significant accumulations associated with pathology, e.g., Alzheimer's disease.
      (5) More selective cell loss in basal ganglia (substantia nigra and putamen), cerebellum, hippocampus, locus coeruleus; brain stem minimally affected.

c. Decreased cerebral blood flow and energy metabolism.
d. Changes in synaptic transmission.
(1) Decreased synthesis and metabolism of major neurotransmitters, e.g., acetylcholine, dopamine.
(2) Slowing of many neural processes, especially in polysynaptic pathways.
e. Changes in spinal cord/peripheral nerves.
(1) Neuronal loss and atrophy: 30–50% loss of anterior horn cells, 30% loss of posterior roots (sensory fibers) by age 90.
(2) Loss of motoneurons results in increase in size of remaining motor units (development of macro motor units).
(3) Slowed nerve conduction velocity: sensory greater than motor.
(4) Loss of sympathetic fibers: may account for diminished, autonomic stability, increased incidence of postural hypotension in older adults.
f. Age-related tremors (essential tremor, ET).
(1) Occur as an isolated symptom, particularly in hands, head, and voice.
(2) Characterized as postural or kinetic, rarely resting.
(3) Benign, slowly progressive; in late stages may limit function.
(4) Exaggerated by movement and emotion.

2. Clinical implications.
a. Effects on movement.
(1) Overall speed and coordination are decreased; increased difficulties with fine motor control.
(2) Slowed recruitment of motoneurons contributes to loss of strength.
(3) Both reaction time and movement time are increased.
(4) Older adults are affected by the speed/accuracy trade off.
(a) The simpler the movement, the less the change.
(b) More complicated movements require more preparation, longer reaction and movement times.
(c) Faster movements decrease accuracy, increase errors.
(5) Older adults typically shift in motor control processing from open to closed loop: e.g., demonstrate increased reliance on visual feedback for movement.
(6) Demonstrate increased cautionary behaviors, an indirect effect of decreased capacity.
b. General slowing of neural processing: learning and memory may be affected.
c. Problems in homeostatic regulation: stressors (heat, cold, excess exercise) can be harmful, even life-threatening.

3. Strategies to slow or reverse changes.
a. Correct medical problems: improve cerebral blood flow.
b. Improve health: diet, smoking cessation.
c. Increase levels of physical activity: may encourage neuronal branching, slow rate of neural decline, and improve cerebral circulation.
d. Provide effective strategies to improve motor learning and control.
(1) Allow for increased reaction and movement times: will improve motivation, accuracy of movements.
(2) Allow for limitations of memory: avoid long sequences of movements.
(3) Allow for increased cautionary behaviors: provide adequate explanation, demonstration when teaching new movement skills.
(4) Stress familiar, well-learned skills; repetitive movements.

Sensory Systems Changes and Adaptations in the Older Adult

1. Age-related changes: older adults experience a loss of function of the senses.
a. May lead to sensory deprivation, isolation, disorientation, confusion, appearance of senility and depression.
b. May strain social interactions and decrease ability to interact socially and with the environment.
c. May lead to decreased functional mobility and increased risk of injury.
d. Alters quality of life.

2. Vision.
a. Aging changes: there is a general decline in visual acuity; gradual prior to sixth decade, rapid decline between ages 60 and 90; visual loss may be as much as 80% by age 90; changes include:
(1) Presbyopia: visual loss in middle and older ages characterized by inability to focus properly and blurred images, due to loss of accommodation, elasticity of lens.
(2) Decreased ability to adapt to dark and light.
(3) Increased sensitivity to light and glare.
(4) Loss of color discrimination, especially for blues and greens.
(5) Decreased pupillary responses, size of resting pupil increases.
(6) Decreased sensitivity of corneal reflex: less sensitive to eye injury or infection.
(7) Oculomotor responses diminished: restricted upward gaze, reduced pursuit eye movements; ptosis may develop.

b. Additional vision loss with pathology.
   (1) Cataracts: opacity, clouding of lens due to changes in lens proteins; results in gradual loss of vision: central first, then peripheral; increased problems with glare; general darkening of vision; loss of acuity, distortion.
      (a) Surgery is an effective treatment.
   (2) Glaucoma: increased intraocular pressure, with degeneration of optic disc, atrophy of optic nerve; results in early loss of peripheral vision (tunnel vision).
      (a) If untreated, it can progress to total blindness.
      (b) If diagnosis is made early, surgery and/or medications are effective treatments.
   (3) Macular degeneration: loss of central vision associated with age-related degeneration of the macula compromised by decreased blood supply or abnormal growth of blood vessels under the retina; typically individuals retain some peripheral vision; increased sensitivity to glare, and difficulty adjusting to light change; may progress to total blindness.
   (4) Diabetic retinopathy: damage to retinal capillaries, growth of abnormal blood vessels and hemorrhage leads to retinal scarring and finally retinal detachment; central vision is impaired, vision is blurred; complete blindness is rare.
      (a) A complication of diabetes mellitus.
   (5) CVA, homonymous hemianopsia: loss of ½ visual field in each eye (nasal half of one eye and temporal half of other eye); produces an inability to receive information from right or left side; corresponds to side of sensorimotor deficit.
   (6) Medications: impaired or fuzzy vision may result with antihistamines, anti-psychotics, anti-depressants, steroids.

c. Clinical implications/compensatory strategies.
   (1) Assess for visual deficits: acuity, peripheral vision, light and dark adaptation, depth perception; diplopia, eye fatigue, eye pain.
   (2) Maximize visual function: assess for use of glasses, need for environmental adaptations. (See Chapter 16.)
   (3) Sensory thresholds are increased: allow extra time for visual discrimination and response.
   (4) Work in adequate light, increase intensity, reduce glare; avoid abrupt changes in light, e.g., light to dark.
   (5) Use large, high contrast print for written materials.
   (6) Provide magnifying glasses (either portable or attached to a stand/work table) to view objects and complete tasks.
   (7) Provide an eye patch for diplopia.
   (8) Decreased peripheral vision may limit social interactions; therefore, stand directly in front of the person at eye level when communicating with him/her.
   (9) Assist in color discrimination: use warm colors (yellow, orange, red) for identification and color coding.
   (10) Provide other sensory cues when vision is limited, e.g., verbal descriptions to new environments, touching to communicate you are listening, "talking" clocks, and watches.
   (11) Provide safety education; reduce fall risk.

3. Hearing.

a. Aging changes: occur as early as fourth decade; affects a significant number of elderly (23% of individuals aged 65–74 have hearing impairments and 40% over age 75 have hearing loss; rate of loss in men is twice the rate of women, also starts earlier).
   (1) Outer ear: buildup of cerumen (ear wax) may result in conductive hearing loss; common in older men.
   (2) Middle ear: minimal degenerative changes of bony joints.
   (3) Inner ear: significant changes in sound sensitivity, understanding of speech, and maintenance of equilibrium may result with degeneration and atrophy of cochlea and vestibular structures, loss of neurons.

b. Types of hearing loss.
   (1) Conductive: mechanical hearing loss from damage to external auditory canal, tympanic membrane or middle ear ossicles; results in hearing loss (all frequencies); tinnitus (ringing in the ears) may be present.
   (2) Sensorineural: central or neural hearing loss from multiple factors, e.g., noise damage, trauma, disease, drugs, arteriosclerosis, etc.
   (3) Presbycusis: sensorineural hearing loss associated with middle and older ages; characterized by bilateral hearing loss, especially at high frequencies at first, then all frequencies; poor auditory discrimination and comprehension, especially with background noise; tinnitus.

c. Additional hearing loss with pathology.
   (1) Otosclerosis: immobility of stapes results in profound conductive hearing loss.
   (2) Paget's disease.
   (3) Hypothyroidism.

d. Clinical implications/compensatory strategies.
   (1) Assess for hearing: acuity, speech discrimination/comprehension; tinnitus, dizziness, vertigo, pain.
   (2) Assess for use of hearing aids; check for proper functioning.

(3) Minimize auditory distractions, work in quiet environment.
(4) Speak slowly and clearly, directly in front of person at eye level.
(5) Use nonverbal communication to reinforce your message; e.g. gesture, demonstration.
(6) Provide written and demonstrated directions/guidelines for activities.
(7) Orient person to topics of conversation he/she cannot hear to reduce paranoia, isolation.
(8) Provide assistive devices to compensate for functional effects of hearing loss and to ensure person's safety; e.g., vibrating and flashing smoke alarms, telephones, doorbells, and clocks.

4. Vestibular/balance control.
  a. Aging changes: degenerative changes in otoconia of utricle and saccule; loss of vestibular hair-cell receptors; decreased number of vestibular neurons; VOR gain decreases; begins at age 30, accelerating decline at ages 55–60 resulting in diminished vestibular sensation.
    (1) Diminished acuity, delayed reaction times, longer response times.
    (2) Reduced function of vestibular ocular reflex (VOR); affects retinal image stability with head movements, produces blurred vision.
    (3) Altered sensory organization: older adults more dependent upon somatosensory inputs for balance.
    (4) Less able to resolve sensory conflicts when presented with inappropriate visual or proprioceptive inputs due to vestibular losses.
    (5) Postural response patterns for balance are disorganized: characterized by diminished ankle torque, increased hip torque, increased postural sway.
  b. Additional loss of vestibular sensitivity with pathology.
    (1) Mèniére's disease: episodic attacks characterized by tinnitus, dizziness, and a sensation of fullness or pressure in the ears; may also experience sensorineural hearing loss.
    (2) Benign paroxysmal positional vertigo (BPPV): brief episodes of vertigo (less than 1 minute) associated with position change; the result of degeneration of the utricular otoconia that settle on the cupula of the posterior semicircular canal; common in older adults.
    (3) Medications: antihypertensives (postural hypotension); anticonvulsants; tranquilizers, sleeping pills, aspirin, NSAIDS.
    (4) Cerebrovascular disease: vertebrobasilar artery insufficiency (TIAs, strokes); cerebellar artery stroke, lateral medullary stroke.
    (5) Cerebellar dysfunction: hemorrhage, tumors (acoustic neuroma, meningioma); degenerative disease of brain stem and cerebellum; progressive supranuclear palsy.
    (6) Migraine.
    (7) Cardiac disease.
  c. Clinical implications/compensatory strategies.
    (1) Increased incidence of falls in older adults.
    (2) See Chapter 16 for information on falls prevention.

5. Somatosensory.
  a. Aging changes.
    (1) Decreased sensitivity of touch associated with decline of peripheral receptors, atrophy of afferent fibers: lower extremities more affected than upper.
    (2) Proprioceptive losses, increased thresholds in vibratory sensibility, beginning around age 50: greater in lower extremities than upper extremities, greater in distal extremities than proximal.
    (3) Loss of joint receptor sensitivity; losses in lower extremities, cervical joints may contribute to loss of balance.
    (4) Cutaneous pain thresholds increased: greater changes in upper body areas (upper extremities, face) than for lower extremities.
  b. Additional loss of sensation with pathology.
    (1) Diabetes, peripheral neuropathy.
    (2) CVA, central sensory losses.
    (3) Peripheral vascular disease, peripheral ischemia.
  c. Clinical implications/compensatory strategies.
    (1) Assess carefully: check for increased thresholds to stimulation, sensory losses by modality, area of body.
    (2) Allow extra time for responses with increased thresholds.
    (3) Use touch to communicate: maximize physical contact, e.g., rubbing, stroking, and tapping.
    (4) Provide augmented feedback through appropriate sensory channels, e.g., using kitchen utensils with wide textured grips may be easier than narrow smooth handles.
    (5) Teach compensatory strategies to prevent injury to anesthetic limbs.
    (6) Provide assistive devices and environmental modifications as needed for fall prevention.
    (7) Provide biofeedback devices as appropriate (e.g., limb load monitor).
    (8) See Chapter 16 for further information.

6. Taste and smell.
  a. Aging changes.
    (1) Gradual decrease in taste sensitivity.
    (2) Decreased smell sensitivity.
  b. Conditions resulting in additional loss of sensation.
    (1) Smoking.

(2) Chronic allergies, respiratory infections.
(3) Dentures.
(4) CVA, involvement of hypoglossal nerve.

c. Clinical implications/compensatory strategies.
(1) Assess for identification of odors, tastes (sweet, sour, bitter, salty); somatic sensations (temperature, touch).
(2) Decreased taste, enjoyment of food leads to poor diet and nutrition.
(3) Older adults frequently increase use of taste enhancers: e.g., salt or sugar.
(4) Decreased home safety; e.g., gas leaks, smoke.

Cognitive Changes and Adaptations in the Older Adult

1. Age-related changes.
a. No uniform decline in intellectual abilities throughout adulthood.
(1) Changes do not typically show up until mid 60s; significant declines affecting everyday life do not show up until early 80s.
(2) Most significant decline in measures of intelligence occurs in the years immediately preceding death (termed "terminal drop").
b. Tasks involving perceptual speed show early declines (by age 39); require longer times to complete tasks.
c. Numeric ability (tests of adding, subtracting, and multiplying): abilities peak in mid-40s, well maintained until 60s.
d. Verbal ability: abilities peak at age 30, well maintained until 60s.
e. Memory.
(1) Impairments are typically noted in short-term memory; long-term memory retained.
(2) Impairments are task dependent; e.g., deficits primarily with novel conditions, new learning.
f. Learning: all age groups can learn. Factors affecting learning in older adults.
(1) Increased cautiousness.
(2) Anxiety.
(3) Sensory deficits.
(4) Pace of learning: fast pace is problematic.
(5) Interference from prior learning.
2. Clinical implications.
a. Older adults utilize different strategies for memory: context-based strategies vs. memorization (young adults).
3. Strategies to slow or reverse changes.
a. Improve health.
(1) Correct medical problems: imbalances between oxygen supply and demand to CNS, e.g., cardiovascular disease, hypertension, diabetes, hypothyroidism.
(2) Assess needed pharmacological changes: drug reevaluation; decrease use of multiple drugs; monitor closely for drug toxicity.
(3) Reduce chronic use of tobacco and alcohol.
(4) Correct nutritional deficiencies.
b. Increase physical activity.
c. Increase mental activity.
(1) Keep mentally engaged, "Use it or Lose it"; e.g., chess, crossword puzzles, book discussion groups, reading to children.
(2) Maintain an engaged lifestyle: socially active; e.g., clubs, travel, work, volunteerism; allow for personal choice in activity.
(3) Use cognitive training activities.
d. Provide multiple sensory cues to compensate for decreased sensory processing and sensory losses and to maximize learning; e.g., provide visual demonstrations, written instructions, and verbal cues.
e. Provide stimulating, 'enriching' environment; avoid environmental dislocation; e.g., hospitalization or institutionalization may produce disorientation and agitation in some elderly.
f. Reduce stress; provide counseling and family support.

Cardiopulmonary System Changes and Adaptations in the Older Adult

1. Cardiovascular age-related changes.
a. Changes due more to inactivity and disease than aging.
b. Degeneration of heart muscle with accumulation of lipofuscins (characteristic brown heart); mild cardiac hypertrophy left ventricular wall.
c. Decreased coronary blood flow.
d. Cardiac valves thicken and stiffen.
e. Changes in conduction system: loss of pace maker cells in SA node.
f. Changes in blood vessels: arteries thicken, less distensible; slowed exchange capillary walls; increased peripheral resistance.
g. Resting blood pressures rise: systolic greater than diastolic.
h. Decline in neurohumoral control: decreased responsiveness of end-organs to beta-adrenergic stimulation of baroreceptors.
i. Decreased blood volume, hemopoietic activity of bone.
j. Increased blood coagulability.
2. Clinical implications for cardiovascular changes.
a. Changes at rest are minor: resting heart rate and cardiac output relatively unchanged; resting blood pressures increase.

b. Cardiovascular responses to exercise: blunted, decreased heart rate acceleration, decreased maximal oxygen uptake and heart rate; reduced exercise capacity, increased recovery time.
c. Decreased stroke volume due to decreased myocardial contractility.
d. Maximum heart rate declines with age.
e. Cardiac output decreases, 1% per year after age 20: due to decreased heart rate and stroke volume.
f. Orthostatic hypotension: common problem in elderly due to reduced baroreceptor sensitivity and vascular elasticity.
g. Increased fatigue; anemia common in elderly.
h. Systolic ejection murmur common in elderly.
i. Possible ECG changes: loss of normal sinus rhythm; longer PR & QT intervals; wider QRS; increased arrhythmias.

3. Pulmonary system age-related changes.
a. Chest wall stiffness, declining strength of respiratory muscles results in increased work of breathing.
b. Loss of lung elastic recoil, decreased lung compliance.
c. Changes in lung parenchyma: alveoli enlarge, become thinner; fewer capillaries for delivery of blood.
d. Changes in pulmonary blood vessels: thicken, less distensible.
e. Decline in total lung capacity: residual volume increases, vital capacity decreases.
f. Forced expiratory volume (air flow) decreases.
g. Altered pulmonary gas exchange: oxygen tension falls with age (at a rate of 4mmHg/decade; PaO2 at age 70 is 75, versus 90 at age 20).
h. Blunted ventilatory responses of chemoreceptors in response to respiratory acidosis: decreased homeostatic responses.
i. Blunted defense/immune responses: decreased ciliary action to clear secretions, decreased secretory immunoglobulins, alveolar phagocytic function.

4. Clinical implications for pulmonary changes.
a. Respiratory responses to exercise: similar to younger adult at low and moderate intensities; at higher intensities, responses include increased ventilatory cost of work, greater blood acidosis, increased likelihood of breathlessness, and increased perceived exertion.
b. Clinical signs of hypoxia are blunted; changes in mentation and affect may provide important cues.
c. Cough mechanism is impaired.
d. Gag reflex is decreased, increased risk of aspiration.
e. Recovery from respiratory illness: prolonged in the elderly.
f. Significant changes in function with chronic smoking, exposure to environmental toxic inhalants.

5. Strategies to slow or reverse changes in cardiopulmonary systems.
a. Complete a cardiopulmonary assessment prior to commencing an exercise program.
(1) This is essential in older adults due to the high incidence of cardiopulmonary pathologies.
(2) Select an appropriate graded exercise testing protocol.
(3) Standardized test batteries and norms for elderly are not available.
(4) Many elderly cannot tolerate maximal testing; submaximal testing commonly used.
(5) Testing and training modes should be similar.
b. Individualized exercise prescription is essential.
(1) Choice of training program is based on: fitness level, presence or absence of cardiovascular disease, musculoskeletal limitations, and the individual's goals, roles, and activity interests.
(2) Prescriptive elements (frequency, intensity, duration, and mode) are the same as for younger adults.
(3) Walking, chair and floor exercises, yoga, tai chi, and modified strength/flexibility calisthenics are well-tolerated by most elderly.
(4) Consider pool programs (exercises, tai chi, walking, swimming) for persons with musculoskeletal and neurological impairments.
(5) Consider multiple modes of exercise on alternate days to maintain interest and reduce likelihood of muscle injury, joint overuse, pain, fatigue, and boredom.
c. Aerobic training programs can significantly improve cardiopulmonary function in the elderly.
(1) Decreases heart rate at a given submaximal power output.
(2) Improves maximal oxygen uptake (VO_2 max).
(3) Greater improvements in peripheral adaptation, muscle oxidative capacity then central changes.
(4) Improves recovery heart rates.
(5) Decreases systolic blood pressure, may produce a small decrease in diastolic blood pressure.
(6) Increases maximum ventilatory capacity: vital capacity.
(7) Reduces breathlessness, lowers perceived exertion.
(8) Psychological gains, improves sense of well-being, self-image.
(9) Improves functional capacity.
d. Improve overall daily activity levels for independent living.
(1) Lack of exercise/activity is an important risk factor in the development of cardiopulmonary diseases.
(2) Lack of exercise/activity contributes to problems of immobility and disability in the elderly.

Other Systems Changes and Adaptations in the Older Adult

1. Integumentary changes.
   a. Changes in skin composition.
      (1) Dermis thins with loss of elastin.
      (2) Decreased vascularity; vascular fragility results in easy bruising (senile purpura).
      (3) Decreased sebaceous activity and decline in hydration.
      (4) Appearance: skin appears dry, wrinkled, yellowed, and inelastic; aging spots appear (clusters of melanocyte pigmentation); increased with exposure to sun.
      (5) General thinning and graying of hair due to vascular insufficiency and decreased melanin production.
      (6) Nails grow more slowly, become brittle and thick.
   b. Loss of effectiveness as protective barrier.
      (1) Skin grows and heals more slowly, less able to resist injury and infection.
      (2) Inflammatory response is attenuated.
      (3) Decreased sensitivity to touch, perception of pain and temperature; increased risk for injury from concentrated pressures or excess temperatures.
      (4) Decreased sweat production with loss of sweat glands results in decreased temperature regulation and homeostasis.
2. Gastrointestinal changes.
   a. Decreased salivation, taste, and smell along with inadequate chewing (tooth loss, poorly fitting dentures); poor swallowing reflex may lead to poor dietary intake, nutritional deficiencies.
   b. Esophagus: reduced motility and control of lower esophageal sphincter; acid reflux and heartburn, hiatal hernia common.
   c. Stomach: reduced motility, delayed gastric emptying; decreased digestive enzymes and hydrochloric acid; decreased digestion and absorption; indigestion common.
   d. Decreased intestinal motility; constipation common.
3. Renal, urogenital changes.
   a. Kidneys: loss of mass and total weight with nephron atrophy, decreased renal blood flow, decreased filtration.
      (1) Blood urea rises.
      (2) Decreased excretory and reabsorptive capacities.
   b. Bladder: muscle weakness; decreased capacity causing urinary frequency; difficulty with emptying causing increased retention.
      (1) Urinary incontinence common (affects over 10 million adults; over half of nursing home residents and one-third of community-dwelling elders); affects older women with pelvic floor weakness and older men with bladder or prostate disease.
      (2) Increased likelihood of urinary tract infections.

Nutrition and the Elderly

Overview and Contributing Factors to Poor Nutrition

1. Many older adults have primary nutrition problems.
   a. Nutritional problems in the elderly are often linked to health status and poverty rather than to age itself.
      (1) Chronic diseases alter the overall need for nutrients, the abilities to take in and utilize nutrients, energy demands, and overall activity levels (e.g., Alzheimer's disease, CVA, and diabetes).
      (2) Limited, fixed incomes severely limit food choices and availability.
2. There is an age-related slowing in basal metabolic rate and a decline in total caloric intake; most of the decline is associated with a concurrent reduction in physical activity.
   a. Both undernourishment and obesity exist in the elderly and contribute to decreased levels of vitality and fitness.
3. Contributing factors to poor dietary intake.
   a. Decreased sense of taste and smell.
   b. Poor teeth or poorly fitting dentures.
   c. Reduced gastrointestinal function.
      (1) Decreased saliva.
      (2) Gastromucosal atrophy.
      (3) Reduced intestinal mobility; reflux.
   d. Loss of interest in foods.
   e. Isolation, lack of social support, no socialization during meals, loss of spouse, loss of friends.
   f. Lack of functional mobility.
      (1) Inability to get to a grocery store to shop.
      (2) Inability to prepare foods.

Outcomes of Poor Nutrition

1. Dehydration is common in the elderly, resulting in fluid and electrolyte disturbances.
   a. Thirst sensation is diminished.
   b. May be physically unable to acquire/maintain fluids.
   c. Environmental heat stresses may be life threatening and should be treated as medical emergencies.
2. Diets are often deficient in nutrients, especially vitamins A and C, B12, thiamine, protein, iron, calcium, vitamin D, folic acid, and zinc.
3. Increased use of alcohol or taste enhancers (e.g., salt and sugar) influences nutritional intake.
4. Drug/dietary interactions influence nutritional intake (e.g., reserpine digoxin, anti-tumor agents, and excessive use of antacids).

Assessment of Nutrition

1. Dietary history: patterns of eating, types of foods.
2. Psychosocial: mental status, desire to eat, depression, grief, social isolation, social supports.
3. Body composition.
   a. Weight/height measures.
   b. Skin fold measurements: triceps/subscapular skin fold thickness.
   c. Upper arm circumference.
4. Olfactory and gustatory sensory function.
5. Dental and periodontal disease, fit of dentures.
6. Ability to feed self: mastication, swallowing, hand/mouth control, posture, physical weakness and fatigue.
7. Integumentary: skin condition, edema.
8. Compliance to special diets.
9. Functional assessment: basic activities of daily living, feeding; overall exercise/activity levels, amount and type of social participation.

Goals and Interventions

1. Assist in monitoring adequate nutritional intake.
2. Assist in maintaining nutritional support.
   a. Refer to dietitian, nutritional consultants, and/or nutritional education programs as needed.
   b. Make recommendations for home health aide to assist with grocery shopping and meal preparation.
   c. Refer to elderly food programs: home delivered, i.e., "meals on wheels"; congregate meals/senior center daily meal programs; federal food stamp programs.
3. Maintain physical function and promote adequate activity levels.
4. Maintain independence in food preparation and self feeding.
   a. Teach work simplification and energy conservation techniques to maximize function.
   b. Modify the environment and adapt activities to enhance mastery and ensure safety.
   c. Refer to Chapters 15 and 16 for more details.

Elder Abuse

Overview: Facts and Statistics

a. Statistics for elder abuse are difficult to accurately assess due to limited reporting. In the United States, the abuse of vulnerable and older adults is a social justice and health care crisis. The below facts are provided to highlight the need for occupational therapists to be vigilant about the potential of abuse, neglect, and exploitation in all interactions with vulnerable and older adults. These statistics will not be on the NBCOT examination.
b. According to the best available estimates, in the United States between 1 and 2 million older adults (age 65 or older) are victims of abuse, neglect, and/or exploitation.
c. Nationally, Adult Protective Services (APS) investigated 565,747 reports of elder and vulnerable adult abuse in 2004. This represents a 19.7% increase from the APS 2000 Survey
   (1) APS substantiated 191,908 reports of elder and vulnerable adult abuse.
d. Most (65.7%) reported elder abuse victims were female.
e. Many (42.8%) were 80 years of age and older.
f. The vast majority (89.3%) of reported elder abuse was about incidences in private homes.

2. Definitions vary; however, there are three basic categories.
   a. Domestic elder abuse.
   b. Institutional elder abuse.
   c. Self-neglect or self-abuse.

Signs and Symptoms of Elder Abuse

1. Physical abuse signs and symptoms.
   a. An elder's report of being physically mistreated.
   b. Bruises, black eyes, welts and/or lacerations.
   c. Rope marks and/or other signs of restraint.
   d. Bone and skull fractures, sprains and/or dislocations.
   e. Open wounds, cuts, and untreated injuries in various stages of healing.
   f. Internal injuries/bleeding.
   g. Broken eyeglasses.
   h. Under- or overdosing of prescribed drugs.
   i. A sudden change in behavior.
   j. The caregiver's refusal to allow visitors to see an elder alone.
2. Sexual abuse signs and symptoms.
   a. An elder's report of sexual assault or rape.
   b. Bruises around the breasts or genital area.
   c. Unexplained venereal disease or genital infection.
   d. Unexplained vaginal or anal bleeding.
   e. Torn, stained, or bloody underclothing.
3. Emotional/psychological abuse signs and symptoms.
   a. An elder's report of being verbally or emotionally mistreated.
   b. Emotionally upset or agitated behavior.
   c. Extremely withdrawn and non-communicative or non-responsive behavior.
   d. Unusual behavior such as sucking, biting, or rocking.
4. Neglect signs and symptoms.
   a. An elder's report of being mistreated.
   b. Dehydration, malnutrition, untreated bedsores, and poor personal hygiene.
   c. Unattended or untreated health problems.
   d. Hazardous or unsafe living conditions.
5. Financial or material exploitation signs and symptoms.
   a. An elder's report of financial exploitation.
   b. Sudden changes in bank account or banking practice.
   c. The inclusion of additional names on an elder's bank signature card.
   d. Unauthorized withdrawal using an ATM card.
   e. Abrupt changes in a will or other financial documents.
   f. Substandard care or unpaid bills despite the availability of funds.
   g. Discovery of a forged signature.
   h. Sudden appearance of relatives claiming rights to decisions, money, or possessions.
   i. Unexplained transfer of funds.
   j. The provision of unnecessary services.

Role of Occupational Therapy

1. Mandatory reporting.
   a. Elder abuse per se may or may not be designated as a specific crime in a state; however, most physical, sexual, and financial/material abuse are crimes in all states.
   b. Health care workers are required to report suspected or observed cases of elder abuse.
   c. Failure to report may be considered a crime.
   d. In most states Adult Protective Services, the area Agency on Aging, or the county Department of Social Services is designated to provide investigation and services.
2. Occupational therapy intervention.
   a. Treat for physical and emotional injuries.
   b. Develop a trusting relationship.
   c. Assist in developing a support system.
   d. Refer to appropriate disciplines and/or agencies.

References

Abrams, W., Beers, M., & Berkow, R. (Eds.). (1995). *The Merck manual of geriatrics*, 2nd ed. Whitehouse Station, NJ: Merck and Co.

Abuse of children: The signs and symptoms. (2001). Cyberparent, Available: www.cyberparent.com/abuse/childabuse.

Amini, D. A. (2007). Motor assessments. In I. E. Asher (Ed.), *Occupational therapy assessment tools: An annotated index*, 3rd ed. (pp. 281–352). Bethesda, MD: AOTA Press.

Anzalone, M. E., & Lane, S. J. (2012). Sensory processing disorder. In S. J. Lane & A. C. Bundy. *Kids can be kids: A childhood occupations approach* (pp. 437–459). Philadelphia: F.A. Davis.

Asher, I. E. (2007). *An annotated index of occupational therapy evaluation tools*, 3rd ed. Bethesda, MD: AOTA Press.

Ayres, A. J. (1998). *Sensory integration and the child*, 13th ed. Los Angeles: Western Psychological Services.

The basics: What is elder abuse. (2001). The Elder Abuse Center, Available: www.elderabusecenter.org/basic/.

Beery, K. E., Buktenica, N. A., & Beery, N. A. (2010). *Beery-Buktenica Developmental Test of Visual-Motor Integration*, 6th ed. (BEERY VMI), San Antonio, TX: Pearson Education.

Bigsby, E., & Vergara, R. (2003). *Developmental and theraputic interventions in the NICU*, 1st ed. Baltimore, MD: Paul H. Brookes.

Bottomley, J. M., & Lewis, C. B. (2003). *Geriatric rehabilitation – A clinical approach*, 2nd ed. Upper Saddle River, NJ: Pearson Education.

Brown, T., & Jackel, A. L. (2007). Perceptual assessments. In I. E. Asher (Ed.), *Occupational therapy assessment tools: An annotated index,* 3rd ed. (pp. 353–419). Bethesda, MD: AOTA Press.

Bundy, A. C., & Murray, E. A., (2002). Sensory integration: A. Jean Ayres' theory revisited. In A. C. Bundy, S. J. Lane, & E. A. Murray, (Eds.), *Sensory integration: Theory and practice,* 2nd ed. (pp. 3–33). Philadelphia: F.A. Davis.

Case-Smith, J. (Ed.). (2001). *Occupational therapy for children,* 4th ed. St. Louis, MO: Mosby.

Case-Smith, J., Allen, A., & Pratt, P. N. (1996). *Occupational therapy for children,* 3rd ed. St. Louis, MO: Mosby.

Case-Smith, J., & Humphry, R. (2005). Feeding intervention. In J. Case-Smith (Ed.), *Occupational therapy for children,* 5th ed. (pp. 485–520). St. Louis, MO: Elsevier Mosby.

Case-Smith, J., & Shortridge, S. (1996). The developmental process. In J. Case-Smith, A. Allen, & P. N. Pratt (Eds.), *Occupational therapy for children,* 3rd ed. (pp. 44–66). St Louis, MO: Mosby.

Case-Smith, J., & O'Brien, J. C. (2010). *Occupational therapy for children,* 6th ed. Maryland Heights, MO: Mosby Elsevier.

Child help. (2010). *National child abuse statistics.* Retrieved February 19, 2010, from http://www.childhelp.org/resources/learning-center/statistics.

Child Welfare Information Gateway. (2006). *Child abuse and neglect fatalities: Statistics and interventions.* Washington, DC: Author.

Crist, P. (2007). Psychological assessments. In I.E. Asher (Ed.), *Occupational therapy assessment tools: An annotated index,* 3rd ed. (pp. 571–614). Bethesda, MD: AOTA Press.

D'Amico, M., & Mortera, M. H. (2007). Assessments of coping and adaptive behaviors. In I. E. Asher (Ed.), *Occupational therapy assessment tools: An annotated index,* 3rd ed. (pp. 633–671). Bethesda, MD: AOTA Press.

D'Amico, M., & Mortera, M. H. (2007). Assessments of disability status. In I. E. Asher (Ed.), *Occupational therapy assessment tools: An annotated index,* 3rd ed. (pp. 673–707). Bethesda, MD: AOTA Press.

Deitchman, G., & Puttkammer, C. (2001). *Preschool Visual Motor Integration Assessment* (PVMIA). Framingham, MA: Therapro.

Dunbar, S. B. (2007). Theory, frame of reference and model: A differentiation for practice considerations. In S. B. Dunbar (Ed.), *Occupational therapy models for intervention with children and families* (pp. 1–9). Thorofare, NJ: Slack.

Elder and vulnerable adult abuse. (2001). Available: www.ccastle.net/~mcpo/elder.

Erhardt, R. P. (1994). *The Erhardt Developmental Prehension Assessment.* Maplewood, MN: Erhardt Developmental Products.

Escolar, D. M., & Toisi, L. L. (2005). Muscles, bones and nerves. In M. L. Batshaw, L. Pellegrino, & N. J. Roizen (Ed.), *Children with disabilities,* 6th ed. (pp. 203–215). Baltimore, MD: Paul H. Brooks.

Exner, C. E. (2005). Development of hand skills. In J. Case-Smith (Ed.), *Occupational therapy for children,* 5th ed. (pp. 304–355). St. Louis, MO.: Elsevier Mosby.

Fisher, A. G., Murray, E. A., & Bundy, A. C. (1991). *Sensory integration theory and practice.* Philadelphia: F.A. Davis.

Gench, B., Hinson, M., & McNurlen, G. (1996). *Human reflexes and reacting resource cards.* Dubuque, IA: Eddie Bowers Publishing.

Haynes, C. J. (2007). Sensory assessments. In I. E. Asher (Ed.), *Occupational therapy assessment tools: An annotated index,* 3rd ed. (pp. 421–454). Bethesda, MD: AOTA Press.

Humphry, R., & Womack, J. (2014). Transformations of occupations: A life course persepctive. In B. A. B. Schell, G. Gillen, & M. E. Scaffa (Eds.), *Willard & Spackman's occupational therapy,* 12th ed. (pp. 60–71). Philadelphia: Lippincott Williams & Wilkins.

Hunter, J. G. (2005). Neonatal intensive care unit. In J. Case-Smith (Ed.), *Occupational therapy for children,* 5th ed. (pp. 688–754). St. Louis, MO: Elsevier Mosby.

Kaplan, H. I., & Sadock, B. J. (2007). *Synopsis of clinical psychiatry: Behavioral sciences/clinical psychiatry,* 10th ed. Philadelphia: Mosby.

Klein, M. (1987). *Pre-scissor skills,* rev. ed. Tucson, AZ: Therapy Skill Builders.

Knox. S. (2008). Development and current use of the Knox Preschool Play Scale. In L. D. Parham & L. S. Fazio (Eds.), *Sensory integration: Theory and practice,* 2nd ed. (pp. 55–70). St. Louis, MO: Elsevier.

Lane, S. J. (2002). Structure and function of the sensory systems. In A. C. Bundy, S. J. Lane, & E.A. Murray (Eds.), *Sensory integration: Theory and practice,* 2nd ed. (pp. 35–68). Philadelphia: F.A. Davis.

Lane, S. J. (2002). Sensory modulation. In A.C. Bundy, S. J. Lane, & E. A. Murray, (Eds.), *Sensory integration: Theory and practice,* 2nd ed. (pp. 101–122). Philadelphia: F.A. Davis.

Law, M., Missiuna, C., Pollock, N., & Stewart, D. (2005). Foundations for occupational therapy practice with children. In J. Case-Smith, (Ed), *Occupational therapy for children,* 5th ed. (pp. 53–87). St. Louis, MO: Elsevier Mosby.

Leech, S. W. (2007). Play assessments. In I. E. Asher (Ed.), *Occupational therapy assessment tools: An annotated index,* 3rd ed. (pp. 177–191). Bethesda, MD: AOTA Press.

Linder, T. (1994). *Transdisciplinary play-based assessment,* rev. ed. Baltimore: Paul H. Brookes.

Liptak, G. S. (2005). Neural tube defects. In M. L. Batshaw, L. Pellegrino, & N. J. Roizen (Eds.), *Children with disabilities,* 6th ed. (pp. 419–438). Baltimore, MD: Paul H. Brooks.

Martin, L. M. (2007) Assessments of social participation and quality of life. In I. E. Asher (Ed.), *Occupational therapy assessment tools: An annotated index,* 3rd ed. (pp. 215–216). Bethesda, MD: AOTA Press.

Miller, L. J. (2006). *Sensational kids hope and help for children with sensory processing disorders* (SPD). New York: G.P. Putnam's Sons.

Mosey, A. C. (1996). *Psychosocial components of occupational therapy.* Philadelphia: Lippincott-Raven.

National Center on Elder Abuse. (2005). *Fact sheet: Elder abuse prevalence and incidence.* Washington, DC.

Kahn-D'Angelo, L. (2013). Theories of development, motor control, and motor learning. In S. B. O'Sullivan & R. P. Siegelman, (Eds.). *National physical therapy examination review & study guide,* 16th ed. (pp. 283–299). Evanston, Il: Therapy Ed.

Participation Scale Development Team (2010). *Participation Scale v6.0*, Amsterdam, Netherland.

Parham, L. D., & Mailoux, Z. (2005). Sensory integration. In J. Case-Smith (Ed.), *Occupational therapy for children*, 5th ed. (pp. 356–409). St. Louis, MO: Elsevier Mosby.

Reeves, G. D., & Cermak, S. A. (2002). Disorders of praxis. In A. C. Bundy, S. J. Lane, & E. A. Murray, (Eds.), *Sensory integration: Theory and practice*, 2nd ed. (pp. 71–100). Philadelphia: F.A. Davis.

Rogers, S. (2005). Common conditions that influence children's participation. In J. Case-Smith (Ed), *Occupational therapy for children*, 5th ed. (pp. 160–215). St. Louis, MO: Elsevier Mosby.

Schultz-Krohn, W. (2007). Assessments of occupational performance. In I. E. Asher (Ed.), *Occupational therapy assessment tools: An annotated index*, 3rd ed. (pp. 33, 51–52). Bethesda, MD: AOTA Press.

Shepherd, J. (2005). Activities of daily living and adaptations for independent living. In J. Case-Smith, (Ed.), *Occupational therapy for children*, 5th ed. (pp. 521–570). St. Louis, MO: Elsevier Mosby.

Smith, S. K. *Mandatory reporting of child abuse and neglect* (2001). Available: www.smithlawfirm.com/mandatoryreporting.

Teaster, P., Dugar, T., Mendiondo, M., Abner, E., & Cecil, K. (2006). *The 2004 survey of state Adult Protective Services: Abuse of adults 60 years of age and older.* Boulder, CO: National Adult Protective Services Association.

United States Census Bureau. (2102). *Expectation of life at birth, and projections*. Retreived September 12, 2013 from http://www.census.gov/compendia/statab/cats/births_deaths_marriages_divorces/life_expectancy.html.

Vergara, E. (1993). *Foundations for practice in the neonatal intensive care unit and early intervention, Volume 2* (pp. 34–35). Baltimore, MD: AOTA Press.

Weinstein, S. L., & Gaillard, W. D. (2005). Epilepsy. In M. L. Batshaw, L., Pellegrino, & N. J. Roizen (Eds.), *Children with disabilities*, 6th ed. (pp. 439–460). Baltimore, MD: Paul H. Brooks.

Review Questions

Human Development Across the Lifespan: Pediatric Through Geriatric Considerations for Occupational Therapy Practice

Below are five questions about key content covered in this chapter. These questions are not inclusive of the entirety of content about human development across the lifespan and pediatric through geriatric considerations for occupational therapy practice that you must know for success on the NBCOT exam. These questions are provided to help you "jump start" the thought processes you will need to apply your studying of content to the answering of exam questions; hence they are not in the NBCOT exam format. Exam items in the NBCOT format which cover the depth and breadth of content you will need to know to pass the NBCOT exam are provided on this text's disc. The answers to the below questions are provided in Appendix 4.

1. You are part of an intraprofessional screening team to determine children's readiness for kindergarten. A 5-year-old child whom you are evaluating has performed at or above level on every aspect of the screening and has not demonstrated any fine motor, visual motor, or gross motor delays. The child has no cognitive deficits. The child performed well on the Beery-Buktenica Developmental Test of Visual-Motor Integration. Given the child's performance so far, which of Erhardt's developmental levels of prewriting skills would you expect the child to use for writing tasks? Explain your answer.

2. A typically developing child with no developmental delays independently creates a building made of blocks from a mental image. Identify the child's age range and describe the skills the child would use during this play activity.

3. A 15-year-old has a group of friends who have recently become involved in experimenting with drugs, alcohol and other risky behaviors. The teen is torn between wanting to remain friends with this group and not wanting to join them in these behaviors. The teen decides to join another group of teens who are engaged a competitive soccer league in order to meet and become connected to a new group of friends. According to Erikson's eight stages of man, what stage of development is the teenager undergoing? Describe the charisteristics of this stage.

4. A 16-month-old toddler is brought to occupational therapy for an evaluation. The parents are concerned with the frequency of the toddler's falls which result in bangs to the head. The child demonstrates delayed motor skills. You notice that the toddler has not yet integrated primitive reflexes. Which primary primitive reflex is most likely absent in this toddler? Explain its relevance to the toddler's health status, safety, and its impact on occupational performance.

5. You provide wellness and prevention services to older adults who attend a community-based senior center. What strategies to slow, reverse, and/or compensate for age-related changes to their muscular, skeletal, and neurological systems can you can share with these older adults?

6

Musculoskeletal System Disorders

COLLEEN MAHER

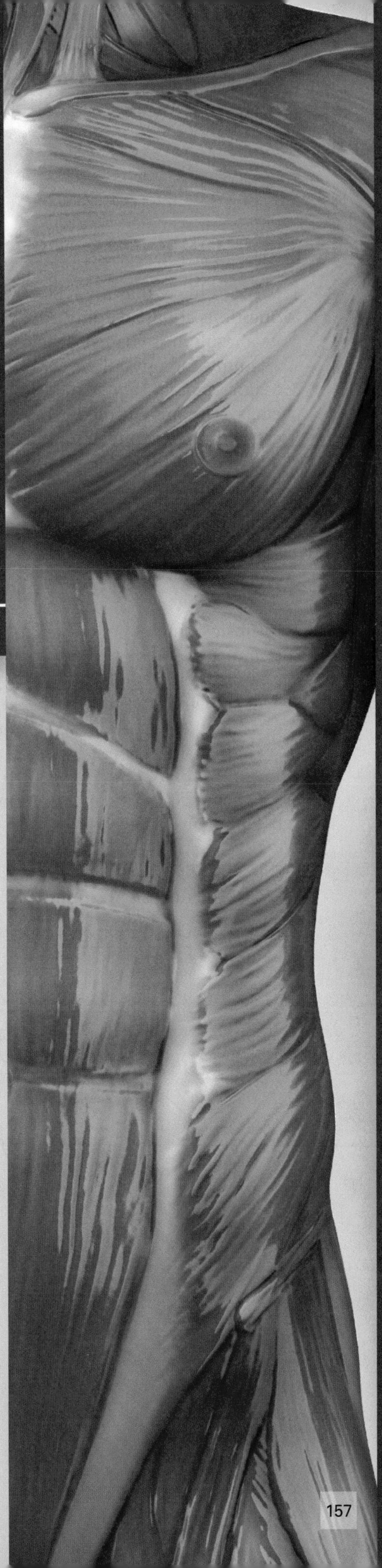

Chapter Outline

Anatomy of the Musculoskeletal System

Relationship to the Examination

1. It is not likely that the NBCOT exam will ask direct questions about anatomy or physiology.
2. As a result, this chapter does not provide a complete anatomy and physiology review.
3. Major structures and functions of the musculoskeletal system are outlined because knowledge of these can help determine the best answer. For example, damage to the opponens pollicis would result in the need to use activities that do not require opposition.

Anatomy of the Hand

1. Intrinsic muscles innervated by the median nerve (Figure 6-1).
   a. Abductor pollicis brevis.
      (1) Origin: scaphoid, trapezium, flexor retinaculum, and tendon of the abductor pollicis longus.
      (2) Insertion: base of proximal phalanx, radial side of thumb.
      (3) Function: palmar abduction.
   b. Opponens pollicis.
      (1) Origin: trapezium and flexor retinaculum.
      (2) Insertion: first metacarpal.
      (3) Function: opposition.
   c. Flexor pollicis brevis: superficial head.
      (1) Origin: trapezium, trapezoid, capitate and flexor retinaculum.
      (2) Insertion: base of proximal phalanx, radial side of thumb.
      (3) Function: thumb MCP flexion, deep head innervated by ulnar nerve.
   d. Lumbricals (radial side).
      (1) Origin: tendons of flexor digitorum profundus, index and middle fingers (radial and palmar sides).
      (2) Insertion: radial side of digits II and III into extensor expansion.
      (3) Function: MCP flexion and extension of IP joints.
2. Intrinsic muscles innervated by the ulnar nerve (Figure 6-2).
   a. Abductor digiti minimi.
      (1) Origin: pisiform and tendon of flexor carpi ulnaris.
      (2) Insertion: proximal phalanx of the 5th digit.
      (3) Function: abduction of the 5th digit.
   b. Opponens digiti minimi.
      (1) Origin: hook of hamate and flexor retinaculum.
      (2) Insertion: 5th metacarpal.
      (3) Function: opposition of the 5th digit.
   c. Flexor digiti minimi.
      (1) Origin: hook of hamate and flexor retinaculum.
      (2) Insertion: proximal phalanx of 5th digit.
      (3) Function: flexion of MCP joint and opposition of the 5th digit.

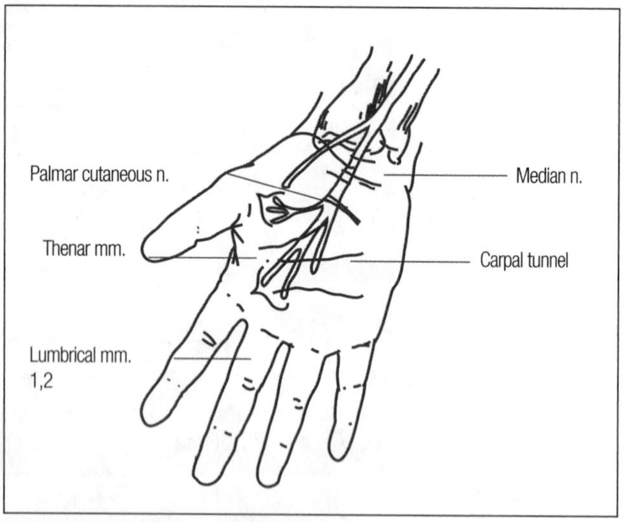

Figure 6-1 Median Nerve

Malick, M., & Kasch, M. (1984). *Manual on management of specific hand problems.* Pittsburgh, PA: AREN. Reprinted with permission.

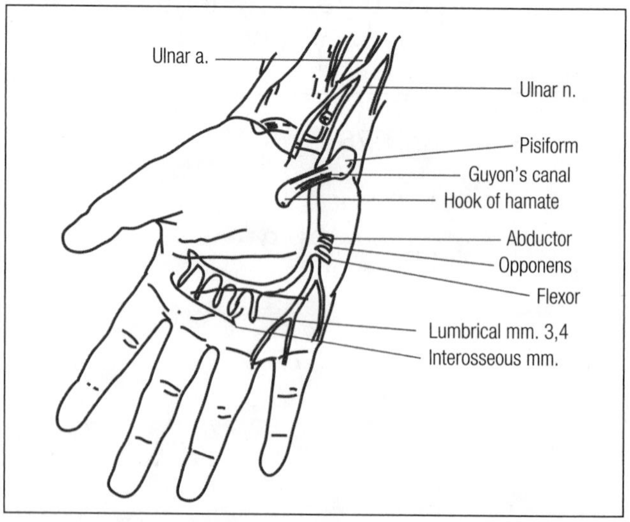

Figure 6-2 Ulnar Nerve

Malick, M., & Kasch, M. (1984). *Manual on management of specific hand problems.* Pittsburgh, PA: AREN. Reprinted with permission.

d. Adductor.
  (1) Origin: oblique head: base of the 2nd and 3rd metacarpal, trapezoid and capitate. Transverse head: palmar border and shaft of 3rd metacarpal.
  (2) Insertion: sesamoid, base of proximal phalanx, tendon of extensor pollicis longus.
  (3) Function: adducts CMC joint of thumb.
e. Lumbricals (ulnar side).
  (1) Origin: tendons of flexor digitorum profundus for digits IV and V.
  (2) Insertion: radial side of digits IV and V into extensor expansion.
  (3) Function: MCP flexion and extension of IP joints of digits IV and V.
f. Palmar interossei.
  (1) Origin: first palmar: ulnar surface of 2nd metacarpal; second palmar: radial surface of 4th metacarpal; third palmar: radial surface of 5th metacarpal.
  (2) Insertion: first palmar: ulnar surface of 2nd proximal phalanx; second palmar: radial surface of 4th proximal phalanx; third palmar: radial surface of 5th proximal phalanx.
  (3) Function: adduction and assistance with MCP flexion and extension of IP joints of digits II through V.
g. Dorsal interossei.
  (1) Origin: all four muscles arise from the adjacent sides of the metacarpals.
  (2) Insertion: proximal phalanx on the radial aspect of the index, radial and ulnar sides of middle finger, and ulnar side of ring finger (all into extensor digitorum).
  (3) Function: abduction and assists with MCP flexion and extension of IP joints of digits II through V.

3. Extrinsic flexor muscles of the hand innervated by the median nerve (Figure 6-3).
  a. Flexor digitorum superficialis (sublimis) (FDS).
    (1) Origin: medial epicondyle.
    (2) Insertion: middle phalanx (two slips).
    (3) Function: flexion of PIP joints.
  b. Flexor digitorum profundus (FDP).
    (1) Origin: proximal 2/3 of the ulna and interosseous membrane.
    (2) Insertion: distal phalanx.
    (3) Function: flexion of DIP joints to digits II and III. (See ulnar nerve for digits IV and V.)
  c. Flexor pollicis longus (FPL).
    (1) Origin: radius, middle 1/3.
    (2) Insertion: distal phalanx of thumb.
    (3) Function: flexion of IP joint of thumb.

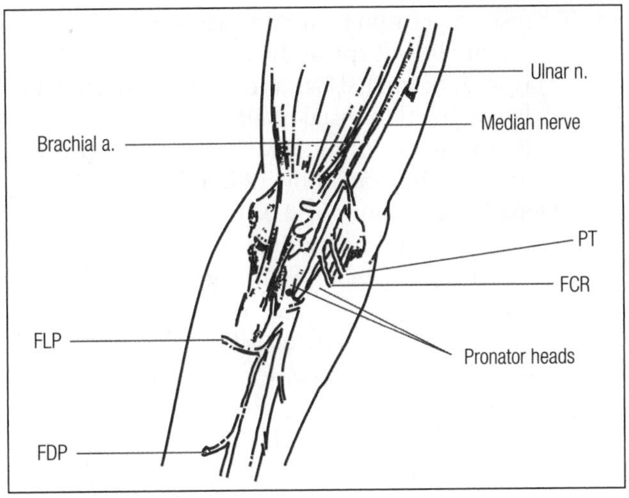

Figure 6-3 Median Nerve

Malick, M., & Kasch, M. (1984). *Manual on management of specific hand problems.* Pittsburgh, PA: AREN. Reprinted with permission.

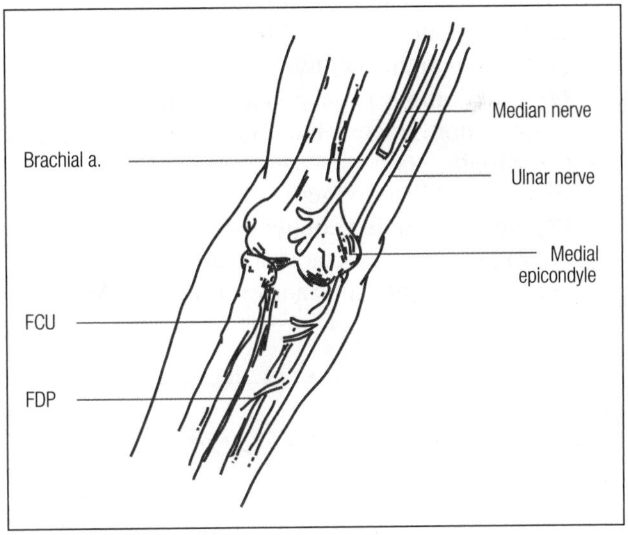

Figure 6-4 Ulnar Nerve

Malick, M., & Kasch, M. (1984). *Manual on management of specific hand problems.* Pittsburgh, PA: AREN. Reprinted with permission.

4. Extrinsic flexors of the hand innervated by the ulnar nerve (Figure 6-4).
  a. Flexor digitorum profundus.
    (1) Origin: proximal 2/3 of the ulna and interosseous membrane.
    (2) Insertion: distal phalanx.
    (3) Function: flexion of DIP joints to digits IV and V.
5. Extrinsic extensor muscles of the hand innervated by the radial nerve (Figure 6-5).

a. Extensor digitorum communis (EDC).
   (1) Origin: lateral epicondyle.
   (2) Insertion: medial band to middle phalanx and lateral band to distal phalanx.
   (3) Function: extension of MCP joints and contributes to extension of the IP joints.

b. Extensor digiti minimi (EDM).
   (1) Origin: lateral epicondyle.
   (2) Insertion: inserts into EDC at MCP level of the 5th digit.
   (3) Function: extension of MCP joint of the 5th digit and contributes to extension of the IP joints.

c. Extensor indicis proprius (EIP).
   (1) Origin: ulna, middle 1/3.
   (2) Insertion: inserts into EDC at MCP level.
   (3) Function: extension of MCP joint of the 2nd digit and contributes to extension of the IP joints.

d. Extensor pollicis longus (EPL).
   (1) Origin: ulna, middle 1/3.
   (2) Insertion: distal phalanx of thumb.
   (3) Function: extension of IP joint of thumb.

e. Extensor pollicis brevis (EPB).
   (1) Origin: radius, middle 1/3.
   (2) Insertion: proximal phalanx of thumb.
   (3) Function: extension of MCP and CMC joints of thumb.

f. Abductor pollicis longus (APL).
   (1) Origin: middle 1/3 of ulna and radius.
   (2) Insertion: first metacarpal, radial side.
   (3) Function: abduction and extension of CMC joint.

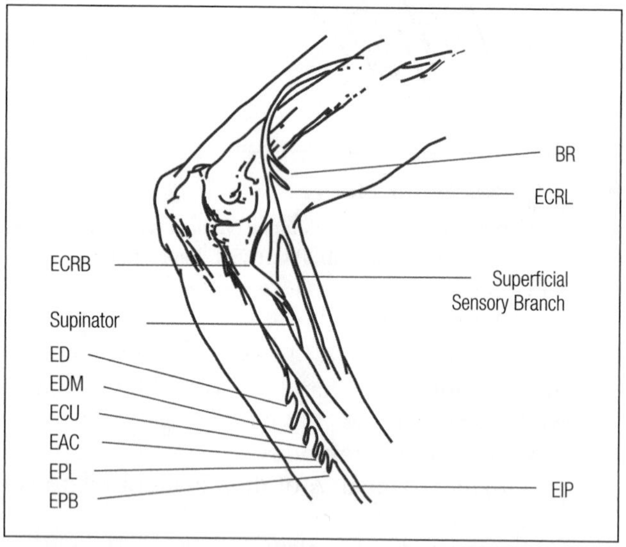

Figure 6-5 Radial Nerve

Malick, M., & Kasch, M. (1984). *Manual on management of specific hand problems*. Pittsburgh, PA: AREN. Reprinted with permission.

Anatomy of the Wrist

1. Wrist flexors innervated by the median nerve (Figure 6-3).
   a. Flexor carpi radialis (FCR).
      (1) Origin: medial epicondyle.
      (2) Insertion: 2nd and 3rd metacarpal, base.
      (3) Function: flexion of wrist and radial deviation.
   b. Palmaris longus (PL).
      (1) Origin: medial epicondyle.
      (2) Insertion: palmar aponeurosis.
      (3) Function: flexion of wrist.
2. Wrist flexors innervated by the ulnar nerve (Figure 6-4).
   a. Flexor carpi ulnaris (FCU).
      (1) Origin: medial epicondyle and proximal 2/3 of the ulna.
      (2) Insertion: pisiform and 5th metacarpal.
      (3) Function: flexion of wrist and ulnar deviation.
3. Wrist extensors innervated by the radial nerve (Figure 6-5).
   a. Extensor carpi radialis brevis (ECRB).
      (1) Origin: lateral epicondyle.
      (2) Insertion: 3rd metacarpal, base.
      (3) Function: extension of wrist and radial deviation.
   b. Extensor carpi radialis longus (ECRL).
      (1) Origin: supracondylar ridge of the humerus.
      (2) Insertion: 2nd metacarpal, base.
      (3) Function: extension of wrist and radial deviation.
   c. Extensor carpi ulnaris (ECU).
      (1) Origin: lateral epicondyle.
      (2) Insertion: 5th metacarpal.
      (3) Function: extension of wrist and ulnar deviation.

Anatomy of the Forearm

1. Volar forearm muscles innervated by the median nerve.
   a. Pronator teres.
      (1) Origin: medial epicondyle and coronoid process of ulna.
      (2) Insertion: lateral surface of radius.
      (3) Function: forearm pronation.
   b. Pronator quadratus.
      (1) Origin: distal ulna.
      (2) Insertion: distal radius.
      (3) Function: forearm pronation.
2. Dorsal forearm muscles innervated by the radial nerve.
   a. Supinator.
      (1) Origin: lateral epicondyle and ulna.
      (2) Insertion: radius.
      (3) Function: forearm supination.

Anatomy of the Elbow

1. Elbow flexion: biceps and brachialis innervated by musculocutaneous nerve; brachioradialis innervated by radial nerve.
   a. Biceps.
      (1) Origin: coracoid process and supraglenoid tubercle.
      (2) Insertion: radial tuberosity.
      (3) Function: elbow flexion with forearm supinated.
   b. Brachialis.
      (1) Origin: distal ⅔ of humerus.
      (2) Insertion: ulnar tuberosity.
      (3) Function: elbow flexion with forearm pronated.
   c. Brachioradialis.
      (1) Origin: supracondylar ridge.
      (2) Insertion: distal radius.
      (3) Function: elbow flexion with forearm neutral.
2. Elbow extension: triceps and anconeus innervated by radial nerve.
   a. Triceps.
      (1) Origin: long head; infraglenoid tuberosity. Lateral head; posterior humerus. Medial head; distal to lateral head.
      (2) Insertion: olecranon.
      (3) Function: elbow extension.
   b. Anconeus.
      (1) Origin: lateral epicondyle and capsule of elbow joint.
      (2) Insertion: olecranon and upper ¼ of dorsal ulna.
      (3) Function: elbow extension.

Anatomy of the Shoulder

1. Rotator cuff muscles.
   a. Subscapularis innervated by the subscapular nerve.
      (1) Origin: anterior surface of scapula.
      (2) Insertion: lesser tuberosity.
      (3) Function: internal rotation.
   b. Supraspinatus innervated by the suprascapular nerve.
      (1) Origin: supraspinatus fossa.
      (2) Insertion: greater tuberosity.
      (3) Function: abduction and flexion.
   c. Infraspinatus innervated by the suprascapular nerve.
      (1) Origin: infraspinatus fossa.
      (2) Insertion: greater tuberosity.
      (3) Function: external rotation.
   d. Teres minor innervated by the axillary nerve.
      (1) Origin: axillary border of scapula.
      (2) Insertion: greater tuberosity.
      (3) Function: external rotation.
2. Shoulder flexion muscles.
   a. Anterior deltoid innervated by axillary nerve.
      (1) Origin: clavicle.
      (2) Insertion: deltoid tuberosity.
   b. Coracobrachialis innervated by the musculocutaneous nerve.
      (1) Origin: coracoid process.
      (2) Insertion: medial aspect of deltoid.
   c. Supraspinatus (as above).
3. Shoulder abduction muscles.
   a. Middle deltoid innervated by the axillary nerve.
      (1) Origin: acromion.
      (2) Insertion: deltoid tuberosity.
   b. Supraspinatus (as above).
4. Horizontal abduction muscles.
   a. Posterior deltoid innervated by the axillary nerve.
      (1) Origin: spine of scapula.
      (2) Insertion: deltoid tuberosity.
5. Horizontal adduction muscles.
   a. Pectoralis major innervated by the lateral pectoral nerve.
      (1) Origin: medial clavicle, sternum, and ribs 1–7.
      (2) Insertion: greater tuberosity.
6. Shoulder extension muscles.
   a. Latissimus dorsi innervated by the thoracodorsal nerve.
      (1) Origin: T6–T12, L1–L5, sacral vertebrae, ribs 9–12, iliac crest and inferior angle of scapula.
      (2) Insertion: intertubercular groove of the humerus.
   b. Teres major innervated by the subscapular nerve.
      (1) Origin: inferior angle of scapula.
      (2) Insertion: intertubercular groove of the humerus.
   c. Posterior deltoid (as above).

Anatomy of the Scapula

1. Upward rotation muscles.
   a. Trapezius (upper, middle, and lower) innervated by the spinal accessory nerve (CNXI).
      (1) Origin.
         (a) Upper fibers: occiput and ligamentum nuchae.
         (b) Middle fibers: spinous processes of T1 to T5.
         (c) Lower fibers: spinous processes of T6 to T12.
      (2) Insertion.
         (a) Upper fibers: lateral ⅓ of the clavicle.
         (b) Middle fibers: acromion and spine of scapula.
         (c) Lower fibers: medial end of spine of scapula.

b. Serratus anterior innervated by the long thoracic nerve.
(1) Origin: ribs 1–8 and aponeurosis of intercostals.
(2) Insertion: superior and inferior angles of scapula and vertebral border of scapula.

2. Downward rotation muscles.
a. Levator scapulae innervated by C3–C4 nerves.
(1) Origin: C1–C4 transverse processes.
(2) Insertion: vertebral border of scapula.
b. Rhomboids (major and minor) innervated by the dorsal scapular nerve.
(1) Origin: C7–T5 spinous processes.
(2) Insertion: vertebral border, distal to the spine of the scapula.
c. Serratus anterior (as above).
d. Latissimus dorsi (as above).
3. Scapula adduction muscles.
a. Middle trapezius (as above).
b. Rhomboid major (as above).
4. Scapula abduction muscles.
a. Serratus anterior (as above).
5. Scapula elevation muscles.
a. Trapezius (upper) (as above).
b. Levator scapulae (as above).
6. Scapula depression muscles.
a. Trapezius (lower) (as above).

Dermatome Distribution

1. Refer to Table 11-3.
2. Refer to Figure 6-6.

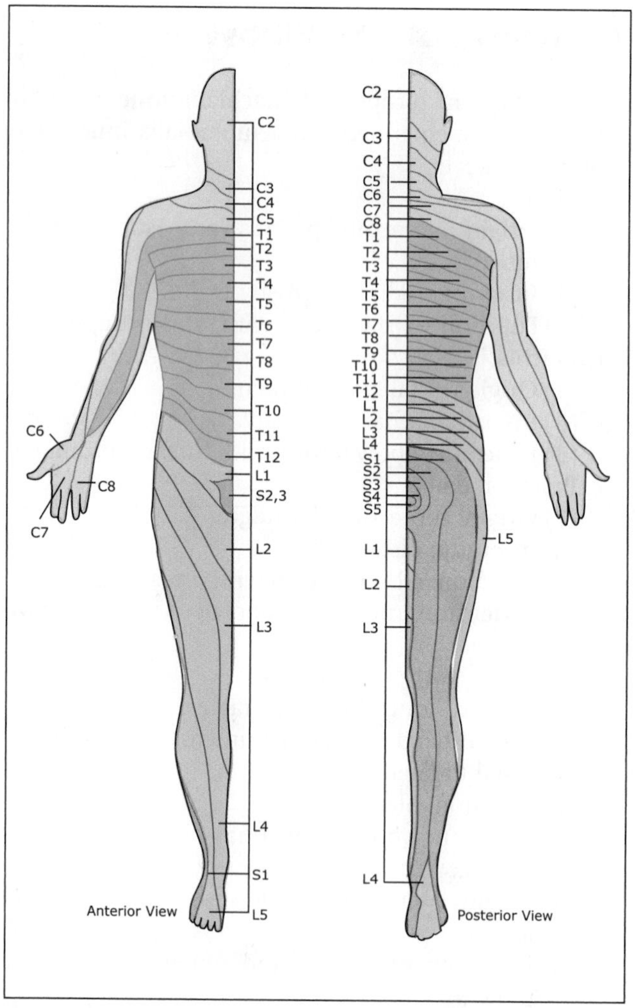

Figure 6-6 **Dermatomes**

Hand and Upper Extremity Disorders and Injuries

Dupuytren's Disease

1. Disease of the fascia of the palm and digits.
a. The fascia becomes thick and contracted. Develops cords and bands that extend into the digits.
b. Results in flexion deformities of the involved digits (Figure 6-7).
2. Etiology: unknown.
3. Conservative treatment has not been successful.
4. Surgical release is required.
a. Fasciotomy with Z plasty.
b. Aponeurotomy.
c. McCash Procedure (open palm).
5. Occupational therapy intervention.
a. Wound care: dressing changes.
b. Edema control: elevation above the heart.

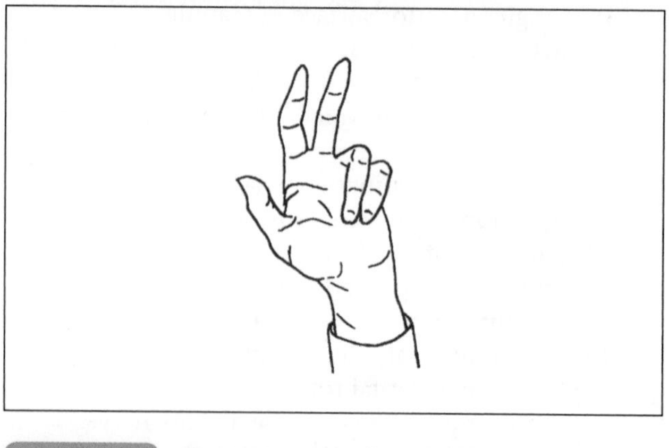

Figure 6-7 **Dupuytren's Contractures**
Adapted from Magee DJ: Orthopedic Physical Assessment, 2nd ed. Saunders, 1992.

c. Extension splint: initially at all times except to remove for ROM and bathing.
d. A/PROM, and progress to strengthening, when wounds are healed.
e. Scar management (massage, scar pad, and compression garment).
f. Purposeful and occupation-based tasks that emphasize flexion (gripping) and extension (release).

Skier's Thumb (Gamekeeper's Thumb)

1. Rupture of the ulnar collateral ligament of the MCP joint of the thumb.
2. Etiology: most common cause is a fall while skiing with the thumb held in a ski pole.
3. Occupational therapy intervention.
   a. Conservative treatment including a thumb splint (for 4 to 6 weeks).
   b. AROM and pinch strengthening (at 6 weeks).
   c. Focus on ADL that require opposition and pinch strength.
   d. Post-operative treatment includes thumb splint for 6 weeks, followed by AROM. PROM can begin at 8 weeks and strengthening at 10 weeks.

Complex Regional Pain Syndrome (CRPS)

1. Type I formerly known as reflex sympathetic dystrophy (RSD).
2. Type II formerly known as causalgia.
3. Vasomotor dysfunction as a result of an abnormal reflex.
4. It can be localized to one specific area or spread to other parts of the extremity.
5. Etiology: may follow trauma (e.g., Colles' fracture) or surgery, but actual cause is unknown.
6. Symptoms include severe pain, edema, discoloration, osteoporosis, sudomotor changes, temperature changes, trophic changes, and vasomotor instability.
7. Occupational therapy intervention.
   a. Modalities to decrease pain.
   b. Edema management: elevation, manual edema mobilization, compression glove.
   c. AROM to involved joints.
   d. ADL to encourage pain-free active use.
   e. Stress loading (weight bearing and joint distraction activities, including scrubbing and carrying activities).
   f. Splinting to prevent contractures and enable ability to engage in occupation-based activities.
   g. Encourage self management.
   h. Interventions to avoid or to proceed with caution include passive range of motion, passive stretching, joint mobilization, dynamic splinting, and casting.

Fractures

1. Types of fractures.
   a. Intraarticular versus extraarticular.
   b. Closed versus open.
   c. Dorsal displacement versus volar displacement.
   d. Midshaft versus neck versus base.
   e. Complete versus incomplete.
   f. Transverse versus spiral versus oblique.
   g. Comminuted.
2. Medical treatment.
   a. Closed reduction: types of stabilization include short arm cast (SAC), long arm cast (LAC), splint, sling, or fracture brace.
   b. Open reduction internal fixation (ORIF): types include nails, screws, plates, or wire.
   c. External fixation.
   d. Arthrodesis: fusion.
   e. Arthroplasty: joint replacement.
3. Most common UE fractures.
   a. Colles' fracture: fracture of the distal radius with dorsal displacement.
   b. Smith's fracture: fracture of the distal radius with volar displacement.
   c. Carpal fractures: most common is scaphoid fracture (60% of carpal fractures). The proximal scaphoid has a poor blood supply and may become necrotic.
   d. Metacarpal fractures: classified according to location (head, neck, shaft, or base). A common complication is rotational deformities. A Boxer's fracture is a fracture of the 5th metacarpal (requires an ulnar gutter splint).
   e. Proximal phalanx fractures: most common with thumb and index. A common complication is loss of PIP A/PROM.
   f. Middle phalanx fractures: not commonly fractured.
   g. Distal phalanx fracture: most common finger fracture. May result in mallet finger (which involves terminal extensor tendon).
   h. Elbow fracture: involvement of the radial head may result in limited rotation of the forearm.
   i. Humerus fractures: nondisplaced vs. displaced fractures.
      (1) Etiology: fall onto an outstretched upper extremity.
      (2) Fractures of the greater tuberosity may result in rotator cuff injuries.
      (3) Humeral shaft fractures may cause injury to the radial nerve resulting in wrist drop.

4. Occupational therapy evaluation.
   a. History should include mechanism of injury and fracture management.
   b. Results of special tests (x-rays, MRI, and CT scan).
   c. Edema.
   d. Pain.
   e. AROM.
      (1) Do not assess PROM or strength until ordered by physician.
      (2) Exceptions are humerus fractures which often begin with PROM or AAROM.
   f. Sensation.
   g. Roles, occupations, ADL and activities related to roles.
5. Occupational therapy intervention.
   a. Immobilization phase: stabilization and healing are the goals.
      (1) AROM of joints above and below the stabilized part.
      (2) Edema control: elevation, retrograde massage, and compression garments.
      (3) Light ADL and role activities with no resistance, progress as tolerated.
   b. Mobilization phase: consolidation is the goal.
      (1) Edema control: elevation, retrograde massage, contrast baths, and compression garments.
      (2) AROM.
         (a) Progress to PROM when approved by physician (4–8 weeks).
         (b) Exceptions are humerus fractures which often begin with PROM or AAROM.
      (3) Light purposeful or occupation-based activities.
      (4) Pain management: positioning and physical agent modalities.
      (5) Strengthening: begin with isometrics when approved by physician.

Cumulative Trauma Disorders (CTD)

1. Also known as repetitive strain injuries (RSI), overuse syndromes, and/or musculoskeletal disorders.
2. Risk factors: repetition, static position, awkward postures, forceful exertions, and vibration.
3. Non-work risk factors: acute trauma, pregnancy, diabetes, arthritis, and wrist size and shape.
4. Most common types.
   a. de Quervain's.
      (1) Stenosing tenosynovitis of the abductor pollicis longus (APL) and the extensor pollicis brevis (EPB) (Figure 6-8).
      (2) Pain and swelling over the radial styloid.
      (3) Positive Finkelstein's Test.

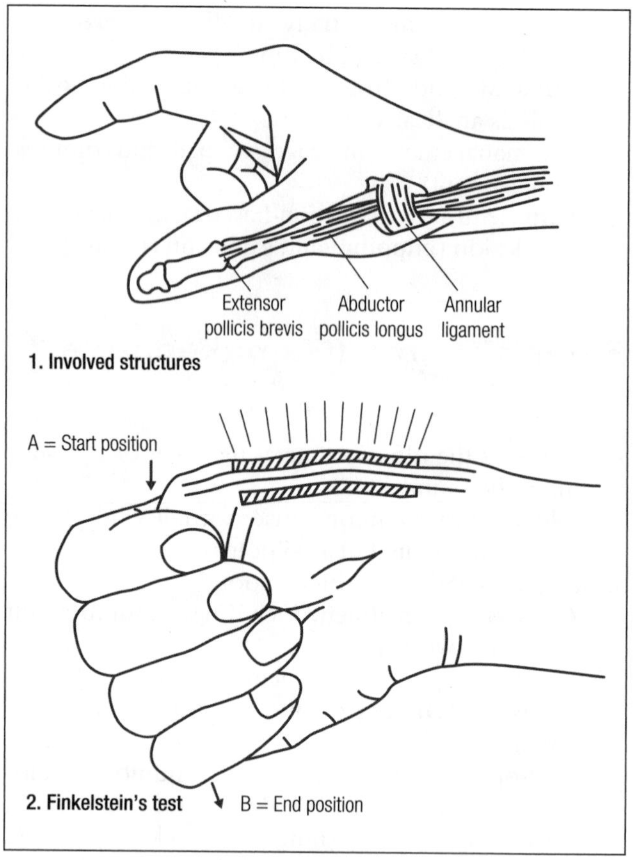

Figure 6-8 **de Quervain's**

      (4) Conservative treatment.
         (a) Thumb spica splint (IP joint free).
         (b) Activity/work modification.
         (c) Ice massage over radial wrist.
         (d) Gentle AROM of wrist and thumb to prevent stiffness.
      (5) Post operative treatment.
         (a) Thumb spica splint and gentle AROM (0–2 weeks).
         (b) Strengthening, ADL, and role activities (2–6 weeks).
         (c) Unrestricted activity (6 weeks).
   b. Lateral and medial epicondylitis.
      (1) Degeneration of the tendon origin as a result of repetitive microtrauma.
      (2) Lateral epicondylitis: overuse of wrist extensors, especially the extensor carpi radialis brevis. Also called tennis elbow.
      (3) Medial epicondylitis: overuse of wrist flexors. Also called golfer's elbow.
      (4) Conservative treatment.
         (a) Elbow strap, wrist splint.
         (b) Ice and deep friction massage.
         (c) Stretching.

(d) Activity/work modification.
(e) As pain decreases, add strengthening. Begin with isometric exercises and then progress to isotonic and eccentric exercises.

c. Trigger finger.
(1) Tenosynovitis of the finger flexors: most commonly is the A1 Pulley.
(2) Caused by repetition and the use of tools that are placed too far apart.
(3) Conservative treatment.
(a) Hand based trigger finger splint (MCP extended, IP jts free).
(b) Scar massage.
(c) Edema control.
(d) Tendon gliding.
(e) Activity/work modification: avoid repetitive gripping activities and using tools with handles too far apart.

d. Nerve compressions: refer to section on peripheral nerve injuries.

Tendon Repairs

1. Rationale for early mobilization.
a. Prevents adhesion formation.
b. Facilitates wound/tendon healing.
2. Occupational therapy goals.
a. Increase tendon excursion.
b. Improve strength at repair site.
c. Increase joint ROM.
d. Prevent adhesions.
e. Facilitate resumption of meaningful roles, occupations, and activities.
3. Early mobilization programs for flexor tendons.
a. As surgical techniques have improved, multiple early mobilization protocols have been developed.
(1) The Kleinert and the Duran Protocols are the most common.
b. Kleinert: passive flexion using rubber band traction and active extension to the hood of the splint. (Figure 6-9).
(1) Protocol.
(a) 0–4 weeks (early phase): dorsal block splint. Wrist is positioned in 20°–30° of flexion, MCP joints in 50°–60° of flexion and IP joints extended. Passive flexion and active extension within limits of splint.
(b) 4–7 weeks (intermediate phase): Continue dorsal block splint, but adjust the wrist to neutral. Place/hold exercises and differential flexor tendon gliding exercises (see Figure 11-2). Scar management.

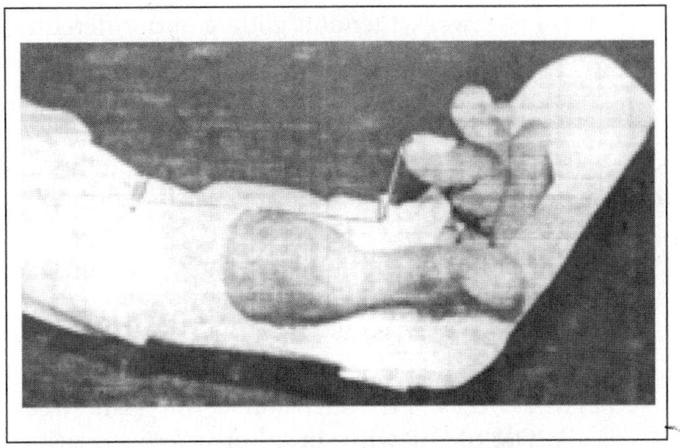

Figure 6-9 A simple palmar pulley can be provided by a safety pin attached to a palmar strap at DPC level. The line passes through the "eye" of the safety pin to direct the pull precisely

Hunter, J.M., MacKin, E.J., & Callahan, A.D. *Rehabilitation of the hand: Surgery and therapy*, 4th ed. (p. 451). St. Louis, MO: Mosby. Reprinted with permission.

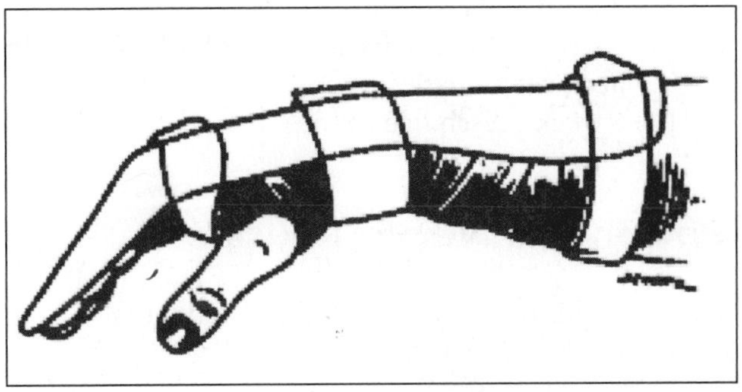

Figure 6-10 Dorsal blocking splint used for "modified Duran" protocol. Wrist and MP joints are flexed, and fingers are strapped in IP joint extension when not exercising

Hunter, J.M.; MacKin, E.J.; & Callahan, A.D. *Rehabilitation of the hand: Surgery and therapy*, 4th ed. (p. 448). St. Louis, MO: Mosby. Reprinted with permission.

(c) 6–8 weeks: AROM. Differential tendon gliding. Light purposeful and occupation-based activities. D/C splint.
(d) 8–12 weeks: strengthening and work and leisure activities.

c. Duran: passive flexion and extension of digit.
(1) Protocol.
(a) 0–4½ weeks: dorsal blocking splint. Exercises in splint include passive flexion of PIP joint, DIP joint and to DPC. 10 reps every hour (Figure 6-10).
(b) 4½–6 weeks: active flexion and extension within limits of splint.

(c) 6–8 weeks: tendon gliding and differential tendon gliding, scar management, and light purposeful and occupation-based activities.
(d) 8–12 weeks: strengthening and work activities.
4. Early mobilization programs for extensor tendons.
a. Zone I and II.
(1) Mallet finger deformity.
(2) 0–6 weeks: DIP extension splint.
b. Zone III and IV.
(1) Boutonniere deformity.
(2) 0–4 weeks: PIP extension splint (DIP free). AROM of DIP while in splint.
(3) 4–6 weeks: begin AROM of DIP and flexion of digits to the DPC.
c. Zone V, VI, and VII.
(1) 0–2 weeks: volar wrist splint with wrist in 20°–30° of extension, MCPs in 0°–10° of flexion, and IP joints in full extension.
(2) 2–3 weeks: shorten splint to allow flexion and extension of IP joints.
(3) 4 weeks: remove splint to begin MCP active flexion and extension.
(4) 5 weeks: begin active wrist ROM. Wear splint in between exercise sessions.
(5) 6 weeks: discharge splint.

Peripheral Nerve Injuries

1. Three major nerves: median, ulnar, and radial.
2. Two types of nerve injuries.
a. Compression.
b. Laceration: partial or complete.
3. Carpal tunnel syndrome (CTS): a median nerve compression.
a. Etiology: repetition, awkward postures, vibration, anatomical anomalies, and pregnancy.
b. Symptoms: numbness and tingling of the thumb, index, middle, and radial half of the ring fingers.
(1) Paresthesias usually occur at night (most characteristic).
(2) Person will complain of dropping things.
(3) Positive Tinel's sign at wrist. Positive Phalen's sign.
(4) Advanced stage of CTS can result in muscle atrophy of the thenar eminence.
c. Conservative treatment.
(1) Wrist splint in neutral: should be worn at night and during the day if performing repetitive activity.
(2) Median nerve gliding exercises and differential tendon gliding exercises.
(3) Activity modification: avoid activities with extreme positions of wrist flexion, wrist flexion with repetitive finger flexion, and wrist flexion with a static grip.
(4) Ergonomics: appropriate workstation design. CTS is the most common work related injury of the upper extremity.
d. Surgical intervention: carpal tunnel release (CTR).
e. Post-operative treatment of CTR.
(1) Edema control: elevation, retrograde massage, compression glove and/or contrast bath.
(2) AROM.
(3) Nerve and tendon gliding exercises.
(4) Sensory reeducation.
(5) Strengthening of thenar muscles (usually 6 weeks post operative).
(6) Work/activity modification.
4. Pronator teres syndrome (proximal volar forearm): a median nerve compression between the two heads of pronator teres.
a. Etiology: repetitive pronation and supination and excessive pressure on volar forearm.
b. Symptoms: same as CTS and also aching pain in proximal forearm.
(1) Positive Tinel's sign at the forearm.
(2) No night symptoms.
c. Conservative treatment.
(1) Elbow splint at 90° with forearm in neutral.
(2) Avoid activities that include repetitive forearm pronation and supination.
d. Surgical intervention: decompression.
e. Post-operative treatment.
(1) AROM.
(2) Nerve gliding.
(3) Strengthening (2 weeks post-operative).
(4) Sensory reeducation.
(5) Work/activity modification.
5. Guyon's canal: an ulnar nerve compression at the wrist.
a. Etiology: repetition, ganglion, pressure, and fascia thickening.
b. Symptoms.
(1) Numbness and tingling in the ulnar nerve distribution of the hand.
(2) Motor weakness of ulnar nerve-innervated musculature.
(3) Positive Tinel's sign at Guyon's canal.
(4) Advanced stages can lead to atrophy of ulnar nerve-innervated musculature in the hand.
c. Conservative treatment.
(1) Wrist splint in neutral.
(2) Work/activity modification.
d. Surgical intervention: decompression.
e. Post-operative intervention.
(1) Edema control.
(2) AROM.
(3) Nerve gliding.

(4) Strengthening (2–4 weeks): focus on power grip.
(5) Sensory reeducation.

6. Cubital tunnel syndrome: an ulnar nerve compression at the elbow.
   a. Etiology: second most common compression; pressure at elbow (leaning on elbow) and extreme elbow flexion.
   b. Symptoms.
      (1) Numbness and tingling along ulnar aspect of forearm and hand.
      (2) Pain at elbow with extreme position of elbow flexion.
      (3) Weakness of power grip.
      (4) Positive Tinel's sign at elbow.
      (5) Advanced stages can lead to atrophy of FCU, FDP to digits IV and V and ulnar nerve-innervated intrinsic muscles of the hand.
   c. Conservative treatment.
      (1) Elbow splint to prevent positions of extreme flexion (especially at night).
      (2) Elbow pad to decrease compression of nerve when leaning on elbows.
      (3) Activity/work modification.
   d. Surgical intervention: decompression or transposition.
   e. Post-operative treatment.
      (1) Edema control.
      (2) Scar management.
      (3) AROM and nerve gliding (2 weeks post-operative).
      (4) Strengthening (4 weeks post-operative).
      (5) MCP flexion splint if clawing noted.
7. Radial nerve palsy: a radial nerve compression.
   a. Etiology: Saturday night palsy, a term used to describe sleeping in a position that places stress on the radial nerve. Also, compression as a result of a humeral shaft fracture.
   b. Symptoms: weakness or paralysis of extensors to the wrist, MCPs, and thumb; wrist drop.
   c. Conservative treatment.
      (1) Dynamic extension splint.
      (2) Work/activity modification.
      (3) Strengthening wrist and finger extensors when motor function returns.
   d. Surgical intervention: decompression.
   e. Post-operative treatment.
      (1) ROM.
      (2) Nerve gliding.
      (3) Strengthening (6–8 weeks post-operative).
      (4) ADL and meaningful role activities.
8. Median nerve laceration.
   a. Sensory loss.
      (1) Central palm (thumb to radial ½ of ring finger).
      (2) Palmar surface of thumb, index, middle, and radial ½ of ring fingers.
      (3) Dorsal surface of index, middle, and radial ½ of ring fingers (middle and distal phalanges).
   b. Motor loss for a low lesion at the wrist.
      (1) Lumbricals I & II (MCP flexion of digits II & III).
      (2) Opponens pollicis (opposition).
      (3) Abductor pollicis brevis (abduction).
      (4) Flexor pollicis brevis (flexion of thumb MCP).
   c. Motor loss for a high lesion at or proximal to the elbow.
      (1) All of the above in b.
      (2) FDP to index and middle fingers, and FPL (flexion of tip of index, middle fingers, and thumb).
      (3) FCR (inability to flex to radial aspect of wrist).
   d. Deformity.
      (1) Flattening of thenar eminence, "ape hand" (Figure 6-11).
      (2) Clawing of index and middle fingers for a low lesion.
      (3) Benediction sign for a high-lesion (Figure 6-12).
   e. Functional loss.
      (1) Loss of thumb opposition.
      (2) Weakness of pinch.
   f. Occupational therapy intervention.
      (1) Dorsal protection splint with wrist positioned in 30° flexion if a low lesion. Include elbow (90° flexion) if a high lesion.
      (2) Begin A/PROM of digits with wrist in flexed position at two weeks post-operative.
      (3) Scar management.
      (4) AROM of wrist 4 weeks; include elbow if a high lesion.
      (5) Begin strengthening at nine weeks.
   g. Splinting considerations: C-bar to prevent thumb adduction contracture.
   h. Sensory reeducation: begin when individual demonstrates a level of diminished protective sensation (4.31) on Semmes-Weinstein.

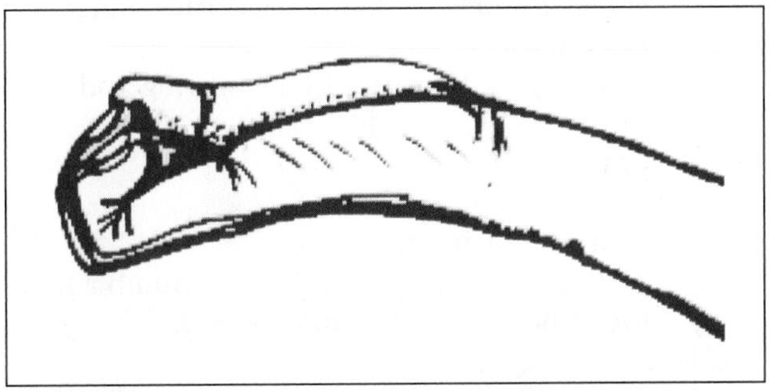

Figure 6-11 **Ape Hand: Due to injury of the distal median nerve**

Darlington, Vicki, OTR/L, CHT with permission.

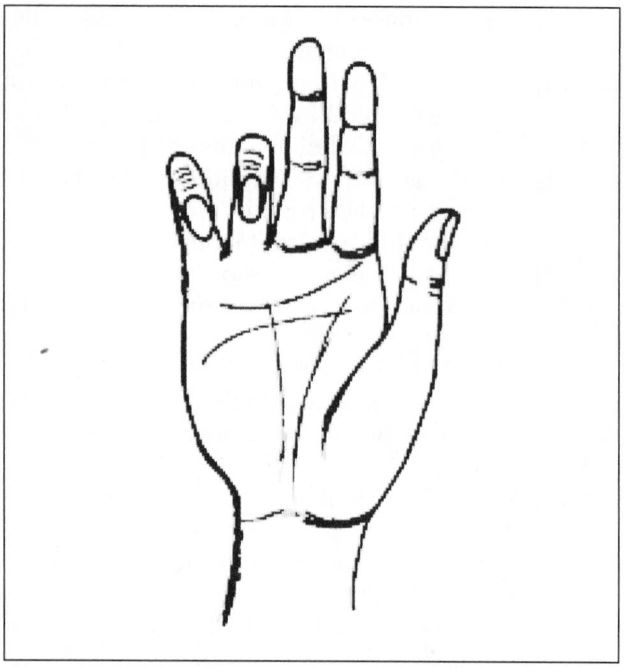

Figure 6-12 **Benediction Sign: Due to a high injury of the median nerve**

Darlington, Vicki, OTR/L, CHT with permission.

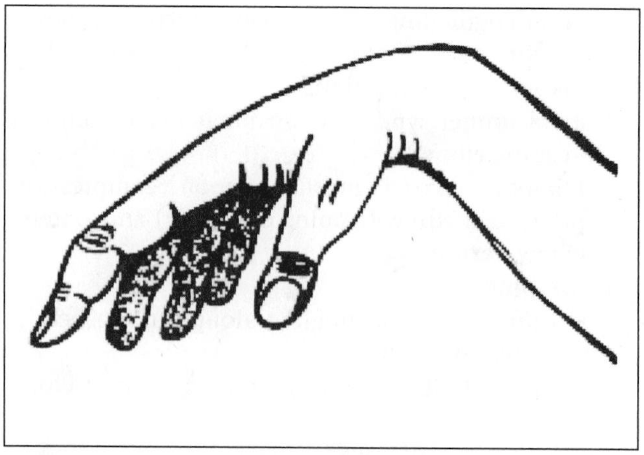

Figure 6-13 **Wrist Drop: Due to injury of the radial nerve**

Darlington, Vicki, OTR/L, CHT with permission.

9. Ulnar nerve laceration.
   a. Sensory loss.
      (1) Ulnar aspects of palmar and dorsal surfaces.
      (2) Ulnar ½ of ring and little fingers on palmar and dorsal surfaces.
   b. Motor loss: low lesion at the wrist.
      (1) Palmar and dorsal interossei (adduction and abduction of MCP joints).
      (2) Lumbricals III & IV (MCP flexion of digits 4 & 5).
      (3) FPB and adductor pollicis (flexion and adduction of thumb).
      (4) ADM, ODM, FDM (abduction, opposition, and flexion of 5th digit).
   c. Motor loss: high lesion wrist or above.
      (1) Same as above, including FCU (flexion toward ulnar wrist).
      (2) FDP IV & V (flexion of DIPs of ring and little fingers).
   d. Deformity.
      (1) Claw hand.
      (2) Flattened metacarpal arch.
      (3) + Froment's sign (assessment of thumb adductor while laterally pinching paper).
   e. Functional loss.
      (1) Loss of power grip.
      (2) Decreased pinch strength.
   f. Occupational therapy intervention.
      (1) See median nerve repair.
      (2) Splinting consideration: MCP flexion block splint.
      (3) Sensory reeducation: same as median nerve.
10. Radial nerve laceration.
   a. Sensory loss: high lesions at the level of the humerus.
      (1) Medial aspect of dorsal forearm. Radial aspect of dorsal palm, thumb, and index, middle and radial ½ of ring phalanges.
   b. Motor loss: low lesion at the level of the forearm.
      (1) Loss of wrist extension due to absent or impaired innervation to ECU.
      (2) EDC, EI, EDM (MCP extension).
      (3) EPB, EPL, APL (thumb extension).
   c. Motor loss: high lesion at the level of the humerus.
      (1) All of the above, including ECRB, ECRL, and brachioradialis.
      (2) If level of axilla, loss of triceps (elbow extension).
   d. Functional loss.
      (1) Inability to extend digits to release objects.
      (2) Difficulty manipulating objects.
   e. Deformity.
      (1) Wrist drop (Figure 6-13).
   f. Occupational therapy intervention.
      (1) Dynamic extension splint.
      (2) ROM.
      (3) Sensory reeducation if needed.
      (4) Instruct in home program.
      (5) Activity modification.

Rotator Cuff Tendonitis

1. Anatomy of rotator cuff.
   a. Supraspinatus.
      (1) Function: abduction and flexion.

b. Infraspinatus and teres minor.
   (1) Function: external rotation.
c. Subscapularis.
   (1) Function: internal rotation.
d. The rotator cuff functions together to control the head of the humerus in the glenoid fossa.
e. Site of impingement: coracoacromial arch (acromion, coracoacromial ligament, and coracoid process).

2. Etiology.
   a. Repetitive overuse.
   b. Curved or hook acromion.
   c. Weakness of rotator cuff.
   d. Weakness of scapula musculature.
   e. Ligament and capsule tightness.
   f. Trauma.
3. Occupational therapy conservative intervention.
   a. Activity modification: avoid above shoulder level activities until pain subsides.
   b. Educate in sleeping posture: avoid sleeping with arm overhead or combined adduction and internal rotation.
   c. Decrease pain: positioning, modalities, and rest.
   d. Restore pain free ROM.
   e. Strengthening: below shoulder level.
   f. Occupation and role specific training.
4. Surgical interventions.
   a. Arthroscopic surgery.
   b. Open repair: small, medium, large, and massive tears.
5. Occupational therapy post-operative intervention.
   a. PROM (0 to 6 weeks); progress to AA/AROM.
   b. Decrease pain: begin with ice, progress to heat.
   c. Strengthening (6 weeks post-operative): begin with isometrics, progress to isotonic (below shoulder level).
   d. Activity modification: light ADL and meaningful role activities; progress as tolerated.
   e. Leisure and work activities (8–12 weeks post-operative).

Adhesive Capsulitis

1. Also known as frozen shoulder.
2. Restricted passive shoulder range of motion.
   a. Greatest limitation is external rotation, then abduction, internal rotation, and flexion.
3. Anatomy: glenohumeral ligaments and joint capsule.
4. Etiology.
   a. Inflammation and immobility.
   b. Linked to diabetes mellitus and Parkinson's disease.
5. Occupational therapy conservative intervention.
   a. Encourage active use through ADL and role activities.
   b. PROM.
   c. Modalities.
6. Surgical interventions: manipulation and arthroscopic surgery.
7. Occupational therapy post-operative intervention.
   a. PROM immediately following surgery.
   b. Pain relief: modalities.
   c. Encourage use of extremity for all ADL and role activities.

Shoulder Dislocations

1. Anterior dislocation most common.
2. Etiology.
   a. Trauma.
   b. Repetitive overuse.
3. Occupational therapy intervention.
   a. Regain ROM: avoid combined abduction and external rotation with anterior dislocation.
   b. Pain free ADL and role activities.
   c. Strengthen rotator cuff.

Arthritis

Definition

1. An inflammation of a joint or joints.

Types

1. Rheumatoid arthritis.
   a. Systemic, symmetrical and affects many joints.
      (1) Most commonly attacks the small joints of the hands.
      (2) Characterized by remissions and exacerbations.
      (3) Begins in the acute phase as an inflammatory process of the synovial lining.
   b. Etiology is unknown but there are two main theories.
      (1) Infection theory.
      (2) Autoimmune theory.

c. Symptoms.
   (1) Pain.
   (2) Stiffness.
   (3) Limited range of motion.
   (4) Fatigue.
   (5) Weight loss.
   (6) Limited activities of daily living status, diminished ability to perform role activities.
   (7) Swelling.
   (8) Deformities.
d. Types of deformities common with rheumatoid arthritis.
   (1) Ulnar deviation and subluxation of the wrists and MCP joints.
   (2) Boutonniere deformity: flexion of PIP joint and hyperextension of DIP joint (Figure 6-14).
   (3) Swan neck deformity: hyperextension of PIP joint and flexion of DIP joint (Figure 6-15).

2. Osteoarthritis.
   a. Degenerative joint disease.
      (1) Not systemic but wear and tear.
      (2) Commonly affects large weight bearing joints.
      (3) Attacks hyaline cartilage.
   b. Etiology.
      (1) Genetic.
      (2) Trauma.
      (3) Inflammation.
      (4) Cumulative trauma.
      (5) Endocrine and metabolic diseases.

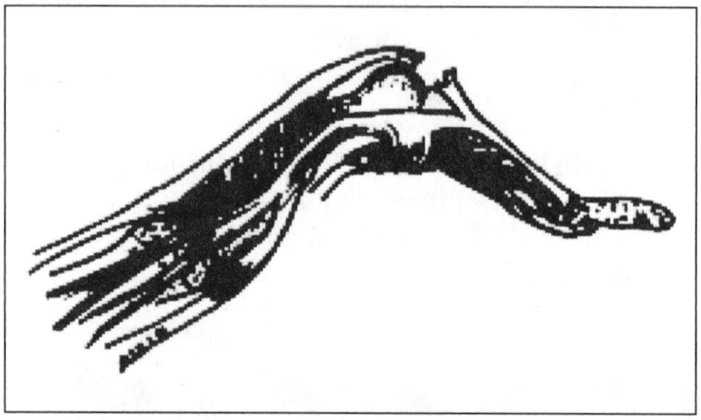

Figure 6-14 **Boutonniere Deformity**
Darlington, Vicki, OTR/L, CHT with permission.

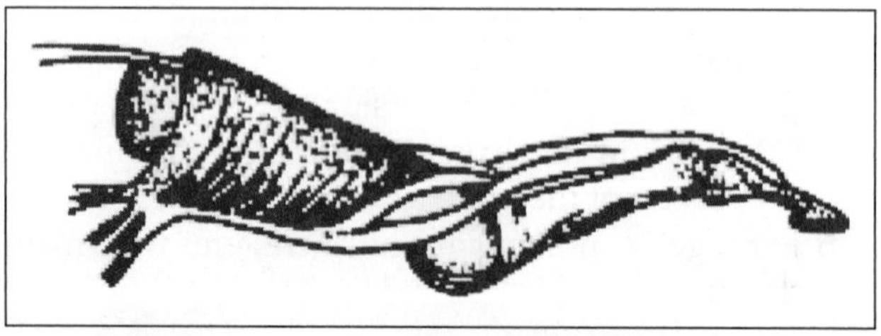

Figure 6-15 **Swan Neck Deformity**
Darlington, Vicki, OTR/L, CHT with permission.

   c. Symptoms.
      (1) Pain.
      (2) Stiffness.
      (3) Limited range of motion.
      (4) Bone spurs.
   d. Types of bone spurs.
      (1) Heberden's nodes at the DIP joints.
      (2) Bouchard's nodes at the PIP joints.

Occupational Therapy Evaluation

1. Occupational Profile.
2. ROM: focus on AROM.
   a. PROM should be avoided, especially in the inflammatory stage.
   b. Note deformities and nodules.
3. Muscle strength.
   a. Avoid muscle testing unless requested by physician.
   b. Document strength in relation to function.
4. Grip strength: use sphygmomanometer.
5. ADL and role activities: note if ADL and role activity deficits are related to pain, limitation in motion, deformity, weakness, or fatigue.
6. Pain: use pain scales.
7. Edema: volumeter or tape measure.

Occupational Therapy Intervention

1. Splinting.
   a. Resting hand splints in the acute stage.
   b. Wrist splint only if arthritis specific to wrist.
   c. Ulnar drift splint to prevent deformity.
   d. Silver ring splints to prevent boutonniere and swan neck deformities.
   e. Dynamic MCP extension splint with radial pull for post-operative MCP arthroplasties.
   f. Hand base thumb splint for CMC arthritis.
2. Joint protection techniques.
3. Energy conservation techniques.
4. ROM: focus on AROM.
   a. Gentle PROM if person unable to perform AROM.
   b. All exercises should be pain free.
5. Heat modalities.
   a. Hot packs can be used before exercise but avoid during the inflammatory stage.
   b. Paraffin is recommended for the hands.
6. Strengthening.
   a. Avoid during inflammatory stage.
   b. Gentle strengthening while avoiding positions of deformity.

7. Purposeful and occupation-based activities.
   a. Joint protection and energy conservation techniques should be incorporated.
   b. Adaptive equipment should be provided to prevent deformity, decrease stress on small joints, and extend reach.
   c. Refer to Chapter 16.

Osteogenesis Imperfecta[1]

Etiology

1. Disorder caused by the dysfunction of one of several genes responsible for producing collagen to strengthen bones.
2. The genes responsible for OI can be inherited from one or both parents.
3. In some cases, the OI genes responsible for collagen begin to malfunction after the child is conceived.

Signs and Symptoms

1. Malformed bones.
   a. Short, small body.
   b. Triangular face.
   c. Barrel-shaped rib cage.
   d. Brittle bones that fracture easily.
   e. Multiple fractures as the child grows.
   f. Developmental growth problems.
2. Loose joints.
3. Sclera of the whites of the eyes look blue or purple.
4. Brittle teeth.
5. Hearing loss (often starting in the 20s or 30s).
6. Respiratory problems.
7. Insufficient collagen.

Classification

1. Eight main types of osteogenesis imperfecta: classified by the genes that are involved.
   a. Types 2, 3, 7, and 8: severe symptoms.
   b. Types 4, 5, and 6: moderate symptoms.
   c. Type 1: mild symptoms.

Diagnosis

1. Family and medical history.
2. Results from a physical examination and medical including x-rays, collagen and blood test.

[1]Marge E. Moffett Boyd contributed this section on osteogenesis imperfecta.

Medical Management

1. Care for broken bones.
   a. See this chapter's section on the medical treatment of fractures.
2. Dental care for brittle teeth.
3. Medication for pain.
4. Surgery.
   a. Fix bone malformations.
   b. Prevent bone malformations.
   c. "Rodding" in which metal rods are put inside the long bones.

Occupational Therapy Evaluation

1. Activity interests that can be safely pursued.
2. Environmental risk factors.
3. See this chapter's sections on occupational therapy evaluation for fractures and the assessment of pain.

Occupational Therapy Intervention

1. Activity adaptation and assistive device prescription and fabrication to facilitate safe participation in daily occupations.
2. Environmental modifications to maintain safety.
3. Preventive positioning and protective splinting/padding.
4. Activities to increase muscle strength.
5. Weightbearing activities to facilitate bone growth.
6. Health education to promote a healthy lifestyle.
   a. Healthy diet and weight control.
   b. Avoid smoking, caffeine, alcohol, steroids.
   c. Exercise: swimming, water therapy, walking.
7. Family, caregiver and teacher education about proper handling, positioning, activity adaptations, environmental modifications, and the need to observe all safety precautions.
8. See this chapter's section on occupational therapy intervention for fractures and musculoskeletal pain.

Hip Fractures

Etiology

1. Trauma.
2. Osteoporosis.
3. Pathological fractures (i.e., cancer).

Types

1. Femoral neck fracture.
2. Intertrochanteric fracture.
3. Subtrochanteric fracture.

Medical Management

1. Closed reduction for minimally displaced fractures.
2. Open reduction internal fixation (ORIF).
3. Joint replacement.

Occupational Therapy Evaluation

1. Review precautions and weight bearing status before initiating evaluation.
2. Occupational role requirements and expectations.
3. ADL: focus on dressing, bathing, and transfers.
4. ROM and strength of upper extremities.
5. Conduct other assessments as needed (e.g., cognitive).

Occupational Therapy Intervention

1. Bed mobility and bedside ADL.
2. Upper extremity strengthening.
3. Functional ambulation and transfers with appropriate weight bearing status and appropriate ambulation device (i.e., walker, crutches).
   a. The type of ambulation device is determined by the person's weight bearing status.
4. Instruct in and practice use of assistive devices for use in the home (e.g., shower chair, elevated commode seat).
5. Practice occupation-based activities (e.g., small meal preparation) using proper weight bearing status and ambulatory device.

Precautions

1. Weight-bearing status and the amount of ROM allowed at the hip will be determined by the surgeon.
2. Time frames for beginning OT intervention are also determined by the surgeon.

Complications

1. Avascular necrosis.
2. Non-union.
3. Degenerative joint disease.

Total Hip Replacement/Total Hip Arthroplasty

Etiology

1. Trauma, from hip fracture.
2. Disease, most often arthritis; surgery is then elective.

Types

1. Total hip joint implant: replaces acetabulum and femoral head.
2. Austin Moore: partial hip replacement. Replaces femoral head.
3. See Figure 6-16.

Surgical Procedures

1. Cemented or uncemented.
2. Anterolateral or posterolateral (more common).

Occupational Therapy Evaluation

1. Review precautions and weight bearing status before initiating evaluation.
2. Complete an Occupational Profile.

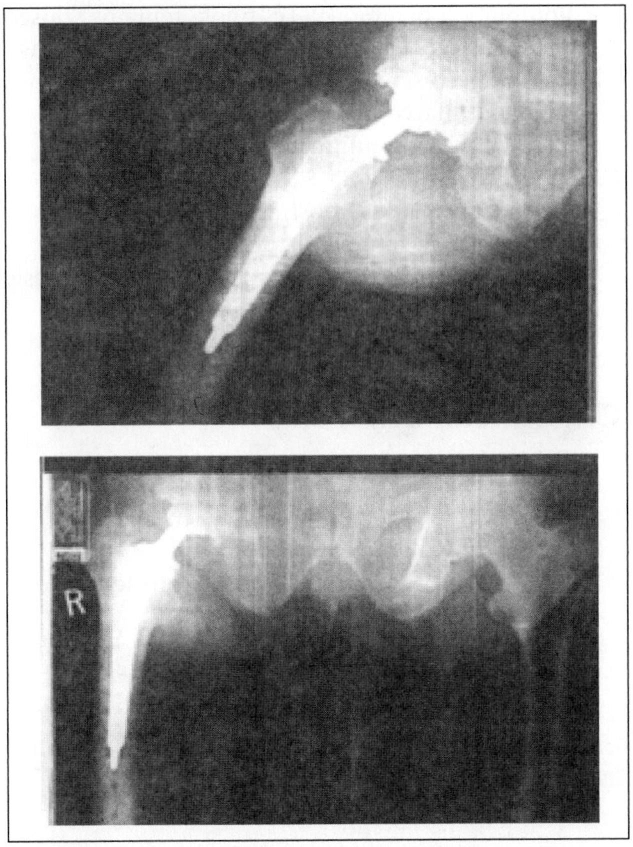

Figure 6-16 Hybrid cemented total hip arthroplasty (Biomet Integral Design, Warsaw, IN)

From Maxey, L., & Magnusson, J. (2006). *Rehabilitation for the postsurgical orthopedic patient* (p. 173). Mosby Publications. Reprinted with permission.

3. Assess ADL; focus on dressing, bathing, and transfers.
4. Assess ROM and strength of upper extremities.
5. Conduct other assessments as needed (e.g., cognitive).

Occupational Therapy Intervention

1. Educate the individual in hip precautions.
   a. Posterolateral.
      (1) Do not flex beyond 90°.
      (2) Do not adduct or cross legs.
         (a) Do not internally rotate.
      (3) Do not pivot at hip.
      (4) Sit only on raised chair and raised toilet seat.
      (5) Transfer sit to stand by keeping operated hip in slight abduction and extended out in front.
   b. Antereolateral.
      (1) Do not externally rotate.
      (2) Do not extend hip.
      (3) Precautions vary for anterior THR. Some surgeons follow a no restriction protocol.
2. Instruct in and practice use of long handled equipment.
3. Provide transfer training.
   a. Practice with tub bench, raised toilet seat.
   b. Practice car transfers.
   c. Practice bed to chair transfers.
4. Practice occupation-based activities (e.g., small meal preparation) using proper weight bearing status and ambulatory device.

Amputations

Etiology

1. Congenital, peripheral vascular disease, trauma, cancer, and infection.

Classification of Amputations

1. Upper extremity level of amputation.
   a. Forequarter: loss of clavicle, scapula and entire upper extremity.
   b. Shoulder disarticulation: loss of entire upper extremity.
   c. Above-elbow (AE) (long or short): amputation above the elbow at any level on the upper arm.
   d. Elbow disarticulation: amputation of the upper extremity distal to the elbow joint.
   e. Below-elbow (BE) (long or short): amputation below the elbow at any level of the forearm.
   f. Wrist disarticulation: amputation distal to the wrist joint. Loss of entire hand.
   g. Finger amputation: amputation of digit(s) at any level.
   h. See Figure 6-17.
2. Lower extremity level of amputation.
   a. Hemipelvectomy: amputation of half of pelvis and entire lower extremity.
   b. Hip disarticulation: amputation at the hip joint. Loss of the entire lower extremity.
   c. Above-knee amputation (transfemoral): amputation above knee at any level on the thigh.

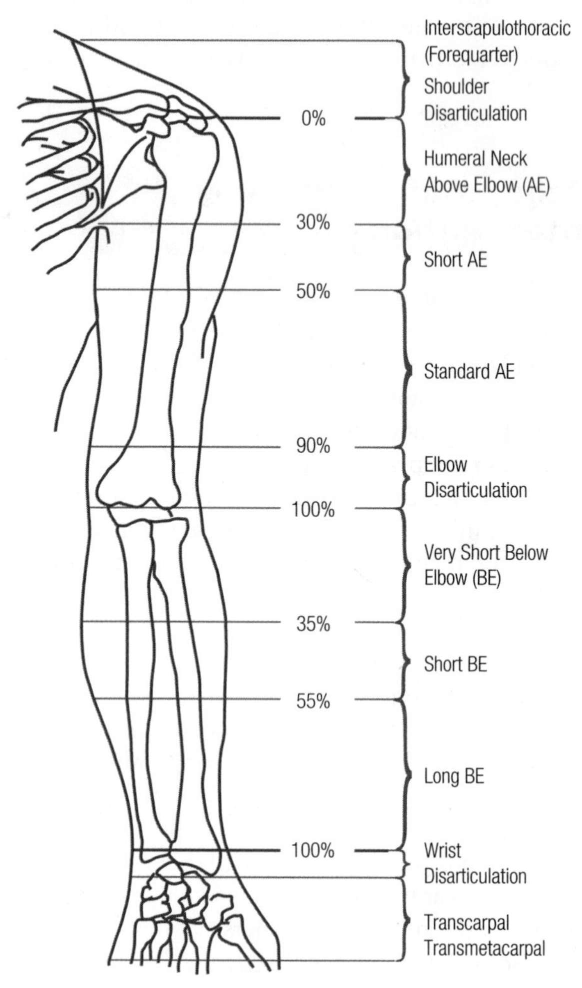

Figure 6-17 **Levels of Amputation**

Celikyol, F. (1995). Amputation and prosthetics. In C. A. Trombly (Ed.). *Occupational therapy for physical dysfunction* (p. 850). Baltimore, MD: Williams and Wilkins. Reprinted with permission.

d. Knee disarticulation: amputation at the knee joint.
e. Below-knee amputation (transtibial): amputation below knee at any level on the calf. This is the most common.
f. Complete tarsal: amputation at the ankle.
g. Partial tarsal: amputation of metatarsals and phalanges.
h. Complete phalanges: amputation of toe(s).

Terminal Devices (TDs)

1. Function to grasp and maintain hold on an object.
2. The two main types of TDs are the hook and the hand.
   a. Voluntary opening (VO): hook remains closed until tension is placed on cable and then it opens.
   b. Voluntary closing (VC): hook remains opened until tension is placed on cable and then it closes.
   c. Cosmetic device: minimal function.
3. Refer to Table 6-1.
4. Determination of the most appropriate TD is based upon the person's interests, roles, and preferences.
   a. TDs can be interchangeably used with a prosthesis if the shaft size is the same.

Complications

1. Neuromas: nerve endings adhered to scar tissue.
   a. These can be very painful and hypersensitive.
2. Skin breakdown.
3. Phantom limb syndrome: sensation of the presence of the amputated limb.
4. Phantom limb pain: sensation of the presence of the amputated limb but is also painful.
5. Infection.
6. Knee flexion contractures in transtibial amputation.
7. Psychological impairments due to shock/grief.

Preprosthetic Treatment

1. Change of dominance activities, if needed.
2. ROM of uninvolved joints.
3. Prepare limb for a prosthesis.
4. Desensitization.
5. Wrapping to shape and shrink the residual limb.
   a. Wrap distal to proximal.
   b. Tension should decrease with proximal wrapping.
6. ADL training, including education in skin care.
7. Supportive counseling to facilitate adjustment.
8. Individualize treatment to enhance physical and psychological adjustment.

Prosthetic Treatment

1. Functional training with prosthesis.
   a. Practice engagement in activities of interest and occupational role activities.
   b. Refer to Table 6-2.
2. Donning and doffing the prosthesis.
3. Increase prosthetic wearing tolerance.
4. Individualize treatment to enhance physical and psychological adjustment.

Chapter 6

Table 6-1

Hooks and Hands Compared

FEATURES	HOOKS VO (BODY POWER)	VC TRS GRIP (BODY POWER)	HANDS (EXTERNAL POWER)	HANDS VO (BODY POWER)	GREIFER (EXTERNAL POWER)
Cosmesis	**Unfavorable**	**Unfavorable**	**Favorable**	**Favorable**	**Unfavorable**
Pinch Force	1 lb/rubber band; more rubber bands yield stronger grip but require more effort to open	Controlled strong grip >40 lb dependent on force exerted on cable	Strong grip, 22 lb; may have proportional control	Pinch stronger than VO hook but weaker than externally powered TD; relies on internal springs, adjustable	Strong pinch, 32 lb
Prehension pattern	Precise, exact pinch	Pinch more precise than hand, less than hook	Cylindrical grasp 3-point pinch; configuration same as BP hand	Cylindrical grasp, 3-point pinch; configuration same as external powered hand	Precise pinch and cylindrical grasp
Weight	Lighter than hands; aluminum to stainless steel; 3–8.7 oz	Aluminum, polymer, stainless steel; 4–16 oz	Heavy; 16.2 oz	Heavy; 10.5–14 oz	Heavy; 19oz
Durability	Durable; stainless steel is strongest	Durable and rugged; especially stainless	Not durable; delicate inner electronics and glove	Not durable; delicate inner spring mechanism and glove	Durable and rugged
Reliability	Very good; requires minimal service	Very good; requires minimal service	Good if not used for rugged activities	Good if not used for rugged activities	Very good
Feedback	Some proprioceptive feedback from tension on harness and limb in socket when operating TD/elbow	Better proprioceptive feedback, as tension on cable must be maintained for sustained grasp	Some feedback through intensity of muscle contraction, particularly for proportional control	Feedback similar to VO hook	Same as externally powered hand
Ease of use	Effort increases with more rubber bands	More effort to sustain grasp; lock available	Low effort to activate	More effort to open; can relax for grasp	Same as externally powered hand
Use in various planes	Difficult for high planes	Similar to VO hook	Very good for transradial amputation	Similar to VO hook/ hand because of harness	Same as externally powered hand
Visibility of items grasped	Very good	Good; less than VO	Poor for small items	Poor for small items	Poor for small items
Cost	Lowest	Higher than hook, less than hand	Highest cost	Higher than hooks; lower than externally powered hand	About the same as externally powered hand

Radomski, M. V., & Trombly-Latham, C. A. (2008). *Occupational therapy for physical dysfunction,* 6th ed. (Chapter 46, p. 1272, Amputations and Prosthetics by Kathy Stubblefield and Anne Armstrong). Baltimore, MD: Lippincott Williams and Wilkins. Reprinted with permission.

Treatment for LE Amputations

1. Wrapping to shape residual limb and decrease swelling.
2. Desensitization.
3. Strengthening (UE) with the focus on triceps.
4. Transfer training, stand pivot.
5. ADL training; LE dressing is the most difficult.
6. Standing tolerance.
7. Wheelchair mobility.

Table 6-2

Procedures for Practice Controls Training for Body Powered Prostheses

COMPONENT	MOVEMENT	INTERVENTION
Terminal device	Humeral flexion with scapular abduction (protraction) on side of amputation; bilateral scapular abduction for midline use of TD or when strength is limited.	Manually guide patient through motions. For transhumeral prostheses, keep elbow unit locked in 90 degree flexion; teach TD control first.
Wrist unit	Rotate TD to supination (fingers of hook up), midposition (fingers toward midline), or pronation (fingers down). For unilateral amputation, patient uses sound hand to rotate TD. For bilateral amputation, rotate TD against stationary object, between knees, or with contralateral TD.	Have patient analyze the task and determine the most efficient approach for grasp, avoiding excessive or awkward movements. Examples: TD in midposition for carrying a tray, in pronation for grasping small box from table.
Elbow unit	Depress arm while extending and abducting humerus to lock or unlock elbow mechanism. Practice flexing and locking elbow in several planes.	Manually guide patient through motions. Begin with elbow unlocked. Patient listens for click as lock activates. Have patient exaggerate movements initially. Use a mirror. Use humeral flexion to flex the elbow; go beyond desired height, since the arm will drop with gravity pull as patient is in process of locking the elbow unit.
Turntable	Rotate elbow turntable toward or away from body using sound hand. With bilateral amputations, push or pull against stationary object to rotate.	Teach patient to analyze task to determine need to use this component for more efficiency.

Radomski, M. V., & Trombly-Latham, C. A. (2008). *Occupational therapy for physical dysfunction*, 6th ed. (Chapter 46, p. 1280, Amputations and Prosthetics by Kathy Stubblefield and Anne Armstrong). Baltimore, MD: Lippincott Williams and Wilkins. Reprinted with permission.

Burns

Classification

1. Superficial (first degree burn) involves the epidermis only.
   a. Minimal pain and edema, but no blisters.
   b. Healing time is 3 to 7 days.
2. Superficial partial thickness burn.
   a. Second degree burns involve the epidermis and upper portion of dermis (e.g., sunburn).
   b. Appearance: red, blistering, and wet.
   c. Painful, no grafting necessary, heals on its own.
   d. Healing time is 7–21 days.
3. Deep partial thickness burn.
   a. Deep second degree burn involving the epidermis and deep portion of dermis; hair follicles and sweat glands.
   b. Appearance: red, white, and elastic.
   c. Sensation may be impaired.
   d. Potential to convert to full thickness burn due to infection.
   e. Healing time is 21–35 days.
4. Full thickness burn.
   a. Third degree burn involving the epidermis and dermis; hair follicles, sweat glands, and nerve endings.
   b. Appearance: white, waxy, leathery, and non-elastic.
   c. Sensation is absent, requires skin graft.
   d. Hypertrophic scar.
   e. Healing time can take months.
5. Fourth degree burn.
   a. Involves fat, muscle, and bone.
   b. Electrical burn: destruction of nerve along pathway.
6. Rule of nines is a method of assessing burn wound size.
   a. Refer to Figure 6-18.

Occupational Therapy Evaluation and Intervention

1. Superficial partial-thickness burns.
   a. Evaluation.
      (1) Occupational Profile.
      (2) ROM, 72 hours post-operative.
      (3) Sensation, when wounds are healed.
      (4) Strength, when wounds are healed.
      (5) ADL and meaningful role activities, as soon as possible.
   b. Intervention.
      (1) Wound care and debridement, sterile whirlpool, and dressing changes.
      (2) Gentle AROM and PROM to individual's tolerance.
      (3) Edema control.
      (4) Splinting, if necessary.
      (5) ADL and role activities.

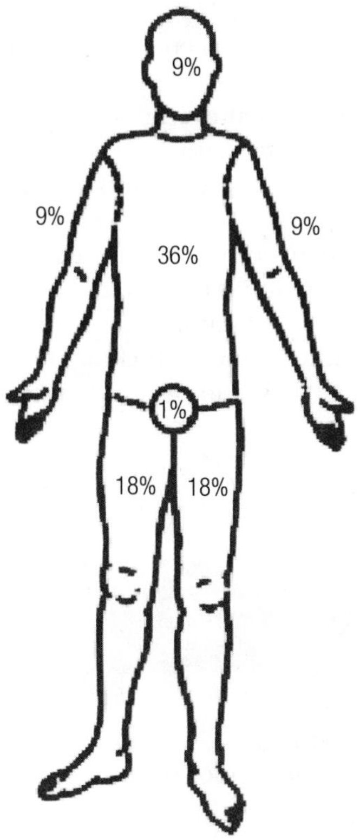

Figure 6-18 Rule of Nines

Adult Pedretti, L.W. (1996). *Occupational therapy: Practice skills for physical dyscunction*, 4th ed. (p. 615). St. Louis, MO: Mosby. Reprinted with permission.

2. Deep partial-thickness burns.
   a. Evaluation.
      (1) Same as superficial partial-thickness burns.
   b. Intervention.
      (1) Wound care and debridement, sterile whirlpool, and dressing changes.
      (2) Gentle AROM and PROM to individual's tolerance.
      (3) Edema control.
      (4) Splinting.
      (5) Occupational role activities and ADL.
      (6) Strengthening (when wounds are healed).
3. Full thickness burn—requires grafting.
   a. Evaluation.
      (1) ROM (5–7 days post-operative).
      (2) All other evaluations same as above.
   b. Post-operative intervention.
      (1) 72 hours: dressing changes, splint at all times.
      (2) Five to seven days: begin AROM, light ADL and meaningful activities, sterile whirlpool.
      (3) Over seven days: PROM as tolerated, ADL and meaningful activities.
      (4) When wounds are healed, use massage.
      (5) Order compression garments.
      (6) Provide otoform/elastomer inserts.
      (7) Strengthening.

Antideformity Positions Following Burn Injury

1. See Table 6-3.

Table 6-3

Anti-Contracture Positioning by Location of Burn

LOCATION OF BURN	CONTRACTURE TENDENCY	ANTI-CONTRACTURE POSITIONING AND/OR TYPICAL SPLINT
Anterior neck	Neck flexion	Remove pillows; use half-mattress to extend the neck; neck extension splint or collar
Axilla	Adduction	120-degree abduction with slight external rotation; axilla splint or positioning wedges; watch for signs of brachial plexus strain
Anterior elbow	Flexion	Elbow extension splint in 5–10 degrees flexion
Dorsal wrist	Wrist extension	Wrist support in neutral
Volar wrist	Wrist flexion	Wrist cockup splint in 5–10 degrees flexion
Hand dorsal	Claw hand deformity	Functional hand splint with MP joints 70–90 degrees, IP joints fully extended, first web open, thumb in opposition
Hand volar	Palmar contracture	Palm extension splint
	Cupping of hand	Myofascial pain syndrome (MPS) in slight hyperextension
Hip-anterior	Hip flexion	Prone positioning; weights on thigh in supine; knee immobilizers
Knee	Knee flexion	Knee extension positioning and/or splints; prevent external rotation, which may cause peroneal nerve compression
Foot	Foot drop	Ankle at 90 degrees with foot board or splint; watch for signs of heel ulcer

Radomski, M. V., & Trombly-Latham, C. A. (2008). *Occupational therapy for physical dysfunction*, 6th ed. (Chapter 45, p. 1249, Burn Injuries by Monica Pessina & Amy Orroth). Baltimore, MD: Lippincott Williams and Wilkins. Reprinted with permission.

Hand Splints

1. Burns to the hand.
   a. Wrist in 20°–30° extension.
   b. MCP joints in 70° flexion.
   c. IP joints in full extension.
   d. Thumb abducted and extended.
2. If burns to volar surface of hand develop flexion contractures. Palmar extension splint:
   a. Wrist in 0°–30° extension.
   b. MCP joints in neutral to slight extension and abducted (monitor collateral ligaments).
   c. IP joints in full extension.
   d. Thumb abducted and extended.
3. Web space burn.
   a. C-splint.

Hypertrophic Scar

1. Most common with deep second and third degree burns.
2. Appears 6–8 weeks after wound closure.
3. One to two years to mature.
4. Compression garments should be worn 24 hours daily.
   a. Applied when wounds are healed.
   b. Recommendation is to wear 24 hours a day for 1–2 years until scar is matured.
5. Additional interventions include ROM, skin care, ADL, role activities, and patient/family education.

Pain

Definition

1. Personal sensation of hurt that can significantly affect an individual's quality of life.

Types of Pain

1. Acute pain has a recent onset and usually lasts for a short duration.
2. Chronic pain is of a long duration and can lead to depression.
3. Myofascial pain is specific to muscles, tendons, or fascia.
   a. Myofascial pain syndrome (MPS).
      (1) Persistent, deep aching pains in muscle, nonarticular in origin.
      (2) Characterized by well-defined, highly sensitive tender spots (trigger points).
4. Fibromyalgia syndrome (FMS) is a musculoskeletal pain and fatigue disorder that can vary in intensity.
   a. Widespread pain accompanied by tenderness of muscles and adjacent soft tissues.
   b. A nonarticular rheumatic disease of unknown origin.
5. Low back pain.
   a. Most common work-related injury.
   b. Location: lumbar lordosis.
   c. Etiology.
      (1) Poor posture: seated and standing.
      (2) Repetitive bending using poor body mechanics.
      (3) Heavy lifting.
      (4) Sleeping with poor posture.
   d. Symptoms.
      (1) Pain.
      (2) Difficulty with self-care activities and other role activities (especially lower extremity activities).
      (3) Difficulty sleeping.

Assessment of Pain

1. Determine location of pain.
   a. Localized or diffuse.
2. Evaluate intensity of pain.
   a. Pain intensity scale of 0–10 is most commonly used.
   b. Identify the time of day the pain is most intense.
3. Determine the onset and duration of pain.
   a. Gradual or sudden onset.
   b. The length of time pain has been experienced.
4. Description of pain.
   a. Common descriptors include sharp, throbbing, tender, burning, and shooting.
5. Functional assessment of pain.
   a. Pain scales that commonly address function.
      (1) McGill Pain Questionnaire.
      (2) Pain Disability Index.
      (3) Functional Interference Estimate.
   b. Refer to pain management section in Chapter 7.

Occupational Therapy Intervention

1. Utilize physical agent modalities and massage in preparation for functional activities.
2. Teach proper positioning techniques.
3. Splint in the resting position.
4. Gentle ROM.
5. Teach relaxation exercises.
6. Utilize proper body mechanics during self-care, leisure, and work activities.
7. Correct environmental factors.
8. Correct standing and seated posture.
9. Modify activities and provide ADL training and adaptive equipment, as needed.
10. Provide alternative exercise programs (e.g., aquatic therapy, ai chi, tai chi).
11. Refer to pain management section in Chapter 7.

References

American Occupational Therapy Association. (2005). Standards of practice for occupational therapy. *American Journal of Occupational Therapy, 59*, 663–665.

American Society of Hand Therapists. (1992). *Clinical assessment recommendations* (2nd ed.). Chicago, IL: Author.

Batshaw, M. L., & Perret, Y. M. (1995). *Children with disabilities: A medical primer.* (4th ed.). Baltimore, MD: Paul Brooke.

Clark, G., Wilgis, E. F., Aiello, B., Eckhaux, D., & Eddington, L. (1993). *Hand rehabilitation: A practical guide,* Orlando, FL: Churchill Livingstone.

Cooper, C. (2007). *Fundamentals of hand therapy.* St. Louis: Mosby.

Falkenstein, N., & Weiss-Lessard, S. (1999). *Hand rehabilitation: A quick reference guide and review.* St. Louis, MO: Mosby.

Greene, D. P., & Roberts, S. L. (2005). *Kinesiology: Movement in the context of activity.* St. Louis, MO: Elsevier Mosby.

Gulick, D. (2005). *Ortho notes: Clinical examination pocket guide.* Philadelphia: F.A. Davis.

Hopkins, H., & Smith, H. (Eds.). (2003). *Willard and Spackman's occupational therapy* (10th ed.). Philadelphia: J.B. Lippincott.

Hunter, J., Mackin, E., & Callahan, A. (1995). *Rehabilitation of the hand: Surgery and therapy* (4th ed.). St. Louis, MO: Mosby.

Jacobs, K. (1997). *Quick reference dictionary for occupational therapy.* Thorofare, NJ: Slack.

Kendall, F. P., McCreary, E. K., & Provance P. G. (2005). *Muscles: Testing and function* (5th ed.). Baltimore: Lippincott Williams & Wilkins.

Malick, M., & Kasch, M. (1984). *Manual on management of specific hand problems.* Pittsburgh, PA: AREN.

Manning, D. C. (2000). Reflex sympathetic dystrophy, sympathetically maintained pain and complex regional pain syndrome: Diagnosis of inclusion, exclusion, or confusion? *Journal of Hand Therapy, 13*(4), 260–268.

Neer, C. (1990). *Shoulder reconstruction.* Orlando, FL: W.B. Saunders.

Pendeleton, H. M., & Schultz-Krohn, W. (2013). *Pedretti's occupational therapy: Practice skills for physical dysfunction* (6th ed.). St. Louis: Mosby

Radomski, M. V., & Trombly-Latham, C. A. (2008). *Occupational therapy for physical dysfunction* (6th ed.). Baltimore, MD: Lippincott Williams and Wilkins.

Restrepo, C., Javad Mortazavi, S. M., Brothers, J., Parvizi, J., & Rothman, R. H. (2011). Hip dislocations: Are hip precautions necessary in anterior approaches. *Clinical Orthopedics Related Research, 469*(2), 417–422.

Semmler, C. J., & Hunter, J. G. (1990). *Early occupational therapy intervention, neonates to three years.* Gaithersberg, MD: Aspen.

Stoykov, M. E. (2001, August 20). OT treatment for complex regional pain syndrome. *OT Practice*, 10–14.

Weiss, S., & Falkenstein, N. (2005) *Hand rehabilitation: A quick reference guide and review.* St. Louis, MO: Elsevier Mosby.

Review Questions

Musculoskeletal System Disorders

Below are six questions about key content covered in this chapter. These questions are not inclusive of the entirety of content related to musculoskeletal system disorders that you must know for success on the NBCOT exam. These questions are provided to help you "jump start" the thought processes you will need to apply your studying of content to the answering of exam questions; hence they are not in the NBCOT exam format. Exam items in the NBCOT format which cover the depth and breadth of content you will need to know to pass the NBCOT exam are provided on this text's disc. The answers to the below questions are provided in Appendix 4.

1. You provide post-operative occupational therapy for clients who have undergone tendon repair surgery. You receive a referral for a client diagnosed with a Zone 1 extensor tendon repair. What is this diagnosis typically termed? According to established protocol, what is your diagnostic-specific intervention for the first six weeks? What are the overall goals for tendon repair surgeries that you will use to guide your intervention?

2. A client incurred a right Colles' fracture. One week ago, the client's cast was removed. You have worked with this client since the initial evaluation and during several intervention sessions. When arriving for the current therapy session, the client is tearful and holding the right arm in a protected position. The client reports that severe pain developed over the weekend in the wrist, hand and shoulder and that it has not gone away. The right hand is swollen and skin is shiny. On a pain scale of 0–10, the client reports a 10+. The client describes an inability (over the past two days) to complete exercises and basic self-care activities due to the pain. What do you suspect is causing the client's increase in symptoms? How would you address the client's new presenting symptoms?

3. A client is referred to you with a diagnosis of (R) de Quervain's. The client's major complaint is pain when lifting (e.g., the client's newborn child, grocery bags). Pain is reported as 8/10. What findings will you expect upon formal evaluation? What interventions should you implement?

4. You receive a referral for a client with a third-degree burn to the hand which includes a prescription for a splint. What is the optimal anti-deformity position you should use to guide your splint construction? Explain your reasoning.

(*Continued*)

Review Questions

Musculoskeletal System Disorders (*Continued*)

5. You receive a referral for a person with a diagnosis of carpal tunnel syndrome (CTS). What conservative treatment methods are indicated for this diagnosis?

6. A child with a diagnosis of osteogenesis imperfecta receives occupational therapy services. What should be the primary foci of occupational therapy intervention? Describe how safety precautions should be integrated into the treatment of a child with osteogenesis imperfecta.

7

Neurological System Disorders

GLEN GILLEN, SUSAN B. O'SULLIVAN, JAN G. GARBARINI, AND MARGE E. MOFFETT BOYD

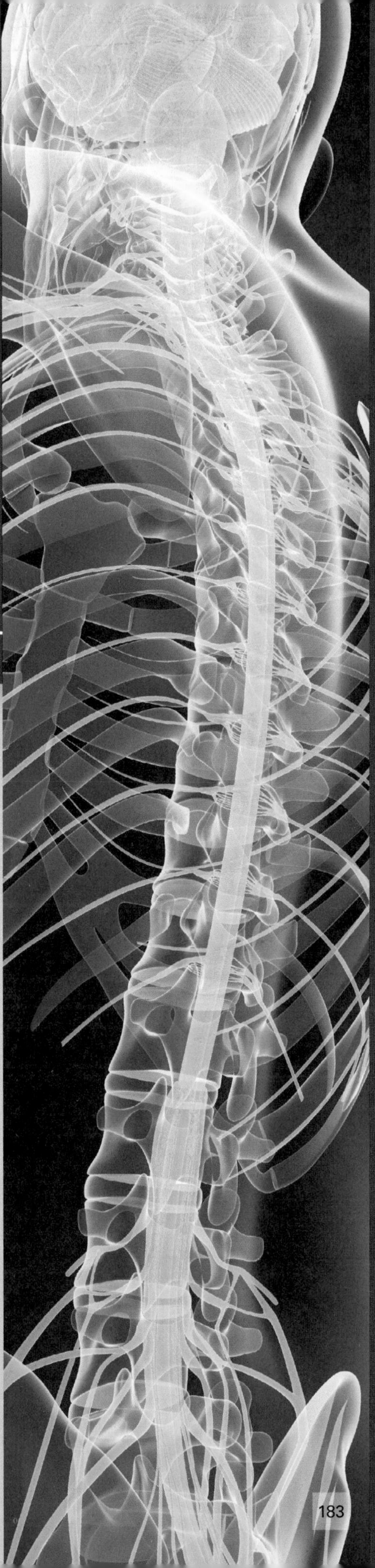

Chapter Outline

Anatomy and Physiology of the Nervous System

Relationship to the Examination

1. It is not likely that the NBCOT exam will ask direct questions about anatomy or physiology.
   a. As a result, this chapter does not provide a complete anatomy and physiology review.
2. Major structures and functions of the nervous system are outlined because knowledge of these can help determine the best answer. For example, damage to the left temporal lobe would result in the need to communicate nonverbally.
3. See Figure 7-1.

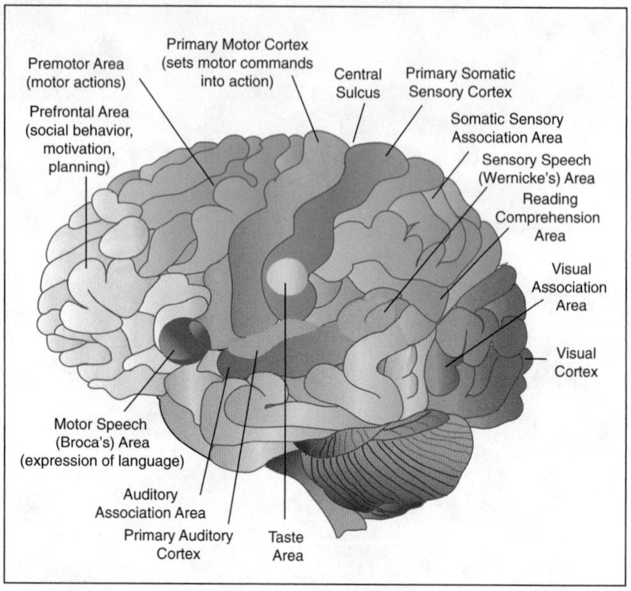

Figure 7-1 **Functional areas of the brain.**

Brain

1. Cerebral hemispheres (telencephalon).
   a. Convolutions of gray matter composed of gyri (crests) and sulci (fissures).
      (1) Lateral central fissure (Sylvian fissure) separates temporal lobe from frontal and parietal lobes.
      (2) Longitudinal cerebral fissure separates the two hemispheres.
      (3) Central sulcus separates frontal lobe from the parietal lobe.
   b. Paired hemispheres, consisting of 6 lobes on each side: frontal, parietal, temporal, occipital, insular, and limbic.
      (1) Frontal lobe.
         (a) Precentral gyrus: primary motor cortex for voluntary muscle activation.
         (b) Prefrontal cortex: controls emotions, judgments, higher order cognitive functions such as ideation and abstraction.
         (c) Premotor cortex related to planning of movements including Broca's area: controls motor aspects of speech.
      (2) Parietal lobe.
         (a) Postcentral gyrus: primary sensory cortex for integration of sensation.
         (b) Receives fibers conveying touch, proprioceptive, pain and temperature sensations from opposite side of body.
      (3) Temporal lobe.
         (a) Primary auditory cortex: receives/processes auditory stimuli.
         (b) Associative auditory cortex: processes auditory stimuli.
         (c) Wernicke's area: language comprehension.
      (4) Occipital lobe.
         (a) Primary visual cortex: receives/processes visual stimuli.
         (b) Visual association cortex: processes visual stimuli.
      (5) Insula: deep within lateral sulcus, associated with visceral functions.
      (6) Limbic system.
         (a) Consists of the limbic lobe (cingulate, parahippocampal, and subcallosal gyri), hippocampal formation, amygdaloid nucleus, hypothalamus, anterior nucleus of thalamus.
         (b) Phylogenetically oldest part of the brain, concerned with instincts and emotions contributing to preservation of the individual.
         (c) Basic functions include feeding, aggression, emotions, endocrine aspects of sexual response, and long-term memory formation.
   c. White matter: myelinated nerve fibers located centrally.
      (1) Transverse (commissural) fibers: interconnect the two hemispheres, including the corpus callosum (the largest), anterior commissure, and hippocampal commissure.
      (2) Projection fibers: connect cerebral hemispheres with other portions of the brain and spinal cord.
      (3) Association fibers: connect different portions of the cerebral hemispheres (within the same hemisphere), allowing cortex to function as an integrated whole.

d. Basal ganglia.
   (1) Masses of gray matter deep within the cerebral hemispheres, including the corpus striatum (caudate nucleus and lenticular nuclei), amygdaloid nucleus, and claustrum. The lenticular nuclei are further subdivided into the putamen and globus pallidus.
   (2) Forms an associated motor system (extrapyramidal system) with other nuclei in the subthalamus and midbrain.
   (3) Has numerous fiber interconnections.
      (a) Caudate loop (complex loop) functions in association with association cortex in the formation of motor plans.
      (b) Putamen loop (motor loop) functions in association with sensorimotor cortex to scale and adjust movements.

2. Diencephalon.
   a. Thalamus.
      (1) Sensory nuclei: integrate and relay sensory information from body, face, retina, cochlea, and taste receptors to cerebral cortex and subcortical regions; smell (olfaction) is the exception.
      (2) Motor nuclei: relay motor information from cerebellum and globus pallidus to precentral motor cortex.
      (3) Other nuclei: assist in integration of visceral and somatic functions.
   b. Subthalamus: involved in control of several functional pathways for sensory, motor, and reticular function.
   c. Hypothalamus.
      (1) Integrates and controls the functions of the autonomic nervous system and the neuroendocrine system.
      (2) Maintains body homeostasis: regulates body temperature, eating, water balance, anterior pituitary function/sexual behavior, and emotion.
   d. Epithalamus.
      (1) Habenular nuclei: integrate olfactory, visceral, and somatic afferent pathways.
      (2) Pineal gland: secretes hormones that influence the pituitary gland and several other organs; influences circadian rhythm.

3. Brain stem.
   a. Midbrain (mesencephalon).
      (1) Connects pons to cerebrum; superior peduncle connects midbrain to cerebellum.
      (2) Contains cerebral peduncles (two lateral halves), each divided into anterior part or basis (crus cerebri and substantia nigra) and a posterior part (tegmentum).
      (3) Tegmentum contains all ascending tracts and some descending tracts; the red nucleus receives fibers from the cerebellum, and is the origin for the rubrospinal tract, important for coordination; contains cranial nerve nuclei: oculomotor and trochlear.
      (4) Substantia nigra is a large motor nucleus connecting with the basal ganglia and cortex; it is important in motor control and muscle tone.
      (5) Superior colliculus is an important relay station for vision and visual reflexes; the inferior colliculus is an important relay station for hearing and auditory reflexes.
      (6) Periaqueductal gray contains endorphinproducing cells (important for the suppression of pain) and descending autonomic tracts.
   b. Pons.
      (1) Connects the medulla oblongata to the midbrain, allowing passage of important ascending and descending tracts.
      (2) Anterior basal part acts as bridge to cerebellum (middle cerebellar peduncle).
      (3) Midline raphe nuclei project widely and are important for modulating pain and controlling arousal.
      (4) Tegmentum contains several important cranial nerve nuclei: abducens, trigeminal, facial, vestibulocochlear.
   c. Medulla oblongata.
      (1) Connects spinal cord with pons.
      (2) Contains relay nuclei of dorsal columns (gracilis and cuneatus); fibers cross to give rise to medial lemniscus.
      (3) Inferior cerebellar peduncle relays dorsal spinocerebellar tract to cerebellum.
      (4) Corticospinal tracts cross (decussate) in pyramids.
      (5) Medial longitudinal fasciculus arises from vestibular nuclei and extends throughout brain stem and upper cervical spinal cord; important for control of head movements and gaze stabilization (vestibulo-ocular reflex).
      (6) Olivary nuclear complex connects cerebellum to brain stem and is important for voluntary movement control.
      (7) Contains several important cranial nerve nuclei: hypoglossal, dorsal nucleus of vagus, and vestibulocochlear.
      (8) Contains important centers for vital functions: cardiac, respiratory, and vasomotor centers.

4. Cerebellum.
   a. Located behind dorsal pons and medulla in posterior fossa.
   b. Structure.
      (1) Joined to brain stem by 3 pairs of peduncles: superior, middle, and inferior.
      (2) Comprised of 2 hemispheres and midline vermis; have cerebellar cortex, underlying white matter, and 4 paired deep nuclei.

(3) Archicerebellum (flocculonodular lobe) connects with vestibular system and is concerned with equilibrium and regulation of muscle tone.
(4) Paleocerebellum (anterior lobes and vermis) receives input from proprioceptive pathways and is concerned with modifying muscle tone and synergistic actions of muscles; it is important in maintenance of posture and voluntary movement control.
(5) Neocerebellum (middle lobes) receives input from corticopontocerebellar tracts and olivocerebellar fibers; it is concerned with the smooth coordination of voluntary movements; ensures accurate force, direction, and degree of movement.

Spinal Cord

1. General structure.
   a. Cylindrical mass of nerve tissue extending from the foramen magnum in skull continuous with medulla to the lower border of first lumbar vertebra in the conus medullaris.
   b. Divided into 30 segments: 8 cervical, 12 thoracic, 5 lumbar, 5 sacral, a few coccygeal segments.
2. Central gray matter contains: 2 anterior (ventral) and 2 posterior (dorsal) horns united by gray commissure with central canal.
   a. Anterior horns contain cell bodies that give rise to efferent (motor) neurons: alpha motor neurons to effect muscles and gamma motor neurons to muscle spindles.
   b. Posterior horns contain afferent (sensory) neurons with cell bodies located in the dorsal root ganglia.
   c. Two enlargements, cervical and lumbosacral, for origins of nerves of upper and lower extremities.
   d. Lateral horn is found in thoracic and upper lumbar segments for preganglionic fibers of the autonomic nervous system.
3. White matter: anterior (ventral), lateral, and posterior (dorsal) white columns or funiculi.
   a. Ascending fiber systems (sensory pathways).
      (1) Dorsal columns/medial lemniscal system: convey sensations of proprioception, vibration, and tactile discrimination; divided into fasciculus cuneatus (upper extremity tracts, laterally located) and fasciculus gracilis (lower extremity tracts, medially located); neurons ascend to medulla where fibers cross (lemniscal decussation) to form medial lemniscus, ascend to thalamus and then to somatosensory cortex.
      (2) Spinothalamic tracts: convey sensations of pain and temperature (lateral spinothalamic tract), and crude touch (anterior spinothalamic tract); tracts ascend 1 or 2 ipsilateral spinal cord segments (Lissauer's tract), synapse and cross in spinal cord to opposite side and ascend in ventrolateral spinothalamic system.
      (3) Spinocerebellar tracts: convey proprioception information from muscle spindles, Golgi tendon organs, touch, and pressure receptors to cerebellum for control of voluntary movements; dorsal spinocerebellar tract ascends to ipsilateral inferior cerebellar peduncle while ventrospinocerebellar tract ascends to contralateral and ipsilateral superior cerebellar peduncle.
      (4) Spinoreticular tracts: convey deep and chronic pain to reticular formation of brain stem via diffuse, polysynaptic pathways.
   b. Descending fiber systems (motor pathways).
      (1) Corticospinal tracts: arise from primary motor cortex, descend in brain stem, cross in medulla (pyramidal decussation), via lateral corticospinal tract to ventral gray matter (anterior horn cells); 10% of fibers do not cross and travel in anterior corticospinal tract to cervical and upper thoracic segments; important for voluntary motor control.
      (2) Vestibulospinal tracts: arise from vestibular nucleus and descend to spinal cord in lateral (uncrossed) and medial (both crossed and uncrossed) vestibulospinal tracts; important for control of muscle tone, antigravity muscles, and postural reflexes.
      (3) Rubrospinal tract: arises in contralateral red nucleus and descends in lateral white columns to spinal gray; assists in motor function.
      (4) Reticulospinal system: arises in the reticular formation of the brain stem and descends (both crossed and uncrossed) in both ventral and lateral columns, terminates both on dorsal gray (modifies transmission of sensation, especially pain) and on ventral gray (influences gamma motor neurons and spinal reflexes).
      (5) Tectospinal tract: arises from superior colliculus (midbrain) and descends to ventral gray; assists in head turning responses in response to visual stimuli.
4. Autonomic nervous system (ANS).
   a. Concerned with innervations of involuntary structures: smooth muscle, heart, glands; helps maintain homeostasis (constant internal body environment).
   b. Divided into 2 divisions: sympathetic and parasympathetic; both have afferent and efferent nerve fibers; preganglionic and postganglionic fibers.
      (1) Sympathetic (thoracolumbar) division: prepares body for fight or flight, emergency responses, raises heart rate and blood pressure,

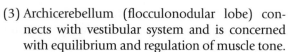

constricts peripheral blood vessels and redistributes blood; inhibits peristalsis.
   (2) Parasympathetic (craniosacral) division: conserves and restores homeostasis; slows heart rate and reduces blood pressure, increases peristalsis and glandular activity.
  c. Autonomic plexuses: cardiac, pulmonary, celiac (solar), hypogastric, pelvic.
  d. Modulated by brain centers.
   (1) Descending autonomic system: arises from control centers in hypothalamus and lower brain stem (cardiac, respiratory, vasomotor) and projects to preganglionic ANS segments in thoracolumbar (sympathetic) and craniosacral (parasympathetic) segments.
   (2) Cranial nerves: visceral afferent sensations via glossopharyngeal, and vagus nerves; efferent outflow via oculomotor, facial, glossopharyngeal, and vagus nerves.

CNS Support Structures

1. Bony structure.
  a. Skull (cranium): rigid bony chamber that contains the brain and facial skeleton, with an opening (foramen magnum) at its base.
2. Meninges: three membranes that envelop the brain.
  a. Dura mater: outer, tough, fibrous membrane attached to inner surface of cranium; forms falx and tentorium.
  b. Arachnoid: delicate, vascular membrane.
  c. Subarachnoid space: formed by arachnoid and pia mater, contains cerebrospinal fluid and cisterns, major arteries.
  d. Pia mater: thin, vascular membrane that covers the brain surface; forms tela choroidea of ventricles.
3. Ventricles: four cavities or ventricles that are filled with cerebrospinal fluid and communicate with each other and with the spinal cord canal.
  a. Lateral ventricles: large, irregularly shaped, with anterior (frontal), posterior (occipital) and inferior (temporal) horns; communicates with third ventricle through foramen of Monro.
  b. Third ventricle: located posterior and deep between the two thalami; cerebral aqueduct communicates third with fourth ventricle.
  c. Fourth ventricle: pyramid-shaped cavity located in pons and medulla; foramina (openings) of Luschka and Magendie communicate fourth ventricle with subarachnoid space.
4. Cerebrospinal fluid: provides mechanical support (cushions brain), controls brain excitability by regulating ionic composition, aids in exchange of nutrients and waste products.
  a. Produced in choroid plexuses in ventricles.
  b. Normal pressure: 70–180 mm/H2O.
  c. Total volume: 125–150 cc.
5. Blood-brain barrier: the selective restriction of blood borne substances from entering the CNS; associated with capillary endothelial cells.
6. Blood supply: brain is 2% of body weight with a circulation of 18% of total blood volume.
  a. Carotid system: internal carotid arteries arise off of common carotids and branch to form anterior and middle cerebral arteries; supplies a large area of brain and many deep structures.
  b. Vertebrobasilar system: vertebral arteries arise off of subclavian arteries and unite to form the basilar artery; this vessel bifurcates into two posterior cerebral arteries; supplies the brain stem, cerebellum, occipital lobe, and parts of thalamus.
  c. Circle of Willis: formed by anterior communicating artery connecting the two anterior cerebral arteries and the posterior communicating artery connecting each posterior and middle cerebral artery.
  d. Venous drainage: includes cerebral veins, dural venous sinuses.

Neurons

1. Structure.
  a. Neurons vary in size and complexity.
   (1) Cell bodies (genetic center) with dendrites (receptive surface area to receive information via synapses).
   (2) Axons conduct impulses away from the cell body (one-way conduction).
   (3) Synapses allow communication between neurons; chemical neurotransmitters are released (chemical synapses) or electrical signals pass directly from cell to cell (electrical synapses).
  b. Neuron groupings and types.
   (1) Nuclei are compact groups of nerve cell bodies; in the peripheral nervous system these groups are called ganglia.
   (2) Projection neurons carry impulses to other parts of the CNS.
   (3) Interneurons are short relay neurons.
   (4) Axon bundles are called tracts or fasciculi; in spinal cord, collections of tracts are called columns, or funiculi.
  c. Neuroglia: support cells that do not transmit signals; important for myelin and neuron production; maintenance of K+ levels and re-uptake of neurotransmitters following neural transmission at synapses.

Table 7-1

Motor Neuron Systems	
LOWER MOTOR NEURON SYSTEM	**UPPER MOTOR NEURON SYSTEM**
Structures: cell bodies in the anterior horn of the spinal cord, spinal nerves, the cranial nerve fibers that travel to target muscles.	Structures: any nerve cell body or nerve fiber in the spinal cord (except the anterior horn cells), all superior structures (gray and white matter affecting motor function and descending nerve tracts), cranial nerve nuclei.
Symptoms of a lesion: flaccidity, decreased or absent deep tendon reflexes, atrophy.	Symptoms of a lesion: increased deep tendon reflexes, spasticity, clonus, emergence of primitive reflexes including Babinski's sign, exaggerated cutaneous reflexes, autonomic dysreflexia, flaccidity may occur at the level of the lesion.

2. Function: neuronal signaling.
   a. Resting membrane potential: positive on outside, negative on inside (about –70mV).
   b. Action potential: increased permeability of Na+ and influx into cell with outflow of K+ results in polarity changes (inside to about +35mV) and depolarization; generation of an action potential is all-or-none.
   c. Conduction velocity is proportional to axon diameter; the largest myelinated fibers conduct the fastest.
   d. Repolarization results from activation of K+ channels.
   e. Myelinated axons: many axons are covered with myelin with small gaps (nodes of Ranvier) where myelin is absent; the action potential jumps from one node to the next, termed saltatory conduction; myelin functions to increase speed of conduction and conserve energy.
   f. Nerve fiber types.
      (1) A fibers: large, myelinated, fast conducting.
         (a) Alpha – proprioception, somatic motor.
         (b) Beta – touch, pressure.
         (c) Gamma – motor to muscle spindles.
         (d) Delta – pain, temperature, touch.
      (2) B fibers: small, myelinated, conduct less rapidly; preganglionic autonomic.
      (3) C fibers: smallest, unmyelinated, slowest conducting.
         (a) Dorsal root: pain, reflex responses.
         (b) Sympathetic: post-ganglionic sympathetics.
   g. Refer to Table 7-1.

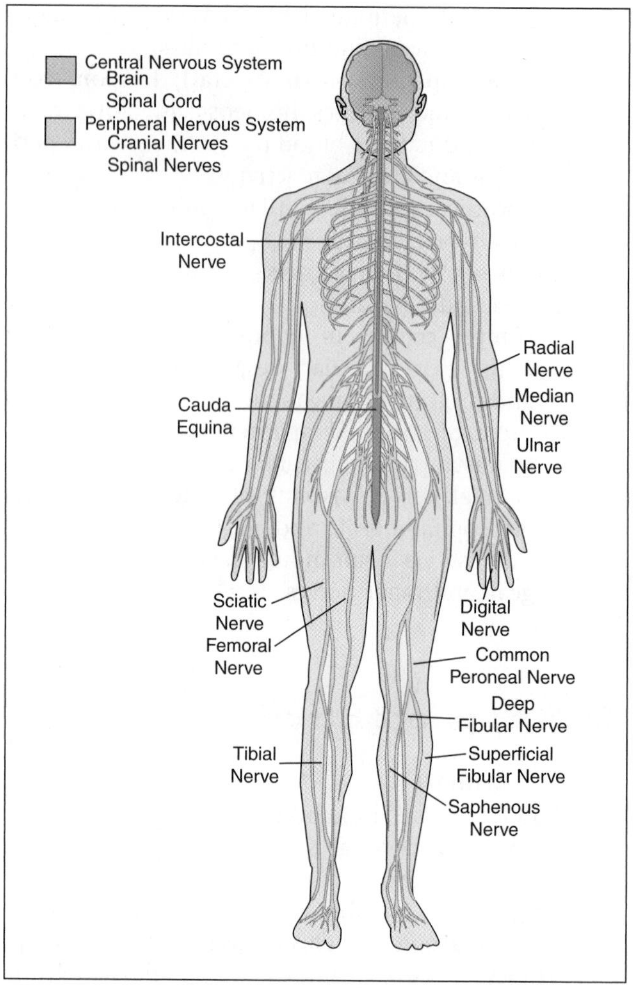

Figure 7-2 **Overview of nervous system.**

Peripheral Nervous System

1. Peripheral nerves are referred to as lower motor neurons (LMN). See Figure 7-2. Functional components include:
   a. Motor (efferent) fibers originate from motor nuclei (cranial nerves) or anterior horn cells (spinal nerves).
   b. Sensory (afferent) fibers originate in cells outside of brain stem or spinal cord with sensory ganglia (cranial nerves) or dorsal root ganglia (spinal nerves).
   c. Autonomic nervous system fibers: sympathetic fibers at thoracolumbar spinal segments and parasympathetic fibers at craniosacral segments.
2. Cranial nerves: 12 pairs of cranial nerves, all nerves are distributed to head and neck except C.N. X which is distributed to thorax and abdomen.
   a. C.N. I, II, VIII are pure sensory, carry special senses of smell, vision, hearing and equilibrium.

b. C.N. III, IV, VI are pure motor, controlling eye movements and pupillary constriction.
c. C.N. XI, XII are pure motor, innervating sternocleidomastoid, trapezius, and tongue.
d. C.N. V, VII, IX, X are mixed: motor and sensory; involved in chewing (V), facial expression (VII), swallowing (IX, X), vocal sounds (X), sensations from head (V, VII, IX), alimentary tract, heart, vessels, and lungs (IX, X), and taste (VII, IX, X).
e. C.N. III, VII, IX, X carry parasympathetic fibers of ANS; involved in control of smooth muscles of inner eye (III), salivatory and lacrimal glands (VII), parotid gland (IX), muscles of heart, lung, and bowel (X).
f. Refer to Chapter 12 for additional information on cranial nerves.

3. Spinal nerves: 31 pairs of spinal nerves; spinal nerves are divided into groups (8 cervical, 12 thoraces, 5 lumbar, 5 sacral, coccygeal) and correspond to vertebral segments; each has a ventral root and a dorsal root.
   a. Ventral (anterior) root: efferent (motor) fibers to voluntary muscles (alpha motoneurons, gamma motoneurons), and to viscera, glands and smooth muscles (preganglionic ANS fibers).
   b. Dorsal (posterior) root: afferent (sensory) fibers from sensory receptors from skin, joints, and muscles; each dorsal root possesses a dorsal root ganglion (cell bodies of sensory neurons); there is no dorsal root for C1.
   c. The term dermatome refers to a specific segmental skin area innervated by sensory spinal axons (Refer to Chapter 11.) See Figure 6-6 and Table 11-3.
   d. The term myotome refers to the skeletal muscles innervated by motor axons in a given spinal root.
   e. A motor unit consists of the alpha motoneuron and the muscle fibers it innervates.
   f. Nerve roots exit from the vertebral column through intervertebral foramina.
      (1) In cervical spine, numbered roots exit above the corresponding vertebral body, with C8 exiting below C7 and above T1.
      (2) In the thoracic and lumbar segments, the roots exit below the corresponding vertebral body.
   g. Spinal cord ends at the level of L1; below L1, nerve roots descend vertically to form the cauda equina.

Spinal Level Reflexes

1. Involuntary responses to stimuli; basic, specific and predictable; dependent upon intact neural pathway (reflex arc).
   a. Reflexes may be monosynaptic or polysynaptic (involving interneurons).
   b. Provide basis for unconscious motor function and basic defense mechanisms.
2. Stretch (myotatic) reflexes.
   a. Stimulus: muscle stretch.
   b. Reflex arc: afferent Ia fiber from muscle spindle to alpha motoneuron projecting back to muscle of origin (monosynaptic).
   c. Functions to maintain muscle tone, support agonist muscle contraction, and to provide feedback about muscle length.
   d. Clinically, sensitivity of the stretch reflex and intactness of spinal cord segment are tested by applying stretch to the deep tendons (DTR).
   e. Reciprocal inhibition: via an inhibitory interneuron the same stretch stimulus inhibits the antagonist muscle.
   f. Reciprocal innervation: describes the responses a stretch stimulus can have on agonist (autogenic facilitation), antagonist (reciprocal inhibition) as well as on synergistic muscles (facilitation).
3. Inverse stretch (myotatic) reflex.
   a. Stimulus: muscle contraction.
   b. Reflex arc: afferent Ib fiber from Golgi tendon organ via inhibitory interneuron to muscle of origin (polysynaptic).
   c. Functions to provide agonist inhibition, diminution of force of agonist contraction.
4. Gamma reflex loop.
   a. Stretch reflex forms part of this loop.
   b. Allows muscle tension to come under control of descending pathways (reticulospinal, vestibulospinal and others).
   c. Descending pathways excite gamma motor neurons, causing contraction of the muscle spindle, and in turn increased stretch sensitivity and increased rate of firing from spindle afferents; impulses are then conveyed to alpha motor neurons.
5. Flexor (withdrawal) reflex.
   a. Stimulus: cutaneous sensory stimuli.
   b. Reflex arc: cutaneous receptors via interneurons to largely flexor muscles; multi-segmental response involving groups of muscles (polysynaptic).
   c. Functions as a protective withdrawal mechanism to remove body part from harmful stimuli.
6. Crossed extension reflex.
   a. Stimulus: noxious stimuli and reciprocal action of antagonists; flexors of one side are excited causing extensors on same side to be inhibited; opposite responses occur in opposite limb.
   b. Reflex arc: cutaneous and muscle receptors diverging to many spinal cord motor neurons on same and opposite side (polysynaptic).
   c. Function: coordinates reciprocal limb activities such as gait.

Chapter 7

Stroke/Cerebral Vascular Accident (CVA)

Specific Types and Etiology

1. The term CVA or stroke applies to clinical syndromes that accompany ischemic or hemorrhagic lesions.
   a. Cerebral insufficiency: due to transient disturbances of blood flow, e.g., transient ischemic attack (TIA).
      (1) A transient ischemic attack (TIA) is a transitory stroke that for the most part lasts only a few minutes.
         (a) TIAs occur when the blood supply to part of the brain is briefly interrupted.
         (b) TIA symptoms, which usually occur suddenly, are similar to those of stroke but do not last as long. Most symptoms of a TIA disappear within an hour, although they may persist for up to 24 hours.
         (c) Symptoms can include: numbness or weakness in the face, arm, or leg, especially on one side of the body; confusion or difficulty in talking or understanding speech; trouble seeing in one or both eyes; difficulty with walking, dizziness, and/or loss of balance and coordination.
         (d) TIAs are often warning signs that a person is at risk for a more serious and debilitating stroke. About one-third of those who have a TIA will have an acute stroke some time in the future.
   b. Cerebral infarction: due to either embolism or thrombosis of the intra or extracranial arteries.
   c. Cerebral hemorrhage: bleed secondary to hypertension or aneurysm.
   d. Cerebral arteriovenous malformation (AVM): abnormal, tangled collections of dilated blood vessels that result from congenitally malformed vascular structures.

Prevalence, Onset, and Prognosis

1. On average, a US citizen incurs a stroke every 40 seconds; every 4 minutes someone dies of a stroke.
2. It is the third-largest cause of death, ranking behind "diseases of the heart" and all forms of cancer.
3. Stroke is a leading cause of serious, long-term disability in the United States.
4. The prevalence of stroke is 6,400,000 based on data collected from 2007–2010.
5. Data show that about 795,000 people incur a new or recurrent stroke each year. About 610,000 of these are first attacks and 185,000 are recurrent attacks.

Symptoms of CVA

1. Abrupt onset of usually unilateral neurological signs (e.g., weakness, vision loss, sensory changes).
2. Symptoms progress over several hours to two days.
3. Specific symptoms are determined by the site of the infarct and the involved artery.
   a. Middle cerebral artery (MCA) stroke results in contralateral hemiplegia, hemianesthesia, homonymous hemianopsia, aphasia (usually left MCA), and/or apraxia (usually left MCA), unilateral neglect (usually right MCA), spatial dysfunction (usually right MCA).
   b. Internal carotid artery (ICA) stroke results in symptoms similar to those associated with MCA CVA.
   c. Anterior cerebral artery (ACA) stroke results in contralateral hemiplegia, grasp reflex, incontinence, confusion, apathy, and/or mutism.
   d. Posterior cerebral artery (PCA) stroke results in homonymous hemianopsia, thalamic pain, hemisensory loss, and/or alexia.
   e. Vertebrobasilar system results in pseudobulbar signs (dysarthria, dysphagia, emotional instability), tetraplegia.
   f. Refer to Table 7-2 for hemispheric specialization information which is based on lateralization in most individuals.
      (1) Hemispheric asymmetry and functional localization can vary in individuals.

Table 7-2

Hemispheric Specialization*

LEFT HEMISPHERE	RIGHT HEMISPHERE
Movement of right side of body Processing of sensory information from right side of body	Movement of left side of body Processing of sensory information from left side of body
Visual reception from right field	Visual reception from left field
Visual verbal processing	Visual spatial processing
Bilateral motor praxis	Left motor praxis
Verbal memory	Nonverbal memory
Bilateral auditory reception	Attention to incoming stimuli
Speech	Emotion
Processing of verbal auditory information	Processing of nonverbal auditory information
	Interpretation of abstract information
	Interpretation of tonal inflections

*Based on hemispheric lateralization in most clients. It must be recognized that hemispheric asymmetry and functional localization varies in individuals.

Risk Factors

1. Modifiable risk factors.
   a. Hypertension.
   b. Cardiac disease.
   c. Atrial fibrillation.
   d. Diabetes mellitus.
   e. Smoking.
   f. Alcohol abuse.
   g. Hyperlipidemia.
2. Nonmodifiable risk factors.
   a. Age: relative risk increases with age.
   b. Gender: males are at higher risk.
   c. Race: African-American and Latino are at greater risk.
   d. Heredity.

Diagnosis

1. Usually diagnosed clinically using symptoms as a guide to lesion location.
2. Infarction visualized via computerized axial tomography (CT) scan (may initially read as negative).
3. Arteriography.
4. Positron emission tomography (PET) and single photon emission computerized tomography (SPECT) scanning to distinguish between infarcted and noninfarcted tissue.
5. Magnetic resonance imaging (MRI) to rule out other conditions and screen for acute bleeding.
6. Diagnostic testing.
   a. Transcranial and carotid Doppler for noninvasive visualization of plaque or occlusion of the cerebral vessels.
   b. Electrocardiogram (ECG) to detect arrhythmias.
   c. Echocardiography to evaluate presence of cardiac emboli and cardiac disease.
   d. Blood work to rule out metabolic abnormalities.

Medical Management

1. Immediate care.
   a. Airway maintenance.
   b. Adequate oxygenation.
   c. Nutritional intervention (IV fluids, alternative feeding routes).
   d. Decubiti prevention.
   e. Treatment of underlying cardiac dysfunction (dysrhythmias).
2. Pharmacologic therapies.
   a. Antithrombotic therapy (antiplatelet and anticoagulation) is used for rapid recanalization and reperfusion of occluded vessels to reduce infarction area, e.g. aspirin, heparin.
   b. Thrombolytic therapy is used in acute strokes to open occluded cerebral vessels and restore blood flow to ischemic areas, e.g., t-PA.

Trauma

Traumatic Brain Injury

1. Etiology.
2. Damage results from penetration of the skull (open TBI), from rapid acceleration or deceleration of the brain (closed TBI), or blunt external force (closed TBI).
   a. Injury occurs in the tissue at the point of impact (coup), at the opposite pole (contrecoup), and diffusely along the frontal and temporal lobes.
   b. Injury can result from a variety of occurrences.
      (1) Skull fractures.
      (2) Closed head injuries.
      (3) Penetrating wounds of the skull and brain.
      (4) Traumatic injury to extracranial blood vessels.
      (5) Nerve tissues, blood vessels, and meninges are sheared, torn, or ruptured, resulting in hemorrhage, edema, and ischemia.
3. Prevalence, onset, and prognosis.
   a. Responsible for more deaths and disabilities than any other neurologic cause in the population under age 50.
   b. Males are twice as likely to incur a TBI with the highest risk group being 15- to 29-year-olds.
   c. Between 2.5 and 6.5 million Americans alive today have had a TBI.
   d. 1.7 million new head injuries are reported each year.
4. Symptoms.
   a. Concussion characterized by post-traumatic loss of consciousness.
   b. Cerebral contusion/laceration/edema accompanied by surface wounds and skull fractures.
   c. A variety of symptoms can result.
      (1) Hemiplegia or monoplegia and abnormal reflexes.
      (2) Decorticate or decerebrate rigidity.
      (3) Fixed pupils.
      (4) Coma.
      (5) Changes in vital signs.
5. Diagnostic testing.
   a. Administration of the Glasgow Coma Scale.
      (1) A neurological scale which provides an objective method to record the conscious state of a person.

(2) It is used for initial evaluation and continuing assessment to determine a person's level of consciousness after head injury.
(3) A client is assessed against the scale's criteria which delineate a range of points for three tests: eye, verbal and motor responses.
- The resulting total points comprise the Glasgow Coma Score (or GCS).
- The score sum as well as the three separate values is considered.
- The highest total GCS is 15 (i.e., a fully conscious person).
- The lowest possible total GCS is 3 (i.e., deep coma or death),
- The GCS is interpreted as severe with GCS <8, moderate with GCS 9–12, and minor with GCS > 13.

(4) See Table 7-3.
(5) Individual test scores as well as the total GCS score are documented (e.g., "GCS 11 = E4 V3 M4 at 11:30pm").

b. Administration of the Rancho Los Amigos Levels of Cognitive Functioning. Refer to Table 7-4.
c. CT scan and MRI to visualize intracranial structure damage.

6. Medical management.
a. Resuscitation.
b. Management of respiratory dysfunction.
c. Cardiovascular monitoring.
d. Surgical, pharmacologic, or mechanical means to decrease intracranial pressure.
e. Neurosurgery to manage lacerated vessels and depressed skull fractures.
f. Pharmacologic interventions.
(1) Antibiotics.
(2) Anticonvulsants.
(3) Sedatives.
(4) Antidepressants.

Table 7-3

Glasgow Coma Scale

Best eye response (E)	Eyes opening spontaneously	4
	Eyes opening to speech	3
	Eyes opening in response to pain	2
	No eye opening	1
Best verbal response (V)	Oriented (patient responds coherently and appropriately to questions such as the patient's name and age, where they are and why, the year, month, etc.)	5
	Confused (patient responds to questions coherently but there is some disorientation and confusion)	4
	Inappropriate words (random or exclamatory speech, but not conversational exchange)	3
	Incomprehensible sounds (moaning but no words)	2
	None	1
Best motor response (M)	Obeys commands (the person does simple things as asked.)	6
	Localizes to pain. (purposeful movements towards changing painful stimuli)	5
	Withdraws from pain (pulls part of body away when pinched)	4
	Flexion in response to pain (decorticate response)	3
	Extension to pain (decerebrate response)	2
	No motor response	1

Reprinted from *The Lancet*, 304., Teasdale G, Jennett B. Assessment of coma and impaired consciousness. A practical scale, 81–84. Copyright 1974, with permission from Elsevier.

Spinal Cord Injury (SCI)

1. Etiology.
a. Trauma to the spinal cord as a result of compression, shearing force, contusion secondary to motor vehicle accident, diving accident, penetration wound (gunshot or knife), sports injury, or fall.
b. Non-traumatic cord injuries may be a result of tumor, progressive degenerative disease.

2. Classification of injury/signs and symptoms.
a. Degree of impairment and severity of injury is graded using the ASIA Impairment Scale:
(1) A = complete, no sensory or motor function is preserved in the sacral segments S4–S5.
(2) B = incomplete, sensory but no motor function is preserved below the neurological level and extends through the sacral segments.
(3) C = incomplete, motor function is preserved below the neurological level, and the majority of key muscle groups below the neurological level have a muscle grade less than 3/5.
(4) D = incomplete, motor function is preserved below the neurological level, and the majority of key muscle groups below the level have a muscle grade greater than or equal to 3/5.
(5) E = normal, sensory and motor function are normal.

3. Specific symptoms.
a. Spinal shock (4–8 weeks), all reflex activity is obliterated below the level of the injury presenting as flaccid paralysis.
b. Sensory deficits may be partial loss or complete.
c. Loss of bowel/bladder control.
d. Loss of temperature control below the lesion.
e. Decreased respiratory function.
f. Sexual dysfunction.

Table 7-4

Rancho Level of Cognitive Functioning
Level I - No Response: Total Assistance
• Complete absence of observable change in behavior when presented visual, auditory, tactile, proprioceptive, vestibular or painful stimuli.
Level II - Generalized Response: Total Assistance
• Demonstrates generalized reflex response to painful stimuli. • Responds to repeated auditory stimuli with increased or decreased activity. • Responds to external stimuli with physiological changes generalized, gross body movement and/or not purposeful vocalization. • Responses noted above may be same regardless of type and location of stimulation. • Responses may be significantly delayed.
Level III - Localized Response: Total Assistance
• Demonstrates withdrawal or vocalization to painful stimuli. • Turns toward or away from auditory stimuli. • Blinks when strong light crosses visual field. • Follows moving object passed within visual field. • Responds to discomfort by pulling tubes or restraints. • Responds inconsistently to simple commands. • Responses directly related to type of stimulus. • May respond to some persons (especially family and friends) but not to others.
Level IV - Confused/Agitated: Maximal Assistance
• Alert and in heightened state of activity. • Purposeful attempts to remove restraints or tubes or crawl out of bed. • May perform motor activities such as sitting, reaching and walking but without any apparent purpose or upon another's request. • Very brief and usually non-purposeful moments of sustained alternatives and divided attention. • Absent short-term memory. • May cry out or scream out of proportion to stimulus even after its removal. • May exhibit aggressive or flight behavior. • Mood may swing from euphoric to hostile with no apparent relationship to environmental events. • Unable to cooperate with treatment efforts. • Verbalizations are frequently incoherent and/or inappropriate to activity or environment.
Level V - Confused, Inappropriate Non-Agitated: Maximal Assistance
• Alert, not agitated but may wander randomly or with a vague intention of going home. • May become agitated in reponse to external stimulation, and/or lack of environmental structure. • Not oriented to person, place or time. • Frequent brief periods, non-purposeful sustained attention. • Severely impaired recent memory, with confusion of past and present in reaction to ongoing activity. • Absent goal directed, problem solving, self-monitoring behavior. • Often demonstrates inappropriate use of objects without external direction. • May be able to perform previously learned tasks when structured and cues provided. • Unable to learn new information. • Able to respond appropriately to simple commands fairly consistently with external structures and cues. • Responses to simple commands without external structure are random and non-purposeful in relation to command. • Able to converse on a social, automatic level for brief periods of time when provided external structure and cues. • Verbalizations about present events become inappropriate and confabulatory when external structure and cues are not provided.
Level VI - Confused, Appropriate: Moderate Assistance
• Inconsistently oriented to person, time and place. • Able to attend to highly familiar tasks in non-distracting environment for 30 minutes with moderate redirection. • Remote memory has more depth and detail than recent memory. • Vague recognition of some staff. • Able to use assistive memory aide with maximum assistance. • Emerging awareness of appropriate response to self, family and basic needs. • Moderate assist to problem solve barriers to task completion. • Supervised for old learning (e.g., self care). • Shows carry over for relearned familiar tasks (e.g., self care). • Maximum assistance for new learning with little or nor carry over. • Unaware of impairments, disabilities and safety risks. • Consistently follows simple directions. • Verbal expressions are appropriate in highly familiar and structured situations.
Level VII - Automatic, Appropriate: Minimal Assistance for Daily Living Skills
• Consistently oriented to person and place, within highly familiar environments. Moderate assistance for orientation to time. • Able to attend to highly familiar tasks in a non-distraction environment for at least 30 minutes with minimal assist to complete tasks. • Minimal supervision for new learning.

(*Continued*)

Chapter 7

Table 7-4

Rancho Level of Cognitive Functioning (*Continued*)
Level VII - Automatic, Appropriate: Minimal Assistance for Daily Living Skills (*Continued*)
• Demonstrates carry over of new learning. • Initiates and carries out steps to complete familiar personal and household routine but has shallow recall of what he/she has been doing. • Able to monitor accuracy and completeness of each step in routine personal and household ADL and modify plan with minimal assistance. • Superficial awareness of his/her condition but unaware of specific impairments and disabilities and the limits they place on his/her ability to safely, accurately and completely carry out his/her household, community, work and leisure ADL. • Minimal supervision for safety in routine home and community activities. • Unrealistic planning for the future. • Unable to think about consequences of a decision or action. • Overestimates abilities. • Unaware of others' needs and feelings. • Oppositional/uncooperative. • Unable to recognize inappropriate social interaction behavior.
Level VIII - Purposeful, Appropriate: Stand-By Assistance
• Consistently oriented to person, place and time. • Independently attends to and completes familiar tasks for 1 hour in distracting environments. • Able to recall and integrate past and recent events. • Uses assistive memory devices to recall daily schedule, "to do" lists and record critical information for later use with stand-by assistance. • Initiates and carries out steps to complete familiar personal, household, community, work and leisure routines with stand-by assistance and can modify the plan when needed with minimal assistance. • Requires no assistance once new tasks/activities are learned. • Aware of and acknowledges impairments and disabilities when they interfere with task completion but requires stand-by assistance to take appropriate corrective action. • Thinks about consequences of a decision or action with minimal assistance. • Overestimates or underestimates abilities. • Acknowledges others' needs and feelings and responds appropriately with minimal assistance. • Depressed. • Irritable. • Low frustration tolerance/easily angered. • Argumentative. • Self-centered. • Uncharacteristically dependent/independent. • Able to recognize and acknowledge inappropriate social interaction behavior while it is occurring and takes corrective action with minimal assistance.
Level IX - Purposeful, Appropriate: Stand-By Assistance on Request
• Independently shifts back and forth between tasks and completes them accurately for at least two consecutive hours. • Uses assistive memory devices to recall daily schedule, "to do" lists and record critical information for later use with assistance when requested. • Initiates and carries out steps to complete familiar personal, household, work and leisure tasks independently and unfamiliar personal, household, work and leisure tasks with assistance when requested. • Aware of and acknowledges impairments and disabilities when they interfere with task completion and takes appropriate corrective action but requires stand-by assist to anticipate a problem before it occurs and take action to avoid it. • Able to think about consequences of decisions or actions with assistance when requested. • Accurately estimates abilities but requires stand-by assistance to adjust to task demands. • Acknowledges others' needs and feelings and responds appropriately with stand-by assistance. • Depression may continue. • May be easily irritable. • May have low frustration tolerance. • Able to self monitor appropriateness of social interaction with stand-by assistance.
Level X - Purposeful, Appropriate: Modified Independent
• Able to handle multiple tasks simultaneously in all environments but may require periodic breaks. • Able to independently procure, create and maintain own assistive memory devices. • Independently initiates and carries out steps to complete familiar and unfamiliar personal, household, community, work and leisure tasks but may require more than usual amount of time and/or compensatory strategies to complete them. • Anticipates impact of impairments and disabilities on ability to complete daily living tasks and takes action to avoid problems before they occur but may require more than usual amount of time and/or compensatory strategies. • Able to independently think about consequences of decisions or actions but may require more than usual amount of time and/or comepensatory strategies to select the appropriate decision or action. • Accurately estimates abilities and independently adjusts to task demands. • Able to recognize the needs and feelings of others and automatically respond in appropriate manner. • Periodic periods of depression may occur. • Irritability and low frustration tolerance when sick, fatigued and/or under emotional stress. • Social interaction behavior is consistently appropriate.

Reprinted with permission from the author Chris Hagen.

g. Changes in muscle tone.
   (1) Spasticity in upper motor neuron lesions.
   (2) Flaccidity in lesions below L1.
h. Loss of motor function resulting in tetraplegia (quadriplegia) or paraplegia; may be complete or incomplete.

4. Clinical syndromes.
   a. Central cord: resulting from hyperextension injuries and presenting as more upper extremity deficits vs. lower extremities.
   b. Brown-Séquard (hemi-section of cord): this injury causes disruption of the descending lateral corticospinal tracts, the ascending dorsal columns (both of which cross in the medulla), and the ascending lateral spinothalamic tracts, which cross within one or two levels of the dorsal root entrance.
      (a) The result is ipsilateral paralysis, ipsilateral loss of position sense, ipsilateral loss of discrimitive touch, contralateral loss of pain, and contralateral loss of thermal sense.
   c. Anterior cord: caused by flexion injuries; motor function, pain, pinprick, and temperature sensation are lost bilaterally below the lesion while proprioception and light touch are preserved.
   d. Posterior cord: least frequent syndrome, injury to the posterior columns results in proprioceptive loss. Pain, temperature, touch are preserved. Motor function is preserved to varying degrees.
   e. Conus medullaris: injury of the sacral cord and lumbar nerve roots resulting in lower extremity motor and sensory loss and an areflexic bowel and bladder.
      (1) If the lesion is in the sacral segments, reflexes may be occasionally preserved.
   f. Cauda equina syndrome: injury at the L1 level and below resulting in a lower motor neuron lesion; flaccid paralysis with no spinal reflex activity; an areflexic bowel and bladder.

5. Complications.
   a. Respiratory complications, decreased vital capacity, pneumonia.
   b. Decubitus ulcer formation.
   c. Orthostatic hypotension: an excessive fall in blood pressure upon assuming the upright position.
   d. Deep vein thrombosis.
   e. Autonomic dysreflexia[1]: an abnormal response to a noxious stimulus that results in an extreme rise in blood pressure, pounding headache, and profuse sweating. This complication is deemed a medical emergency if not reversed by removing the irritating stimulus quickly.
      (1) Irritants that would normally cause pain to areas below the spinal injury specific to the bowel include bowel irritation or over-distention (e.g., constipation/impaction, distention during bowel program [digital stimulation], hemorrhoid infection or irritation).
      (2) Irritants specific to the bladder include bladder infection or over distention (e.g., urinary tract infection [UTI], urinary retention, blocked catheter, overfilled urine collection bag, non-compliance with intermittent catheterization program).
      (3) Skin-related irritants can include any skin irritation below area of injury (e.g., decubitus ulcers, ingrown toenails, burns, tight or restrictive clothing or pressure to skin from clothing restrictions or wrinkles in clothing).
      (4) Sexual activity irritants can include over-stimulation during sex, stimuli to the pelvic region that would be felt as pain if sensation were intact, menstrual cramps, labor and delivery.
      (5) Other irritants can include heterotopic ossification/myositis ossificans, skeletal fractures and appendicitis.
      (6) Management of autonomic dysreflexia.
         (a) Identify the offending stimulus and relieve the underlying issue immediately.
         (b) Medications if no impact can be made by removing the irritant.
      (7) Prevention of autonomic dysreflexia.
         (a) Teach person/caregiver frequent pressure relief principles.
         (b) Ensure compliance with intermittent catheterization.
         (c) Practice well-balanced diet habits.
         (d) Ensure medication compliance.
         (e) Educate the person with the condition (and/or at risk) and caregivers on how to use prevention methods; recognize the cause, signs, and symptoms (i.e., sweating, headache); and initiate first aid procedures to deal effectively with the occurrence of this condition.
   f. Urinary tract infection.
   g. Heterotopic ossification, the formation of bone in abnormal anatomical locations.

6. Medical management.
   a. Prevention of further cord damage via stabilization.
   b. Traction and rest for unstable injuries.
   c. Surgery with internal or external fixation.
   d. Diuretic prescription to decrease inflammation.
   e. Bladder care.
   f. Decubiti prevention.
   g. Control of autonomic dysreflexia and orthostatic hypotension.
   h. Prevention of thrombus formation.
   i. Treatment for heterotopic ossification.

[1]Ann Burkhardt contributed to this section on autonomic dysreflexia.

Cerebral Palsy (CP)

1. Etiology.
   a. Caused by an injury and/or disease prior to, during, or shortly after birth resulting in brain damage and secondary neurological and muscular deficits.
   b. Common causes during the perinatal period include lack of oxygen, intracranial hemorrhage, meningitis, chronic alcohol abuse, toxicosis, infections, genetic factors, endocrine and metabolic disorders.
2. Onset, prevalence, and prognosis.
   a. Occurs in 3.3 per 1,000 births.
      (1) In the United States, 1200–1500 preschool children are diagnosed each year.
   b. Prognosis is dependent on the severity of the brain injury and the location.
   c. It is nonprogressive; however, deformities and contractures may develop depending on the level of involvement.
   d. It may be accompanied with seizure, intellectual and/or behavioral disorders.
   e. The individual can have normal intelligence, which is masked by significant motor deficits.
   f. An increase in the number of infants surviving prematurely and an increase in low birth weight have resulted in a higher incidence of the spastic diplegia type of CP.
3. Diagnosis.
   a. Detected usually by 12 months of age.
   b. Sometimes diagnosis may not be identified in early infancy.
      (1) An infant may initially present with hypotonia.
      (2) As the child's neuromotor status evolves spasticity may develop.
      (3) The child may present with primitive reflexes and automatic reactions, hyperresponsive reflexes, clonus, variable tone, asymmetry, involuntary movements, feeding difficulties due to oral motor impairments, cognitive, and other developmental delays.
   c. Persistence of primitive reflexes contributes to diagnosis.
      (1) These may extend into adulthood.
   d. The location and severity of the lesion determines the type of cerebral palsy. Types include:
      (1) Spastic cerebral palsy: a lesion of the motor cortex will result in spasticity with flexor and extensor imbalance. Spasticity can express itself as:
         (a) Hypertonia: increased muscle tone.
         (b) Hyperreflexia: increased intensity of reflex responses.
      (2) Dyskinetic cerebral palsy: a lesion in the basal ganglia results in fluctuations in muscle tone. This lesion expresses itself as:
         (a) Dystonia: excessive or inadequate muscle tone.
         (b) Athetosis: writhing involuntary movements which are more distal than proximal.
         (c) Chorea: spasmodic involuntary movements which are more proximal than distal and a lack of cocontractions.
      (3) Ataxic cerebral palsy: a lesion in the cerebellum results in hypotonia and ataxic movements; characterized by a lack of stability so coactivation is difficult, resulting in more primitive total patterns of movement. Classification is according to level of severity.
         (a) Previously classified as mild, moderate and severe.
         (b) Current gross motor classification: the Gross Motor Functional Classification System (GMFCS) which delineates five levels of functional motor performance for children aged 6 to 12 years. See Table 7-5.
         (c) Current manual ability classification: the Manual Ability Classification System (MACS) for Children with Cerebral Palsy which describes five levels of handling objects placed within easy reach and everyday functional tasks. See Table 7-5.
   e. The distribution of the disorder in limbs determines the classification.
      (1) Monoplegia involves one extremity.
      (2) Hemiplegia involves the upper and lower extremity on the same side.
      (3) Paraplegia involves the lower extremities.
      (4) Quadriplegia involves all extremities.
      (5) Diplegia involves less upper extremity involvement and greater lower extremity functional impairment.
4. Complications.
   a. Seizures occur in 50% of children with cerebral palsy.
   b. Language and cognitive deficits occur in 50%–75% of children with cerebral palsy. These include:
      (1) Speech and language deficits.
      (2) Difficulty coordinating breathing with swallowing which is a necessary function for speech.
      (3) Dysarthria.
      (4) Aphasia.
      (5) Cognitive deficits are more typically associated with the presence of seizures.
   c. Visual impairments occur in 40%–50% of children with cerebral palsy.
      (1) Strabismus: deviation of how one eye aligns with the other.
      (2) Nystagmus: a reflexive response of the eyes triggered by head movement.
      (3) Refractive errors:
         (a) Myopia (nearsightedness).

Table 7-5

The Manual Ability Classification System (MACS) for Children with Cerebral Palsy

LEVEL	DESCRIPTION OF FUNCTIONAL MOTOR PERFORMANCE
For Each Level of the Gross Motor Functional Classification System	
I	Walks without restrictions; limitations in more advanced gross motor skills.
II	Walks without assistive devices; limitations walking outdoors and in the community.
III	Walks with assistive mobility devices; limitations walking outdoors and in the community.
IV	Self-mobility with limitations; children are transported or use power mobility outdoors and in the community.
V	Self-mobility is severely limited, even with the use of assistive technology.
For Each Level of the Manual Ability Classification System for Children With Cerebral Palsy	
I	Handles objects easily and successfully.
II	Handles most objects but with somewhat reduced quality and/or speed of achievement.
III	Handles objects with difficulty; needs help to prepare and/or modify activities.
IV	Handles a limited selection of easily managed objects in adapted situations.
V	Does not handle objects and has severely limited ability to perform even simple actions.

Missiuna, C., Polatajko, H., Pollock, N., & Cameron, D. (2012). Neuromotor disorders, p. 463. In Lane & Bundy (Eds.). *Kids can be kids: A childhood occupation.* Philadelphia: FA Davis.

(b) Hyperopia (farsightedness).
(c) Presbyopia: decreased elasticity of the lenses causing difficulty in accommodation when focusing on objects nearby and when shifting focus from near to far.

d. Feeding disturbances (e.g., difficulty swallowing, chewing).
e. Diminished sensation is common in spastic hemiplegia.

5. Medical management.
   a. Antispasticity drugs (e.g., benzodiazepines).
   b. Medication to reduce tremors and relax muscles (e.g., baclofen pumps).
   c. Medication to relax muscles to decrease muscle stiffness and increase controlled movement (e.g., botulinum toxin [Botox]).
   d. Orthopedic management to address development of scoliosis and joint contractures.
   e. Surgery may be indicated to decrease contractures and improve functional movement (e.g., dorsal rhizotomy surgery).
   f. Medications for seizures if present.
   g. Dietary interventions and special feeding techniques for regularity in elimination and/or other medical complications.
6. Occupational therapy evaluation and intervention.
   a. See Chapter 5: Human Biopsychosocial Growth and Development Across the Lifespan.
   b. See Chapter 12: Neurological Approaches: Evaluation and Intervention.
   c. See Chapter 15: Evaluation and Intervention for Performance in Areas of Occupation.

Disorders of Movement/Neuromuscular Diseases

Classification of Symptoms

1. Tremor: rhythmic, alternating, oscillatory movements produced by repetitive patterns of muscle contraction and relaxation.
   a. Tremors are classified by rate, rhythm, and distribution.
   b. Tremors are identified as to whether they occur at rest (resting tremor) or during activity (action or intention tremor).
2. Dyskinesias: involuntary, nonrepetitive, but occasionally stereotyped movements affecting distal, proximal, and axial musculature in varying combinations. Most dyskinesias are representative of basal ganglia disorders.
3. Myoclonus: a brief and rapid contraction of a muscle or group of muscles.
4. Tics: brief, rapid, involuntary movements, often resembling fragments of normal motor behavior. They tend to be stereotyped and repetitive, but not rhythmic.

5. Chorea: brief, purposeless, involuntary movements of the distal extremities and face; usually considered to be a manifestation of dopaminergic overactivity in the basal ganglia.
6. Dystonia: results in sustained abnormal postures and disruptions of ongoing movement resulting from alterations of muscle tone. Dystonias may be generalized or focal.
7. Ataxia: describes a lack of coordination while performing voluntary movements. It may appear as clumsiness, inaccuracy, or instability. Movements are not smooth and may appear disjointed or jerky.
8. Hemiballismus: usually characterized by involuntary flinging motions of the extremities. The movements are often violent and have wide amplitudes of motion. They are continuous and random and can involve proximal and/or distal muscles on one side of the body.

Parkinson's Disease

1. Etiology: a hypokinetic CNS movement disorder that is idiopathic, slowly progressive, and degenerative.
2. Prevalence, onset, and prognosis.
   a. Onset of the disease is usually after age 40, with increasing incidence in older age groups.
   b. Occurs in 1% of the population over 50.
   c. Rate of deterioration ranges from 2 to 20 years.
3. Symptoms.
   a. Begins insidiously with a resting "pill-rolling" tremor of one hand.
   b. Cardinal signs include tremor, rigidity, resistance to passive motion that is not velocity dependent (cogwheel or lead pipe), akinesia, postural instability, festinating gait, falling backwards (retropulsion) or forwards (propulsion), mask face, micrographia.
4. Diagnostic testing.
   a. Presence of cardinal signs.
   b. Degeneration in dopaminergic pathways in the basal ganglia, primarily in the substantia nigra.
   c. Positive response to Sinemet (Levodopa/Carbidopa).
   d. Stage of disease progression is diagnosed using Hoehn and Yahr's five-stage scale.
      (1) Stage I = unilateral tremor, rigidity, akinesia, minimal or no functional impairment.
      (2) Stage II = bilateral tremor, rigidity or akinesia, with or without axial signs, independent with ADL, no balance impairment.
      (3) Stage III = worsening of symptoms, first signs of impaired righting reflexes, onset of disability in ADL performance, can lead independent life.
      (4) Stage IV = requires help with some or all ADL, unable to live alone without some assistance, able to walk and stand unaided.
      (5) Stage V = confined to a wheelchair or bed, maximally assisted.
5. Medical management.
   a. Surgical interventions: thalamotomy, pallidotomy, fetal tissue transplant, deep brain stimulators.
   b. Pharmacology: Levodopa (the metabolic precursor of dopamine), Sinemet (Levodopa/Carbidopa), dopamine agonists, anticholinergics (Benadryl, Artane, Cogentin) for rigidity and tremors, dopamine releasers (Amantadine).
   c. Side effects are common when the disease is being managed pharmacologically.
      (1) During early treatment, side effects from carbidopa-levodopa therapy are usually not a major problem.
      (2) As the disease progresses, the drug works less evenly and predictably.
         (a) As a result, some people may experience involuntary movements (dyskinesia), primarily when the medication is having its peak effects.
         (b) The length of time for which each dose is effective may begin to shorten (wearing-off effect), leading to more frequent doses.
      (3) The on-off effect, of long-term carbido-palevodopa usage may cause Parkinson's-related movement problems to appear and disappear suddenly and unpredictably.
      (4) Other side effects may include:
         (a) Hallucinations.
         (b) A drop in blood pressure when standing (orthostatic hypotension).
         (c) Nausea.
   d. Despite the above potential side effects, carbidopa-levodopa typically allows people with Parkinson's disease to extend the time that they are able to lead relatively normal lives and in many cases is effective for a number of years.

Spina Bifida

1. Etiology is unknown.
   a. Genetic, intrauterine, and/or environmental factors contribute to the failure of the spinal column's vertebral arches to fully form to enclose and to protect the neural tube. This defect may result in a protrusion of the neural tube.
   b. Some studies suggest certain medications and a lack of folic acid may induce neural tube defects.
2. Onset, prevalence, and prognosis.
   a. Occurs in about 1 in every 1,000 births.
      (1) The most common neural tube disorder.
      (2) Incidence has decreased with folic acid being prescribed to women before and during pregnancy.
         (a) Selective abortion has also decreased incidence.

(3) The first year survival rate for infants has increased to over 92%.
(4) The survival rate of infants with encephalocele is over 75%.

b. The prognosis and degree of impairment is dependent on the level of the lesion and the extent of the neural tube defect of the vertebral arches and the spinal column.
(1) Lesions usually occur in the thoracic or lumbar spine.

3. Diagnosis.
a. Detected prenatally through amniocentesis for levels of alpha-fetoprotein (AFP) and acetylcholinesterase, and ultrasound if indicated.
b. A less reliable means of prenatal detection involves determining the amount of AFP the unborn baby produces in the mother's blood.

4. Classification of spina bifida is dependent on the level of the leision and the extent of tissue involved.
a. Spina bifida occulta: a bony malformation with separation of vertebral arches of one or more vertebrae with no external manifestations; may not be discovered until late childhood.
(1) Occult spinal dysraphism (OSD): when external manifestations such as a red birthmark (hemangioma or flame nevus), patch of hair, a dermal sinus (opening in skin), a fatty benign tumor (lipoma), or dimple covering the site are present.
b. Spina bifida cystica: an exposed pouch comprised of the spinal cord and meninges.
(1) Spina bifida with meningocele: protrusion of a sac through the spine, containing cerebral spinal fluid and meninges; however, does not include the spinal cord.
(2) Spina bifida with myelomeningocele: protrusion of a sac through the spine, containing cerebral spinal fluid and meninges as well as the spinal cord or nerve roots.
(a) Most commonly located in the lumbar region, however it can occur at any point along the spinal column.

5. Specific symptoms.
a. Spina bifida occulta usually does not result in any symptoms.
(1) Occasionally slight instability and neuromuscular impairments, such as mild gait involvement and bowel or bladder problems may occur.
b. Occult spinal dysraphism may result in the spinal cord being split (diplomyelia) or being tied down and tethered (diastematomyelia) which may lead to neurological damage and developmental abnormality as the child grows.
c. Spina bifida meningocele usually does not present with symptoms impacting on function as the spinal cord itself is not entrapped.
(1) Occasionally slight instability and neuromuscular impairments, such as mild gait involvement and bowel or bladder problems may occur.
d. Spina bifida with a myelomeningocele results in sensory and motor deficits occurring below the level of the lesion, and may result in lower extremity paralysis and/or deformities, bowel and bladder incontinence, decubitus ulcer and deep vein thrombosis.
(1) The level of lesions determine the impact leg movements.
(2) Lesions of S2–S4 results in bladder and bowel problems.
(a) A neurogenic bladder impacts on the sensation to urinate and the control of the urinary sphincter.
(b) Incomplete emptying of the bladder results; this often leads to infections.
(c) A neurogenic bowel causes constipation and incontinence.

6. Tethered cord syndrome occurs in the tail end of the spinal cord when the cord is stretched as a result of compression, being trapped with a fatty mass or scar tissue, developmental abnormality, or an injury.
a. Visible signs include a hairy patch of skin, a hemangioma, and/or a dimple of the lower spine.
b. Difficulties with bowel and bladder control, gait disturbances, and/or deformities of the feet, low back pain, scoliosis, may result.
c. May go undiagnosed until the above symptoms emerge.
d. Symptoms may be exacerbated with pregnancy or with age due to spinal stenosis.

7. Medical management.
a. During the neonatal period precautions are taken to protect the sac from rupturing and from infection which may result in meningitis.
(1) All or part of the sac may be removed 24 to 48 hours after birth.
b. A ventriculoperitoneal or other type of shunt is indicated should the complication of hydrocephalus occur, in which the cerebral spinal fluid is not absorbed resulting in an increase in size of the ventricles and the infant's head.
(1) Brain damage as a result of increased intracranial pressure can cause mental retardation.
(2) Increased pressure may also result in Arnold-Chiari Syndrome in which a portion of the cerebellum and medulla oblongata slip down through the foramen magnum to the cervical spinal cord.
(3) Shunts can become blocked resulting in increased intra-cranial pressure.
(a) Signs and symptoms during the first year of life include extreme head growth and often a soft spot on the forehead.

(b) Signs and symptoms by the second year of life include severe headache, vomiting, and/or irritability.
(c) Intracranial pressure can possibly lead to paralysis of the sixth cranial nerve resulting in visual impairments.
(d) Intracranial pressure may contribute to seizure disorders and deterioration of physical and/or cognitive functioning.
(4) Shunts can become infected.
(a) Signs and symptoms include vomiting, lethargy, and/or fever.
(b) Seizures and deterioration of physical and/or cognitive functioning may result.
(5) Early identification is vital, as these conditions are life threatening.
(a) Immediate notification of signs and symptoms to the child's/facility's neurosurgeon is required.
(b) Blocked shunts are revised by removing the blocked section and replacing it with a catheter.
(c) Infections are treated by withdrawing fluid through or replacing the tubing. Intravenous antibiotics are also administered.
(d) Medications to reduce cerebrospinal fluid production and intra-cranial pressure are sometimes used as an interim measure.

c. Urological management, and if indicated intermittent catheterization.
d. Orthopedic management for motor deficits.
e. Surgical intervention may be indicated for tethered cord syndrome.

Muscular Dystrophies/Atrophies

1. Etiology: a group of degenerative disorders resulting in muscle weakness and decreased muscle mass due to a hereditary disease process.
   a. Muscular dystrophies are due to an absent muscle protein product, dystrophin.
   b. In muscular dystrophies blood tests demonstrating a highly elevated level of creatine kinase (CK) provide a differential diagnosis to congenital myopathies in which levels of creatine kinase are normal or just slightly elevated.
   c. The responsible genes and biochemical abnormalities can be tested through a muscle biopsy to determine the level or absence of dystrophin.
2. Onset, prevalence, and prognosis.
   a. Muscular dystrophies/atrophies can begin in infancy, childhood, or adulthood.
   b. First symptoms may not be apparent until 2.5 years of age.
   c. Average age of diagnosis is 5 years, unless there is a known family history; whereby, earlier detection is more likely to occur.
   d. Prevalence of muscular dystrophy: 1 in 5,600 to 1 in 7,700 males aged 5 to 24 years.
      (1) Prenatal testing and selective abortion accounts for a decrease in the number of children born with muscular dystrophies.
   e. Progress may be rapid and fatal, or may remain stable throughout life.
      (1) Those starting early in life tend to be more severe and to progress more rapidly.
3. Diagnosis.
   a. Detection is confirmed by blood tests for muscle enzymes or muscle proteins, nerve conduction velocity, electromyography, and, if indicated muscle or nerve biopsy.
   b. In muscular dystrophies blood tests demonstrate a high elevated level of creatine kinase (CK).
   c. Common symptoms include hypotonia, muscle weakness, and atrophy.
4. Major types.
   a. Duchenne's muscular dystrophy is the most common form of muscular dystrophy.
      (1) It is detected between two and six years of age.
      (2) It is inherited, sex-linked and recessive occurring in males 1 per 3,500 to 6,000 male births.
      (3) Symptoms include pseudohypertrophy which is enlargement of calf muscles, and at times enlargement of the forearm and thigh muscles, giving an appearance the child is is muscular and healthy.
      (4) Weakness of the proximal joints progresses to the point that the child has significant functional mobility impairments. These include:
         (a) Ambulating with a trendelenburg (i.e., waddling) gait with frequent falls.
         (b) Difficulty getting up from the floor to a standing position; uses hands to crawl up the thighs to get to the standing position, known as Gower's sign.
      (5) Weakness occurs in all voluntary muscles, including the heart and diaphragm.
      (6) Behavioral and learning difficulties and delayed speech may occur.
      (7) Individuals rarely survive beyond their early 20s due to respiratory problems, infections, and/or cardiovascular complications.
   b. Becker muscular dystrophy.
      (1) A variant of of Duchenne muscular dystrophy that is slower to progress, less severe, and less predictable.
      (2) Presenting symptoms include:
         (a) Loss of motor function of the hips, thighs, pelvic area, and shoulders.
         (b) Enlarged calves.
         (c) Cardiac system can be involved.

(3) Survival can be into late adulthood.
(a) A normal lifespan can be attained if there is minimal cardiac involvement.

c. Arthrogryposis multiplex congenita.
(1) It is detected at birth and associated with loss of anterior horn cells.
(2) Presence of weakness, deformities, and associated joint contractures.
(3) Position of rest for the upper extremities tends to be internal rotation of the shoulders, extension of the elbows, and flexion of the wrists; for the lower extremities, there is flexion and internal rotation of the hips and clubfeet.
(4) It may be stable, mildly progressive, or may improve.
(5) Related problems include congenital heart defects, spinal defects, torticollis, and involvement of the diaphragm.

d. Limb-girdle muscular dystrophy.
(1) Onset begins between the first and third decades of life.
(2) Proximal muscles of the pelvis and shoulder are initially affected.
(3) Typically progresses slowly.

e. Fascioscapulohumeral muscular dystrophy.
(1) Occurs in early adolescence.
(2) Involves the face, upper arms, and scapular region, causing masking, weakness, decreased mobility of the face, and the inability to lift the arms above shoulder level.
(3) As it progresses, the weakness can extend to the abdominal muscles and sometimes the hip muscles.
(4) Progresses slowly and rarely affects the cardiac or respiratory systems; thus, life expectancy can be relatively normal.

f. Spinal muscular atrophy.
(1) Caused by a decrease of a motor neuron protein called Survival of Motor Neuron (SMN), Chromosone 5.
(2) Weakness of the voluntary muscles of the shoulders, hips, thighs, and upper back which can result in spinal curvatures.
(3) Muscles for breathing and swallowing can be affected.
(4) The earlier the age of diagnosis, the greater the severity of functional deficits and the shorter the life expectancy.
(a) Type I, birth or infancy: the infantile form known as Werdnig-Hoffman disease has a life expectancy up to approximately two years of age.
(b) Type II, children: the intermediate form is detected six months to three years of age and progresses rapidly with a life expectancy of early childhood.
(c) Type III, older children: later onset, less severe form.
(d) Types IV, adolescent or adult: later onset, less severe form.

g. Congenital myasthenia gravis.
(1) A disorder involving transmission of impulses in the neuromuscular junction.
(2) Onset starting near birth and occurring more frequently in males.

h. Charcot-Marie-Tooth disease.
(1) A disease involving the peripheral nerves marked by progressive weakness, primarily inperoneal [fibular] and distal leg muscles.
(2) Typically occurs in the teenage years or earlier.

i. Myopathies.
(1) Symptoms are similar to dystrophies; however, myopathies progress slowly; resulting in a better prognosis.
(2) Weakness of the face, neck and limbs is characteristic.

5. Specific symptoms.
a. Low muscle tone and weakness contributes to abnormal movement patterns and delayed developmental milestones.
b. There may be difficulty with oral motor feeding, necessitating a nasogastric or gastrostomy tube.
c. Weakness contributes to deformities of the extremities and spine.
d. Difficulty with breathing may require tracheostomies or mechanical ventilators, and frequently results in death.

6. Medical management.
a. Prescribed medications to decrease pulmonary and cardiac complications and prolong life.
b. Nutritional management for difficulties with feeding and the tendency to gain weight secondary to inactivity.
c. Prevention of skin breakdown and decubitus ulcers.
d. Steroids to help delay or reverse muscle weakness; however, the undesirable side effects associated with steroids bring their use into question.

Progressive Supranuclear Palsy

1. Etiology: manifested by loss of voluntary, but preservation of reflexive eye movements, bradykinesia, rigidity, axial dystonia, pseudobulbar palsy, and dementia.
2. Onset, prevalence, and prognosis.
a. Occurs in later middle life.
b. Affects 6.5 per 100,000 people.
c. Death occurs approximately 15 years after onset.

Huntington's Chorea

1. Etiology: an autosomal dominant disorder.
2. Onset, prevalence, and prognosis.
   a. Begins in middle-age.
   b. Onset of this disease process is insidious.
   c. Occurs in 1 in 10,000.
   d. Characterized by choreiform movements and progressive intellectual deterioration.
   e. Psychiatric disturbance (personality change, manic-depressive symptoms, and schizophreniform illness) may precede the onset of the movement disorder.

Cerebellar/Spinocerebellar Disorders

1. Etiology: characterized by ataxia, dysmetria, dysdiadochokinesia, hypotonia, movement decomposition tremor, dysarthria, and nystagmus.

Structural Cerebellar Lesions

1. Etiology: includes vascular lesions (stroke) and tumor deposits, producing symptoms and signs appropriate to their locus within the cerebellum.
   a. Demyelinating plaques of multiple sclerosis may also arise in the cerebellum white matter and give rise to cerebellar symptoms.
   b. Alcoholism and nutritional deprivation can cause degeneration of the vermis and anterior cerebellum.

Spinocerebellar Degenerations

1. Etiology: a group of degenerative disorders, characterized by progressive ataxia due to the degeneration of the cerebellum, brain stem, spinal cord, peripheral nerves, and the basal ganglia.
2. These disorders are grouped as spinal ataxias, cerebellar ataxias, and multiple system degeneration.
   a. Friedrich's ataxia.
      (1) Etiology: autosomal recessive inheritance.
      (2) Onset occurs in childhood or early adolescence.
      (3) Symptoms: the prototype of spinal ataxia.
         (a) This process is characterized by gait unsteadiness, upper extremity ataxia, and dysarthria.
         (b) Tremor may be a minor feature.
         (c) Presentation also includes areflexia and loss of large fiber sensory modalities.
         (d) As the disease progresses scoliosis and cardiomyopathy are common.
   b. Cerebellar cortical degeneration.
      (1) Etiology: pathologic changes are seen in the cerebellum and the inferior olives.
      (2) Onset begins between ages 30 and 50.
      (3) Symptoms: cerebellar symptoms are the only signs detectable.
   c. Multiple systems degeneration (olivopontocerebellar atrophies).
      (1) Etiology: characterized by spasticity, extrapyramidal, sensory, lower motor neuron, and autonomic dysfunction.
      (2) Onset occurs in young to middle life.
3. Medical management for movement disorders is limited in many cases.
   a. Pharmacologic intervention may be able to dampen effects of the movement disorders.
   b. Agents utilized for this population include propranolol, clonazepam, clonidine, and anticholinergic agents depending upon symptomatology.

Disorders of the Peripheral Nervous System/Neuromuscular Diseases

Amyotrophic Lateral Sclerosis (ALS)

1. Etiology: motor neuron disease of unknown etiology characterized by progressive degeneration of corticospinal tracts and anterior horn cells or bulbar efferent neurons.
2. Onset, prevalence, and prognosis.
   a. The disease is more prevalent in men than women at a ratio of 1.2:1.
   b. Onset occurs at an average age of 57.
   c. Death usually occurs in 2–5 years.
3. Symptoms.
   a. Muscle weakness and atrophy, evidence of anterior horn cell destruction, often begins distally and asymmetrically.
   b. Cramps and fasciculations precede weakness.

c. Signs usually begin in the hands.
d. Lower motor neuron signs are soon accompanied by spasticity, hyperactive deep tendon reflexes, and evidence of corticospinal tract involvement.
e. Dysarthria and dysphagia are evident.
f. Sensory systems, eye movements, and urinary sphincters are often spared.
g. Symptom severity is documented by scores on the ALS Functional Rating Scale. (1) Symptoms that are quantifed include speech, salivation, swallowing, handwriting, cutting food, dressing/hygiene, turning in bed, walking, climbing stairs, dyspnea, orthopnea, respiratory insufficiency, number of years with symptoms.

4. Diagnosis.
   a. Usually clinical, with generalized motor involvement unaccompanied by sensory abnormalities.
   b. Electromyography can support the diagnosis.
   c. Other processes such as spinal cord tumors and myopathies must be ruled out.
5. Medical management.
   a. There is no specific treatment to slow the disease process.
   b. Treatment is aimed at treating secondary complications such as spasticity (treated with antispasmodics), prevention of aspirations (gastrostomy and modified diets), prevention of decubiti, prevention of contracture, and pain management.

Brachial Plexus Disorder

1. Etiology: secondary to traction during birth, invasion of metastatic cancer, after radiation treatment secondary to fibrosis, or traction injury.
2. Symptoms.
   a. Mixed motor and sensory disorders of the corresponding limb.
   b. Rostral injuries produce shoulder dysfunction while caudal injuries produce dysfunction in the hand.
3. Diagnosis.
   a. Made via CT scanning of the plexus in cases where a mass is present.
   b. EMG/nerve conduction velocities are used to localize the plexus lesion.
4. Common injuries of the brachial plexus seen in children include:
   a. Erb's palsy: a paralysis of the upper brachial plexus including the fifth and sixth cervical nerves; C7 may also be involved in some cases.
      (1) Muscles most often paralyzed include the supraspinatus and infraspinatus as well as the deltoid, biceps, brachialis, and subscapularis.
      (2) The arm cannot be raised, elbow flexion is weakened and weakness in retraction and protraction of scapula may be noted.
      (3) The arm grossly presents with the arm straight and wrist fully bent (the "waiter's tip" position).
      (4) After the age of 6 months, contractures may begin to develop (adduction and internal rotation contractures).
         (a) Supination deformity of the forearm may also develop from the imbalance between the supinator and the paralyzed pronator muscles.
      (5) Positioning and ROM exercises are necessary to retain external rotation, abduction, and flexion at the shoulder as well as distal flexibility.
   b. Klumpke's Palsy: a paralysis of the lower brachial plexus including the seventh and eighth cervical and first thoracic nerves.
      (1) Relatively rare when compared to the prevalence of Erb's Palsy.
      (2) It results in paralysis of the hand and wrist, often with ipsilateral Horner's syndrome (miosis, ptosis, and facial anhidrosis).
      (3) Characteristic signs are that the hand is limp and the fingers do not move.

Peripheral Neuropathies

1. Etiology: peripheral neuropathy of a single nerve may be the result of trauma, pressure paralysis, forcible overextension of a joint, hemorrhage into a nerve, exposure to cold or radiation, or ischemic paralysis.
   a. Multiple nerves may be affected in cases of collagen vascular disease, metabolic diseases (diabetes mellitus), or infectious agents (Lyme disease).
   b. Other causes include nutritional deficiency, malignancy, microorganisms, exposure to toxic agents, and chronic alcohol abuse.
2. Diagnosis.
   a. Focused on the cause of the symptoms.
   b. Specific tests utilized include electromyography, nerve conduction velocity, muscle biopsy, and examinations to identify systemic disorders.
3. Symptoms.
   a. A syndrome of sensory, motor, reflex, and vasomotor symptoms.
   b. Symptoms include pain, weakness, and paresthesias in the distribution of the affected nerve.
4. Medical management.
   a. Guided by the underlying disease process, not the symptoms of the neuropathy.
   b. Treatment of the underlying systemic disorder (diabetes, tumor, multiple myeloma), may slow progression, although recovery is slow.

Guillain-Barré Syndrome

1. Etiology is unknown. May occur after an infectious disorder, surgery, or an immunization.

2. Onset, prevalence, and prognosis.
   a. Affects both sexes at any age.
   b. Onset of recovery is 2–4 weeks after first symptoms.
   c. Long-term prognosis.
      (1) 50% exhibit mild neurological deficits.
      (2) 15% exhibit residual functional deficits.
      (3) 80% are ambulatory in 6 months.
      (4) 5% die of complications.
3. Diagnosis.
   a. Diagnosis is based on clinical symptoms.
   b. Lumbar puncture reveals increased protein without cells in the cerebrospinal fluid.
   c. Electromyography and nerve conduction studies may support the diagnosis.
   d. Segmental demyelination is apparent and in severe cases, axonal degeneration accompanies the demyelination.
4. Symptoms.
   a. Acute, rapidly progressive form of polyneuropathy characterized by symmetric muscular weakness and mild distal sensory loss/paresthesias.
   b. Weakness is always more apparent than sensory findings and is at first more prominent distally.
   c. Relatively minor sensory signs and symptoms occur.
      (1) The patient may complain of painful extremities.
      (2) Subjective and objective sensory disturbances are common initially.
         (a) Most commonly occurring in a distal (stocking-glove) distribution.
   d. Deep tendon reflexes are lost and sphincters are spared.
   e. Respiratory failure and dysphagia may be seen in some cases.
5. Medical management.
   a. Severe cases constitute a medical emergency requiring constant monitoring of vital signs.
   b. Respiratory support may be necessary in some cases.
   c. Plasmapheresis may be utilized to slow symptoms or halt progression.
   d. Intravenous immunoglobulin has been utilized effectively.

Myasthenia Gravis

1. Etiology: the disease is caused by an autoimmune attack on the acetylcholine receptor of the postsynaptic neuromuscular junction.
   a. This process is considered a disorder of neuromuscular transmission.
   b. The initiating event leading to antibody production is unknown.
2. Onset, prevalence, and prognosis.
   a. Occurs at any age but most often affects younger women and older men.
   b. Occurs in 14 per 100,000.
   c. Prognosis varies, but usually is a progressive disabling process.
   d. Death may occur from respiratory complications.
3. Diagnosis.
   a. Diagnosis is often missed because of the rarity of the disease and the vagueness of symptoms.
   b. Characterized by episodic muscle weakness, chiefly in muscles innervated by cranial nerves.
   c. The possibility of myasthenia gravis is suggested by any of the below symptoms and is confirmed by response to anticholinesterase drugs.
4. Symptoms.
   a. Common symptoms include ptosis, diplopia, muscle fatigue after exercise, dysarthria, dysphagia, and proximal limb weakness.
   b. Sensation and deep tendon reflexes are intact.
   c. Symptoms fluctuate over the course of the day.
   d. In relapsing periods, quadriparesis may develop.
   e. Life threatening respiratory muscle involvement may occur.
5. Medical management.
   a. Treatment includes cholinesterase inhibitors, corticosteroids, immunosuppressive agents, and plasmapheresis.
   b. The anticholinergics and plasmapheresis treat current symptoms.
   c. Corticosteroids and immunosuppressives may alter the disease course by interfering with autoimmune pathogenesis.

Post-Polio Syndrome (PPS)

1. Etiology: some motor neurons infected with the polio virus die (leaving paralyzed muscle cells), others survive. Recovered motor neurons develop new terminal axon sprouts that reinnervate muscle cells. After years of stability, these motor units break down, causing new muscle weakness.
   a. Degeneration of the axon sprouts explains the new weakness and fatigue, but the mechanism remains controversial.
   b. A current explanation is related to the overuse of individual motor neurons over time.
2. Onset, prevalence, and prognosis.

a. 250,000 people live with post-polio syndrome.
b. Onset is typically 15 years after recovery from polio.
c. Progress is slow with a good prognosis unless breathing or swallowing difficulties occur.
3. Diagnosis.
a. Based on clinical symptoms.
b. Characterized by the onset of new muscle weakness after years of stable functioning.
c. Disuse weakness should be ruled out.
4. Symptoms.
a. New onset of weakness.
b. Easily fatigued.
c. Muscle pain.
d. Joint pain.
e. Cold intolerance.
f. Atrophy.
g. Loss of functional skills.
5. Medical management.
a. Bracing with orthoses and pacing daily activity.
b. Stretching programs.
c. Exercise program.
d. Low doses of tricyclic antidepressants to relieve muscle pain.
e. Pyridostigmine to reduce fatigue and improve strength.

Demyelinating Disease

Multiple Sclerosis (MS)

1. Etiology: the exact cause is unknown.
a. The myelin damage is probably mediated by the immune system.
b. Postulated etiologies include infection by a slow or latent virus and the possibility of environmental factors contributing to the disease.
2. Onset, prevalence, and prognosis.
a. More prevalent in areas further north of the equator.
b. Approximately 300,000 people are living with MS in the United States; 2.1 million people worldwide.
(1) A significantly higher incidence of the disease is found in the northernmost latitudes of the northern and the southern hemispheres compared to southernmost latitudes.
c. Occurs most often between the ages of 20 and 50; it is most often diagnosed when persons are in their 30s.
d. Overall prognosis is variable with an unpredictable disease course.
3. Diagnosis.
a. Diagnosis is largely based on symptoms.
b. Slowly progressive CNS disease characterized by patches of demyelination in the brain and spinal cord.
c. Basic diagnostic criteria are evidence of multiple CNS lesions and evidence of at least two episodes of neurological disturbance in an individual between 10 and 59 years.
d. Diagnostics may include MRI to detect lesions, evoked potentials to measure conduction along sensory pathways, and cerebrospinal fluid examination.
4. Symptoms.
a. Multiple and varied neurologic symptoms and signs, usually with remissions and exacerbations.
b. Onset of symptoms is usually insidious.
c. Paresthesias in one or more extremities, on the trunk, or in the face.
d. Weakness or clumsiness in the leg or hand is common.
e. Visual disturbance (diplopia, partial blindness, nystagmus, eye pain, etc.).
f. Emotional disturbances (lability, euphoria, and reactive depression).
g. Balance loss and/or vertigo.
h. Bladder dysfunction.
i. Cognitive features may include apathy, memory loss, lack of judgment, and inattention.
j. Sensorimotor findings may include: spasticity, increased reflexes, ataxia, weakness, gait instability, easy fatigue, hemiplegia or quadriplegia.
k. The course of the symptoms is highly variable and may follow one of four patterns.
(1) Relapsing remitting.
(2) Secondary progressive.
(3) Primary progressive.
(4) Progressive relapsing.
5. Medical management is symptom-specific.
a. During acute exacerbation, anti-inflammatory drugs are used to control symptoms.
b. Antispasmodics (Baclofen) may be effective to counteract spasticity.
c. Management of bowel and bladder dysfunction may require pharmacologic intervention. Catheterization (indwelling or intermittent) is necessary in many cases of bladder dysfunction.
d. Disease modifying drugs are used to slow progression. Examples include Avonex, Betaseron, Copaxone, and Rebif.

Overview of Occupational Therapy Evaluation and Intervention for Neurological System Disorders

Occupational Profile

1. The initial step in the evaluation process that provides an understanding of the client's occupational history and experiences, patterns of daily living, interests, values, and needs.
2. The client's problems and concerns about performing occupations and daily life activities are identified and the client's priorities are determined.

Analysis of Performance in Areas of Occupation

1. Basic activities of daily living (BADL).
2. Instrumental activities of daily living (IADL).
3. Education.
4. Work.
5. Play and leisure.
6. Rest and sleep.
7. Social participation.
8. See Chapter 15 for more information on the evaluation of occupational performance.

Evaluation of Client Factors and Performance Skills

1. Determine sensory and motor dysfunction and strengths.
   a. Extent of paralysis/weakness.
   b. Severity and distribution of spasticity.
   c. Gross and fine motor coordination loss.
   d. Evaluation of sensory modalities: light touch, pain, pressure, proprioception, kinesthesia, temperature, gustatory, olfactory, auditory.
   e. Postural control evaluation.
   f. Range of motion testing.
   g. Manual muscle testing.
   h. Skin integrity.
2. Determine cognitive/perceptual dysfunction and strengths.
   a. Evaluation of foundation visual skills: acuity, visual fields, ocular range of motion, accommodation, pursuits, saccades.
   b. Evaluation of pervasive impairments: decreased arousal, decreased alertness, loss of selective/sustained attention, concrete thinking, decreased insight, impaired judgment, confusion, disorientation, language dysfunction, impaired motivation, and impaired initiative.
   c. Evaluation of the impact of specific deficits on basic and instrumental activities of daily living and mobility including apraxia, spatial neglect, body neglect, perseveration, spatial relations dysfunction, various agnosias, organization and sequencing dysfunction, and memory loss.
3. Determine psychosocial dysfunction and strengths.
   a. Evaluation of emotional/affective disturbances: lability, euphoria, apathy, depression, aggression, irritability, frustration tolerance.
   b. Coping mechanisms.
   c. Adaptation to change in occupational role functioning or to difficulty in assuming occupational roles.
4. See subsequent evaluation chapters for more information on each of the above areas.

Performance Context Evaluation

1. Cultural barriers.
2. Architectural barriers.
3. Societal limitations.
   a. Financial barriers.
   b. Stigma.
4. Home evaluation.
5. School/work site evaluations.
6. See Chapter 16 for more information on the evaluation of environmental contexts.

General Intervention/Treatment Guidelines

1. Positioning.
   a. Seating and wheeled mobility prescription.
   b. Bed positioning.
   c. Pressure reduction and pressure relief techniques.
2. Postural control training for seated and standing activities.
3. Motor learning approaches.
4. Motor control retraining/relearning for functional integration of affected limbs.
5. Specific ADL training/retraining/adaptation.
6. Prescription of assistive devices and technology.
7. Splinting for contracture prevention and/or enhancement of function (e.g., tenodesis splint).
8. Family/caregiver education.
9. Cognitive-perceptual retraining/compensation in the context of functional activities.
10. Visual skills retraining and/or adaptation (e.g., visual occlusion for diplopia).

11. Intervention for sexual dysfunction.
12. Bowel and bladder training with adaptive techniques and equipment.
13. Skin care education.
14. Durable medical equipment prescription.
15. Sensory re-education, compensation, and safety training for those without return of sensation.
16. Assistance with the development of coping strategies.
17. Community re-integration.
18. Return to work or work hardening programs for adults.
19. Collaboration with educational team for children.
20. See subsequent intervention chapters for more information on each of the above areas.

Pain

Definition

1. The sensory and emotional experience associated with actual or potential tissue damage.

Pain Pathways/Neurophysiology

1. Fast pain: transmitted over A delta fibers.
   a. Processed in spinal cord dorsal horn lamina (I & V).
   b. Crosses to excite lateral (neo) spinothalamic tract.
   c. Terminates in brain stem reticular formation and thalamus with projections to cortex.
   d. Functions for localization, discrimination of pain.
2. Slow pain: transmitted over C fibers.
   a. Processed in spinal cord lamina (II & III to V).
   b. Crosses to excite anterior (paleo) spinothalamic tract.
   c. Terminates in brain stem reticular formation.
   d. Excites reticular activating system (RAS).
   e. Functions for diffuse arousal (protective/aversive reactions), affective and motivational aspects of pain.
   f. Also terminates in thalamus with projections to cortex.
3. Intrinsic inhibitory mechanisms.
   a. Gate control theory: transmission of sensation at spinal cord level is controlled by balance between large fibers (A alpha, A beta) and small fibers (A delta, C).
      (1) Activity of large fibers at the level of first synapse can block activity of small fibers and pain transmission (counter-irritant theory).
   b. Descending analgesic systems: endogenous opiates (endorphins, enkephalins) produced throughout CNS in periaqueductal gray, raphe nuclei, and pituitary gland/hypothalamus; can depress pain transmission at various sites through mechanisms of presynaptic inhibition.

Acute Pain

1. Pain provoked by noxious stimulation.
2. Associated with an underlying pathology (injury or acute inflammation/disease).
3. Signs include sharp pain and sympathetic changes (increased heart rate, increased blood pressure, pupillary dilation, sweating, hyperventilation, anxiety, protective/escape behaviors).

Chronic Pain

1. Pain that persists beyond the usual course of healing.
2. Symptoms present for greater than 6 months for which an underlying pathology is no longer identifiable or may never have been present.

Pain Syndromes

1. Neuropathic pain: pain as a result of lesions in some part of the nervous system (central or peripheral); usually accompanied by some degree of sensory deficit.
   a. Thalamic pain: continuous, intense pain occurring on the contralateral hemiplegic side; the result of a stroke involving the ventral posterolateral thalamus; poor rehabilitation potential.
   b. Complex Regional Pain Syndrome Type I (formerly known as reflex sympathetic dystrophy, [RSD]): pain maintained by efferent activity of sympathetic nervous system.
      (1) Characterized by abnormal burning pain (causalgia), hypersensitivity to light touch, and sympathetic hyperfunction (coldness, sweating, etc.).
      (2) Usually associated with traumatic injury.
   c. Disorders of peripheral roots and nerves.
      (1) Complex Regional Pain Syndrome Type II (formerly known as neuralgia): pain occurring along the branches of a nerve; frequently paroxysmal.
      (2) Radiculalgia: neuralgia of nerve roots.
      (3) Paresthesias, allodynia: with nerve injury or transection.
   d. Herpes Zoster (shingles): an acute, painful mononeuropathy caused by the varicella-zoster virus.

(1) Characterized by vesicular eruption and marked inflammation of the posterior root ganglion of the affected spinal nerve or sensory ganglion of the cranial nerve; ventral root involvement (motor weakness) in 5%–10% of cases.
(2) Infection can last from 10 days to 5 weeks.
(3) Pain may persist for months (post-herpetic neuralgia).

e. Phantom limb pain: pain in a limb following amputation of that limb; differentiated from far more common phantom limb sensation.
f. Musculoskeletal pain: see Chapter 6.
g. Psychosomatic pain: the origin of the pain experience is due to mental or emotional disorders.
h. Headache and craniofacial pain, e.g., temporomandibular joint syndrome (TMJ).
i. Referred pain: pain arising from deep visceral tissues that is felt in a body region remote from the site of pathology, resulting in tenderness and cutaneous hyperalgesia; e.g., medial left arm pain with heart attack; right subscapular pain from gallbladder attack.

Assessment of Chronic Pain

1. History: determine chief complaints, description of onset, and mechanism of injury.
2. Determine localization: chronic pain is poorly localized, not well defined.
3. Identify nature of pain: constant, intermittent.
4. Determine irritating stimuli/activities.
5. Determine subjective assessment using pain intensity rating scales.
   a. Simple descriptive scales: verbal report, (e.g., select the words that best describe your pain).
   b. Semantic differentiation scales (e.g., McGill Pain Questionnaire).
   c. Numerical rating scales (rate pain on a scale of 1 to 10, e.g., 8/10).
   d. Visual analog scale (e.g., bisect line where your pain falls, from mild to severe pain).
   e. Spatial distribution of pain: using drawings to plot location, type of pain.
   f. Visual scales (e.g., Wong-Baker FACES® Pain Rating Scale).
6. Physical examination: identification of underlying pathology (cause of pain); objective physical findings are usually not readily identified.
   a. Assess all systems: musculoskeletal, neurologic, and cardiopulmonary. Check for muscle guarding.
   b. Check for postural stress syndrome (PSS): chronic muscle lengthening and/or shortening that causes postural malalignment and stress to soft tissues.
   c. Check for movement adaptation syndrome (MAS): habituated movement dysfunction.
   d. Check for autonomic changes (sympathetic activity): typically present with acute pain but not with chronic pain.
   e. Assess for abnormal movements.
7. Assess degree of suffering.
   a. Verbal complaints are out of proportion to degree of underlying pathology; include emotional content.
   b. The person exhibits a stooped posture, antalgic gait.
   c. The person exhibits facial grimacing.
8. Assess for functional changes.
   a. Check for self-imposed limited activity; disrupted lifestyle; disuse syndrome.
   b. Check for avoidance of work, home management, leisure, social, and/or sexual activity.
9. Assess for consequences of pain, behavioral impact, and secondary gains.
   a. Monetary benefits (malingering, insurance claims).
   b. Sympathy and attention.
   c. Avoidance of undesirable tasks.
10. Assess for depression and anxiety.
11. Assess for prescription drug misuse.
12. Assess for dependence on health care system: multiple health care providers, clinical services; "shopping around" behaviors.
13. Determine responsiveness of pain to physiological interventions/treatments: chronic pain is often unresponsive.
14. Determine motivational/affective components.
    a. Previous experience with pain.
    b. Learned responses to pain.
    c. Perception of control over pain.
    d. Ethnic/cultural aspects of pain.
    e. Familial response to pain behavior.

Occupational Therapy Intervention

1. Educate the individual about contributing factors.
2. Assist the individual in identifying and responding adaptively to pain behaviors.
   a. Remove behavioral reinforcers.
   b. Establish a behavior contract.
   c. Provide positive reinforcers, educational support.
   d. Demonstrate change, allow person to experience success.
   e. Practice well behaviors.
3. Assist the individual in developing strategies and using techniques to manage pain.
   a. Teach coping skills/stress management/assertive communication.
   b. Provide relaxation training.
      (1) Progressive relaxation techniques (e.g., Jacobson's), deep breathing exercises.
      (2) Guided imagery.

(3) Yoga, tai chi, ai chi.
(4) Biofeedback.

4. Refer to other professionals for direct pain/symptom control interventions.
5. Establish a realistic daily activity program.
   a. Improve overall level of conditioning: daily walking program.
   b. Improve overall functional capacity, independence in functional mobility skills, activities of daily living and meaningful occupations.
   c. Prescribe assistive devices as appropriate.
   d. Teach energy conservation techniques.
   e. Provide meaningful diversional activities.
6. Provide family education.

Sensory Processing Disorders

Etiology

1. Unknown.
2. Subtle, primarily subcorticala, neural dysfunction with impaired processing of sensory information and modulation of multisensory systems.

Symptom Classification

1. Ayre's Sensory Integration© model: see Chapter 12.
2. Dunn's model: symptoms are classified according to the interaction of sensory stimuli that are needed to stimulate a behavioral response.
   a. There are two types of neurological threshold: high neurological threshhold and low neurological threshhold.
      (1) High neurological threshold: failure to register or respond to routine environmental sensation or sensation must be experienced over a prolonged time period to elicit a behavioral response.
      (2) Low neurological threshold: the minial stimulous facilitates a behavioral over-response.
   b. There are two types of behavioral responses.
      (1) Passive behavioral response: the individual makes no attempt to change the intensity or duration of sensory input.
      (2) Active behavioral response: the individual avoids or seeks to avoid sensory stimuli.
   c. Neurological thresholds and behavioral responses combine to form four categories. These include:
      (1) Poor registration: high neurological thresholds and passive behavioral responses.
      (2) Sensory seeking: low neurological thresholds and active behavioral responses.
      (3) Sensory sensitivity: low neurological thresholds and passive behavioral responses.
      (4) Sensory avoiding: low neurological thresholds and active behavioral responses.
3. Ecological Model of Sensory Modulation Disorder describes individuals' unique response to interactions between external and internal dimensions of sensory processing in the context of their lives.
   a. External dimensions include culture, relationships, and chosen tasks.
   b. Internal dimensions include sensation, emotion, and attention.
   c. Difficulty with modulation either can result in:
      (1) Difficulties with social and environmental interactions.
      (2) Difficulties with self-regulation due to a mismatch between internal capabilities and external environment and activities.
4. Sensory processing nosology has been put forth for inclusion in diagnostic manuals which classify symptoms under the categories of:
   a. Sensory modulation disorder (SMD) in any sensory system.
      (1) Sensory overresponsivity (SOR).
      (2) Sensory underresponsivity (SUR).
      (3) Sensory seeking/craving (SS).
   b. Sensory-based motor disorder (SBMD) includes underlying sensory discrimination disorder as well as possible sensory modulation disorder.
      (1) Dyspraxia.
      (2) Sensory-based postural disorders.
   c. Sensory discrimination disorder (SDD).
      (1) Visual.
      (2) Auditory.
      (3) Tactile.
      (4) Vestibular.
      (5) Proprioceptive.
      (6) Taste/smell.

Presenting Signs and Symptoms

1. Fluctuating or extreme responsiveness while engaging in everyday activities (e.g., stress and frustration demonstrated in performance of everyday activities).
2. Difficulties in interacting with the environment in play, learning, and social situations, and while engag-

ing in other developmental and health promoting activities.
3. Difficulty with conceiving, planning, sequencing, or executing novel actions (dyspraxia).
   a. Tendency to avoid or reject simple motor challenges.
4. Poor initiation of activities as demonstrated in some children due to difficulty generating ideas (ideation).
5. Difficulty with goal-directed action on the environment, known as an adaptive response.
6. Responses may present along a continuum of under-responsivity to over-responsivity of multisensory processing and sensory seeking.
7. Tactile processing dysfunction manifestations.
   a. Deficits in modulation (regulation and organization).
      (1) Tactile defensiveness: over-responsivity to ordinary touch sensations.
         (a) The individual may demonstrate irritation and discomfort from a variety from textures such as clothing, sand, grass, glue, water, paint and/or food.
         (b) The individual may dislike brushing his/her teeth or hair.
         (c) The individual may demonstrate various behavioral responses including distractibility, anger, hostility, temper tantrums, fear, and/or distress.
      (2) Under-responsivity to tactile stimuli as demonstrated by diminished sensory registration and responsiveness.
         (a) The individual may not respond to normal levels of tactile input and may seek disproportionate amounts of stimuli to gain environmental information (eg. excessive touching of people and objects).
   b. Deficits in tactile discrimination.
      (1) Difficulty interpreting tactile information in a precise and efficient manner.
         (a) Contributes to impaired body scheme and somatodyspraxia (a disorder in motor planning due to poor tactile perception and proprioception).
         (b) Contributes to awkwardness in fine and gross motor tasks and impaired manipulation skills, visual perception, and eye-hand coordination.
         (c) Hinders ability to learn about properties and substances.
      (2) Difficulty with localizing tactile stimuli.
         (a) Impaired stereognosis and decreased fine motor and eye-hand coordination skills may be demonstrated in difficulties with writing and cutting with a scissors and knife.
8. Proprioceptive processing disorder manifestations.
   a. Deficits in modulation.
   b. Discrimination deficits demonstrated by poor awareness of position of body, body parts and body schema.
   c. Clumsiness, awkwardness.
   d. Distractibility.
   e. Motor planning and movement difficulties.
   f. Reliance on visual cues or other cognitive strategies to motor plan, guide movements, and perform tasks.
   g. Use of too much or too little force, e.g., stomping when walking, breaking objects unintentionally.
   h. Poor awareness of personal space.
   i. Seeks heavy resistance and pressure.
9. Vestibular processing disorder manifestations.
   a. Deficits in modulation.
      (1) Hypersensitivity to movement, characterized by aversion to movement impacting on the sympathetic system.
      (2) Hyposensitivity to movement characterized by the individual seeking intense vestibular stimulation without complaints of feeling dizzy, and by a tendency to be a thrill seeker unaware of potential danger.
      (3) Gravitational insecurity characterized by excessive fear during typical activities, especially when the individual's feet are off the ground, when moving backwards or upwards in space, walking on uneven terrain, jumping, getting on/off elevators, using any playground equipment involving movement, and when handling even minimal heights.
   b. Vestibular discrimination deficits, characterized by the above symptoms; however, symptoms are demonstrated on a subtle level.
   c. Low muscle tone.
   d. Postural-ocular deficits.
   e. Decreased balance and equilibrium reactions.
   f. Deficits in bilateral coordination.
   g. Low endurance.
   h. Deficient motor planning and sequencing.
   i. Behavior responses include difficulty with attention, organization of behavior, communication.
10. Sensory-based motor disorder.
   a. Deficits in proprioceptive and vestibular systems.
   b. Dyspraxia: difficulty with planning movements, particularly those that are complex or new.
   c. Postural disorders: decreased muscle tone impacting on stability.

Medical Management

1. Possible pharmacology intervention to decrease activity level.

Occupational Therapy Evaluation

1. Parent/caregiver interview regarding medical and developmental history.
2. Teacher interview regarding school performance, play, and behaviors (e.g., Sensory Processing Measure [SPM]; see Chapter 12).
3. Formal assessment of sensory processing (e.g., the Sensory Profile; see Chapter 5).
4. Informal observations of performance and behavior in a variety of settings (e.g., classroom, playground, home, and work).
5. Formal assessment of clinical observations using Ayres' unpublished and nonstandardized tools. See Chapter 12.
   a. Items to be observed include specific reflexes, crossing body midline, bilateral coordination, muscle tone.
6. Standardized tests for tactile processing, vestibular-proprioceptive processing, visual perception, practic ability and their impact on occupational functioning (e.g., SPM; see Chapter 12).

Occupational Therapy Intervention

1. See Chapter 12 for information on the sensory integration (SI) frame of reference and SI intervention approaches.

Seizure Disorders

Etiology

1. Seizure disorders must be differentiated from epilepsy.
   a. Epilepsy is a chronic state of recurrent seizures.
   b. Seizure disorder refers to a temporary disturbance in brain activity causing a group of nerve cells to fire excessively, interfering with normal brain function.
2. Seizures are typically idiopathic; they also can be hereditary.
   a. In almost two-thirds of all epilepsy cases, the cause remains unknown.
3. Seizures are often associated with other conditions. These include:
   a. Oxygen deprivation (e.g., during childbirth).
   b. Severe head injuries or brain hemorrhage.
   c. Cerebral palsy.
   d. Stroke.
   e. Brain tumors.
   f. Other neurological disorders (e.g., Alzheimer disease).
   g. Hydrocephalus.
   h. Metabolic disorders.
   i. Infections, meningitis, encephalitis, congenital infections.
   j. Rubella.

Prevalance

1. 2.3 million adults and 467,711 children in the United States have epilepsy.
2. Nearly 150,000 Americans develop the condition each year.

Specific Classifications of Seizures and Presenting Signs and Symptoms

1. Two broad groups.
   a. Primary generalized seizures: seizures begin with widespread involvement of both sides of the brain.
   b. Partial seizures seizures begin with involvement of a smaller, localized area.
      (1) The disturbance can still spread within seconds or minutes to widespread areas of the brain (known as secondary generalized seizure).
2. Generalized seizures.
   a. Tonic-clonic seizures/grand mal seizures.
      (1) Most common type of seizure disorder in children.
      (2) A brief warning/aura such as numbness, taste, smell, or other sensation occurs.
      (3) Tonic phase includes a loss of consciousness, stiffening of the body, heavy and irregular breathing, drooling, skin pallor, and occasional bladder and bowel incontinence for a few seconds before the clonic phase begins.
      (4) Clonic phase includes alternating rigidity and relaxation of muscles.
      (5) Postictal state follows the clonic phase, and includes a period of drowsiness, disorientation, or fatigue.
   b. Myoclonic-akinetic seizure.
      (1) Myoclonic seizures are not the same as infantile myoclonic seizures.

(2) Myoclonic seizures are brief, involuntary jerking of the extremities, with or without loss of consciousness.
(3) Akinetic seizures include a loss of tone.
(4) Myoclonic-akinetic seizures are difficult to control.

c. Petit mal seizures, also called absence seizures.
(1) Typically occur between ages of 4 and 12 years.
(2) A loss of consciousness without loss of muscle tone occurs.
(3) Rapid blinking or staring into space.
(4) The child does not fall down, but does not recall the episode or any lapse in time.

3. Partial focal seizures.

a. Simple partial seizures.
(1) Abnormal electrical impulses occur in a localized area of the brain, often in the motor strip of the frontal lobe.
(2) Involuntary, repetitive jerking of the left hand and arm occurs, but the individual can maintain interaction with his/her environment.
(3) Focal seizures may become generalized, and result in a loss of consciousness.

b. Complex partial or psychomotor seizures.
(1) Symptoms vary.
(2) There are alterations in consciousness and unresponsiveness.
(3) May appear confused or dazed, unable to respond to questions or directions.
(4) Automatic motions, such as lip smacking, chewing and swallowing, and nervous movement of the hands/fingers, and repetitive movements occur.
(5) Visual or auditory sensations occur just before the seizure.

4. Selected seizure syndromes.

a. Infantile spasms or West syndrome, infantile myoclonic seizures or jackknife epilepsy.
(1) Begins at 3 to 9 months of age.
(2) Dropping of the head and flexion of the arms occurs.
(3) Seizures may occur hundreds of times per day.
(4) Prognosis is generally poor.
(5) Spasms sometimes decrease after several years, but are often replaced by other seizure disorders.
(6) These seizures often indicate an underlying disorder such as tuberous sclerosis.

b. Lennax-Gastaut syndrome.
(1) Children with severe seizures, mental retardation, and a specific EEG pattern.
(2) Seizures of different types begin during the first three years of life and are difficult to control.
(3) Associated with various brain disorders from structural abnormalities to birth asphyxia.
(4) A regression of developmental status can occur in some cases.

c. Landau-Kleffer syndrome or acquired epileptic aphasia.
(1) Progressive encephalopathy.
(2) Loss of language skills.
(3) Auditory agnosia (inability to distinguish different sounds).
(4) Behavioral disturbances such as inattention.

5. Simple febrile seizures.

a. Most common type of seizure, occurring in 5%–10% of children under the age of five, precipitated by a fever.
b. The seizure lasts less than 10 minutes and it includes a loss of consciousness and involuntary, generalized jerking of a grand mal seizure.
c. These seizures usually do not cause damage and they do not lead to epilepsy.

6. Status epilepticus: prolonged seizures or seizures in rapid succession.

a. Can be life threatening, sometimes triggered when medication is stopped abruptly.
b. Rarely does sudden death occur; however, it is possible due to resulting erratic heart rhythm.
(1) Typically occurs with tonic-clonic seizures that are not well-controlled.

Diagnostic Criteria

1. Clinical observations of the obvious manifestations associated with the specific seizure disorder.
2. The EEG alone is not sufficient to diagnose a seizure disorder since the disorder does not always show up on the EEG and conversely abnormal EEG patterns may appear when there is no clinical evidence of seizures.

Impact on Occupational Performance

1. The seizure disorder and/or the anticonvulsive medication(s) prescribed to control the seizures may affect the individual's alertness and learning potential.
2. The amount of brain damage incurred by the seizures and associated conditions and the effects of medication can influence performance in all areas of occupation.

Medical Management

1. A neurologist is most often required to medically manage seizures.
2. Seizure disorders are treated with anticonvulsive medications.

a. Phenobarbital (Luminal), carbamazepine (Tegretol), Phenytoin (Dilantin) and valproic acid (Depakene) are used with grand mal seizures.
b. Ethosuximide (Zarontin) is used with petit mal seizures.
c. Carbamazepine and primidone are used with psychomotor seizures.
d. Clonazepam (Clonopin), steroids, and CTH (hormone secreted by the pituitary gland) are used with myoclonic seizures.

Intervention for Seizure Disorders

1. First aid procedures for seizures.
   a. Remain calm.
      (1) In the case of status elepticus, have someone call for immediate medical attention.
   b. Remove dangerous objects from the area.
   c. Protect the individual from harm, without interfering with the individual's movements.
   d. If the person is in a hospital bed, raise the bed rails.
   e. Do not place anything in the mouth.
   f. Turn the individual on his/her side if there is a risk of aspiration (e.g., person is salivating or vomiting).
   g. Allow the seizure to happen, protecting the head and/or extremities if injury could occur from violent shaking.
   h. Once the clonus activity is over (for tonic-clonic type), place the person in the recovery position (side-lying).
   i. Attempt placement in recovery position during seizure if person is salivating or vomits and could aspirate fluid.
   j. Monitor for improving mental state post-ictal.
   k. Do not be alarmed if the individual seems to stop breathing momentarily.
      (1) If breathing actually stops, use standard rescue breathing techniques.
   l. Call for medical attention during seizures:
      (1) If this is the individual's first seizure.
      (2) The person has a seizure in water.
      (3) If the person has a second seizure.
      (4) If the individual does not regain consciousness within 5 or 10 minutes following the seizure.
      (5) If the seizure lasts 5 minutes or more.
      (6) If the individual is diabetic or pregnant.
2. Post-seizure care.
   a. Allow the individual to rest or sleep after the seizure.
   b. Call a physician if this is the individual's first seizure, if the seizure is followed by another seizure (status epilepticus), or if the seizure lasts more than 5 minutes.
   c. Notify the parents/guardians/caregivers or designated emergency contact person that a seizure has occurred.
   d. Observe safety precautions if the individual seems groggy, confused, or weak following the seizure.
3. Occupational therapy evaluation and intervention.
   a. Assess and intervene for developmental delays as necessary.
   b. Observe all medical and safety precautions.
   c. Document and report any seizure activity, medication side effects, or behavioral changes.
   d. Refer to Chapter 15 for information on evaluation and intervention for deficits in performance in areas of occupation.

References

Anzalone, M. E., & Lane, S. J. (2012). Sensory processing disorder. In S. J. Lane & A. C. Bundy. *Kids can be kids: A childhood occupations approach* (pp. 437–459). Philadelphia: F.A. Davis.

Blackman, J. A. (1997). Spina bifida. In J. A. Blackman, *Medical aspects of developmental disabilities in children birth to three,* 3rd ed. (pp. 36–39). Gaithersberg, MD: Aspen.

Blackman, J. A. (1997). Seizure disorders. In J. A. Blackman, *Medical aspects of developmental disabilities in children birth to three,* 3rd ed. (pp. 238–246). Gaithersberg, MD: Aspen.

Bundy, A. C., & Murray, E. A. (2002). Sensory integration: A. Jean Ayres' theory revisited. In A. C. Bundy, S. J. Lane, & E. A. Murray (Eds.), *Sensory integration: Theory and practice,* 2nd ed. (pp. 3–33). Philadelphia: F.A. Davis.

Case-Smith, J. (Ed.). (2005). *Occupational therapy for children,* 5th ed. St. Louis, MO: Elsevier Mosby.

Centers for Disease Control and Prevention, (2013). *Data and statistics, muscular dystrophy – NCBDDD.* Retrieved August 4, 2013 from http://www.cdc.gov/ncbddd/musculardystrophy.data.html.

Centers for Disease Control and Prevention, (2013). *Epilepsy - Frequently asked questions.* Retrieved August 4, 2013 from http://www.cdc.gov/epilepsy/basics/faqs.htm.

Centers for Disease Control and Prevention, (2013). *Facts about muscular dystrophy.* Retrieved August 4, 2013 from http://www.cdc.gov/ncbdd/musculardystrophy/facts.html.

Centers for Disease Control and Prevention, (2013). *Spina bifida - Facts.* Retrieved August 4, 2013 from http://www.cdc.gov/ncbdd/spinalbifida/facts.html.

Centers for Disease Control and Prevention. (2013). *Treatments - muscular dystrophy.* Retrieved August 4, 2013 from http://www.cdc.gov/ncbdd/musculardystrophy/treatment.html.

Escolar, D. M., & Toisi, L. L. (2007). Muscles, bones and nerves. In M. L. Batshaw, L. Pellegrino, & N. J. Roizen (Eds.), *Children with disabilities,* 6th ed. (pp. 203–215). Baltimore: Paul H. Brooks.

Gillen, G. (Ed.). (2011). *Stroke rehabilitation: A function-based approach,* 3rd ed. St. Louis, MO: Elsevier/Mosby.

Gutman, S. A. (2007). *Quick reference neuroscience for rehabilitation professionals: The essential neurologic principles underlying rehabilitation practice,* 2nd ed. Thorofare, NJ: Slack.

Gutman, S. A., & Schonfeld, A. B. (2009). *Screening adult neurologic populations: A step-by-step instruction manual,* 2nd ed. Bethesda, MD: AOTA Press.

Humphry, R., & Wakeford, L. (2006). An occupation-centered discussion of development and implications for practice. *American Journal of Occupational Therapy, 60,* 258–267.

Kandell, E. R., Schwartz, T. H., & Tessel, T. M. (Eds.), (2012). *Principles of neural science,* 5th ed. New York: McGraw Hill.

Lane, S. J. (2002). Sensory modulation. In A. C. Bundy, S. J. Lane, & E. A. Murray (Eds.), *Sensory integration: Theory and practice,* 2nd ed. (pp. 101–122). Philadelphia: F.A. Davis.

Lane, S. J. (2002). Structure and function of the sensory systems. In A. C. Bundy, S. J. Lane, & E. A. Murray (Eds.), *Sensory integration: Theory and practice,* 2nd ed. (pp. 35–68). Philadelphia: F.A. Davis.

Liptak, G. S. (2005). Neural tube defects. In M. L. Batshaw, L. Pellegrino, & N. J. Roizen (Eds.), *Children with disabilities,* 6th ed. (pp. 419–438). Baltimore: Paul H. Brooks.

Madsen, J. H. *Tethered cord syndrome: Questions and answers.* Retrieved July 30, 2001 from www.boston-neurosurg.org/amphitheater/tetheredcord.html

Memorial Eye Center. (2013). *Refractive errors.* Retrieved August 4, 2013 from: http://www.memoriaeyecenter.com/disordersrefractive.shtml.

Miller, L. J. (2006). *Sensational kids hope and help for children with sensory processing disorders (SPD).* New York: G.P. Putnam & Sons.

Miller, L. S., Anzalone, M. E., Lane, S. J., Cermak, S. A., & Osten, E. T. (2007). Concept evolution in sensory integration: A proposed nosology for diagnosis. *American Journal of Occupational Therapy 61,* 135–140.

Missiuna, C., Polatajko, H., Pollock, N., & Cameron, D. (2012). Neuromotor disorders. In S. J. Lane and Anita C. Bundy (Eds.), *Kids can be kids: A childhood occupations approach.* Philadelphia: FA Davis.

Muscular Dystrophy Association, (2013). *Diseases.* Retrieved August 4,2013 from http://mdausa.org/disease.

National Institutes of Neurological Disorders and Stroke, (2012). *NINDS tethered spinal cord syndrome information page.* Retrieved August 4, 2013 from http://www.ninds.nih.gov/disorders/tethered_cord/tethered_cord.h.

Parham, L. D. & Mailoux, Z. (2005). Sensory integration. In J. Case-Smith (Ed.), *Occupational therapy for children,* 5th ed. (pp. 356–409). St. Louis, MO: Elsevier Mosby.

Pellegrino, L. (2007). Cerebral palsy. In M. L. Batshaw, L. Pellegrino, & N. J. Roizen (Eds.), *Children with disabilities,* 6th ed. (pp. 387–408). Baltimore: Paul H. Brooks.

Pendleton, H., & Schultz-Krohn, W. (Eds.). (2013). *Pedretti's occupational therapy: Practice skills for physical dysfunction,* 6th ed. St. Louis, MO: Elsevier Science/Mosby.

Reeves, G. D., & Cermak, S. A. (2002). Disorders of praxis. In A. C. Bundy, S. J. Lane, & E. A. Murray (Eds.), *Sensory integration: Theory and practice,* 2nd ed. (pp. 71–100). Philadelphia: F.A. Davis.

Rogers, S. (2005). Common conditions that influence children's participation. In J. Case-Smith (Ed), *Occupational therapy for children,* 5th ed. (pp. 160–215). St. Louis, MO: Elsevier Mosby.

Shaf, R., & Lane, S. (2009). Neuroscience foundations of vestibular, proprioceptive, and tactile sensory strategies. *OT Practice, 14*(22), CE1–CE8.

United Cerebral Palsy (UCP). (2010). *Cerebral palsy information.* Retrieved August 4, 2013 from www.ucp.org.

Vining-Radomski, M., & Trombly-Latham, C.A. (2007). *Occupational therapy for physical dysfunction,* 6th ed. Baltimore: Williams & Wilkins.

Weinstein, S. L., & Gaillard, W. D. (2005). Epilepsy. In M. L. Batshaw, L. Pellegrino, & N. J. Roizen (Eds.), *Children with disabilities,* 6th ed. (439–460). Baltimore: Paul H. Brooks.

Review Questions

Neurological System Disorders

Below are five questions about key content covered in this chapter. These questions are not inclusive of the entirety of content related to neurological disorders that you must know for success on the NBCOT exam. These questions are provided to help you "jump start" the thought processes you will need to apply your studying of content to the answering of exam questions; hence they are not in the NBCOT exam format. Exam items in the NBCOT format which cover the depth and breadth of content you will need to know to pass the NBCOT exam are provided on this text's disc. The answers to the below questions are provided in Appendix 4.

1. You will be evaluating two persons who have survived strokes. One incurred a left MCA stroke and one incurred a right MCA stroke. What symptoms might each patient present during his/her respective evaluation session?

2. You are working on a spinal cord unit. You are about to evaluate a client who has an injury classified as ASIA A. The injury is at the C5 level. What is the expected sensory and motor status of your client?

3. You have just completed your first evaluation session with a client that sustained a TBI two weeks ago. Your findings include that the patient was alert and in heightened state of activity (easily overstimulated) and attempting to pull out the IV and feeding tube. The patient could not remember directions exhibiting poor short-term memory. The patient screamed out for no reason several times during the session and was observed to be aggressive (e.g., attempting to hit you and the nurse). The patient required maximum assist for BADL. Your facility requires you to document each TBI patient's Rancho Level of Cognitive Function. What is the appropriate level for you to record?

4. During an occupational therapy evaluation of a toddler, you observe that the child tends to sit or lay as placed, without moving. The parent reports that the child shows interest in toys, but never seems to reach out to them or handle them. The child is reported to be a "picky eater" who shows no interest in self-feeding. When you attempt to approach or make eye contact, the child cries. Based on this information, how would you describe the child's disorder to the parent?

5. You are working with a child who suddenly has a series of seizures that occur in rapid succession and are prolonged. When the parents are contacted, they report that they ran out of the child's medicine the day before. What type of seizure do these symptoms represent? How should you have responded to this situation?

8

Cardiovascular and Pulmonary System Disorders

REGINA M. LEHMAN, SUSAN B. O'SULLIVAN, JULIA ANN STARR, AND JOSEPHINE DOLERA

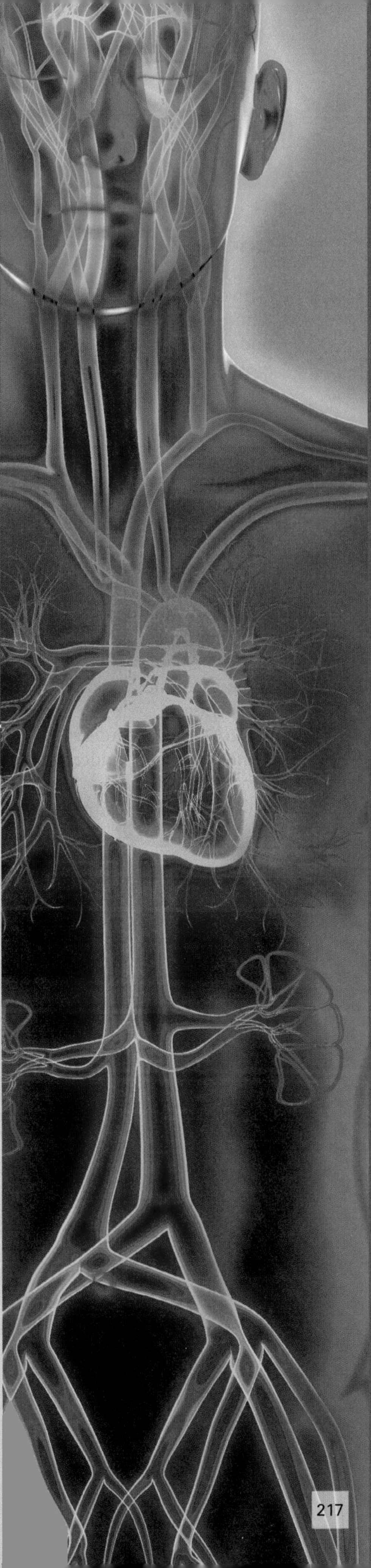

Chapter Outline

Cardiovascular System

Function

1. Delivers oxygen to organs and tissues.
2. Removes carbon dioxide and other by-products from body.
3. Assists in the regulation of core body temperature.

Cardiovascular Anatomy and Physiology

1. Relationship to the examination.
   a. It is not likely that the NBCOT exam will ask direct questions about anatomy and physiology.
   b. As a result, this chapter does not provide a complete anatomy and physiology review.
   c. Major structures and functions are outlined and specific figures are provided because knowledge of these can increase understanding of cardiovascular function.
   d. Knowledge of cardiovascular function will improve the ability to understand pathology, presenting symptoms, medical interventions, and occupational therapy treatment rationales.

The Heart and Circulation

1. Heart tissue.
   a. Pericardium: fibrous protective sac enclosing heart.
   b. Epicardium: inner layer of pericardium.
   c. Myocardium: heart muscle, the major portion of the heart.
   d. Endocardium: smooth lining of the inner surface and cavities of the heart.
2. Heart chambers.
   a. Four chambers arranged in pairs, functioning as two pumps working in sequence.
      (1) Right atrium (RA): receives blood from systemic circulation (from the superior and inferior cavae); during systole (contraction) blood is sent into right ventricle.
      (2) Right ventricle (RV): pumps blood via the pulmonary artery to the lungs for oxygenation; the low-pressure pulmonary pump.
      (3) Left atrium (LA): receives oxygenated blood from the lungs and the four pulmonary veins; during systole, blood is sent into the left ventricle.
      (4) Left ventricle (LV): pumps blood via the aorta throughout the entire systemic circulation; walls of left are thicker and stronger than right ventricle and form most of the left side and apex of the heart; the high-pressure systemic pump.
   b. See Figure 8-1.
   c. Blood flow.
      (1) Systemic circulation to RA to RV then to lungs for oxygenation.
      (2) LA receives oxygenated blood from the lungs, sends blood to LV.
      (3) LV pumps blood to the body via the aorta.
3. Valves: ensure unidirectional blood flow through the heart; provide one-way flow of blood into, out of, and within heart.

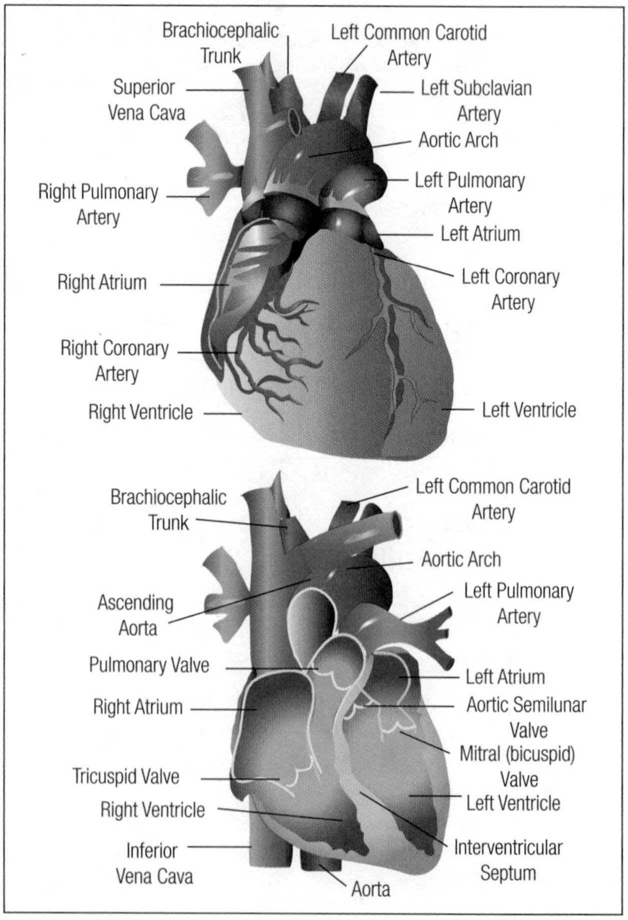

Figure 8-1 **The heart.**

a. Atriventricular valves: prevent backflow of blood into the atria during ventricular systole; valves close when ventricular walls contract.
   (1) Tricuspid valve (three cusps of leaflets): right heart valve.
   (2) Bicuspid or mitral valve (two cusps or leaflets): left heart valve.

b. Semilunar valves: prevent backflow of blood from aorta and pulmonary arteries into the ventricles during diastole.
   (1) Pulmonary valve: prevents right backflow.
   (2) Aortic valve: prevents left backflow.

4. Cardiac cycle.
   a. The rhythmic pumping action of the heart.
   b. Systole: the period of ventricular contraction.
   c. Diastole: the period of ventricular relaxation and filling of blood.
   d. Atrial contraction occurs during the last third of diastole and completes ventricular filling.

5. Coronary circulation.
   a. Right coronary artery (RCA): supplies right atrium, most of right ventricle, and in most individuals the inferior wall of left ventricle, atrioventricular (AV) node, and bundle of His; 60% of the time supplies the sinoatrial (SA) node.
   b. Left coronary artery (LCA): supplies most of the left ventricle; has two main divisions.
      (1) Left anterior descending (LAD) supplies the anterior wall of the left ventricle.
      (2) Circumflex supplies the lateral and inferior walls of the left ventricle and portions of the left atrium; supplies SA node 40% of the time.
   c. Veins: parallel arterial system.
   d. See Figure 8-2.

6. Conduction: specialized tissue allows rapid transmission of electrical impulses in the myocardium; includes nodal tissue and Purkinje fibers.
   a. Sinoatrial (SA) node: main pacemaker of the heart; initiates sinus rhythm; has sympathetic and parasympathetic innervation affecting both heart rate and strength of contraction.
   b. Atrioventricular (AV) node: has sympathetic and parasympathetic innervation; merges with bundle of His.
   c. Purkinje tissue: specialized conducting tissue of the ventricles.
   d. Conduction of heart beat.
      (1) Impulse originates in SA node and spreads throughout both atria, which contract together.
      (2) Impulse stimulates AV node, is transmitted down bundle of His to the Purkinje fibers; impulse spreads throughout the ventricles, which contract together.

7. Myocardial fibers: striated muscle tissue/fibers which exhibit rhythmicity of contraction; fibers contract as a functional unit; myocardial metabolism is primarily aerobic, sustained by continuous O_2 delivery from the coronary arteries.

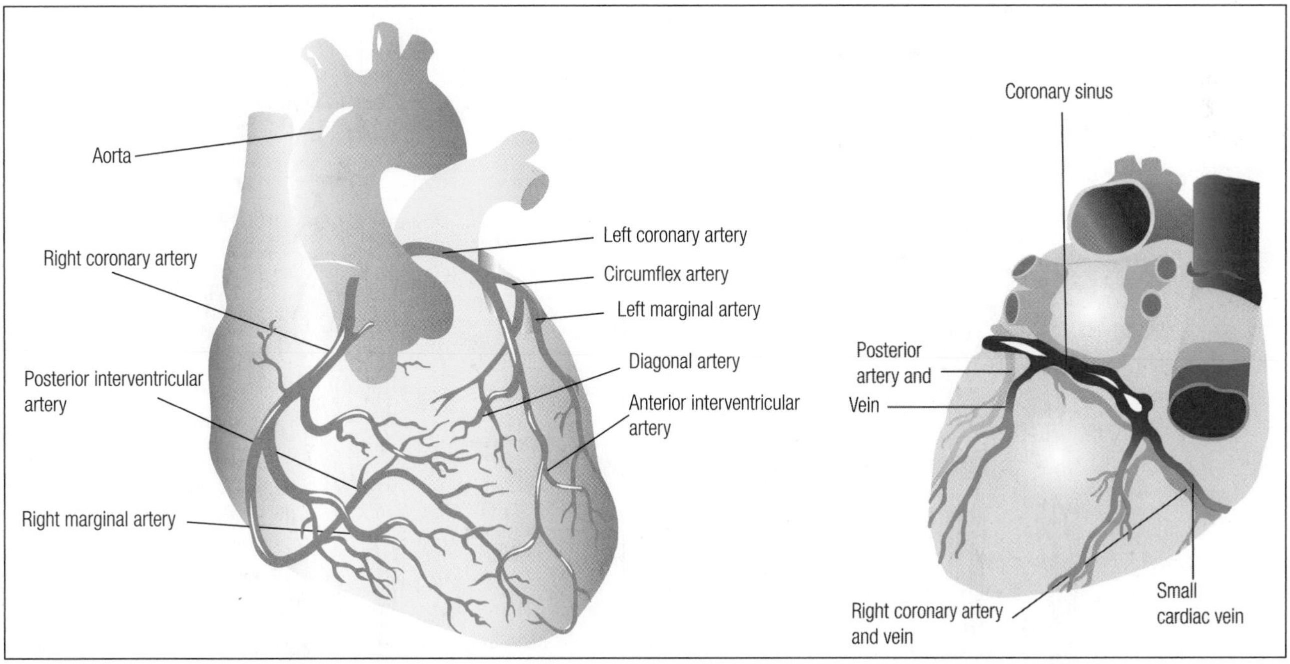

Figure 8-2 **Coronary arteries.**

8. Hemodynamics.
   a. Cardiac output: amount of blood ejected from the heart per minute; dependent upon heart rate and stroke volume.
   b. Stroke volume: average amount of blood ejected per heart beat.
   c. Ejection fraction: percentage of blood emptied from the ventricle during systole; a clinically useful measure of left ventricle (LV) function.

Peripheral Circulation

1. Arteries.
   a. Transport oxygenated blood from areas of high pressure to lower pressures in the body tissues.
   b. Arterial circulation maintained by heart pump.
   c. Influenced by elasticity and extensibility of vessel walls, peripheral resistance, and amount of blood in body.
   d. See Figure 8-3.
2. Capillaries.
   a. Minute blood vessels that connect the ends of arteries (arterioles) with the beginning of veins (venules); forms an anastomosing network.
   b. Function for the exchange of nutrients and fluids between blood and tissues.
   c. Capillary walls are thin, permeable.
3. Veins.
   a. Transport dark, unoxygenated blood from tissues back to the heart.
   b. Larger capacity, thinner walls than arteries, greater number.
   c. One-way valves to prevent backflow.
   d. Venous system includes both superficial and deep veins (deep veins accompany arteries, while superficial ones do not).
   e. See Figure 8-4.
4. Lymphatic system.
   a. Includes lymphatics (superficial, intermediate, and deep), lymph fluid, lymph tissues, and organs (lymph nodes, tonsils, spleen, thymus, and the thoracic duct).
   b. Drains lymph from bodily tissues and returns it to venous circulation.
   c. Lymph travels from lymphatic capillaries to lymphatic vessels to ducts to left subclavian vein. Lymphatic contraction occurs by:
      (1) Parasympathetic, sympathetic, and sensory nerve stimulation.
      (2) Contraction of adjacent muscles.
      (3) Abdominal and thoracic cavity pressure changes during normal breathing.
      (4) Mechanical stimulation of dermal tissues.
      (5) Volume changes within each lymphatic vessel.

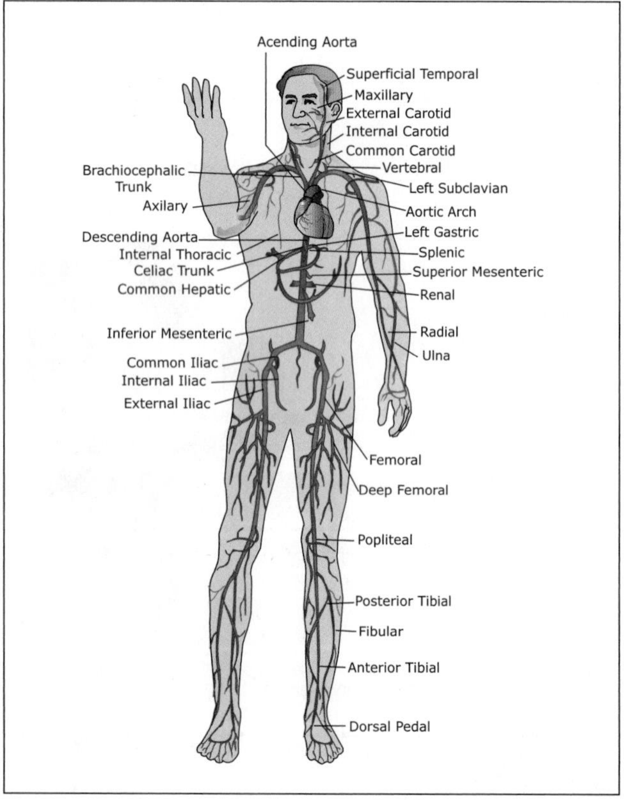

Figure 8-3 **Circulatory system: Arteries.**

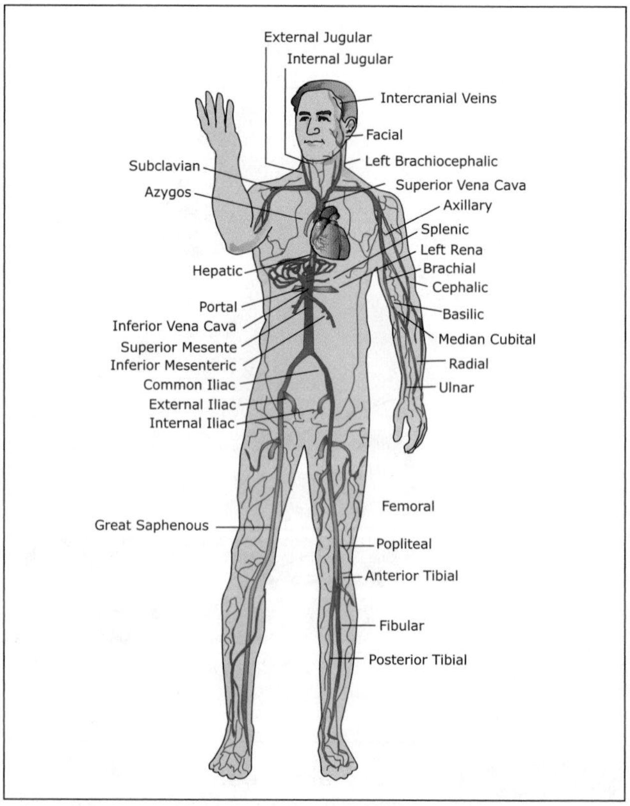

Figure 8-4 **Circulatory system: Veins.**

d. Major lymph nodes are submaxillary, cervical, axillary, mesenteric, iliac, inguinal, popliteal, and cubital.
e. Contributes to immune system function; lymph nodes collect cellular debris and bacteria; remove excess fluid, blood waste, and protein molecules; and produce antibodies.
f. See Figure 8-5.

Neorohumoral Influences

1. Neural control of heart rate and blood vessels.
2. Parasympathetic control (cholinergic): cardioinhibitory center; slows rate and force of myocardial contraction; decreases myocardial metabolism; causes coronary artery vasoconstriction.
3. Sympathetic control (adrenergic): cardioacceleratory center; causes an increase in the rate and force of myocardial contraction and myocardial metabolism; causes coronary artery vasodilation.
4. Additional control mechanisms.
   a. Baroreceptors: main mechanism controlling heart rate; respond to changes in blood pressure.
   b. Chemoreceptors: sensitive to changes in blood chemicals (O_2, CO_2, lactic acid).
   c. Body temperature: heart rate changes analogously to temperature.
   d. Ion concentrations.
      (1) Hyperkalemia: increased potassium ions, decreases the rate and force of contraction, and produces EKG changes.
      (2) Hypokalemia: decreased potassium ions, produces EKG changes; arrhythmias, may progress to ventricular fibrillation.
      (3) Hypercalcemia: increased calcium concentration; increases heart rate.
      (4) Hypocalcemia: decreased calcium concentration; depresses heart action.
   e. Peripheral resistance.
      (1) Increased peripheral resistance increases arterial blood volume and pressure.
      (2) Decreased peripheral resistance decreases arterial blood volume and pressure.
      (3) Influenced by arterial blood volume: viscosity of blood and diameter of arterioles and capillaries.

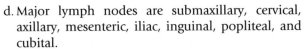

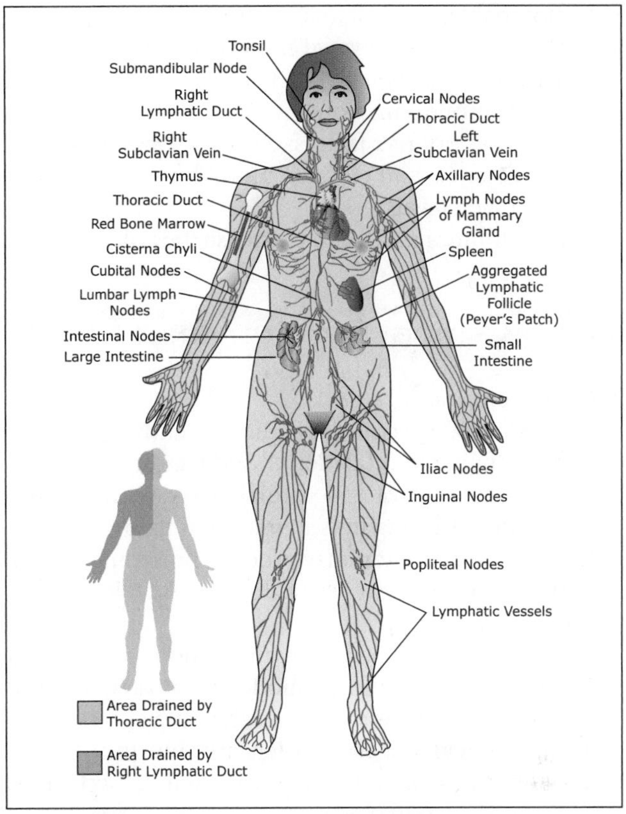

Figure 8-5 Lymphatic system.

Coronary Artery Disease (CAD)

Definition

1. Atherosclerotic disease process that narrows the lumen of coronary arteries resulting in ischemia to the myocardium.

Atherosclerosis

1. Etiology.
   a. Disease of lipid-laden plaques (lesions) affecting moderate and large-size arteries.
   b. Characterized by thickening of the intimal layer of the blood vessel wall from the focal accumulation of lipids, platelets, monocytes, plaque, and other debris.
2. Onset: variable depending upon presence or absence of risk factors.
3. Prevalence: increases with age and presence of risk factors.
4. Prognosis: good with early detection and treatment.
5. Multiple risk factors.
   a. Non-modifiable risk factors: age, sex, race, family history of CAD.

b. Modifiable risk factors: cigarette smoking, high blood pressure, elevated cholesterol levels and low-density lipoprotein (LDL) levels, elevated blood homocystine, emotional stress.
c. Contributory risk factors: diabetes, obesity, sedentary lifestyle, and elevated blood homocystine and fibrinogen levels.
d. Two or more risk factors increase the risk of CAD.

Main Clinical Syndromes of CAD

1. Characteristics:
   a. Involves a spectrum of clinical entities ranging from angina to infarction to sudden cardiac death.
   b. An imbalance of myocardial oxygen supply and demand resulting in ischemic chest pain.
   c. Subacute occlusion may produce no symptoms.
   d. Symptoms present when lumen is at least 70% occluded.
2. Angina pectoris: clinical manifestation of ischemia characterized by mild to moderate substernal chest pain/discomfort most commonly felt as pressure or dull ache in the chest and left arm but may be felt anywhere in the upper body including neck, jaw, back, arm, epigastric area.
   a. Usually lasts less than 20 minutes due to transient ischemia.
   b. Represents an imbalance in myocardial oxygen supply and demand; brought on by:
      (1) Increased demands on heart: exertion/exercise, emotional upsets, smoking, extremes of temperature (especially cold), overeating, tachyarrhythmias.
      (2) Vasospasm: symptoms may be present at rest.
   c. Types of angina.
      (1) Stable angina: classic exertional angina occurring during exercise or activity; relieved with rest and/or sublingual nitroglycerin.
      (2) Unstable angina (preinfarction, crescendo angina): coronary insufficiency at rest without any precipitating factors or exertion. Chest pain increases in severity, frequency, and duration. Increases risk for myocardial infarction or sudden death (lethal arrhythmia); pain is difficult to control.
      (3) Variant angina (Prinzmetal's angina): caused by vasospasm of coronary arteries in the absence of occlusive disease. Responds well to nitroglycerin or calcium channel blocker long term.
3. Myocardial infarction (MI): prolonged ischemia, injury, and death of an area of the myocardium caused by occlusion of one or more of the coronary arteries; results in necrosis of heart tissue.
   a. Precipitating factors: atherosclerotic heart disease with thrombus formation, coronary vasospasm or embolism; cocaine toxicity.
   b. Symptomology/presenting signs and symptoms.
      (1) Severe substernal pain of more than 20 minutes duration which may radiate to neck, jaw, arm, epigastric area.
      (2) Dyspnea, rapid respiration, shortness of breath.
      (3) Indigestion, nausea, and vomiting.
      (4) Pain may be misinterpreted as indigestion.
      (5) Pain unrelieved by rest and/or sublingual nitroglycerin.
   c. Infarction sites.
      (1) Transmural (Q wave infarction); full thickness of myocardium.
      (2) Nontransmural (non-Q wave infarction); subendocardial, subepicardial, intramural infarctions.
      (3) Coronary artery occlusion.
         (a) Inferior MI, right ventricle infarction, disturbances of upper conduction system: right coronary artery.
         (b) Lateral MI, ventricular ectopy: circumflex artery.
         (c) Anterior MI, disturbances of lower conduction system: left anterior descending artery.
   d. Results of impaired ventricular function.
      (1) Decreased stroke volume, cardiac output and ejection fraction.
      (2) Increased end diastolic ventricular pressure.
   e. Electrical instability, arrhythmias, present in injured and ischemia areas.
4. Heart failure (HF):
   a. A clinical syndrome in which the heart is unable to maintain adequate circulation of the blood to meet the metabolic needs of the body.
   b. Etiology: may be caused by coronary artery disease, valvular disease, congenital heart disease, hypertension, infections.
   c. Physiological abnormalities: decreased cardiac output, elevated end diastolic pressures (preload); increased heart rate; impaired ventricular contractility.
   d. Types of heart failure:
      (1) Left-sided heart failure (congestive heart failure, CHF): blood is not adequately pumped into systemic circulation.
         (a) Characterized by pulmonary congestion, edema, and low cardiac output due to backup of bood from left ventricle (LV) to the left atrium (LA) and lungs.
         (b) Occurs with insult to the left ventricle from myocardial disease; excessive workload of the heart (hypertension, valvular disease, or congenital defects); cardiac arrhythmias, or heart damage.
      (2) Right heart failure: blood is not adequately returned from the systemic circulation to the heart.

Table 8-1

Possible Clinical Manifestations of Cardiac Failure

LEFT VENTRICULAR FAILURE	RIGHT VENTRICULAR FAILURE
Signs and symptoms of pulmonary congestion:	
Dyspnea, dry cough	Dependent edema
Orthopnea	Weight gain
Paroxysmal nocturnal dyspnea (PND)	Ascites
Pulmonary rales, wheezing	Liver engorgement (hepatomegaly)
Signs and symptoms of low cardiac output:	
Hypotension	Anorexia, nausea, bloating
Tachycardia	Cyanosis (nail beds)
Lightheadedness, dizziness	Right upper quadrant pain
Cerebral hypoxia: irritability, restlessness, confusion, impaired memory, sleep disturbances	Jugular vein distension
Fatigue, weakness	Right-sided S_3 heart sounds
Poor exercise tolerance	Murmurs of pulmonary or tricuspid insufficiency
Enlarged heart on chest x-ray	
S_3 heart sound, possibly S_4	
Murmurs of mitral or tricuspid regurgitation	

(a) Characterized by increased pressure load on the right ventricle (RV) with higher pulmonary vascular pressures.

(b) Occurs with insult to the right ventricle (RV) from LV failure, mitral valve disease of chronic lung disease (cor pulmonale); produces hallmark signs of jugular vein distension and peripheral edema.

(3) Biventricular failure: severe LV pathology producing back up into the lungs, increased PA pressure, and RV signs of HF.

e. Associated symptoms: muscle wasting, myopathies, osteoporosis.

f. Possible clinical manifestations of heart failure. See Table 8-1.

Classification of Heart Failure

1. The New York Heart Association (NYHA) Functional Classfication is the most commonly used classification system to assess the stage of heart failure.
   a. Relates symptoms to everyday activities and the patient's quality of life.
   b. Places patients into categories based on limitations during physical activity.
2. Functional capacity: how a patient with cardiac disease feels during physical activity.
   a. Class I: Patients with cardiac disease but resulting in no limitation of physical activity. Ordinary physical activity does not cause undue fatigue, palpitation, dyspnea, or angina pain.
   b. Class II: Patients with cardiac disease resulting in slight limitation of physical activity. They are comfortable at rest. Ordinary physical activity results in fatigue, palpitation, dyspnea, or angina pain.
   c. Class III: Patients with cardiac disease resulting in marked limitation of physical activity. They are comfortable at rest. Less than ordinary activity causes fatigue, palpitation, dyspnea, or angina pain.
   d. Class IV: Patients with cardiac disease resulting in inability to carry on any physical activity without discomfort. Symptoms of heart failure or the angina syndrome may be present even at rest. If any physical activity is undertaken, discomfort increases.
3. Objective assessment: based on measurements such as electrocardiograms, stress tests, x-rays, echocardiograms, and radiological images.
   a. Class A: no objective evidence of cardiovascular disease. No symptoms and no limitation in ordinary physical activity.
   b. Class B: objective evidence of minmal cardiovascular disease. Mild symptoms and slight limitation during ordinary activity. Comfortable at rest.
   c. Class C: objective evidence of moderately severe cardiovascular disease. Marked limitation in activity due to symptoms, even during less-than-ordinary activity. Comfortable only at rest.
   d. Class D: objective evidence of severe cardiovascular disease. Severe limitations. Experiences symptoms even while at rest (Criteria Committee of the NY Heart Association, 1994, 253–256).

Medical and Surgical Management/Relevant Pharmacology

1. Diagnostic procedures.
   a. Chest x-ray: done to evaluate evidence of congestion in lungs, heart chamber hypertrophy, and structural abnormalities.
   b. Electrocardiogram (ECG): done to identify cardiac arrhythmias, assess amount and location of damage to myocardium, determine adequacy of oxygenation of myocardium.
   c. Holter monitor: records ECG signals over a 24-hour period while person engages in normal daily routine to determine heart function during various activities.
   d. Echocardiogram: ultrasound used to record size, structure, and motion of the heart and vessels; reveals valvular defects and structural abnormalities.
   e. Cardiac stress test: records cardiac activity during graded exercise; used to determine the extent to which cardiac disease affects functional capacity; provides guidelines related to the type and amount of physical activity that a person can engage in safely.
   f. Cardiac catheterization: invasive procedure used to visualize coronary circulation to determine the degree of CAD, congenital heart defect, valvular disease, myocardial damage.
   g. Pulmonary function test: used to determine cause of dyspnea, degree of lung disease; provides information related to endurance potential for functional activities.
2. Dietary interventions: low salt, low cholesterol, weight reduction.
3. Medical therapy: medications designed to manage specific aspects of cardiovascular function to prevent or decrease the risk of cardiac events and the progression of related diseases; drugs aimed at reducing oxygen demand on the heart and increasing coronary blood flow.
   a. Nitrates/vasodilators/ACE inhibitors: (nitroglycerin, Nitrostat, Minoxidil, Vasotec, Capoten, and Monopril) decrease preload through peripheral vasodilation, reduce myocardial oxygen demand, reduce chest discomfort (angina); may also dilate coronary arteries, improve coronary blood flow.
   b. Beta blockers (e.g., Inderal, Coreg, Labetalol, Atenolol) reduce myocardial demand by reducing heart rate and contractility; control arrhythmias, chest pain; reduce blood pressure.
   c. Calcium channel blockers (e.g., Cardizem, Procardia) inhibit flow of calcium ions; decrease heart rate, decrease contractility, dilate coronary arteries, reduce BP, control arrhythmias, chest pain.
   d. Antiarrhythmics (numerous drugs, 4 main classes) alter conductivity, restore normal heart rhythm, control arrhythmias, and improve cardiac output (e.g., quinidine, procainamide, Procainamide, Inderal, and Cordarone).
   e. Antihypertensives (numerous drugs, 4 main types) control hypertension; goal is to maintain a diastolic pressure less than 90 mmHg; decrease afterload, reduce myocardial oxygen demand (e.g., Inderal, Lopressor, propranolol, reserpine).
   f. Digitalis (cardiac glycosides) increase contractility and decrease heart rate; mainstay in the treatment of CHF (e.g., Digoxin).
   g. Diuretics decrease myocardial work (reduce preload and afterload), control hypertension (e.g., Lasix, Esidrix, Microzide).
   h. Antithrombitics: aspirin decreases platelet aggregation and reduce clot formation, may prevent myocardial infarction.
   i. Tranquilizers decrease anxiety, sympathetic effects.
   j. Hypolipidemic agents (6 major cholesterol-lowering drugs) reduce serum lipid levels when diet and weight reduction are not effective (e.g., Colestid, Zocor, and Mevacor).
   k. Anticoagulants: work to prevent blood clot formation that may interfere with blood circulation or cause venous thrombosis.
      (1) Injectables: enter bloodstream and take effect immediately (e.g., Fragmin, Lovenox).
      (2) Oral: take 3–5 days to take full effect (e.g., Warfarin/Coumadin).
4. Surgical interventions.
   a. Angioplasty (percutaneous transluminal coronary angioplasty [PCTA]): under fluoroscopy, surgical dilation of a blood vessel using a small balloon-tipped catheter inflated inside the lumen.
      (1) Catheter is inserted into the femoral artery and guided through the arterial system into the coronary arteries.
      (2) Relieves obstructed blood flow in acute angina or acute MI.
      (3) Results in improved coronary blood flow, improved left ventricular function, anginal relief.
   b. Intravascular stents: an endoprosthesis (pliable wire mesh) implanted postangioplasty to prevent restenosis and occlusion in coronary or peripheral arteries.
   c. Revascularization surgery (coronary artery bypass grafting, CABG): surgical circumvention of an obstruction in a coronary artery using an anastomosing graft (saphenous vein, internal mammary artery).
      (1) Multiple grafts may be necessary.
      (2) Results in improved coronary blood flow and left ventricular function, anginal relief.
      (3) Surgery results in deconditioning.

d. Transplantation: used in end-stage myocardial disease, e.g., cardiomyopathy, ischemic heart disease, valvular heart disease.
   (1) Heterotopic: involves leaving the natural heart and piggy-backing the donor heart.
   (2) Orthotopic: involves removing the diseased heart and replacing it with a donor heart.
   (3) Heart and lung transplantation: involves removing both organs and replacing them with donor organs.
   (4) Major problems post-transplantation: rejection, infection, complications on immunosuppressive therapy.
e. Ventricular assistive devices (VADs).
   (1) Implanted device (accessory pump) that improves tissue perfusion and maintains cardiogenic circulation.
   (2) Used with severely involved patients (e.g., cardiogenic shock, unresponsive to medications, severe ventricular dysfunction; those awaiting heart transplant).
   (3) Often called the "bridge to transplantation."

5. Thrombolytic therapy for acute myocardial infarction.
   a. Medications administered to activate body's fibrinolytic system, dissolve clot, and restore coronary blood flow (e.g. Streptokinase, Tissue plasminogen [TPA], Urokinase).

Peripheral Vascular Disease (PVD)

1. Arterial disease.
   a. Occlusive peripheral arterial disease (PAD). See Table 8-2.
      (1) Chronic, occlusive arterial disease of medium and large-sized vessels.
      (2) Associated with hypertension and hyperlipidemia; patients may also have CAD, diabetes, cerebrovascular disease, metabolic syndrome, history of smoking.
      (3) Diminished blood supply to affected extremities with pulses decreased or absent.
      (4) Early stages: patients exhibit intermittent claudication. Pain is described as burning, searing, aching, tightness, or cramping. Occurs regularly and predictably with walking and is relieved by rest.
      (5) Late stages: patients exhibit rest pain, muscle atrophy, trophic changes (i.e., hair loss, skin, and nail changes).
      (6) Affects primarily lower extremities.
   b. Thromboangiitis obliterans (Buerger's disease): chronic inflammatory vascular occlusive disease of small arteries and also veins.
      (1) Most common in young males who smoke.
      (2) Begins distally and progresses proximally in both lower and upper extremities.
      (3) Symptoms include pain, paresthesias, cold extremities, diminished temperature sensation, fatigue; risk of ulceration and gangrene.
   c. Diabetic angiopathy: inappropriate elevation of blood glucose levels and accelerated atherosclerosis; neuropathies a major problem; ulcers may lead to gangrene and amputation.
   d. Raynaud's phenomenon: episodic spasm of small arteries and arterioles abnormal vasoconstriction reflex exacerbated by exposure to cold or emotional stress; tips of fingers develop pallor, cyanosis, numbness, and tingling; affects largely females.
2. Venous disease.
   a. Varicose veins: distended, swollen superficial veins; tortuous in appearance; may lead to varicose ulcers.
   b. Superficial vein thrombophlebitis: clot formation and acute inflammation in a superficial vein; localized pain usually in saphenous vein.
   c. Deep vein thrombosis (DVT): inflammation of a vein in association with the formation of a thrombus; usually occurs in lower extremities.
      (1) Associated with venous stasis (bed rest, lack of leg exercise), hyperactivity of blood coagulation, and vascular trauma.
      (2) Early mobility (out of bed activities) after surgery helps to eliminate venous stasis.
      (3) May be a contributing factor to or a complication of cerebral vascular accident (CVA) or the result of prolonged bed rest during serious illness.
      (4) Signs and symptoms: may be asymptomatic early; progressive inflammation with tenderness to palpation; change in lower extremity temperature, color circumference, appearance, or tenderness/pain. These require immediate medical attention. May be life threatening.
   d. Chronic venous insufficiency (Table 8-2).
      (1) Chronic leg edema; skin pigmentation changes, scaly appearance, itchy.
3. Lymphedema.
   a. Chronic disorder with excessive accumulation of fluid due to obstruction of lymphatics.
   b. Causes swelling if the soft tissues in arms and legs.
   c. Results from mechanical insufficieny of the lymphatic system.
   d. Primary lymphedema: congenital condition with abnormal lymph node or lymph vessel formation (hypoplasia or hyperplasia).
   e. Secondary lymphedema: acquired, due to injury of one or more parts of the lymphatic system. Possible causes include:

Table 8-2

Differential Diagnosis: Peripheral Vascular Diseases

	CHRONIC ARTERIAL INSUFFICIENCY	CHRONIC VENOUS INSUFFICIENCY	CHRONIC LYMPHATIC INSUFFICIENCY
Etiology	Atherosclerosis Thrombosis Emboli Inflammatory process	Thrombophlebitis Trauma Vein obstruction (clot) Vein incompetence	Primary lymphedema Secondary lymphedema
Risk factors	Age: > 60 years Smoking Diabetes mellitus Gender: slightly higher in men Dyslipidemia Hypertension Hyperhomocysteinemia Race (African American)	Venous hypertension Varicose veins Inherited trait Gender: female Age Increased BMI Sedentary lifestyle/prolonged sitting Ligamentous laxity	Lymphadenectomy Radiation treatment Inflammatory arthritis Obesity
Signs and symptoms: determined by location and degree of vascular involvement			
Pain	Severe muscle ischemia/intermittent claudication Worse with exercise, relieved by rest Rest pain indicates severe involvement Muscle fatigue, cramping, numbness Paresthesias over time	Minimal to moderate steady pain Aching pain in lower leg with prolonged standing or sitting (dependency) Superficial pain along course of vein	Heaviness, tightness, aching or discomfort
Location of pain	Usually calf, lower leg or dorsum of foot May occur in thigh, hip or buttock	Muscle compartment tenderness	Edematous limb
Vascular	Decreased or absent pulses Pallor of forefoot on elevation Dependent rubor	Venous dilatation or varicosity Edema: moderate to severe, especially after prolonged dependency	Rare complications unless severe and untreated edema
Skin changes	Pale, shiny, dry skin Loss of hair Nail changes Coolness of extremity	Hemosiderin deposition: Dark, cyanotic, thickened, brown skin Lipodermatosclerosis: fibrosing of the subcutaneous tissue May lead to stasis dermatitis, cellulitis	Cutaneous fibrosis May lead to cellulitis, lymphangitis
Acute	Acute arterial obstruction: distal pain, paresthetic, pale, pulseless, sudden onset	Acute thrombophlebitis (deep venous thrombosis, DVT): Calf pain, aching, edema, muscle tenderness, 50% asymptomatic	Rarely acute, usually progressive over time except with changes in pressure to limb altering flow (repeated blood pressure measurements, airplane flights)
Ulceration	May develop in toes, feet or areas of trauma; pale or yellow to black eschar, gangrene may develop; regular in shape and may appear punched out	May develop at sides of ankles, especially medial malleolus along the course of veins; gangrene absent; painful, shallow, exudative and have granulation tissue in the base; irregular borders	Unusual

Adapted from Bickley, L., Szilagyi, P. Bates, *Guide to physical examination and history taking*, 8th ed., Philadelphia, Lippincott Williams & Wilkins, 2003.

(1) Surgery: e.g., radical mastectomy, femoropopliteal bypass, lymph node removal.
(2) Tumors, trauma or infection affecting the lymph nodes.
(3) Radiation therapy with fibrosis of tissues.
(4) Chronic venous insufficiency.
(5) In tropical and subtropical areas, filariasis (nematode worm larvae in the lymphatic system).

f. Initiating factors that can trigger lymphedema.
(1) Inactivity and changes in cabin pressure during air flight.
(2) Fluctuation in weight gain and fluid volumes.
(3) Hyperemia.
(4) Hypoproteinemia.

g. Stages of lymphedema; it is a progressive disease.
(1) Stage 1, reversible lymphedema: limb is soft and pitting; swelling may increase overnight.
(2) Stage 2, spontaneously irreversible lymphedema: swelling with increase in fibrotic tissue; risk for infection.
(3) Stage 3, lymphostatic elephantiasis: extreme increase in swelling skin changes (fibrosis, sclerosis, papillomas).

Pulmonary System

Function

1. Respiration, delivers oxygen to cardiovascular system.
2. Removes carbon dioxide and other by-products from body.

Anatomy and Physiology

1. Bony thorax: anterior border is the sternum, lateral border is the ribcage, posterior border is the vertebral column; shoulder girdle can affect the motion of the thorax.
2. Airways.
   a. Upper airways: nose, pharynx, larynx.
   b. Lower airways: conducting airways (trachea to terminal bronchioles) and the respiratory unit (respiratory bronchioles, alveolar ducts, alveolar sacs and alveoli).
3. Lungs.
4. Pleura.
5. Muscles of ventilation.
   a. Primary muscles of inspiration: diaphragm, intercostals.
   b. Accessory muscles of inspiration: used when a more rapid or deeper inhalation is required or in disease; include sternocleidomastoid, scalenes, levator costarum, serratus, trapezius, and pectorals.
   c. Expiratory muscles.
      (1) Resting expiration: done by passive relaxation of inspiratory muscles and elastic recoil tendency of lungs.
      (2) Expiratory muscles used when quicker, fuller expiration is desired or in disease; include quadratus lumborum, intercostals, rectus abdominis, triangularis sterni.
6. Mechanics of breathing: forces acting upon the rib cage include elastic recoil of lungs, bony thorax, muscles.
7. Ventilation and perfusion: the movement of gas in and out of the pulmonary system.
   a. Measurements include volumes, capacities, flow rates.
   b. Optimal respiration occurs when ventilation and perfusion (blood flow to lungs) are matched.
   c. Body position/gravity affects distribution of ventilation and perfusion.
8. Respiration: diffusion of gas across the alveolocapillary membrane.
9. Control of ventilation.
   a. Receptors: baroreceptors, chemoreceptors, irritant receptors, stretch receptors.
   b. Central control centers: brain and autonomic nervous system.
   c. Ventilatory muscles.

Pulmonary Dysfunction

Acute Diseases

1. Bacterial pneumonia: an intra-alveolar bacterial infection.
   a. Gram positive bacteria usually acquired in the community; pneumococcal pneumonia (streptococcal) is the most common type.
   b. Gram negative bacteria usually develop in host who has underlying chronic condition, acute illness, recent antibiotic therapy; usually results in early tissue necrosis and abscess formation.
2. Viral pneumonia: an interstitial or interalveolar inflammatory process caused by viral agents (influenza, adenovirus, cytomegalovirus, herpes, parainfluenza, respiratory syncytial virus, measles).
3. Aspiration pneumonia: aspirated material causes an acute inflammatory reaction within the lungs; usually found in patients with impaired swallowing ability (dysphagia).
4. Tuberculosis: See subsequent section.
5. Pneumocystis pneumonia (PCP): pulmonary infection caused by a fungus (Pneumocystis carinii) in immunocompromised hosts; most often found in patients following transplantation, neonates, and those infected with HIV.
6. SARS (severe acute respiratory syndrome).
   a. An atypical respiratory illness caused by a coronavirus. Initial outbreak in southern mainland China with worldwide spread to other areas such as Singapore, Toronto, Vietnam, and Hong Kong.

Tuberculosis (TB)[1]

1. Etiology: an airborne infection caused by a bacterium (Mycobacterium tuberculosis).
2. Risk factors.
   a. A person with TB of the throat or chest can pass the infection by sneezing or coughing.
   b. People most at risk for infection are those who live around or are in close contact with an infected individual every day (e.g., family members, friends, coworkers, health care personnel).
   c. People who have weakened immune systems are at greater risk for rapid onset of TB disease, such as people with:
      (1) HIV/AIDS.
      (2) Substance abuse.
      (3) Diabetes.
      (4) Scoliosis.
      (5) Cancer of the head or neck.
      (6) Leukemia or Hodgkin's disease.
      (7) Severe kidney disease.
      (8) Low body weight.
      (9) Certain medical conditions receiving special treatments (e.g., steroid users or organ recipients).
   d. People who have had a TB infection within 2 years of treatment are at high risk for re-infection.
   e. Babies, young children, and elderly people have a higher risk.
   f. Intravenous drug users have a higher risk.
3. People who breathe in TB bacteria and become infected may be able to fight the infection. The TB cells become inactive, but remain alive in the body. This is called TB infection. People with TB infection:
   a. Are asymptomatic.
   b. Do not feel ill.
   c. Are not contagious.
   d. Do usually have a positive TB skin test.
   e. Can develop full-blown TB later, if they do not get drug treatment for the TB infection.
4. Signs and symptoms of TB.
   a. A bad cough for more than 2 weeks.
   b. Chest pain.
   c. Blood tinged sputum or phlegm.
   d. Weakness or fatigue.
   e. Weight loss.
   f. Loss of appetite.
   g. Chills/fever.
   h. Night sweats.
5. Prevention, detection and early intervention.
   a. Avoid high risk situations that contribute to possible exposure.
      (1) Spending time with a person who is infected with TB.
      (2) Traveling to countries where TB is prevalent.
      (3) Residence in a setting where TB is common.
         (a) Homeless shelters.
         (b) Migrant farm shelters.
         (c) Prisons and jails.
         (d) Some nursing homes.
   b. Get checked frequently (every 1–2 years) for TB by having a skin test if person has no history of a positive skin test.
   c. Get a chest x-ray if person is TB positive or if person was injected with BCG (a vaccine for TB that is given outside of the United States).
   d. Frequent checkups are essential if:
      (1) Immune system is impaired or weakened (e.g., HIV/AIDS, lupus, cancer, MS).
      (2) Person lives in an area of the United States where TB is common.
   e. It takes 10–12 weeks after exposure to TB for a skin test to detect infection.
      (1) BCG vaccination can make a skin test appear positive. Individuals who were given BCG can still get TB infected.
         (a) If they become TB infected, they may have a large skin reaction.
      (2) Additional reasons individuals who have been vaccinated may become infected with TB.
         (a) Vaccination was many years before being skin tested.
         (b) Someone in their family has TB.
         (c) Their origin is from a country where TB is common.
6. Medical treatment.
   a. Drug therapy is frequently used to treat TB infection or prevention after an exposure.
   b. Persons who have TB disease may need to take several different drugs to do a better job of killing the bacteria.
   c. If a person stops taking the drugs before the prescribed interval, the drugs may become ineffective in fighting the infection.
   d. Development of multi-drug resistant TB (MDR TB) can occur.
   e. Types of drugs.
      (1) Isoniazid (INH) which must be taken for 6 months.
         (a) People with weakened or undeveloped immune systems may have to take INH longer.
         (b) All of the INH pills prescribed must be taken.
         (c) A person on INH must see the doctor/nurse regularly or they may develop a resistance to the drug therapy.
         (d) Side effects of INH therapy include loss of appetite, nausea, vomiting, jaundice, and fever lasting more than 3 days, abdominal pain, tingling in the fingers or toes.

[1] This section was completed by Ann Burkhardt.

(e) A person receiving INH should avoid alcoholic beverages while receiving drug therapy.
(2) Rifampin.
(a) Side effects include orange tint to urine, saliva, or tears; inability to wear contact lenses; sun sensitivity.
(b) Affects birth control pills and implants, rendering them ineffective.
(c) Lessens effectiveness of methadone therapy for drug addiction.
(3) Pyrazinamide.
(4) Ethambutol.
(5) Streptomycin.
f. Serious side effects of all of the above drug therapies.
(1) No appetite.
(2) Nausea, vomiting.
(3) Jaundice.
(4) Fever lasting more than 3 days.
(5) Abdominal pain.
(6) Tingling in the fingers or toes.
(7) Easy bruising.
(8) Blurred vision.
(9) Tinnitus, hearing loss.
7. Sequelae of TB.
a. Once the infection settles into a person's lungs, it can spread to other parts of the body.
(1) Kidney dysfunction can occur.
(2) Spine: Rood's disease can occur, which is vertebral collapse caused by TB resulting in compression of the spinal cord.
(a) Spinal structural integrity can be compromised.
(b) Cervical spinal lesions can result in hand functional impairment, sensory impairment, postural changes.
(c) Thoracic spinal lesions can result in paraparesis, neurogenic bowel/bladder, altered mobility, and altered activity of daily living activities.
(3) Space-occupying lesions in the brain produce stroke-like symptoms.

Chronic Obstructive Diseases

1. Chronic obstructive pulmonary disease (COPD): a disorder characterized by poor expiratory flow rates.
a. Peripheral airways disease: inflammation of the distal conducting airways; association with smoking.
b. Chronic bronchitis: chronic inflammation of the tracheobronchial tree with cough and sputum production lasting at least 3 months for 2 consecutive years.
c. Emphysema: permanent abnormal enlargement and destruction of air spaces distal to terminal bronchioles; may result in destruction of acini, the functional units for gas exchange in the lungs.
(1) Etiology: based on the assumption that there is an imbalance between protease and antiprotease enzymes.
(a) Causes tissue breakdown, and antiprotease enzymes.
(b) Leads to loss of lung parenchyma, elastic recoil during exhalation and normal airway resistance during inspiration.
(c) Results in airway dilation, premature airway closure, air trapping, and increased residual air volume or hyperinflation.
(2) Signs and symptoms: patients present with a mixture of clinical features. These include the following.
(a) Primary complaint of dyspnea on exertion.
(b) Diminished breath sounds, wheezing (typically associated with exertion).
(c) Prolonged expiratory phase.
(d) Pursed lip breathing.
(e) Physical presentation may include: enlarged anterior/posterior dimensions of the chest wall (barrel chest), hypertrophied accessory muscle from overuse, use of accessory muscles for breathing, forward leaning posture.
(f) Presence of a chronic cough and sputum production will vary and depend on the infectious history of the patient.
(g) Disease advancement may result in patient becoming cachectic (emaciated), signs of right heart failure due to secondary pulmonary hypertension.
(3) Interventions.
(a) Smoking cessation.
(b) Short-acting and long-acting β2 agonists/bronchodilators.
(c) Anticholinergic drugs to block brocho-constriction (e.g., Atrovent, Ventolin, Proventil, Maxair); not the first line of medications.
(d) Xanthine Derivatives (e.g., theophylline) for bronchodilation, limitation of inflammatory response.
(e) Corticosteroids for anti-inflammatory effects.
(f) Preventive vaccination against influenza and pneumococcus.
(g) Oxygen therapy to
- reduce level of dyspnea.
- improve/decrease maximal voluntary ventilation, polycythemia, by correcting hypoxemia.

- decrease pulmonary HTN.
- improve quality and quantity of sleep.
- improve cognitive function and exercise tolerance.

(h) Surgeries may include bullectomy, volume reduction, lung transplantation.

(4) Prognosis: varies depending upon degree of obstruction, presence of hypercapnia (increased levels of CO_2), recurrence of infections, and development of right heart failure.

2. Asthma: an increased reactivity of the trachea and bronchi to various stimuli (allergens, exercise, cold).
   a. Etiology: unknown.
      (1) Factors associated with the development of asthma include maternal smoking, early infections (respiratory syncytial virus), and genetics.
   b. Risk factors: childhood asthma, family history, maternal smoking, occupational exposures, environmental exposure, exposure to secondhand smoke.
   c. Manifests by widespread narrowing of the airways due to inflammation, smooth muscle constriction, and increased secretions.
   d. Sign and symptoms: wheezing, dyspnea, chest pain, facial distress, non-productive cough with acute exacerbation where airways may become obstructed with vicious, tenacious mucous (more severe in children than adults).
      (1) Symptoms in adults may include paroxysmal nocturnal dyspnea, morning chest pain and increased symptoms with exposure to cold.
   e. Intervention.
      (1) Prevention.
      (2) Smoking cessation and minimizing exposure to second hand smoke for pregnant women.
      (3) Annual flu shot.
      (4) Avoidance of stimulants that precipitate asthmatic episode.
      (5) Use of short- and long-acting dilators.
      (6) Common medications: Albuterol (e.g., Ventolin, Proventil) Atrovent, w/albuteral, Combivent).
      (7) Establishment of a routine exercise program.
   f. Reversible in nature.
3. Cystic fibrosis. (See section on pediatric pulmonary disorders.)
4. Hyaline membrane disease/respiratory distress syndrome. (See pediatric pulmonary disease section.)

Chronic Restrictive Diseases

1. Etiologies vary.
2. Diseases are all characterized by difficulty expanding the lungs causing a reduction in lung volumes.
3. Restrictive disease due to alterations in lung parenchyma and pleura: fibrotic changes within the pulmonary parenchyma or pleura due to idiopathic pulmonary fibrosis, asbestosis, radiation pneumonitis, oxygen toxicity.
4. Restrictive disease due to alteration in the chest wall: restricted motion of the bony thorax, with diseases such as ankylosing spondylitis, arthritis, scoliosis, pectus excavatum, arthrogryposis, or the integumentary changes of the chest wall such as thoracic burns or scleroderma.
5. Restrictive disease due due to alteration in the neuromuscular apparatus: decreased muscular strength results in an inability to expand rib cage, seen in disease states such as multiple sclerosis, muscular dystrophy, Parkinson's disease, spinal cord injury, or cerebrovascular accident (CVA).

Carcinomas

1. Refer to Chapter 9.

Other Pulmonary Conditions

1. Pulmonary edema: excessive seepage of fluid from the pulmonary vascular system into the interstitial space; may eventually cause alveolar edema.
2. Pulmonary emboli: a thrombus from the peripheral venous circulation becomes embolic and lodges in the pulmonary circulation. Small emboli do not necessarily cause infarction.
3. Pleural effusion: excessive fluid between the visceral and parietal pleura, caused mainly by increased pleural permeability to proteins from inflammatory diseases (pneumonia, rheumatoid arthritis, systemic lupus), neoplastic disease, increased hydrostatic pressure within pleural space (congestive heart failure), decrease in osmotic pressure (hypoproteinemia), peritoneal fluid within the pleural space (ascites Cirrhosos), or interference of pleural reabsorption from a tumor invading pleural lymphatics.
4. Atelectasis: collapsed or airless alveolar unit, caused by hypoventilation secondary to pain during the ventilator cycle (pleuritis, postoperative pain, rib fracture), internal bronchial; obstruction (aspiration, mucus plugging), external bronchial compression (tumor or enlarged lymph nodes), low tidal volumes (narcotic overdose, inappropriately low ventilator settings), or neurologic insult.

Occupational Therapy Cardiopulmonary Assessment

Medical Status and History

1. Review medical record.
2. Interview patient and/or family/caregiver.
3. Presenting symptoms.
   a. Pain/angina: note location, severity, type. See Table 8-3.
   b. Dyspnea (shortness of breath): note severity, position, or times at which discomfort is experienced. See Table 8-4.
   c. Fatigue/perceived exertion: note severity, time of occurrence, association with activities.
   d. Palpitations: note person's awareness of heart rhythm abnormalities including pounding, fluttering, racing heart beat, skipped beats.
   e. Dizziness: note time of occurrence and association with postural changes during activity.
   f. Edema.
      (1) Fluid retention may be identified by swelling, especially in the lower extremities, or sudden weight gain.
      (2) Note location, measurements, time of day when edema is most prominent, resolution with activity.
4. Past medical history.
   a. Onset of incident, concomitant diagnoses, chronic conditions; diagnosis, prognosis.
   b. Review to determine premorbid status/functional level for occupational therapy treatment implications, long term goal planning, selection of modalities/activities, and potential level of independence at discharge.
   c. List of current medications.
5. Diagnostic tests (see medical and surgical management).
   a. Review results to determine implications for occupational therapy intervention including activity restrictions, vital sign parameters, and prognosis.
6. Social history.
   a. Information used to determine implications for occupational therapy intervention including activity selection, educational/learning needs, social supports, discharge needs.
   b. Areas include educational history, vocational/avocational history, leisure pursuits and activities history, presence/absence of substance abuse, diet, family configuration, and social supports.
7. Discharge environment and anticipated level of activity.

Table 8-3

Intermittent Claudication Rating Scale	
0	No claudication pain
1	Initial, minimal pain
2	Moderate, bothersome pain
3	Intense pain
4	Maximal Pain, cannot continue

Williams, M. (Ed.): AACVPR: (2004). *Guidelines for cardiac rehabilitation and secondary prevention programs,* 4th ed. (p. 81). Champaign, IL: Human Kinetics. Reprinted with permission.

Table 8-4

Common Angina and Dyspnea Rating Scales	
5-GRADE ANGINA SCALE	
0	No angina
1	Light, barely noticeable
2	Moderate, bothersome
3	Severe, very uncomfortable
4	Most pain ever experienced
5-GRADE DYSPNEA SCALE	
0	No dyspnea
1	Mild, noticeable
2	Mild, some difficulty
3	Moderate difficulty, but can continue
4	Severe difficulty, cannot continue
10-GRADE ANGINA/DYSPNEA SCALE	
0	Nothing
0.5	Very, very slight
1	Very slight
2	Slight
3	Moderate
4	Somewhat severe
5	Severe
6	
7	Very severe
8	
9	
10	Very, very severe
	Maximal

Williams, M. (Ed.): AACVPR: (2004). *Guidelines for cardiac rehabilitation and secondary prevention programs,* 4th ed. (p. 81). Champaign, IL: Human Kinetics. Reprinted with permission.

Chapter 8

Vital Signs

1. Important and reliable indicator of activity tolerance/ response to evaluation and treatment.
   a. Refer to Table 8-5 for normal vital sign values for infants and adults.
2. Pulse/heart rate: rhythmical throbbing of arterial wall as a result of each heartbeat; influenced by force of contraction, volume and viscosity of blood, diameter and elasticity of vessels, emotions, exercise, blood temperature, and hormones.
   a. Assessment: done by palpation of peripheral pulses; with normal rhythm palpate 30 seconds; with irregular rhythm palpate 1–2 minutes; taken prior to activity, during activity, and post activity.
   b. Palpation sites.
      (1) Radial: most common monitoring site; radial artery, radial wrist at base of thumb.
      (2) Temporal: superior and lateral to eye.
      (3) Carotid: on either side of anterior neck between sternocleidomastoid muscle and trachea; best reflects cardiac function.
      (4) Brachial: medial aspect of the antecubital fossa; used to monitor blood pressure.
      (5) Femoral.
      (6) Popliteal.
      (7) Pedal.
3. Pulse/heart rate (HR) parameters.
   a. Normal adult HR is 70 beats per minute (bpm); range 60–100 bpm.
      (1) As an individual ages, the normal resting heart rate range may increase up to 100 bpm.
   b. Pediatric: newborn is 120 bpm; range 70–170 bpm.
   c. Tachycardia: greater than 100 bpm.
   d. Bradycardia: less than 60 bpm.
   e. Irregular: force and frequency vary; may be due to arrhythmia, myocarditis.
   f. Weak, thready pulse.
   g. Bounding, full pulse.

Table 8-5

Normal Values for Infants and Adults

PARAMETER	INFANT	ADULT
Heart Rate	120 bpm	60–100 bpm
Blood Pressure	75/50 mmHg	< 120/80 mmHg
Respiratory Rate	40 br/min	12–20 br/min
PaO_2	75–80 mmHg	80–100 mmHg
$PaCO_2$	34–54 mmHg	35–45 mmHg
pH	7.26–7.41	7.35–7.45
Tidal Volume	20 ml	500 ml

   h. Bruit: abnormal sound or murmur; associated with atherosclerosis.
4. Auscultation of heart: done with stethoscope to assess heart sounds. Note the addition of extra, abnormal heart sounds.
5. Blood pressure (BP).
   a. Monitor at rest, during evaluation/activity, post activity.
   b. Normal adult BP is < 120/80 mmHg (systolic/ diastolic); range between 110–140 systolic, 60–80 diastolic.
   c. Pediatric: 1 month–80 systolic, 45 diastolic, 6 years–105–125 systolic, 60–80 diastolic.
   d. Increased BP may be related to stress, pain, hypoxia, drugs, and disease.
   e. Decreased BP may be related to bed rest, drugs, arrhythmias, blood loss/shock, and myocardial infarction.
   f. Hypertension: BP above 120/80.
6. Respiration.
   a. Monitor at rest, during evaluation/activity, post activity.
   b. Rate and depth of breathing: normal is 12–18 breaths per minute.
   c. Auscultation of lungs/respiratory sounds.
      (1) Normal: soft, rustling sound heard throughout all inspiration and start of expiration.
      (2) Abnormal: crackles/rales.
         (a) Rattling, bubbling sounds; may be due to secretions in lungs.
         (b) Wheezes, whistling sounds.

Condition of Extremities

1. Diaphoresis: excessive sweating associated with decreased cardiac output.
2. Pulses: decreased or absent pulses associated with peripheral vascular disease (PVD). See Table 8-6.
3. Skin color and vascular status.
   a. Cyanosis: bluish color related to decreased cardiac output or cold; especially lips, fingertips, nail beds.

Table 8-6

Grading Scale for Peripheral Pulses

0	Absent pulse, not palpable
1+	Pulse diminished, barely perceptible
2+	Easily palpable, normal
3+	Full pulse, increased strength
4+	Bounding pulse

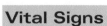

Table 8-7

Grading Scale for Edema	
1+	Mild, barely perceptible indentation; < ¼ inch pitting
2+	Moderate, easily identified depression; returns to normal within 15 seconds; ¼–½ inch pitting
3+	Severe, depression takes 15–30 seconds to rebound; ½–1 inch pitting
4+	Very severe, depression lasts for > 30 seconds or more; > 1 inch pitting

b. Pallor: absence of rosy color in light skinned individuals, associated with decreased peripheral blood flow, PVD.
c. Rubor: dependent redness with PVD.
d. Temperature.
e. Skin changes: clubbing of fingernails; pale, shiny, dry, abnormal pigmentation; ulceration, dermatitis; gangrene.
f. Intermittent claudication: pain, cramping, fatigue occurring during exercise and relieved by rest, associated with PVD; pain is typically in calf.
g. Edema. See Table 8-7.

Mobility Assessment

1. Bed mobility.
2. Transfers.
3. Wheelchair mobility.
4. Ambulation status.
5. Refer to Chapter 16.

Cognition

1. Provides baseline of person's ability to understand, process, retain, and apply information taught during rehabilitation.
   a. Orientation.
   b. Memory.
   c. Concentration.
   d. Judgment.
2. Refer to Chapter 13.

Activities of Daily Living/ Instrumental Activities of Daily Living

1. Self care.
2. Household management tasks.
3. Leisure activities.
4. Community activities.
5. Note level of function and type of assistance required.
6. Note level of dyspnea and angina reported during activities. See Tables 8-3 and 8-4.
7. See Chapter 15 for more information on evaluation of ADL and IADL.

Activity Tolerance

1. Graded exercise test done by exercise physiologist or physical therapist (6 Minute Walk Test, physical performance tests).
2. Observation of activities with monitoring of vital signs (heart rate, blood pressure, respiration rate, rate of perceived exertion).
3. Periodic monitoring of dyspnea, angina and claudication pain. See Tables 8-3 and 8-4.
4. Periodic monitoring of exertion.
   a. Borg rate of perceived exertion: a self-report rating scale which ranges from no exertion at all (e.g., sitting or lying) to maximal exertion (e.g., hard work that is not advisable to engage in).
5. Metabolic equivalent levels (METs). See Tables 8-8 and 8-9.
   a. The use of METs during the assessment of activity tolerance must take into consideration the physical status of the patient and their pattern of activities prior to the cardiac event.

Psychosocial Assessment

1. Overt signs and symptoms of depression, anxiety, and/or stress and the observed effects on the individual's ability to complete/engage in activities.
2. Stress management/coping styles and psychosocial, family/caregiver and spiritual supports.
3. Refer to Chapter 10 and Chapter 14.

Environmental Assessment

1. Accessibility issues related to safety, risk for falls, and environmental barriers in the discharge environment.
2. Physical demands of the discharge environment. Presence of stairs, airborne irritants.
3. Refer to Chapter 16.

Table 8-8

Approximate Metabolic Cost of Activities[a]

ENERGY LEVEL	OCCUPATIONAL	RECREATIONAL
1.5–2 MET[b] 4–7 mL O²/ min/kg 2–2.5 kcal/ min[d]	Desk work Auto driving[c] Typing Electric calculat- ing machine operation	Standing Walking (strolling 1.6 km or 1 mile/hr) Flying,[c] motorcycling[c] Playing cards[c] Sewing, knitting
2–3 MET 7–11 mL O²/ min/kg 2.5–4 kcal/min[d]	Auto repair Radio, TV repair Janitorial work Typing, manual Bartending	Level walking (3.25 km or 2 miles/hr) Level bicycling (8 km or 5 miles/hr) Riding lawn mower Billiards, bowling Skeet,[c] shuffleboard Woodworking (light) Powerboat driving[c] Golf (power cart) Canoeing (4 km or 2.5 miles/hr) Horseback riding (walk) Playing piano and many muscial instruments
3–4 MET 11–14 mL O²/ min/kg 4–5 kcal/min[d]	Brick laying, plastering Wheelbarrow (220 lb or 100 kg load) Machine as- sembly Trailer-truck in traffic Welding (mod- erate load) Cleaning windows	Walking (5 km or 3 miles/hr) Cycling (10 km or 6 miles/hr) Horseshoe pitching Volleyball (6 person noncompetitive) Golf (pulling bag cart) Archery Sailing (handling small boat) Fly fishing (standing in waders) Horseback (sitting to trot) Badminton (social doubles) Pushing light power mower Energetic musician
4–5 MET 14–18 mL O²/ min/kg 5–6 kcal/min[d]	Painting, masonry Paperhanging Light carpentry	Walking (5.5 km or 3.5 miles/hr) Cycling (13 km or 8 miles/hr) Table tennis Golf (carrying clubs) Dancing (foxtrot) Badminton (singles) Tennis (doubles) Raking leaves Hoeing Many calisthenics
5–6 MET 18–21 mL O²/ min/kg 6–7 kcal/min[d]	Digging garden Shoveling light earth	Walking (6.5 km or 4 miles/hr) Cycling (16 km or 10 miles/hr) Canoeing (6.5 km or 4 miles/hr) Horseback (posting to trot) Stream fishing (walking in light current in waders) Ice or roller skating (15 km or 9 miles/hr)

(Continued)

Table 8-8

Approximate Metabolic Cost of Activities[a] (Continued)

ENERGY LEVEL	OCCUPATIONAL	RECREATIONAL
6–7 MET 21–25 mL O²/ min/kg 7–8 kcal/min[d]	Shoveling 10 min (22 lb or 10 kg)	Walking (8 km or 5 miles/hr) Cycling (17.5 km or 11 miles/hr) Badminton (competitive) Tennis (singles) Splitting wood Snow shoveling Manual lawn mowing Folk (square) dancing Light downhill skiing Ski touring (4 km or 2.5 miles/hr), loose snow Water skiing
7–8 MET 25–28 mL O²/ min/kg 8–10 kcal/min[d]	Digging ditches Carrying 175 lb or 80 kg Sawing hard- wood	Jogging (8 km or 5 miles/hr) Cycling (19 km or 12 miles/hr) Horseback (gallop) Vigorous downhill skiing Basketball Mountain climbing Ice hockey Canoeing (8 km or 5 miles/hr) Touch football Paddleball
8–9 MET 28–32 mL O²/ min/kg 10–11 kcal/ min[d]	Shoveling 10 min (31 lb or 14 kg)	Running (9 km or 5.5 miles/hr) Cycling (21 km or 13 miles/hr) Ski touring (6.5 km or 4 miles/hr), loose snow Squash (social) Handball (social) Fencing Basketball (vigorous)
10+ MET 32+ mL O²/ min/kg 11+ kcal/min[d]	Shoveling 10 min (35 lb or 16 kg)	Running 6 mph = 10 MET 7 mph = 11.5 MET 8 mph = 13.5 MET 9 mph = 15 MET 10 mph = 17 MET Ski touring (8+ km or 5+ miles/hr), loose snow Handball (competitive) Squash (competitive)

[a] Includes resting metabolic needs.

[b] 1 MET is the energy expenditure at rest, equivalent to approximately 3.5 mL O²/kg body weight/min.

[c] A major increase in metabolic requirements may occur because of excitement, anxiety, or impatience, which are common responses during some activities. The patient's emotional reactivity must be assessed when prescribing or sanctioning certain activities.

[d] Based on a 70 kg person.

Atchison, B. (1995). Cardiopulmonary diseases. In Trombly, C.A. (Ed.). *Occupational therapy for physical dysfunction* (4th ed., pp. 881–882). Baltimore, MD: Williams & Wilkins. Reprinted with permission.

Table 8-9

Metabolic Equivalent (MET) Activity Chart

INTENSITY (70-KG PERSON)	ENDURANCE PROMOTING	ACTIVITY
1.5–2 METs	Too low in energy level	Standing, walking slowly (1 mph)
2–3 METs	Too low in energy level, unless capacity is very low	Level walking (2 mph), level bicycling (5 mph)
3–4 METS	Yes, if continuous and if target heart rate reached	Level walking (3 mph), bicycling (6 mph)
4–5 METs	Recreational activities must be continuous, lasting longer than 2 minutes	Walking (3½ mph), bicycling (8 mph)
5–6 METs	Yes	Walking at brisk pace (4 mph), bicycling (10 mph)
6–7 METs	Yes	Walking at very brisk pace (5 mph), bicycling (11 mph), swimming leisurely (20 yd/min)
7–8 METs	Yes	Jogging (5 mph), bicycling (12 mph)
8–9 METs	Yes	Running (5.5 mph), bicycling (13 mph), swimming (30 yd/min)
>10 METs	Yes	Running 6 mph = 10 METs, 7 mph = 11.5 METs, 8 mph = 13.5 METs, 9 mph = 15 METs, 10 mph = 17 METs; swimming moderate/hard (> 40 yd/min)

Adapted from: Fox, Naughton, Gorman. Mod Concepts Cardiovas Dis 1972, 4:25. American Heart Association.

Occupational Therapy Cardiopulmonary Rehabilitation

Phase 1: Inpatient Rehabilitation/Hospitalization Stage (Acute)

1. Begins when the patient is determined to be medically stable following the cardiac or pulmonary event (MI, CABG, angioplasty, valve repair/replacement, CHF, etc).
   a. Typically after 24 hours or until the patient is stable for 24 hours.
2. Program focus.
   a. Patient and family education regarding disease process and recovery.
      (1) Increase knowledge of energy conservation and work simplification principles and techniques (see Chapter 11).
      (2) Increase knowledge of the approximate metabolic cost of activities (See Tables 8-8 and 8-9).
   b. Improve ability to carry out self care and low level functional activities.
   c. Decrease anxiety.
   d. Promote risk factor modification (i.e., support smoking cessation and dietary modification efforts if warranted).
   e. Discharge to home.
3. Evaluation and intervention.
   a. Initiated at bedside with a monitored, functional assessment of self care and mobility.
   b. If person is pain free, exhibits no arrhythmia, and has regular pulse of 100 or less, an activity program is initiated.
   c. Intense monitoring during activity especially in CCU.
   d. Beginning activities at MET level = 1–2.
      (1) Bed mobility, static standing.
      (2) Transfer from bed to chair/bedside commode.
      (3) Bed bath, feeding, grooming at sink in sitting.
      (4) AROM/warm-up exercises.
      (5) Wheelchair mobility/ambulation in room.
   e. All activities use energy conservation techniques. General principles of energy conservation and work simplification include:
      (1) Pace oneself.
      (2) Monitor body position during activities.
      (3) Organize daily activities and work areas.
      (4) Delegate responsibilities.
   f. Breathing exercises.
      (1) Abdominal diaphragmatic breathing: strengthens diaphragm, decreases need to use neck and shoulder muscles, decreases energy required for activity.
      (2) Pursed lip breathing: controls respiratory rate; decreases rate of breathing, helps remove trapped air from lungs.
      (3) Techniques are done during all exercises and activities.

Chapter 8

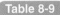

g. Vital signs are monitored prior to each activity, at peak of each activity, immediately upon cessation of activity and 4–5 minutes post activity.

h. Exertion scales are monitored prior to each activity, at the peak of each activity, 30 seconds before the cessation of activity, immediately upon cessation of activity, and 3–5 minutes post activity.
   (1) To ensure the validity of the person's responses on exertion scales, clear and accurate instructions must be provided.
      (a) The therapist must make sure that the person has a clear understanding of what the ratings mean (i.e., all ratings should reflect the person's perceptions of how the exercise is making him/her feel; how hard he/she is working to perform the exercise).

i. Adhere to activity guidelines and MET levels. See Tables 8-8 and 8-9.
   (1) As the patient's activity tolerance improves, more strenuous, higher MET level activities are added in progression from basic ADL to IADL.

j. Observe any contraindications/precautions as per physician orders.
   (1) Observe/monitor for shortness of breath, (SOB), chest pain, nausea, vomiting, dizziness, and/or fatigue.
   (2) Adhere to activity guidelines and MET levels. See Tables 8-8 and 8-9.
   (3) Observe for decrease in systolic BP greater than 20 mmHg.
   (4) Observe facial expression; be alert to facial changes.
   (5) Monitor heart rate (use facility specific guidelines, if available).
      (a) Max HR 100 very light activity–very high risk.
      (b) Max HR 120 light activity–less than 6 weeks after MI, surgery.
      (c) Max HR 130 recent bypass surgery, cardiomyopathy, CHF.
      (d) Target HR 60%–80% patient's max HR - treadmill test.
   (6) Monitor BP also for resting diastolic BP 120 mmHg; systolic 200 mmHg.
   (7) Monitor oxygen saturation (O_2 sat); below 86% for pulmonary patients, below 90% for cardiac patients.
   (8) Monitor ECG for signs and symptoms of myocardial ischemia.
   (9) Monitor exertion scales for signs and symptoms of distress during activity, speed of recovery. See Tables 8-3 and 8-4.
   (10) Avoid isometric muscle work, straining, breath holding (Valsalva).
   (11) Avoid overhead exercises or holding UEs over head for extensive time periods.
   (12) Avoid lateral arm movements and exercises that stretch chest and pull incision.

k. There may be clinical signs/symptoms or diagnoses for which therapy should either be stopped or is contraindicated.
   (1) Uncontrolled atrial/ventricular arrhythmias.
   (2) Recent embolism/thrombophlebitis.
   (3) Dissecting aneurysm.
   (4) Severe aortic stenosis.
   (5) Acute systemic illness.
   (6) Acute MI.
   (7) Digoxin toxicity.
   (8) Acute hypoglycemia or metabolic disorder.
   (9) Third degree heart block.
   (10) Unstable angina.

l. Patients are generally discharged to Phase 2 when they are able to carry out activities at MET level 3.5. See Tables 8-8 and 8-9.
   (1) Tables should be used as a general reference to determine the approximate level of energy required to perform an activity.
   (2) MET levels are used to quantify the amount of energy required to perform an activity and to provide the therapist with a guideline for grading activities used in treatment.
      (a) Selection of activities based on MET level must take into consideration the patient's physical status and activity patterns prior to the cardiac or pulmonary event, as well as the patient's subjective report of level of exertion during activity performance.

m. Educate individual about heart disease and the recovery process, provide emotional support.

4. Length of stay 5–14 days in the hospital.
   a. Commonly 3–5 days for uncomplicated MI (no post-MI angina, malignant arrhythmias, or heart failure).
   b. Continued inpatient services may be required in a transitional setting for up to 6 weeks post cardiac event, surgery, or pulmonary disease exacerbation.

5. See Box 8-1 and Box 8-2 for indications and contraindications for inpatient cardiac rehabilitation and adverse responses to inpatient exercise leading to exercise termination.

BOX 8-1 Contraindications for Inpatient and Outpatient Cardiac Rehabilitation

Absolute Contraindications

- Acute MI (within 2 days)
- Unstable angina not previously stabilized by medical therapy
- Uncontrolled cardiac arrhythmias causing symptoms or hemodynamic compromise
- Acute PE or pulmonary infarction
- Acute myocarditis or pericarditis
- Acute aortic dissection

Relative Contraindications

- Left main coronary stenosis
- Moderate stenotic valvular heart disease
- Electrolyte abnormalities
- Severe arterial hypertension
- Tachyarrhythmias or bradyarrhythmias
- Hypertrophic cardiomyopathy and other forms of outflow tract obstruction
- Mental or physical impairment leading to inability to exercise adequately
- High-degree atrioventricular block

Adapted from Gibbons et al, 2002.

BOX 8-2 Possible Effects of Physical Training/Cardiac Rehabilitation

- Decreased HR at rest and during exercise; improved HR recovery after exercise.
- Increased stroke volume.
- Increased myocardial oxygen supply and myocardial contractility; myocardial hypertrophy.
- Improved respiratory capacity during exercise.
- Improved functional capacity of exercising muscles.
- Reduced body fat, increased lean body mass; successful weight reduction requires multifactorial interventions.
- Decreased serum lipoproteins (cholesterol, triglycerides).
- Improved glucose tolerance.
- Improved blood fibrinolytic activity and coagulability.
- Improvement in measures of psychological status and functioning: self-confidence and sense of well-being.
- Increased participation in exercise; improved outcomes with adherence to rehabilitation programming.
  - Decreased angina in patients with CAD: anginal threshold is raised secondary to decreased myocardial oxygen consumption.
  - Reduced total and cardiovascular mortality in patients following myocardial infarction.
  - Decreased symptoms of heart failure, improved functional capacity in patients with left ventricular systolic dysfunction.
  - Improved exercise tolerance and function in patients with cardiac transplantation.

Phase 2: Outpatient Rehabilitation/Convalescence Stage (Subacute)

1. Begins as early as 24 hours after discharge from the hospital.
   a. Frequency of visits depends on the clinical needs of the patient.
2. Program focus.
   a. Educate patient on the importance of continued exercise.
   b. Build up activity tolerance.
   c. Improve ability to carry out IADL and community tasks.
   d. Improve ability to perform work activities.
   e. Support person's efforts in smoking cessation and lifestyle changes as needed.

3. Evaluation and intervention.
   a. Home evaluation.
   b. Consumer and family education.
   c. Graded exercise program with slow and gradual increase of weight.
   d. Begin with activities at MET level 4–5, gradually increasing as patient's tolerance improves.
   e. Resumption of sexual activity usually at 5–6 MET level as per physician recommendation.
   f. Practice of functional activities in the discharge environment.
   g. Use of energy conservation techniques and compensatory techniques in daily tasks.
   h. Community activities.
   i. Work site evaluation if applicable.
4. Length of outpatient program is dependent upon several factors including patient's physical and mental status post event and/or surgery, progress through MET levels, activity tolerance, and prognosis.
5. See Box 8-1 and Box 8-2 for indications and contraindications for outpatient cardiac rehabilitation.

Phase 3: Maintenance/Training Stage (Community Exercise Programs)

1. Patients generally attend maintenance/training sessions once a week following the completion of Phase 2.
2. Groups may be integrated into individual exercise programs.
3. Occupational therapy intervention is provided as necessary for IADL, leisure pursuits, and work.
4. Maintenance gym program.
   a. Weight training to maintain upper and lower body strength.
   b. Cardiovascular training to maintain cardiopulmonary health.
5. See Table 8-10 for the recommended continuum of care for cardiac rehabilitation services and lifelong maintenance.

Rehabilitation Guidelines for Lymphatic Disease

1. Phase I, Management: edema secondary to lymphatic dysfunction.
   a. Short-stretch compression bandages, worn 24 hours/day.
   b. Manual lymph drainage (MLD) with complete decongestive therapy.
      (1) Massage and passive range of motion (PROM) to assist lymphatic flow.
      (2) Emphasis on decongesting proximal segments first (trunk quadrant), then extremities, directing flow distal to proximal.
      (3) Compression using multi-layered padding and short-stretch bandages.
      (4) Certified specialists (cettified lymphedema therapist).
   c. Functional activities.
      (1) ADL.
      (2) Adaptation of IADL, work, and leisure activities.
      (3) Energy conservation techniques to minimize exacerbation of swelling.
      (4) Patient and family education for skin care, donning and doffing compression garments, environmental changes to improve mobility and function.
      (5) Address psychosocial issues including stress, distress, depression, anxiety.
2. Phase II Management (self-management).
   a. Skin care.
   b. Compression bandages.
   c. Exercise.
   d. Lymphadema bandaging at night.
   e. MLD as needed.
   f. Compression pumps: use with caution; limited benefits.

Table 8-10

Recommended Continuum of Care for Cardiac Rehabilitation

WEEKS													
0	1	2	3	4	5	6	7	8	9	10	11	12	Beyond
Inpatient – hospital clinical pathway													
		Transitional care – subacute facility, home care, pretraining at home											
		Outpatient programming – cardiac rehabilitation center											
			Maintenance – lifelong – community facility or at home										

Williams, M. (Ed.): AACVPR: (2004). *Guidelines for cardiac rehabilitation and secondary prevention programs*, 4th ed., (p. 32). Champaign, IL: Human Kinetics. Reprinted with permission.

Table 8-11

Summary of Key Basic Life Support (BLS) Components for Adults, Children and Infants

	RECOMMENDATIONS		
COMPONENT	ADULTS	CHILDREN	INFANTS
Recognition	Unresponsive (all ages) No breathing, not breathing normally (e.g., only gasping)	Same as for adults	Same as for adults
CPR Sequence	CAB	CAB	CAB (ABC for neonates)
Compression Rate	At least 100/minute	Same as for adults	Same as for adults
Compression Depth	At least 2 inches (5 cm)	At least 1/3 AP depth, about 2 inches (5 cm)	At least 1/3 AP depth, about 1½ inches (4 cm)
Chest Wall Recall	Allow complete recoil between compressions, HCPs rotate compressors every 2 minutes	Same as for adults	Same as for adults
Compression Interruption	30:2 (1 or 2 rescuers)	30:2 single rescuer, 15:2 2 HCP rescuers	30:2 single rescuer, 15:2 2 HCP rescuers
Airway	Head tilt-chin lift (HCP suspected trauma: jaw thrust)	Same as for adults	Same as for adults
Compression to Ventilation Ratio (until advanced airway placed)	30:2 (1 or 2 rescuers)	30:2 single rescuer or 15:2 2 HCP rescuers	30:2 single rescuer or 15:2 2 HCP rescuers
Ventilations: when rescuer untrained or trained and not proficient	Compressions only	Compressions only	Compressions only
Ventilations with Advanced Airway (HCP)	1 breath every 6–8 seconds (8–10 breaths/min) Asynchronous with chest compressions About 1 second per breath Visible chest rise	Same as for adults	Same as for adults
Defibrillation	Attach and use AED as soon as available. Minimize interruptions in chest compressions before and after shock, resume CPR, beginning with compressions immediately after each shock	Same as for adults	Same as for adults

Key: CAB: compressions, airway, breathing; HCP: health care provider; CPR: cardiopulmonary resuscitation; AED: automatic electronic defibrillator.
From 2010 American Heart Association Guidelines for CPR and ECG. Downloaded from circ.ahajournals.org on July 5, 2011.

3. Education.
   a. Skin and nail care.
   b. Self-bandaging, garment care.
   c. Infection management.
   d. Maintain exercise while preventing lymph overload.
   e. Incorporation of home management program into daily routine.

Basic Life Support and Cardiopulmonary Resuscitation (CPR)

1. Current CPR Guidelines.
   a. Compressions come first, then focus on airway and breathing (CAB). Only exception is newborn babies.
   b. No more looking, listening, and feeling. Call 911 immediately.
   c. Push a little harder for adult CPR: at least 2 inches deep on chest.
   d. Push a little faster: about 100 compressions/minutes.
   e. Hands-only CPR for untrained lay rescuers.
   f. Don't stop pushing, no interuptions.
   g. See Table 8-11.

First Aid

1. External bleeding.
   a. Minor bleeding.
      (1) Usually clots within 10 minutes.
      (2) If patient/client is taking aspirin or nonsteroidal anti-inflammatory drugs (NSAIDS), clotting may take longer.

b. Severe bleeding characteristics.
(1) Blood spurting from a wound.
(2) Blood fails to clot even after measures to control bleeding have been taken.
(3) Arterial bleed: high pressure, spurting, red.
(4) Venous bleed: low pressure, steady flow, dark red or maroon blood.
(5) Capillary bleed: low pressure, oozing, dark red blood.
c. Controlling external bleeding.
(1) Use standard precautions such as wearing gloves.
(2) Apply gauze pads using firm pressure. If no gauze available, use a clean cloth, towel, a gloved hand, or patient's own hand. If blood soaks through, do not remove any gauze, add additional layers.
(3) Elevate the part if possible unless it is deformed or it causes significant pain when elevated.
(4) Apply a pressure bandage, such as roller gauze, over the gauze pads.
(5) If necessary, apply pressure with the heel of your hand over pressure points. The femoral artery in the groin and the brachial artery in the medial aspect of the upper arm are two such points.
(6) Monitor A, B, Cs and overall status of the patient. Administer supplemental oxygen if nearby. Seek more advanced care as necessary.
2. Internal bleeding.
a. The possible result of a fall, blunt force trauma, or a fracture rupturing a blood vessel or organ.
b. Severe internal bleeding may be life-threatening.
c. Severe internal bleeding characteristics.
(1) Ecchymosis (black and blue) in the injured area.
(2) Body part, especially the abdomen, may be swollen, tender, and firm.
(3) Skin may appear blue, gray, or pale and may be cool or moist.
(4) Respiratory rate is increased.
(5) Pulse rate is increased and weak.
(6) Blood pressure is decreased.
(7) Patient may be nauseated or vomit.
(8) Patient may exhibit restlessness or anxiety.
(9) Level of consciousness may decline.
d. Management of internal bleeding.
(1) If minor, follow RICE procedure: rest, ice, compression, elevation.
(2) Major internal bleeding.
(a) Summon advanced medical personnel.
(b) Monitor A, B, Cs and vital signs.
(c) Keep the patient comfortable and quiet. Keep the patient from getting chilled or overheated.
(d) Reassure patient or victim.
(e) Administer supplemental oxygen if available and nearby.
3. Shock (hypoprefusion).
a. Failure of the circulatory system to perfuse vital organs.
b. At first, blood is shunted from the periphery to compensate.
(1) The victim may lose consciousness as the brain is affected.
(2) The heart rate increases, resulting in increaded oxygen demand.
(3) Organs ultimately fail when deprived of oxygen.
(4) Heart rhythm is affected, ultimately leading to cardiac arrest and death.
c. Types and causes of shock.
(1) Hemorrhagic: severe internal or external bleeding.
(2) Psychogenic: emotional stress causes blood to pool away from the brain.
(3) Metabolic: loss of body fluids from heat ir severe vomiting or diarrhea.
(4) Anaphylactic: allergic reaction form drugs, food, or insect stings.
(5) Cardiogenic: MI or cardiac arrest results in pump failure.
(6) Respiratory: respiratory illness or arrest results in insufficient oxygenation of the vlood.
(7) Septic: severe infections cause blood vessels to dilate.
(8) Neurogenic: traumatic brain injury (TBI), spinal cord injury (SCI), or other neural trauma causes disruption of autonomic nervous system resulting in disruption of blood vessel dialation/constriction.
d. Signs and symptoms.
(1) Pale, gray, or blue, cool skin.
(2) Increased, weak pulse.
(3) Increased respiratory rate.
(4) Decreased blood pressure.
(5) Irritability or restlessness.
(6) Dimishing level of consciousness.
(7) Nausea or vomiting.
e. Care for shock.
(1) Obtain history if possible.
(2) Examine the victim for airway, breathing, circulation, and bleeding.
(3) Assess level of consciousness.
(4) Determine skin characteristics and perform capillary refill test of fingertips.
(a) Capillary refill test: squeeze fingernail for 2 seconds.
(b) In healthy individuals, the nail will blanch and turn pink when pressure is released.
(c) If nail bed does not refill and turn pink within 2 seconds, the cause could be that blood is beign shunted away from the periphery to vital organs to maintain core temperature.
(5) Treat any specific condition if possible: control bleeding, splint a fracture, EpiPen for anaphylaxis, and so on.

(6) Keep the victim from getting chilled or overheated.
(7) Elevate the legs 12 inches unless there is suspected spinal injury or painful deformities of the lower extremities.
(8) Reassure the victim and continue to monitor A, B, Cs.
(9) Administer supplemental oxygen if nearby.
(10) Do not give any food or drink.

Pediatric Pulmonary Disorders[2]

Cystic Fibrosis (CF)

1. Etiology.
   a. Genetically inherited autosomal recessive trait, gene mutation.
   b. Both parents must be carriers. Neither parent will have the disease.
2. Prevalence and prognosis.
   a. 30,000 children and adults in the United States (70,000 worldwide).
   b. Currently, individuals with CF can expect to live into their 30s, 40s, and beyond.
3. Diagnosis.
   a. Chronic, progressive lung disease characterized by production of abnormal mucous.
   b. Salt concentration in the sweat.
   c. Decreased release of certain enzymes by the pancreas.
   d. Certain abnormalities revealed on x-rays.
   e. Failure to grow properly.
4. Complications.
   a. Reduced life expectancy.
      (1) The abnormal mucous clogs the lungs and leads to life-threatening lung infections.
      (2) The mucous obstructs the pancreas and stops natural enzymes from helping the body break down and absorb food.
   b. Cardiac symptoms are a possible complication of CF.
   c. Diabetes, cirrhosis, and rectal prolapse are rare complications of CF.
   d. 5%–10% of children with CF present with intestinal blockage.
5. Medical management/relevant pharmacology.
   a. Aerosol (mist).
   b. Chest physical therapy to loosen secretions that block lung airways.
   c. Vitamin and mineral supplements, enzymes.
   d. Antibiotics.
6. Effect on function.
   a. Exercise intolerance.
   b. Poor nutrition due to malabsorption may contribute to developmental delays.
7. Occupational therapy evaluation.
   a. Assess for developmental delays related to decreased strength and endurance and decreased attention due to pain.
   b. Assess the environment to determine adaptations for energy conservation and possible equipment needs.
   c. Assess psychosocial status.
      (1) Child and family stress related to frequent hospitalizations, school absences, social isolation, and ongoing home treatment.
      (2) Fatigue related to the level of care that is required.
      (3) Emotional stress related to the pain and prognosis.
8. Occupational therapy intervention.
   a. Energy conservation.
   b. Environmental adaptations to enhance performance.
   c. Positioning to promote postural drainage.
   d. Neurodevelopmental treatment to improve endurance and postural stability.
   e. Facilitation of fine, gross, visual motor, cognitive, and psychosocial development.
   f. Parent education.
      (1) Treatment protocols for the above interventions.
      (2) Advocacy skills to obtain necessary services and equipment for the child.
      (3) Advocacy skills to obtain respite services.
   g. Teacher education.
      (1) Energy conservation techniques.
      (2) Encourage physical activity within reason.
      (3) Use precautions for playground play and participation in other healthful physical activities.
         (a) Use the above mentioned medical precautions and energy conservation techniques during play.
   h. Observe medical precautions during occupational therapy sessions (i.e., respiratory/cardiac contraindications).

[2] This section was completed by Marge E. Moffet Boyd and Jan G. Garbarini.

Respiratory Distress Syndrome (RDS)

1. Etiology.
   a. Premature birth.
   b. Insufficient production of surfactant to keep alveoli (air pockets of the lungs) open.
2. Diagnosis.
   a. Lungs collapse after each breath.
   b. X-ray of lungs reveals "ground glass" appearance.
   c. Collapsed alveoli are dense and appear white on the x-ray as opposed to the black appearance on an x-ray of air filled alveoli.
   d. RDS is also called Hyaline Membrane Disease (HMD).
3. Prenatal management.
   a. To stimulate surfactant production and to reduce the risk of RDS, the mother is treated prophylactically with steroid medication 24–36 hours before delivery of a premature infant.
4. Medical management/relevant pharmacology.
   a. Mild case.
      (1) Supplemental oxygen alone, or in combination with positive airways pressure (CPAP), a mixture of oxygen and air provided under pressure through short, two-pronged tubes placed in the nose.
   b. Severe case.
      (1) Intubation and a mixture of oxygen and air provided by a ventilator under positive end expiration pressure (PEEP).
   c. To reduce the severity of RDS and the risk of chronic lung disease, a single dose of surfactant replacement is given within 6 hours of development of RDS.
5. Complications/secondary diagnosis.
   a. Risk of severe intracranial hemorrhage (approximately 35%).
   b. Risk of bronchopulmonary dysplasia (BPD) (approximately 35%).
   c. Risk for developmental delay; severe developmental delay (less than 15%).
   d. The risk for these complications is far greater for infants who do not receive the above mentioned treatments.
6. Effect on function.
   a. The future intellectual development of the premature infant who had RDS and who received the latest treatments appears to be good.
   b. The functional effects for infants who develop BPD or who incur a severe intracranial hemorrhage may include motor, sensory, cognitive, and/or language impairments.
   c. For premature infants with RDS, functional effects may include visual defects, hypotonia, and other health issues that can impact on development.
7. Occupational therapy evaluation.
   a. Assess for developmental delays.
   b. Assess the environment.
8. Occupational therapy intervention.
   a. Monitor development.
   b. Facilitate sensori-motor and cognitive development.
   c. Address psychosocial issues that arise.
   d. Provide parent education regarding handling, positioning, energy conservation, and methods to facilitate normal development.
   e. Adapt environment as needed.
   f. Observe medical precautions.
   g. Refer as necessary to ophthalmologist and other relevant services.

Bronchopulmonary Dysplasia (BPD)

1. Etiology.
   a. Respiratory disorder often as a result of barotrauma.
      (1) High inflating pressures.
      (2) Infection.
      (3) Meconium aspiration.
      (4) Asphyxia.
   b. A complication of prematurity.
   c. The walls of the immature lungs thicken, making the exchange of oxygen and carbon dioxide more difficult.
   d. The mucous lining of the lung is reduced along with the airway diameter.
2. Diagnosis.
   a. Infant must work harder than normal to obtain sufficient oxygen for survival.
3. Medical management/relevant pharmacology.
   a. Months or years of oxygen therapy and artificial ventilation.
   b. Bronchodilators and diuretics to keep the airways and lungs dry.
4. Complications.
   a. Greater risk for hypotonia and gross motor delays.
   b. Feeding problems can lead to poor nutrition.
      (1) Malabsorption problems.
      (2) Fragile bones with an increased risk of fractures.
   c. Central nervous system problems, such as damage to parts of the brain, can lead to delays or impairments in motor, sensory, speech, and cognitive function.
   d. Recurrent otitis media can lead to conductive hearing loss that can affect the development of speech and language as well as cognition.
5. Effect on function.
   a. Poor autonomic and sensory state regulation, can impact on the alert state which is necessary for proper feeding.
   b. Poor exercise/activity tolerance due to illness and compromised respiration.
   c. Reduced ability to socialize due to long periods of poor health and the increased susceptibility to infection.

d. Isolation and stress on the child and family members can lead to psychosocial problems.
e. Greater risk for attachment disorder, affecting the child's ability to relate to others due to isolation and dependence on technological equipment.

6. Occupational therapy evaluation.
   a. Assess for developmental delays/deficits.
   b. Assess the environment to determine adaptations related to energy conservation, positioning, and enhanced occupational performance.
7. Occupational therapy intervention.
   a. Facilitate sensori-motor and cognitive development.
   b. Address psychosocial issues that arise.
   c. Adapt environment.
   d. Provide parent education regarding handling, positioning, feeding, energy conservation and appropriate environmental adaptations.
   e. Parent advocacy related to acquiring necessary services and equipment.
   f. Observe all medical precautions.

References

American Association of Cardiovascular and Pulmonary Rehabilitation (AACVPR). (2004). *Guidelines for cardiac rehabilitation and secondary prevention programs,* 4th ed. Champaign, IL: Human Kinetics.

American Occupational Therapy Association. (2008). Occupational therapy practice: Domain and process, 2nd ed. *American Journal of Occupational Therapy,* 62, 625–683.

Atchison, B. (1995). Cardiopulmonary diseases. In Trombly, C. A. (Ed.), *Occupational therapy for physical dysfunction,* 4th ed. (pp. 884–885). Baltimore: Williams & Wilkins.

Batshaw, M. L., Pellegrino, L., & Roizen, N. J. (2007). *Children with disabilities: A medical primer* 6th ed. (p. 638). Baltimore: Paul H. Brookes.

Centers for Disease Control and Prevention: Division of Tuberculosis Elimination. (2007). Retrieved February 15, 2008 from http://www.cdc.gov/TB/pubs/tbfactsheets/TBTrends.htm.

Ciccone, C. (2004). Medication. In W. DeTurk & L. Cahalin (Eds.), *Cardiovascular and pulmonary physical therapy: An evidence-based approach* (pp. 189–218). New York: McGraw-Hill.

Collins, S., & Cocanour, B. (2004). Anatomy of the cardiopulmonary system. In W. DeTurk & L. Cahalin (Eds.), *Cardiovascular and pulmonary physical therapy: An evidence-based approach* (pp. 73–94). New York: McGraw-Hill.

Criteria Committee of the New York Heart Association. (1994). *Nomenclature and criteria for diagnosis of diseases of the heart and great vessels,* 9th ed. Boston: Little, Brown & Co.

Hillegass, E., and Sadowsky, S. (2001). *Essentials of cardiopulmonary physical therapy,* 2nd ed. Philadelphia: Saunders.

Huntley, N. (2008). Cardiac and pulmonary diseases. In M.V. Radomski & C. A. Trombly Latham (Eds.), *Occupational therapy for physical dysfunction,* 6th ed. (pp. 1295–1330). Baltimore: Lippincott Williams & Wilkins.

Matthews, M. (2013). Cardiac and pulmonary diseases. In Pendleton, H., & Schultz-Krohn, W. (Eds.), *Pedretti's occupational therapy: Practice skills for physical dysfunction,* 7th ed. (pp. 1194–1214). St. Louis, MO: Elsevier Science/Mosby.

McIntyre, M. (2007, March 5). Keeping VAD patients functional. *Advance for Occupational Therapy Practitioners,* 43–44, 56.

National Institutes of Health. Accessed on September 10, 2013 at http://www.nhlbi.nih.gov/health/health-topics/topics/bpd/.

Rais-Bahrami, K., & Short, B. L. (2007). Premature and small-for-dates infants. In M. L. Batshaw, L. Pellegrino, & N. J. Roizen (Eds.), *Children with disabilities* 6th ed. (pp. 107–122). Baltimore, MD: P.H. Brooks.

Rogers, S. L. (2005). Common conditions that influence children's participation. In J. Case-Smith (Ed.), *Occupational therapy for children,* 6th ed. (pp. 160–215). St. Louis, MO: Elsevier Mosby.

Sandhu, S. (2009). *AOTA comments on lymphedema for meeting of Medicare Evidence Development and Coverage Advisory Committee on November 18, 2009.* Retrieved September 26, 2013 from http://www.aota.org/~/media/Corporate/Files/Advocay/Reim/News/Archives/Archived-Letters/Lymphadema%20letter%20to%20MedCAC.ashx.

Vining-Radomski, M., & Trombly-Latham, C. A. (Eds). (2007). *Occupational therapy for physical dysfunction,* 6th ed. Baltimore: Williams & Wilkins.

Wells, C. (2004). Pulmonary pathology. In W. DeTurk & L. Cahalin (Eds.), *Cardiovascular and pulmonary physical therapy: An evidence-based approach* (pp. 151–188). New York: McGraw-Hill.

Review Questions

Cardiovascular and Pulmonary System Disorders

Below are five questions about key content covered in this chapter. These questions are not inclusive of the entirety of content related to cardiovascular and pulmonary system disorders that you must know for success on the NBCOT exam. These questions are provided to help you "jump start" the thought processes you will need to apply your studying of content to the answering of exam questions; hence they are not in the NBCOT exam format. Exam items in the NBCOT format which cover the depth and breadth of content you will need to know to pass the NBCOT exam are provided on this text's disc. The answers to the below questions are provided in Appendix 4.

1. An adult with a diagnosis of left ventricular failure congestive heart failure (CHF) has been referred to occupational therapy for Phase I cardiac rehabilitation during an acute hospitalization. What are the primary goals of inpatient cardiac rehabilitation? What symptoms of CHF does the occupational therapist need to be aware of that might manifest during therapeutic activities?

2. What are the clinical indications that may lead an occupational therapist to stop an activity during a cardiac rehabilitation intervention session? How does the occupational therapist monitor the patient during activity for signs/symptoms of distress?

3. An older adult status-post myocardial infarction (S/P MI) has been referred to occupational therapy for Phase II outpatient cardiac rehabilitation. The client is able to carry out all basic ADL independently and has fair tolerance for activities that require standing and overhead movements. The client lives with a spouse and identifies being a partner, home maintainer, and gardener as primary roles. The client would like to be able to resume role-related activities. The occupational therapy prescription calls for activities beginning at MET level 3 and increasing to MET level 5 according to the patient's activity tolerance. Taking into consideration the therapy prescription, the patient's current status, desired occupational roles, and activity preferences, which treatment approaches and activities should the occupational therapist include in intervention?

4. You have been asked to consult with a teacher to discuss precautions for a student who has a diagnosis of cystic fibrosis. What precautions should you discuss with the teacher? Provide a rationale for your recommendations.

5. You are completing an evaluation on a 20-month-old toddler who was diagnosed with Bronchopulmonary Dysplasia (BPD) shortly after birth. What are the typical deficits resulting from BPD that the child may exhibit during the occupational evaluation? Provide an explanation for your answers.

9

Gastrointestinal, Renal-Genitourinary, Endocrine, Immunological, and Integumentary Systems Disorders

ANN BURKHARDT AND RITA P. FLEMING-CASTALDY

Chapter Outline

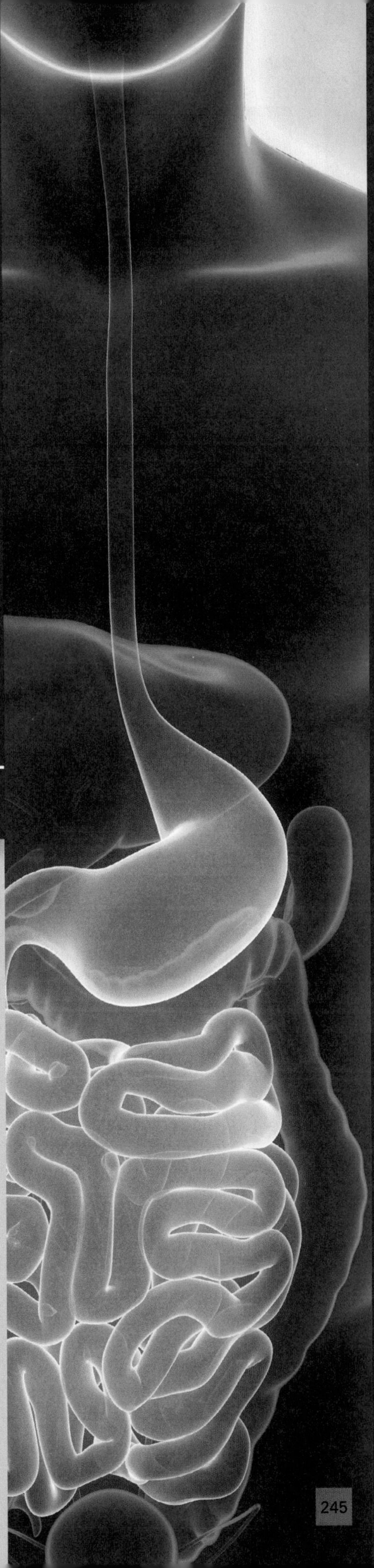

Gastrointestinal System

Dysphagia and Swallowing Disorders

1. Structures involved.
   a. Oral facial musculature.
   b. Pharyngeal and laryngeal structures.
   c. Piriform sinuses.
   d. Vocal folds.
   e. Bronchioles/bronchi.
   f. Lungs.
   g. Esophagus.
2. Facial paralysis.
   a. Incomplete closure of the mouth.
   b. Loss of the bolus out of the front of the oral cavity.
3. Praxis/motor planning deficits.
   a. Inability to effectively chew and coordinate tongue movements to propel the bolus toward the base of the tongue.
   b. Residual food centrally located in the oral cavity.
   c. Difficulty forming a bolus with smoother consistencies.
4. Sensory impairment of the oral cavity.
   a. Lack of awareness of residual food on the side of the mouth that has decreased sensation.
      (1) Pocketing of food.
      (2) Spillage of residual food into the airway at a time when the vocal cords are open; timing of the swallow sequence is off.
5. Weakness of the tongue/base of tongue structures.
   a. Inefficient propulsion of bolus at an efficient rate of speed past the base of the tongue into the pharyngeal cavity.
   b. Lack of closure at the cricopharyngeal junction.
      (1) Sub-optimal propulsion of the bolus.
      (2) Interference with the normal timing of the swallow sequence.
      (3) Failure to trigger closure of the vocal folds during swallow; aspiration.
6. Weakness of the elevation of the pharynx during swallow.
   a. Incomplete triggering (diminished neural stimulation) of the pharyngeal phase of swallowing.
7. Vocal cord paralysis.
   a. Inefficient closure of the vocal folds during the pharyngeal phase of swallow.
      (1) Vocal cords are in paramedian position; swallow may be safe.
      (2) Vocal cords fail to meet/close to protect airway; aspiration may occur.
8. Penetration of the bronchioles/bronchi by the bolus when aspiration occurs.
   a. Food enters the lung; true aspiration occurs.
      (1) Bacteria can cause pneumonia (aspiration pneumonia).
      (2) If the person's immune system is functioning well, he/she may not experience pneumonia.
9. Clinical aspiration.
   a. Food enters the airway.
      (1) Person can clear airway by coughing (reflex intact).
      (2) Person silently aspirates.
         (a) Bolus enters lung and person does not react.
         (b) Bolus enters the lung and person experiences respiratory distress without a cough.
         (c) Person coughs too weakly to raise the bolus in order to expel it.
10. Diminished esophageal motility.
   a. Bolus sits in the esophagus and can slowly either move toward the stomach or upward toward the pharynx.
      (1) Person may feel that food is stuck in the esophagus.
      (2) Person aspirates when food propels upward and he/she cannot swallow it.
11. Clinical exams and functional findings.
   a. Staff report questioning swallowing dysfunction.
      (1) Person coughs during or after drinking water or other thin liquid.
   b. The person's face changes color during or after eating.
      (1) Flushed/reddened color, ashened appearance for persons with darker skin.
      (2) Blanches.
   c. Person gasps for breath, but has a partial or complete airway obstruction.
      (1) To clear the obstruction and raise the bolus that has been aspirated, the Heimlich maneuver is used as long as the person is awake and responsive.
      (2) If the person loses consciousness, basic life support procedures are used to continue to try to reestablish the airway.
         (a) This includes abdominal thrusts and back blows, plus periodically looking in the oral cavity to try to visualize the object. If visualized, it may be possible to remove the object and restore respiratory function.

d. Bedside swallowing evaluation.
 (1) Assess level of alertness, ability to follow directions, level of awareness of impairment, orientation to activity.
 (2) Assess sensory and motor components of swallowing.
 (3) Asses ability to manage own secretions.
  (a) Auscultation of neck to hear elongation of the oropharyngeal structures and to listen for wetness/gurgling which could be a sign of insufficient swallowing.
  (b) Clinical observation of person.
 (4) Assess swallowing function using trial boluses.
  (a) Suggest diet modification, as indicated.
  (b) Recommend further testing if needed.
e. Modified barium swallow (MBS).
 (1) In diagnostic radiology suite.
 (2) Done with swallowing team and radiologist.
  (a) Person seated at uprighted edge of radiology table.
  (b) Person must have adequate sitting balance.
  (c) Person must be supervised at all times.
 (3) Person administered trial boluses laced with barium.
  (a) Person should be given boluses mixed with food consistencies, purees, thick liquids, solids, and thin liquids.
  (b) If the person aspirates, the test ceases.
 (4) Video records moving x-ray of swallow. A copy of the video is kept as part of the record.
 (5) Still x-ray shots are taken if aspiration is observed.
f. Flexible endoscopic esophageal swallow (FEES).
 (1) May be done at bedside or in an office setting.
 (2) Food consistencies are laced with green food coloring.
 (3) A flexible endoscopic catheter containing a miniature video camera is passed through the nasal cavity into the pharyngeal cavity.
 (4) The person is given a variety of consistencies to swallow and observation is made to determine whether the swallow is intact or impaired.
 (5) Sensation for light touch in the pharyngeal cavity can be tested by forcing air through the endoscopic tube generating a light touch stimulus.

12. Relationship of swallowing dysfunction to occupation.
 a. Disruption of the person's role relative to his/her family unit/decreased ability to comfortably eat at the dinner table.
  (1) Modified diet could be infantilizing.
  (2) Tube feeding may preempt person's ability to partake in the family meal in cultural/social context.
 b. Disruption of ability/decreased comfort level for eating out in public.
  (1) Person may choose not to dine in a public social context.
  (2) If business lunches or dinners are part of a vocational role, the person may not be able to resume his/her vocation without modification of expectations regarding how participation in social meals relates to vocational performance.
 c. Alteration of self-concept concerning life roles and appearance.
  (1) If person is tube fed, how does that alter how he/she perceives self?
   (a) Sex appeal can be questioned.
   (b) Self image as it impacts on life roles (e.g., a jet-setter or fashion plate) can be altered.
  (2) If tube fed, how does that alter how others perceive him/her?
   (a) Accepted, feared, or pitied by children, grandchildren, family, and friends.

13. Intervention.
 a. Provide family-centered intervention to determine an acceptable dinner table alternative to interaction.
 b. Work with person toward developing new roles and occupations to transition from old role (i.e., head of table).
 c. Provide ongoing education and information to family regarding person's feeding/nutrition.
 d. See Chapters 14 and 15 for further information on psychosocial interventions and interventions for performance in areas of occupation.

Gastric Esophageal Reflux Disease (GERD)

1. Structures involved include the lower esophageal sphincter and gastric sphincter.
 a. Food enters stomach and mixes with stomach acid/digestive juices.
 b. Lower esophageal sphincter inefficiently closes; stomach contraction propels acid/acidic bolus back into the esophagus.
  (1) Person reports heartburn sensation, indigestion, or dull chest pain.
 c. Positional elevation of the head above the stomach, when the person is reclined, may discourage upward retropulsion of the bolus from the stomach.
2. Frequent complaints of people who have GERD.
 a. Heartburn/indigestion.
 b. Swallowing problems.
  (1) A sensation of feeling that something is getting stuck in their 'throat.'
  (2) Chest pressure or pain.
  (3) Regurgitation after swallowing.

3. Tests.
   a. Barium swallow (observing below the pharynx). Visualize external to airway in profile via x-ray.
   b. Flexible endoscopy (observing at the pharynx and descending to the esophagus directly).
4. Intervention.
   a. Sleeping with more than one pillow (elevating the head to discourage regurgitation associated with body posture).
   b. Drug therapy.
   c. Diet modification.
      (1) Less spice.
      (2) Small meals on a more frequent basis.
      (3) Lower alcohol intake.
   d. Stress management.

Small Bowel Obstruction

1. Etiology.
   a. Secondary to scar tissue.
   b. Secondary to radiation of the abdomen (long-term effect).
   c. Result of tumor obstruction.
2. Surgical treatment.
   a. Resection with open stoma (colostomy).
   b. Closed abdominal surgery.
3. Rehabilitation issues.
   a. Self-care aspects of stoma care must be addressed for persons with decreased fine motor skills (e.g., individuals with peripheral neuropathy secondary to chemotherapy treatment).
   b. Decrease mobility of gross movements that cause traction on the healing scar.
      (1) Bending.
      (2) Stooping.
      (3) Foot/lower leg related self-care.
         (a) Dressing.
         (b) Bathing.
         (c) Nail and foot care.
   c. Altered appetite in post-operative phase.

Neurogenic Bowel

1. Etiology: sympathetic nerve impairment, generally occurring in persons who have spinal cord injury above the (thoracic) T-6 level.
   a. Loss of control of anal sphincter.
   b. Sensory loss resulting in a lack of awareness of feces in the bowel.
   c. Motor loss, decreased or lost ability to self-initiate or control a bowel movement.
2. Flaccidity of muscles results in incontinence.
3. Autonomic dysreflexia, an extreme rise in blood pressure can result.
   a. This is a medical emergency if not reversed.
   b. See Chapter 7's section on the complications of spinal cord injury for more information.

Renal-Genitourinary System

Kidney Disease

1. Risk factors.
   a. Diabetes.
      (1) 3 of every 10 individuals with diabetes develop kidney failure.
      (2) 60%–65% of all persons with diabetes also have high blood pressure.
      (3) 10%–40% of people with Type 2 diabetes develop severe kidney disease and End Stage Renal Disease (ESRD).
      (4) Diabetes can contribute to development of nephrotic syndrome.
   b. Hypertension (HTN).
      (1) Uncontrolled or poorly controlled hypertension is the primary diagnosis for 26% of all new cases of chronic kidney failure each year.
      (2) Hypertension is a serious problem among African-Americans.
      (3) 65% of HTN in women and 78% of HTN in men can be directly attributed to obesity.
   c. Systematic lupus erythematosus.
      (1) Lupus can contribute to development of nephrotic syndrome.
2. Treatment for renal disease.
   a. Prevention, early intervention, and control of hypertension.
      (1) Diet.
      (2) Medication.
      (3) Exercise.
      (4) Stress reduction.
      (5) Smoking cessation.
   b. Prevention, early detection, and control of diabetes. See this chapter's section on diabetes.
   c. Medical treatment of lupus.
      (1) Control symptoms to prevent complications.
      (2) Treat with diuretics and drugs that prevent spillage of protein in the urine (angiotensin converting enzyme-ACE).

d. Medical treatment of nephrotic syndrome.
  (1) Treat with diuretics and drugs that prevent spillage of protein in the urine.
  (2) Drug control of fluid overload and/or spillage of protein into the urine (proteinuria).
  (3) Encourage compliance with drug therapy, dietary and exercise recommendations.
e. Medical treatment of acute renal failure.
  (1) Drug control of underlying medical contributory conditions.
  (2) Emergent, acute dialysis.
f. Medical treatment of end stage renal disease (ESRD).
  (1) Dialysis required to stay alive.
    (a) Hemodialysis.
    (b) Peritoneal dialysis: inpatient treatment, continuous ambulatory peritoneal dialysis (CAPD).
  (2) Transplantation.
    (a) Cadaver.
    (b) Living related.
    (c) Living unrelated.

3. Impact on performance skills/and client factors.
  a. Motor dysfunction.
    (1) Fatigue.
    (2) Muscle pain.
    (3) Edema limiting mobility.
    (4) Weakness.
  b. Sensory system function.
    (1) Neuropathy (diabetes related, toxicity related, cyclosporin, anti-rejection drug related).
    (2) Vision loss (diabetes related).
  c. Cognitive dysfunction.
    (1) Alteration of body image due to dialysis (tied to equipment/schedule) or post transplant (foreign tissue).
    (2) Delusions due to sepsis or toxicity.
    (3) Dementia, multi-infarct or metabolic.
  d. Perceptual/neurobehavioral dysfunction.
    (1) Dementia/infarct related.
    (2) Stroke related.
  e. Psychological/emotional dysfunction.
    (1) Anxiety disorder.
    (2) Depression.
    (3) Mood/adjustment disorder.
    (4) Poor management of psychosocial disorders can increase the risk of cardiac arrest.
    (5) Supportive counseling and social support are indicated.
    (6) Drug therapy and complementary medicine.

4. Impact on performance in areas of occupation.
  a. Self-care.
    (1) Alteration in urination.
    (2) Need for meticulous sanitary technique with self dialysis.
    (3) Strict adherence to a disease specific/highly restrictive diet.
    (4) Alteration in sexuality.
      (a) Impotence.
      (b) Alteration of self esteem/body image.
      (c) Feeling less desirable.
    (5) Need for use of adapted equipment.
      (a) Tub/toilet bench.
      (b) Build-ups.
      (c) Reaching assistive devices.
      (d) Fine motor assistive devices (button hooks, etc.).
    (6) Energy conservation and work simplification; fatigue is an issue.
    (7) Altered mobility.
      (a) Wheeled mobility.
      (b) Use of assistive devices to walk such as an ankle-foot orthosis, walker, cane.
  b. Instrumental activities.
    (1) Housekeeping.
      (a) Need for lighter work load and housekeeping assistance.
      (b) Altered role in the family.
    (2) Community mobility.
      (a) Adapted vehicles.
      (b) Access to transit passes and/or accessible parking spaces.
      (c) Special planning for long distance travel.
    (3) Meal preparation.
      (a) Training to change usual habits to cook appropriately for dietary limitations.
      (b) Planning to budget and purchase appropriate supplies.
      (c) Safety in cooking.
    (4) Management of personal finances.
      (a) Ability to do banking.
      (b) Ability to budget funds.
      (c) Ability to prioritize goals.
      (d) Ability to achieve goals or problem solve solutions.
    (5) Leisure/sports activities.
      (a) Ability to participate.
      (b) Ability to pace self/self regulate.
      (c) Choice of activities that allow participation with minimum risk.
      (d) Awareness of precautions for participation.
      (e) Access to sports facilities that have adaptive possibilities or sources for adaptations.

5. Impact on performance contexts.
  a. Social context.
    (1) How disease affects role in the family.
    (2) How disease affects role in the workplace.
    (3) How disease affects role in the community, including spiritual communities, social groups, special interests.

b. Cultural context.
(1) How cultural group accepts condition and/or treatment.
(2) Relative taboo of treatment options/choices.
(3) Acceptance of individual in view of impairment/disease.

Neurogenic Bladder/UTI

1. See this chapter's gastrointestinal system section.

Stress Incontinence

1. Etiology: local damage to bladder sphincter associated with the aftereffects of bearing children, morbid obesity, and weakening of accessory musculature associated with normal aging.
2. Intervention.
a. Kegel exercises to strengthen pelvic floor.
b. Timed routines for emptying bladder before it is full enough to cause spillage.
c. Lifestyle adjustments to use incontinence supporting garments for a socially acceptable solution and to decrease public attention to the incontinence.
d. Medications may be used when the physician feels the client can tolerate the side effects of drug therapy support.
e. Electric stimulation may be used, if client fits the parameters of recovery for the condition.

Immunological System

Cancer

1. Etiology: unknown for some cancers, strong link to risk factors for others.
2. Risk factors for cancer.
a. Heredity.
(1) Some tumors seem to have a high hereditary risk.
(a) Breast cancer.
(b) Prostate cancer.
(c) Skin cancer.
(d) Colon cancer.
b. Environmental.
(1) Cluster patterns related to chemical pollution.
c. Habit or lifestyle related.
(1) Smoking and use of smokeless/chewing tobacco can contribute to lung cancer and head and neck cancer.
(2) Drinking alcohol contributes to some head and neck cancers.
(3) Obesity/high fat diets may be linked to an increased risk of some cancers.
3. Prevention, early intervention, and control.
a. Specific to type of cancer.
(1) Mammograms are recommended for women beginning at age 40, yearly after age 50.
(a) Recently, it has been recommended that ultrasound screening may be better in women who have dense breasts.
(b) Insurers continue to recommend mammography as the preferred screening method.
(2) Prostate and testicular exams are indicated for all adult males.
(a) The Prostate Specific Antigen (PSA) blood test has recently been criticized as having insufficient evidence to uphold its efficacy in screening for prostate cancer.
(3) Skin checks should be done regularly for people who have a family history of skin cancer or those who have a high exposure to the sun (e.g., construction workers, fishermen, landscapers, etc.).
(4) Those with a family history of colon cancer should have screening and follow-up colonoscopies throughout adulthood and interventional colonoscopy if they are symptomatic.
(a) Routine screening for colon cancer via colonoscopy is recommended for all adults over the age of 50.
(5) Women should have regular pap smears to detect vaginal/cervical/uterine cancer.
(6) Women who have a risk for ovarian cancer should be screened by blood test and abdominal ultrasound.
b. Avoid environmental contributing factors (e.g., chemically contaminated land, lead paint).
c. Avoiding contributory habits.
(1) Health care professionals should coach people who want to quit or change habits (e.g., cease smoking).
(a) Promote self-regulatory behaviors/willpower to change habits.
(b) Recommend help-seeking assistance to increase compliance (e.g., 12-step programs, support groups, individual treatment).

4. Diagnostic staging of cancer.
   a. Stage 1: tumor present, no perceived spread of disease.
      (1) Lesion operable.
      (2) Prognosis good (70%–90% mean survival at 5 years).
         (a) No spread of disease to the lymph nodes.
         (b) No metastatic lesions.
   b. Stage 2: localized spread of the tumor.
      (1) Lesion is operable and can be removed with margins.
      (2) Spread is limited and usually responds well to treatment (chemo/radiation/immuno-therapy).
      (3) Mean 5-year survival rate is 50% ± 5%.
   c. Stage 3: extensive evidence of a primary tumor that has spread to other organs in the body.
      (1) Tumor can be surgically debulked, but some cells may remain behind.
      (2) There is deeper spread of the tumor cells in the lymphatics.
      (3) Widespread evidence of cancer throughout multiple organs of the body.
      (4) Mean 5-year survival rate is 20% ± 5%.
   d. Stage 4: inoperable primary lesion.
      (1) Survival dependent on depth and extent of the tumor spread as well as the ability to have the tumor respond to therapy (mean 5-year survival rate is < 5%).
      (2) Multiple metastases.
5. Medical treatment.
   a. Surgery.
      (1) Lumpectomy.
      (2) En bloc resection.
      (3) Reconstruction.
      (4) Amputation.
   b. Chemotherapy.
      (1) Intravenous.
      (2) Shunt.
      (3) Oral.
   c. Radiation.
      (1) External beam.
         (a) Wide beam.
         (b) Cone down.
      (2) Brachytherapy.
         (a) Seed implantation, flexible rods.
   d. Immunotherapy.
      (1) Interferon.
      (2) Monoclonal antibodies.
   e. Hormonal therapy.
   f. Transplantation.
      (1) Bone marrow.
6. Rehabilitation.
   a. Pre-operative.
      (1) Pre-operative functional assessments and preparation of the client for post-operative phase and care.
      (2) Client and caregiver education concerning recovery and follow up care/functional expectations and client engagement.
   b. Post-operative.
      (1) Intervention planning based on a client's medical status and blood value guidelines that can affect safety during activity (platelets, hemoglobin level).
      (2) Post-operative precautions related to structural change from surgery.
         (a) This will be dependent on the location of the tumor and the procedure done (e.g., if a joint is replaced with an en bloc resection and shoulder indwelling prosthetic; abdominal precautions when the tumor is in the abdominal cavity; regional precautions when there is an incision near a joint, etc).
   c. Convalescence.
      (1) Rehabilitation of motor impairments.
      (2) Rehabilitation of sensory impairments.
      (3) Rehabilitation of cognitive impairments.
      (4) Rehabilitation of neurobehavioral impairments.
      (5) Psychological support to enhance coping ability during recovery from cancer treatment phase.
         (a) Liminality: self recognition of vulnerability and self sense of mortality.
         (b) Occupational role and body image adjustment.
         (c) Obtainment of social support.
      (6) Development of health supporting behaviors with follow-up support (diet, exercise, stress management, vocational skill support, or assistance to change job skills).
   d. Palliative care.
      (1) Prevent and relieve suffering for persons with life-threatening illness through early identification, assessment, and treatment of pain.
      (2) Address physical, psychosocial, and spiritual needs.
      (3) Enhance quality of life by supporting clients' engagement in daily life occupations that they find meaningful and purposeful.
      (4) Consider environmental and contextual factors (e.g., accessibility of objects or places in the environment, social contacts available to prevent isolation) and client factors (e.g., decreased endurance, increased anxiety) that may limit a client's abilities and satisfaction when performing desired occupations.
      (5) Collaborate with the client and family members throughout the occupational therapy process to identify occupations that are meaningful, incorporate strategies that support occupational engagement, and provide caregiver training as needed.

e. End of life care (hospice).
   (1) Support quality of life as disease advances and functional status declines.
   (2) Provide client with as much control as they can and desire to have to their day to day life and lifestyle-support.
   (3) Be present, be accountable, listen and counsel as possible concerning progression of disease and sense of liminality.
   (4) Encourage planning for death, control over goodbyes, funeral arrangements, advanced directives, etc.
   (5) Empower life celebration and life reflection (journaling, scrapbooks, phone call contact and recontact, letter writing).
   (6) Refer for legal support, if needed and requested).
   (7) See Chapter 14 for additional information on psychosocial issues related to the end of life and adjustment to death and dying.

Scleroderma

1. Rheumatic, connective tissue disease associated with impaired immune response.
2. Etiology: unknown.
   a. Three main components.
      (1) Vascular.
         (a) Raynaud's phenomenon.
         (b) Constant recurrent constriction of small blood vessels leading to pulmonary hypertension.
         (c) Decreased esophageal motility.
      (2) Fibrotic.
         (a) Scar tissue resulting from excess collagen (protein) causing thickness of skin and a burning sensation in the skin.
         (b) Fibrosis of the lungs causing restrictive lung disease.
      (3) Autoimmunity.
         (a) B Cell-produced antibodies (anti-centromere, anti-topisomerase I antibodies).
   b. Two basic types of the disease.
      (1) Limited.
         (a) Skin involvement (with a good prognosis).
         (b) Linear scleroderma (bands of thicker skin, with a good prognosis).
      (2) Systemic.
         (a) Systemic sclerosis of internal organs, which is life threatening.
         (b) CREST Syndrome with a good prognosis.
            • Calcinosis, or calcium in the skin.
            • Raynaud's phenomenon.
            • Esophageal dysfunction.
            • Sclerodactyly of fingers and toes.
            • Telangiectasis or red spots covering the hands, feet, forearms, face and hips.
         (c) General morphea.
3. Risk factors: unknown, two main theories.
   a. Genetic.
   b. Environment.
4. Prevalence in the United States.
   a. 80% of scleroderma victims are women 30–50 years old at diagnosis.
   b. 300,000 cases in the United States, but only about 49,000 have the systemic form of the disease.
5. Prevention.
   a. Control symptoms of Raynaud's phenomenon.
   b. Have screening echocardiograms to rule out pulmonary hypertension.
   c. Smoking cessation.
6. Intervention.
   a. Raynaud's phenomenon.
      (1) Keep fingers and toes warm.
      (2) Dress in layers.
      (3) Drug therapy: vasodilators: Procardia XL, Altace, Norvasc, Trental, Cardizem.
      (4) Biofeedback.
   b. Pulmonary artery problems.
      (1) Drug therapy: Procardia SL, anti-coagulation therapy.
      (2) Oxygen: nasal.
   c. Gastrointestinal problems.
      (1) Drug therapy: antacids, e.g., Maalox, Mylanta, Tums, Tagamet, etc.
      (2) Dietary modifications: soft diet, avoidance of alcoholic beverages and spicy foods.
      (3) Treatment of infection: erythromycin, tetracycline, doxycycline.
   d. Fibrosis of the skin.
      (1) Protective gloves: cotton, insulated, mildly compressive.
      (2) Drug therapy: Cuprimine, Relaxin (under investigation).
   e. Myositis: inflammatory muscle disease.
      (1) Cessation of exercise.
      (2) Drug therapy: low dose of oral steroids.
   f. Fibrosis of the lungs.
      (1) Drug therapy: Cytoxan, or Cuprimine and Methotrexate.
7. Sequelae of scleroderma and recommendations.
   a. Poor circulation, as in Raynaud's phenomenon.
      (1) Use of dressing in layers of clothing and clothing style modifications for neutral warmth.
      (2) Biofeedback: guided imagery to concentrate on improving distal circulation.
      (3) Education to encourage skin inspection.
      (4) Activity modifications to prevent trauma to fingers and toes.

b. Contractures.
  (1) Splinting at optimal resting length for hands/wrists to attempt to slow progressive development of contractures.
  (2) Use of silicone gel in the palms of the hands.
  (3) Use of electrical/mechanical vibration (muffled) to stimulate rapidly adapting-type A-nerve fibers and decrease burning sensation in hands.
c. Facial disfigurement and alteration in body image and self-identity.
  (1) 'Look good/feel better' programs.
  (2) Work with people to help them choose adaptations and new accessories to ease their adjustment to their changing appearance.
  (3) Support groups: in person and on-line.
d. Thoracic spinal lesions can result in paraparesis, neurogenic bowel/bladder, altered mobility, and altered activity of daily living activities.
  (1) Neuro rehabilitation and biomechanical approaches as indicated.
e. Space occupying lesions in the brain produce stroke-like symptoms.
  (1) Rehabilitation for functional deficits.

Acquired Immunodeficiency Syndrome (AIDS)

1. Etiology: infection by the human immunodeficiency virus (HIV).
2. Risk factors for infection.
  a. Unprotected sex.
  b. Contact with blood or body fluids.
3. Prevention.
  a. Avoid unprotected sex via abstinence or use of condoms.
  b. Avoid contact with body fluids.
    (1) Blood procedures.
    (2) Breast feeding.
    (3) Secretions of vagina/rectum, during birth (protection of baby), during sex, during hygiene.
    (4) Urine or feces.
    (5) Tears (low % of infection).
  c. Practice standard precautions with all persons. Refer to Table 3-2 and Table 3-3 in Chapter 3.
4. Human immunodeficiency virus (HIV) infection.
  a. Retrovirus.
    (1) The RNA of the virus combines with recombinant RNA of human cells.
    (2) The new DNA has 1 strand of normal RNA/1 strand of virus.
    (3) The virus can eclipse into the cell, remaining dormant until stimulated by the body.
  b. HIV attacks the lymphatic system, the system that protects the body's immunity to opportunistic infections.
    (1) The T-cells (also known as CD4+ cells) attack the cells of the body including central nervous system cells, gastrointestinal tract cells, uterine/cervical cells.
  c. Four stages of infection.
    (1) Acute infection: flu-like response to initial contact with the virus.
    (2) Asymptomatic disease: HIV replicates and affects the immune system, but no visible signs other than blood abnormalities are detectable.
    (3) Symptomatic HIV: signs and symptoms appear.
    (4) Advanced disease, or AIDS: severely compromised immunity; CD4+ level drops to below 1000/mm3.
  d. Sequelae of HIV infection.
    (1) Generalized lymphadenopathy/enlarged lymph nodes.
      (a) Fatigue.
      (b) Weight loss, malabsorption of nutrients (wasting syndrome).
      (c) General malaise.
    (2) Fever.
    (3) Diarrhea.
    (4) All of the above result in decreased tolerance for activity participation and lack of energy.
    (5) Neurological impairment.
      (a) Cognitive impairment (i.e., safety issues, communication and expression impairments, alteration of personality, decreased ability to engage as before in interpersonal relationships).
      (b) Affective changes.
      (c) Sensory changes (associated with dementia).
      (d) Basic ADL impairments such as inability to hold and manipulate objects for use (money, combs, tooth brushes, writing implements, feeding utensils, telephone, remote control, etc.).
      (e) Myelopathy (spinal cord pathology).
      (f) Peripheral neuropathy.
      (g) Visual impairment (i.e., peripheral: cytomegaloviral (CMV) infection, retinopathy, central: neurobehavioral loss/impairment).
  e. Drug therapy.
    (1) Protease inhibitors work to suppress the viral load in the bloodstream.
      (a) Must be taken consistently on time or effectiveness is lost.
      (b) Has shown a dramatic change in the management, treatment, and survivability of persons with a diagnosis of HIV/AIDS.
    (2) Chemotherapy.
      (a) Less effective than protease inhibitors.
      (b) Loaded with side effects (specific to drugs used).

(c) Drugs used related to neoplastic processes observed. Examples include Kaposi's sarcoma, lymphoma.
(d) Drugs used to treat Hodgkin's, non-Hodgkin's (highly differentiated type, non-differentiated type).
(e) Drugs used to treat opportunistic infections. Examples include Foscarnet.

Hepatitis

1. Etiology: a viral infection.
2. Risk factors.
   a. Type A.
      (1) Contaminated seafood.
      (2) Protective immunization possible.
   b. Type B, C, and other identified forms.
      (1) Body and blood borne exposure.
      (2) Protective immunization possible for type B.
         (a) Health care workers are most susceptible to hepatitis B.
         (b) It is estimated that many people in the US population may have undetected Hepatitis C infections which they can potentially (and unknowingly) communicate to others.
3. Prevention.
   a. Practice standard precautions with all persons to prevent contact with blood or body fluids. Refer to Table 3-2 and Table 3-3 in Chapter 3.
4. Sequelae.
   a. Fever.
   b. Fatigue.
   c. The above contribute to decreased tolerance for activity participation and lack of energy.
   d. Hepatitis C infections can cause life threatening cirrhosis over time and may contribute to chronic fatigue and disability.

Tuberculosis (TB)

1. See Chapter 8.

Methicillin-Resistant Staphylococcus aureus (MRSA)

1. Etiology: usually mild infections (pimples or boils) on the skin; or more serious infections on skin; or infection in surgical wounds. The infection can be locally confined or systemic (entering the bloodstream and affecting primarily the lungs or the urinary tract).
2. Risk factors.
   a. Having a weakened immune system.
   b. Confinement in a hospital or other health care institutions.
   c. Living in close quarters (military, college, etc.).
   d. Direct skin contact with an infected body part of another person (contact sports).
   e. Secondary skin contact from something used by someone with an infection (e.g., shared towels during sports activities).
3. The infection resists treatment from known antibiotics, even broad spectrum antibiotics. Some antibiotics still work to fight it.
4. Signs and symptoms.
   a. Redness accompanied by swelling and pain in the area of the wound.
   b. Drainage such as pus in the local area of the wound.
   c. Fever.
   d. Skin abscess.
   e. Chest pain.
   f. Cough.
   g. Fatigue.
   h. Head ache.
   i. Muscle ache.
   j. Rash.
   k. Shortness of breath.
5. Testing.
   a. Cultures of blood, sputum, skin, or urine.
6. Prevention, detection, and early intervention.
   a. Avoid high risk situations that contribute to possible exposure.
   b. Take preventative measures.
      (1) Wash your hands.
      (2) Avoid sharing personal items (e.g., razors or towels).
      (3) Keep any wounds or cuts covered.
      (4) Avoid communal bathing/swimming where infected persons may have been.
      (5) Assure facilities you use are clean.
7. Medical treatment for MRSA.
   a. Draining of a skin sore by an MD.
   b. Antibiotic treatment.
   c. Additional measures depending on severity and location of infection.
      (1) Intravenous fluids.
      (2) Oxygen.
      (3) Dialysis (if kidney failure occurs).
8. Sequelae of MRSA.
   a. Chance of recurrence of infection in the future.
   b. Any organ system damage that occurs as a result from untreated or unmanaged infections.

Rehabilitation for Immunological System Disorders

1. Overall goals and approaches can be preventive, restorative, supportive, and/or palliative depending

on treatment setting, diagnosis, stage of illness, and expected outcomes.

2. Interventions for impairment level problems.
   a. Counsel people to be compliant with screening and treatment regimens.
   b. Set personal goals to invest behaviorally in one's health.
   c. Provide support to those dealing with immunological system disorders that are chronic illnesses (i.e., AIDS).
   d. Provide supportive counseling and social support for psychological disorders that can develop (e.g., anxiety disorder, depression, and/or adjustment disorders).
   e. Refer to physician for drug therapy and complementary medicine as indicated for accompanying physical and/or psychiatric disorders (e.g., kidney disease, depression).
3. Interventions for activity level problems.
   a. Self-care.
      (1) Adaptations and training to do self-care tasks with greatest ease while conserving energy. For example, for an individual with scleroderma:
         (a) Alter grasp and pinch patterns and level of demand and upper extremity demand.
         (b) Alter size of feeding utensils and tooth brushes to accommodate decreased ability to open mouth.
         (c) Prevent shearing forces on skin during specific personal activities of daily living tasks.
   b. Work.
      (1) Work capacity evaluations.
      (2) Modifications to work site to allow participation in component tasks and activities.
      (3) Counseling and intervention for transition to disability status when work is no longer possible.
   c. Leisure/sports.
      (1) Modify specific tasks and activities (e.g., to protect body parts involved by sclerodermic changes).
      (2) Evaluate interests and skills to introduce new leisure or sports activities of interest to the person to transition to less physically demanding tasks as a disease progresses.
   d. Rest.
      (1) Monitor and intervene to maximize the ability to be well positioned during sleep.
      (2) Monitor sleep habits and patterns and intervene when strategies are needed to relax and unwind or to schedule time and opportunity for relaxation.
4. Interventions for participation problems.
   a. Needs assessment to determine individual issues the person has with mobility, social, or political access to their personal, home, or community environments.
   b. Identification and facilitation of procurement of system changes to allow person access and ability to participate as a contributing member of society.
5. Acute hospitalization phase.
   a. Early mobilization.
   b. Preservation of function.
   c. Positioning.
   d. Psychological/emotional support.
   e. Prevention of long-term disability.
6. Inpatient rehabilitation.
   a. Evaluation and restoration of functional abilities.
      (1) Self-care, basic ADL.
      (2) Instrumental ADL.
      (3) Energy conservation and work simplification.
      (4) Use of the Pizzi Assessment of Productive Living for Adults with HIV (PAPL) for persons with HIV.
   b. Restoration of activity/exercise tolerance.
   c. Achievement and maintenance of quality of life.
   d. Role readjustment intervention.
   e. Planning to return to community.
      (1) Access to environment.
      (2) Participation issues.
7. Home care.
   a. Use of a collaborative assessment (e.g., Canadian Occupational Performance Measure [COPM]) to set client goals.
   b. Evaluation and restoration of functional ability.
   c. Restoration of activity/exercise tolerance.
   d. Community mobility.
      (1) To inner and outer boundaries of home environment.
      (2) Into the street/block.
      (3) Further ability to venture out into the community (i.e., marketing, use of transportation, medical/business appointments, leisure access).
8. Community-based care.
   a. School related.
      (1) Transition from home schooling back to school for the child returning.
      (2) Transition of having student return to class for the classmates.
   b. Work related.
      (1) Participatory as per Americans with Disabilities Act (ADA).
   c. Population-related intervention.
      (1) Coalition-related and grant funded initiatives for prevention and outreach programs.

Chapter 9

Endocrine System

Diabetes

1. Prevalence.
   a. There are 20.8 million children and adults in the United States, or 7% of the population, who have diabetes.
   b. While an estimated 14.6 million have been diagnosed, 6.2 million people (or nearly one-third) are unaware that they have the disease.
2. Types, etiology, and risk factors.
   a. Type 1 diabetes (insulin-dependent) (5%–10% of all diagnosed cases of diabetes).
      (1) Autoimmune.
      (2) Genetic.
      (3) Environmental factors.
   b. Type 2 diabetes (non-insulin-dependent) (90%–95% of all diabetes).
      (1) Older age.
      (2) Obesity.
      (3) Family history.
      (4) Prior history of gestational diabetes.
      (5) Impaired glucose tolerance.
      (6) Physical inactivity.
      (7) Race/ethnicity.
         (a) African-Americans.
         (b) Hispanic/Latino Americans.
         (c) American Indians.
         (d) Asian-Americans (non-Japanese).
         (e) Pacific Islanders.
   c. Gestational diabetes (2%–5% of all pregnancies; 40% may go on later to develop Type 2 diabetes in later life).
      (1) Usually resolves after pregnancy.
      (2) Occurs at a greater frequency in people in race/ethnicity risk groups.
      (3) Obesity is another risk factor.
   d. Other types of diabetes (1%–2% of all cases of diabetes).
      (1) Genetic syndromes.
      (2) Surgery.
      (3) Drugs (e.g., steroids).
      (4) Malnutrition.
      (5) Infections.
3. Signs and symptoms.
   a. Frequent urination.
   b. Excessive thirst.
   c. Unexplained weight loss.
   d. Extreme hunger.
   e. Visual changes.
   f. Sensory changes (tingling/numbness) in the hands or feet.
   g. Fatigue.
   h. Very dry skin.
   i. Slow healing wounds.
   j. Increased rate of infections.
4. Prevention.
   a. Regular physical activity may reduce the risk of type 2 diabetes.
   b. Maintaining normal body weight may be preventive.
5. Sequelae/complications.
   a. Fatigue/decreased activity tolerance.
   b. Urinary disturbance.
   c. Visual loss, low vision, blindness.
   d. Peripheral neuropathy.
      (1) Amputations.
   e. Propensity to develop wounds.
   f. Poor general health/increased rate of infections disrupting life roles and activity participation.
   g. Hypoglycemia.
      (1) Symptoms include vagueness, dizziness, tachycardia, pallor, weakness, diaphoresis, seizures, and/or coma.
      (2) If person is conscious, immediately provide carbohydrates in the form of hard candy, fruit juice, or honey.
      (3) If person is unconscious, immediately call for emergency medical care.
   h. Hyperglycemic crisis.
      (1) Ketoacidosis: signs include dehydration, rapid and weak pulse, and acetone breath.
      (2) Hyperosmolar coma: signs include stupor, thirst, polyuria, and neurologic abnormalities.
      (3) Call for emergency medical services as IV fluids and insulin are required.
6. Rehabilitation.
   a. Preventive exercise.
   b. Education concerning compliance and need for medical management of condition.
   c. Psychological and emotional support to improve self-care habits.
   d. Lifestyle readjustment to complications when and if they occur.
      (1) Low vision.
      (2) Safety assessment and intervention.
      (3) Physical adaptations.
   e. Protective issues regarding peripheral neuropathy.
      (1) Safety assessment.
      (2) Education concerning risk associated with sensory loss.
      (3) Skin care.
      (4) Pain management.

(5) Adapted equipment/techniques to facilitate participation in lifestyle.
(6) Instrumental activities supporting compliance of self management.

f. Early attention to wound management.
(1) Teach skin care and inspection techniques.
(2) Teach person to self advocate quickly when changes are observed.

g. Assistance in problem solving and modifying self-care as changes occur in the medical status of the condition.
(1) Problem solve resources for specialized treatment.
(2) Teach person to recognize changes in their functional status that warrant further attention and intervention.

Obesity and Bariatric Issues[1]

1. Obesity is defined as a condition characterized by excess body fat.
2. Body mass index (BMI): a formula for determining obesity. BMI is calculated by dividing an individual's weight in kilograms by the square of the person's height in meters.
   a. World Health Organization Classification (adopted by National Institutes of Health):
      (1) Overweight defined as BMI ranging from 25 to 29.9.
      (2) Obesity defined as BMI $\geq$ 30.
      (3) Morbidly obese defined as BMI > 40.
3. A national health problem: overweight (65% of Americans) and obesity (31% of Americans).
   a. Health risks associated with obesity: metabolic syndrome, hypertension, hyperlipidemia, type 2 diabetes, cardiovascular disease, stroke, glucose intolerance, sleep apnea, gallbladder disease, menstrual irregularities and infertility, cancer (endometrial, breast, prostate, and colon), chronic low back pain.
      (1) The result is an increased mortality rate.
   b. Waist circumference is used to determine distribution of body fat. Abdominal obesity (central accumulation of fat) is an independent predictor of morbidity and mortality.
   c. Childhood obesity: most prevalent nutritional disorder affecting children in United States.
4. Etiology: health disparity; result of complex social, behavioral, cultural, environmental, physiological, and genetic factors.
   a. Social.
      (1) Education and income level.
      (2) Occupation.
      (3) Family background.
   b. Behavioral.
      (1) Eating on the run/fast food.
      (2) Eating alone.
      (3) Eating for comfort/"comfort foods."
      (4) Binge eating.
   c. Cultural.
      (1) "Food and love" cultures (food given as a sign of affection).
      (2) Larger body size is more highly valued (e.g., West African cultures).
      (3) Post depression-era eating (i.e., consuming more because there is money to buy).
      (4) "Restaurant cultures" (larger proportions/food diversity/higher fat content).
   d. Environmental.
      (1) Lack of time to devote to meal planning and preparation.
      (2) Lack of time to develop and maintain a proper exercise routine (sandwich generation: caregiving their parents and children simultaneously/perceived lack of time for self).
      (3) Lack of access to resources.
         (a) No facilities in which to exercise.
         (b) No exercise coach/partners.
   e. Physiological.
      (1) A nutritionally related imbalance that occurs resulting in excess body fat.
         (a) Poor diet and nutrition.
         (b) Eating processed foods.
         (c) Excessive food consumption: excess calories are consumed that are not expended by work or exercise.
            - Activity level: lack of exercise; poor choice of exercise in proportion to what is consumed.
            - Compulsive over-eating: psychiatric disorder.
      (2) Excess body fat that occurs from a metabolic imbalance.
         (a) Gestational diabetes (passively introduced to fetus: results in oversized infants at birth).
         (b) Adrenal disorders: cortisol and stress.
      (3) Side effects of the atypical second-generation anti-psychotic (SGAs) medications.
         (a) SGAs effect the metabolism process, alter resting metabolic rate, and increase cravings for carbohydrates.
         (b) The rate of metabolic syndrome is substantially higher for persons with mental illness as compared to the general population.
5. Prevention.
   a. Education.
      (1) Raising awareness of behavioral factors that contributes to obesity (e.g. sedentary lifestyle).

[1] Susan O'Sullivan contributed to this section.

(2) Community driven group intervention focused on health promotion and wellness.

b. Habit intervention with occupations and activities that contribute to obesity (e.g. choose this/not that approaches, not eating while stressed, mindful eating).

c. Tertiary intervention when overcoming obesity is not the issue-focus on occupational needs of the client.

6. Sequelae.

a. Decreased ability in performance areas of occupations (BADL, IADL, mobility, social participation).

b. Symptomatology related to larger body size: musculoskeletal pain, limited mobility, lower activity tolerance.

7. Rehabilitation.

a. Lifestyle redesign: combination of changes in daily habits, patterns, and routines to reduce body weight through nutritional changes (e.g., emphasis on fruits, vegetables, whole grains, and lean protein), changes in activity time engagement combined with increased physical activity.

(1) Personalized plan to change lifestyle habits that contribute to obesity risk.

(2) Personalized activity-focused exercise program combining personal interests, desired participation, goals, and positive meaning (e.g., OT walks with NAMI).

(3) Instruction in self-monitoring of exercise responses (heart rate, perceived exertion).

(4) Supportive coaching/counseling to improve compliance and make long term life altering change.

b. Inpatient rehabilitation tertiary care.

(1) Access devices and equipment to maximize client participation in daily activities of meaning (BADL, IADL, mobility, and participation).

(a) Bariatric equipment: wheeled mobility, assistive devices, lifters, seating adaptations, clothing adaptations. See Chapter 15.

(2) Activity participation to relearn lifestyle modifications and to offer practice in altering habits and patterns that require adjustment in order to maximize the individual client's participation and meaningful engagement.

c. Co-morbidities.

(1) Cardiopulmonary compromise is typically exhibited (i.e., shortness of breath, elevated blood pressure, and angina).

(2) Altered biomechanics affects hips, knees, ankle/foot; back and joint pain.

(a) Increased risk of orthopedic injury.

(3) Increased risk of pressure ulcers due to shear forces and immobility.

(4) Increased occurrence of lymphedema, cellulitis, skin fold dermatitis, and other skin infections.

(5) Increased heat intolerance, risk of hyperthermia and heat exhaustion.

(6) Increased risk of practitioner injury when using poor body mechanics or inadequate assistance during transfers and lifts.

Lyme Disease

1. Etiology and risk factors.

a. Tick bites.

(1) Ticks attach to people as they brush by the object to which the tick is attached.

(a) Tick attaches to hidden and hairy areas such as groin, armpits, and scalp.

2. Prevention.

a. Ticks are usually found on animals, on the tips of grasses and shrubs, in woody areas, and on the fringes of gardens, especially those surrounding new homes that were built in formerly wooded areas.

b. Avoid tick-infested areas especially in May, June, and July.

c. Wear light-colored clothing, so ticks can be easily seen.

d. Tuck pants legs into socks or boots and shirt into pants.

e. Tape the area where pants and socks meet.

f. Spray insect repellent containing DEET on clothes and exposed skin, excluding the face.

g. Use permethrin (kills ticks on contact) on clothes.

h. Wear a hat and long-sleeved shirt.

i. Walk in the center of trails and avoid contact with grass and brush.

j. After being outdoors, change clothes and inspect skin for the presence of ticks.

k. Remove any ticks with tweezers, grasping the tick as close to the skin surface as possible and pull straight back.

l. Save the live tick (if retrieved) in a plastic container and take it to a local health department for identification.

3. Sequelae and symptoms.

a. Impairs the immune response and affects the neurological and orthopedic systems.

b. Early symptoms.

(1) Fatigue.

(2) Headache.

(3) Chills and fever.

(4) Muscle and joint pain.

(5) Swollen lymph nodes.

(6) Rash, erythema migrans: a circular red patch occurring 3 days–1 month after the bite from an infected tick.

(a) Commonly in the groin, thigh, trunk and armpits.

(b) The center of the rash may clear as it enlarges, resembling a bulls-eye.

c. Late symptoms.

(1) Arthritis: brief bouts of pain and swelling in one or more of the large joints.

(a) Knees are most commonly affected joints.

(2) Nervous system abnormalities.

(a) Numbness.

(b) Pain.

(c) Bell's palsy.

(d) Meningitis.

(3) Heart rate irregularities.

4. Diagnosis.

a. Presence of symptoms and signs.

b. History of exposure to ticks, especially in geographic areas where Lyme disease is known to occur.

c. Blood titer to determine whether antibodies for Lyme disease are present.

5. Medical treatment.

a. Antibiotics, oral or intravenous.

b. Management of joint-related symptoms from the accompanying arthritis.

6. Rehabilitation.

a. Treat joint pain and swelling.

(1) Provide education regarding acute arthritic flares.

(a) Rest.

(b) Anti-inflammatory medicine compliance.

(c) Splinting or wrapping to protect inflamed joints and prevent over-stretching of enlarged joint.

(d) Teach energy conservation and work simplification.

(2) Following flare, in sub-acute phase, provide gradual re-introduction of normal performance of daily tasks and activities.

b. Treat nervous system abnormalities.

(1) Numbness.

(a) Safety assessment and intervention to preserve safety and prevent injury.

(b) Management of aesthesias that are perceived as painful.

(c) Occupation-based interventions to encourage and preserve function and to cope with chronic pain conditions.

(2) Pain.

(a) Use of physical agent modalities to reduce pain.

(b) Use of stress management (complementary care) techniques to control the intensity of the pain and to increase coping ability.

(c) Use of neutral warmth to decrease intensity of pain.

(d) Use of adapted techniques to avoid triggering of movements that exacerbate pain during activity (e.g., sit on higher seat to decrease stress load in sit or stand).

(3) Bell's palsy.

(a) Make a facial splint to prevent long-term asymmetry of facial muscles. Clip or pincer mold of the inside and outer lip of the mouth on the involved side. Elastic attaching mouth mold to ear piece (similar to eyeglass ear rim).

(b) Use electric stimulation to stimulate denervated muscles.

(c) Teach person to use their fingers to assist buccal closure and prevent spillage of the bolus through the lips.

(d) Provide counseling concerning alteration in body image, since the individual is coping with a facial deformity.

(4) Meningitis.

(a) Acute care: positioning, splinting, supportive care while hospitalized.

(b) Rehabilitation if there is recovery-related sequelae (i.e., neurological impairment, motor impairment, sensory impairment, cognitive impairment, or activity of daily living impairment).

(5) Heart rate irregularities.

(a) Telemetry during daily performance of tasks and activities that support role performance.

(b) Pulse oximetry measurements, if oxygenation is poor during performance of daily tasks and activities.

(c) Work simplification, adaptation, and modification to prevent further complications associated with arrythmia.

Integumentary System

Pressure/Decubitus Ulcers

1. Etiology and risk factors.

a. Pressure that interrupts normal circulation causing localized areas of cellular necrosis.

(1) Greatest risk is over bony prominences (e.g., ischial tuberosity).

(2) Intensity and duration of the pressure determines the severity of the decubiti.

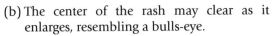

b. Conditions that predispose an individual to the formation of decubitus ulcers include immobility or altered mobility, weight loss, edema, incontinence, sensory deficiencies, circulatory abnormalities, dehydration, inadequate nutrition, obesity, pathological conditions/multiple comorbidities, and/or changes in skin condition due to aging.

c. The presence of substance abuse, cognitive deficits, and/or psychological impairments can jeopardize the individual's ability to understand and complete the required daily ulcer prevention regimen.

2. Types, signs, and symptoms.
   a. The National Pressure Ulcer Advisory Panel has updated the definitions and stage classifications of pressure ulcers.
      (1) This revision includes the original four stages and two additional stages of deep tissue injury and unstageable pressure ulcers.
      (2) Pressure ulcers and decubiti are often called bedsores by lay persons.
   b. Suspected deep tissue injury.
      (1) Localized discoloration of intact skin (purple or maroon) or a blister filled with blood resulting from damage of underlying soft tissue.
         (a) Deep tissue injury may be difficult to detect in individuals with darkly pigmented skin.
      (2) This stage may further evolve and can rapidly expose additional layers of tissue.
   c. Stage I pressure ulcer.
      (1) Skin is intact with visible nonblanchable redness over a localized area, typically over a bony prominence.
         (a) Visible blanching may not be evident in darkly pigmented skin; the color may appear different than from the surrounding area.
      (2) The area may be soft or firm and/or cooler or warmer when compared to adjacent skin.
      (3) The area may be painful or itchy.
      (4) This stage may indicate 'at risk' persons but can be difficult to detect.
   d. Stage II pressure ulcer.
      (1) Involves the dermis with partial thickness loss which presents as a shallow open ulcer that can be shiny or dry.
         (a) A Stage II ulcer can also present as a blister that is intact or open/ruptured.
      (2) The wound bed is a red pink color without slough or bruising.
   e. Stage III pressure ulcer.
      (1) Involves full thickness tissue loss with subcutaneous fat possibly visible.
         (a) The depth of tissue loss is not obscured if slough (i.e., dead matter/necrotic tissue) is present.
         (b) Bone, tendon or muscle are not exposed or directly palpable.
      (2) The depth of a Stage III pressure ulcer can vary according to anatomical location and can range from shallow in areas that do not have subcutaneous tissue (e.g., the nose, ear) to very deep in areas with significant fat (e.g., the buttocks).
   f. Stage IV pressure ulcer.
      (1) Involves full thickness tissue loss with bone, tendon, or muscle visible or directly palpable.
      (2) The depth of a Stage IV pressure ulcer can vary according to anatomical location and can range from shallow in areas that do not have subcutaneous tissue (e.g., the nose, ear) to very deep in areas with significant fat (e.g., the buttocks).
      (3) Osteomyelitis is possible if Stage IV ulcers extend into muscle, fascia, tendon and/or the joint capsule.
   g. Unstageable pressure ulcers.
      (1) Involves full thickness tissue loss in which the wound bed has slough and/or eschar (i.e., a scab or dark crusted ulcer) which covers the base of the ulcer.

3. Evaluation.
   a. Early assessment is critical to prevent pressure ulcers from developing and/or progressing.
      (1) The skin integrity of all patients should be assessed.
      (2) The presence of risk factors for pressure ulcers should be assessed to determine the patient's potential for developing an ulcer.
   b. While nursing staff in medical model settings typically assume the responsibility for skin and risk assessments, OT practitioners can (and should) contribute to this process.
      (1) In non-medical model settings (e.g., home care), the OT practitioner may need to take a more active role in the evaluation process.
   c. Persons determined to be at a high risk for developing pressure ulcers should be re-evaluated every 12 hours.
      (1) In non-medical model settings, caregivers should be trained to perform this assessment.
   d. Persons determined to be at a low risk for developing pressure ulcers should be re-evaluated whenever there is a change in their status.

4. Intervention.
   a. Prevention is the most effective intervention.
      (1) Use wheelchair cushions, flotation pads, and pressure-relief bed aids to distribute pressure over a larger skin surface. CMS has divided pressure-reducing devices into three categories for reimbursement purposes. These are:
         (a) Group 1: cushions or mattresses that use non-electrical means (e.g., air, foam, gel, or water) to distribute pressure.
         (b) Group 2: dynamic, electric-powered devices (e.g., alternating and low air loss mattresses) for persons with full thickness ulcers or those at moderate to high risk.

(c) Group 3: dynamic, electric-powered devices (e.g., air-fluidized beds) for persons with nonhealing full thickness ulcers.

(2) Train the individual and/or caregivers in positioning and weight-shifting techniques and schedules and in proper skin care.

(a) Full push-ups, lateral leans, forward leans, or wheelchair tilt/recline options are common techniques used depending upon the abilities of the individual.

(b) Weight shifts should occur every 30 minutes for 30 seconds or every 60 minutes for 60 seconds.

(c) Integrate weight-shifting into daily activities (e.g., lean forward to pick up the phone, lean sideways when reading the mail).

(3) Train in proper skin care.

(a) Keep skin free of excessive moisture, dryness, and heat.

(b) Check skin at least two times per day for any evidence of breakdown.

- Most individuals perform this in bed in the morning before arising and in the evening before sleep.
- Target for inspection the scapula, elbows, ischia, sacrum/coccyx, trochanters, heels, ankles, and knees.

(4) Encourage adequate intake of fluids and food to maintain nutrition, promote healing, and achieve a recommended body weight.

b. Medical management including occlusive dressings, debridement, surgery and/or grafting may be needed depending upon the severity of the decubitus ulcer.

c. Encourage participation in meaningful and productive activities.

(1) Individuals who pursue active lifestyles have fewer decubiti.

Whole Body System Disorders

Heat Syndromes/Hyperthermia

1. Etiology and risk factors.

a. Heat production increases with infection, exercise, and/or drugs.

b. Heat loss decreases with high humidity and/or temperature, excess clothing, obesity, cardiovascular disease, dehydration, sweat gland dysfunction, lack of acclimatization, and/or drugs.

c. When an individual's heat loss is not sufficient to offset his/her heat production, his/her body will retain heat and a heat syndrome can develop.

d. Individuals who are elderly, obese, or taking drugs are at increased risk.

2. Prevention.

a. In hot weather, wear light-weight, loose-fitting clothing.

b. Avoid hot places; seek shade, use fans, and air conditioners.

c. Rest frequently.

d. Increase fluid intake.

3. Types, signs and symptoms.

a. Heat cramps are characterized by a normal body temperature, nausea, diaphoresis, muscle twitching or spasms, weakness, and/or severe muscle cramps.

b. Heat exhaustion is characterized by a rapid pulse, decreased blood pressure, nausea, vomiting, cool pallid skin, mental confusion, headache, and/or giddiness but no fever.

c. Heat stroke is characterized by hot, dry red skin; a body temperature higher than 104 degrees; slow, deep respiration; tachycardia; dilated pupils; confusion; progressing to seizures and possibly loss of consciousness.

4. Intervention.

a. Heat stroke is a medical emergency and hospitalization is required.

(1) Immediately call emergency medical services.

(2) Lower person's body temperature by getting the person to a cooler area, placing ice packs on arterial pressure points, and/or spraying body with a cool mist.

(3) Hypothermia blankets, IV infusions, and medications are necessary.

b. Heat cramps and heat exhaustion usually do not require hospitalization.

(1) Loosen clothing and have the person lie in a cool place.

(2) Replace fluid and electrolytes with fruit juice or a balanced electrolyte drink. If these are not available, give fluids and seek additional medical care.

(3) Massage muscles if cramps are severe.

(4) IV infusions and oxygen may be indicated if symptoms are severe.

References

American Cancer Society (2013). *Cancer facts & figures 2013.* Atlanta: American Cancer Society, Retrieved August 18, 2013 from http://www.cancer.org/acs/groups/content/@epidemiologysurveilance/documents/document/acspc-036845.pdf

American Diabetes Association (2013). *Fast facts: Data and statistics about diabetes,* Retrieved August 18, 2013 from http://professional.diabetes.org/admin/UserFiles/020-Sean/FastFactsMarch2013.pdf

American Occupational Therapy Association. (2007). Specialized knowledge and skills in feeding, eating, and swallowing for occupational therapy practice. *American Journal of Occupational Therapy, 61,* 686–700.

American Occupational Therapy Association. (2007). Position paper: Obesity and occupational therapy. *American Journal of Occupational Therapy, 61,* 701–703.

American Occupational Therapy Association. (2011). The role of occupational therapy in end-of-life care. *American Journal of Occupational Therapy, 65*(Suppl.), S66–S75.

Balasundaram, I., et al. (2013). Rehabilitation interventions and their effect on quality of life in patients following major head and neck cancer surgery: Part 1. *Face Mouth & Jaw Surgery,* 2(2).

Balducci, L., & Fossa, S. D. (2013). Rehabilitation of older cancer patients. *Acta Oncologica, 52*(2), 233–238.

Balsara, Z., Ross, S. S., Dolber, P. C., Wiener, J. S., Tang, Y., & Seed, P. (2013). Enhanced susceptibility to urinary tract infection in the spinal cord-injured host with neurogenic bladder. *Infection and immunity, 81*(8), 3018–26.

Bergholdt, S. H., Søndergaard, J., Larsen, P. V., Holm, L. V., Kragstrup, J., & Hansen, D. G. (2013). A randomised controlled trial to improve general practitioners' services in cancer rehabilitation: Effects on general practitioners' proactivity and on patients' participation in rehabilitation activities. *Acta Oncologica, 52*(2), 400–409.

Blanchard, S. A. (2009). Variables associated with obesity among African-American women in Omaha. *American Journal of Occupational Therapy, 63,* 58–68.

Brody, J. (2007). *Science Times: Swallowing difficulty.* Retrieved February 8, 2008 from http://health.nytimes.com/health/guides/symptoms/swallowing-difficulty/overview.html

Buenaver, L., McGuire, L., & Haythornthwaite, J. (2006). Cognitive-behavioral self-help for chronic pain. *Journal of Clinical Psychology; 62,* 1389–96.

Burkhardt, A. (2006). Oncology in W. Schultz-Krohn & H. Pendleton (Eds.), *Occupational therapy: Practice skills for physical dysfunction,* 6th ed. (pp. 1157–1168) St. Louis, MO: Elsevier Science/Mosby.

Burkhardt, A., & Joachim, J. (1996). *A therapist's guide to oncology: Medical issues affecting management.* San Antonio, TX: Therapy Skill Builders.

Casale, R., Buounocore, M., & Matucci-Cerinic, M. (1997). Review article: Systemic sclerosis (scleroderma): An integrated challenge in rehabilitation. *Archives of Physical Medicine and Rehabilitation, 78,* 767–773.

Centers for Disease Control. (2013, May 10). Testing for hepatitis C virus (HCV) infection: An update of guidance for clinicians and laboratorians. *Weekly, 62*(18), 362–365. Retrieved May 7, 2013 from http://www.cdc.gov/mmwr.

Centers for Disease Control. (2013). *Lyme Disease Statistics.* Retrieved September 8, 2013 from http://www.cdc.gov/lyme/stats/index.html.

Centers for Disease Control. (2009). *Healthcare-associated methicillin resistant staphylococcus aureus (HA-MRSA).* Retrieved September 8, 2013 from http://www.cdc.gov/ncidod/dhqp/ar_ MRSA.html

Centers for Disease Control and Prevention. (2010). *HIV/AIDS statistics and surveillance.* Retrieved August 22, 2010 from http://www.cdc.gov/hiv/topics/surveillance/

Centers for Disease Control. (2010). *US Government Web, subsection on diabetes.* [On-line]. Available: http://www.cdc.gov/diabetes/

Cohen, S. D., Norris, L., Acquaviva, K., Peterson, R. A., & Kimmel, P.L. (2007) Screening, diagnosis, and treatment of depression in patients with end-stage renal disease. *Clinical Journal of the American Society of Nephrology, 2,* 1332–42.

Colodny, N. (2002). Interjudge and intrajudge reliabilities in fiberoptic endoscopic evaluation of swallowing (FEES) using the penetration-aspiration scale: A replication study. *Dysphagia, 17,* 308–15.

Cox, M., Holm, S., Kurfuerst, S., Lynch, A., & Schuberth, L. (2007). Specialized knowledge and skills in feeding, eating, and swallowing for occupational therapy practice. *American Journal of Occupational Therapy, 61,* 686–700.

Curtin, R., Mapes, D., Schatell, D., Burrows-Hudson, S. (2005). Self-management in patients with end stage renal disease: Exploring domains and dimensions. *Nephrology Nursing Journal, 32,* 389–95.

Dickman, R., Green, C., Fass, S., Quan, S., Dekel, R., Risner-Adler, S., Fass, R. (2007). Relationships between sleep quality and pH monitoring findings in persons with gastroesophageal reflux disease. *Journal of Clinical Sleep Medicine, 15,* 505–13.

Dorsher, P. T., & McIntosh, P. M. (2012). Neurogenic bladder. *Advances in urology, 2012.*

Dunn, L. Rovner, E., Bozeman, E., Chancellor, M., and Nicolson, P. (2007). *Healthwise: Electrical stimulation for urinary incontinence.* Retrieved February 8, 2008 from http://www.webmd.com/urinary-incontinence-oab/oab-8/living-with

Eades, M., Murphy, J., Carney, S., Amdouni, S., Lemoignan, J., Jelowicki, M., & Gagnon, B. (2012). Effect of an interdisciplinary rehabilitation program on quality of life in patients with head and neck cancer: Review of clinical experience. *Head & Neck, 35*(3), 343–349.

Ekberg, O., Hamdy, S., Woisard, V., Wuttge-Hannig, A., & Ortega, P. (2002). Social and psychological burden of dysphagia: Its impact on diagnosis and treatment. *Dysphagia, 17*(2), 139–46.

Farri, A., Accornero, A., & Burdese, C. (2007) Social importance of dysphagia: Its impact on diagnosis and therapy. *Acta Otorhinolaryngol Italia, 27,* 83–6.

Foley, R. N., & Collins, A. J. (2007) End-stage renal disease in the United States: An update from the United States Renal Data System. *Journal of the American Society for Nephrology, 18,* 2644–2648.

Forhan, M., Bhambhani, Y., Dyer, D., Ramos-Salas, X., Ferguson-Pell, M., Sharma, A. (2010) Rehabilitation in bariatrics: Opportunities for practice and research. *Disability & Rehabilitation, 32*(11), 952–959.

Furusawa, K., Sugiyama, H., Ikeda, A., Tokohiro, A., Koyoshi, H., Takahashi, M., & Tajima, F. (2007) Autonomic dysreflexia during a bowel regimen program in patients with cervical spinal cord injury. *Acta Medica Okayama, 61,* 221–227.

George, B., & Malkenson, G. (2008, December). Pressure ulcers: A clinical review. *Rehabilitation Management,* 16–19.

Go, A. S., Mozaffarian, D., Roger, V. L., Benjamin, E. J, Berry, J. D., Borden, W. B., Bravata, D. M., et al. (2013). *Heart disease and stroke statistics—2013 update: A report from the American Heart Association. Diabetes Mellitus - 2013 Statistical Fact Sheet. Circulation. 127,* e6-e245.

Haig, A. J. (2007). Developing world rehabilitation strategy II: Flex the muscles, train the brain, and adapt to the impairment. *Disability and Rehabilitation, 29,* 977–9.

Kaiser, F., Spiridigliozzi, A. M., & Hunt, M. P. (2001). Promoting shared decision-making in rehabilitation: development of a framework for situations when patients with dysphagia refuse diet modification recommended by the treating team. *Dysphagia,* 27(1), 81–87.

Karlsson, A. K. (1999). Scientific review: Autonomic dysreflexia. *Spinal Cord, 37,* 383–391.

Kielhofner, G., Braveman, B., Fogg, L., et al. (2008). A controlled study of services to enhance productive participation among people with HIV/AIDS. *American Journal of Occupational Therapy; 62,* 36–45.

King, J. M., & Ligman, K. (2011). Patient noncompliance with swallowing recommendations: Reports from speech-language pathologists. *Contemporary Issues In Communication Science And Disorders, 38,* 53–60.

Lin, Y. H., & Pan, P. J. (2012). The use of rehabilitation among patients with breast cancer: a retrospective longitudinal cohort study. *BMC Health Services Research, 12*(1), 282.

McDevitt, J., Wilbur, J., Kogan, J., & Briller, J. (2005). A walking program for outpatients in psychiatric rehabilitation: pilot study. *Biological Research for Nursing, 7*(2), 87–97.

Mewes, J. C., Steuten, L. M., IJzerman, M. J., & van Harten, W. H. (2012). Effectiveness of multidimensional cancer survivor rehabilitation and cost-effectiveness of cancer rehabilitation in general: A systematic review. *The Oncologist, 17*(12), 1581–1593.

Mittalhenkle, A., Stehman-Breen, C., Shlipak, M., Fried, L., Katz, R., Young, B., Seliger, S., Gillen, D., Newman, A., Psaty, B., & Siscovick, D. (2008). Cardiovascular risk factors and incident acute renal failure in older adults: The cardiovascular health study. *Clinical Journal of the American Society of Nephrology, 3*(2), 450–456.

Moinuddin, I., and Leehey, D. J. (2008). A comparison of aerobic exercise and resistance training in patients with and without chronic kidney disease. *Advances in Chronic Kidney Disease, 15,* 83–96.

National Kidney Foundation. (2010). *Nephrotic syndrome.* Retreived August 8, 2013 from http://www.kidney.org/atoz/content/nephrotic.cfm.

National Pressure Ulcer Advisory Panel (NPUAP). (2007). *Pressure ulcer stages revised by NPUAP.* Retrieved February 3, 2011 from http://www.npuap.org/pr2.htm.

OTs Walk With NAMI (2011). Retieved February 3, 2011 from http://www.downstate.edu/CHRP/ot/nami.html.

Padilla, R. (2003). Clara: A phenomenology of disability. *American Journal of Occupational Therapy, 57,* 413–423.

Patil, N. J., Nagaratna, R., Garner, C., Raghuram, N. V., & Crisan, R. (2012). Effect of integrated Yoga on neurogenic bladder dysfunction in patients with multiple sclerosis: A prospective observational case series. *Complementary Therapies in Medicine, 20*(6), 424–430.

Pizzi, M., & Burkhardt, A. (2003) Adult immunological diseases. In E. Crepeau, B. Schell, & E. Cohn (eds.), *Willard & Spackman's occupational therapy,* 10th ed. (pp. 821–834) Philadelphia: Lippincott.

Poole, J. L. (2010) Musculoskeletal rehabilitation in the person with scleroderma. *Current Opinions in Rheumatology, 22,* 205–12.

Prieto, L., Thorsen, H., & Juul, K. (2005). Development and validation of a quality of life questionnaire for patients with colostomy or ileostomy. *Health and Quality of Life Outcomes, 12,* 62.

Roberts, P., Cox, M. S., Holm, S., Kurfurst, S. T., Lynch, A. K., & Schuberth, L. M. (2007). Specialized knowledge and skills in feeding, eating, and swallowing for occupational therapy practice. *American Journal of Occupational Therapy, 61,* 686–700.

Salyers, W. J., Mansour, A., El-Haddad, B., Golbeck, A. L., & Kallail, K. J. (2007). Lifestyle modification counseling in patients with gastroesophageal reflux disease. *Gastroenterological Nursing, 30,* 302–4.

Silver, J. K., Baima, J., & Mayer, R. S. (2013). Impairment-driven cancer rehabilitation: An essential component of quality care and survivorship, *7,* 16. *A Cancer Journal for Clinicians.*

Siracusa, G., Sparacino, A., & Lentini, V. L. (2013). Neurogenic bladder and disc disease: A brief review. *Current Medical Research & Opinion, 29*(8), 1–19.

Stenzelius, K., Westergren, A., & Hallberg, I. R. (2007). Bowel function among people 75+ reporting fecal incontinence in relation to help seeking, dependency and quality of life. *Journal of Clinical Nursing, 16,* 458–68.

Toalson, P., Ahmed, S., Hardy, T., & Kabinoff, G.(2004). The metabolic syndrome in patients with severe mental illnesses. *Primary Care Companion to the Journal of Clinical Psychiatry* 6(4),152–158.

Tubaro, A., Puccini, F., De Nunzio, C., Digesu, G. A., Elneil, S., Gobbi, C., & Khullar, V. (2012). The treatment of lower urinary tract symptoms in patients with multiple sclerosis: A systematic review. *Current Urology Reports,13*(5), 335–342.

Wilson, H., & Vincent, R. (2006). Autoimmune connective tissue disease: Scleroderma. *British Journal of Nursing. 15,* 805–9.

World Health Organization. (2013). Definition of palliative care. Retrieved September 10, 2013 from http://www.who.int/cancer/palliative/definition/en/.

Yiping, W., Tianwen, H., Xiuyu, Y., Xia, S., & Li'e, C. (2012). Effect of rehabilitation nursing on postoperative functional recovery of neurogenic bladder in patients with tethered cord syndrome. *Modern Clinical Nursing, 1,* 016.

Review Questions

Gastrointestinal, Renal-Genitourinary, Endocrine, Immunological, and Integumentary Systems Disorders

Below are five questions about key content covered in this chapter. These questions are not inclusive of the entirety of content related to disorders of the gastrointestinal, renal-genitourinary, endocrine, immunological, and integumentary systems that you must know for success on the NBCOT exam. These questions are provided to help you "jump start" the thought processes you will need to apply your studying of content to the answering of exam questions; hence they are not in the NBCOT exam format. Exam items in the NBCOT format which cover the depth and breadth of content you will need to know to pass the NBCOT exam are provided on this text's disc. The answers to the below questions are provided in Appendix 4.

1. You work with clients who have dysphagia and swallowing disorders to develop their feeding skills. What would you do if a client chokes and cannot clear his/her airway during the activity?

2. If clients have a colostomy or a stoma due to surgery to their bowel, must they have intact fine motor functioning to learn to manage their stoma independently? What can an occupational therapy practitioner do to work with clients to develop their ability to manage their stoma care independently?

3. What intervention options are useful for someone who has bladder urgency with stress urinary incontinence and a diagnosis of non-insulin dependent diabetes mellitus? Describe these.

4. You are treating an adult client with a diagnosis of scleroderma and colon cancer who was referred to occupational therapy because soft tissue/connective tissue changes are affecting hand function. Would it be appropriate to have a restorative goal for evolving contractures? Describe your rationale.

5. You work in a community that has people living and working in it who have spinal cord injuries. A primary care doctor refers clients to you who have reddening of skin in their sacral regions.What could you do to work with these clients to improve their skin integrity and prevent decubiti?

10

Psychiatric and Cognitive Disorders

WILLIAM L. LAMBERT, RITA P. FLEMING-CASTALDY, AND JANICE ROMEO

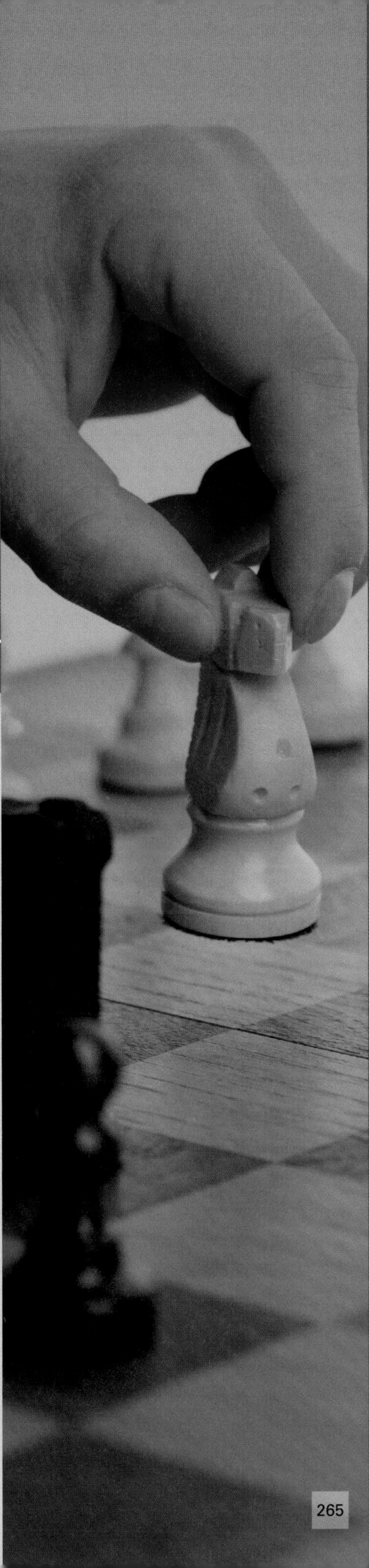

Chapter Outline

Signs and Symptoms of Psychiatric Illness and/or Cognitive Disorders

Consciousness

1. A state of awareness that responds to external stimuli.
2. Disturbances of consciousness.
   a. These disturbances are usually a result of brain pathology.
   b. Disorientation is a disturbance of orientation to person, place, or time. Situation is sometimes used as a fourth consideration.
   c. Delirium is an acute, reversible disorder that presents as a disoriented reaction with confusion, lability, and disturbances in behavior; e.g., aggression.
      (1) It may be associated with fear and hallucinations.
   d. Confusion involves inappropriate reactions to environmental stimuli, manifested by a disordered orientation in relation to person, place, and time.
   e. Sundowner syndrome occurs in the late afternoon and at night in older people, often seen in individuals with dementia.
      (1) Characterized by drowsiness, confusion, ataxia, falling, agitation, and sometimes aggression.
      (2) It is associated with sedation/over sedation, dementia, and changes in orienting cues such as light, familiar people, and objects.

Attention

1. The ability to remain focused on the various aspects of an activity or experience or the ability to concentrate.
2. Disturbances of attention.
   a. Distractibility is the inability to concentrate one's attention without attention being drawn to unimportant or irrelevant stimuli.
   b. Selective inattention is blocking out those activities, objects, or concepts that produce anxiety.
   c. Hypervigilance is excessive attention and alertness that guards against potential danger.

Emotion

1. A feeling state associated with affect and mood that consists of psychological and physical components (e.g., fear, anger, joy).
   a. Physiological disturbances associated with mood are frequently autonomic in nature.
2. Affect is the observable component of emotions.
   a. Appropriate affect is consistent/congruent with the accompanying idea, thought, or speech.
   b. Disturbances of affect.
      (1) Inappropriate affect is inconsistent/incongruent with the accompanying idea, thought, or speech.
      (2) Blunted affect is a severe lack of affect. As seen clinically, an affect that does not demonstrate the ability to change is observed.
      (3) Restricted or constricted affect is observed as reduced affect, but less so than blunted affect.
      (4) Flat affect is the absence of any affective signs of emotion.
      (5) Labile affect is rapid and abrupt changes in affect.
3. Mood is a pervasive and sustained emotion manifested by thoughts and actions (e.g., elation, anger, depression).
   a. Rapid changes in affect (lability) are usually accompanied by rapid changes in mood.
   b. These rapid changes are frequently referred to as "mood swings."
4. Other emotions.
   a. Anxiety is a feeling of apprehension or worry associated with anticipation of future danger.
      (1) Free-floating anxiety is a pervasive anxiety that does not have a specific focus.
   b. Fear is an anxiety that is focused on a real danger.

Motor Behavior

1. Behavioral and motoric expressions of impulses, drives, wishes, motivations, and cravings.
2. Disturbances of motor behavior.
   a. Echopraxia is the meaningless imitation of another person's movements.
   b. Catatonia is characterized by immobility or rigidity.
   c. Stereotypy is the repetition of fixed patterns of movement and speech (e.g., echolalia).
   d. Psychomotor agitation is excessive motor and cognitive activity, usually nonproductive and in response to inner tension.
   e. Hyperactivity is restless, sometimes aggressive, or destructive activity, often associated with brain pathology.
   f. Psychomotor retardation is decreased or slowed motor and cognitive activity.
   g. Aggression is forceful, angry, or destructive speech or behavior.
   h. Acting out is the physical expression of thoughts and impulses.

i. Akathisia is the state of restlessness characterized by an urgent need for movement, usually as a side effect of medication.
j. Ataxia is the irregularity or failure of muscle coordination upon movement.

Thought

1. Thinking is a goal-directed reasoned flow of ideas and associations.
   a. When thinking follows a logical sequence, it is considered normal.
2. Disturbances in form of thought.
   a. Circumstantiality is speech that is delayed in reaching the point and contains excessive or irrelevant details.
   b. Tangentiality is the abrupt changing of focus to a loosely associated topic.
   c. Perseveration is a persistent focus on a previous topic or behavior after a new topic or behavior has been introduced.
   d. Flight of ideas refers to rapid shifts in thoughts from one idea to another.
   e. Thought blocking is the interruption of a thought process before it is carried through to completion.
   f. Loosening of associations is a disorder of the logical progression of thoughts where seemingly unrelated and unconnected ideas shift from one subject to another.
3. Disturbances in content of thought.
   a. Delusions are false beliefs about external reality without an appropriate stimulus that cannot be explained by the individual's intelligence or cultural background.
   b. Compulsions are a need to act on specific impulses to relieve associated anxiety.
   c. Obsessions constitute a persistent thought or feeling that cannot be eliminated by logical thought.
   d. Concrete thinking is characterized by actual things, events and immediate experience; the inability to think abstractly.

Speech

1. The expression of ideas, thoughts, and feelings through language.
2. Disturbances in speech.
   a. Pressured speech is rapid and increased in amount. It may be difficult to understand and/or interrupt.
   b. Poverty of speech is limited in amount; i.e., one word answers to questions.
   c. Poverty of content in speech is speech that is adequate in amount but conveys little information due to vagueness, lack of specificity, and limited detail.
   d. Nonspontaneous speech consists of responses that are given only when spoken to directly.
   e. Stuttering consists of the repetition or prolongation of sounds or syllables.
   f. Perseveration in speech is continued, persistent repetition of a word or phrase, often in response to different stimuli or different questions.
3. Disturbances in language output.
   a. Expressive aphasia (i.e., Broca's) is a disturbance in which the individual knows what he/she wants to say, but cannot say it.
   b. Receptive aphasia (i.e., Wernicke's) is an organic loss of the individual's ability to comprehend what has been said to him/her.
   c. Nominal aphasia (also known as anomial or amnestic) is the inability to name objects.
   d. Global aphasia involves all forms of aphasia.

Perception

1. The process of interpreting sensory information received from the environment.
2. Disturbances of perception.
   a. Hallucinations are false sensory perceptions that are not in response to an external stimulus.
      (1) Often referred to clinically as "responding to internal stimuli."
   b. Illusions are misperceptions or misinterpretations of real sensory events.
   c. Disturbances associated with cognitive disorders.
      (1) Agnosia is the inability to understand and interpret the significance of sensory input.
         (a) Visual agnosia is the inability to recognize people and objects.
      (2) Astereognosis is the inability to identify objects through touch.
      (3) Apraxia is the inability to carry out specific motor tasks in the absence of sensory or motor impairment.
      (4) Adiadochokinesia is the inability to perform rapidly alternating movements.
      (5) See Chapter 13 for additional information about cognitive-perceptual deficits.
4. Disturbances associated with conversion and dissociative phenomena.
   a. These disturbances are in response to repressed material and involve physical symptoms and distortions that are not under voluntary control or associated with a physical disorder.
   b. Depersonalization is a subjective sensation of unreality about oneself or the environment.
   c. Derealization is a subjective sense that the environment is unreal.
   d. Fugue is a state of serious depersonalization, often involving travel or relocation, in which the

individual takes on a new identity with amnesia for his/her old identity.
e. Dissociative identity disorder involves the appearance that an individual has developed two or more distinct personalities.
f. Dissociation involves the separation of a group of mental or behavioral processes from the rest of the person's psychic activity.
(1) It may involve separating an idea from its emotional tone.

Memory

1. A process where what has been experienced or learned is registered and stored, can be retained to varying degrees, and can be recalled at will.
2. Levels of memory.
a. Immediate memory is the ability to recall material within seconds or minutes, also known as short term memory.
b. Recent memory is the ability to recall events of the past few days.
c. Recent past memory is the ability to recall events of the past few months.
d. Remote memory is the ability to recall events of the distant past, also known as long-term memory.
e. Procedural memory is an automatic sequence of behavior such as conditioned responses.
f. Declarative memory is recall specific to consciously learned facts, such as school subjects.
g. Semantic memory is knowing the meaning of words and the ability to classify information.
h. Episodic memory is the knowledge of one's personal experiences.
i. Prospective memory is the capacity to remember to carry out actions in the future, such as knowing you have appointments scheduled, to turn off the stove and to pay bills on time.
(1) Prospective memory is clinically important, especially with regard to an individual's ability to live safely and independently.
3. Disturbances of memory.
a. Amnesia is an inability to recall past experiences or personal identity.
(1) It may be caused by organic or emotional dysfunction.
(2) Retrograde amnesia is the inability to remember events that occurred prior to the precipitating event.

Diagnosis of Psychiatric Disorders

Determination of Diagnosis by the Psychiatrist

1. The individual's psychiatric history and physical status is reviewed.
2. A clinical interview, which includes a mental status examination, is conducted.
3. Clinical observation of the individual. This includes:
a. Appearance.
b. Speech.
c. Actions.
d. Thoughts.

The Mental Status Examination

1. General description of the individual.
a. Appearance.
b. Behavior and psychomotor activity.
c. Attitude toward examiner.
2. Mood and affect.
a. Mood (pervasive, sustained emotion).
b. Affect (observable expression of mood).
c. Appropriateness of mood and affect.
3. Speech.
4. Perceptual disturbances.
5. Thought.
a. Process or form of thought.
b. Content of thought.
6. Sensorium and cognition.
a. Alertness and level of consciousness.
b. Orientation to person, place, time, and situation.
c. Memory.
d. Concentration and attention.
e. Capacity to read and write.
f. Abstract thinking.
g. Fund of information and intelligence.
7. Impulse control.
8. Judgment and insight.
9. Reliability.

Shortened Forms of the Mental Status Examination

1. The Folstein Mini-Mental.
2. The Short Portable Mental.

3. Occupational therapy practitioners often use the above shortened forms as a screening tool to assess cognitive functioning.
4. See Chapter 14 for mental status examination specifics.

Diagnostic Information According to DSM-IV-TR

1. The Diagnostic and Statistical Manual of Mental Disorders, 4th edition, text revision (DSM-IV-TR) has been the primary source used to diagnose psychiatric disorders since 2000; thus, it is the reference source for current (i.e., 2014) NBCOT exam items.
   a. Terminology related to several mental health disorders (e.g., schizophrenia, autism-related disorder) has changed with the publication of the fifth edition of Diagnostic and Statistical Manual of Mental Disorders (DSM-5).
      (1) According to the NBCOT, certification examinations administered in the near future will continue to use language from the DSM-IV-TR.
      (2) The certification examination items will begin to transition to DSM-5 terminology as OT education programs incorporate the new language into their curricula.
         (a) As of the publication of this text, the NBCOT has not made public a more specific time frame for this change.
   b. Major changes in the DSM-5 are presented throughout the chapter to prepare readers for changes they may encounter in clinical settings such as fieldwork placements and entry level positions that may be transitioning to the new manual.
2. The DSM-IV-TR uses a multiaxial format for diagnosing mental disorders.
   a. Axis I identifies the clinical disorders and other conditions that may be a focus of clinical attention.
   b. Axis II includes personality disorders and mental retardation.
      (1) In DSM-5, mental retardation is reclassified as intellectual disability/intellectual disorder and falls under the classification of neurodevelopmental disorders, which has replaced disorders usually first diagnosed in infancy, childhood or adolescence.
         (a) Many advocacy rights groups, practice settings, and professional organizations and publications have already adopted this change in terminology.
   c. Axis III identifies general medical conditions.
   d. Axis IV lists psychosocial and environmental problems.
      (1) Problems with primary support group.
      (2) Problems related to the social environment.
      (3) Educational problems.
      (4) Occupational problems.
      (5) Housing problems.
      (6) Economic problems.
      (7) Problems with access to health care services.
      (8) Problems related to interaction with the legal system/crime.
      (9) Other psychosocial and environmental problems.
   e. Axis V provides a global assessment of functioning (GAF) (coded 0-100).
      (1) The GAF is based on the clinicians' assessment of the person's psychological, social, and occupational functioning on a proposed mental health continuum that is coded from 0-100.
         (a) 0 designates there is inadequate information upon which to make an assessment.
         (b) The subsequent codes are provided in increments of 10 (e.g., 10-1, 20 -11, etc).
         (c) The code of 1-10 designates a person who has completed a serious suicide act or who presents a persistent danger to self or others. This danger can be physical harm or the complete inability to care for self.
         (d) The code of 100-91 designates a person who functions at a superior level and has no mental health symptoms.
      (2) Along the GAF's hypothetical continuum, the code descriptions include:
         (a) The functional impact of psychiatric symptoms (e.g., code 30-21: behavior is seriously influenced by hallucinations, code 90-81: anxiety impedes performance on a test).
         (b) The level of impairment in occupational functioning (e.g., code 40-31: major impairments result in inability to work or failure at school, code 70-61: some difficulties at work or school such as occasional truancy).
         (c) The level of impairment in social functioning (e.g., 20-11: severe communication impairments such as mutism, 50-41: serious impairments that result in having no friends).
      (3) The occupational therapist can provide valuable information to the clinical team about a client's occupational and social functioning to help obtain an accurate GAF diagnostic code.
3. DSM-IV-TR diagnoses are made when the following criteria are met.
   a. The behavior is not caused by other medical conditions, substance abuse, or medications.
   b. The symptoms cause significant distress and impairments in function.
   c. The symptoms cannot be better accounted for by another diagnosis.

Chapter 10

Overview of DSM-5 Changes

1. DSM-5 remains a categorical classification of separate disorders, but it no longer uses the multiaxial system.
   a. The multiaxial system has been replaced by a process of looking at an appropriate dimensional diagnosis for each disorder in addition to the categorical diagnosis. The categorical diagnoses are presented in a revised organization of the chapters.
   b. DSM-5 consists of three sections:
      (1) "DSM-5 Basics" highlights how to use the new manual.
      (2) "Diagnostic Criteria and Codes" contains a reorganization of the chapters describing each diagnosis.
      (3) "Emerging Measures and Models" presents information on assessment, looking at cultural issues and conditions that require further research and study.
2. New to the DSM-5.
   a. Consolidation of Autistic Disorder, Asperger's Disorder, and Pervasive Developmental Disorder into Autism Spectrum Disorder.
   b. The elimination of the section "Disorders Usually First Diagnosed in Infancy, Childhood, Or Adolescence."
   c. A new chapter "Neurodevelopmental Disorders" that includes some disorders previously in "Disorders First Diagnosed in Infancy, Childhood, or Adolescence" such as intellectual disabilities (formerly mental retardation) and attention deficit/hyperactivity disorder.
   d. Revised classification of bipolar and depressive disorders.
   e. Restructuring of substance abuse disorders to now include "Gambling Disorder."
   f. A new chapter Neurocognitive Disorders that includes dementia, delirium and Alzheimer's disease.
   g. Personality disorders are now included with all disorders due to the elimination of Axis I and Axis II diagnoses.
   h. The subtypes of schizophrenia such as paranoid or disorganized are no longer used.
   i. "NOS" (Not otherwise specified) is no longer used.
   j. "General Medical condition" is repaced by "another medical condition."
   k. A new chapter titled "Disruptive-Impulse-Control and Conduct Disorder" has been added that includes Oppossitional Defiant Disorder, Conduct Disorder and Intermittent Explosive Disorder.
   l. A chapter titled Trauma and Stressor Related Disorders has been added that includes Acute Stress Disorder, Adjustment Disorder, Posttraumatic Stress Disorder and Reactive Attachment Disorder.
3. Additional information about major diagnostic DSM-5 changes is provided in this chapter's subsequent diagnostic-specific sections.

Psychotic Disorders[1]

Schizophrenia

1. Diagnostic criteria.
   a. Criterion A: the presence of two or more of the following symptoms.
      (1) Delusions.
      (2) Hallucinations.
      (3) Disorganized speech.
      (4) Grossly disorganized or catatonic behavior (positive symptoms).
      (5) Negative symptoms (see below).
   b. Criterion B: disturbance in one or more areas of function such as work, interpersonal relations, or self care.
   c. Criterion C: continuous signs of the illness for 6 months including at least one month of symptoms that meet criterion A.
   d. Positive symptoms are the excesses or distortions of normal function as found in criterion A.
   e. Negative symptoms represent a loss or absence of function.
      (1) Restricted emotion (affective flattening).
      (2) Difficulty in experiencing pleasure (anhedonia).
      (3) Decreased thought and speech (alogia).
      (4) Lack of energy (anergia) and initiative, which is often misinterpreted as lack of motivation.
      (5) Inability to relate to others.
2. Subtypes of schizophrenia.
   a. Paranoid type.
      (1) Characterized by preoccupation with one or more delusions of persecution or grandeur.
      (2) Auditory hallucinations are frequently present.
      (3) Individuals with paranoid type schizophrenia tend to exhibit fewer of the negative symptoms.
   b. Disorganized type.
      (1) Distinguished by marked regression demonstrating primitive, disinhibited, and disorganized behavior.

[1] *Psychotic* is often used interchangeably with *thought disorder*. A *thought disorder* is any disturbance of thinking that affects language, communication or thought content and is a predominate feature of schizophrenia.

c. Catatonic type.
   (1) Characterized by severe disturbances in motor behavior involving stupor, negativism, rigidity, excitement, or posturing.
d. Undifferentiated type.
   (1) Used to classify those patients who do not clearly fit into one of the other categories.
e. Residual type.
   (1) Used when there is continued evidence of schizophrenic behavior in the absence of a complete set of diagnostic criteria.
3. Onset, prevalence, and prognosis.
   a. The onset of schizophrenia is usually between early adolescence and the mid thirties with a life time prevalence of 0.6%–1.9%. Recovery is possible with effective intervention.
      (1) 50% of diagnosed cases have been found to sustain a good outcome of either a complete recovery or sufficient recovery to live an independent, satisfying life.
      (2) 25% are able to lead satisfying lives with ongoing supports.
      (3) The prognosis is poorer for the remaining 25% of individuals with schizophrenia who have repeated hospitalizations, periods of exacerbation, and episodes of major mood disorders.

Other Psychotic Disorders

1. Schizophreniform disorder.
   a. The individual meets the criteria for schizophrenia; however, the episode lasts more than one month but less than the six months required for a diagnosis of schizophrenia.
2. Schizoaffective disorder.
   a. The person has an uninterrupted period of illness during which, at some time, there is a major depressive episode, a manic episode, or a mixed episode concurrent with symptoms that meet criterion A symptoms for schizophrenia.
3. Delusional disorder.
   a. The individual's predominant symptoms are nonbizarre delusions with the absence of other criterion A symptoms of schizophrenia.
4. Brief psychotic disorder.
   a. The individual experiences at least one day but less than one month with one or more criterion A symptoms of schizophrenia which result from severe psychosocial stress.

Impact on Function

1. Many individuals with psychotic disorders demonstrate deficits in cognitive-perceptual and social interaction skills that affect all areas of function.
   a. The deficits in the processing of sensory information which are experienced by some individuals make interaction with the environment difficult and frightening.
   b. Individuals who have difficulty with their own ego boundaries often exhibit socially inappropriate, sometimes intrusive, behaviors.
   c. Some individuals have lost or failed to develop the social and communication skills necessary for effective and satisfying interpersonal interactions and relationships.
   d. Deficits in cognitive function due to thought disorders and difficulties with the performance of basic skills interfere with all areas of occupation from personal activities of daily living and leisure pursuits to social participation, education, and work activities.
   e. It is important to assess and continue to monitor the degree of assistance and structure needed to maintain optimum independence in all areas of occupation.

Symptom Management

1. Treatment consists primarily of the use of antipsychotic medications and the provision of a structured supportive environment.
2. Psychopharmacology.
   a. Traditional antipsychotic medications.
      (1) Thorazine, Prolixin, Haldol, and Navane. Mellaril, Stelazine, and Trilafon. These are infrequently used, but occasionally still prescribed.
      (2) Long-acting injections are available for Haldol (once a month) and Prolixin (once every two weeks).
         (a) Long-acting injections improve/assist in medication compliance.
      (3) Side-effects may include: dry mouth, blurry vision, photosensitivity, constipation, orthostatic hypotension, Parkinsonism, dystonias (i.e., impaired tonicity), akathisia (i.e., restless, anxiety provoking need for movement), and cardiovascular disorders.
      (4) Complications may include:
         (a) Neuroleptic malignant syndrome: an autonomic emergency leading to increased blood pressure, tachycardia, sweating, convulsions, and coma.
         (b) Tardive dyskinesia: a neurological disorder resulting from long-term or high-dose use of antipsychotic medications characterized by abnormal, involuntary, irregular movements of the head, limbs and trunk, often presenting as slow, rhythmic, automatic, stereotyped movements.
         (c) Neuroleptic-induced Parkinsonism (pseudo-Parkinson's): a disorder that presents

with muscle stiffness, cog-wheel rigidity, shuffling gait, stooped posture and drooling. The pill-rolling tremor of idiopathic Parkinsonism is rare, but regular, coarse tremors may be present, and tremors of the lips and mouth can also be seen with this disorder which also results from use of antipsychotic medications. Atypical antipsychotics are not as problematic as the use of older medications such as Stelazine, Thorazine and Mellaril.

b. Atypical antipsychotics.
   (1) Clozaril, Risperdal, Zyprexa, Seroquel, Geodon, Sphris, Fanapt, Latuda, Symbyax, Invega and Abilify.
      (a) Long-acting atypical injections are available for Risperdal Consta (once every 2 weeks) and Invega Sustenna (once every 4 weeks).
         - Long-acting injections assist and improve medication compliance.
   (2) Side-effects vary with individual medications.
   (3) Complications of Clozaril may include agranulocytosis, which is a decrease in certain white blood cells that is potentially fatal.
      (a) A result of this potentiality necessitates weekly blood count monitoring initially, biweekly after 6 months, and monthly after a year of treatment.
   (4) The resulting disruptions in lifestyle can be problematic for those on this medication which can effect medication compliance.

c. Neuromuscular side-effects of antipsychotics may be treated by Cogentin, Artane, Benadryl, and Symmetrel.
   (1) Side effects include dry mouth, blurry vision, sedation, dizziness, hypotension, insomnia, and confusion.

Diagnostic-Specific Considerations for Occupational Therapy

1. When working with persons with psychotic disorders, the presence of disordered thinking requires the occupational therapy practitioner to communicate simply, clearly, and concretely.
2. External structure and consistency to organize the individual's thinking, environment, and daily activities is often required.
3. The provision of supports and tools to enable recovery is essential (e.g., WRAP – Wellness and Recovery Action Plan; see Chapter 14).
4. See this chapter's sections on occupational therapy mental health evaluation and occupational therapy mental health intervention for additional guidelines.
5. Chapter 14 provides further information on general OT psychosocial evaluation and intervention approaches and specific interventions to manage psychotic behaviors (i.e., delusions and hallucinations).

Major DSM-5 Changes

1. Schizophrenia Spectrum and Other Psychotic Disorders is the new diagnostic category.
   a. This now includes Schizotypal personality disorder, although it is not coded here and is still represented in and coded in Personality Disorders.
2. Catatonia has its own distinct coding and its own diagnostic category.
3. Subtypes of schizophrenia such as paranoid, disorganized, catatonic, undifferentiated and residual types are deleted.
4. Delusional disorder no longer has the requirement that the delusions must be non-bizzare.

Mood Disorders

Overview

1. Mood disorders are diagnosed based on the incidence of manic, hypomanic, major depressive, and mixed episodes. (See below for descriptions of specific episodes.)
2. Mood episodes are not coded diagnoses in and of themselves.
3. Treatment addresses the symptoms of the episode experienced by the person.
   a. Interventions will vary with shifts in mood.

Diagnostic Criteria for Specific Mood Disorders

1. Major depressive disorder.
   a. One or more depressive episodes.
   b. May be a single episode or recurrent episodes.
2. Bipolar I disorder.
   a. One or more manic episodes.
   b. May be combined with depressive episodes.
3. Bipolar II disorder.
   a. One or more major depressive episodes.

b. There must be at least one hypomanic episode.
c. There is no history of a manic episode.
4. Other mood disorder diagnoses.
a. Dysthymia is characterized by at least two years of a depressed mood, most days, with depressive symptoms that are not severe enough to meet the criteria for a major depressive episode.
b. Cyclothymic disorder is characterized by at least two years with numerous periods of hypomanic and depressive symptoms that do not meet the criteria for a manic episode or a major depressive episode.

Onset, Prevalence, and Prognosis

1. While major depressive disorder can develop at any age, the median age at onset is 32.
2. The median age of onset for bipolar disorder is 25 years, although the illness can start in early childhood or as late as the 40s and 50s.
3. The lifetime prevalence of depressive disorders is 20%–26% in women and 8%–12% in men.
4. Bipolar disorders have a lifetime prevalence of 1.0%–2.4%.
5. While the prognosis for recurrences of mood disorders is poor, recovery is possible.
a. Early intervention is more effective than later intervention.
b. The use of effective medications and interventions based on a recovery model have increased the number of individuals with mood disorders who are able to maintain satisfying life-styles, resulting in a more favorable overall prognosis.
c. Minimizing the frequency of episodes helps with recovery.

Manic Episode

1. Diagnostic criteria.
a. A distinct period of abnormally and persistently elevated, expansive, or irritable mood lasting at least one week.
b. During this period, three or more of the following symptoms have persisted.
(1) Inflated self-esteem or grandiosity.
(2) Decreased need for sleep.
(3) More talkative than usual or pressured speech.
(4) Flight of ideas or feeling that thoughts are racing.
(5) Distractibility.
(6) Increase in goal-directed activity or psychomotor agitation.
(7) Excessive involvement in pleasurable activities that have a high potential for painful consequences.
c. Behaviors often associated with a manic episode.
(1) Treatment-resistance resulting from failure to recognize illness.
(2) Suggestive or flamboyant dress.
(3) Gambling, promiscuity, excessive spending, or giving things away.
(4) Irritable, assaultive, or suicidal behavior.
2. Impact on function.
a. The lack of inhibition experienced during a manic phase may lead to excessive spending, impulsive travel, flamboyant and promiscuous dress and/or behavior, etc.
b. Individuals may be euphoric in early phases, but may become labile, threatening, and assaultive.
c. Individuals may have high, often undirected, energy levels and require little sleep.
d. Poor judgment can lead to dangerous situations, poor self care, problems in relationships, and decreased or irresponsible work performance.
e. The incidence of substance abuse is increased.
3. Symptom management.
a. Antipsychotics (refer to prior section on psychotic disorders).
b. Mood stabilizing medications (first line of psychopharmacological treatment).
(1) Lithium: Eskalith, Lithobid, and time-released forms.
(a) Side effects include excessive thirst, tremors, excessive urination, weight gain, nausea, diarrhea, and cognitive impairment.
(b) Precautions include the monitoring of blood levels to maintain the narrow therapeutic window.
- High levels may cause nerve damage and death.
- Early symptoms of toxicity include motoric disturbances.

(2) Anticonvulsants.
(a) Depakote, Tegretol, Lamictal, Topamax, Neurontin, and Trileptal.
(b) Side effects include dizziness, drowsiness, ataxia, weight gain, and sedation.
(3) Mood stabilizers are also used to prevent bipolar disorder.
(4) Anti-psychotic medications such as Zyprexa, Seroquel, Risperdal, Geodon and Abilify are also used to treat symptoms of bipolar disorder.
4. Diagnostic-specific considerations for occupational therapy.
a. Limit-setting to set and improve boundaries, reduce the individual's fears of losing control, increase participation in the intervention process, and promote safety.
b. Engagement in activities that provide structure and the opportunity for release of excess energy in a positive and therapeutic manner.
c. Periods between episodes should be used to educate the individual, the family, and significant others on symptom management.

d. See this chapter's sections on occupational therapy mental health evaluation and occupational therapy mental health intervention for additional guidelines.
e. Chapter 14 provides additional information on general OT psychosocial evaluation and intervention approaches and specific intervention approaches for managing manic or monopolizing behaviors.

Major Depressive Episode

1. Diagnostic criteria.
   a. A 2-week period of depressed mood or loss of interest or pleasure.
   b. Five or more of the following symptoms.
      (1) Depressed mood most of the day.
      (2) Markedly diminished interest or pleasure.
      (3) Weight loss/gain, increase/decrease in appetite.
      (4) Insomnia/hypersomnia.
      (5) Psychomotor retardation/agitation.
      (6) Fatigue, loss of energy.
      (7) Feelings of worthlessness or guilt.
      (8) Diminished ability to concentrate/make decisions.
      (9) Recurrent thoughts of death/suicide (with or without a plan), suicide attempt.
   c. Behaviors often associated with depressive episodes.
      (1) Irritability, anxiety, phobias, and obsessive thinking.
      (2) Difficulties in social interactions, relationships, and sexual functioning.
      (3) Self-destructive behavior including suicide and substance abuse.
      (4) May be manifested as somatic complaints.
      (5) There may be an increased use of medical services.
2. Impact on function.
   a. Individuals are often tearful, brooding, and isolative.
   b. Anxiety leads to excessive concerns about physical health, complaints of pain, and alcohol abuse.
   c. Hopelessness, lack of energy, and slow thought processing lead to limited interest in activity and difficulty performing tasks in all areas of occupation, including personal and instrumental activities of daily living, leisure, social participation, education, and work activities.
3. Symptom management.
   a. Antidepressant medications.
      (1) Selective Serotonin Reuptake Inhibitors (SSRIs) include Prozac, Zoloft, Paxil, Celexa, and Lexapro.
         (a) Side effects include nausea, headache, sexual dysfunction, and insomnia.
      (2) Tricyclics include Elavil, Tofranil, Norpramin, and Pamelor. However, these are rarely used secondary to the efficacy of the SSRIs and SNRIs.
         (a) Side effects include dry mouth, blurred vision, sedation, postural hypotension, and other anticholinergic effects.
      (3) Selective norepinephrine or serotonin and norepinephrine inhibitors (SNRIs) include Effexor, Cymbalta.Wellbutrin is similar in effect and has fewer sexual side effects.
         (a) Side effects vary but may include hypertension, anxiety, dizziness, sedation, nervousness, weight gain, nausea, and sweating.
      (4) Monoamine Oxidase Inhibitors (MAOIs) include Nardil and Parnate.
         (a) Side-effects include weight gain, hypotension, insomnia, and liver damage.
         (b) Precautions include dietary restrictions for individuals taking MAOIs.
            - Ingesting foods or beverages that contain the amino acid tyramine can suddenly increase blood pressure and may lead to stroke or other serious cardiac reactions.
            - Foods and beverages with tyramine must be completely avoided. These include aged cheeses, pickled foods (e.g., sauerkraut, herring), cured or smoked meats (e.g., salami, sausage, pepperoni, hot dogs), liver, yogurt, sour cream, fruits that must ripen to eat (e.g., avocados, bananas), fava beans, peapods, chocolate, beer and red wine (including non-alcoholic and alcohol-reduced), meat tenderizers, soy products (soy sauce, tofu), yeast extracts, and any product that has been improperly stored, over-ripened, not fresh, and/or past an expiration date.
            - Many over the counter drugs also contain ingredients that can cause a serious interaction with MAOIs. These include cold, sinus, and hay fever medications, nasal decongestants, asthma inhalants, "pep" pills, and appetite suppressants.
         (c) Severe headaches or palpitations can be the first sign of a hypertensive crisis.
            - The medication should be stopped immediately and a physician consulted.
   b. The most effective treatment involves antidepressant medication combined with psychotherapy.
   c. Cognitive approaches (i.e., cognitive behavioral therapy [CBT]) are helpful for those who demonstrate self-awareness, intact cognitive skills, and the ability to actively participate in the intervention process. See Chapter 14.

d. Electroconvulsive therapy (ECT) is very effective and the treatment of choice for those who have been unresponsive to trials on medications and other interventions.
(1) How ECT works is not fully understood.
(a) A limiting factor is that ECT often produces memory loss and confusion for the period surrounding treatment. Both are reversible, and evolution of ECT over the past decades has produced innovations that diminish cognitive effects while maintaining benefits.
4. Diagnostic-specific considerations for occupational therapy.
a. The provision of a safe environment and the management of behaviors that threaten the safety and well-being of the individual are paramount.
(1) Individuals must be closely monitored for self-destructive and/or suicidal behavior.
(2) The most dangerous time may be when the depression begins to lift and the person becomes mobilized.
(a) This includes the days after inpatient admission and just prior to discharge.
b. See this chapter's sections on occupational therapy mental health evaluation and occupational therapy mental health intervention for additional guidelines.
c. Chapter 14 provides further information on general OT psychosocial evaluation and intervention approaches and specific interventions to manage suicidal behaviors and other depressive symptoms.

Mixed Episode

1. The criteria are met for both a manic episode and a major depressive episode for at least one week.

Hypomanic Episode

1. Symptoms are the same as for a manic episode; however, they are not severe enough (i.e., they last for four days rather than one week) to cause marked impairment in social or occupational function or to require hospitalization.

Major DSM-5 Changes

1. Bipolar Disorder and Depressive Disorders are now separate diagnostic categories and the chapter categorizing "Mood Disorders" has been eliminated.
2. Several new depressive disorders, including disruptive mood dysregulation disorder and premenstrual dysphoric disorder are included.
3. Dysthymia now falls under the category of persistent depressive disorder.
4. Core criterion symptoms for the diagnosis of major depressive episode are unchanged.

Substance-Related Disorders

Overview

1. Substance-related disorders are diagnosed based upon the taking of a drug of abuse (including alcohol and prescription medications), the side-effects of medication(s), and/or exposure to toxins (inhalants, lead).
2. Substance-related disorders are categorized into two groups.
a. Substance use disorders include dependence and abuse.
b. Substance-induced disorders include a multitude of diagnoses including intoxication, withdrawal, and substance-induced anxiety, affective, and psychotic disorders.
(1) These disorders are generally treated medically and therefore will not be further described.

Substance Dependence

1. Diagnostic criteria.
a. There must be evidence of tolerance and withdrawal.
(1) Tolerance to a substance results in diminished effects from taking the same amount of a substance and the need to use increasing amounts to experience the desired effect.
(2) Withdrawal refers to the symptoms (specific to the substance) that occur with decrease or discontinuation.
(a) The substance is then used not for pleasure, but to prevent or relieve the withdrawal symptoms.
b. Individual continues to use the substance despite serious consequences.

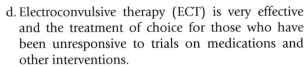

Substance Abuse

1. Diagnostic criteria.
   a. There must be continued use despite serious consequences.

Onset, Prevalence, and Prognosis

1. The onset of substance abuse is starting earlier and earlier. While it often begins in adolescence, it may begin anytime from childhood through seniority.
2. Recent statistics reveal the prevalence for substance abuse or dependence.
   a. 9.3% for adolescents aged 12 to 17 years.
   b. 19.6% for young adults aged 18 to 25.
   c. 5.9% for adults ages 26 or older.
3. According to a 2008 study, drinking alcohol is a prevalent activity in the United States.
   a. Among youths aged 12 to 17, the percentage of males who were current drinkers (14.2%) was similar to the rate for females (15.0%).
   b. Among adults aged 18 to 25, an estimated 58.0% of females and 64.3% of males reported current drinking in 2008.
4. Prognosis varies depending on several factors including motivation, substance used, and degree and type of support.

Impact on Function

1. The impact substance use has on the individual depends on the type of substance used and on whether the individual is abusing the substance, or is dependent upon it.
2. Results of disorders of use.
   a. Disinterest and inability to care for self and others.
   b. Difficulty with and loss of personal relationships.
   c. Inability to be productive and/or maintain employment.
   d. Absence of leisure and/or social pursuits that do not involve substance use.
   e. Involvement with the legal system.
3. Prolonged use may lead to severe physical, cognitive, and psychiatric problems and can result in death.

Medical Management

1. Medications to help the individual refrain from substance use can be provided.
2. This medical management is typically supplemented with psychotherapy and support groups, (e.g., Alcoholics Anonymous, Narcotics Anonymous).
3. Methadone clinics and the use of methadone for detoxification and maintenance for opiod dependence is the most accepted approach for heroin addiction.

Diagnostic-Specific Considerations for Occupational Therapy

1. Due to the presence of learned "survival skills," the individual's abilities and potential may be overestimated.
   a. The occupational therapist apprises the team and the individual of the person's actual skills and deficits as evident during evaluation and intervention.
   b. The occupational therapist assists the team and the person in identifying realistic expectations and discharge plans.
2. The individual's identification of the reasons for substance use is important to address during the evaluation process.
3. The development of the skills necessary to cope with life stressors without substance use is critical for a substance-free lifestyle. Skills needed include:
   a. Communication and social skills to support substance-free social participation.
   b. Skills to engage productively in work, education, and/or other productive activities (e.g., volunteering).
   c. Skills to use leisure time without using substances.
4. Life-long patterns of denial, resistance, and other defensive behaviors can make treatment challenging and difficult.
5. Referrals to support groups, including Alcoholics Anonymous, Narcotics Anonymous, and others can sustain recovery.
6. See this chapter's sections on occupational therapy mental health evaluation and occupational therapy mental health intervention for additional guidelines.
7. Chapter 14 provides further information on general OT psychosocial evaluation and intervention approaches.

Major DSM-5 Changes

1. The substance-related disorder chapter now includes Gambling Disorder.
2. The diagnoses of substance abuse and dependence are not separate as in the past.

Anxiety Disorders

Overview

1. Anxiety disorders include a range of disorders that include episodic periods of intense anxiety to chronic periods of lower levels anxiety.
2. Anxiety is an internal sense of apprehension and psychological distress. It may or may not have a specific focus.

Panic Attacks and Agoraphobia

1. Panic attacks are symptoms of anxiety.
   a. They are not coded diagnoses.
2. Panic attacks are discrete periods of intense fear or discomfort, in which four or more symptoms develop abruptly and reach a peak within 10 minutes.
   a. Palpitations, or accelerated heart rate.
   b. Sweating.
   c. Trembling or shaking.
   d. Sensations of shortness of breath or smothering.
   e. Feelings of choking.
   f. Chest pain or discomfort.
   g. Nausea or abdominal stress.
   h. Feeling dizzy, unsteady, lightheaded, or faint.
   i. Derealization or depersonalization.
   j. Fear of losing control or going crazy.
   k. Fear of dying.
   l. Paresthesias.
   m. Chills or hot flashes.
3. Agoraphobia associated with panic attack.
   a. Anxiety about being in places or situations from which escape may be difficult or embarrassing, or in which help may not be available if needed.
   b. Situations are avoided or endured with anxiety about having a panic attack.

Specific Anxiety Disorders

1. Panic disorder.
   a. Recurrent panic attacks followed at least once by concern for recurrence.
2. Specific phobia.
   a. A clinically significant anxiety from a specific object or situation leading to avoidant behavior.
3. Social phobia.
   a. A clinically significant anxiety from certain types of social or performance situations leading to avoidance.
4. Obsessive-compulsive disorder.
   a. Obsessions are recurrent and persistent thoughts, images, or impulses that are disturbing, intrusive, and inappropriate.
   b. Compulsions are repetitive behaviors that the person is driven to perform to reduce anxiety or prevent a dreaded event of situation.
   c. The obsessions or compulsions are time-consuming and distressing despite the individual's awareness of their irrationality.
5. Post-traumatic stress disorder.
   a. The persistent re-experiencing (for more than one month) of an extremely traumatic event that produces symptoms of increased arousal.
   b. Results in avoidance of stimuli associated with the traumatic event.
6. Acute stress disorder.
   a. Similar to post-traumatic stress disorder; however, it immediately follows the event.
   b. The symptoms do not persist beyond one month.
7. Generalized anxiety disorder.
   a. Consists of 6 months of persistent and excessive unfocused anxiety and worry.

Onset, Prevalence, and Prognosis

1. Anxiety disorders often begin in childhood but may develop at any time.
2. Post-traumatic stress disorder and acute stress disorder follow the stressful event.
3. Prevalence and prognosis vary with the specific disorder.

Impact on Function

1. The degree of impact varies with the severity and type of anxiety disorder.
2. Reactions may vary from temporary discomfort to severely avoidant and paralyzing behavior.

Symptom Management

1. Psychotherapy to explore psychodynamic issues.
2. Cognitive-behavioral therapy to develop skills to manage symptoms.

3. Several types of medications may be helpful depending on the specific disorder.
   a. Anxiolytic medications include Xanax, Valium, Librium, Ativan, Klonopin, and BuSpar.
      (1) Side effects include drowsiness, ataxia, headache, nausea, depression, and dependence.
   b. Antidepressant medications are helpful in some cases.
      (1) Refer to mood disorder section for side-effect profiles.
   c. Anti-obsessional medications (Anafranil, Paxil, Prozac, and Zoloft, at high doses) reduce obsessional thinking. Luvox is rarely used due to potentiating effects.
      (1) Side effects are similar to that of the Selective Serotonin Reuptake Inhibitors.
   d. In some cases hypnotic medications to induce sleep may be used briefly.
      (1) Hypnotic medications include Restoril, Dalmane, Ambien, and Benadryl.
      (2) Side effects are similar to those of the anxiolytics.

Diagnostic-Specific Considerations for Occupational Therapy

1. Skills training and using cognitive behavioral approaches may reduce avoidant behavior.
2. Developing relaxation and stress management skills may decrease the incidence and severity of symptoms.
3. Providing graded activities designed to promote self-efficacy may increase self-confidence, motivation, and participation in intervention.
4. See this chapter's sections on occupational therapy mental health evaluation and occupational therapy mental health intervention for additional guidelines.
5. Using systematic desensitization, which involves incremental exposure in attempts to diminish anxiety related to specific fears through the use of imagery and relaxation, and then contact with the image or actual object.
   a. Used most often with phobic disorders and requires special training.
6. Chapter 14 provides further information on general OT psychosocial evaluation and intervention approaches.

Major DSM-5 Changes

1. The chapter on anxiety disorder no longer includes obssessive-compulsive disorder or posttraumatic stress disorder.
   a. OCD is now in the chapter "Obsessive-Compulsive and Related Disorders."
   b. PTSD is now classified in the chapter on "Trauma and Stressor-Related Disorders."
2. Separation Anxiety Disorder is now classified here rather than in the former DSM-IV-TR section on "Disorders Usually First Diagnosed in Infancy, Childhood or Adolsesence.

Personality Disorders

Diagnostic Criteria

1. Evidence of characteristics and patterns of inner experience and behavior that deviate markedly from the culturally accepted norms in cognition, affect, impulse control, and interpersonal relating.
2. Behavior must be inflexible and maladaptive across a broad range of personal and social situations.
3. There must be evidence of onset in late childhood or adolescence.
4. Personality disorders are grouped in clusters according to their impact on behavior.
   a. Cluster A.
      (1) Paranoid, schizoid, and schizotypal.
      (2) Individuals with these disorders are often perceived as odd and eccentric.
   b. Cluster B.
      (1) Antisocial, borderline, histrionic, and narcissistic.
      (2) Individuals with these disorders are often perceived as dramatic, emotional, and erratic.
   c. Cluster C.
      (1) Avoidant, dependent, obsessive-compulsive, and those not otherwise specified.
      (2) Individuals with these disorders are often perceived as anxious or fearful.

Specific Personality Disorders

1. Paranoid personality disorder.
   a. Persons with this disorder are characterized by long-standing suspiciousness and mistrust of people in general.
   b. They refuse responsibility for their own feelings and assign responsibility for them to others.
   c. They can often appear hostile, irritable, and angry.

2. Schizoid personality disorder.
   a. This is frequently diagnosed in individuals who display a lifelong pattern of social withdrawal.
   b. Their discomfort with human interaction, their introversion, and their bland, constricted affect are noteworthy.
   c. Persons with schizoid personality disorder are often seen by others as eccentric, isolated, or lonely.
3. Schizotypal personality disorder.
   a. Persons with this disorder appear odd or strange in their thinking and behavior to those who come in contact with them.
   b. Magical thinking, peculiar ideas, ideas of reference, illusions, and derealization are part of this individual's everyday world.
4. Antisocial personality disorder.
   a. This disorder is characterized by continual antisocial or criminal acts, but it is not synonymous with criminality.
   b. It is an inability to conform to social norms that involves many aspects of the individual's adolescent and adult development.
   c. Persons with antisocial personality disorder have no regard for the safety or feelings of others and they lack remorse.
   d. Individuals diagnosed with a conduct disorder that does not respond to treatment or is untreated can be a precursor to developing this disorder.
5. Borderline personality disorder.
   a. Individuals with borderline personality disorder experience extraordinarily unstable affect, mood, behavior, relationships, and self-image.
   b. Fear of real or imagined abandonment leads to frantic efforts to avoid it.
   c. Recurrent self-destructive or self-mutilating behavior may be threatened or carried out.
   d. Majority of patients have a history of trauma (i.e., physical, sexual, emotional abuse).
6. Histrionic personality disorder.
   a. This disorder is characterized by colorful, dramatic, extroverted behavior in excitable, emotional persons.
   b. An inability to maintain deep, long-lasting attachments with accompanying flamboyant presentation is often characteristic.
7. Narcissistic personality disorder.
   a. Persons with this disorder are characterized by a heightened sense of self-importance and a grandiose feeling that they are special in some way.
8. Avoidant personality disorder.
   a. Persons with this disorder show an extreme sensitivity to rejection, which may lead to a socially withdrawn life.
   b. These individuals are not, however, asocial. They show a great desire for companionship but consider themselves inept or unworthy.
   c. Individuals with avoidant personality disorder need unusually strong and repeated guarantees of uncritical acceptance.
   d. These persons are commonly referred to as having an inferiority complex.
9. Dependent personality disorder.
   a. Persons with this disorder subordinate their own needs to those of others and need others to assume responsibility for major areas in their lives.
   b. Individuals with dependent personality disorder lack self-confidence.
   c. They may experience discomfort when alone for more than a brief period.
10. Obsessive-compulsive personality disorder.
   a. Characterized by emotional constriction, orderliness, perseverance, stubbornness, and indecisiveness.
   b. The essential feature is a pervasive pattern of perfectionism and inflexibility.
   c. It should not be confused with obsessive-compulsive disorder.
11. Personality disorders not otherwise specified (NOS).
   a. Passive-aggressive.
   b. Depressive.
   c. Sadomasochistic.
   d. Sadistic.

Onset, Prevalence, and Prognosis

1. Symptoms of personality disorders usually begin in childhood or early adolescence.
2. The prevalence of personality disorders varies with the specific disorder from rare to approximately 9.1%.
3. The prognosis for individuals with personality disorders varies, with the condition often remaining unchanged.
   a. There is an increased risk of the development of depressive disorders among persons with personality disorders.
   b. There is some evidence that the symptoms of avoidant, borderline, and antisocial personality disorders may decrease with age.

Impact on Function

1. The type and degree of impact on areas of occupation, personal relationships, and daily life depend on the severity and type of personality disorder.

Symptom Management

1. Psychotherapy and certain medications may reduce symptomatology for some patients.
2. Dialectical behavior therapy (DBT) has demonstrated success in the treatment of borderline personality disorder.
3. Monitoring, supervision, and hospitalization may be required during periods of increased symptoms, and/or aggressive or self-destructive behavior.

Diagnostic-Specific Considerations for Occupational Therapy

1. Assistance to the individual in identification of the above issues may increase commitment to treatment and the pursuit of behavioral change.
2. Cognitive behavioral approaches (including dialectical behavioral therapy) can increase functional and coping skills and may decrease symptomatic behavior.
3. See this chapter's sections on occupational therapy mental health evaluation and occupational therapy mental health intervention for additional guidelines.
4. Chapter 14 provides further information on general OT psychosocial evaluation and intervention approaches.

Major DSM-5 Changes

1. The criteria for personality disorders have not changed.
2. Because the multiaxial system has been eliminated, they are now included with the other diagnoses and are no longer known as Axis II disorders.

Delirium, Dementia, and Amnestic and Other Cognitive Disorders

Diagnostic Criteria

1. Conditions for which the primary symptoms are cognitive deficits. This may be from substance abuse, medical conditions, or other known or unknown causes.
2. Delirium.
   a. A disturbance of consciousness (awareness of environment) with a decreased ability to attend.
   b. There is a change from previous cognition and/or perception.
   c. It covers a short period of time (hours to days) and tends to fluctuate.
   d. There are many causes.
      (1) Brain dysfunction.
      (2) Medication.
      (3) Endocrine disorders.
      (4) Cardiac disorders.
      (5) Fever.
      (6) Liver function disorders.
3. Dementia.
   a. Disturbances of memory and multiple cognitive deficits.
      (1) Aphasia.
      (2) Apraxia.
      (3) Agnosia.
      (4) Disturbance of executive function (i.e., planning, organization, sequencing).
   b. Dementia often includes personality changes.
   c. Dementia must lead to functional problems.
   d. It represents a decline in the person's previous level of cognitive skills.
   e. Alzheimer's type and vascular dementia account for 75% of all cases.
   f. Other causes include AIDS, Pick's disease, Huntington's chorea, Parkinson's disease, and alcoholism.
   g. Although symptoms of Alzheimer's and vascular dementia are the same, vascular dementia requires evidence of a vascular cause.
   h. Mental confusion due to reversible causes must be ruled out. See Table 10-1.
4. Amnesic disorders.
   a. Difficulty with memory only, but sufficient to cause functional difficulty.
   b. Causes and types.
      (1) Cerebrovascular accident.
      (2) Multiple sclerosis.
      (3) Korsakoff's syndrome.
      (4) Alcoholic blackouts.
      (5) Electroconvulsive therapy.
      (6) Traumatic brain injury.
      (7) Transient global amnesia.

Table 10-1

Reversible Causes of Mental Confusion
Sensory changes and problems
• Age-related losses in hearing, vision, touch, etc.
• Unavailable or inadequate prostheses such as hearing aids, glasses, dentures, etc.
• Sensory overload; too much, too long, too fast.
• Sensory deprivation; too little stimulation, isolation, restraints.
• Loss of cues to aid orientation and memory such as clocks, magazines, calendars, and strict adherence to routines and rituals.
DEPRESSION
Drug use and misuse
• Drug interactions, side effects, and build-up from longer absorption and elimination times.
• Over-the-counter cold, sleeping, and pain remedies; often taken without the physician's knowledge and which react with prescribed drugs.
Infections/Inflammation
• Viral or bacterial infections; may be accompanied by fever.
• Urinary tract infections, pneumonia, etc.
• Gallbladder disease.
Metabolic problems caused by
• Liver or kidney disease.
• Thyroid disorders (hyperthyroidism and hypothyroidism).
• Dehydration from diuretics, low fluid intake, hot weather.
• Poorly controlled diabetes.

Onset, Prevalence, and Prognosis

1. Delirium occurs in 10%–25% of hospitalized individuals depending on the related medical condition.
   a. It may resolve quickly or take several days.
   b. It is more severe with advanced age.
   c. It may indicate a poor prognosis over time.
2. Dementia is present in 5% of those over 65 and increases with age.
   a. There may be periods of plateauing with a gradual decline over time.
3. The prevalence of and prognosis for amnesic disorders varies with the cause.
   a. It is most often associated with alcohol use disorders and head injury.

Impact on Function

1. The degree of impact varies according to the nature and severity of the symptoms.
2. The individual may require intervention varying from education in compensatory strategies to the need for total care.
3. Reisburg's stages of mental confusion describe the progressive impact of dementia on functional abilities. See Table10-2.

Symptom Management

1. Differential diagnosis to ensure that symptoms are not pseudodementia due to a reversible cause. See Table 10-1.
2. Medical treatment involves resolution of the causes of the disorder if possible.
3. There are a limited number of newer medications that appear to maintain or slow the decline of cognitive function (e.g., Aricept, Cognex).
4. If causes of the disorder are not treatable, attempts are made to mitigate symptoms where possible.

Diagnostic-Specific Considerations for Occupational Therapy

1. Maintenance of quality of life through activity adaptation and environmental modification. See Chapters 15 and 16.
2. Family education to understand the nature of the person's disorder and improve the management of its symptoms and functional effects.
3. See this chapter's sections on occupational therapy mental health evaluation and occupational therapy mental health intervention for additional guidelines.
4. Chapter 14 provides further information on general OT psychosocial evaluation and intervention approaches and specific interventions to manage the effects of cognitive disorders and Alzheimer's disease.

Major DSM-5 Changes

1. This section has been renamed "Neurocognitive Disorders."
   a. Under this category falls delirium with updated criteria.
   b. The diagnoses of dementia and amnestic disorder now are subsumed under the newly named entity "Major Neurocognitive Disorder."

Table 10-2

Reisburg's Stages for Dementia	
Stage 1: No disability is noted	
Stage 2: The person complains about forgetting normal age-related information (location of objects: keys, wallet, etc.)	
Stage 3: Beginning signs and deficits are noted in this stage	
THE PERSON'S STRENGTHS	**THE PERSON'S WEAKNESSES**
1. Remains independent in IADL	1. Forgets important information for first time in one's life
2. Can recognize challenging situations to avoid, in order to minimalize manifested deficits	2. Experiences difficulty completing complex tasks
3. Can utilize compensation as an adaptive mechanism	3. Experiences difficulty negotiating directions to new location
Stage 4: Deficits are noted in all IADL	
THE PERSON'S STRENGTHS	**THE PERSON'S WEAKNESSES**
1. Can still perform simple, repetitive ADL independently	1. Becomes increasingly forgetful
2. Can live at home with support	2. Becomes unable to follow and sequence written cues
3. Can follow simple verbal and demonstrational cues	3. Becomes unable to perform familiar, challenging activities
	4. Experiences difficulty in word finding
	5. Cannot manage at home without assistance
Stage 5: Person cannot function independently	
THE PERSON'S STRENGTHS	**THE PERSONS WEAKNESSES**
1. Can perform ADL and some IADL with correct cues and assistance	1. Demonstrates poor judgment
2. Can respond to encouragement	2. Experiences difficulty with all decision making
3. Becomes unable to safely drive an automobile	3. Forgets to take care of hygiene
Stage 6: Person cannot perform ADL without cues	
THE PERSON'S STRENGTHS	**THE PERSON'S WEAKNESSES**
1. Can perform components of familiar tasks	1. Demonstrates significant deficits in following 2 steps of a task
2. Can follow demonstration/hand over hand cues	2. Cannot sequence steps of ADL tasks
	3. Cannot speak in full sentences
	4. Becomes incontinent of bowel and bladder
Stage 7: The person can be in a vegetative state. He/she is usually bedbound and unable to respond verbally or non-verbally to questions or commands	

Reproduced with permission from *Dementia: A Systematic Approach to Identifying Reversible Causes.* Geriatrics: 41:430–446, 1986. Copyright by Advanstar Communications Inc. Advanstar Communications Inc. retains all rights to this article.

Eating Disorders

Anorexia Nervosa

1. Diagnostic criteria.
   a. Refusal to maintain body weight at or above normal weight for age and height, or failure to make expected weight gain during a period of growth leading to a body weight less than 85% of that expected.
   b. Intense fear of gaining weight or becoming fat, even though underweight.
   c. Disturbance in the way in which one's body weight or shape is experienced.
      (1) Undue influence of body weight or shape on self-evaluation.
      (2) Denial of the seriousness of the current low body weight even when hospitalized or gravely ill.
   d. In postmenarchical females, amenorrhea, the absence of at least three consecutive menstrual cycles.
   e. Anorexia includes a food restrictive type and a binge eating/purging type.

2. Onset, prevalence, and prognosis.
   a. Anorexia most commonly begins in the mid-teens.
      (1) It occurs in 5% of adolescent girls.
      (2) It is 10 to 20 times more common in girls.
   b. The long-term prognosis may not be good, with mortality rates from 5%–18%.
3. Behavioral characteristics.
   a. Individuals often exhibit obsessive/compulsive behavior, depression, anxiety, rigidity, perfectionism, and poor sexual adjustment.

Bulimia Nervosa

1. Diagnostic criteria.
   a. Recurrent episodes of binge eating defined as a lack of control over discrete periods of excessive eating of an abnormally large amount of food.
   b. The purging type includes recurrent, inappropriate compensatory behavior in order to prevent weight gain.
      (1) Self-induced vomiting.
      (2) Use of laxatives and/or diuretics.
      (3) Fasting.
      (4) Excessive exercising.
   c. Binge eating and purging behaviors both occur, on average, at least twice a week for three months.
   d. Self-evaluation is unduly influenced by body shape and weight.
   e. The disturbance does not occur exclusively during episodes of anorexia nervosa.
2. Onset, prevalence, and prognosis.
   a. The usual age of onset of bulimia is later than that of anorexia.
      (1) It begins in adolescence or in early adulthood.
      (2) It is present in 1%–3% of women.
      (3) It is significantly more common in women.
   b. The prognosis is better than for anorexia, with 80% of individuals not meeting the criteria for diagnosis after 10 years.
3. Behavioral characteristics.
   a. Individuals are often obsessed with their appearance and attractiveness to the opposite sex.
   b. They are likely to be sexually active and maintain a normal weight.

Eating Disorders Not Otherwise Specified

1. Includes several types.
   a. Binge-eating disorder (BED) is the one that will be most typically seen in OT practice due to the co-morbidities caused by the obesity that result from this disorder (e.g., diabetes).
      (1) Recurrent episodes of binge eating until uncomfortably full without purging.
         (a) Eating is more rapid than typical and is often initiated when not hungry and/or when alone due to embarrassment about the amount of food being consumed.

Impact on Function

1. ADL such as self-care, eating, and feeding can be severely disrupted.
2. IADL such as shopping for clothing and food, meal preparation and cleanup, and health management and maintenance can be significantly affected.
3. Work skills can be intact unless food-restricting behaviors and/or medical problems interfere with work performance or prevocational/vocational skill development.
   a. Focus on weight control may interfere with pursuit of vocational goals and/or the development of prerequisite skills.
4. Leisure skills can be intact unless affected by food-restricting behaviors and/or medical complications.
   a. Activities may focus mainly on appearance, rather than on those that have meaning or purpose.
   b. Exercise activities previously done for fun (e.g., running, swimming, cycling) may now be done excessively without enjoyment to decrease weight.
5. Social participation (including family, community, and peer/friend) can be greatly impacted by the excessive use of food-restricting behaviors, the need to maintain secrecy about the behaviors, and feeling ashamed, guilty, embarrassed, and/or depressed about atypical and disturbed eating habits and patterns.

Symptom Management

1. The use of antidepressant medications may be used in anorexia nervosa, but they are more effective for individuals with bulimia.
   a. Antipsychotics can be used as well to improve distorted thinking and perceptions.
2. Treatment of any of the resulting medical complications such as cardiac disturbances (hypotension, slow heart rate), reduced thyroid metabolism, osteoporosis, seizures, severe dehydration, electrolyte imbalances, irregular bowel movements, pancreatitis, peptic ulcers, gastric and/or esophageal inflammation and possible rupture, tooth decay, etc., may also be necessary.
3. Treatment most often takes place in outpatient or day care programs.
4. Hospitalization may be necessary if the individual has medical difficulties, is suicidal, cannot care for

him/her self, or needs to be removed from his/her environment.

5. Behavioral programs designed around a privileging system are often used.
   a. Consistency among staff is crucial for program effectiveness.
6. Medical management also typically includes individual psychotherapy, family counseling, and behavioral and/or cognitive therapies.

Diagnostic-Specific Considerations for Occupational Therapy

1. The building of trust is essential to effective intervention due to the secrecy, guilt, anger, resistance, and ego fragility often associated with the disorder and its stages of recovery.
2. The occupational therapist must be honest, supportive, and gently confrontational when indicated.
3. Evaluation and intervention must include the identification of the socio-emotional needs the eating disorder had fulfilled for the person so that health-promoting occupation-based alternatives can be explored and developed.
   a. Non-food related areas of interest and meaningful purposeful activities should be pursued to promote a reality-based body image and foster improved coping.
4. Education about nutritional food management and the development of healthy leisure time (i.e., does not involve excessive exercise) are key.
5. See this chapter's sections on occupational therapy mental health evaluation and occupational therapy mental health intervention for additional guidelines.
6. Chapter 14 provides further information on general OT psychosocial evaluation and intervention approaches.

Major DSM-5 Changes

1. Several of the feeding and eating disorders of infancy or early childhood from DSM-IV-TR are now included in the DSM-5 chapter "Feeding and Eating Disorders."
2. While the core diagnostic criteria for anorexia nervosa are basically unchanged, the requirement for amenorrhea has been eliminated.
3. The only change to Bulimia Nervosa is a reduction in the required minimum average frequency of binge eating and inappropriate compensatory behavior frequency from twice to once weekly.

Disorders Usually First Diagnosed in Infancy, Childhood, or Adolescence

Diagnostic Criteria

1. Oppositional defiant disorder.
   a. Negativistic, hostile, and defiant behaviors that result in functional impairment.
2. Conduct disorder.
   a. Disregard for the rights of others leading to aggression toward people and animals, destruction of property, deceitfulness, theft, or serious violation of rules.
3. Disruptive Behavior Disorder, NOS.
   a. Children who do not meet the criteria for Conduct Disorder or Oppositional Defiant Disorder; however, they display significant functional impairment and conduct and oppositional behaviors are present.

Onset, Prevalence, and Prognosis

1. Oppositional defiant disorder.
   a. Oppositional, negative behavior begins in early childhood and may be seen in 1%–16% of school-age children.
   b. The course and prognosis depend on the severity of behaviors, the presence of other disorders, and the intactness of the family.
   c. It is most likely to progress into a conduct disorder if aggression is prominent.
   d. Lifetime prevalence of ODD is estimated to be 10.2% (males = 11.2%; females = 9.2%).
2. Conduct disorder.
   a. It is estimated that 6%–16% of boys and 2%–9% of girls under the age of 18 have a conduct disorder.
   b. Prognosis is related to the age of onset and the severity of symptoms and behavior.
      (1) Severe conduct disorder is often associated with the development of other disorders and substance abuse later in life.
   c. Assaultive behavior and parental criminality correlate highly with future incarceration.
3. Disruptive behavior disorder, NOS.
   a. This category is for those children that do not meet the criteria for Conduct Disorder nor Oppositional Defiant Disorder, however significant behavioral impairment is demonstrated and conduct and oppositional behaviors are present. It can be a

convenient diagnostic category for children who display problematic, disruptive behaviors yet do not fit into any other category.

Impact on Function

1. Children with disruptive behavior disorders have difficulty at school and with the formation of healthy social and familial relationships.
2. Difficulties within the family affect not only the child but all family members, impacting on their role performance.

Symptom Management

1. Behavioral techniques are often the most effective forms of intervention with adolescents.
2. The identification and treatment of other disorders, (e.g., attention-deficit/hyperactivity disorder, learning disorders, substance use, depression) is important.
3. The use of medications such as antipsychotics, antidepressants, anxiolytics, and mood stabilizers may be helpful.
4. A consistent approach from all team members is essential.

Diagnostic-Specific Considerations for Occupational Therapy

1. Contributing disorders (e.g., attention deficit/hyperactivity disorder, mood disorders, learning disorders) and their effect on the performance skills and areas of occupation must be evaluated and addressed in intervention.
2. The child's goals, stressors, and family and social relationships should be considered.
3. Skill development may improve emotional adjustment.
4. Behavioral approaches must be consistent throughout all programming.
5. The therapist should assist the parents, other family members, teachers, and other school personnel to understand the nature of the child's condition and to develop strategies for behavior management.
6. See this chapter's sections on occupational therapy mental health evaluation and occupational therapy mental health intervention for additional guidelines.
7. Chapter 14 provides further information on general OT psychosocial evaluation and intervention approaches and specific interventions to manage offensive, intrusive, and escalating behaviors.

Major DSM-5 Changes

1. The chapter "Disorders Usually First Diagnosed in Infancy, Childhood and Adolescence" no longer exists.
2. Diagnoses formerly found in the chapter above such as "Oppositional Defiant Disorder and Conduct Disorder" have been placed in the new chapter "Disruptive, Impulse-Control, and Conduct Disorders."

Pervasive Developmental Disorders/Autism Spectrum Disorders[2]

Autism

1. Etiology.
   a. Organic brain pathology.
   b. May or may not be seen with other disorders.
2. Onset, prevalence, and prognosis.
   a. May occur from birth up to three years of age.
   b. Occurs in one out of 88 live births in the United States (1 in 54 boys and 1 in 252 girls) about 6 times as many boys as girls.
   c. The prognosis for functional independence is poor with 70% of children needing a supervised living setting (although the life expectancy is normal).
3. Diagnostic characteristics.
   a. Presence of at least six items from the listing below, including two or more from (1) and at least one from (2) and (3).
      (1) Impaired social interaction and in most cases cognitive disabilities.
         (a) Impaired nonverbal behaviors; e.g., infrequent/poor eye contact, impaired attachment behavior, anxiety with changes in typical routines.
         (b) Difficulty relating to others and forming relationships at an age appropriate level.
         (c) Lack of spontaneous social seeking behavioral interactions with others and lack of awareness of others who are seeking interactions (e.g., sharing a snack, pointing at an object of interest).

[2] Jan Garbarini contributed this section on Pervasive Developmental Disorders.

(d) Lack of social reciprocation due to decreased ability to infer feelings and intentions of others (e.g., the child does not understand that sharing is expected; the child does not point at an object to have the parents name the object or point to pictures in a book and look to the reader for a response).

(2) Difficulty with communication.
(a) Lack of initiation, reflection, development of spoken language or alternative means for communication.
(b) If speech is developed, difficulty in initiating or engaging in conversation and lack of appropriate context.
(c) Stereotyped echolalia and/or use of indiscernible language.
(d) Lack of spontaneous pretend, imitative, or exploratory play.

(3) Repetitive and stereotyped behaviors and movements in one or more of the following.
(a) Ritualistic nonfunctional routines, preoccupation.
(b) Rigid observance of nonfunctional routines or behavioral patterns.
(c) Repetitive motor action (e.g., flapping and wiggling of fingers, head banging, rocking of the head or body).
(d) Restrictive fixation on parts of a whole object (e.g., wheel of a toy car).

b. Prior to three years of age, delay or impairment in social interaction and/or language and/or play (symbolic or imaginative).
c. Not better described as Rett's syndrome or childhood disintegrative disorder.
d. Difficulty with sensory processing and perception of various sensory stimuli; difficulty in modulation of stimuli at various levels of the continuum, e.g., hyper- or hypo-responsiveness.
e. Common associated behaviors may include unanticipated mood swings, temper tantrums, lack of ability to focus, insomnia, and enuresis.
f. Deficits tend to be more severe in verbal sequencing and abstraction versus abilities in visuospatial and rote memory skills (e.g., calculation, musical abilities).

Asperger's Disorder

1. Etiology is unknown; however, studies indicate a strong relation to autism. It is hypothesized to be due to genetic, metabolic, infectious, or perinatal causes.
2. Onset, prevalence, and prognosis.
   a. Little is known, and course and prognosis are variable.
   b. Those individuals with a normal IQ and high level social skills appear to have a good prognosis, although they tend to be socially uncomfortable and demonstrate illogical thinking.
3. Diagnostic characteristics.
   a. Difficulty with social interaction.
   b. Restricted interests and behaviors.
   c. Characterized by clumsiness.
   d. Delayed developmental motor milestones.
   e. Differentiated from autism by adequate language and the level of social interaction and engagement in activities with others.

Rett's Syndrome

1. Etiology is unknown; however, since deterioration occurs after a period of normal development it is thought to be attributed to a genetic metabolic disorder.
2. Onset, prevalence, and prognosis.
   a. Motor and social skills are age appropriate from 6 months to 2 years of development when the onset of progressive encephalopathy develops.
   b. Occurs in one in 10,000 girls.
   c. Development of physical growth and head circumference plateau resulting in progressive encephalopathy.
   d. A child may live for over 10 years following the onset.
3. Diagnostic characteristics and sequelae.
   a. Deterioration of language, receptive and expressive communication skills and social skills may plateau at a six-month to one-year developmental level.
   b. Motor deterioration is characterized by a loss of purposeful hand movements with the development of stereotypical movements, such as hand wringing and licking, biting, and slapping of fingers.
      (1) Deterioration of the integrity of the skin results-from these repetitive stereotypical movements
   c. Muscle tone becomes hypotonic and then progresses to spasticity and then rigidity.
      (1) The result is an ataxic, uncoordinated, and stiff gait.
   d. Muscle wasting can make these children prone to scoliosis and eventually may necessitate the use of a wheelchair.
   e. Breathing patterns become irregular, marked by hyperventilation, apnea, and holding of breath.
   f. Regression occurs in cognition and praxis.
   g. EEGs are abnormal and seizures are common.

Pervasive Developmental Disorder, Unspecified

1. Disorders are similar with impairments seen in the above Pervasive Developmental Disorders.

2. Impairments are evident in social interaction, communication, motor behavior, interests, and activities; however, they cannot be classified as indicative of a pervasive developmental disorder since not all diagnostic criteria are met.

Symptom Management

1. Medications prescribed will depend on the presenting symptoms of a specific PDD.
   a. Seizure medications.
   b. Medication for muscle deterioration and/or complications due to abnormal tone.
   c. Medications to increase alertness.
   d. Medications to modulate behaviors.

Diagnostic-Specific Considerations for Occupational Therapy

1. Evaluate developmental and functional levels. See Chapter 5.
2. Develop sensorimotor, social interaction, vocational readiness, and community participation skills relevant to the child's level. See Chapter 5.
3. Provide sensory integrative intervention, if indicated. See relevant sections in Chapter 5 and Chapter 12.
4. If indicated, prescribe and train in technologically-based augmentive communication.
5. Provide adaptive and positioning equipment to facilitate function, e.g., the stereotypical movements of licking, biting and slapping of the hands in a child with Rett's Syndrome may require adaptations to maintain the integrity of the skin, such as dynamic elbow splints that inhibit a hand-to-mouth pattern by limiting full elbow flexion.
6. Collaborate with the family and interdisciplinary team to promote occupational performance and social participation.
7. See this chapter's sections on occupational therapy mental health evaluation and occupational therapy mental health intervention for additional guidelines.
8. Chapter 14 provides further information on general OT psychosocial evaluation and intervention approaches and specific interventions to manage behaviors.

Major DSM-5 Changes

1. Autism was changed to "Autism Spectum Disorders" which encompasses previous DSM-IV diagnoses of "Autistic Disorder (Autism)," "Aspergers Disorder," "Childhood Disintegrative Disorder" and "Pervasive Developmental Disorder (NOS)."
2. The diagnoses in this section formerly were contained in the DSM-IV-TR chapter "Disorders Usually First Diagnosed in Infancy, Childhood, or Adolesence.

Reactive Attachment Disorder (RAD) of Infancy or Early Childhood

Etiology

1. Exact cause is unknown.
2. Early poor experiences with initial caregivers and/or pathogenic care may contribute to the disorder.
   a. Indicators of pathogenic care:
      (1) Persistent disregard of the child's basic emotional needs.
      (2) Persistent disregard of the child's basic physical needs.
      (3) Repeated changes of primary caregiver or a succession of caregivers prevents the establishment of stable, appropriate attachments.

Onset, Prevalence, and Prognosis

1. Onset begins before five years of age.
2. Exact prevalence or incidence of Reactive Attachment Disorder is unknown.
3. There is a high risk of prevalence for toddlers and children in foster care and orphanages and for children with frequently changing caregivers.
4. Prognosis: unknown.

Diagnostic Criteria

1. There are two types of Reactive Attachment Disorder.
   a. Reactive Attachment Disorder, Inhibited type, characterized by:
      (1) Persistent failure to initiate or respond in a developmentally appropriate fashion to most social interactions.
      (2) Interactions are excessively inhibited, hypervigilant, or highly ambivalent and contradictory in nature.

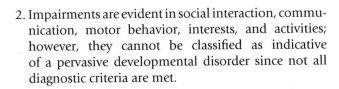

b. Reactive Attachment Disorder, Disinhibited type, characterized by:
   (1) Indiscriminate sociability with inability to exhibit appropriate selective attachments.
   (2) Demonstrated by excessive familiarity with relative strangers or lack of selectivity.

Impact on Function

1. Children with RAD exhibit challenging behaviors. These include:
   a. A high need to be in control.
   b. Frequent lying.
   c. Affectionate and overly related with strangers.
   d. Frequent episodes of hoarding or gorging on food without physical need.
   e. Denial of responsibility.
   f. Projecting blame for their actions on others.
2. Due to the above behaviors, children with RAD can be frustrating to work with and difficult to parent.

Symptom Management

1. No one standard treatment for Reactive Attachment Disorder is apparent in the literature.
2. Interventions that may be efficacious:
   a. Nondirective play therapy.
   b. Sensory integrative therapy. See Chapter 12.
   c. Attachment therapy (somewhat controversial).
   d. Psychotherapy combined with psychoeducation.

Diagnostic-Specific Considerations for Occupational Therapy

1. Close and ongoing collaboration with the child's family facilitates successful outcomes.
2. Actively involve parents in treatment.
3. Assist children to form a more secure sense of self.
4. Limit the child's exposure to multiple caregivers.
5. Provide high levels of structure and consistency.
6. Goals need to be specific, realistic and attainable.
7. See this chapter's sections on occupational therapy mental health evaluation and occupational therapy mental health intervention for additional guidelines.
8. Chapter 14 provides further information on general OT psychosocial evaluation and intervention approaches and specific interventions to manage behaviors.

Major DSM-5 Changes

1. Reactive Attachment Disorder has been placed in the chapter "Trauma- and Stressor-Related Disorders."
2. Reactive Attachment Disorder no longer includes "Inhibited Type" and "Disinhibited Type."
3. "Disinhibited Social Engagement Disorder" has been added as a separated disorder based on "Reactive Attachment Disorder, Disinhibited Type" and is also included in the chapter "Trauma- and Stressor-Related Disorders."

Attention-Deficit/Hyperactivity Disorders

Etiology

1. Unknown, however, there are suggested contributing factors. These include:
   a. Genetic factors include higher occurrence in monozygotic twins than in dizygotic twins, and twice the occurrence in siblings of hyperactive children.
   b. Neurological factors include the possibility of minimal or subtle brain damage due to circulatory, toxic, metabolic, or mechanical effects during fetal or perinatal periods; and infection, inflammation, and/or trauma during early childhood.
   c. Neurochemical dysfunction related to neurotransmitters in the adrenergic and the dopaminergic systems.
   d. Psychosocial factors include stress, anxiety, or predisposing factors such as temperament.

Subtypes of Attention-Deficit/Hyperactivity Disorder

1. DSM-IV-TR delineates three subtypes.
   a. Predominantly inattentive type.
   b. Predominantly hyperactive-impulsive type.
   c. Combined type.

Onset, Prevalence, and Prognosis

1. Symptoms are often noted during the toddler years, usually by the age of three.
   a. Caution is advised to not make a diagnosis in early childhood years.

   b. Diagnosis is most often made during elementary school years when behavior interferes with adjustment to school.
2. Occurs in 5%–8% of elementary school children.
   a. Incidence in boys to girls is a 3 to 1 ratio, most common in firstborn boys.
3. Partial remission may occur between the ages of 12 and 20, allowing for a productive adolescence and adulthood.
   a. Although hyperactivity may disappear, distractibility and impulsivity can persist.
4. Symptoms persist into adulthood in 60% of cases.

Diagnostic Criteria

1. The presence of six or more symptoms in the inattention domain, the hyperactivity-impulsivity domain, or both.
2. Symptoms in the inattention domain or hyperactivity-impulsivity domain that interfere with occupational activities are present for at least 6 months or more.
3. Symptoms of the inattention domain may include lack of attention to detail, poor listening, limited follow through of tasks, difficulty with organization, and avoidance of tasks that require sustained attention, tendency to lose things, distractibility, and forgetfulness.
4. Symptoms of the hyperactivity domain may include fidgeting, inability to remain seated, inappropriate activity level for a given situation, difficulty with quiet sedentary activities, frequent movement, and excessive talking.
5. Symptoms of impulsivity include answering questions before they are fully stated, difficulty with turn taking, and interrupting the conversations or activities of others.
6. Visual-perceptual, auditory-perceptual, language, and/or cognitive problems may be present.
7. Some of the symptoms that result in impairment were evident before 7 years of age.
8. Symptoms that result in impairment are present in two settings, such as school, home, and/or work.
9. A detailed developmental history to confirm behavior patterns and the meeting of six or more symptoms of inattention or hyperactivity-impulsivity of the DSM-IV-TR diagnostic criteria.

Impact on Function

1. Infants are over-active, difficult to soothe when crying, and demonstrate poor sleeping habits.
2. Defensiveness to environmental stimuli, frequent irritability, aggressive behavior, emotional lability, and fluctuating and unpredictable performance.
3. Difficulty with delayed gratification in the school and home.
4. Deficits in perceptual motor tasks with disorders in reading, mathematics, written expression, and general coordination resulting.
5. Disorders of memory, thinking, speech, and hearing.
6. Depression secondary to frustration and difficulty with learning.
   a. This often leads to low self-esteem and conduct disorders.
7. Individuals with symptoms remaining in adolescence and adulthood are prone to antisocial personality disorders, and are at risk for substance-related disorders.

Symptom Management

1. Prescribed medications depend on presenting symptoms.
   a. Stimulants.
      (1) Most commonly used include dextroamphetamine (e.g., Dexedrine, Focalin) for children 3 years and older, and methylphenidate (e.g., Concerta, Ritalin, Adderall, Metadate) for children 6 years and older.
      (2) Side effects include loss of appetite, weight loss, loss of appetite, disturbed sleep patterns, and slow growth.
   b. Antidepressants.
      (1) Imipramine.
      (2) Used when stimulants are unable to be used.
      (3) Careful monitoring of cardiac functioning is required.
   c. Anxiolytics.
      (1) Clonidine (Catapres).
      (2) Guanfacine (Tenex).
      (3) Require careful dosing and competent adults for administration.
         (a) Medications cannot be stopped suddenly because this could medically compromise the child.
2. Monitoring of medication and its impact on cognitive and psychosocial function (e.g., learning and self-esteem).
3. Psychotherapy, behavior modification, parent and individual counseling may be indicated.

Diagnostic-Specific Considerations for Occupational Therapy

1. Behavior's impact on school, home, play/leisure, and social participation must be considered.

2. Environmental modifications and activity adaptations to structure the client's home environment can enhance function.
3. Environmental modifications and activity adaptations to structure the child's environment at school and the adult's environment at work can support more successful outcomes (e.g., the elimination of sensory distracters, the use of lists, datebooks, and/or texted reminders).
4. Training in social skills and self-management (i.e., the use of humor, personally initiated time-outs) can improve adaptive behaviors.
5. Interventions to promote sensory modulation are emphasized. See Chapter 12.
6. Consultation is provided to parents, family members, teachers, and employees regarding strategies for the provision of structure and expectations in a manner that fosters the person's psychosocial adaptation.
7. In school-based practice, ongoing collaboration with individualized education planning team members and parents is vital.
8. See this chapter's sections on occupational therapy mental health evaluation and occupational therapy mental health intervention for additional guidelines.
9. Chapter 14 provides further information on general OT psychosocial evaluation and intervention approaches and specific interventions to manage problem behaviors.

Major DSM-5 Changes

1. "Attention Deficit/Hyperactivity Disorder" is now classified under "Neurodevlopmental Disorders."
2. A diagnosis of ADHD may now be given to adolescents and adults as well as children.

Intellectual Disorders

Etiology

1. Genetic conditions such as chromosomal abnormalities (e.g., Down syndrome, Fragile X Syndrome, Prader-Willi Syndrome, and Klinefelter's Syndrome).
2. Metabolic conditions such as phenylketonuria, hypothyroidism, and Tay-Sachs disease.
3. Prenatal infections such as rubella, toxoplasmosis, AIDS.
4. Maternal substance abuse.
5. Perinatal factors such as trauma and prematurity.
6. Acquired conditions including infections such as encephalitis, meningitis.
7. Head trauma sustained in motor vehicle accidents, falls, child abuse, etc.

Diagnostic Classification and Functional Implications

1. In DSM-IV-TR, intellectual disorders are classified as mental retardation. This is no longer the accepted taxonomy and has changed with the publication of DSM-5.
2. Diagnosis is based on the measurement of intelligence or IQ tests.
   a. Individuals, who score more than two standard deviations below the norm, or below an IQ of 70, are considered to have an intellectual disability.
3. An IQ range of 55 to 69 indicates a mild intellectual disability.
   a. Focus is placed on the individual acquiring social and vocational skills to function independently in desired occupational roles.
   b. Minimal support is required.
   c. Additional intermittent support may be required in special circumstances.
4. An IQ range of 40 to 54 indicates a moderate intellectual disability.
   a. Focus is usually placed on the individual acquiring independence in routine daily skills and skills necessary to perform in desired occupational roles with supports and structure (e.g., work in a vocational rehabilitation [sheltered] workshop).
   b. Limited support and assistance may be required in specific occupational performance areas on a daily basis.
   c. Supervised living is required.
5. An IQ range of 25 to 39 indicates a severe intellectual disability.

a. Focus is usually placed on the individual acquiring communication skills and some basic health habits.
b. Assistance is required for performance of most tasks in all areas of occupation on a daily basis.
c. Supervised living is required.
d. Significant impairments in motor functioning and physical development are typical.

6. IQ of 25 or below indicates a profound intellectual disability.
a. Assistance and ongoing supervision are required for basic survival skills.
b. Significant impairments in motor functioning and physical development are typical.
c. Supervised living is required.

7. Multiple disabilities such as hearing and other sensory impairments, seizures, and other neurological abnormalities may be associated with various syndromes (e.g., fetal alcohol syndrome).

Impact on Development

1. The developmental impact of intellectual disability can vary greatly.
a. The impact is greatest in children with severe and profound intellectual disability.

2. Cognitive development.
a. Slower learning ability.
b. Shorter attention span.
c. Difficulty with problem-solving and critical thinking.
d. Difficulty generalizing information and mastering abstract thinking.
e. Increased distractibility.

3. Motor development.
a. Slower development with the attainment of physical milestones occurring at a later age than typical.
b. Uncoordinated appearance and movements.
c. Low muscle tone.

4. Sensory development.
a. Diminished sensory modulation abilities.
b. Hyper- or hypo-sensitivity to all sensory stimuli.

5. Language development.
a. Decreased ability in recalling and retrieving words secondary to cognitive deficits (e.g., inattention and impaired memory).
b. Difficulty grasping and expressing concepts secondary to cognitive deficits (e.g., impaired abstract thinking).
c. Difficulty with the motor aspects of creating language secondary to motor deficits (e.g., low tone).

6. Psychosocial development.
a. Impaired ability to respond to social cues can result in a number of behavioral outcomes. These can include:
(1) Excessive shyness.
(2) Aggressiveness.
b. Hyperactivity and distractibility can also impede psychosocial development.

Symptom Management

1. Dependent upon presenting symptoms and complications.
2. Psychological, audiological, and speech evaluations and interventions may be indicated.
3. Intermittent support may be required in special circumstances.

Diagnostic-Specific Considerations for Occupational Therapy

1. Self-determination and person-centered planning within the person's capabilities should be a priority.
2. Support and assistance may be required to address performance skills and patterns in areas of occupation.
3. Development of community and social participation skills are a major focus.
4. Interdisciplinary team and family collaboration is helpful to support the development of the person's functional and social skills and to promote participation in areas of occupation.
5. If individual is of school age, collaboration with the educational team is needed to develop a comprehensive educational program. See Chapter 4.

Major DSM-5 Changes

1. A new chapter, "Neurodevelopmental Disorders" includes Intellectual Disability, formerly known as Mental Retardation.
2. Severity of intellectual disabilities is now determined by level of adaptive functioning rather than IQ score in an attempt for assessment to include cognitive capacity (IQ) as well as adaptive functioning.

Chapter 10

Occupational Therapy Mental Health Evaluation

Evaluation Focus

1. Determination of values, interests, desired occupational roles, and self-determined goals.
2. Identification of cognitive, perceptual, and psychosocial strengths and skills and their ability to facilitate recovery.
3. Identification of cognitive, perceptual, and psychosocial deficits and limitations and their impact on function and lifestyle.
4. Determination of functional problems associated with psychiatric symptoms (e.g., safety awareness and judgment).
5. Treatment history and ability and interest to engage in recovery.
6. Identification of coping skills, stressors, and environmental and social supports,

Role of the OTA

1. The OTA can contribute to the evaluation process in collaboration with the occupational therapist.
   a. Supervision by an occupational therapist is required,
   b. The level of supervision required will be determined by the OTA's experience.
2. Service competency must be established.
3. The OTA cannot independently evaluate or interpret evaluation results.

Occupational Therapy Mental Health Intervention

Intervention Focus

1. The focus of intervention during periods of acute hospitalization includes:
   a. Management of all behaviors that threaten the safety and well being of the individual as well as that of others on the unit.
   b. Stabilization of behavior to enable engagement in intervention.
   c. Engagement in activities that are "do-able" (e.g., brief and structured) to enable success and promote reality-based thinking.
      (1) Graded activities are designed to promote self-efficacy which can increase self-confidence, motivation, and participation in treatment.
   d. Engagement of the person in the treatment process.
   e. Development of relaxation and stress management skills to help decrease the incidence and severity of symptoms and facilitate recovery.
   f. Development of the skills needed to pursue desired occupational roles and attain self-determined goals.
   g. Engagement in activities to improve communication skills and self-expression.
   h. The gathering and sharing of ongoing assessment information with the treatment team.
      (1) The person's status typically changes drastically during the course of an acute hospitalization due to the stabilizing effects of psychotropic medications.
         (a) The input of OT practitioners about a patient's observed symptoms and functional behaviors is critical in assisting with the effective titration of psychotropic medications.
   i. Assistance with discharge planning to support recovery and a healthy life style.
2. The focus of intervention during periods of long-term hospitalization includes:
   a. Development and implementation of a plan for self-determined goal achievement.
   b. Provision of a normalizing environment that enables participation in meaningful and desired occupational roles.
   c. Engagement of the person in the treatment process.
   d. Provision of graded activities to develop the skills needed for competence in ADL, IADL, social participation, leisure, school, and/or work.
   e. Development of relaxation and stress management skills to help decrease the incidence and severity of symptoms and facilitate recovery.
   f. Continuation of assessment to determine realistic and meaningful discharge goals.
   g. Development of the skills and external supports needed to pursue desired post-discharge occupational roles, participate in the anticipated discharge environment, and attain self-determined discharge goals.
3. The focus of intervention in community settings.

a. Provision of services that facilitate recovery and assist in the maintenance of existing skills.
b. Assistance with the continued development of skills needed for community living, social participation, and the pursuit of valued occupational roles.
c. Development of skills and supports to enable ongoing recovery (e.g., WRAP – Wellness and Recovery Action Plan, NAMI – National Alliance for the Mentally Ill).
d. Development of skills and the provision of assistance, if needed, to obtain concrete practical resources to support community living (e.g., supplemental social security [SSI], affordable housing, and food stamps).
e. Monitoring of the individual for changing clinical, personal, and social needs.

Role of the OTA

1. The OTA implements intervention with supervision of the occupational therapist.
   a. The level of supervision required depends upon the OTA's experience and established service competence.
2. During the implementation of intervention, the OTA informs the supervising occupational therapist of any change in the individual's status and any other relevant information that may affect treatment.

References

American Academy of Child and Adolescent Psychiatry. (2009). *Facts for families: Children with oppositional defiant disorder.* Retrieved March 25, 2010 from http://www.aacap.org/galleries/FactsForFamilies/72_children_with_oppositional_ defiant_disorder.pdf.

American Occupational Therapy Association. (2010b). The scope of practice of occupational therapy service for individuals with autism spectrum disorders across the life span. *American Journal of Occupational Therapy, 64*(6), 467–468.

American Occupational Therapy Association. (2007.) Societal statement on family caregivers. *American Journal of Occupational Therapy, 61*(6), 710.

American Psychiatric Association. (2013). *Desk reference to the diagnostic criteria from DSM-5.* Arlington, VA: Author.

American Psychiatric Association (2013). *Diagnostic and statistical manual of mental disorders: DSM 5,* 5th ed. Arlington, VA: Author.

American Psychiatric Association. (2000). *DSM-IV-TR: Diagnostic and statistical manual of mental disorders, text revision,* 4th ed. Washington, DC: Author.

American Psychiatric Association. (2000). *Quick reference to the diagnostic criteria from DSM-IV-TR.* Arlington, VA: Author.

Autism Speaks. (2010). *What is autism?* Retrieved March 25, 2010 from http://www.autismspeaks.org/whatisit/index.php.

Ayd, F. J. (1995). *Lexicon of psychiatry, neurology, and the neurosciences.* Baltimore: William and Wilkins.

Batshaw, M. L., & Perret, Y. M. (2000). *Children with disabilities: A medical primer,* 4th ed. Baltimore: Paul H. Brookes.

Bonder, B. (1991). *Psychopathology and function.* Thorofare, NJ: Slack.

Cara, E., & MacRae, A. (Eds.). (2005). *Psychosocial occupational therapy: A clinical practice,* 2nd ed. Clifton Park, NY: Thomson Delmar Learning.

Cara, E., & MacRae, A. (Eds.). (2013). *Psychosocial occupational therapy: An evolving practice,* 3rd ed. Clifton Park, NY: Delmar Cengage Learning.

Case-Smith, J. (Ed.). (2005). *Occupational therapy for children,* 5th ed. St. Louis, MO: Elsevier Mosby.

Cornell, C., & Hamrin, V. (2008). Clinical interventions for children with attachment problems. *Journal of Child and Adolescent Psychiatric Nursing, 21*(1), 35–47.

Costa, D. (2009, June 29). Eating disorders: Occupational therapy's role. *OT Practice,* 13–16.

Cutler, J. L., & Marcus, E. R. (1999). *Psychiatry.* Philadelphia: W.B. Saunders.

Depression and Bipolar Support Alliance. (2009). *Bipolar statistics.* Retrieved March 25, 2010 from http://www.dbsalliance.org/site/PageServer?pagename=about_statistics_bipolar

Depression and Bipolar Support Alliance. (2009). *Statistics on depression.* Retrieved March 25, 2010 from http://www.dbsalliance.org/site/PageServer?pagename=about_statistics_ depression

Fleming-Castaldy, R. (2009). Activities, human occupation, participation, and empowerment. In J. Hinojosa & M. L. Blount (Eds.), *The texture of life: Purposeful activities in occupational therapy,* 3rd ed. (pp. 483–521). Bethesda, MD: AOTA Press.

Glanzman, M. M., & Nathan J. Blum. (2007). Attention deficits and hyperactivity. In M. L. Batshaw, L. Pellegrino, & N. J. Roizen (Eds.), *Children with Disabilities,* 6th ed. (pp. 345–365). Baltimore, MD: Paul H. Brooks.

Hardy, L. (2007). Attachment theory and reactive attachment disorder: Theoretical perspectives and treatment implications. *Journal of Child & Adolescent Psychiatric Nursing, 20*(1), 27–39.

Hopkins, H. L., & Smith, H. D. (2003). *Willard and Spackman's occupational therapy,* 10th ed. Philadelphia: Lippincott.

Hyman, S. L., & Towbin, K. E. (2007). Autism spectrum disorders. In M. L. Batshaw, L. Pellegrino, & N. J. Roizen (Eds.), *Children with Disabilities,* 6th ed. (pp. 345–365). Baltimore, MD: Paul H. Brooks

Kaplan, J.I., & Sadock, B.J. (2007). *Synopsis of psychiatry,* 10th ed. Philadelphia: Mosby.

Lenzenweger, M., Lane, M., Loranger, A., & Kessler, R. (2007). DSM-IV personality disorders in the National

Comorbidity Survey Replication. *Biological Psychiatry, 62*(6), 553–64.

Livneh, H., & Antonak, R. F. (1997). *Psychosocial adaptation to chronic illness and disability.* Gaithersburg, MD: Aspen.

Merikangas, K., Akiskal, H., Angst, J., Greenberg, P., Hirschfeld, R., Petukhova, M., & Kessler, R. (2007). Lifetime and 12-month prevalence of bipolar spectrum disorder in the national comorbitity survey replication. *Archives of General Psychiatry, 64*(5), 543–552.

Myers, D. G. (1993). *Exploring psychology,* 2nd ed. New York: Worth.

National Institute of Mental Health. (2012). *Bipolar, depression and anxiety disorders.* Retrieved July 20, 2013 from http://www.nimh.nih.gov/index.shtml.

Nock, M., Kazdin, A., Hiripi, E., & Kessler, R. (2007). Lifetime prevalence, correlates, and persistence of oppositional defiant disorder: Results from the National Comorbidity Survey Replication. *Journal of Child Psychology and Psychiatry, 48*(7), 703–713.

Physicians' desk reference, 53rd Ed. (1999). Montvale, NY: Medical Economics.

Physicians desk reference, 62nd Ed. (2007). Montvale, NY: Medical Economics.

Rett Syndrome Research Trust. (2008). *Prevalence of Rett and related disorders.* Retrieved March 25, 2010 from http://www.rsrt.org/about-Rett/prevelance-of-Rett-and-related-disorders.html

Right Health. (2010). *Prevalence of autism.* Retrieved 3/8/2020 from: http://www.righthealth.Com.

Rogers, S. (2005). Common conditions that influence children's participation. In J. Case-Smith (Ed.), *Occupational therapy for children,* 5th ed. (pp. 160–215). St. Louis, MO: Elsevier Mosby.

Sadock, B. J., & Sadock, V. A. (2008).*Kaplan and Sadock's concise textbook of clinical psychiatry,* 3rd ed. Philadelphia: Lippincott Williams & Wilkins

Sheperis, C., Renfro-Michel, E., & Doggett, R. (2003). In-home treatment of reactive attachment disorder in a therapeutic foster care system: A case example. *Journal of Mental Health Counseling, 25*(1), 76–88.

Venes, D. (Ed.). (1991). *Taber's cyclopedic medical dictionary,* 20th ed. Philadelphia: F.A. Davis.

Review Questions

Psychiatric and Cognitive Disorders

Below are five questions about key content covered in this chapter. These questions are not inclusive of the entirety of content related to psychiatric and cognitive disorders that you must know for success on the NBCOT exam. These questions are provided to help you "jump start" the thought processes you will need to apply your studying of content to the answering of exam questions; hence they are not in the NBCOT exam format. Exam items in the NBCOT format which cover the depth and breadth of content you will need to know to pass the NBCOT exam are provided on this text's disc. The answers to the below questions are provided in Appendix 4.

1. You are asked to provide consultation services for an individual who lives in a group home. The resident has become dehydrated and inconsistent in taking oral medications. You interview the resident about his/her daily habits and routines and learn that the resident will not drink the tap water in the group home. The resident states, "The water is poisoned. They are trying to poison me. If I drink the water I will die." Identify the psychiatric symptom that is preventing this person from drinking the water. Describe an intervention approach you would use to help the resident hydrate and take presecribed medications. Explain the importance of this person staying hydrated and taking prescribed medications.

2. Upon evaluation of an adolescent you find that the teen has great difficulty reading the various nonverbal behaviors of others (e.g., eye contact, facial expression, gestures and body language) that are needed to regulate social interactions. The adolescent has not been able to develop relationships with a peer group. The teen is preoccupied and intensely interested in World War II, its history, battles, and generals and talks about nothing else. The teen's bedroom is filled with World War II memorabilia and books about the war. This adolescent's cognitive, language and communication skills, and ADL development has been age-appropriate; however the teen has not developed age-appropriate social interaction skills. Based on this information, what diagnosis is most reflective of this teen's functional status? What intervention goals would be helpful to work on with this adolescent?

3. You are conducting an evaluation of a 16-month-old toddler. The parent reports that the toddler has frequent tantrums with no clear precipitant. The parent thinks these behaviors may be the result of the toddler's frustration due to language delays. When unable to reach a toy, the toddler pulled the parent's hand toward the toy without pointing. The toddler also did not point to pictures in books. When playing with blocks or cars, the toddler lined them up, but did not spontaneously manipulate or move them. The toddler exhibited a rigid and limited repertoire of play and interaction skills. What diagnosis is most consistent with the toddler's presenting behaviors? Explain your rationale.

(Continued)

4. You are a home health therapist providing services to an elderly client. The client's caregiver reports that the client is having trouble remembering things, sustaining attention, and making decisions. The caregiver reports the client seems mentally confused and asks whether the symptoms are indicative of dementia. As a therapist, you know that there are possible reversible causes of mental confusion. What are the reversible causes of mental confusion that you should consider during your intervention and inform the caregiver to consider for further evaluation?

5. You observe that a very thin client in your outpatient partial hospital program has been losing weight. The individual has no medical problems.The physician supervising the program states the client is well below the normal weight for age and height. The client participates in cooking groups with peers, but will not eat whatever is prepared other than salad without dressing. When encouraged to try other foods, the client says "I don't want to get fat, and I already need to lose a few pounds." You are concerned that the individual has anorexia nervosa. What signs of this eating disorder are being exhibited? What additional symptoms would you expect to see that would indicate this diagnosis?

11

Biomechanical Approaches: Evaluation and Intervention

COLLEEN MAHER AND RITA P. FLEMING-CASTALDY

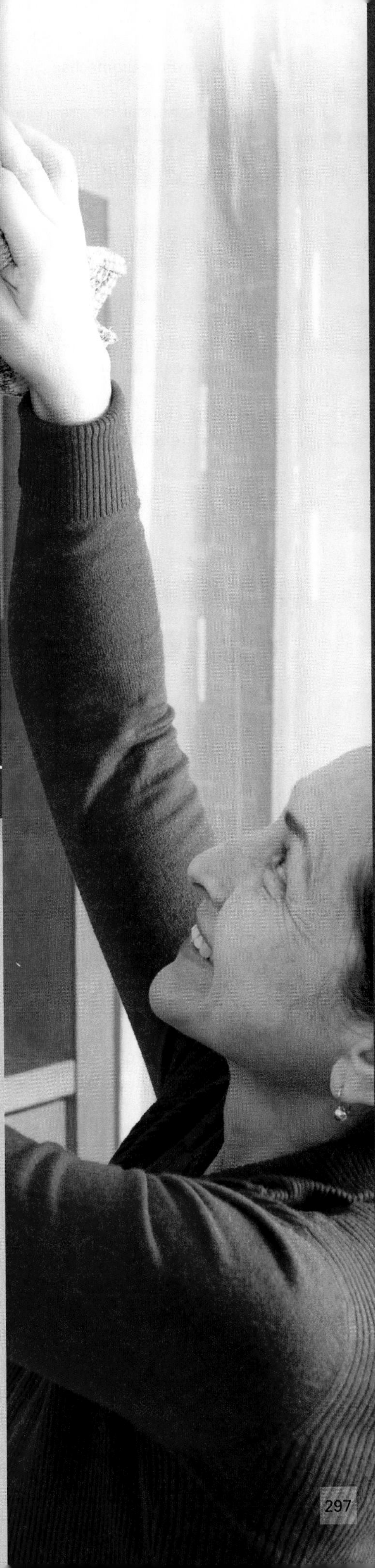

Chapter Outline

Chapter 11

Biomechanical Approach

Overview

1. The biomechanical frame of reference is based on the works of Bird T. Baldwin (reconstruction model), Marjorie Taylor (orthopedic model), Dr. Sydney Licht, and William Dunton, Jr. (kinetic model).
2. The biomechanical approach focuses on the range of motion, strength, and endurance required to perform an occupation.
3. It is most commonly used to treat patients with lower motor neuron deficits and orthopedic problems.
4. The biomechanical approach should *not* be used in isolation.
   a. This approach is *most* effective when used in combination with other occupational therapy treatment approaches which focus on the client's engagement in meaningful occupations and desired purposeful activities.
5. Settings that most commonly use the biomechanical approach.
   a. Hand clinics.
   b. Work programs.
   c. Physical medicine and rehabilitation (PM&R) departments.
   d. Ergonomic programs.

Evaluation

Range of Motion (ROM)

1. Measurement tool: goniometer consisting of an axis, stationary and movable arms.
2. Types of range of motion.
   a. Functional ROM: ROM needed to perform functional movements (e.g., reach to top of head, small of back, etc.).
   b. AROM: active ROM (contractile structures) movement produced by one's own muscle.
   c. PROM: passive ROM (noncontractile structures) movement produced by an external force.
   d. AAROM: active assistive ROM, movement produced by one's own muscles and assisted by an external force.
   e. Finger ROM: total active motion (TAM) and total passive motion (TPM).
      (1) Measures tendon excursion.
      (2) Add extension deficits and subtract from flexion measurement, e.g.:
         Digit #2 (Index)
         MCP 10°–50°
         PIP 15°–75°
         DIP 0°–10°
         TAM 110°
3. Recording measurements.
   a. Starting position/ending position (e.g., 0°–150°).
   b. Do not use negatives.
   c. Within functional limits (WFL): ROM is functional.
   d. Within normal limits (WNL): ROM achieves normal ranges (e.g., shoulder flexion 0°–180°).
4. Review bony landmarks and normal ranges. Refer to Table 11-1.

Muscle Strength

1. Types of manual muscle tests (MMT).
   a. Break test is the most common MMT.
      (1) Test position: gravity eliminated (lessened) or against gravity.
      (2) Stabilization: usually proximal to the joint the muscle crosses over. Do not hold over the muscle belly being tested.
      (3) Resistance: applied in opposite direction of movement; should be gradual.
      (4) Muscle grades: refer to Table 11-2.
   b. Resistance test.
      (1) Resistance is applied throughout the range.
      (2) The individual can compensate easily.
      (3) Requires experienced therapist.

Grip Strength

1. Measurement tool: dynamometer.
2. Position of upper extremity: shoulder adducted to side, elbow flexed to 90° and forearm in neutral.
3. Types of grip strength tests.
   a. Dynamometer handle placed on position #2. The mean of three trials of each hand is compared to the norms.
   b. One trial in all five positions for each hand. A bell curve is observed if the individual is applying maximal effort.
   c. Sphygmomanometer cuff or vigorometer/bulb dynamometer should be used to evaluate the grip strength of a person with arthritis.

Table 11-1

Average Normal Rom (180° Method)

JOINT	ROM	ASSOCIATED GIRDLE MOTION
Cervical Spine		
Flexion	0°–45°	
Extension	0°–45°	
Lateral flexion	0°–45°	
Rotation	0°–60°	
Thoracic and Lumbar Spine		
Flexion	0°–80°	
Extension	0°–30°	
Lateral flexion	0°–40°	
Rotation	0°–45°	
Shoulder		
Flexion	0°–170°	Abduction, lateral tilt, slight elevation, slight upward rotation
Extension	0°–60°	Depression, adduction, upward tilt
Abduction	0°–170°	Upward rotation, elevation
Adduction	0°	Depression, adduction, downward rotation
Horizontal abduction	0°–40°	Adduction, reduction of lateral tilt
Horizontal adduction	0°–130°	Abduction, lateral tilt
Internal rotation		Abduction, lateral tilt
Arm in abduction	0°–70°	
Arm in adduction	0°–60°	
External rotation		Adduction, reduction of lateral tilt
Arm in abduction	0°–90°	
Arm in adduction	0°–80°	
Elbow		
Flexion	0°–135°–150°	
Extension	0°	
Forearm		
Pronation	0°–80°–90°	
Supination	0°–80°–90°	
Wrist		
Flexion	0°–80°	
Extension	0°–70°	
Ulnar deviation (adduction)	0°–30°	
Radial deviation (abduction)	0°–20°	

(*Continued*)

Table 11-1

Average Normal Rom (180° Method) (*Continued*)

JOINT	ROM	ASSOCIATED GIRDLE MOTION
Thumb*		
DIP flexion	0°–80°–90°	
MP flexion	0°–50°	
Adduction, radial and palmar	0°	
Palmar abduction	0°–50°	
Radial abduction	0°–50°	
Opposition	composite motion	
Fingers*		
MP flexion	0°–90°	
MP hyperextension	0°–15°–45°	
PIP flexion	0°–110°	
DIP flexion	0°–80°	
Abduction	0°–25°	
Hip		
Flexion	0°–120° (bent knee)	
Extension	0°–30°	
Abduction	0°–40°	
Adduction	0°–35°	
Internal rotation	0°–45°	
External rotation	0°–45°	
Knee		
Flexion	0°–145°	
Ankle And Foot		
Plantar flexion	0°–50°	
Dorsiflexion	0°–15°	
Inversion	0°–35°	
Eversion	0°–20°	

*DIP, distal interphalangeal; MP, metacarpophalangeal; PIP, proximal interphalangeal.

Data adapted from American Academy of Orthopaedic Surgeons. (1965). *Joint motion: method of measuring and recording.* Chicago: The Association; Esch, D., & Lepley, M. (1974). *Evaluation of joint motion: Methods of measurement and recording.* Minneapolis: University of Minnesota Press.

Pedretti, L. W. (1996). *Occupational therapy: Practice skills for physical dysfunction*, 4th ed. (p. 84). St. Louis, MO: Mosby. Reprinted with permission.

Table 11-2

Muscle Testing Grading System

GRADE	DEFINITION	DESCRIPTION
5	Normal	The part moves through full ROM against gravity and takes maximal resistance.
4	Good	The part moves through full ROM against gravity and takes moderate resistance.
4–	Good minus	The part moves through full ROM against gravity and takes less than moderate resistance.
3+	Fair plus	The part moves through full ROM against gravity and takes minimal resistance before it breaks.
3	Fair	The part moves through full ROM against gravity and is unable to take any added resistance.
3–	Fair minus	The part moves less than full range of motion against gravity.
2+	Poor plus	The part moves through full ROM in a gravity-eliminated plane and then takes minimal resistance and breaks.
2	Poor	The part moves through full range of motion in a gravity eliminated plane with no added resistance.
2–	Poor minus	The part moves less than full ROM in a gravity-eliminated plane.
1	Trace	Tension is palpated in the muscle or tendon, but no motion occurs at the joint.
0	Zero	No tension is palpated in the muscle or tendon.

Radomski. M. V., & Trombly Latham, C. A. (2008). *Occupational therapy for physical dysfunction*, 6th ed. Baltimore: Lippincott Williams and Wilkins. Reprinted with permission.

Pinch Strength

1. Measurement tool: pinchmeter.
2. Position of upper extremity: shoulder adducted to side, elbow flexed to 90° and forearm in neutral.
3. Types of pinch strength test.
   a. Key or lateral pinch: thumb pulp to the lateral aspect of the index middle phalanx.
   b. Three jaw chuck (palmar pinch): pulp of thumb to pulps of index and middle fingers.
   c. Tip to tip: thumb pulp to pulp of index finger.
4. Three trials on each hand are obtained for all pinch strengths. The mean of three trials on each hand is compared to the norms.

Endurance/Activity Tolerance

1. Count number of repetitions per unit of time.
2. Determine percent of maximum heart rate.
3. Measure time until fatigue.
4. Use metabolic equivalent (METS) levels. See Chapter 8.

Edema

1. The body's initial response to injury.
   a. It is the transfer of exudate in which the fluid from the blood stream moves to the interstitial tissue.
   b. Edema can be localized or diffuse.
2. Types.
   a. Pitting - acute.
   b. Brawny - chronic.
3. Evaluation of circumference.
   a. Measurement tool: tape measure, recorded in centimeters.
   b. Compare extremities, document landmarks.
   c. To measure the entire hand, use the figure-of-eight method; this is the most reliable method.
4. Evaluation of hand and arm mass.
   a. Measurement tool: volumeter, recorded in milliliters.
   b. Significant change in edema would be more than 10 mL.
   c. The only true objective tool.

Sensation

1. Demonstrate sensory test with vision; then occlude vision for actual testing.
2. Test uninvolved side first. Apply stimulus to volar and dorsal surfaces (exceptions will be noted).
3. Spinal cord injuries are tested proximal to distal following dermatome pattern.
4. Neurological disorders assess for dermatome pattern.
5. Peripheral nerve injuries are tested distal to proximal following peripheral nerves.
6. Peripheral nerve injuries assess for peripheral nerve involvement. Order of return: pain, moving touch, static light touch, and touch localization.
7. Types of sensory testing.
   a. Light touch: cotton swab. Person responds "yes" or "touched" when touched. Scoring: + (intact), – (impaired), or 0 (absent).
   b. Localization: cotton swab. Person responds "yes" when touched and then with vision points to area touched. Scoring +, –, 0.
   c. Pain: paper clip. Person responds "sharp" or "dull." Scoring: S+, D+, D, S, S–, or D–.
   d. Temperature sensation: test tubes or thermal kit. Person responds "hot" or "cold." Scoring: +, –, 0.

e. Stereognosis: recognition by touch of common objects. Scoring: number of correct objects.
   (1) A second set of identical common objects should be used for individuals with expressive aphasia.
f. Moving two point discrimination: disk-criminator or caliper.
   (1) Testing begins with points 5–8mm apart.
   (2) Applied proximal to distal on fingertips in a horizontal orientation.
   (3) Person responds to the number of points he/she feels - "one" or "two."
   (4) Seven out of ten responses must be correct before decreasing the distance of the two points.
   (5) Scoring: normal = 2mm.
g. Static two point discrimination: disk-criminator or caliper.
   (1) Test begins at 5mm.
   (2) Applied to fingertips in a longitudinal orientation.
   (3) Person states "one" or "two" in response to the number of points he/she feels.
   (4) Distance between points is increased until seven out of ten responses are correct.
   (5) Test is stopped at 15mm.
   (6) Scoring.
      (a) Normal = 5mm.
      (b) Fair = 6–10mm.
      (c) Poor = 11–15mm.
      (d) Protective = one point perceived.
      (e) Anesthetic = no points perceived.
h. Proprioception: position sense.
   (1) Therapist positions involved extremity.
   (2) Person duplicates position with contralateral extremity.
i. Kinesthesia: movement sense.
   (1) Therapist moves segment.
   (2) Person responds up or down.

8. Refer to Figure 6 in Chapter 6 and Table 11-3 for dermatome distribution.

Table 11-3

Dermatomes

SPINAL SEGMENT	DERMATOME LOCATION	MUSCLES FACILITATED	FUNCTION
CN V	Anterior facial region	Mastication	Ingestion
C3	Neck region	Sternocleidomastoid, upper trapezius	Head control
C4	Upper shoulder region	Trapezius (diaphragm)	Head control
C5	Lateral aspect of shoulder	Deltoid, biceps, rhomboid major and minor	Elbow flexion
C6	Thumb and radial forearm	Extensor carpi radialis, biceps	Shoulder abduction, wrist extension
C7	Middle finger	Triceps, extensors of wrist and fingers	Wrist flexion, finger extension
C8	Little finger, ulnar forearm	Flexor of wrist and fingers	C8 finger flexion
T1	Axilla and proximal medial arm	Hand intrinsics	Abduction and adduction of fingers
T2–12	Thorax	Intercostals	Respiration
T4–T6	Nipple line	Intercostals	Respiration
T11	Midchest region, lower rib	Abdominal wall, abdominal muscles	T5–7 superficial abdominal reflex
T10	Umbilicus	Psoas, iliacus	Leg flexion
L1–2	Inside of thigh	Cremasteric reflex, accessory muscles	Elevation of scrotum
L2	Proximal anterior thigh	Iliopsoas, adductors of thigh	Reflex voiding
L3–4	Anterior knee	Quadriceps, tibialis anterior, detrusor urinae	Hip flexion, extensors of knee, abductors of thigh
L5	Great toe	Lateral hamstrings	Flexion at knee, toe extension
L5–S1	Foot region	Gastrocnemius, soleus, extensor digitorum longus	Flexor withdrawal, urinary retention
S2	Narrow band of posterior thigh	Small muscles of foot (flexor digitorum, flexor hallucis)	Bladder retention

McCormack, G. (1996). The Rood approach to treatment of neuromuscular dysfunction. In L.W. Pedretti (Ed.). *Occupational therapy: Practice skills for physical dysfunction*, 4th ed. (p. 383), St. Louis, MO: Mosby.

Coordination/Dexterity

1. The NBCOT examination may include a description of evaluation methods and/or the names of specific commercial assessment tools; therefore, a review of major coordination assessments is important for examination preparation.
   a. This can increase understanding and knowledge of common approaches in the evaluation of co-ordination.
   b. This can further strengthen the clinical reasoning skills needed to answer examination questions that address the evaluation of coordination.
2. As of the publication of this text, NBCOT has not made public the names of all of the specific evaluations that may be on the examination.
   a. The evaluations included in this chapter are based on the author's review of NBCOT self-assessment tools, major OT textbooks, and feedback obtained from OT practitioners regarding measures used in practice.
3. Purdue Pegboard.
   a. Test of fingertip dexterity and assembly job simulation.
   b. Subtests.
      (1) Thirty-second test: right hand, left hand, both hands, R+, L+, both.
      (2) One-minute test: assembly.
   c. Scoring: thirty second test is the number of pins placed in the board in 30 seconds. Assembly is the number of parts assembled during one minute.
4. Minnesota Manual Dexterity Test.
   a. Test of gross hand and arm movements.
   b. Subtests.
      (1) Placing test: measures rate of hand movement (one hand only).
      (2) Turning test: measures rate of finger manipulation (bilateral).
   c. Scoring: time to complete board. One practice trial and four scored trials.
5. O'Connor Tweezer Test.
   a. Test of eye-hand coordination using tweezers.
   b. Scoring: the number of seconds to place all pins in board using tweezers.
6. Crawford Small Parts Dexterity Test.
   a. Test of fine motor dexterity using small tools (tweezers and screwdriver).
   b. Scoring: time to complete assembly.
7. Nine Hole Peg Test.
   a. Measures finger dexterity.
   b. Scoring: time for each hand to place nine pegs in a square board and remove them.
   c. The Purdue Pegboard is preferred over the Nine Hole Peg Test because it is unilateral and bilateral. It is also more reliable.
8. Jebson Hand Function Test.
   a. Test of hand function.
   b. Seven subtests.
      (1) Writing.
      (2) Simulated page turning.
      (3) Picking up common objects.
      (4) Simulated feeding.
      (5) Stacking.
      (6) Picking up large light objects.
      (7) Picking up large heavy objects.
   c. Scoring: time to complete each subject.
9. Informal assessment of coordination should include:
   a. Fine motor: observation of routine task performance.
      (1) Handwriting, manipulation of various sized objects, handling money, cutting food, and buttoning are examples of daily tasks to observe to assess fine motor coordination.
   b. Gross motor: observation of activities that include gross motor movements.
      (1) Tossing a ball, reaching into cabinets for specific items, and dressing are examples of activities to observe to assess gross motor coordination.

Intervention

Increasing Range of Motion

1. Passive ROM and passive stretching.
   a. PROM is moving the joint to the desired range using an external force.
      (1) PROM can be performed by the therapist gently moving the extremity to the desired range or when resistance is felt.
   b. Passive stretching is PROM with overpressure.
   c. A careful review of the physician's orders is paramount to distinguish the type of passive exercise being requested.
   d. Heat prior to stretch increases extensibility.
   e. Joint mobilization requires special training. More effective if performed before passive ROM.
   f. Manual stretching within individual's tolerance. Also, contract/relax and hold/relax increase ROM.

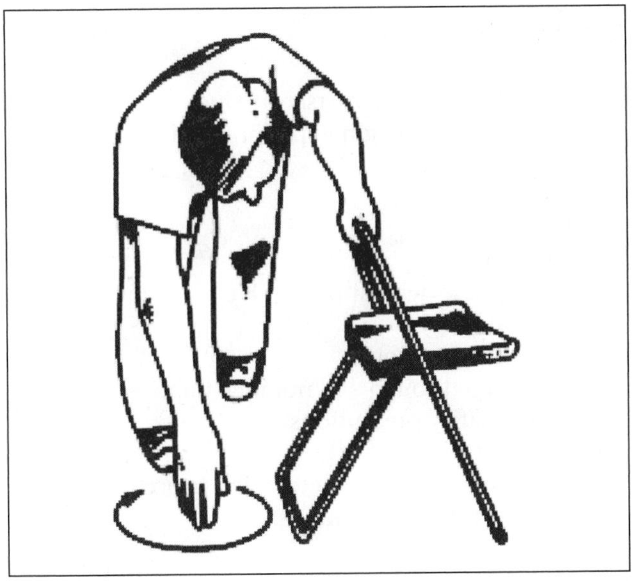

Figure 11-1 **Codman's exercise.**

Hawkins R. J., Bell R. H., & Lippitt S. B. (1996). *Atlas of shoulder surgery*. St Louis: Mosby. Reprinted with permission.

g. Codman's exercise: common form of PROM used for post surgical shoulder patients.
   (1) See Figure 11-1.
h. Instruction in home exercises. Stress the importance of home exercises to facilitate change in tissue length.
i. Splinting: dynamic and serial splinting.
j. Exercise equipment: continuous passive movement (CPM), pulleys, etc.

2. Active ROM.
   a. Should be performed when PROM is greater than AROM.
   b. Differential tendon gliding exercises: differentiates tendon movement and increases tendon excursion.
      (1) See Figure 11-2.
   c. Blocking exercises: used to isolate individual joint motion.
   d. Emphasize functional use; encourage use for ADL and role activities.
   e. Preparatory interventions: wall walking, AROM, cane exercises, etc.
   f. Purposeful and occupation based activities: ADL, work activities, crafts, games, and sports. Incorporate individual's leisure interests.
3. Precaution: myositis ossificans may result from overstretching (especially noted in elbow flexors).

Increasing Strength

1. High resistance, low repetitions.
2. Type of contractions.
   a. Isometrics: contraction without movement.
      (1) Sometimes can produce more forceful contraction.
      (2) Isometrics are contraindicated for persons with hypertension and cardiovascular problems. They can increase blood pressure (BP) and heart rate (HR), so they should be avoided.
   b. Isotonic: contraction with movement.
      (1) eccentric = lengthening.
      (2) concentric = shortening.

Increasing Endurance

1. Work at 50% of maximal resistance or less.
2. Increase repetitions, and duration, not resistance.
3. Use energy conservation methods.

Edema Reduction Techniques

1. Elevation: extremity should be placed above the heart.
   a. This is contraindicated if the individual has circulation problems.
2. Manual edema mobilization: hands on technique that activates the lymphatic system to remove edema.
   a. This technique requires specialized training.

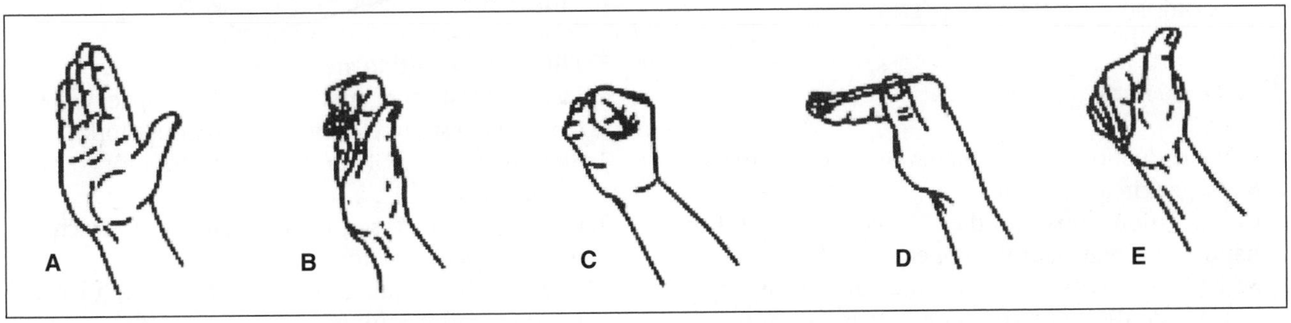

Figure 11-2 **Tendon gliding exercises.**

The five positions: A. Straight. B. Hook. C. Fist. D. Tabletop. E. Straight fist. Adapted with permission from Rozmaryn, L. M., Dovelle, S., Rothman, E. R., Gorman, K., Olvey, K. M., & Bartko, J. J. (1998). Nerve and tendon gliding exercises and the conservative management of carpal tunnel syndrome. *Journal of Hand Therapy*, 11, 171–179. Reprinted with permission.

3. Retrograde massage assists the return of blood and lymphatic fluids to the venous system.
   a. This type of massage is still being used but is slowly being replaced by manual edema mobilization. Instructions:
      (1) Stroking is applied in centripetal direction.
      (2) Massage should be performed with the extremity elevated.
4. Manual edema mobilization and retrograde massage are contraindicated when cardiac edema is present.
5. Compression garments prevent re-accumulation of fluids following retrograde massage.
   a. Common types.
      (1) Isotoner glove.
      (2) Tubigrip (stockinet with elastic).
      (3) Ace wraps.
      (4) Custom made compression garments.
      (5) Coban wrap (digit is wrapped distal to proximal).
         (a) Effective for decreasing edema in a digit.
         (b) Avoid too much tension.
         (c) The individual can exercise and use his/her hand for ADL and role activities while wearing Coban.
6. Cold packs: most effective when combined with elevation.
   a. Monitor vascular status.
7. Contrast bath.
   a. Technique of immersing the hand in warm (temperature of bath water) and cold water. Evidence is conflicting as to its effectiveness in reducing hand edema.
8. Other edema techniques: string wrapping, ace bandage wraps, and intermittent compression pump.
   a. These techniques are not as common.
9. Heat is commonly contraindicated. However, if the effects of heat are needed in a mild case of edema it could be cautiously used and combined with elevation.
10. Precautions/contraindications.
    a. Infection.
    b. Grafts or wounds.
    c. Vascular damage.
    d. Unstable fractures.
    e. Congestive heart failure (CHF).

Scar Management

1. ROM: early mobilization programs are most effective.
2. Massage (circles and friction).
3. Compression: coban for digits, isotoner glove for the hand and tubigrip for the upper extremity.
4. Scar pad with compression (otoform, elastomer and topigel are the most common scar pads). Scar pads can be purchased at health supply stores.
5. Splinting: to prevent contractures resulting from scar.
6. Edema control: especially in acute phase.

Sensory Training

1. Desensitization for hypersensitivity.
   a. If post-surgery, begin in periphery of the scar and as tolerated work over the scar.
   b. Massage.
   c. Textures.
   d. Vibration.
   e. Three-phase desensitization kit.
   f. Fluidotherapy.
2. Sensory re-education.
   a. Same as b through e in number 1 above.
   b. Review safety precautions.
3. Compensation.
   a. Avoid use of hands where vision is occluded.
   b. Observe safety precautions.

Improving Coordination

1. Begin with gross motor activities and gradually grade up to fine motor activities.
2. Select activities in which the ROM required is within the person's reach and yet challenging.
3. Focus on accuracy and speed. Begin with slow gross movements and gradually progress to faster precise movements.
4. Focus on accuracy and speed.

Energy Conservation and Work Simplification Principles and Methods

1. Plan short rest periods (5–10 minutes) during daily routine.
2. Schedule tasks for the day, week, and month to alternate and balance heavy and light work tasks.
3. Organize tasks; gather all necessary items and equipment before beginning task.
4. Avoid multiple trips to obtain items by using a utility cart, a bucket, walker bag, backpack, etc. to carry all items needed in one trip.
5. Eliminate tasks that are non-essential.
6. Delegate tasks that are beyond one's capacity.
7. Combine tasks to eliminate extraneous work.
8. Sit to work at a table or use a high stool for countertop work.
9. Organize cabinets so that items are easy to reach and in convenient locations.
10. Use adaptive equipment (e.g., reachers) to avoid bending and stooping.
11. Use electrical appliances (e.g., mixers) to decrease personal effort.
12. Slide rather than lift heavy items.

13. Use lightweight equipment, tools, and utensils.
14. Rest before fatigue sets in; intermittent rest during an activity is more effective than resting after exhaustion has occurred.

Joint Protection Principles and Methods

1. Maintain joint ROM by using maximal ROM during daily activities.
2. Maintain muscle strength by using maximal strength during daily activities.
3. Use the strongest and largest joint that is possible for task completion.
   a. Use knees and hips for lifting, not the back.
   b. Push large items that need to be moved with a full body rather than pulling.
   c. Lift objects with both hands, palms pointed upward.
   d. Carry purses, bags on the forearm rather than wrist; most preferred is use of an ergonomically designed back pack.
4. Use each joint in its most stable and functional position.
   a. Stand directly in front of item to be reached for, opened or closed, rather than to the side.
   b. Keep wrists and fingers in proper alignment.
5. Avoid holding joints in one position or sustaining muscle contractions for extended periods of time.
   a. Use adaptive equipment to hold items for long periods of time (e.g., a book holder).
   b. Take breaks from extended activities.
6. Avoid positions of deformity and activities in the direction of deformity (e.g., ulnar drift).
   a. Perform movements in the direction opposite the potential deformity (e.g., opening a door with the right hand and closing it with the left hand to prevent ulnar drift).
   b. Use adaptive equipment that is ergonomically designed (e.g., tools and utensils with angled handles that eliminate deviations at the wrist).
7. Do not start an activity that cannot be immediately stopped if it requires capacities beyond existing capabilities.
8. Recognize that discomfort may be a reality of activity but that pain is a warning sign indicating that an activity should be modified or stopped.

Body Mechanics Principles and Methods

1. Do not move items that are too heavy; ask for assistance.
2. Slide or push an object along the surface rather than lift it, if possible.
3. Directly face the object about to be lifted. Do not face the direction in which the item is going to move.
4. Keep object close to the body during lifting and carrying.
5. Hold object centered at waist level.
6. Feet should be kept flat on the floor; balancing on toes should be avoided.
7. Maintain a firm and broad base of support. Maintain the body balanced over a wide stance.
8. Bend at the knees and hips, not at the waist.
9. Keep the back as straight as possible.
10. Breathe while lifting.
11. Lift by straightening legs; do not pull upward with arms and back.
12. Move smoothly; do not jerk.
13. Do not rotate the trunk. Pick up the object completely and then pivot the entire body.
14. Lower the body to the level of work.

Splinting

1. Types of splints.
   a. Static: has no resilient components and immobilizes a joint or part.
   b. Dynamic: includes a resilient component (elastic, rubber band, or spring) which the individual moves.
      (1) Designed to increase PROM or to augment AROM.
2. Purposes of splinting.
   a. Rest.
   b. Prevent deformities and contractures.
   c. Increase joint ROM.
   d. Protect bone, joint, and soft tissue.
   e. Increase functional use.
3. Hand splinting design standards.
   a. Maintain arches of the hand.
      (1) Proximal transverse arch.
      (2) Distal transverse arch.
      (3) Longitudinal arch.
   b. Do not impinge upon creases of the hand.
      (1) Distal and proximal palmar creases.
      (2) Distal and proximal wrist creases.
      (3) Thenar crease.
4. Mechanical principles of splinting.
   a. Decrease pressure: wide, long splint base is the most desirable. Round edges are needed.
   b. Use sling applied with a 90° angle of pull.
   c. Use low load to increase duration.
   d. Maintain three-point pressure versus circumference.
   e. Avoid the position of deformity.
      (1) Wrist flexion.
      (2) MCP hyperextension.
      (3) IP joints flexed.
      (4) Thumb adducted.

f. Select the appropriate splinting position.[1]
(1) Resting hand splint: functional position.
(a) Wrist 20°–30° extension.
(b) MCPs 30°–45° flexion.
(c) IPs 0°–20° flexion (may be referred to as slight flexion).
(d) Thumb abducted (may be referred to as opposition).
(2) Safe position splint (may be referred to as intrinsic-plus or anti-deformity splint).
(a) Wrist 20°–30° extension.
(b) Several texts suggest 30°–40°. The therapist must be cautious due to the resultant increased carpal canal pressure.
(c) MCPs 70°–90° flexion.
(d) IPs in extension.
(e) Thumb abducted and extended.

5. Precautions and education.
a. Check individual's skin condition before and after making splint.
b. Instruct splint wearer in procedures for splint maintenance and routine skin inspection and care.
(1) Check skin when donning and doffing.
(2) Provide wear and care form.
c. Ensure individual accepts and understands the purpose(s), function(s), and limitation(s) of the splint.
d. Teach proper technique for donning and doffing splint.
e. Provide functional training in use of splint in role activities (e.g., use of tenodesis splint to do schoolwork).
f. Reevaluate individual's use of splint at periodic intervals.

6. Occupational therapist/OTA role.
a. Occupational therapist/OTA team must carefully assess for most appropriate splint.
b. Occupational therapist must set splinting goals.
c. Experienced OTAs can fabricate static splints and assist with dynamic splints.

7. Splints for common diagnoses.
a. Brachial plexus injury: flail arm splint.
b. Radial nerve palsy: dynamic wrist, finger, and thumb extension splint.
c. Median nerve injury: opponens splint, C-Bar or thumb post splint.
d. Ulnar nerve injury: dynamic/static splint to position MPs in flexion.
e. Combined median ulnar: figure-of-eight or dynamic MCP flexion splint.
f. Spinal cord (C6–C7): tenodesis splint.
g. Carpal tunnel syndrome: wrist splint positioned in neutral.
h. Cubital tunnel syndrome: elbow splint positions at 30° of flexion.
i. DeQuervains: thumb splint, includes wrist, IP joint free.
j. Skier's thumb: (UCL) hand-based thumb splint.
k. CMC arthritis: hand-based thumb splint.
l. Ulnar drift: ulnar drift splint.
m. Flexor tendon injury: dorsal protection splint.
n. Swan neck: silver rings or buttonhole splint.
o. Boutonniere: silver rings or PIP extension splint.
p. Arthritis: functional splint or safe splint, depending on stage.
q. Flaccidity: resting splint.
r. Spasticity: spasticity splint or cone splint.
s. Muscle weakness (ALS, SCI, Guillain-Barré): balanced forearm orthosis (BFO), deltoid sling/suspension sling.
(1) Mounts to wheelchair.
(2) Individuals must have shoulder or trunk movement.
t. Hand burns: Wrist 15°–30° extension, MCP 50°–70° flexion, and IPs in full extension.

Physical Agent Modalities (PAMs)

1. Physical agent modalities (PAMs) can be used as preparatory interventions in preparation for purposeful and occupation-based activities.
a. PAMs are *not* an appropriate occupational therapy intervention *if* they are used in isolation of purposeful or occupation based activities.
b. PAMs *are* an appropriate occupational therapy intervention *if* they precede, support, and/or enable the individual's ability to perform purposeful activities and meaningful occupations.
c. PAMs are, therefore, preparatory intervention methods for they add to and complement the primary OT intervention methods of purposeful activity and meaningful occupation.
d. Many states require specialized training to use PAMs as an OT intervention.
2. Common types of PAMs used by entry level occupational therapists.
a. Superficial thermal.
(1) Paraffin.
(2) Hot packs.
(3) Fluidotherapy.

[1]There are slight variations reported in occupational therapy and splinting textbooks in regards to the exact degrees for resting hand (functional) splints and safe (anti-deformity) spints. Thus, it is unlikely that the NBCOT exam will include items that have two possible correct answers which include these subtle variations.

b. Superficial cooling agents.
  (1) Cold packs.
  (2) Ice massage.
c. Mechanotherapy.
  (1) Ultrasound.
  (2) Whirlpool.
d. Electrical stimulation units.
  (1) Neuromuscular electrical stimulation (NMES).
  (2) Transcutaneous electrical nerve stimulator (TENS).
  (3) High volt galvonic stimulation (HVGS).
  (4) Iontophoresis.

3. Types of heat transfer.
  a. Conduction (hot packs, whirlpool, and paraffin). Heats superficial structures up to 1 cm.
  b. Convection (fluidotherapy).
  c. Radiation (laser).
  d. Conversion (ultrasound). Heats deeper structures up to 4–5cms.
4. Benefits of superficial heat therapy.
  a. Relieves pain.
  b. Increases tissue extensibility (increases ROM).
  c. Assists with wound healing (increased blood flow).
  d. Decreases muscle spasms.
5. Precautions and contraindications for heat. Do not use with.
  a. Postsurgical repairs.
  b. Acute injuries.
  c. Impaired sensation.
  d. Impaired vascular supply.
6. Application of superficial heat modalities.
  a. Hotpacks.
    (1) Check skin prior to and after application.
    (2) Check temperature of hydrocollator; 165° F is the standard.
    (3) Place hot pack in cover and add 4 layers of a folded towel (1 towel) in between the patient's skin and the hot pack cover. For fragile skin, an additional towel should be considered.
    (4) Check skin after 5 minutes to assess for burn or any other skin issues.
    (5) Hot pack is removed after a total of 20 minutes.
  b. Paraffin.
    (1) Check skin prior to and after application.
    (2) Check temperature of paraffin; 125°–130°F is the standard.
    (3) After washing and thoroughly drying the hand, dip the hand into paraffin and quickly pull out. Repeat this process 8–12 times, forming a glove of paraffin over the hand.
    (4) Following the dip method, the hand should be wrapped with cellophane and then covered with a towel.
    (5) The immersion method (which is not as common), the person keeps his/her hand immersed in the paraffin for the duration of the treatment.
  c. Fluidotherapy.
    (1) Preheat the fluidotherapy machine (temperature can range between 102°–118°F).
    (2) Adjust the blowers according to the person's sensitivity (if the person is hypersensitive, begin with turning the blowers down).
    (3) Place the person's hand in the fluidotherapy via a sleeve on the machine for 20 minutes. During this time the person can exercise his/her hand and wrist.
    (4) Treatment is for 20 minutes. The person's hand is slowly removed from the machine making certain no particles of ground cornhusk spills out.
  d. Whirlpool.[2]
    (1) To clean and debride wounds:
      (a) Fill tank with water at 100°–108°F if treating burns, water should be set at body temperature.
      (b) Maintain sterile technique.
      (c) Adjust turbine and turn it on. Check temperature again.
      (d) Slowly lower the extremity into the whirlpool.
    (2) Treatment will be for 20 minutes.
7. Benefits of cryotherapy.
  a. Relieves pain.
  b. Controls edema.
  c. Decreases abnormal tone.
  d. Facilitates muscle tone.
  e. Commonly used to treat acute injuries and post surgical repairs.
8. Precautions and contraindications for cryotherapy. Do not use with:
  a. Sensory deficits including hypersensitivity.
  b. Impaired circulation.
  c. Raynaud's disease.
9. Application of cryotherapy.
  a. Ice pack.
    (1) Check skin prior to and after application.
    (2) Apply a dry or wet towel between the client's skin and the cold pack.
    (3) Check skin after 3–5 minutes.
    (4) Cold pack remains cold for up to 10 minutes.
  b. Another commonly used type of cryotherapy includes ice massage (used for smaller areas; applied directly to the skin for 3–5 minutes).
10. Electrical stimulation.
  a. Benefits of electrical stimulation.
    (1) Pain control.
    (2) Decreases swelling.

---

[2]Whirlpool (WP) is not as commonly used as in the past; now used on a case by case basis. WP replaced by more advanced wound management interventions. WP requires strict cleaning and disinfecting procedures; refer to CDC for recommendations.

(3) Stimulates and strengthens muscles.
(4) Muscle reeducation.
(5) Stimulates denervated muscle.

b. Contraindications for electrical stimulation.
(1) Cardiac pacemaker.
(2) Phrenic or urinary bladder stimulators.
(3) Presence of thrombosis or thrombophlebitis.
(4) Over carotid sinus.

11. Ultrasound.
a. Types: continuous (thermal effects) and pulsed (nonthermal effects).
b. Benefits of continuous ultrasound.
(1) Increases tissue extensibility (increases ROM, decreases joint stiffness).
(2) Reduces pain.
(3) Increases blood flow and tissue permeability.
(4) Reduces muscle spasms.
(5) Reaches deeper tissues (up to 5cms).
c. Benefits of pulsed ultrasound.
(1) Decreases inflammation.
(2) Heals tissue.
d. Contraindications of ultrasound.
(1) Active malignant tumor.
(2) Pregnancy.
(3) Area near pacemaker.
(4) Some joint replacements (cemented or plastic).
(5) Thrombophlebitis.
(6) Precautions: fractures, growth plates and breast implants.

12. Guidelines for competent and ethical use of PAMs in occupational therapy.
a. PAMs should be used when they can benefit the individual's treatment program.
b. PAMs should be not be used when they will not benefit the individual's treatment program.
c. Indications, contraindications, and precautions for use of PAMs must be adhered to strictly.
(1) General contraindications for PAMs. Do not use if a person has:
(a) Cancer.
(b) Pacemaker.
(c) Pregnancy.
(d) Cognitive impairment.
(e) Sensory impairment.
(f) Vascular impairment.
(g) Deep vein thrombophlebitis.
(2) Prior to using PAMs with an individual, diagnostic and age considerations must be carefully reviewed. For example, ultrasound is never used over a growth plate.
d. Practitioner competence must be established for any and all PAMs used in OT intervention.

References

American Occupational Therapy Association. (2005). Standards of practice for occupational therapy. *American Journal of Occupational Therapy*, 59, 663–665.

American Society of Hand Therapists. (1992). *Clinical assessment recommendations*, 2nd ed. Chicago: Author.

Bain, B., & Leger, D. (1997). *Assistive technology: An interdisciplinary approach*. Orlando, FL: Churchill Livingstone.

Cameron, M. (1999). *Physical agents in rehabilitation: From research to practice*. Orlando, FL: W.B. Saunders.

Clark, G.,Wilgis, E. F., & Aiello, B. (1993). *Hand rehabilitation and upper extremity rehabilitation: A practical guide*. Orlando, FL: Churchill Livingstone.

Evan, R. B. (2002). Therapist's management of carpal tunnel syndrome. In E.J. Mackin, A.D. Callahan, & T.M. Skirven (Eds.), *Rehabilitation of the hand and upper extremity*, 5th ed. (pp. 660–661). St Louis: Mosby.

Falkenstein, N., & Weiss-Lessard, S. (1999). *Hand rehabilitation: A quick reference guide and review*. St. Louis, MO: Mosby.

Greene, D., & Roberts, S. (1999). *Kinesiology movement in the context of activity*. St. Louis, MO: Mosby.

Hislop, H., & Montgomery, J. (1995). *Daniel's and Worthingham's muscle testing*, 6th ed. Orlando, FL: W.B. Saunders.

Hopkins, H., & Smith, H. (Eds.). (2003). *Willard and Spackman's occupational therapy*, 10th ed. Philadelphia: J.B. Lippincott.

Jacobs, M. L., & Austin, N. M. (2014). *Orthotic intervention for the hand and upper extremity: Splinting principles and process*. Baltimore: Lippincott Williams & Wilkins.

Kendall, F. (1995). *Muscle testing and function*, 4th ed. Baltimore: Williams and Wilkins.

Knight, K. L., & Draper, D. O. (2013). *Therapeutic modalities: The art and science*. Baltimore: Lippincott Williams and Wilkins.

Lashgari, D., & Yasuda, Y. L. (2013). Orthotics. In H. M. Pendleton & W. S. Schultz-Krohn (Eds.), *Occupational therapy practice skills for physical dysfunction*, 7th ed. (pp. 755–795), St. Louis: Mosby.

Malick, M., & Kasch, M. (1984). *Manual on management of specific hand problems*. Pittsburgh, PA: AREN Publications.

Manning, D. C. (2000). Reflex sympathetic dystrophy, sympathetically maintained pain and complex regional pain syndrome: Diagnosis of inclusion, exclusion, or confusion? *Journal of Hand Therapy, 13*(4), 260–268

Michlovitz S. L., & Nolan T. P. (2005), *Modalities for therapeutic intervention*, 4th ed. Philadelphia: F.A. Davis.

Minnesota Manual Dexterity Test. (1969). Lafayette Instrument, PO Box 5729, Lafayette, WI 47903.

Neer, C. (1990). *Shoulder reconstruction*. Orlando, FL: W.B. Saunders.

O'Connor Tweezer Dexterity Test. (1986). Smith & Nephew Roylan, Inc. Menomonee Falls, WI 53051.

Pedretti, L., Smith, R., Hammel, J., Rein, J., Anson, D., & McGuire, M. J. (1996). Use of adjunctive modalities in occupational therapy. In R. P. Cottrell (Ed.), *Perspectives on purposeful activity: Foundation and future of occupational therapy* (pp. 451–458). Bethesda, MD: AOTA.

Pendeleton, H. M., & Schultz-Krohn, W. (2013). *Pedretti's occupational therapy: Practice skills for physical dysfunction.* St. Louis: Mosby.

Purdue Pegboard Procedure Manual. Lafayette Instrument, PO Box 5729, Lafayette, IN 47903.

Radomski. M. V. & Trombly. Latham, C. A. (2008). *Occupational therapy for physical dysfunction*, 6th ed. Baltimore: Lippincott Williams and Wilkins.

Weiss, S., & Falkenstein, N. (2005). *Hand rehabilitation a quick reference guide and review*, 2nd ed. St. Louis: Elsevier Mosby.

Review Questions

Biomechanical Approaches: Evaluation and Intervention

Below are six questions about key content covered in this chapter. These questions are not inclusive of the entirety of content related to biomechanical approaches that you must know for success on the NBCOT exam. These questions are provided to help you "jump start" the thought processes you will need to apply your studying of content to the answering of exam questions; hence they are not in the NBCOT exam format. Exam items in the NBCOT format which cover the depth and breadth of content you will need to know to pass the NBCOT exam are provided on this text's disc. The answers to the below questions are provided in Appendix 4.

1. You work in a practice setting which serves many clients with musculoskeletal disorders. The majority of clients have decreased ROM. What are the different types of ROM you should consider during assessment? How should you document your evaluation and its results?

2. A new client is admitted into an intensive care unit with a diagnosis of a spinal cord injury. The physician requests an evaluation to aide in determining the level of injury. How would you perform a light touch sensory test? How does this method of testing differ from the procedures used during sensory testing for other major diagnostic categories?

3. An adult client is having difficulty performing daily activities due to decreased ROM and pain in both shoulders. You decide to treat the client with preparatory interventions followed by an occupation-based intervention. What interventions can you use to increase ROM and decrease pain?

4. You provide consultation services to a Center for Independent Living which serves persons with a diversity of disabilities. You are scheduled to conduct an educational session on energy conservation and work simplification. What key principles and methods should you be sure to include in your presentation?

5. Your client is diagnosed with rotator cuff tendonitis and is experiencing severe pain. The physician has ordered the use of transcutaneous electrical nerve stimulator (TENS), gentle ROM, and below shoulder level ADL. During your evaluation, you review the client's past medical history. You learn that the person has a history of cardiac issues that required the implantation of a pacemaker. Which of the prescribed interventions will you use with this client? What are additional interventions you can use with this client to decrease pain and prepare the person for occupation-based interventions?

6. Your client is status post a below knee amputation. You assess the strength of the client's triceps in preparation for transfer training. The results of the MMT reveal that the client can take moderate resistance and then break. What muscle grade would you document the client possesses?

12

Neurological Approaches: Evaluation and Intervention

GLEN GILLEN

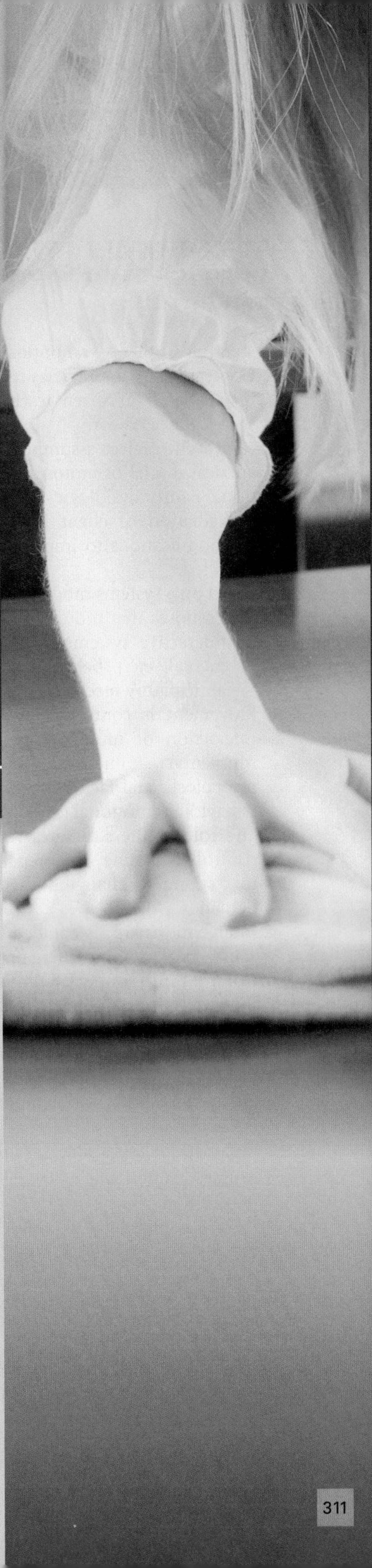

Chapter Outline

Neurological Frames of Reference Related to Motor Performance

Contemporary Task-Oriented Approaches to Motor Control Training

1. General principles/assumptions.
   a. Contemporary approaches to motor control training are based on current research and knowledge of the motor behavior.
   b. Approaches reject assumptions of the reflex-hierarchical model of motor control and of the traditional neurophysiologic therapies.
   c. Remediation of client factors and environmental modifications to improve task performance is included.
   d. Based on a systems model of motor control.
      (1) Proposes that motor control is determined by interactive systems (motor, cultural, environmental, etc.), behavioral tasks, and adaptive/anticipatory mechanisms.
   e. Movement is controlled by the integration and interaction of multiple systems including environmental influences, sensorimotor factors, musculoskeletal factors, regulatory functions, and behavioral/emotional goals.
   f. The role of the structures responsible for motor control is to tune and prepare the motor system to respond to changing environmental and task demands.
   g. Interventions are also guided by therapist's understanding of motor learning principles.
   h. Control is not simply over muscle actions, but over the interactions of kinematic variables.
   i. Movement dysfunction following CNS damage reflects the system's best effort to accomplish task goals.
2. Principles of the Contemporary Task-Oriented Approach.
   a. Occupational performance emerges from the interaction of multiple systems including personal and performance contexts.
   b. Personal and environmental systems, including the central nervous system, are heterarchically organized.
   c. An individual's behavioral changes reflect his/her attempts to compensate and to achieve functional goals.
   d. Individuals must practice with varied strategies to find optimal solutions for motor problems and develop skill in performance.
   e. Functional tasks help organize motor behavior.
   f. The therapist must determine which control parameters or systems (personal, environmental, etc.) have positive or negative influences on motor behavior.
   g. Practice opportunities are provided which are appropriate to the person's stage of learning.
   h. The therapist conducts the evaluation using a top-down approach.
   i. Evaluation efforts focus initially on role performance and occupational performance tasks because they are the goals of motor behavior.
   j. After a patient has identified the most important role and occupational performance limitations, the therapist uses task analysis to identify which subsystem(s) of the person and/or environmental factor(s) are limiting functional performance.
   k. Interventions are focused on:
      (1) Helping patients adjust to role and task performance limitations.
      (2) Creating an environment that utilizes the common challenges of everyday life.
      (3) Practicing functional tasks or close simulations to find effective and efficient strategies for performance.
      (4) Providing opportunities for practice outside of therapy time.
      (5) Remediating a client factor.
      (6) Minimizing inefficient of ineffective movement patterns.
      (7) Adapting the environment.
      (8) Modifying the task.
      (9) Using assistive technology.
3. Principles of Carr and Shepherd's Motor Relearning Program (MRP).
   a. The person is an active participant whose goal is to relearn effective strategies for performing functional movement.
   b. Postural adjustments and limb movements are linked together in the learning process.
   c. Successful task relearning has occurred when activities are performed automatically and efficiently.
   d. The learning of skills does not follow a developmental sequence.
   e. Continued practice of compensatory strategies limits functional recovery.
   f. Intervention is not focused on learning specific movements but instead on learning general strategies for solving motor problems.

g. Obstacles to efficient movement include loss of soft tissue extensibility, balance loss, fixation patterns due to postural insecurity, and muscle weakness.

h. Abnormal movement patterns are attributed to the repeated practice of compensatory movement strategies that become overlearned.

4. Principles of Motor Learning.
   a. Contemporary approaches to treating motor dysfunction incorporate principles of motor learning during interventions focused on remediating motor control in persons with CNS dysfunction. See Table 12-1.

Table 12-1

Summary of Motor Learning Principles/Considerations

PRINCIPLES/CONSIDERATIONS	EXAMPLES
Classification of tasks to be learned: Learning is contingent on the type of task that is being learned.	
– Discrete tasks: Tasks with a recognizable beginning and end.	Kick a ball, push a button
– Continuous tasks: There is no recognizable beginning and end. Tasks are performed until they are arbitrarily stopped.	Jogging, driving, swimming
– Serial tasks: Comprised of a series of movements linked together to make a "whole."	Play an instrument, dressing, light a fireplace
– Closed tasks: Performed in a predictable and stable environment. Movements can be planned in advance.	Oral care, signing a check, bowling
– Open tasks: Performed in a constantly changing environment that may be unpredictable.	Driving in traffic, catching an insect, soccer
– Variable motionless tasks: Involve interacting with a stable and predictable environment, but specific features of the environment are likely to vary between performance trials.	Performance of ADL outside of the usual home environment.
– Consistent motion tasks: An individual must deal with environmental conditions that are in motion during activity performance; the motion is consistent and predictable between trials.	Stepping onto an escalator, assembly line work, retrieving luggage from an airport baggage carousel
Practice conditions: The law of practice refers to performance changing linearly with the amount of time spent in practice.	
– Massed practice: Rest time is much less than practice time.	Constraint Induced Movement Therapy
– Distributed practice: Practice time is equal to or less that rest time.	Practice sessions of a tub transfer are spaced to include rest breaks.
– Blocked practice: Repetitive practice of the same task, uninterrupted by practice of other tasks.	Practicing moving from sit to stand multiple times in a row. Practice sequence of tasks "A," "B," "C": AAAAABBBBBBCCCCC
– Random or Variable practice: Tasks being practiced are ordered randomly. Attempt multiple tasks or variations of a task before mastering any one of the tasks.	Practice transferring to multiple surfaces (couch, toilet, bench, chair, stool, car) in one OT session.
– Whole practice: The task is practiced in its entirety and not broken into parts.	Practice sequence of tasks "A," "B," "C": ACBACABCCBACABCACABBACCACB
– Part practice: The task is broken down into its parts for separate practice.	Practicing dressing.
	Don/doff shirt.
Feedback: A key feature of practice is the information the learner receives about their attempts to learn a skill.	Knowing you made an error as you spill water when trying to pour from a pitcher to a cup.
– Inherent (intrinsic) feedback: feedback normally received while performing a task.	A therapist provides feedback related to task performance. "You need to lock your wheelchair brakes."
– Augmented feedback: Information about task performance that is supplemental to inherent feedback.	While practicing reaching the therapist says "Don't hike your shoulder."
– Concurrent feedback: Given during task performance.	After practice of reaching the therapist says "You didn't open your hand wide enough."
– Terminal feedback: Given after task performance.	
– Immediate feedback: Given immediately after performance.	Right after an attempt at a tub transfer the therapist says "That was perfect."
– Delayed feedback: Feedback is delayed by some amount of time.	The OT says "You did better this morning but keep checking your brakes."
– Knowledge of results (KR): Feedback given after task performance about the outcome.	The OT says: "Your shirt is on backwards" or "You dropped the cup."
– Knowledge of Performance (KP): Feedback given after task about the nature of performance.	The OT says: "Next time, dress your right arm first" or "Your elbow was bent."

Gillen G. (2014). Motor function and occupational performance. In B.A.B. Schell, G. Gillen, & M. E. Scaffa. (Eds). *Willard and Spackman's occupational therapy*, 12th ed. Philadelphia: Lippincott Williams & Wilkins. Reprinted with permission.

b. The ultimate goal of utilizing motor learning theory is the acquisition of functional skills that can be generalized to multiple situations and environments.

c. Stages of motor learning.

(1) Skill acquisition stage (cognitive stage) occurs during initial instruction and practice of a skill.

(2) Skill retention stage (associated stage) involves 'carry-over,' as individuals are asked to demonstrate their newly acquired skill after initial practice.

(3) Skill transfer stage (autonomous stage) involves the individual demonstrating the skill in a new context.

(4) Refer to Table 12-2 for further description of these stages.

d. Practice.

(1) Random (or variable) practice involves practice of several tasks that are presented in a random order encouraging reformulation of the solution to the presented motor problem.

Table 12-2

Motor Learning Stages and Training Strategies
COGNITIVE STAGE CHARACTERISTICS
• The learner develops an understanding of task; cognitive mapping assesses abilities, task demands; identifies stimuli, contacts memory; selects response; performs initial approximations of task; structures motor program; modifies initial responses. • "What to do" decision.
Training Strategies
• Highlight purpose of task in functionally relevant terms. • Demonstrate ideal performance of task to establish a reference of correctness. • Have patients verbalize task components and requirements. • Point out similarities to other learned tasks. • Direct attention to critical task elements. • Select appropriate feedback. – Emphasize intact sensory systems, intrinsic feedback systems. – Carefully pair extrinsic feedback with intrinsic feedback. – High dependence on vision: have patient watch movement. – Knowledge of Performance (KP): focus on errors as they become consistent; do not cue on large number of random errors. – Knowledge of Results (KR): focus on success of movement outcome. • Ask learner to evaluate performance, outcomes; identify problems, solutions. • Use reinforcements (praise) for correct performance, continuing motivation. • Organize feedback schedule. – Feedback after every trial improves performance during early treatment. – Variable feedback (summed, fading, bandwidth designs) increases depth of cognitive processing, improves retention; may decrease performance initially. • Organize initial practice. – Stress controlled movement to minimize errors. – Provide adequate rest periods (distributed practice) if task is complex, long, or energy costly or if learner fatigues easily, has short attention, poor concentration. – Use manual guidance to assist as appropriate. – Break complex tasks down into component parts, teach both parts as integrated whole. – Utilize bilateral transfer as appropriate. – Use blocked (repeated) practice of same task to improve performance. – Use variable practice (serial or random practice order) of related skills to increase depth of cognitive processing and retention; may decrease performance initially. – Use mental practice to improve performance and learning, reduce anxiety.

(Continued)

Table 12-2

Motor Learning Stages and Training Strategies (*Continued*)
COGNITIVE STAGE CHARACTERISTICS (*Continued*)
• Assess, modify arousal levels as appropriate. – High or low arousal impairs performance and learning. – Avoid stressors, mental fatigue. • Structure environment. – Reduce extraneous environmental stimuli, distracters to ensure attention, concentration – Emphasize closed skills initially gradually progressing to open skills.
ASSOCIATED STAGE CHARACTERISTICS
• The learner practices movements, refines motor programs: spatial and temporal organization; decreases errors and extraneous movements. • Dependence on visual feedback decreases, increases for use of proprioceptive feedback; cognitive monitoring decreases. • "How to do" decisions.
Training Strategies
• Select appropriate feedback. – Continue to provide KP, intervene when errors become consistent. – Emphasize proprioceptive feedback, "feel of movement" to assist in establishing an internal reference of correctness. – Continue to provide KR; stress relevance of functional outcomes. – Assist learner to improve self evaluation, decision making skills. – Facilitation techniques, guided movements may be counterproductive during this stage of learning. • Organize feedback schedule. – Continue to provide feedback for continuing motivation; encourage patient to self-assess achievements. – Avoid excessive augmented feedback. – Focus on use of variable feedback (summed, fading, bandwidth) designs to improve retention. • Organize practice. – Encourage consistency of performance. – Focus on variable practice order (serial or random) of related skills to improve retention. • Structure environment. – Progress toward open, changing environment. – Prepare the learner for home, community, work environments.
AUTONOMOUS STAGE CHARACTERISTICS
• The learner practices movements, continues to refine motor responses, spatial and temporal highly organized, movements are largely error-free, minimal level of cognitive monitoring. • *"How to succeed"* decision.
Training Strategies
• Assesses need for conscious attention, automaticity of movements. • Select appropriate feedback. – Learner demonstrates appropriate self evaluation, decision-making skills. – Provide occasional feedback (KP, KR) when errors evident. • Organize practice. – Stress consistency of performance in variable environments, variations of tasks (open skills). – High levels of practice (massed practice) are appropriate. • Structure environment. – Vary environments to challenge learner. – Ready the learner for home, community, work environments. • Focus on competitive aspects of skills as appropriate, e.g., wheelchair sports.
O'Sullivan, S. & Schmitz, T. (2007). *Physical rehabilitation,* 5th ed. Philadelphia: F.A. Davis Company. Reprinted with permission.

(2) Blocked practice involves repeated performance of the same motor skill.
(3) Practice of the whole task.
(4) Practice of parts of the task.
(5) Variable conditions involve practice of skills in various contexts to improve transfer of learning and retention of skills.
(6) Mental practice involves cognitive rehearsal of a skill without actually moving.

e. Intrinsic feedback.
(1) Information received by the learner as a result of performing the task.
(2) Information is received from tactile, vestibular, and visual systems during and after the task.

f. Extrinsic feedback.
(1) Feedback provided from an outside source (i.e., the therapist or a mechanical device).
(2) Includes knowledge of performance, which is verbal feedback about the process or performance itself.
(3) Includes knowledge of results, which is the therapist's provision of feedback about the outcome or end product or results of the motor action.

g. Factors/conditions that promote generalization of motor learning.
(1) Capacity to generate intrinsic feedback.
(2) High feedback regarding knowledge of performance.
(3) Low extrinsic feedback regarding knowledge of results.
(4) Practice conditions that are variable, random.
(5) Whole task performance as opposed to breaking activities into contrived parts.
(6) High contextual interference utilizes environmental conditions that increase the difficulty of learning such as noise distractions, crowded environments, and random practice.
(7) Practice in naturalistic settings, i.e. the setting in which the skill being taught will be utilized or an environment that closely resembles the one in which the skill will be performed.

h. Treatment sequence to promote generalization of learning.
(1) The initial task is the first activity performed by the patient.
(2) Near transfer is an alternate form of the initial task.
(3) Intermediate transfer has a moderate number of changes in task parameters but still has some similarities to the initial task.
(4) Far transfer introduces an activity that is conceptually the same as but physically different from the initial task.
(5) Very far transfer requires spontaneous use of the new strategy in daily functional activities.

i. Task categories.
(1) Closed tasks are activities in which the environment is stable and predictable and methods of performance are consistent over time.
(2) Variable motionless tasks also involve interacting with a stable and predictable environment, but specific features of the environment are likely to vary between performance trials.
(3) Consistent motion tasks require an individual to deal with environmental conditions that are in motion during activity performance; the motion is consistent and predictable between trials.
(4) Open tasks require people to make adaptive decisions about unpredictable events because objects within the environment are in random motion during task performance.

j. Refer to Table 12-3 for training strategies appropriate for each stage of motor learning.

Review of Neurophysiologic Frames of Reference

1. Also known as sensorimotor approaches.
   a. They include the neurodevelopmental treatment approach (NDT), proprioceptive neuromuscular facilitation (PNF), Brunnstrom's approach, and Margaret Rood's approach.
   b. See Table 12-3 for a summary and comparison of these traditional approaches.
2. Utilized for persons with central nervous system dysfunction.
3. Approaches developed in the 1940s and 1950s based on the understanding of nervous system pathology at that time.
   a. They are outlined in this chapter only because this information is included in key occupational therapy textbooks that NBCOT identifies as the references for the composition of NBCOT exam items.
   (1) Consequently, some NBCOT exam items may reflect these traditional perspectives.
4. General assumptions/principles/treatment foundations.
   a. Controlled movement is preceded by stereotypic reflex responses.
   b. Sensory input regulates motor output and sensation is necessary for movement to take place.
   c. Normal movements are governed by hierarchical centralized motor programs that determine muscle activation patterns.
   (1) The cerebral cortex controls the middle levels (basal ganglia, brainstem, etc.) which in turn control the spinal cord.
   d. Damage to higher control centers release lower level or primitive reflexes and movement patterns from inhibition.

Table 12-3

Comparison of Key Treatment Strategies Used in the Traditional Sensorimotor Approaches

KEY TREATMENT STRATEGIES	ROOD APPROACH	BRUNNSTROM APPROACH (MOVEMENT THERAPY)	PROPRIOCEPTIVE NEUROMUSCULAR APPROACH	NEURODEVELOPMENTAL TREATMENT
Sensory stimulation used to evoke a motor response	YES (Uses direct application of sensory stimuli to muscles and joints)	YES (Movement occurs in response to sensory stimuli)	YES (Tactile, auditory, visual sensory stimuli promote motor responses)	YES (Abnormal muscle tone occurs, in part, because of abnormal sensory experiences)
Reflexive movement used as a precursor for volitional movement	YES (Reflexive movement achieved initially through the application of sensory stimuli)	YES (Move patient along a continuum of reflexive to volitional movement patterns)	YES (Volitional movements can be assisted by reflexive supported postures)	NO
Treatment directed toward influencing muscle tone	YES (Sensory stimuli used to inhibit or facilitate tone)	YES (Postures, sensory stimuli used to inhibit or facilitate tone)	YES (Movement patterns used to normalize tone)	YES (Handling techniques and postures can inhibit or facilitate muscle tone)
Developmental patterns/sequences used for the development of motor skills	YES (Ontogenic motor patterns used to develop motor skills)	YES (Flexion and extension synergies; proximal to distal return)	YES (Patterns used to facilitate proximal to distal motor control)	YES
Conscious attention is directed toward movement	NO	YES	YES	YES
Treatment directly emphasizes development of skilled movements for task performance	NO	NO	NO	YES

Schultz-Krohn, W. et al. (2006). Traditional Sensorimotor Approaches to Intervention. In W. Schultz-Krohn & H. Pendelton (Eds.), *Pedretti's Occupational Therapy: Practice skills for physical dysfunction*, 6th ed. St. Louis: Elsevier Science/Mosby. Reprinted with permission.

e. When basic movements and postures are normalized, skilled movement would occur automatically.

f. "Integration" of lower level spinal and brainstem reflexes occurs by eliciting higher level righting and equilibrium responses.

g. Controlled sensory input applied by the therapist can influence motor responses (i.e., a reflex model of control).

h. The use of "facilitation" and "inhibition" techniques can improve motor performance.

Neurodevelopmental Treatment (NDT)/The Bobath Technique

1. Principles/assumptions.
   a. Normalization of postural and limb tone is prerequisite to normal movement.
      (1) Tone abnormalities include flaccidity (low tone) or spasticity (high tone).
   b. Avoidance of movements and activities that increase tone.
   c. Inhibition of primitive reflexes and abnormal postural and limb movements.
   d. Development of normal patterns of posture and movement.
   e. Improvement of the quality of movement and performance of the involved side.
   f. Associated reactions (nonfunctional and involuntary changes in the uninvolved limb position and tone) should be avoided.
   g. Postural reactions are considered the basis for control of movement.
      (1) These reactions include righting, equilibrium, and protective responses.
   h. Loss of postural control results in overuse of the sound side and limits functional movements.
   i. The stereotypical patterns of the trunk and limbs observed in persons with CNS dysfunction are viewed as abnormal patterns of motor coordination.

j. Focus is on improving the quality of movement.
  (1) Normalization of movement patterns.
  (2) Integration of both sides of the body/re-establishment of symmetry of the sides of the body to increase functional use.
  (3) Establishment of the ability to weight bear and weight shift through the limbs.
  (4) Establishment of normal righting and equilibrium patterns.

k. Handling is the primary intervention to promote normal movement.

Proprioceptive Neuromuscular Facilitation (PNF)

1. Principles/assumptions.
  a. The response of the neuromuscular mechanisms can be hastened through stimulation of the proprioceptors.
    (1) Utilized for neurologic and orthopedic populations throughout the lifespan.
  b. Techniques are superimposed on patterns of movement (diagonals) and posture, focusing on sensory stimulation from manual contacts, visual cues, and verbal commands.
  c. Normal motor development proceeds in a cervicocaudal and proximodistal direction.
  d. Early motor behavior is dominated by reflex activity.
    (1) Mature motor behavior is supported or reinforced by postural reflexes that are integrated throughout the lifespan.
  e. Early motor behavior is characterized by spontaneous movement, which oscillates between extremes of flexion and extension.
    (1) These movements are rhythmic and reversing in character.
  f. Developing motor behavior is expressed in an orderly sequence of total patterns of movement and posture.
  g. In development, there are shifts between flexor and extensor dominance.
  h. Locomotion depends on reciprocal contraction of flexors and extensors.
  i. The maintenance of posture requires continual adjustment for nuances of imbalance.
  j. Frequency of stimulation and repetitive activity are used to promote and retain motor learning, and to develop strength and endurance.
  k. Goal-directed activities coupled with techniques of facilitation are used to hasten learning of total patterns of walking and self-care activities.
  l. Goal-directed activity is made up of reversing movements.
  m. Diagonal patterns or mass movement patterns are utilized during functional activities.
    (1) All patterns cross midline and encourage rotary components to movement.
    (2) Upper extremity patterns are identified as D1 or D2, flexion or extension.
      (a) D1 flexion.
        - Scapula: abducted and upwardly rotated.
        - Shoulder: flexed, adducted, externally rotated.
        - Elbow: slightly flexed.
        - Forearm: supinated.
        - Wrist: flexed toward radial side.
        - Fingers: flexed, adducted.
        - Thumb: flexed, adducted.
      (b) D1 extension.
        - Scapula: adducted, downwardly rotated.
        - Shoulder: extended, abducted, internally rotated.
        - Elbow: extended.
        - Forearm: pronated.
        - Wrist: extended toward ulnar side.
        - Fingers: extended, abducted.
        - Thumb: extended, abducted.
      (c) D2 flexion.
        - Scapula: adducted and upwardly rotated.
        - Shoulder: flexed, abducted, externally rotated.
        - Elbow: extended.
        - Forearm: supinated.
        - Wrist: extended toward radial side.
        - Fingers: extended, abducted.
        - Thumb: extended, abducted.
      (d) D2 extension.
        - Scapula: abducted and downwardly rotated.
        - Shoulder: extended, adducted, internally rotated.
        - Elbow: toward flexion.
        - Forearm: pronated.
        - Wrist: flexed toward ulnar side.
        - Fingers: flexed, adducted.
        - Thumb: flexed, abducted, opposed.

Brunnstrom's Movement Therapy

1. Principles/assumptions.
  a. Brunnstrom's approach focused on facilitating recovery through a specific sequence.
  b. Treatment is focused on the promotion of movement from reflexive to volitional.
    (1) Seven stages of motor recovery following the onset of hemiplegia that the individual

progresses through in a stereotypical fashion were identified by Brunnstrom.

(2) This recovery pattern includes the identification of developing synergies.

Margaret Rood's Approach

1. Principles/assumptions.
   a. Sensorimotor control is developmentally based.
      (1) Treatment must begin at the person's current level and progress sequentially.
   b. Rood proposed four sequential phases of motor control.
      (1) Reciprocal inhibition/innervation.
         (a) An early mobility pattern that is primarily a reflex governed by spinal and supraspinal centers.
      (2) Co-contraction.
         (a) Defined as a simultaneous contraction of the agonist and antagonist that provides stability in a static pattern.
         (b) Utilized to hold a position or object for a long duration.
      (3) Heavy work.
         (a) Also termed "mobility superimposed on stability."
         (b) In these patterns, proximal muscles contract and move and the distal segments are fixed.
      (4) Skill.
         (a) Considered the highest level of control and combines stability and mobility.
         (b) These patterns consist of a stabilized proximal segment while the distal segments move in space.
   c. Muscular responses of the agonists, antagonists, and synergists are believed to be reflexively programmed according to a purpose or plan.
   d. Rood described a sequence of motor development termed "ontogenic motor patterns" that includes eight different patterns in sequence (i.e., supine withdrawal, rollover, prone extension, neck co-contraction, prone on elbows, quadruped, standing).
   e. Rood proposed that the motor response that is achieved is dependent on the type of sensory stimulation that the therapist applies.

Evaluation of Motor Control Dysfunction

Assessment for Components of Motor Control

1. Spasticity is evaluated by the elicitation of velocity-dependent stretch reflexes.
   a. The limb is quickly stretched in a direction opposite the pull of the muscle group being tested.
      (1) Objectively measured by the five-point Ashworth Scale (1 = normal tone and 5 = severe hypertonus/rigidity) or the Modified Ashworth Scale (0 = no increase in muscle tone and 4 = the affected part is rigid in flexion or extension).
      (2) Quick stretch is applied in a direction opposite the pull of the muscle group being tested and graded utilizing a "minimal/moderate/severe" rating scale depending on which point in the range elicits a stretch reflex (minimal if "catch" is felt at end of range and severe if "catch" is felt at the beginning of the range).
2. Reflex testing.
   a. Utilized to evaluate involuntary stereotyped responses to a particular stimulus.
   b. Responses develop during fetal life and persist through early infancy.
   c. Reflexes may be released after brain injury or not integrated during early development secondary to CNS pathology.
   d. Intensity and quality of the response in monitored.
   e. A response to stimulus is termed 'positive' and no response to stimulus is 'negative.'
   f. Therapist notes the highest level of reflex control achieved.
   g. Examples of reflexes that are tested.
      (1) Grasp.
         (a) Stimulus: pressure to palm of hand.
         (b) Response: finger flexion that resists object removal.
      (2) Flexor withdrawal.
         (a) Stimulus: stimuli to sole of foot.
         (b) Response: flexion of stimulated leg.
      (3) Crossed extension.
         (a) Stimulus: passively flex extended leg while opposite leg is flexed.
         (b) Response: extension of opposite leg with adduction and internal rotation.
      (4) Asymmetrical tonic neck reflex.
         (a) Stimulus: rotate head 90°.
         (b) Response: limb extension on face side, flexion dominated on skull side.

(5) Symmetrical tonic neck reflex.
  (a) Stimuli: flexion of the head followed by head extension.
  (b) Response: flexion of head results in flexion of arms/extension of legs. Extension of head results in extension of arms/flexion of legs.
(6) Tonic labyrinthine.
  (a) Stimulus: prone position followed by supine position.
  (b) Response: prone results in flexor posturing of arms/legs. Supine results in extensor posturing of arms/legs.
(7) Positive supporting reaction.
  (a) Stimulus: contact to ball of foot in an upright position.
  (b) Response: extension of the legs.
(8) Associated reactions.
  (a) Stimulus: resisted voluntary movements of the less involved limb.
  (b) Response: involuntary movement of the contralateral resting limb (i.e., "overflow").
(9) Neck righting acting on the body.
  (a) Stimulus: head rotation to one side.
  (b) Response: body rotates to align with head.
(10) Body righting acting on the body.
  (a) Stimulus: limb[1] (usually lower) rotation to one side.
  (b) Response: segmental rotation of the trunk.
(11) Optical righting.
  (a) Stimulus: alter body position in all directions.
  (b) Response: head orients to vertical with mouth horizontal.
(12) Protective extension.
  (a) Stimulus: displace center of gravity outside the base of support.
  (b) Response: arms and legs respond to protect against falling.
(13) Equilibrium reactions.
  (a) Stimulus: displace center of gravity by tipping support surface.
  (b) Response: righting of head/trunk/limbs.

h. Therapist must be aware of the age range that is considered normal for each reflex. (See Chapter 5.)
i. Treatment is planned to progress individual to an age-appropriate level of reflex hierarchy.

[1]Note: some sources also identify head rotation to one side as a stimulus for the body acting on body reflex.

3. Qualitative descriptions of motor control.
  a. Evaluation of motor control should include observations of the quality of movement during performance of functional tasks.
  b. Examples of motor control issues resulting in observable poor quality of movement.
    (1) Intention tremor is the worsening of action tremor as the limb approaches a target in space.
    (2) Dysmetria is the undershooting (hypometria) or overshooting (hypermetria) of a target.
    (3) Dyssynergia is a breakdown in movement resulting in joints being moved separately to reach a desired target as opposed to moving in a smooth trajectory; decomposition of movement.
    (4) Dysdiadochokinesia is impaired ability to perform rapid alternating movements.
    (5) Ataxia is loss of motor control including tremors, dysdiadochokinesia, dyssynergia, and visual nystagmus.
    (6) Resting tremor is an involuntary tremor noted in resting postures.
    (7) Rigidity is an increased resistance to passive movement throughout the range; may be "cogwheel" (alternative contraction/relaxation of muscles being stretched) or "lead pipe" (consistent contraction throughout range).
    (8) Bradykinèsia is an overall slowing of movement patterns.
    (9) Akinesia is the inability to initiate movements.
    (10) Athetosis is a dyskinetic condition that includes inadequate timing, force, and accuracy of movements in the trunk/limbs; movements are writhing and worm-like.
    (11) Dystonia is an involuntary sustained distorted movement or posture involving contraction of groups of muscles.
    (12) Chorea consists of involuntary movements of the face and extremities which are spasmodic and of short duration.
    (13) Hemiballismus is a unilateral chorea characterized by violent, forceful movements of the proximal muscles.
4. Assessment for glenohumeral joint subluxation.
  a. Allow the person's arm to dangle into gravity.
  b. Palpate the space underneath the acromion process with your index finger.
  c. Compare to the intact side and document the width of the space in terms of finger breadths.

Orthotic/Splinting Interventions for Neuromotor Dysfunction

Purposes of Orthoses/Splints

1. Orthoses may be utilized in the population with neuromuscular dysfunction to meet the following goals.
   a. Prevent/correct deformity via prolonged stretch and proper alignment.
   b. Control spasticity by aligning joints and providing prolonged stretch to spastic muscles.
   c. Prevent/decrease/accommodate contractures of the joint or soft tissue.
   d. Correct biomechanical malalignment by external force.
   e. Position the hand in a functional posture to promote engagement in activities.
   f. Compensate for weakness to allow intact muscle groups to function.
   g. Provide proximal support.
   h. Support a painful joint.
   i. Promote distal mobility.
   j. Enhance a specific activity, e.g., fabrication of a typing or writing splint or utilization of a cock-up splint for feeding.
   k. Immobilize joints and soft tissues to promote healing.
   l. Prevent or reduce scarring via prolonged pressure and appropriate stretch.

Types of Orthoses/Splints

1. Splint classification.
   a. Static (no moving parts) splints are utilized for external support, prevention of motion, stretching of contractures, aligning joints for healing, resting joints, or reducing pain.
   b. Dynamic (moving parts are included) splints have a resilient component (elastic bands or spring) and are utilized to increase passive motion, assist weak motions, or substitute for lost motion.
   c. Serial splints are utilized to achieve a slow, progressive increase in motion by progressive remolding.
2. Hand/wrist based splints may be dorsal or volar.
   a. Cock-up splints.
      (1) Supports the wrist in 10°–20° of extension to prevent contracture.
      (2) Allows the digits to function (e.g., to support flaccid wrist).
   b. Resting hand splint.
      (1) Utilized for persons who need to have their wrist, digits, and thumb supported in a functional position for prolonged periods, i.e., when developing contracture of the long flexors.
   c. Opponens splints.
      (1) May be short or long.
      (2) Designed to support the thumb in a position of abduction and opposition.
      (3) Utilized during functional activities to compensate for weakness patterns.
3. Types of inhibitory/tone normalizing orthoses.
   a. Based on the neurophysiologic frames of reference.
   b. Bobath finger spreader (abduction splint).
      (1) This soft splint positions the digits and thumb in abduction in an effort to reduce tone.
   c. Rood cone.
      (1) Based on Rood's inhibitory principles of sustained deep pressure.
      (2) This cone-shaped splint is utilized to reduce flexor spasticity in the hand.
   d. Orthokinetic splints.
      (1) This type of splint utilizes tactile input (e.g., via elastic bandages) to facilitate and/or inhibit appropriate muscle groups.
   e. Spasticity reduction splint.
      (1) This splint places the spastic distal extremity on submaximal stretch to reduce spasticity.
4. Types of supportive orthoses.
   a. Overhead suspension sling.
      (1) This orthotic device incorporates an arm support that is supported by a sling and suspended by an overhead rod.
      (2) Persons presenting with proximal weakness (amyotrophic lateral sclerosis, Guillian-Barré syndrome, muscular dystrophy) with muscle grades in the 1/5 to 3/5 range are appropriate candidates.
   b. Balanced forearm orthoses (mobile arm supports or ball-bearing forearm orthoses).
      (1) Consists of an arm trough, proximal and distal arms, and a support bracket.
      (2) Allows a patient with weak proximal musculature to utilize available control of the trunk and shoulder to engage in functional tasks.
   c. Shoulder slings.
      (1) Utilized to support a flaccid arm after neurologic insult for short and controlled periods of time.
      (2) Long-term use may be detrimental in terms of soft-tissue contracture, edema, and the development of pain syndromes.
   d. Supports may be utilized on a wheelchair to position a flaccid arm (e.g., lapboards, arm troughs, etc.).

Splinting Considerations

1. Wearing schedules must be prescribed to enhance the function of the splint.
   a. Splints that are utilized to decrease spasticity or reverse contractures require longer wearing times.
2. Splints must be monitored for pressure over bony prominences.
3. Donning/doffing procedures should be reviewed with individuals and caretakers and be documented.
4. The appropriate material must be chosen by the inclusion of necessary characteristics including resistance to stretch, memory, conformability/drape, rigidity/flexibility, and self-adherence.
5. Refer to Chapter 11 for additional splinting information.

Oral Motor Dysfunction

Presenting Characteristics

1. May result in speech impairments (dysarthria), swallowing impairments (dysphagia), or psychosocial stresses related to facial asymmetry and/or drooling.

Evaluation

1. Range of motion, strength, and tone of the lips, cheeks, and tongue.
2. Extra- and intra-oral sensation.
3. Dentition (e.g., integrity of teeth, denture fit, etc.).
4. Oral control of bolus includes the following abilities.
   a. Contain the bolus in the oral cavity.
   b. Form a cohesive bolus.
   c. Propel the bolus posteriorly into the pharynx.
5. The presence of a swallow reflex.
   a. Laryngeal elevation when the larynx rises to approximate the epiglottis and protect the airway.
   b. Soft-palate elevation when the soft palate rises to close off the naso-pharynx to prevent food/liquid from entering the nasal cavity.
   c. Pharyngeal peristalsis when peristaltic "waves" of muscle contraction propel food through the pharynx.
6. Airway protection via the following mechanisms.
   a. Gag reflex which expels a bolus that is too large from entering the pharynx.
   b. Volitional and spontaneous cough is utilized to clear the pharynx of residual material.
   c. Vocal fold adduction closes off the airway and prevents food from entering the larynx.
   d. Reflexive inhibition of respiration which prevents inhalation of food into the airway.
7. Relaxation of the esophageal sphincter.
8. Primitive reflexes.
   a. Rooting reflex.
      (1) Tested by lightly stroking from the corner of the mouth along the cheek in a direction toward the ear.
      (2) A normal response is no reaction.
      (3) A pathological response includes head turning and tongue protrusion toward the direction of the stimulus.
   b. Jaw jerk.
      (1) The center of the mandible is firmly tapped 1–2 times.
      (2) A normal response is no reaction.
      (3) A pathological response is a reflexive jaw closure/opening response.
   c. Bite reflex.
      (1) A tongue depressor is placed lightly between the upper and lower teeth.
      (2) A reflexive bite indicates pathology.
   d. ATNR/STNR.
9. Cranial nerve testing (Table 12-4).
10. Objective testing; i.e., Modified Barium Swallow/Videofluoroscopy, FEES (fiberoptic endoscopic evaluation of swallowing) may be required depending on consistency of bedside evaluation and/or departmental procedures.

Intervention

1. Direct therapy involves techniques that utilize a bolus.
   a. Modification of consistency, amount, and pacing of solids and liquids.
   b. Utilizing postural interventions to increase swallowing efficiency during meals.
      (1) Chin tuck.
      (2) Forward head tilt/chin tuck.
      (3) Head turn.
   c. Utilizing specific swallowing adaptations.
      (1) Supraglottic swallow technique to voluntarily close/protect the airway during food intake.
      (2) Mendlesohn's maneuver (voluntarily prolonging the rise of the larynx by prolonging tongue contraction).

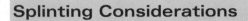

Table 12-4

Cranial Nerves

NUMBER/NAME	FUNCTION	TESTING PROCEDURE
I. Olfactory	Sensory: Carries impulse for sense of smell.	Person is asked to sniff various aromatic substances.
II. Optic	Sensory: Carries impulses for vision.	Eye-chart testing, visual field testing.
III. Oculomotor	Motor: Fibers to the superior, inferior, and medial rectus muscles of the eye and to the smooth muscle controlling lens shape. Medial and vertical eye movements. Sensory: Proprioception of the eye.	Pupil sizes are compared for shape and equality, pupillary reflex is tested; visual tracking is tested.
IV. Trochlear	Proprioceptor and motor fibers for superior oblique muscle of the eye. Downward and inward eye movements.	Tested with cranial nerve III relative to following moving objects.
V. Trigeminal	Motor and sensory for face, conducts sensory impulses from mouth, nose, eyes; motor fibers for muscles of mastication. Control of jaw movements.	Pain, touch, and temperature are tested with proper stimulus; corneal reflex tested with a wisp of cotton; person is asked to move jaw through full ranges of motion.
VI. Abducens	Motor and proprioceptor fibers to/from lateral rectus muscle. Lateral eye movements.	Tested in conjunction with cranial nerve III relative to moving eye laterally.
VII. Facial	Mixed (sensory and motor): sensory fibers to taste buds and anterior ⅔ tongue; motor fibers to muscles of facial expression and to salivary glands.	Check: symmetry of face, ask person to attempt various facial expressions; sweet, salty, sour, and bitter substances are applied to tongue to test tasting ability.
VIII. Vestibulocochlear	Sensory: Transmits impulses for senses of (Acoustic) equilibrium and hearing.	Hearing is checked with a tuning fork.
IX. Glossopharyngeal	Motor fibers for pharynx and salivary glands; sensory fibers for pharynx and posterior tongue. Taste sensation for sweet, bitter, and sour.	Gag and swallow reflexes are checked; posterior one third of tongue is tested for taste.
X. Vagus	Sensory/motor impulses for larynx and pharynx; parasympathetic motor fibers supply smooth muscles of abdominal organs; sensory impulses from viscera.	Tested in conjunction with cranial nerve IX.
XI. Spinal Accessory	Sensory/motor fibers for sternocleidomastoid, trapezius muscles, muscles of soft palate, pharynx, and larynx. Movement of neck and shoulders.	Sternocleidomastoid and trapezius muscle testing.
XII. Hypoglossal	Motor/sensory fibers to/from tongue. Movement of tongue.	Ask person to stick out tongue, positional abnormalities are noted.

2. Indirect therapy involves procedures that do not include use of a bolus.
   a. Thermal (cold) stimulation provides sensory input to the inferior faucial arches via a chilled dental examination mirror to elicit a swallow reflex.
   b. Reflex facilitation.
   c. Strengthening, facilitation, and coordination of oral movements.
   d. Airway adduction procedures.
   e. Positioning to maintain the trunk/head/neck in correct postures.
3. See Chapter 9 for further information on dysphagia and swallowing disorders.

Limb and Postural Control Impairments

Overview of Constraint Induced Movement Therapy (CIMT)

1. A task oriented approach that utilizes constraint induced movement therapy for those who present with control of the wrist and digit can be used.
2. Current and past protocols have used the following motor control inclusion criteria for the more affected side.
   a. 20° of extension of the wrist and 10° of extension of each finger or
   b. 10° extension of the wrist, 10° abduction of the thumb, and 10° extension of any two other digits, or
   c. Able to lift a wash rag off a table top using any type of prehension and then release it.

CIMT Intervention Guidelines

1. Massed practice and shaping of the affected limb during repetitive functional activities is the main focus of therapeutic intervention.
   a. In addition, the less affected upper extremity is constrained via a splint, sling, or glove to remind the person who is undergoing the intervention to utilize the more affected side throughout the day and in therapy.
      (1) In essence, intervention is designed to "force use" of the more affected side.
2. An environment that utilizes the common challenges of everyday life is created by the therapist.
   a. In this environment, the practicing of functional tasks or close simulations that have been identified as important by participants is used to find effective and efficient strategies for performance.
3. Opportunities for practice outside of therapy time (e.g., homework assignments, circuit training, etc.) are provided.
4. Adaptations to the environment, task modifications, assistive technology, and/or a reduction in the effects of gravity are used to enhance occupational performance.
5. Use contemporary motor learning principles in training or retraining skills such as using random and variable practice within natural contexts in treatment, providing decreasing amounts of physical and verbal guidance, helping the client develop problem-solving skills so that he/she can find their own solutions to occupational performance problems are also used.
6. For persons with poor control of movement (e.g., incoordination, tremor, ataxia, dysmetria, etc.), the degrees of freedom are constrained to enhance performance.

Ayres Sensory Integration® Approach for Sensory Processing Disorders[2]

Overview

1. A sensory integrative approach to view the neural organization of sensory information for an adaptive response.
2. The Ayres sensory integration approach was developed by A. Jean Ayres.

Principles/Assumptions of Ayres Sensory Integration® Approach

1. Plasticity (structural changes) of the central nervous system (CNS) allows for modification of the CNS.
2. Sensory integration occurs in a developmental sequential manner.
3. Higher cortical processing functions are dependent on adequate processing and organization of sensory stimuli by lower brain centers.
4. Adequate modulation of sensory stimuli must occur for an adaptive response to occur.
   a. Sensory stimuli can be either facilitory or inhibitory, and each sensory system influences other sensory systems.
5. Adaptive responses facilitate the integration of sensory stimuli.
6. Individuals seek out sensorimotor experiences that have an organizing effect.

[2] Jan Garbarini and Marge Boyd contributed this section on Ayres sensory integration approach.

Evaluation for Sensory Processing Disorders

1. Sensory Integration and Praxis Tests (SIPT).
   a. Standardized tests for children 4 to 8.11 years of age.
      (1) Seventeen tests primarily address the relationship among tactile processing, vestibular-proprioceptive processing, visual perception, and practic ability.
      (2) Test scoring requires either computerized scoring by the publishing company or use of a software program purchased from the publisher.
   b. Categorized into four overlapping groups.
      (1) Measures of tactile and vestibular-proprioceptive sensory processing.
      (2) Tests of form and space perception and visual-motor coordination.
      (3) Tests of practic ability.
      (4) Measures of bilateral integration and sequencing.
   c. Administration and interpretation of the SIPT *requires* certification.
2. DeGangi-Berk Test of Sensory Integration (TSI).
   a. A standardized test for children 3 to 5 years of age.
   b. Measures sensory integrative function with focus on the vestibluar system.
   c. Categorized into three areas: bilateral motor coordination, postural control, and reflex integration.

3. Test of Sensory Functions in Infants.
   a. A standardized test for children 1–18 months of age.
   b. Assesses the level of an infant's sensory responsiveness to a variety of sensory stimuli.
4. Sensory Processing Measure (SPM).
   a. A test for elementary school age children.
   b. Measures sensory processing, praxis, and social participation across different environments.
   c. Assesses visual, auditory, tactile, olfactory-gustatory, proprioceptive, and vestibular behaviors.
   d. The Home Form is completed by the primary caregiver, the Main Classroom Form is completed by the primary classroom teacher, and the School Environments Form is completed by other school personnel involved with the child in other settings (e.g., art/music/physical education class, bus, cafeteria, playground).
5. Sensory profile.
   a. See Chapter 5.
6. Additional tests assess sensorimotor components indicative of sensory processing deficits.
   a. Informal assessment and observation.
      (1) Consider the context of standardized tests along with informal observations.
      (2) Clinical observations, although unpublished and nonstandardized, are commonly used.
      (3) Classroom, playground, home observations.
   b. Assess certain reflexes, crossing body midline, bilateral coordination, and muscle tone.
   c. Interview parents and teachers.

Intervention

1. General application principles for Ayres Sensory Integration® Approach. The occupational therapist:
   a. Controls sensory input that is child-driven and play-based to improve sensory processing, facilitate sensory integration, and elicit an adaptive response.
   b. Creates an environment to facilitate active participation for the "just right challenge."
   c. Ensures registration of meaningful sensory input to obtain an adaptive response.
   d. Balances structure and freedom, tapping into the child's inner drive to obtain neural organization.
   e. Gradually introduces activities requiring more mature and complex patterns of behaviors.
   f. Promotes organized adaptive responses to enhance a child's general behavioral organization, including socialization.
2. Intervention principles for specific sensory processing deficits.
   a. The occupational therapist generally grades for the appropriate combination of the type of movement, rate of movement, and amount of proprioceptive resistance.
      (1) Firm pressure and resistance is less threatening than light touch; see subsequent proprioceptive section.
      (2) Linear movement is less threatening than angular; see subsequent vestibular section.
      (3) Slow movement is less threatening than rapid movement; see subsequent vestibular section.
   b. A combination of stimuli must be used to elicit an adaptive response and for effective intervention.
      (1) This combination is a starting point for children with severe processing deficits.
   c. The therapist closely observes child's responses and adheres to all precautions.
   d. Intervention for tactile deficits.
      (1) Tactile modulation for tactile defensiveness, hypersensitivity/over-responsivity; hyposensitivity/under-responsivity and sensory seeking.
         (a) Self-applied stimuli are more tolerable than passive application of tactile stimuli.
         (b) Provide firm pressure making sure that the child can see the source of the stimuli that is being applied. Firm pressure tends to be calming, while light touch can be perceived aversive. The face, abdomen, and palmar surfaces of the extremities are particularly sensitive to light touch.
         (c) Provide controlled sensory activities that simultaneously provide tactile and vestibular-proprioceptive information.
         (d) Begin with slow linear movements and deep touch-pressure.
         (e) Apply tactile stimuli in the direction of hair growth which is less aversive.
         (f) Follow tactile stimuli with joint compression.
         (g) Monitor and adjust stimuli that seem to influence modulation of stimuli; e.g., lighting, sound, etc.
         (h) Be alert and assess the child's behavioral responses up to a few hours following treatment when negative impacts may still be demonstrated.
         (i) Tactile defensiveness and sensory-seeking can be reduced if the treatment approach is effective.
      (2) Tactile discrimination.
         (a) Provide deep touch pressure to the hands as well as the body.
         (b) Deficits in tactile discrimination are rarely seen in isolation, and somatodyspraxia is typically seen; therefore, treatment for tactile discrimination is usually performed simultaneously when providing treatment for deficits in motor planning.
         (c) Provide graded activities requiring tactile discrimination activities using a mixture of textures and items.

e. Intervention for proprioception deficits.
   (1) Deficits in modulation demonstrated by over-responsivity, under-responsivity, and sensory seeking.
      (a) Provide firm touch, pressure, joint compression, or traction.
      (b) Provide resistance to active movement to help the child learn the appropriate amount of force to perform tasks.
      (c) Provide activities in various body positions combining vestibular proprioceptive information (e.g., yoga).
      (d) Provide slow linear movement, resistance, and deep pressure.
      (e) Use adaptive techniques (e.g., weighted vests).
   (2) Discrimination deficits.
      (a) Provide treatment as noted above.
      (b) Provide activities requiring the child to demonstrate the ability to grade the force or efforts of movement.
f. Intervention for vestibular deficits.
   (1) Deficits in modulation of vestibular input include over-responsivity, under-responsivity, hypersensitivity (aversion response), sensory seeking, and gravitational insecurity (fear response).
      (a) Grade for type and rate of movement and for the amount of resistance.
         • Precautions must be observed.
      (b) Slowly introduce linear movement with touch pressure in prone and provide resistance to active movements, especially for gravitational insecurity.
      (c) Use linear vestibular stimuli to increase awareness of spatial orientation (otolith organ).
      (d) Provide rapid rotary and angular movements with frequent starts/stops and acceleration/deceleration to increase ability to distinguish the pace of movement (semicircular canals).

3. Special advanced training and knowledge of the effects of various sensory stimuli is required.
   a. A therapist must be well aware of precautions for movements, as their impact may not be apparent for several hours.
   b. Continually ask how the child is feeling and observe for signs involving the autonomic nervous system such as pupil dilation, sweaty palms, and changes in the rate of respiration.
   c. Provide a safe physical and emotionally supportive environment for the child.
4. Provide compensatory skill development; e.g., environmental adaptations, hand writing supports.
5. Reduce environmental barriers and identify facilitators of occupational performance.
6. Use group treatment to develop the social interaction skills needed for improved occupational performance in a classroom, with peer groups, and/or in afterschool programs.
7. Consult with and/or educate teachers and parents.
8. Share strategies to promote the child's occupational performance in the home, school and community.

References

Anzalone, M. E., & Lane, S. J. (2012). Sensory processing disorder. In S. J. Lane & A. C. Bundy. *Kids can be kids: A childhood occupations approach*, (pp. 437–459). Philadelphia: F.A. Davis.

Asher, I. E. (Ed.). (2007). *Occupational therapy assessment tools: An annotated index*, 3rd ed. Bethesda, MD: AOTA Press.

Bundy, A. C., & Murray, E. A. (2002). Sensory integration: A. Jean Ayres' theory revisited. In A. C. Bundy, S. J. Lane, & E. A. Murray (Eds.), *Sensory integration: Theory and practice*, 2nd ed. (pp. 3–33). Philadelphia: F.A. Davis.

Gillen, G. (2009). *Cognitive and perceptual rehabilitation: Optimizing function.* St. Louis, MO: Elsevier/Mosby.

Gillen, G. (Ed.). (2011). *Stroke rehabilitation: A function-based approach*, 3rd ed. St. Louis, MO: Elsevier/Mosby.

Gillen, G. & Scaffa M. E. (Eds.), *Willard and Spackman's occupational therapy*, 12th ed. (pp. 816–868). Philadelphia: Lippincott, Williams & Wilkins.

Gutman, S. A., & Schonfeld, A. B. (2009). *Screening adult neurologic populations: A step-by-step instruction manual*, 2nd ed. Bethesda, MD: AOTA Press.

Haynes, C. J. (2007). Sensory assessments. In I. E. Asher (Ed.), *Occupational therapy assessment tools: An annotated index*, 3rd ed. (pp. 421–454). Bethesda, MD: AOTA Press.

Katz, N. (2011). *Cognition, occupation, and participation across the life span: Neuroscience, neurorehabilitation, and models of intervention in occupational therapy*, 3rd ed. Bethesda, MD: AOTA Press.

Lane, S. J. (2002). Sensory modulation. In A. C. Bundy, S. J. Lane, & E. A. Murray, (Eds.), *Sensory integration: Theory and practice*, 2nd ed. (pp. 101–122). Philadelphia: F.A. Davis.

Lane, S. J. (2002). Structure and function of the sensory systems. In A. C. Bundy, S. J. Lane, & E. A. Murray (Eds.), *Sensory integration: Theory and practice*, 2nd ed. (pp. 35–70). Philadelphia: F.A. Davis.

Lane, S. J., Smith Roley, S., & Champagne, T. (2014). Sensory integration and processing: Theories and applications to occupational performance. In B. Schell, G. Gillen, & M. E. Scaffa (Eds.). *Willard and Spackman's occupational therapy,* 12th ed. (pp. 816–868). Philadelphia: Lippincott, Williams & Wilkins.

Miller, L. J. (2007). *Sensational kids hope and help for children with sensory processing disorder (SPD).* New York: G.P. Putnam & Sons.

Parham, L. D., & Mailoux, Z. (2005). Sensory integration. In J. Case-Smith (Ed.), *Occupational therapy for children,* 5th ed. (pp. 356–409). St. Louis, MO: Elsevier Mosby.

Schmidt, R. A. & Lee, T. D. (2011). *Motor control and learning: A behavioral emphasis,* 5th ed. Champaign, Il: Human Kinetics.

Schultz-Krohn, W., & Pendleton, H. (Eds.) (2013). *Pedretti's occupational therapy: Practice skills for physical dysfunction,* 6th ed. St. Louis, MO: Elsevier Science/Mosby.

Shumway-Cook, A., & Woollacott, M. H. (2012). *Motor control: Translating research into clinical practice,* 4th ed. Baltimore: Lippincott Williams and Wilkins.

Vining-Radomski, M., & Trombly-Latham, C. A. (2007). *Occupational therapy for physical dysfunction,* 6th ed. Baltimore: Williams & Wilkins.

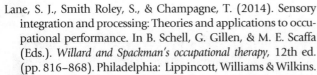

Review Questions

Neurological Approaches: Evaluation and Intervention

Below are five questions about key content covered in this chapter. These questions are not inclusive of the entirety of content about occupational therapy evaluation and intervention approaches for neurological disorders that you must know for success on the NBCOT exam. These questions are provided to help you "jump start" the thought processes you will need to apply your studying of content to the answering of exam questions; hence they are not in the NBCOT exam format. Exam items in the NBCOT format which cover the depth and breadth of content you will need to know to pass the NBCOT exam are provided on this text's disc. The answers to the below questions are provided in Appendix 4.

1. What level of motor control must be present for a person to be a candidate for CIMT?

2. What is the correct procedure to evaluate the severity of spasticity in a muscle or group of muscles?

3. What is the purpose of applying a static orthosis (splint) to an affected body part?

4. You are working with a client with hemiplegia after a brain tumor resection. The client is learning to transfer using a tub bench for the first time. Thus, the person is at the cognitive stage of learning. According to principles of motor learning, what types of interventions would be appropriate to teach this transfer skill at this stage of learning?

5. You receive a referral for occupational therapy services for a toddler. The parents report that the toddler dislikes changes to daily routines, meeting strangers, and being touched. During your evaluation, you observe that the toddler does not like to move or explore unfamiliar objects and toys. Upon analysis of evaluation results, you determine that the toddler is over-responsive to sensory stimuli and avoids all sensory experiences. According to the principles of Ayres Sensory Integration® approach, what types of sensory stimuli should you introduce during interventions with this toddler and how should you structure your initial intervention sessions? Explain your rationale.

13

Cognitive-Perceptual Approaches: Evaluation and Intervention

GLEN GILLEN

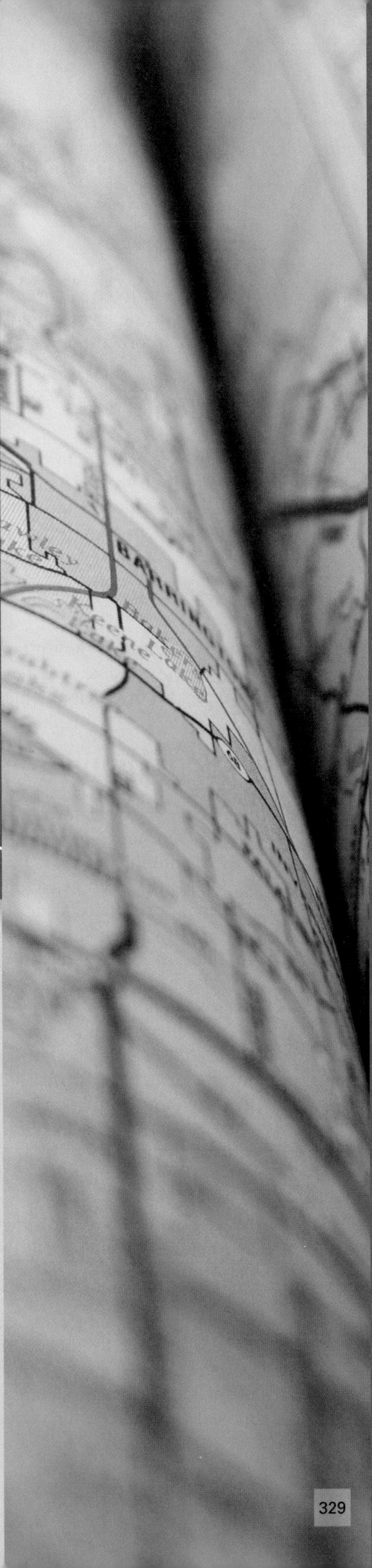

Chapter Outline

Overview of Cognitive-Perceptual Terminology/Symptoms

Perception

1. The integration/interpretation of sensory impressions received from the environment into psychologically meaningful information.

Cognition

1. The ability of the brain to process, store, retrieve, and manipulate information. It involves the skills of understanding and knowing, the ability to judge and make decisions, and an overall environmental awareness.

Cognitive-Perceptual Deficits

1. Occur as a result of multiple pathologies including CVA, TBI, neoplasms, acquired diseases, psychiatric disorders, and/or developmental disabilities.

Functional Impairments

1. Impaired alertness or arousal.
   a. The person has a decreased response to environmental stimuli.
2. Astereognosis, also known as tactile agnosia.
   a. The inability to recognize objects, forms, shapes, and sizes by touch alone.
   b. A failure of tactile recognition although sensation (i.e., touch and proprioception) when tested is intact.
3. Impaired attention.
   a. An inability to attend to or focus on specific stimuli.
   b. May result in distraction by irrelevant stimuli.
   c. Includes difficulty with sustained attention and selective attention in addition to difficulty dividing and alternating/switching attention between two tasks.
4. Ideational apraxia.
   a. A breakdown in the knowledge of what is to be done or how to perform.
   b. A lack of knowledge regarding object use.
   c. The neuronal model about the concept of how to perform is lost although the sensorimotor system may be intact.
5. Motor apraxia/ideomotor apraxia.
   a. Loss of access to kinesthetic memory so that purposeful movement cannot be achieved because of ineffective motor planning although sensation, movement, and coordination are intact.
6. Long-term memory loss.
   a. Lack of storage, consolidation, and retention of information that has passed through working memory.
   b. Includes the inability to retrieve this information.
7. Short-term memory loss.
   a. Lack of registration and temporary storing of information received by various sensory modalities.
   b. Includes the loss of working memory.
8. Impaired organization/sequencing.
   a. The inability to organize thoughts with activity steps properly sequenced.
9. Right-left indiscrimination.
   a. Inability to discriminate between the right and left sides of the body or to apply the concepts of right and left to the environment.
10. Body scheme disorders.
    a. Loss of awareness of body parts, as well as the relationship of the body parts to each other and objects.
    b. Includes body neglect and asomatognosia.
11. Spatial relations impairment.
    a. Difficulty relating objects to each other or to the self secondary to a loss of spatial concepts (up/down, front/back, under/over, etc.).
12. Asomatognosia.
    a. A body scheme disorder that results in diminished awareness of body structure, and a failure to recognize body parts as one's own.
13. Topographical disorientation.
    a. Difficulty finding one's way in space secondary to memory dysfunction or an inability to interpret sensory stimuli.
14. Unilateral body neglect.
    a. Failure to respond to or report unilateral stimulus presented to the body side contralateral to the lesion.
15. Unilateral spatial neglect.
    a. Inattention to, or neglect of, stimuli presented in the extrapersonal space contralateral to the lesion.
       (1) This can include near and/or far extrapersonal space.
    b. May occur independently of visual deficits.
16. Figure/ground dysfunction.
    a. An inability to distinguish foreground from background.
17. Anosognosia.
    a. An unawareness of motor deficit.
    b. May be related to a lack of insight regarding disabilities.

18. Perseveration.
    a. The continuation or repetition of a motor act (premotor perseveration) or task (prefrontal perseveration).
19. Acalculia.
    a. The acquired inability to perform calculations.
20. Alexia.
    a. The acquired inability to read.
21. Agraphia.
    a. The acquired inability to write.
22. Impaired problem solving.
    a. The inability to manipulate a fund of knowledge and apply this information to new or unfamiliar situations.
23. Disorientation.
    a. Lack of knowledge of person, place, situation, and time.
24. Anomia.
    a. Loss of the ability to name objects or retrieve names of people.
25. Broca's aphasia.
    a. Loss of expressive language indicated by a loss of speech production.
26. Wernicke's aphasia.
    a. A deficit in auditory comprehension that affects semantic speech performance, manifested in paraphasia or nonsensical syllables.
27. Global aphasia.
    a. The symptoms of global aphasia are those of severe Broca's aphasia and Wernicke's aphasia combined. There is an almost total reduction of all aspects of spoken and written language, in expression as well as comprehension.
28. Agnosia.
    a. A loss of ability to recognize objects, persons, sounds, shapes, or smells while the specific sense is not defective nor is there any significant memory loss.
29. Executive dysfunction or dysexecutive syndrome.
    a. Impairments related to multiple specific functions; such as, decision making, problem solving, planning, task switching, modifying behavior in the light of new information, self-correction, generating strategies, formulating goals, and sequencing complex actions.

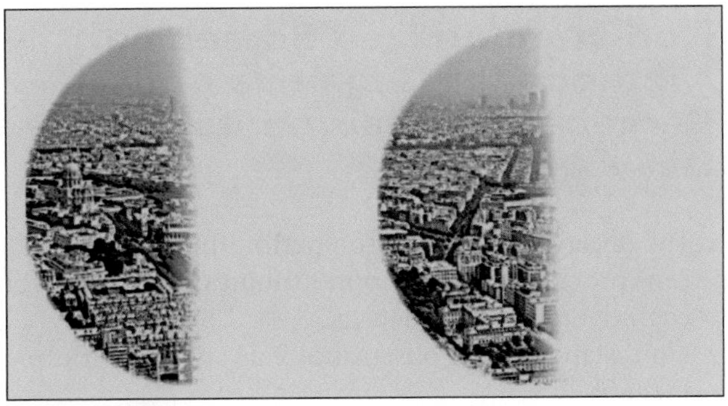

Figure 13-1 Right homonymous hemianopsia. Retrieved from Hemianopsia (2012) http://en.wikipedia.org/wiki/File:Lhvf.png

Visual Foundation Skills

1. These skills must be evaluated to differentiate perceptual dysfunction and visual system deficits.
   a. Visual acuity.
      (1) The clarity of vision both near and far.
   b. Visual fields.
      (1) The available vision to the right, left, superior, and inferior.
      (2) An example of field loss is right homonymous hemianopsia (the right temporal field and left nasal field are affected). See Figure 13-1.
   c. Oculomotor function.
      (1) Control of eye movements.
   d. Scanning.
      (1) Ability to systematically observe and locate items in the environment.

Cognitive-Perceptual Evaluation

Overview

1. The NBCOT examination may include a description of evaluation methods and/or the names of specific assessment tools; therefore, a review of major cognitive-perceptual assessments is important for examination preparation.
   a. This can also increase understanding and knowledge of common approaches in the evaluation of cognition and perception.
   b. This can further strengthen the clinical reasoning skills needed to answer examination questions that address evaluation.
2. As of the publication of this text, NBCOT has not made public the names of all of the specific assessments that may be on the examination.
   a. The assessments included in this chapter are based on the author's review of NBCOT self-assessment tools, major OT textbooks, and feedback obtained from OT practitioners regarding measures used in practice.

Non-standardized Screening Methods for Cognitive and Perceptual Impairments during Daily Activities

1. The observation of a person performing routine tasks can provide multiple opportunities to screen for cognitive-perceptual deficits.
2. Non–standardized observations during daily routine include:
   a. Alertness or arousal: when impaired, the person requires sensory cues to maintain arousal such as a loud voice, tactile stimulation, and/or vestibular input.
      (1) The person appears lethargic or may fall asleep during ADL performance.
   b. Attention: attentional deficits can be observed according to the multiple components of attention.
      (1) Sustained attention: when impaired, the person is not able to attend to long conversations, instructions, class lessons, television shows, or movies.
      (2) Selective attention: when impaired, the person has difficulty processing and filtering of relevant information in the presence of irrelevant stimuli, e.g., studying outside with the noise of traffic and children playing.
      (3) Divided attention: when impaired, the person is unable to do two tasks at the same time, e.g., make toast and tea at the same time.
      (4) Attentional switching: when impaired, the person has difficulty switching attention from one task to another, e.g., going from typing a paper to answering the phone and then back to typing.
   c. Body neglect: when evident, the person does not attend to one side of the body, e.g., the person dresses one side of the body or shaves one side of the face (usually the left).
      (1) The person does not incorporate the involved limbs into activities such as bed mobility or sandwich making.
   d. Ideational apraxia: when evident, the person uses objects incorrectly (e.g., using a hairbrush as a toothbrush), cannot sequence the steps of an activity (e.g., meal preparation), and/or may not engage in task.
   e. Motor/ideomotor apraxia: when evident, the person appears "clumsy," has difficulties crossing midline and with manipulation activities (e.g., manipulating coins), uses awkward grasp pattern to answer the phone, has difficulty with bilateral activities (e.g., folding a sheet).
   f. Perseveration: when evident, the person repeats the same motor act such as continuing to wash one arm or continuing to pull up a sock that already covers the foot, has difficulty terminating a hand to mouth pattern when the plate or bowl is empty, repeats the same task (e.g., dress, undress, dress, undress).
   g. Sequencing and organization: when impaired, steps of the task are not in a logical order (e.g., putting on shoes and socks before pants) or steps of the activity are left out such as washing dishes without soap.
   h. Somatagnosia when impaired, the person attempts to dress the therapist's arm, they may attempt to brush the teeth of his/her mirror image.
   i. Spatial neglect: when evident, the person cannot find food on one side of the plate or the phone on one side of the desk (usually the left side) or cannot balance a check book (e.g., the number $1,550.00 may be perceived as 50.00).
      (1) The person gets lost easily during ambulation or wheelchair mobility due to only responding to only one side of the environment.
   j. Spatial relations dysfunction: when evident, the person has difficulty with dressing (e.g., orienting a shirt to the body; thus, the shirt is put on backwards or upside down) and/or aligning/moving his/her body in space during a transfer.
      (1) The person is observed undershooting or overshooting when reaching for glasses and/or spilling milk when pouring into a glass.
   k. Visual agnosia: when evident, the person cannot recognize objects (e.g., a glass in a sink).
      (1) Other senses such as touch are required to recognize objects.

Allen Cognitive Level Test

1. Utilized for populations with psychiatric disorders, acquired brain injury, and or dementia.
2. Used as a screening tool to estimate an individual's cognitive level.
3. The person performs three leather lacing stitches progressing in complexity.
4. Allen has developed a six level scale of cognitive function (Level 1 = automatic actions to Level 6 = planned actions). See Chapter 14.

Arnadottir Occupational Therapy Neurobehavioral Evaluation (A-ONE)

1. Utilized in the adult population presenting with cognitive/perceptual (neurobehavioral) deficits by evaluators who have completed A-ONE training.
2. Structured observations of BADL and mobility skills are performed to detect underlying neurobehavioral dysfunction.

3. A system of error analysis is utilized to document the underlying performance components (e.g., neglect, spatial dysfunction, body scheme disorder, apraxia) that have a direct impact on daily living tasks.
4. Scoring.
   a. Functional Independence Scale with 0 = unable to perform to 4 = independent.
   b. Neurobehavioral Specific Impairment Scale with 0 = no neurobehavioral impairment is observed to 4 = unable to perform secondary to neurobehavioral dysfunction.

Assessment of Motor and Process Skills (AMPS)

1. May be administered to persons three years of age and older regardless of diagnoses by evaluators who have completed AMPS training.
2. Examines person's functional competence in two or three familiar and chosen BADL or IADL tasks.
3. Individuals choose activities to perform from a list of over 80 standardized tasks.
4. The therapist observes and documents the motor and process skills that interfere with task performance.
5. Sixteen motor and twenty process skills are scored for each task performed.
   a. Skills are scored from 1 = deficit to 4 = competent.
   b. Final scores account for task difficulty and the therapist's rater severity.
6. A test of occupational performance that is appropriate for those living with a variety of impairments including cognitive and perceptual impairments.

Behavioral Inattention Test

1. Utilized with adults presenting with unilateral neglect.
2. Examines the presence of neglect and its impact on functional task performance.
3. Includes nine activity-based subtests (i.e., picture scanning, menu reading, map navigation, address and sentence copying, card sorting, article reading, telephone dialing, coin sorting, and telling/setting the time).
4. Includes six pen/paper subtests (i.e., line crossing, star cancellation, letter cancellation, figure and shape copying, and line bisection).

Catherine Bergego Scale

1. A standardized checklist to detect presence and degree of unilateral neglect during observation of everyday life situations.
2. The scale also measures self-awareness of behavioral neglect.
3. A functional scale consisting of 10 items related to neglect in everyday life (such as dressing, washing, eating, communicating, exploratory activities and moving around) is used.

Cognistat Neurobehavioral Cognitive Status Examination

1. The Cognistat explores, quantifies, and describes performance in central areas of brain-behavior relations.
   a. This includes level of consciousness, orientation, attention, language, constructional ability, memory, calculations, and reasoning.
2. Usually less than 45 minutes is needed for administration.

Executive Function Performance Test (EFPT)

1. Assesses executive function deficits during the performance of real-world tasks.
   a. Tasks include cooking oatmeal, making a phone call, managing medications, and paying a bill.
2. A structured cueing and scoring system is used to assess initiation, organization, safety, and task completion and to develop cuing strategies.
3. The precursor to the EFPT is the Kitchen Task Assessment (KTA). See Chapter 15.

Lowenstein Occupational Therapy Cognitive Assessment (LOTCA)

1. Utilized for persons who have experienced a stroke, TBI, or tumor.
2. Measures basic cognitive functions that are prerequisite for managing everyday tasks.
3. Consists of 20 subtests in five areas: orientation, visual, spatial perception, visual motor organization, and thinking operations.
4. Abilities are scored from 1 = low ability to 4 = high ability.

Mini-Mental State Examination (MMSE) or Folstein Test

1. A brief 30-point questionnaire test that is used to screen for cognitive impairment.
2. It is commonly used to screen for dementia.

Montreal Cognitive Assessment (MOCA)

1. A screening instrument for mild cognitive dysfunction.
2. It assesses different cognitive domains: attention and concentration, executive functions, memory, language, visuoconstructional skills, conceptual thinking calculations, and, orientation.
3. Time to administer the MoCA is approximately 10 minutes.
4. The total possible score is 30 points; a score of 26 or above is considered normal.

Rivermead Behavioral Memory Test

1. Utilized for persons with memory dysfunction.
2. Offers an initial evaluation of the individual's memory function.
3. Indicates appropriate treatment areas.
4. Monitors memory skills throughout the rehabilitation program.
5. Contains 11 categories with nine subtests.
   a. Each subtest presents a series of items that the person is required to memorize and recall in later assessment.
6. Scoring as follows: 0–9 = severely impaired memory, 10–16 = moderately impaired memory, 17–21 = poor memory, 22–24 = normal.

Rivermead Perceptual Assessment Battery

1. For individuals 16 years and older who are experiencing visual-perceptual deficits after head injury or stroke.
2. Consists of 16 performance tests that assess form and color constancy, object completion, figure-ground, body image, inattention, and spatial awareness.
3. Utilizes deficit-specific tasks in isolation from ADL tasks.
4. Scoring is based on accuracy of task completion and the time taken to complete each task.

Cognitive-Perceptual Intervention

Remedial/Restorative/Transfer of Training Approach

1. Focuses on restoration of components to increase skill.
2. Deficit specific.
3. Targets cause of symptoms.
4. Emphasizes performance components.
5. Assumes improvements in performance components will result in increased skill.
6. Assumes the cerebral cortex is malleable and can reorganize.
7. Utilizes tabletop and computer activities (e.g., memory drills, block designs, parquetry) as treatment modalities.

Compensatory/Adaptive/Functional Approach

1. Involves repetitive practice of functional tasks.
2. Emphasizes modification. For example, modifying clothing closures by using Velcro to replace buttons and/or zippers for those with motor apraxia.
3. Activity choice driven by tasks the person needs or wants to perform.
4. Emphasizes intact skill training.
5. Treats symptoms, not the cause.
6. Utilizes techniques of environmental adaptation (e.g., placing a list of morning care activities on the bathroom mirror for those with memory loss or sequencing issues) and compensatory strategies (e.g., taping lectures in school for those with poor sustained attention).
7. The use of compensatory cognitive strategies requires a level of awareness of deficits.
8. Environmental modifications may be caregiver driven.
9. Treatment is task specific.
10. Utilizes functional tasks (i.e., BADL, IADL, work, and leisure tasks) that the individual desires or is required to perform at discharge as the basis of treatment.

Information Processing Approach

1. Provides information on how the individual approaches the task.
2. Investigates how performance changes with cueing.
3. Standardized cues are given to determine their effect on performance. For example, "Try re-reading the recipe" or "Try speaking the steps out loud."

4. Cues or feedback are utilized to draw attention to relevant features of the task.
5. Investigative questions (e.g., "Why do you think it took so long to get dressed?" or "Do you know why I had to help you balance the checkbook?") are used to provide insight to the underlying deficits.

Dynamic Interactional Approach

1. Emphasizes transfer of information from one situation to the next.
2. Utilizes varying treatment environments.
3. Practice of a targeted strategy with varied tasks and situations (i.e., multicontextual).
4. Emphasizes metacognitive skills (i.e., self-awareness of strengths and deficits) as basis of learning and generalization of learning.
5. Transfer of learning must be taught from one situation to the next and does not occur automatically.
6. Transfer of learning occurs through a graded series of tasks that decrease in similarity (e.g., training scanning strategies for a person with a visual neglect to find items in a refrigerator to a less similar task such as scanning to cross the street).
7. The person's processing abilities and self-monitoring techniques are used to facilitate learning for different tasks or environments.
8. The therapist utilizes awareness questioning (e.g., "How do you know this is right?") to help the individual detect errors, estimate task difficulty, and predict outcomes.

The Quadraphonic Approach

1. Based on remediation.
2. Based on information processing theory and teaching/learning theory.
3. Micro-perspective includes evaluation of management of performance component subskills such as attention, memory, motor planning, postural control, and problem solving.
4. Macro-perspective evaluation includes the use of narratives, interview, real-life occupations (e.g., shopping, cooking, other IADL).
5. Makes use of several theories.
   a. Information processing. For example, for those that are minimally responsive after head injury, determine which type of sensory stimulus the person responds to (e.g., a loud voice, painful tactile stimulus, various aromas).
   b. Teaching/learning evaluation. For example, determining which stage of learning a client is in, determining which environment is most appropriate for treatment (i.e., quiet bedside vs. stimulating OT clinic), and/or determining which cues are most effective (e.g., using more visual/gestural cues for those with aphasia).
   c. Neurodevelopmental evaluation. For example, determining level of postural control, symmetry of movement, mobility, and stability.
   d. Biomechanical evaluation. For example, determining amount of AROM, endurance, strength, coordination.

Neurofunctional Approach

1. Based on learning theory.
2. Specifically used for individuals with acquired neurological impairments.
3. Focuses on retraining real world skills rather than cognitive-perceptual processes.
4. Utilizes an overall adaptive approach but incorporates some remediation components.
5. Treatment is focused on training specific functional skills in true contexts.

Cognitive Disabilities Model

1. Originally developed for use with individuals who have psychosocial dysfunction, currently also being utilized with persons with neurologic dysfunction and dementia.
2. Describes cognitive function on a continuum from level 1 (profoundly impaired) to level 6 (normal).
3. Each level describes the extent of a person's disability and difficulty in performing occupations.
4. After the person's level has been established, routine tasks are presented that the person can perform or that have been adapted so that he/she can perform them.
5. Focus is placed on adaptive approaches and strengthening residual abilities.
6. See Chapter 14.

General Intervention Strategies for Specific Deficits

1. Intervention strategies for impaired alertness or arousal.
   a. Increase environmental stimuli.
   b. Use gross motor activities.
   c. Increase sensory stimuli.
2. Intervention strategies for motor/ideomotor apraxia.
   a. Utilize general verbal cues as opposed to specific.
   b. Decrease manipulation demands.

c. Provide hand over hand tactile-kinesthetic input.
d. Utilize visual cues.
3. Intervention strategies for ideational apraxia.
a. Provide step by step instructions.
b. Use hand over hand guiding techniques.
c. Provide opportunities for motor planning and motor execution.
4. Intervention strategies for perseveration.
a. Bring perseveration to a conscious level and train the person to inhibit the behavior.
b. Redirect attention.
c. Engage the individual in tasks that require repetitive action.
5. Intervention strategies for spatial neglect.
a. Provide graded scanning activities.
b. Grade activities from simple to complex.
c. Use anchoring techniques to compensate (e.g., a strip of red tape of placed on the left side of the sink to draw attention to the left hemi-field).
d. Utilize manipulative tasks in conjunction with scanning activities.
e. Use external cues (e.g., colored markers and written directions).
6. Intervention strategies for body neglect.
a. Provide bilateral activities.
b. Guide the affected side through the activity.
c. Increase sensory stimulation to the affected side.
7. Intervention strategies for aphasia.
a. Decrease external auditory stimuli.
b. Give the individual increased response time.
c. Use visual cues and gestures.
d. Use concise sentences.
e. Investigate the use of augmentative communication devices.
8. Intervention strategies for sequencing and organization deficits.
a. Use external cues (e.g., written directions, daily planners).
b. Grade tasks that are increasingly complex in terms of number of steps required.
9. Intervention strategies for spatial relations dysfunction.
a. Utilize activities that challenge underlying spatial skills (e.g., orienting clothing to your body during dressing, wrapping a gift, making a bed).
b. Utilize tasks that require discrimination of right/left (e.g., use cues such as "dress your left arm first" or "the plates are in the right lower cabinets").
10. Intervention strategies for memory loss.
a. Use rehearsal strategies.
b. "Chunk" information (e.g., for recalling a phone number, the person could chunk the digits into three groups: first, the area code (such as 123), then a three-digit chunk (456), and, last, a four-digit chunk (7890).
c. Utilize memory aids (e.g., smart phones, alarm watches, timers).
d. Utilize "temporal tags," focusing on when the event to be remembered occurred.

References

Gillen, G. (2009). *Cognitive and perceptual rehabilitation: Optimizing function.* St. Louis, MO: Elsevier/Mosby.

Gillen, G. (Ed.). (2011). *Stroke rehabilitation: A function-based approach,* 3rd ed. St. Louis, MO: Elsevier/Mosby.

Gutman, S. A., & Schonfeld, A. B. (2009). *Screening adult neurologic populations: A step-by-step instruction manual,* 2nd ed. Bethesda, MD: AOTA Press.

Katz, N. (2011). *Cognition, occupation and participation across the lifespan: Neuroscience, neurorehabilitation, and models for intervention in occupational therapy,* 3rd ed. Bethesda, MD: AOTA Press.

Schultz-Krohn, W., & Pendleton, H. (Eds.). (2013). *Pedretti's occupational therapy: Practice skills for physical dysfunction,* 7th ed. St. Louis, MO: Elsevier Science/Mosby.

Vining-Radomski, M., & Trombly-Latham, C. A. (2007). *Occupational therapy for physical dysfunction,* 6th ed. Baltimore: Williams & Wilkins.

Review Questions

Cognitive-Perceptual Approaches: Evaluation and Intervention

Below are five questions about key content covered in this chapter. These questions are not inclusive of the entirety of content about cognitive-perceptual evaluation and intervention approaches that you must know for success on the NBCOT exam. These questions are provided to help you "jump start" the thought processes you will need to apply your studying of content to the answering of exam questions; hence they are not in the NBCOT exam format. Exam items in the NBCOT format which cover the depth and breadth of content you will need to know to pass the NBCOT exam are provided on this text's disc. The answers to the below questions are provided in Appendix 4.

1. You are observing a client with apraxia eat breakfast. What behaviors would you most likely observe?

2. Your client presents with unilateral spatial neglect and poor awareness. The client has a supportive partner. What environmental modifications will be useful to maximize performance and safety indoors?

3. What are examples of activities you can use to evaluate components of attention?

4. Your client has left-sided body neglect. Describe the behaviors would you expect to see during the person's morning self-care routine.

5. You are working in acute care with a person with low arousal after a head trauma. Describe approaches and activities that would be useful to include during interventions with this person.

14

Psychosocial Approaches: Evaluation and Intervention

WILLIAM L. LAMBERT, RITA P. FLEMING-CASTALDY, AND JANICE ROMEO

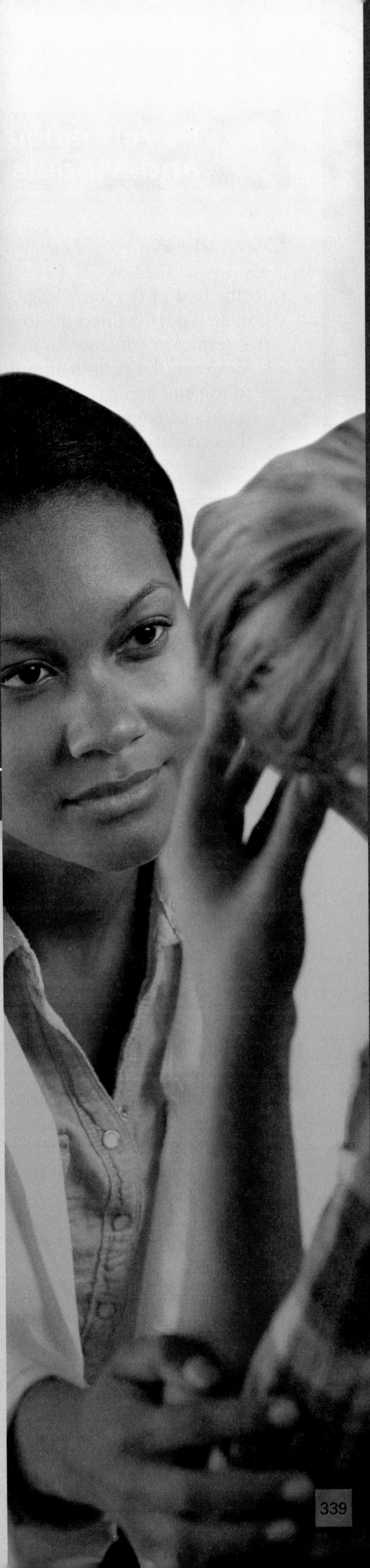

Chapter Outline

Chapter 14

Psychosocial Frames of Reference and Models of Practice

Overview

1. To the best of our knowledge, the NBCOT examination does not ask direct questions about specific theories, frames of reference, or models of practice.
   a. However, the examination does require the ability to use and apply psychosocial theoretical theories, frames of reference, and practice models to guide the occupational therapy process.
2. Information about the major theoretical principles of frames of reference and models of practice is provided because it can be helpful in the analysis of case scenarios and the answering of exam items.
   a. These require clinical reasoning to select assessments, identify factors that enable or limit occupational performance, develop client-centered, occupation based intervention goals, and implement interventions according to a relevant conceptual framework.

Occupational Therapy Frames of Reference

Model of Human Occupation (MOHO)

1. Developed by Gary Kielhofner based on the Occupational Behavior model of Mary Reilly.
2. Principles.
   a. "Occupation is dynamic and context-dependent" (Kielhofner, 2004, p. 151).
   b. Personal occupational choices and engagement in occupation shape the individual.
   c. Three elements are inherent to humans.
      (1) Volition includes thoughts and feelings that motivate people to act and is comprised of personal causation, values, and interests.
      (2) Habituation includes organized, recurring patterns of behavior and is comprised of roles and habits.
      (3) Performance capacity includes the physical and mental skills needed for performance and the subjective experience of engaging in occupation.
   d. The environment impacts on the individual through the opportunities, demands, resources, and constraints it provides.
      (1) The environment is divided into physical and social components.
      (2) Each component is influenced by the culture(s) in which it takes place.
2. Evaluation.
   a. Focuses on exploring the individual's occupational history, goals, volition, habits, and occupational performance.
   b. Many tools have been designed specifically for use with the MOHO (e.g., OCAIRS, OSA); however, any procedure or instrument that provides pertinent information about the environment and the person may be used.
3. Intervention.
   a. Focuses on occupational engagement and includes activities that are purposeful, relevant and meaningful to people and their social context.

Person-Environment-Occupation Model

1. Developed by Charles Christiansen and Carolyn Baum.
2. Principles.
   a. Occupational performance is dynamic in nature.
   b. Occupational performance is considered the outcome of the transactional relationship between people, their occupations, and the environment.
   c. Occupational performance necessarily changes across the lifespan.
3. Evaluation.
   a. Addresses the occupational performance issues that the client identifies.
   b. Emphasizes the environment of the individual to include where he or she lives, works and plays.
   c. Evaluation is client-centered and flexible as there are no specific evaluations.
4. Intervention.
   a. Considers the transactional relationships of occupations with people and their environment to address occupational performance issues and goals.
   b. Recognizes the temporal nature of occupational performance as the person, his or her environment, and occupations are constantly changing.
   c. Offers many avenues for change, as practitioners can be flexible in their choice of intervention strategies.

Life-Style Performance Model

1. Developed by Gail Fidler.
2. Principles.
   a. The Life-Style Performance Model seeks to identify and describe the nature and critical "doing" elements of an environment that support and foster achievement of a satisfying, productive life-style.
   b. It proposes a method for looking at the match between that environment and the individual's needs.
   c. Four hypotheses are proposed.
      (1) "Mastery and competence in those activities that are valued and given priority in one's society or social group have greater meaning in defining one's social efficacy than competence in activities that carry less social significance.
      (2) "A total activity and each of its elements have symbolic as well as reality-based meanings that notably affect individual experiences and motivation.
      (3) "Mastery and competence are more readily achieved, and the sense of personal pleasure and intrinsic gratification is more intense, in those activities that are most closely matched to one's neurobiology and psychological structure.
      (4) "Competence and achievement are most readily seen and verified in the end-product or outcome of an activity; thus, the ability to do, to overcome, and to achieve becomes obvious to self and others" (Fidler, 1996, pp. 115–116).
   d. Performance and quality of life can be enhanced by an environment that provides for ten fundamental human needs.
      (1) Autonomy: self-determination.
      (2) Individuality: self-differentiation.
      (3) Affiliation: evidence of belonging.
      (4) Volition: the having of alternatives.
      (5) Consensual validation: acknowledgment of achievement and verification of perspectives.
      (6) Predictability: discernment and evaluation of cause and effect.
      (7) Self-efficacy: evidence of competence.
      (8) Adventure: exploration of the new and unknown.
      (9) Accommodation: freedom from physical or mental harm and compensation for limitations.
      (10) Reflection: contemplation of events and the meaning of things.
   e. Performance is measured in the quality of functioning in four domains.
      (1) Self-care and maintenance.
      (2) Intrinsic gratification.
      (3) Service to others.
      (4) Reciprocal relationships.
3. Evaluation.
   a. Focuses on obtaining an activity history and a life-style performance profile related to the four skill domains.
   b. Environmental factors are explored.
4. Intervention.
   a. Addresses five main questions that identify the focus of intervention.
      (1) What does the person need to be able to do?
      (2) What is the person able to do?
      (3) What is the person unable to do?
      (4) What interventions are needed, and in what order?
      (5) What are the characteristics and patterns of activity and of the environment that will enhance the person's quality of life?
   b. Any interventions or activities that promote performance in the four domains are acceptable.

Ecology of Human Performance (EHP) Model[1]

1. Developed by Winnie Dunn and colleagues at the University of Kansas Medical Center.
2. Principles.
   a. The EHP model emphasizes the role of an individual's context (i.e., a person's cultural, physical, and social environments) and how the environment impacts a person and his/her task performance.
   b. This model is applicable to people across the life-span.
   c. The four main constructs of this model include the person, tasks, context, and personal-context-task transaction.
   d. There are 11 assumptions of this model.
      (1) Ecology refers to the interaction between a person and his/her environments.
      (2) A person's performance is understood by looking at the relationship between the person, context, and the task.
      (3) Performance occurs when a person acts to engage in tasks within a context.
      (4) Each person is a unique individual with sensorimotor, cognitive, and psychosocial skills and abilities.
      (5) The range of a person's performance is based on the transaction between the person and the context.
      (6) Skills that a person possesses can be increased or decreased due to illness and/or stress; a person's interests and life experiences lead to continually changing variables.

[1]This section was written by Donna Costa, DHS, OTR/L, FAOTA.

(7) Contexts are dynamic rather than static; there is a reciprocal relationship between a person and his/her context where one influences the other.
(8) The roles that a person has in life are made up of tasks; the transactional relationship between the person, task, and context makes up occupations and roles.
(9) There is a difference between a person's performance in his/her natural contexts and simulated experiences.
(10) In the occupational therapy process, people are empowered by increasing their self-determination.
(11) This model defines independence as using the supports in a person's context to meet his/her needs and wants.

3. Evaluation.
   a. Utilizes checklists that were designed along with this model. These include checklists for the person, the environment, task analysis, and personal priorities.
   b. The Sensory Profile. See this chapter's assessment section.
4. Intervention.
   a. Five specific strategies designed to help the person, context, task, or all three are used. These include:
      (1) Establish and restore: enhancing a person's abilities by teaching skills lost due to illness or disability or never learned.
      (2) Alter: assessing a person's contexts to determine which is the best match for the person's abilities.
      (3) Adapt/modify: changing the context or task in some way so that it leads the person to successful performance.
      (4) Prevent: minimizing risks that might develop so that problems in performance do not develop.
      (5) Create: assisting the person by promoting enriching and complex performances in the person's context.

Occupational Adaptation

1. Developed by Janette Schkade and Sally Schultz.
2. Principles.
   a. Occupational adaptation is concerned with the processes that the individual goes through to adapt to his/her environment.
   b. It consists of three elements: the person, the occupational environment, and the interaction between the two.
      (1) The person element consists of the sensorimotor, cognitive, and psychosocial components of the individual.
      (2) The occupation environment is viewed as the physical, social and cultural systems within which work, play/leisure, and self-maintenance take place.
      (3) The outcome of the interaction between the person and the environment is referred to as the occupational response.
   c. The occupational adaptation model makes two basic assumptions.
      (1) "Occupation provides the means by which humans adapt to changing needs and conditions, and the desire to participate in occupation is the intrinsic motivational force leading to adaptation.
      (2) "Occupational adaptation is a normative process that is most pronounced during periods of transition, both large and small. The greater the adaptive transitional needs, the greater the importance of the occupational adaptation process, and the greater the likelihood that the process will be disrupted" (Schkade & Shultz, 1992, pp. 829–830).
3. Evaluation.
   a. Focuses on occupational environment, role expectation, and the individual's potential for adaptation and the best means for adaptation to occur.
4. Intervention.
   a. Focuses on increasing the skills needed for occupational adaptation.
   b. Addresses both the individual and the environment.

Role Acquisition

1. Developed by Ann Mosey.
2. Principles.
   a. The individual employs task and social skills to meet the demands of personally desired and necessary roles.
   b. Performance is addressed through function/dysfunction continuums in seven categories.
      (1) Task skills.
      (2) Interpersonal skills.
      (3) Family interaction.
      (4) Activities of daily living.
      (5) School.
      (6) Work.
      (7) Play/leisure/recreation.
   c. Temporal adaptation addresses the individual's temporal orientation and ability to organize his/her use of time in a need-satisfying manner.
3. Evaluation.
   a. Focuses on gathering data indicative of function/dysfunction in the above categories.
4. Intervention.
   a. Focused on the acquisition of the specific skills an individual needs in order to function in his/her environment.
   b. The principles of learning are used to promote skill development. See Chapter 3's section on tools of practice.

c. General postulates for change are provided to guide the intervention process.
   (1) Long-term goals are set based on the person's expected environment.
   (2) Initially, tasks and interpersonal skills can be taught separately or they can be taught within the context of the learning of social roles.
   (3) An adequate repertoire of behavior is acquired through activities that elicit the desired behavior, are interesting to the client, include socializing, and apply the principles of learning. See Chapter 3.
   (4) Intrapsychic content is shared matter-of-factly with the client and reality testing is provided.
   (5) The occupational therapist must know very specifically what kind of behavior he/she wishes to promote or enhance.

d. Specific postulates are provided for each of the continuums.

e. Any treatment activities or strategies that employ the teaching-learning principles are acceptable.

Cognitive Disabilities

1. Developed by Claudia Allen.
2. Principles.
   a. Based on the stages of cognitive development as described by Piaget and knowledge of the neurobiological sciences at the time of the model's development.
   b. Cognitive ability is determined by biological factors and the potential for improvement is dictated by those factors.
   c. Functional behavior is based on cognition.
   d. If the person's cognitive level cannot change, adapting the activity or task provides opportunities for the individual to succeed.
   e. Once the maximum level has been achieved, compensations must be made biologically, psychologically, or environmentally.
   f. Cognitive performance is placed on a continuum divided into six levels that are further divided into modes.
      (1) Automatic Actions, Level I, are characterized by automatic motor responses and changes in the autonomic nervous system. Conscious response to the external environment is minimal.
      (2) Postural Actions, Level II, are characterized by movement that is associated with comfort. There is some awareness of large objects in the environment, and the individual may assist the caregiver with simple tasks.
      (3) Manual Actions, Level III, are characterized by beginning to use hands to manipulate objects. The individual may be able to perform a limited number of tasks with long-term repetitive training.
      (4) Goal Directed Actions, Level IV, are characterized by the ability to carry simple tasks through to completion. The individual relies heavily on visual cues. He/she may be able to perform established routines but cannot cope with unexpected events.
      (5) Exploratory Actions, Level V, are characterized by overt trial and error problem solving. New learning occurs. This may be the usual level of functioning for 20% of the population.
      (6) Planned Actions, Level VI, are characterized by the absence of disability. The person can think of hypothetical situations and do mental trial-and-error problem solving.
3. Evaluation.
   a. Focus is on identifying the individual's current cognitive abilities and their implications for performance, independence, and the need for assistance.
      (1) The potential for improvement is also considered.
   b. Observation during functional tasks is emphasized.
   c. Several evaluation tools have been developed to assist with the identification of the individual's cognitive level.
      (1) The Allen Cognitive Level Screen-5 (ACLS-5) is a structured task that allows the therapist to observe the individual performing three increasingly complex leather lacing stitches and make determinations about that person's cognitive skill level.
         (a) The Allen Diagnostic Manual provides craft projects that can be used for evaluation as well as treatment that can also be used to determine the individual's level of skills according to the first five levels listed above. (See this chapter's evaluation section.)
      (2) The Routine Task Inventory gathers data about the individual's ADL performance from an informed caregiver. See Chapter 15.
      (3) The Cognitive Performance Test assesses the functional performance of individuals with Alzheimer's disease. The focus is on the identification of the effects that particular deficits have on the performance of ADL.
4. Intervention.
   a. Activities are selected based on the individual's highest cognitive level.
   b. Therapy focuses on maintaining the individual's highest level of function.
   c. Environmental changes and activity adaptations are made to compensate for deficits and allow the greatest degree of independence.

d. The OT practitioner works with the team to develop an appropriate discharge plan.
e. The OT practitioner should meet with the family or other caregivers to develop understanding of the individual's abilities, deficits, and care needs.

Sensory Models[2]

1. This approach in mental health is known by several different terms including sensory integration, sensory processing, sensory motor model, sensory defensiveness, sensory modulation, and sensory based treatment.
2. Based on the work of A. Jean Ayres and originally known as sensory integration.
3. Developed by Lorna Jean King, an occupational therapist who worked with people with schizophrenia and observed that they had disturbances in posture, gait patterns, balance, and hand function.
4. Mildred Ross built upon the work of Lorna Jean King. Ross worked with long-term and regressed psychiatric patients and added movement patterns to the calming and alerting sensory input of King's approach.
   a. Ross' approach is known as the Five Stage Group Model because of the five different kinds of brief activities done within each group. See this chapter's section on intervention groups.
5. Pat and Julia Wilbarger developed an approach for children and adults who they observed exhibiting a specific avoidance pattern which they termed sensory defensiveness.
   a. The Wilbargers developed a treatment protocol that is aimed at reducing these patterns of sensory defensiveness.
      (1) It includes a brushing pattern, along with a sensory diet and education.
6. Winnie Dunn developed the model of sensory processing that looked at how sensory input was processed and then responded to in one of four patterns of neurological thresholds.
   a. Sensory-seeking.
   b. Sensory-avoiding.
   c. Sensory sensitivity.
   d. Low registration.
   e. See Chapter 7 for more detail.
7. Tina Champagne built upon the work of all the above to develop her Sensory Modulation approach for adults.
   a. Sensory modulation approaches are used by occupational therapy practitioners to help prepare, enhance, and/or maintain the person's ability to engage actively in meaningful life roles and activities.
      (1) Approaches include the use of sensory-related assessment tools, sensorimotor activities, sensory modalities, and environmental modifications, and assistance in learning how to self-regulate through the process of self-organization and positive change.
   b. The implementation of a Sensory Modulation Program requires the use of a strengths-based, person-centered and relationship-centered model of care.
      (1) It is essential to assist each individual in recognizing not only symptom(s) and problem areas but also his/her unique strengths which are utilized when following through with the exploration, practice,and integration of sensory modulation approaches into one's daily life.
8. Evaluation.
   a. Assessments used in sensory models include the Adolescent/Adult Sensory Profile and the Allen Cognitive Level Screen. See this chapter's assessment section.
9. Intervention.
   a. The use of sensory based interventions in mental health practice settings is widespread, including an alternative to the use of physical restraints. Methods include:
      (1) Snoezelen rooms, multi-sensory environments, and/or "Comfort Rooms" to calm/alert individuals with psychiatric illness, autism, pervasive developmental disorders, and dementia.
      (2) Therapeutic weighted blankets, dolls, and stuffed animals as a modality for self-soothing.
   b. Psycho-education to increase personal knowledge of how to self-modulate.
   c. Sensory diets including alerting/calming stimuli, and heavy work patterns.

Psychodynamic/Psychoanalytic

1. An early OT frame of reference based on the work of S. Freud, A. Freud, Jung, and Sullivan.
   a. Principle developers were Gail Fidler and Ann Mosey.
   b. Due to the advances in psychiatry, temporal and financial constraints, and the nature of the population served, these approaches are rarely used today.
   c. Proper use of this approach requires further specialized training.
2. Principles.
   a. All behavior is largely determined by unconscious psychological forces and internal processes.
   b. Interaction among these forces creates behavior thoughts and emotions.
   c. Abnormal behavior results when these dynamic forces are in conflict, known as intrapsychic conflict.

[2] This section was written by Donna Costa, DHS, OTR/L, FAOTA.

d. Conflicts are resolved when brought to consciousness and explored.
e. Behavior patterns are believed to begin in early childhood.
f. Individuals may protect themselves from anxiety through the use of defense mechanisms. Some are healthy; some are not.
g. Understanding the function of defensive mechanisms is useful in therapeutic relationships.
h. Defense mechanisms are grouped into a hierarchy according to the phases of maturity associated with them.
   (1) Narcissistic mechanisms.
      (a) Denial: the failure to acknowledge the existence of some aspect of reality that is apparent to others (e.g., an alcohol abuser is unable to acknowledge that his/her problems are a result of drinking).
      (b) Projection: attributing attributes or unacknowledged feelings, impulses or thoughts to others (e.g., someone who feels guilty attributes what others say as blaming him/her).
      (c) Splitting: rigid separating of positive and negative thoughts and of feelings (e.g., staff members may be seen as all good or all bad when variations of behavior are anxiety-provoking).
   (2) Immature mechanisms.
      (a) Passive-aggressive: aggression toward others which is indirectly or unassertively expressed (e.g., a patient is late for a treatment session when he/she is angry with the practitioner).
      (b) Regression: returning to an earlier stage of development to avoid the tension and conflict of the present one (e.g., an individual becomes needy and/or child-like during a period of stress or illness).
      (c) Somatization: the conversion of psychological symptoms into physical illness (e.g., a person who feels stuck in an unhappy marriage develops low back pain).
   (3) Neurotic mechanisms.
      (a) Rationalization: creating self-justifying explanations to hide the real reasons for one's own or another's behavior (e.g., a parent believes a lazy adult child is not working because the job market is poor).
      (b) Repression: blocking from consciousness painful memories and anxiety-provoking thoughts (e.g., an adult child has no memory of being mistreated by a beloved parent).
      (c) Displacement: redirecting an emotion or reaction from one object to a similar but less threatening one (e.g., a child gets angry with his/her parents and hits a younger sibling).
      (d) Reaction formation: the switching of unacceptable impulses into its opposite (e.g., hugging someone you would like to hit).
   (4) Mature mechanisms.
      (a) Humor: using comedy to express feelings and thoughts without provoking discomfort in self and others (e.g., making fun of yourself for coming inappropriately dressed for a specific function).
      (b) Sublimation: redirecting energy from socially unacceptable impulses to socially acceptable activities (e.g., an angry individual channels that anger into aggressive sports play).
      (c) Suppression: consciously or semi-consciously avoiding thinking about disturbing problems, thoughts, or feelings (e.g., cleaning closets and drawers while waiting for the results of medical tests).
i. Appropriate individuals for therapy are non-psychotic with mild to moderate psychopathology, well integrated egos, and the capacity for introspection and insight.

3. Evaluation.
   a. Historically, occupational therapy evaluations using this model included the Fidler Battery, Azima Battery, Goodman Battery, BH Battery, The Magazine Picture Collage and the Comprehensive Assessment Process.
   b. The Magazine Picture Collage continues to be used today, for individual as well as group evaluation. See this chapter's assessment section.
4. Intervention.
   a. Projective and functional tasks are used to promote self-awareness and the identification and exploration of intrapsychic content.
   b. By bringing unconscious conflicts to consciousness, intrapsychic content can lead to intrapsychic conflict resolution.
   c. Due to the advances in psychiatry, the use of more contemporary recovery models, temporal and financial practice setting constraints, and the nature of the population typically served (i.e., people with serious mental illness), these approaches are infrequently used today.
   d. Proper use of this approach requires specialized training and education for those practicing in mental health, including occupational therapists.

Interdisciplinary Mental Health Practice Models

Cognitive Behavioral Frame of Reference/Cognitive Behavioral Therapy (CBT)

1. Relevance to occupational therapy practice.
   a. CBT is widely used in practice today.
      (1) Many of the suggested interventions in this frame of reference fall within the scope of occupational therapists' professional preparation and occupational therapy's domain of practice.
   b. Research has supported CBT as an effective approach for a diversity of clinical populations.
      (1) CBT has been shown to be especially effective in the treatment of individuals with depression.
         (a) Individuals with depression tend to distort reality through dysfunctional thought processes.
         (b) CBT works to alter these individuals' negative thoughts about themselves, the world, and the future by correcting misinterpretations of life events.
      (2) CBT is also used with individuals with schizophrenia, anxiety, bipolar, panic, obsessive-compulsive, personality, somatoform, and eating disorders.
2. Principles.
   a. CBT combines principles of cognitive therapy and behavioral therapy.
      (1) Cognitive therapy looks at a person's thoughts and beliefs, while behavioral therapy looks at a person's actions and attempts to change maladaptive patterns of behavior.
   b. Cognitive restructuring is "a key CBT concept which alters cognitions and cognitive processes in order to facilitate behavioral and emotional changes" (Cara & MacRae, 2005, p. 108).
   c. The three components of cognitive therapy are didactic aspects, cognitive techniques, and behavioral techniques.
      (1) Didactic aspects involve the therapist explaining the basic concepts and principles of CBT to the client.
      (2) Cognitive techniques involve "eliciting automatic thoughts, testing automatic thoughts, identifying maladaptive underlying assumptions, and testing the validity of maladaptive assumptions" (Sadock & Sadock, 2008, p. 462).
      (3) Behavioral techniques are used with cognitive techniques to test and challenge maladaptive and inaccurate cognitions.
   d. A pattern of negative thinking termed the "cognitive triad" is identified.
      (1) This triad is comprised of negative self-evaluation, a pessimistic world view, and a sense of hopelessness regarding the future.
      (2) This triad underlies depression in particular and is evident in other disorders.
   e. Three basic principles of cognitive therapy can help individuals with depression. These include:
      (1) All moods are created by a person's thoughts and the way he/she looks at and interprets situations and events.
      (2) When people are depressed, their thoughts are pervasively negative.
      (3) Research has indicated that negative thoughts which cause emotional distress usually contain distortions.
   f. The development of insight is necessary for growth and change.
      (1) Thinking influences behavior.
      (2) Changing the way a person thinks reduces symptoms.
      (3) Thinking can be self-regulated.
      (4) Change occurs through clients' involvement in learning and developing skills.
3. Evaluation.
   a. The Beck Depression Inventory (BDI-II) is the primary initial evaluation tool.
      (1) The BDI-II s a self-completed questionnaire that assesses level of depression.
      (2) No special training is required to administer this client completed evaluation.
      (3) Interpretation of the results of the BDI-II must be completed by a mental health professional that has completed required training and acquired adequate knowledge about the BDI-II and CBT.
      (4) See this chapter's assessment section.
   b. The evaluation of cognition is frequently completed by occupational therapists.
   c. A variety of evaluation methods and assessments are available for use by occupational therapists in many practice settings. See this chapter's section on assessments and Chapter 13.
4. Intervention.
   a. General postulates for change are used to guide the intervention process.
      (1) Dysfunctional cognitive processes produce psychological disorder.
      (2) Altering a person's cognition can improve psychological health.

(3) Cognitions are the prime cause of psychopathology and therefore are the focus of intervention.
(a) Automatic thoughts cause psychological disorder and through cognitive restructuring these thoughts are brought to awareness to be confronted and facilitate change.

b. Approaches using CBT emphasize the following.
(1) Assisting the client in the identification of current problems and potential solutions.
(2) Using active and collaborative therapist-client interaction as an essential part of the therapeutic process.
(3) Helping the client learn how to identify distorted or unhelpful thinking patterns, recognize and change inaccurate beliefs, and relate to others in more positive ways.
(4) Gaining insight and acquiring skills that "maximize client functioning and quality of life through the development of coping skills and meaningful healthy occupational patterns" (Hemphill-Pearson, 2008, p. 68).
(5) Facilitating the client's active role in the therapeutic process by frequently providing homework and structured assignments as part of the intervention process.
(a) Intervention goals are designed to help the client monitor and refute negative thoughts about themselves.
(6) Scheduling activities.
(a) Increasing mastery and pleasure.
(b) Grading tasks to enable client success.
(7) Cognitive rehearsal.
(8) Self-reliance training.
(a) Self reliance can be facilitated by performing activities of daily living (e.g., making one's bed, doing personal shopping and preparing one's own meals).
(9) Role playing.
(10) Diversion techniques and visual imagery.
(11) Engaging in physical, work, leisure/play, and/or social participation activities.

c. Research in the area of cognitive functioning supports the importance of providing clients with meaningful tasks and therapeutic activities.
(1) Occupational therapy's focus on meaningful occupation and purposeful activities is inherently congruent with the CBT.
(2) Many of the life skills workbook activities used by occupational therapists apply cognitive therapy principles.
(a) Activity gradation, an area of specialization for occupational therapists, is particularly useful in providing effective treatment using the CBT frame of reference.

5. Dialectical Behavior Therapy (DBT).
a. A form of CBT.
b. Focus of DBT.
(1) Addresses suicidal thoughts and actions and self injurious behaviors.
(2) Commonly used with individuals with borderline personality disorder since a feature of this diagnosis is suicidal thinking and behavior.
(3) Also used to treat individuals who have depression, substance abuse issues, and/or eating disorders.

c. Evaluation.
(1) Often begins with an accurate DSM diagnosis by the psychiatrist.
(2) Occupational therapy evaluation tools are not trait or diagnostically based.
(3) A variety of psychological evaluations may be used, including those that address personality.
(4) Occupational therapy assessments that focus on functioning in performance areas and performance contexts can provide relevant information for intervention planning.

d. Intervention.
(1) Programming using DBT teaches assertiveness, coping and interpersonal skills.
(a) Occupational therapy practitioners are often involved in assisting clients develop these skills.
(2) DBT groups address how the acquisition of skills affects occupational performance and provide opportunities to practice new skills.
(3) A strong therapist-client relationship is essential.
(a) Rapport is used for validation as well as confrontation.

Recovery Model[3]

1. Relevance to occupational therapy practice.
a. Recovery principles and approaches are highly congruent with those of occupational therapy.
b. The active use of the recovery model throughout the OT process can help practitioners empower people by fostering their intrinsic motivation to redefine self and establish a sense of hope for the future.
c. The primary focus of the recovery process is to improve quality of life and the ability to attain desired life goals through self-advocacy.

2. Principles.
a. Conceptualizes recovery from illness as a journey of healing and transformation that enables individuals with mental health problems to live a meaningful life in a community of their choice.
b. Individuals with mental illness can strive to meet their potential and find meaning and purpose in their lives.
c. Major concepts which guide recovery.

[3] This section was written by Patricia Wisniewski, MS, OTR/L, CPRP.

Chapter 14

(1) Self-direction: consumers identify their own goals and their own personal track to recovery.
(2) Individualized and person-centered: recovery is unique as dictated by each individuals' personal strengths, needs, past experiences, cultural background, and desires.
(3) Empowerment: people take control over their lives by making educated decisions that impact on their recovery.
(4) Holistic: recovery signifies the interrelatedness of the mind, body, spirit, and community.
(5) Nonlinear: recovery can include episodes that disrupt the track to recovery but individuals learn from set backs and proceed in a manner that supports continued recovery.
(6) Strengths-based: recovery builds upon and exercises an individual's strengths.
(7) Peer support: reciprocal relationships with others who have lived experience in supporting recovery priniciples are formed.
(8) Respect: recovery is based on the premise of social acceptance of self and by others, including society, one's community, and service providers.
(9) Responsibility: personal commitment to self in working towards personal goals, including taking care of oneself to promote overall health and wellness.
(10) Hope: being a change agent in recovery enables the person to embrace an optimistic future.
(11) Family: members play an essential role in a person's recovery. Family remain committed to supporting an individual's potential and personal strengths, despite potential set-backs.
(12) Commmunity: support inclusion and remains steadfast in eliminating barriers to recovery.

3. Evaluation.
   a. Quality of Life Interview.
      (1) Measures the person's level of function using objective-based questions and life satisfaction using subjective-based questions.
      (2) Areas assessed include the person's living situation, daily activities, family and social relationships, finances, work-school issues, legal-safety issues, health issues, leisure activities, and overall quality of life.
      (3) Can be administererd by an occupational therapist.
   b. Oregon Quality of Life Questionnaire.
      (1) Measures adjustment in relation to how an individual's needs are met in combination with the demands society places upon him or her.
      (2) Two versions exist: a self-report interview and a semi-structured interviewer-rated interview.
      (3) Can be administered by an occupational therapist.
   c. The Empowerment Scale.
      (1) Measures a central component of recovery, including the following areas: self-esteem, power, activism, control, and anger.
      (2) Results can be used to develop strategies for regaining control over one's life.
      (3) Can be administered by an occupational therapist.
4. Intervention.
      (1) The development and implementation of a Wellness Recovery Action Plan (WRAP) is an essential part of the recovery process.
      (2) Storytelling is a means of decreasing stigma and supporting others by sharing experiential life experiences.
      (3) Advocacy through the dessimination of knowledge, skill development in activism, and forming support groups to prevent discrimination and improve acceptance in society.

Psychiatric Rehabilitation[4]

1. Relevance to occupational therapy practice.
   a. Psychiatric rehabilitation and the profession of occupational therapy both share the common goal of eliminating barriers and promoting health and wellness.
   b. Both believe recovery from physical, mental, emotional and cognitive disabilities is possible.
      (1) Recovery is not a linear process, rather individuals will experience challenging periods when progress may lapse.
      (2) Recovery is person specific.
   c. The goal of psychiatric rehabilitation is to help individuals develop the skills necessary to compensate for, adapt to, and/or control the influence symptoms have on function, including any disability caused by social or environmental barriers.
2. Principles.
   a. Individualization: any service provided to an individual is structured to support each person's unique needs.
   b. Client involvement: individuals control their recovery.
   c. Partnership with service providers: a mutual rapport between all persons involved nurtures a commitment based on respect and trust for every one.
   d. Community-based services: all services are provided where the individual lives, works, and socializes.
   e. Strengths-focused: build on a person's strengths rather than focusing on his/her weaknesses.

[4] This section was written by Patricia Wisniewski, MS, OTR/L, CPRP.

f. Situational assessments: the focus is on collecting data while observing the individual in the environment where challenges are experienced.
g. Holistic approach: treatment and rehabilitation services are viewed as equal and mutually dependent methods that support recovery.
h. Continued, accessible, coordinated services: services are always available for any given period time.
i. Vocational focus: work is healing; a psychiatric rehabilitation professional partners with individuals (regardless of their abilities) to develop work skills, habits, and resources needed to become successful.
j. Skills training: includes all actions or behaviors necessary to accomplish a task.
    (1) For example, writing an email to a friend includes not only knowing how to organize your thoughts, but also knowing how to use proper grammar and punctuation, operate a computer, practice computer etiquette, and acknowledge a reply.
k. Environmental modification: changing the environment so it supports function.
l. Partnership with family: family is viewed as a consistent source of support; thus, family education is provided to nurture healthy relationships.
m. Evaluation of outcomes: service providers are expected to monitor the services they provide for effectiveness to ensure compatibility with the individuals being served.

3. Evaluation.
    a. Assessments are based on real-life situations that will provide accurate data specific to an individual, environment, and activity at a moment in time.
    b. Evaluation of readiness for change is an essential component of the evaluation process.
        (1) Foremost, individuals with a mental disability have to make a conscious effort to overcome it.
        (2) The effort includes acknowledging one has a mental disability and overcoming stigma or other barriers that may hinder recovery.
4. Intervention.
    a. Goal is to assist individuals with a psychiatric disability to perform the physical, emotional, social, and intellectual skills needed to live and work in the community at their highest functional level with the least amount of professional support as the individual deems necessary.
    b. Assertive Community Treatment uses a variety of interdisciplinary interventions aimed at restoring function and role performance in the community.
    c. Interventions take place where a person chooses to live, work, and socialize.
    d. Day programs that embed pyschiatric rehabilitation principles include clubhouses where the goal is to improve quality of life by instilling self-worth and determination in its members.
        (1) Clubhouse members include individuals who have a psychiatric disability and staff who share all responsibilities in managing the clubhouse.
            (a) Common modules that support the work-ordered day at a clubhouse include outreach, transitional employment, education, meal preparation, and advocacy.
    e. Case management services strive to offer continuity of care, accessibility, accountability, and efficiency.
    f. Vocational rehabilitation is supported as a natural activity where individuals are capable of achieving success.
        (1) Supported employment affords services to the individual where they are needed: on the actual job or as a consultation.
    g. Supported education offers normalization, structure, self-determination, and fosters both hope and empowerment.
        (1) This is important because education is often interrupted when someone experiences a mental disability.

Psychosocial Evaluation

Areas Addressed During Evaluation

1. Performance skills (i.e., cognitive, perceptual, psychological, and social) and their impact on performance in areas of occupation.
2. Client factors and physical conditions or limitations that impact functional behaviors and performance in areas of occupation.
3. The impact of the individual's social, cultural, spiritual, and physical contexts.
4. Identification of the roles and behaviors that are required of the individual either by society or for the achievement of his/her desired goals.
5. Precautions and safety issues such as suicidal and/or aggressive behavior.
6. History of behavior patterns.

7. Individual's goals, values, interests, and attitudes.
8. Consideration and involvement of family, caregivers and significant others.
9. Presenting problems and issues identified by the client.
10. Desired outcomes.
    a. If the person is hospitalized, discharge planning begins on day one of hospitalization.
11. Probable (and possible) living environments of choice.

Assessment Methods

1. Interviews - structured and unstructured.
   a. Occupational profile.
2. Standardized tests.
3. Clinical observation.
4. Rating scales.
5. Questionnaires.
6. Self-report inventories.

Relationship to the NBCOT Examination

1. The NBCOT examination may include a description of evaluation methods and/or the names of specific assessment tools; therefore, a review of major psychosocial assessments is important for examination preparation.
   a. This can also increase understanding and knowledge of common approaches for the evaluation of psychosocial assets and deficits.
   b. This can further strengthen the clinical reasoning skills needed to answer examination items that address the evaluation process within psychosocial domains of OT practice.
2. As of the publication of this text, NBCOT has not made public the names of all of the specific evaluations that may be on the examination.
3. The evaluations included in this chapter are based on the authors' review of NBCOT self-assessment tools, major OT textbooks, and feedback obtained from OT practitioners regarding measures used in practice.

Major Psychosocial Assessments

General Assessments of Mental Status

1. Mini-Mental State Examination (also known as the Folstein Mini-Mental).
   a. Focus: a widely used, quick screening test of cognitive functioning.
   b. Method.
      (1) Structured tasks are presented in an interview format.
      (2) Part one requires verbal responses to assess orientation, memory, and attention.
      (3) Part two assesses the ability to write a sentence, name objects, follow verbal and written directions, and copy a complex polygon design.
   c. Scoring and interpretation.
      (1) Point value of each item ranges from 1 to 5.
      (2) The maximum score is 30 and a score of 24 or below indicates cognitive impairment.
   d. Population: individuals with cognitive or psychiatric dysfunction.
2. Short Portable Mental Status Questionnaire.
   a. Focus: intellectual function.
   b. Method.
      (1) A short questionnaire asks nine questions such as "What day of the week is it?" and "Who is the president of the United States now?"
      (2) A subtraction task requests, "Subtract 3 from 20 and keep subtracting 3 from each new result."
   c. Scoring and interpretation.
      (1) Each item receives one point if response is inaccurate.
      (2) One point is added for education beyond high school and one point is subtracted if education does not go beyond grade school.
      (3) The number of errors is totaled with a potential error score of 10.
         (a) A score of 0 to 2 indicates intact intellectual function.
         (b) A score of 3 to 4 indicates mild intellectual impairment.
         (c) A score of 5 to 7 indicates moderate intellectual impairment.
         (d) A score of 8 to 10 indicates severe intellectual impairment.
   d. Population: individuals with cognitive or psychiatric dysfunction.

Assessments of Cognition, Affect, and/or Sensory Processing

1. Adult/Adolescent Sensory Profile.
   a. Focus: allows clients to identify their personal behavioral responses to daily sensory experiences and develop strategies for enhanced participation.
      (1) There are four quadrants (i.e., sensory sensitivity, sensation avoiding, low registration, sensation seeking) which cover the sensory processing categories of taste/smell, movement, visual, touch, activity level, and auditory.
   b. Method.
      (1) Requires the completion of a 60-item questionnaire about an individual's reactions to daily sensory experiences via the person's self-report.
   c. Scoring and interpretation.
      (1) Cutoff scores indicate typical performance and probable, definite, and significant differences.
         (a) Differences indicate which sensory system is hindering performance.
         (b) Can be used for intervention planning.
   d. Population: 11–65 years.
2. Allen Cognitive Level Screen-5 (ACLS-5).
   a. Focus: assesses the cognitive level of the individual according to the Allen cognitive levels. See this chapter's prior section on the Cognitive Disabilities model.
   b. Method.
      (1) Requires the performance of several leather lacing stitches following instruction and/or demonstration.
      (2) Comparable tasks may be substituted.
      (3) Administration time varies.
   c. Materials: kit contains a leather purse, lacing strip, needle, and manual for wording for standardized instructions and scoring.
      (1) The Large Allen Cognitive Level Screen -5 (LACLS-5) is available to enable this tool to be used by persons who have impairments in hand function and/or vision which may impact their task performance.
   d. Scoring and interpretation.
      (1) The task demands for each stitch are proposed to require the use of abilities associated with Allen's cognitive levels.
         (a) Level 3: running stitch.
         (b) Level 4: whipstitch.
         (c) Level 5: cordovan stitch.
      (2) The ACLS-5 manual provides detailed scoring tables that list specific behaviors which may be observed during task completion and their corresponding level and mode of performance.
         (a) Scores range 3.0 to 5.8 and correspond to their respective mode on the Allen scale.
      (3) Identification of Allen cognitive level yields information about the individual's abilities and limitations.
         (a) The Allen Diagnostic Manual can be used to assess an individual's cognitive level.
            - Consists of twenty-four craft projects.
            - Provides Allen cognitive level ratings from 3.0 to 5.8.
            - Activities are delineated according to the ACL scale.
            - Provides observation criteria for each activity.
   e. Population: adults with psychiatric or cognitive dysfunction.
3. Beck Depression Inventory.
   a. Focus: measurement of the presence and depth of depression.
   b. Method.
      (1) Administered by an interviewer to persons who have language or comprehension difficulties or completed as a questionnaire by the individual.
      (2) The individual rates his/her feelings relative to 21 characteristics associated with depression (i.e., mood, pessimism, sense of failure, lack of satisfaction, guilt, sense of punishment, self-dislike, self accusations, suicidal wishes, crying spells, irritability, social withdrawal, indecisiveness, distortion of body image, work inhibition, sleep disturbance, fatigability, loss of appetite, weight loss, somatic preoccupation, loss of libido).
   c. Scoring and interpretation.
      (1) Items are scored as 0 to 3, with 3 being the most severe.
      (2) The 21 item ratings are totaled with higher scores indicating higher levels of depression.
   d. Population: adolescent and adult.
4. Elder Depression Scale.
   a. Focus: assesses depression in the elderly.
   b. Method: completion of a 30-item checklist that looks at the presence of characteristics associated with depression (somatic concerns, affect, cognitive impairment, feelings of discrimination, impaired motivation, lack of future orientation, lack of self-esteem, etc.).
   c. Scoring and interpretation.
      (1) Items are scored yes or no.
      (2) A score of 10–11 is the threshold most often used to indicate depression.
   d. Population: older adults.
5. Hamilton Depression Rating Scale.
   a. Focus: measures the severity of illness and changes over time in individuals diagnosed with a depressive illness.
   b. Method.

(1) Information is gathered through interview and consultation with family, staff, and other informed individuals.
(2) The clinician rates the information obtained relative to 17 symptoms and characteristics (i.e., depressed mood, guilt, suicide, initial insomnia, middle insomnia, delayed insomnia, work and interest, retardation, agitation, psychic anxiety, somatic anxiety, gastrointestinal somatic symptoms, general somatic symptoms, genital symptoms, hypochondriasis, insight, weight loss).
(3) Also rated are diurnal variation, depersonalization, paranoid symptoms, and obsessional symptoms.

c. Scoring and interpretation.
(1) Items are rated 0–2, with 0 signifying absent, 1 signifying trivial, or 2 signifying present, or are rated 0–4 signifying absent, trivial, mild, moderate, or severe.
(2) The scores for items 1–17 are totaled for a final score.
(3) The significance of the total score is not made. Subsequent changes are noted to determine changes in the individual's status.

d. Population: individuals with a diagnosis of mood disorder.

Assessments of Task Performance

1. Bay Area Functional Performance Evaluation (BAFPE).
a. Focus: assesses the cognitive, affective, performance, and social interaction skills required to perform activities of daily living.
b. Method.
(1) Brief interview prior to assessment to collect basic demographic and clinical information and to familiarize the individual with the evaluation.
(2) The Task Oriented Assessment (TOA).
(a) Measures cognition, performance, affect, qualitative signs, and referral indicators through the completion of 5 standardized, timed tasks (i.e., sorting shells, bank deposit slip, house floor plan, block design, draw-a-person).
(b) Evaluator observes and rates task performance but does not provide guidance for task completion.
(3) The Social Interaction Scale (SIS).
(a) Assesses general ability to relate appropriately to other people within the environment through observations of the individual in 5 situations (i.e., one to one, mealtime, unstructured group, structured activity group, structured verbal group).
(4) Optional self-report social interaction questionnaire.
(5) Perceptual motor screening.
c. Scoring and interpretation of TOA.
(1) Scoring consists of 3 component, 12 parameter, and 5 task scores.
(2) Ten functional components of the 5 tasks are rated (i.e., paraphrase, productive decision-making, motivation, organization of time and materials, mastery and self-esteem, frustration tolerance, attention span, ability to abstract, verbal or behavioral evidence of thought or mood disorder, ability to follow instructions leading to correct task completion).
(3) Norms are presented for comparison with specific adult psychiatric populations.
d. Scoring and interpretation of SIS.
(1) Scoring consists of 7 situation and 5 parameter scores as well as one total SIS score.
(2) Seven categories are rated (i.e., response to authority figures, verbal communication, psychomotor behavior, independence/dependence, socially appropriate behavior, ability to work with peers, participation in group/program activities).
e. The TOA and SIS scores are not combined for a total BAFPE score.
(1) The results of the TOA and SIS are used as indicators of overall functional performance, and provide information about the person's cognitive, affective, social, and perceptual motor skills.
f. Population: adult individuals with psychiatric, neurological, or developmental diagnoses.

2. Comprehensive Occupational Therapy Evaluation Scale (COTE Scale).
a. Focus: a structured method for observing and rating behaviors and behavioral changes in the areas of general, interpersonal, and task skills.
(1) Seven items address general behavior such as appearance, punctuality, and activity level.
(2) Six items address interpersonal behavior such as cooperation, sociability, and attention-getting behavior.
(3) Twelve items address task behavior such as concentration, following directions and problem solving.
(4) It may be used for initial assessment and to record progress.
b. Method.
(1) The individual's behavior is observed during a therapeutic session as the individual completes a task.
(2) Behavior is rated by the therapist according to specific criteria presented for each item.
(3) The tasks used are selected/designed by the therapist.

c. Scoring and interpretation.
(1) Each item is rated on a scale of 0 (normal) to 4 (severe).
(2) Results may be used to plan treatment and assist with discharge planning.
d. Population: adults with acute psychiatric diagnoses.
3. The Kohlman Evaluation of Living Skills (KELS).
a. See Chapter 15's section on the evaluation of activities of daily living.
4. The Milwaukee Evaluation of Daily Living Skills (MEDLS).
a. See Chapter 15's section on the evaluation of activities of daily living.
5. Test of Grocery Shopping.
a. See Chapter 15's section on the evaluation of activities of daily living.

Assessments of Occupational Performance and Occupational Roles

1. Activity Card Sort (ACS).
a. Focus: the identification of a person's level and amount of involvement in instrumental, leisure, and social activities.
b. Method.
(1) The individual is presented with a set of 89 cards which each pictorially represent real people engaging in an activity and asked to manually sort the cards according to level and amount of involvement (i.e., never done, gave up doing, do less than in the past, do the same, do more than in the past).
(2) The real-life activities presented for sorting include 20 instrumental activities, 35 low-physical-demand leisure activities, 17 high-physical-demand leisure activities, and 17 social activities.
c. Scoring and interpretation.
(1) Total scores (current, previous, and % retained) for each of the activity categories (i.e., instrumental, low-physical-demand leisure, high-physical-demand leisure, and social activities) are obtained.
(2) Categorical scores are compiled into Global Scores for Current Activity, Previous Activity, and Percent Retained.
(a) These scores can be used to monitor changes in activity participation over time by comparing previous to current activity participation.
(3) The ACS can be used for initial assessment, goal setting, and intervention planning.
(a) Only activities that a person identifies as part of his/her daily routine are included in the scoring.
(b) The information acquired can help the therapist assist clients in building (or re-building) routines comprised of meaningful and healthy activities.
(4) The person's responses can contribute to the development of an occupational history.
(a) The pictorial representations of the activities often trigger memories and/or associations that when shared by the person can enhance the therapist's understanding of the person's activity engagement and motivation.
d. Population: originally developed for older adults with dementia.
(1) Three versions are currently available to address the unique needs of adults and older adults residing in institutional settings, living in the community, or recovering from an incurred illness, injury, or disability.
2. Activities Health Assessment.
a. Focus: time usage, patterns and configurations of activities, roles, and underlying skills and habits.
b. Method.
(1) The person completes an Idiosyncratic Activities Configuration Schedule by constructing a color-coded chart which depicts the way his/her time is spent during a typical week.
(a) Activities configuration is a term used to denote a measure which asks a person to record his or her daily actitivies for a week and describe the needs the activities satisfy, whether the person wants to or has to do each activity, how well the person does the activity, and how the person feels while engaging in the activity.
(2) The person completes the Idiosyncratic Activities Configuration Questionnaire.
(3) Therapist interviews person using interview guidelines.
c. Administration time.
(1) Time is dependent upon whether schedule is completed retrospectively during a 60-minute session or over the course of a week (7 days).
(2) Questionnaire time is 60 minutes to 2 hours.
(3) Interview time is 45 minutes to 60 minutes.
d. Scoring and interpretation.
(1) Not scored. Activities classified by type and then sub-grouped according to questionnaire and interview guidelines.
(2) A determination of the person's activities health is made by the person and the therapist based on the completed schedule, questionnaire, and interview.
(3) Significance is placed on the person's interpretation of the level of balance, satisfaction, and comfort to which each activity contributes.
e. Population: adults through elders.

3. Adolescent Role Assessment.
   a. Focus: assesses the development of internalized roles within family, school and social settings.
   b. Method: a semi-structured interview that follows an interview guide to generate discussion in the areas of family, school performance, peer interactions, occupational choice and work.
   c. Scoring and interpretation: scoring indicates behavior that is appropriate, marginal or inappropriate.
   d. Population: adolescents age 13 to 17.
4. Barth Time Construction (BTC).
   a. Focus: time usage, roles and underlying skills and habits.
   b. Method.
      (1) The person constructs a color-coded chart, individually or in a group format, which depicts the way his/her time is spent during a typical week.
      (2) A COTE scale may also be completed by the therapist based on observations made during the session.
   c. Scoring and interpretation.
      (1) Not scored. Percentages of time are calculated according to main groupings.
      (2) Significance of information is based on appropriate use of time and discussion with individual.
   d. Population: adolescent through elder.
5. Canadian Occupational Performance Measure (COPM).
   a. Focus: identifies the individual's perception of satisfaction with performance and changes over time in the areas of self-care, productivity, and leisure.
   b. Method.
      (1) A semi-structured interview identifies the individual's perception of his/her occupational performance in:
         (a) Self-care (personal care, functional mobility, community management).
         (b) Productivity (paid/unpaid work, household management, play/school).
         (c) Leisure (quiet recreation, active recreation, socialization).
      (2) Care-givers of children and/or adults who are unable to participate in an interview may answer the COPM questions for their care recipient.
      (3) Problem areas are identified.
      (4) The identified problems are rated by the individual as to performance and satisfaction.
      (5) Reassessment takes place at appropriate intervals.
   c. Scoring and interpretation.
      (1) Items are rated on a scale of 1 to 10, with 10 being the highest.
      (2) Total scores for performance and satisfaction are used to identify treatment focus, treatment outcomes, and individual satisfaction.
   d. Population: individuals over the age 7 or parents of small children.
6. Goal Attainment Scaling (GAS).
   a. Focus: facilitates active participation in the goal-setting process by having the individual and/or caregivers identify desired intervention outcomes for the client that are personally relevant to them.
      (1) Used post-intervention, the GAS assesses the individual's attainment of these goals and relevant changes in occupational performance.
   b. Method: a personal interview is used during goal-setting and post-treatment sessions.
   c. Scoring and interpretation. As a goal setting and program evaluation tool, the GAS does not have a scoring protocol.
      (1) In writing the goals, the practitioner seeks to accurately predict the level of performance the person is expected to achieve after a specified duration of intervention and identify equal increments above and below the expected level of performance.
      (2) For example, a 5-point scale is used for scaling goals with 0 (zero) being used to represent the predicted expected level of performance and –2 to +2 being used to respectfully indicate performance below or above expectations.
   d. Population: Older children, adolescents, adults and care-givers of younger children and/or adults who are unable to participate in an interview.
7. Occupational Circumstances Assessment Interview Rating Scale (OCAIRS), version 4.
   a. Focus.
      (1) The nature and extent of an individual's occupational adaptation.
      (2) Based on the Model of Human Occupation (MOHO), this interview obtains, analyzes, and reports information relevant to intervention and discharge planning.
      (3) Twelve areas of occupational adaptation are explored; these include personal causation, self-perception of past circumstances and experiences, social environment, physical environment, values, interests, roles, habits, skills, readiness for change, and long- and short-term goals.
   b. Method.
      (1) Information is gathered using a semi-structured interview format comprised of guided questions in 12 delineated areas.
      (2) Questions may be adapted to meet the needs and abilities of the individual.
   c. Scoring and interpretation.
      (1) Following the interview, the therapist rates each item on a scale of 1 to 4 (4 being the highest) according to item-specific guidelines.

(2) The person's self-report and perceptions provide qualitative data to explain the rationales for the quantitative ratings.
(3) A case analysis method is used to interpret the data according to the MOHO to obtain a profile of the person's strengths and weaknesses.

d. Population: originally designed for adult through elder persons with psychiatric diagnoses, it is now being used in a broader context.
(1) Three interview formats are currently available to address population-specific issues; these are physical disabilities, mental health, and forensic mental health.

8. Occupational Performance History Interview-II (OPHI-II).
a. Focus: gathers information about an individual's life history, past and present occupational performance, and the impact of the incidence of disability, illness or other traumatic event in the person's life.
b. Method.
(1) Information is gathered using a semi-structured interview format.
(2) Interview questions cover five content areas addressing daily routines; occupational roles, occupation/activity choices, critical life choices, and occupational behavior settings.
c. Scoring and interpretation.
(1) Following the interview, the therapist rates the person's occupational identity and competence and the impact of the person's occupational behavior settings on a scale of 1 to 4 with 1 equaling extreme occupational dysfunction and 4 equaling exceptionally occupational competent.
(2) Ratings are used to identify the individual's life history pattern.
(3) A narrative of the individual's life history pattern is written based on his/her self-report.
d. Population: individuals who are able to participate in a comprehensive interview from adolescents to elders.
(1) The OPHI is not recommended to be used with children less than 12 years old.

9. Occupational Self-Assessment.
a. Focus: self-report checklist of individual's perceptions of efficacy in areas of occupational performance and their importance.
b. Method: two-part self report. Clients are given a list of 21 everyday activities.
c. Scoring and interpretation: clients use a 4-point scale to rate how well they do each activity to assess occupational competence and then complete a 4-point scale to report how important the activity is to assess the value of the occupation.
d. Population: adults 18 years and older.

10. The Role Checklist.
a. Focus: assesses self-reported role participation and the value of specific roles to the individual.
b. Method.
(1) A checklist is completed by the individual alone or with the therapist.
(a) Part One asks the person to identify the major roles that have been part of his/her life in the past, present roles, and anticipated future roles; these roles include student, worker, volunteer, care giver, home maintainer, friend, family member, religious participant, hobbyist/amateur, participant in organizations, other (this last category enables the person to identify a role that is not listed).
(b) Part Two asks the person to identify the degree to which he/she values each role.
c. Scoring and interpretation.
(1) The person's responses are totaled to identify roles that have been continuous in the person's life, roles that have been disrupted or changed, present roles, roles that are desired for the future, and valuable, somewhat valuable, and very valuable roles.
(2) The data collected can be further discussed with the individual and used to address goal identification and treatment planning, quality of life, and discharge planning.
d. Population: adolescent through elder individuals with physical or psychosocial dysfunction.

11. Refer to Chapter 15 for additional information about evaluation tools for the occupational performance areas of ADL, IADL, leisure, and work.

Projective Assessments

1. Focus: based on psychodynamic/psychoanalytic models, these assessments allow clients to project intrapsychic content for discussion and resolution in therapy by bringing unconscious intrapsychic conflicts to consciousness through the completion and processing of an activity.
2. Methods.
a. Several projective assessments (e.g., The House-Tree-Person, Draw-A-Person, and the Kinetic Family Drawing) are currently used by diverse professionals.
b. The Magazine Picture Collage (developed by Carol Learner) is the projective evaluation most typically used by occupational therapy practitioners applying a psychodynamic frame of reference.
(1) During the completion of the Magazine Picture Collage:

(a) Clients are given scissors, glue, and magazines and instructed to select pictures, cut them out and glue them to a sheet of construction paper and to put his or her name, the date, and a title for their collage on the paper's back.

(b) Observing clients during the completion of this task, the therapist can assess a variety of skills (e.g., fine motor, attention span, ability to follow directions, organizational ability) and obtain projective content through the clients' comments and picture selection.

(2) The Magazine Picture Collage can be easily adapted to meet the assessment needs of a client or population beyond the free choice of collage topic by assigning themes (e.g., good day/bad day, likes/dislikes).

(3) Scoring and interpretation.

(a) Interpretation should be based on the client's report of the content and not inferred by the therapist.

(b) Following completion of the collage, the therapist discusses the client's interpretation or description with the individual to facilitate insight and exploration of any pertinent issues that may arise.

3. Population: projective evaluations such as the magazine picture collage can be used with children, adolescents, survivors of traumatic events and any individual with the capacity for insight and a willingness to change through the exploration of intrapsychic issues.

a. Generally not used with persons with psychosis.

Psychosocial Intervention

General Intervention Considerations

1. One-to-one versus group intervention.
   a. Indicators for one-to-one intervention.
      (1) Refusal to attend groups.
      (2) Inability to tolerate group interaction.
      (3) Presence of behaviors that would be disruptive to the goals of the group.
      (4) Individual is on suicide precautions or is a danger to self or others; e.g., on inpatient psychiatric settings.
      (5) The issues that must be addressed are specific to that patient/client only.
   b. Indicators for group intervention.
      (1) More cost effective.
      (2) Effective at assisting members to learn to live in social environments.
      (3) Takes advantage of group dynamics and therapeutic milieu.
         (a) Groups that are facilitated in a therapeutic manner by an occupational therapist are inherently curative.
         (b) See Chapter 3 for a comprehensive review of therapeutic groups and Yalom's curative factors.
2. Factors that influence the effectiveness of intervention.
   a. Skillful therapeutic use of self.
   b. An understanding of the individual's cognitive abilities.
   c. Exploration of the needs and wants of the individual.
   d. The establishment of realistic goals.
   e. Skill with activity analysis.
   f. An understanding of the realities of the treatment conditions and intervention contexts.
   g. Prioritization of the most goal-directed use of the person's time.
3. The relationship of intervention activities to desired goals.
   a. Initial intervention may need to focus on the performance skills needed for desired occupational performance.
   b. Once basic skills are in place, intervention focuses on performance of functional activities specifically relevant to the individual.
      (1) Activities that require the actual desired skills or behaviors, in their natural environment, are often the most effective (e.g., assisting the client to use a checking account to pay bills).
      (2) Activities that simulate desired behaviors in clinical setting may be less effective (e.g., using kits that simulate checking materials).
      (3) Activities that utilize the performance skills of desired behaviors and rely on generalization may be the least effective (e.g., practicing arithmetic calculation).

General Considerations for Group Intervention

1. The taxonomy of groups described by Anne Mosey provides a useful framework for designing OT intervention groups.

a. Evaluation groups.
   (1) Designed to gather information about the individual's task and group interaction skills that can be used to establish goals and plan intervention.
      (a) Although their primary purpose is evaluation, these groups are often therapeutic through their process and/or content and can help establish rapport.
b. Task-oriented groups.
   (1) The purpose is to assist the members in becoming aware of their needs, values, ideas, and feelings through the performance of a shared task.
c. Developmental groups.
   (1) The purpose is to assist the members to acquire and develop group interaction skills.
   (2) Developmental groups offer five levels of interaction.
      (a) Parallel groups use individual tasks with minimal interaction required.
      (b) Project groups consist of common, short-term activities requiring some interaction and cooperation.
      (c) Egocentric cooperative groups require joint interaction on long-term tasks; however, completion of the task is not the focus. The members are beginning to express their needs and address those of others.
      (d) Cooperative groups learn to work together cooperatively, not specifically to complete a task, but to enjoy each other's company and meet emotional needs.
      (e) Mature groups are responsive to all members' needs and can carry out a variety of tasks. There is good balance between carrying out the task and meeting the needs of the members.
   (3) The directive leadership role of the therapist decreases from parallel to mature.
      (a) See Chapter 3.
d. Thematic groups are designed for the learning of specific skills.
e. Topical groups focus on the discussion of activities and issues outside of the group that are current or anticipated.
f. Instrumental groups are concerned with meeting health needs and maintaining function.
g. Refer to Chapter 3 for more detail.

2. The curative factors of groups described by Irving Yalom support the inherent value of OT interventions that use a group format.
   a. Groups and group activities that are designed to facilitate these curative factors are most effective.
   b. Refer to Chapter 3 for a complete listing.
3. Considerations in group planning.
   a. Member demographics including gender, age, culture, and ethnicity.
   b. Individual characteristics of members.
      (1) Cognitive level.
      (2) Functional skill level.
      (3) Individual goals.
      (4) Contraindications and safety issues.
   c. Logistical considerations.
      (1) Number of people in the group.
      (2) Length of sessions.
      (3) Number of sessions.
      (4) Space availability.
      (5) Environmental characteristics.
      (6) Budget and materials required.
      (7) Number of leaders.
      (8) Open group vs. closed group.
   d. Frame of reference.
4. Elements of a group protocol.
   a. Title/name: reflect the purpose or goal of the group (e.g., Communication Skills Group), not the media used (e.g., Crafts Group).
   b. Purpose: a brief statement of what the group hopes to accomplish (e.g., to improve the members' ability to effectively and appropriately communicate to others their needs and feelings and to enter into satisfying interpersonal relationships).
   c. Rationale: explains the value of this group to the members, and why it is important to offer this service to this population.
   d. Theoretical base/frame of reference: explains in brief and readily understandable terms the theory on which this intervention is based and the rationale for its use.
   e. Criteria for membership: explains who should/should not be included in the group, and what will indicate when the member will no longer benefit from participation.
   f. Goals/anticipated outcomes: the expectations of what the members will be able to do as a result of having attended this group.
      (1) A list of "Patient/client will..." statements, (e.g., patient will be able to initiate and sustain social interactions with peers).
   g. Method/format: explains how the group will be carried out.
      (1) Includes the format, scheduling, activities, materials, procedures, etc.
      (2) Includes the information another therapist would need to lead this group.
   h. Role of the therapist: the tasks of the therapist in preparing for and leading the group.
      (1) Includes such things as supplying materials, designing activities, facilitating interaction, providing a safe environment, etc.
      (2) Refer to Chapter 3 for further discussion of leadership roles and styles.
   i. Quality assurance: explains how the need for this intervention and its effectiveness will be monitored.

j. Outcome measures: determine whether the identified goals were met.
k. The actual format used to write protocols varies from setting to setting.

5. Procedure for developing a group.
   a. Conduct a needs assessment to identify intervention needs. (See Chapter 4 for needs assessment procedures).
   b. Develop the protocol.
   c. Present the protocol to the treatment team or program administrators.
   d. Select potential members who would benefit from the group.
   e. Meet with each potential member to explain the purpose and circumstances of the group.
   f. Hold introductory sessions of the group and revise the protocol as needed.
6. Group member leadership roles: (see Chapter 3).
7. Considerations in activity selection.
   a. Degree of structure (inherent or imposed).
   b. Type(s) and degree of instruction provided.
   c. Degree of new learning required.
   d. Complexity of the activity.
   e. Length of time for completion.
   f. Nature and degree of skill required for engagement and completion.
   g. Degree of challenge to the members' skills.

Intervention Group Types

1. ADL/IADL groups.
   a. Focus is on the development of ADL skills (e.g., self-care) and IADL skills (e.g., meal preparation, money management, transportation) to enable independent living.
   b. May be conducted in a modular and/or psychoeducational format.
2. Basic task skills groups.
   a. Include intervention activities designed to develop the basic cognitive skills (e.g., attention, ability to follow multi-step directions, problem solving) necessary for the completion of simple tasks.
      (1) This group uses a skill acquisition approach which differs from the psychodynamic approach used in the task-oriented group described by Fidler and Mosey.
3. Community participation/reintegration groups.
   a. Focuses on the identification and use of community resources (e.g., leisure facilities) and the development of skills (e.g., the use of public transportation) to enable full community participation.
   b. May be conducted in a modular and/or psychoeducational format.
4. Coping skills groups.
   a. Focuses on identifying and implementing the problem-solving and stress-management techniques needed to cope with life stressors.
5. Directive groups as developed by Kathy Kaplan.
   a. These are highly structured groups designed to assist persons with limited abilities in developing basic task and social skills.
   b. Each session is divided into five parts followed by a 15-minute review of the session by the leaders.
      (1) Part I consists of an orientation to the purpose and goals of the group (maximum of 5 minutes).
      (2) Part II involves a review of everyone's name and the introduction of new members (5–10 minutes).
      (3) Part III consists of warm-up activities to make members comfortable and engage them in the group (5–10 minutes).
      (4) Part IV involves one or more activities designed to address the goals of the group and the needs of its members (10–20 minutes).
      (5) Part V includes activities designed to give meaning to the activities and closure to the group (10 minutes).
6. Discharge planning groups.
   a. Focuses on activities to problem-solve potential obstacles and identify resources for successful post-discharge community reintegration.
7. Five Stage groups as developed by Mildred Ross.
   a. Expanded on the sensory integration work of Lorna Jean King which examined the sensory distortions, postural disturbances, and vestibular stimulating activities that were observed in individuals with chronic schizophrenia.
      (1) King proposed that using non-cortical, alerting, stimulating, and pleasurable activities (e.g., parachute games) would normalize movement patterns, increase strength and flexibility, and facilitate adaptive behaviors.
   b. Ross extended the use of sensorimotor approaches to other chronic populations including persons with intellectual disabilities, Alzheimer's disease, and neurological impairments.
   c. Each of the five stages of this group follows a clear structure to attain a specific aim.
      (1) Stage I: Orientation consists of orienting the members to the session and each other.
      (2) Stage II: Movement uses a variety of vigorous gross motor activities designed to be stimulating and alerting.
      (3) Stage III: Perceptual-Motor uses brief (30 minutes or less) activities that utilize perceptual-motor skills designed to be calming and to increase ability to focus.

(4) Stage IV: Cognitive includes activities to provide cognitive stimulation to promote organized thinking.
(5) Stage V: Closure consists of brief discussions to promote a sense of satisfaction and closure.

8. Goal-setting groups.
   a. Consists of activities designed to identify personal objectives and treatment goals and the steps needed for their achievement.
9. Leisure groups.
   a. May include the identification of interests, development of activity specific skills, identification of resources, and recognition of the importance of healthy use of unstructured time for personal well-being.
10. Modular groups.
    a. The focus of each session is rotated in a way that allows an individual to join the group at any time and still cover each topic (e.g., an Independent Living Skills group that addresses nutrition the first session, money management the second, transportation the third, etc. and then begins the cycle again with a session on nutrition).
    b. This approach is similar to the current "treatment mall" approach that allows for patient choice among a variety of treatment topics.
11. Play groups.
    a. Frequently used in pediatric settings for observation, assessment, and to teach and develop a variety of skills.
    b. Play groups provide opportunities to develop play, task, and social skills at the child's developmental level and provide a developmentally-appropriate outlet for children to express thoughts and feelings.
12. Prevocational groups.
    a. Focuses on the identification of personal skills, limitations, and interests and the development of work habits and behaviors.
    b. The desired outcome is the development of the knowledge and skills that are prerequisite for participation in vocational training, vocational rehabilitation or for the acquisition of competitive employment.
13. Psychoeducational.
    a. An intervention approach that uses a classroom format and the principles of learning to provide information to members and to teach skills.
    b. A teacher/student relationship exists.
    c. The use of homework assignments is encouraged to facilitate skill development and generalization of learning.
14. Reminiscence.
    a. Activities are designed to review past life experiences to promote the use of cognitive abilities and foster a sense of personal worth.
    b. Current memory is not necessary nor is it facilitated.
15. Self-awareness.
    a. Includes such activities as values clarification, awareness of personal assets, limitations, and adaptive/maladaptive behaviors; and the individual's impact on others.
16. Sensory awareness.
    a. Includes activities to promote sensory functions and environmental awareness.
17. Social interaction groups.
    a. Include interventions to develop communication skills, socially acceptable behaviors, and interpersonal relationship skills.
    b. May be conducted in a modular and/or psychoeducational format.

Managing Problem Behaviors

1. Hallucinations.
   a. Create an environment free of distractions that trigger hallucinatory thoughts and interfere with reality-based activity.
   b. Use highly structured simple, concrete and tangible activities that hold the individual's attention.
   c. When the person appears to be focusing on a hallucinatory experience, attempt to redirect him/her to reality-based thinking and actions.
2. Delusions.
   a. Do not attempt to refute the delusion.
   b. Redirect the individual's thoughts to reality-based thinking and actions.
   c. Avoid discussions and other experiences that focus on and validate or reinforce delusional material.
3. Akathisia.
   a. Allow the person to move around as needed if it can be done without causing disruption to the goals of the group.
   b. Keep in mind that participation on many levels and in many forms can be beneficial to the individual.
   c. Whenever possible, select gross motor activities over fine motor or sedentary ones.
4. Offensive behavior (physical or verbal).
   a. Set limits and immediately address the behavior during a session.
   b. Reasons the behaviors are not acceptable should be clearly presented in a manner that is not confrontational or judgmental.

c. The consequences of continued offensive behavior should be clearly communicated.
d. It is required that staff protects all patients from the threat of harm or abuse by another patient. The needs of the entire unit and/or group membership must be kept in mind.

5. Lack of initiation/participation.
   a. Together with the individual, identify the reasons for lack of participation, e.g., lack of skill, irrelevance of activity, attention deficits, embarrassment, depression, etc.
   b. Motivational hints.
      (1) Individuals are more likely to participate in activities that address issues that are of interest or concern to them.
      (2) The more ownership patients have of the activity, the more they will participate.
      (3) Success is motivating.
      (4) Fun is motivating.
      (5) Positive feedback and rewards are motivating.
      (6) Everyone has his/her own motivators. It is important to identify what they are.
      (7) Curiosity can be used to motivate.
      (8) Food is often motivating (as per Maslow's hierarchy of needs. (See Chapter 5.)
         (a) Using secondary reinforcers such as praise is usually preferable to using primary reinforcers such as food.
      (9) Offer choices.
      (10) Encourage individual to remain in group and participate when/if they are ready.
6. Manic or monopolizing behavior.
   a. Select or design highly structured activities that hold the individual's attention and require a shift of focus from patient to patient.
   b. Thank the individual for their participation and redirect attention to another group member.
   c. Refer to limit-setting discussed above.
7. Escalating behavior.
   a. Avoid what can be perceived as challenging behavior (e.g., eye contact, standing directly in front of the patient).
   b. Maintain a comfortable distance.
   c. Actively listen.
   d. Use a calm, but not patronizing, tone.
      (1) Speaking in a softer or lower tone than the individual is often effective in decreasing the volume and intensity of the escalating individual.
   e. Speak simply, clearly, and directly. Avoid miscommunication.
   f. Do not make or communicate value judgments about the individual's thoughts, feelings, or behaviors.
   g. Clearly present what you would like the person to do.
   h. Avoid positions where either you or the patient feels trapped.
   i. Individuals most often calm in response to the above interventions. If an individual continues to escalate and is nonresponsive to interventions, additional steps are needed to ensure safety.
      (1) Remove other patients from the area.
      (2) Get or send for other staff.
8. Acting out behavior in children.
   a. Acting out is the expression of thoughts and feelings through maladaptive behavior instead of verbalizing.
   b. Depending on the severity of the situation, therapeutic options include:
      (1) Interpretation: a therapeutic technique where the therapist puts words to observed behavior enabling the child to appropriately express the feelings he or she is experiencing.
      (2) Redirection: a verbal tactic that refocuses the child on the assigned or current activity that provides cues for appropriate participation.
      (3) Limit setting: informing the child of what is permissible and what is unacceptable.
      (4) Time-out: an intervention technique that results in behavioral changes by removing the child from a problematic situation to a specific area.
9. The effects of dementia (e.g., Alzheimer's disease).
   a. Make eye contact and show that you are interested in the person.
      (1) Value and validate what is said by the person.
   b. Maintain a positive and friendly facial expression and tone of voice during all communications.
      (1) Do not give orders.
      (2) Use short, simple words and sentences.
      (3) Do not argue or criticize.
   c. Do not speak about the individual as if he/she was not there.
   d. Use non-verbal communication.
   e. Create a routine that uses familiar and enjoyable activities.
      (1) Use activities that demonstrate and promote personal interests and independence.
      (2) Do not introduce infantilizing activities.
      (3) Analyze and grade activities carefully.
      (4) Do not rush activities.
         (a) It is the process of engaging in an activity that is important; task completion is not needed.
   f. Note the effects of the time of day on behavior and activity performance.
   g. Attend to safety issues at all times.

Special Considerations in Psychosocial Evaluation and Intervention

Domestic Abuse

1. Facts and figures.
   a. In the United States, domestic abuse is a major social justice crisis and health care concern. The below facts and figures are provided to highlight the need for occupational therapists to be vigilant about the potential of domestic abuse during all interactions with all clients and family members, regardless of age. These statistics will not be on the NBCOT examination.
   b. 90% of abuse is committed by men against women.
   c. Four million women are victims of domestic violence each year.
   d. Four women are killed every day by domestic violence.
   e. 70% of men who abuse their partners also abuse their children.
   f. Children who witness domestic violence are 74% more likely to commit assaults against others.
   g. 50% of homeless women and children are homeless because of violence at home.
   h. Many incidents involve alcohol and/or drug use.
   i. Domestic abuse knows no boundaries. It occurs regardless of socioeconomic factors, race, culture, ethnicity, religion, or age.
2. Definition and types.
   a. Definitions vary greatly from state to state.
   b. Definitions involve violence or abuse that is used to control another member of the household.
   c. Domestic abuse can take one or more forms.
      (1) Physical abuse: hitting, kicking, punching, slapping, choking, and/or burning.
      (2) Emotional abuse: criticizing, humiliating, playing mind games, abusing or killing pets, withholding affection, isolating, and/or dominating.
      (3) Economic abuse: making the other ask for money, giving an allowance, and/or preventing the other from taking a job.
      (4) Intimidation and coercion: making the other afraid, breaking things, displaying weapons, threatening to leave or report the other for something, and/or making the other do something illegal.
      (5) Using children: making the other feel guilty about the children, using the children to relay messages, using visitation to harass the other, and/or threatening to take the children away.
      (6) Stalking: following, having followed, invading homes and privacy, and/or creating fear of immediate harm.
      (7) Sexual abuse: performing and/or requiring the other to perform unwanted sexual activities through force, threats, or intimidation.
   d. Patterns of abuse.
      (1) Impulsive abuse, during which the abuser has sudden attacks of rage, which may be regular or random.
      (2) Premeditated abuse, during which the abuser is cool and calculating.
3. Signs of physical abuse.
   a. Bruises at different stages of healing or in unusual places.
   b. Burns suggestive of specific objects.
   c. Lacerations to the face or genitals.
   d. Orthopedic injuries which are inconsistent with the explanations.
   e. Internal injuries of the head and organs.
   f. Head and facial injuries suggestive of hitting, shaking, or pulling.
   g. Reluctance to talk about injuries.
   h. Abuser not wanting to leave victim alone with others.
4. Reasons for failure to report or leave an abusive relationship.
   a. Economic pressure.
   b. Religious beliefs.
   c. Feeling of love for abuser.
   d. Believing the abuse is deserved.
   e. Viewing abuse as normal due to exposure to abuse/violence as a child.
   f. Fear of increasing abuse.
   g. Fear of retaliation.
   h. Belief things will change.
   i. Concern for children.
   j. Nowhere to go.
   k. Lack of support systems.
5. Role of occupational therapy.
   a. Develop a trusting relationship.
   b. Use the RADAR approach to screen for and respond to domestic abuse.
      (1) R = Routinely ask. Inquiring about potential abuse when interviewing all clients can be the first step in intervention; this acknowledges that abuse is not an acceptable secret.
      (2) A = Affirm and ask. Acknowledge and support the person who discloses abuse. Ask direct

questions of all clients to determine risk (e.g., Do you feel safe with your partner?).
(3) D = Document objective findings (e.g., the person has multiple bruises) and record client statements in quotes.
(4) A = Assess and address the person's safety (i.e., Has abuse become more violent? Are there weapons in the home?)
(5) R = Review options and referrals. Refer the person to domestic violence hotlines, domestic violence shelters, and/or safe houses which have staff trained in family violence and safety planning.
(a) The National Hotline is 1-800-799-7233.
(b) The National Sexual Assault Hotline is 1-800-656-4673.
(c) The National Teen Dating Abuse Hotline is 1-866-331-9474.

c. Areas to discuss with the person who has been/is being abused.
(1) Stress and safety.
(2) Fear and abuse.
(3) Family, friends, and support network.
(4) Emergency plan.

d. Provide information about treatment and support programs which enable empowerment of the individual.

e. Provide intervention for physical and emotional injuries and to develop skills needed to live an independent empowered life.

f. Inform supervisor and/or other treatment staff.

g. Mandatory reporting is required in some states, but laws vary.

Child Abuse

1. See Chapter 5.

Elder Abuse

1. See Chapter 5.

Patient/Client Abuse

1. See Chapter 4.

Psychological Reaction to Disability

1. Several factors influence the individual's reaction to disability.
   a. Permanency of the disability.
   b. Sudden vs. chronic onset.
   c. Appraisal of life experiences.
   d. Spiritual beliefs.
   e. Support systems.
   f. Cultural factors.
2. Adjustment.
   a. Active participation in social, vocational, and avocational pursuits.
   b. Successful negotiation of the physical environment.
   c. Awareness of remaining strengths and assets as well as functional limitations.
3. Phases of adjustment.
   a. Shock.
      (1) Initial reaction to a sudden physical or psychological trauma.
      (2) Characterized by emotional numbness, depersonalization, and reduced speech and mobility.
   b. Anxiety.
      (1) A panic-stricken reaction to awareness of the seriousness of the situation.
      (2) Characterized by restlessness, confusion, racing thoughts and psychological symptoms associated with anxiety.
   c. Denial.
      (1) Retreat from the realization of the seriousness and implications of the situation.
      (2) Characterized by minimalism, negation, aloofness, and unrealistic expectations.
   d. Depression.
      (1) Bereavement for the associated losses as the realities of those losses is identified.
      (2) Characterized by hopelessness, helplessness, isolation, and decreased self-esteem.
   e. Internalized anger.
      (1) Resentment and bitterness directed toward self.
      (2) Characterized by blaming of self for the event, the extent of the loss, or the failure to recover.
   f. Externalized anger.
      (1) An attempt to retaliate for the imposed losses, directed against those associated with the onset or rehabilitation of the situation.
      (2) Characterized by aggression, antagonism, demanding and critical attitudes, and passive-aggressive behavior.
   g. Acknowledgement.
      (1) The first step toward acceptance of the situation.
      (2) Characterized by acceptance of a new self-concept and the identification of values and goals.
   h. Adjustment.
      (1) An emotional acceptance of the situation and reintegration into identified roles.
      (2) Characterized by a positive sense of self and potentialities, and achievement of meaningful goals.
4. OT intervention.
   a. Acknowledgement of the individual's losses.
   b. Identification of what the individual is able to do with emphasis on personal accomplishments.

c. Assistance to the individual in his/her assumption of an active role in shaping his/her life.
d. The use of person-centered approaches based on empowerment theory is critical.
e. Reduction of limitations through changes in the physical and social environment.
f. Development of the skills necessary to participate in valued activities and meaningful occupations.
   (1) Stress management and coping skills.
   (2) Cognitive reframing/restructuring: the process of altering cognitions and cognitive processes (usually maladaptive thoughts and thinking) to facilitate changes in emotions and behavior.
g. Acquisition of resources and supports to enable full social participation.
h. Development of peer supports.

Suicide

1. Facts and figures.
   a. In the United States, suicide is a major social-justice crisis and health care concern. The below facts and figures are provided to highlight the need for occupational therapists to be vigilant about the potential of suicide during all interactions with all clients and family members, regardless of age. These statistics will not be on the NBCOT examination.
   b. In the United States, suicide is a leading cause of death.
      (1) A person dies by suicide about every 15 minutes in the United States.
      (2) In 2007 (the latest available data), suicide was the fourth-leading cause of death for adults between the ages of 18 and 65 years, the third-leading cause of death among those 15–24 years old, and the fifth-leading cause of death among those 5–14 years old.
   c. It is estimated that there are 11 nonfatal suicide attempts for every suicide death.
   d. The attempts of men and the elderly are more likely to be more fatal than those of women and youth.
      (1) The suicide rate for men is more than 4 times that of women due to men using firearms at a higher rate than women.
      (2) The elderly commit suicide at twice the rate of younger adults due to the losses associated with age.
   e. The suicide rate is increasing in children and adolescents.
      (1) 1 in 5 high school students and 1 in 10 college students have written a plan.
      (2) 10% of high school students have attempted suicide.
   f. Single individuals who were never married commit suicide at twice the rate of those who are or were married.
2. Identification of risk.
   a. A member of the treatment team (usually a physician) will ask the individual about suicidal thinking.
   b. It is important to identify the degree of risk.
      (1) The person is usually asked, if he/she was to try to hurt him/herself, how he/she would do it.
      (2) The degree of detail given indicates the seriousness of intent.
      (3) The potential for the plan to succeed also indicates the degree of risk.
   c. Risk factors for suicide.
      (1) Previous attempt or fantasized suicide.
      (2) Anxiety, depression, exhaustion, pervasive pessimism or hopelessness.
      (3) Availability of means of suicide; e.g., firearms in the home.
      (4) Concern for effect of suicide on family members.
      (5) Verbalized suicidal ideation, plan, or intent.
      (6) Preparation of a will.
      (7) Resignation after agitated depression.
      (8) Proximal life crisis, such as mourning, divorce, pending surgery, or disciplinary or legal problems.
      (9) Family history of suicide; exposure to suicide of others.
      (10) Family violence, including physical or sexual abuse.
      (11) Clinically diagnosed depression or other mental disorder.
      (12) Co-occurring mental health and/or substance abuse disorders.
      (13) Incarceration.
      (14) Impulsive and/or aggressive tendencies.
3. OT intervention.
   a. Identification of the motivation behind the suicidal intent and the identification of alternatives.
      (1) Development of a *contract for safety*, which can also be called an emergency or contingency plan, that specifies what the individual should do if experiencing suicidal ideation, plan or intent.
         (a) A contract for safety asks the individual to contract or commit to telling appropriate person/persons if he or she is having thoughts of suicide.
   b. Development of problem solving skills and stress management techniques to increase the individual's resilience and ability to manage life stressors.
   c. Identification of positive goals and interests to increase motivation for recovery.
   d. Identification of positive personal attributes and support systems to increase hopefulness.
      (1) This may be facilitated by a review of past successes.
      (2) This may be difficult to facilitate in individuals with depression.
   e. Activities that produce successful outcomes, especially those with a visible end-product, promote positive thinking.

Chapter 14

f. Activities designed for the expression and validation of feelings.
g. Moderate physical activity elevates mood.
h. Development of skills that increase functional performance.
i. Activities that are future-oriented, i.e., going to college, starting a new career, babysitting a grandchild, enjoying family traditions with friends and family over the holidays.
j. Patient/client and family education including:
   (1) Managing relapse and disappointment with a plan in place for dealing with active suicidal ideations.
   (2) Developing strategies for dealing with hopelessness.
   (3) Reinforcing and supporting engagement in treatment.
   (4) Maintaining medication compliance.
   (5) Increasing family involvement.
   (6) Identifying support groups and resources.
   (7) Developing strategies to handle setbacks in recovery.
k. National Suicide Hotline 1-800-273-TALK (8255).

Self-Harm/Self-Mutilation

1. Definition.
   a. "Deliberate destruction or alteration of one's body tissue without conscious suicidal intent" (Favazza, 1996, pp. xviii–xix).
   b. Also known as self-injurious behavior, parasuicide, self-wounding and "cutting."
2. A maladaptive coping skill for dealing with uncomfortable feelings.
3. Role of occupational therapy.
   a. Improving self-management by teaching stress, anger and emotional regulation skills.
   b. Instructing client in the use of alternative coping strategies (ice, rubber bands).
   c. Implementing interventions using CBT principles.
   d. Using DBT techniques if appropriate to the client.
   e. Providing instruction in the use of sensory approaches (tactile stimulation, massage, self-soothing) to manage the feelings that lead to self-harm.
   f. Developing problem solving skills.
   g. Improving communication skills.

Adjustment to Death and Dying

1. Stages of the individual's response as described by Elizabeth Kubler-Ross may include:
   a. Denial.
      (1) A coping strategy that allows the individual to refuse to accept or address the reality of his/her illness (e.g., "There must have been a mistake with the x-rays").
      (2) Denial may lead the individual to see many health professionals, hoping to find the one who will give a different prognosis.
      (3) Denial may be a response to the denial or discomfort experienced by others.
      (4) Denial will end when the individual is psychologically prepared to face the reality of the situation.
      (5) OT intervention includes allowing the person to ask questions and discuss the situation at his/her own pace.
   b. Anger.
      (1) The individual becomes angry as he/she accepts the reality of impending death (e.g., "Get out of here. You don't know what it's like").
      (2) This anger may be projected onto anyone who is seen as healthy or in a better position.
      (3) Rages, outbursts, and hurtful behavior must be identified for the purposes they serve.
      (4) OT intervention allows the individual to vent anger while identifying its source and developing more effective coping strategies.
   c. Bargaining.
      (1) In an attempt to gain control, the individual may bargain with doctors, caretakers, or God (e.g., "Just let me go to my child's graduation and then I'll be okay with this").
      (2) Bargains are an attempt to buy time.
      (3) Bargains are often associated with guilt related to things not done or promises not kept.
      (4) The individual should not be expected to keep to these bargains.
      (5) OT intervention involves responding honestly to questions.
   d. Depression.
      (1) As the individual acknowledges impending death, he/she begins to identify the feelings of loss and become depressed.
      (2) The tendency is to say goodbye to all but a few and isolate oneself as thoughts and feelings turn inward.
      (3) OT intervention assists in providing physical and psychological comfort for both the individual and his/her loved ones.
   e. Acceptance.
      (1) As the individual recognizes impending death, he/she begins to make plans and think about the future for self and family.
      (2) It may be a time of peace without fear or despair.
      (3) As time goes on, the need to communicate diminishes.
      (4) OT intervention is to provide ongoing support to the individual and family.
2. General considerations.
   a. People vary in the way they go through each stage.
   b. They may stop at any stage (e.g., some may stay in denial as their preferred coping strategy).

c. The needs of loved ones must be considered as they are likely going through stages similar to the dying individual.
d. Occupational therapists should assist the individual in coping with each stage without pushing for progression into the next stage.
3. Occupational therapy intervention throughout each stage.
   a. Assist the individual in maintaining as much control and independence as possible.
   b. Respond honestly and at the appropriate depth to questions.
   c. Assist the individual in developing coping skills.
   d. Encourage positive life review and support the legacies the individual leaves.
      (1) Gifts and mementos can be made or selected for significant others.
   e. Assist the individual in pursuing interests and maintaining meaningful roles.
   f. Actively listen.
   g. Incorporate family and friends in the treatment process.
   h. While being realistic, the therapist should not deprive the individual of hope.

References

Allen, C., Austin, S., David, S., Earhart, C., McCraith, C., Riska-Williams, L. (2007). *Manual for the Allen Cognitive Level Screen-5 (ACLS-5) and Large Allen Cognitive Level Screen-5 (LACLS-5)*. Camarillo, CA: ACLS and LACLS Committee.

Allen, C. K., Earhart, C. A., & Blue, T. (1992). *Occupational therapy treatment goals for the physically and cognitively disabled.* Bethesda, MD: American Occupational Therapy Association.

Alzheimer's Association. (2003). www.alz.com.

American Foundation for Suicide Prevention. (2011). *Facts and figures national statistics.* Retrieved April 12, 2011 from http://www.afsp.org/index.

American Occupational Therapy Association. (2007). *Models for community-based psychosocial practice chapter 7: Recovery model* [PDF document]. Retrieved from http://ce.aota.org/workshops/model/Chapter7.asp.

American Occupational Therapy Association. (2008). Occupational therapy practice framework: Domain and process, 2nd ed. *American Journal of Occupational Therapy, 62,* 625–688.

American Psychiatric Association. (2000). *DSM-IV-TR: Diagnostic and statistical manual of mental disorders text revision,* 4th ed. Washington, DC: American Psychiatric Association.

Artemis Center for Alternatives to Domestic Violence. *The facts (2001)*. Available: www.artemiscenter.org/facts.

Asher, I. (2007). *Occupational therapy assessment tools: An annotated index,* 3rd ed. Bethesda, MD: AOTA Press.

Benson, A. M., & Champagne, T. (2009). *Occupational therapy using a sensory integration–based approach with adult populations.* Retreived September 12, 2013 from http://www.aota.org/~/media/Corporate/Files/AboutOT/Professionals/WhatIsOT/MH/Facts/SI%20Fact%20Sheet%202.ashx

Bonder, B. (1991). *Psychopathology and function.* Thorofare, NJ: Slack.

Brown, C. (2011). Cognitive skills. In C. Brown, & V. Stoffel, (Eds.), *Occupational therapy in mental health: A vision for participation* (pp. 241–261). Philadelphia: F.A. Davis.

Brown, C., & Nicholson, R. (2011). Sensory skills. In C. Brown, & V. Stoffel, (Eds.), *Occupational therapy in mental health: A vision for participation* (pp. 280–297). Philadelphia: F.A. Davis.

Bruce, M. & Borg, B. (2002). *Psychosocial frames of reference: Core for occupation-based practice,* 3rd ed. Thorofare, NJ: Slack.

Cara, E., & MacRae, A. (Eds.). (2013). *Psychosocial occupational therapy: An evolving practice,* 3rd ed. Clifton Park, NY: Delmar Cengage Learning.

Cole, M., & Tufano, R. (2008). *Applied theories in occupational therapy: A practical approach.* Thorofare, NJ: Slack.

Cole, M. B. (2005). *Group dynamics in occupational therapy: The theoretical basis and practice application of group dynamics,* 3rd ed. Thorofare, NJ: Slack.

Crepeau, E., Cohn, E., & Schell. (Eds.). (2003). *Willard and Spackman's occupational therapy,* 10th ed. Philadelphia: Lippincott, Williams & Wilkins.

Domestic Abuse. (2001). Metro Nashville Police Department. Available: www.telalink.net/~police/abuse/symptoms.htm.

Drench, M., Noonan, A., Sharby, N., & Ventura, S. (2012). *Psychosocial aspects of health care,* 3rd ed. Upper Saddle River, NJ: Pearson.

Early, M. (2009). *Mental health techniques and concepts for the occupational therapy assistant.* Philadelphia: Lippincott Williams and Wilkins.

Fidler, G.S. (1996). Life-style performance: From profile to conceptual model. In R. P. Cottrell (Ed.), *Perspectives on purposeful activity: Foundation and future of occupational therapy* (pp. 113–121). Bethesda, MD: American Occupational Therapy Association.

Fleming-Castaldy, R. (2009). Activities, human occupation, participation, and empowerment. In J. Hinojosa & M. L. Blount (Eds.), *The texture of life: Purposeful activities in occupational therapy,* 3rd ed., (pp. 483–521) Bethesda, MD: AOTA Press.

Greenward, B. (2001) *Death and dying.* Available: www.uic.edu/orgs/convening/deathdyi.htm.

Helfrich, C. A. (2000). Domestic violence: Implications and guidelines for occupational therapy practitioners. In R. P. Cottrell (Ed.), *Proactive approaches in psychosocial occupational therapy* (pp. 309–316). Thorofare, NJ: Slack.

Hemphill, B. J. (Ed.) (1988). *Mental health assessment in occupational therapy.* Thorofare, NJ: Slack.

Hemphill, B. J. (Ed.) (1981). *The evaluative process in psychiatric occupational therapy.* Philadelphia: Lippincott.

Hemphill-Pearson, B. J. (Ed.) (1999). *Assessments in occupational therapy mental health: An integrative approach.* Thorofare, NJ: Slack.

Hopkins, H., & Smith, H. (Eds.). (2003). *Willard and Spackman's occupational therapy,* 10th ed. Philadelphia: J.B. Lippincott.

Hussey, S., Sabonis-Chafee, B., & O'Brien, J. (2007). *Introduction to occupational therapy,* 3rd ed. St. Louis, MO: Elsevier Mosby.

Kaplan, J. I., & Sadock, B. J. (2007). *Synopsis of psychiatry,* 10th ed. Philadelphia: Mosby.

Kielhofner, G. (2004). *Conceptual foundations of occupational therapy,* 3rd ed. Philadelphia: F.A. Davis.

Lane, S., Scott Roley, S., & Champagne, T. (2013). Sensory intergration and processing theory and application to occupational therapy, In B. A. B. Schell, G. Gillen, & M. E. Scaffa (Eds), *Willard and Spackman's occupational therapy,* 12th ed. (pp. 816–868). Philadelphia: Lippincott Williams & Wilkins.

Lehman, A. F. (1988). A quality of life interview for the chronically mentally ill. *Evaluation and Program Planning 11*(1), 51–62.

Miller, P. J., & Walker, K. F. (Eds.) (1993). *Perspectives on theory for the practice of occupational therapy.* Gaithersburg, MD: Aspen Publishers.

Mosey, A. C. (1996). *Psychosocial components of occupational therapy.* New York: Raven Press.

National Institute of Mental Health (NIMH). (2009). *Suicide in the U.S.: Statistics and prevention.* Retrieved February 24, 2010, from http://www.nimh.nih.gov/health/publications/suicide-in-the-us-statistics-and-prevention/index.shtml#factors.

Pratt, C. W., Gill, K. J., Barrett, N. M., & Roberts, M. M. (2007). *Psychiatric rehabilitation,* 2nd ed. Burlington, MA: Elsevier Academic Press.

Schkade, J. K., & Schultz, S. (1999). Occupational adaptation: Toward a holistic approach for contemporary practice, part 1, *American Journal of Occupational Therapy 46,* 829–837.

Schkade, J. K., & Schultz, S. (1999). Occupational adaptation: Toward a holistic approach for contemporary practice, part 2, *American Journal of Occupational Therapy 46,* 917–925.

Sladyk, K., Jacobs, K., & MacRae, N. (2010). *Occupational therapy essentials for clinical competence.* Thorofare, NJ: Slack.

Substance Abuse and Mental HealthServices Administration. (2012). *10 guiding principles of recovery.* Retrieved from: http://store.samhsa.gov/shin/content/PEP12-RECDEF/PEP12-RECDEF.pdf.

Wora, B. A., & McCarter, R. (1999). Validation of the empowerment scale with an outpatient mental health population. *Pyschiatric Services. 50,* 959–961.

Review Questions

Psychosocial Approaches: Evaluation and Intervention

Below are seven questions about key content covered in this chapter. These questions are not inclusive of the entirety of content related to psychosocial occupational therapy approaches that you must know for success on the NBCOT exam. These questions are provided to help you "jump start" the thought processes you will need to apply your studying of content to the answering of exam questions; hence they are not in the NBCOT exam format. Exam items in the NBCOT format which cover the depth and breadth of content you will need to know to pass the NBCOT exam are provided on this text's disc. The answers to the below questions are provided in Appendix 4.

1. What are key general postulates for change that are used in cognitive behavioral therapy (CBT) to guide the intervention process? How can these be applied throughout the occupational therapy process?

2. Identify three evaluation tools that can be used to assess an individual's cognitive level according to the Cognitive Disabilities model. Describe a practice situation in which each evaluation would be most effectively used.

3. Describe five current intervention approaches that use sensory models to guide treatment and how they can be effectively applied in occupational therapy practice.

4. Describe three interventions that can effectively help individuals experiencing hallucinations and/or delusions manage their symptoms during an occupational therapy group.

5. The RADAR approach is used to screen for and respond to domestic abuse. How would an occupational therapist apply this approach?

(Continued)

Psychosocial Approaches: Evaluation and Intervention (*Continued*)

6. You are watching television with your roommate in the eighth floor apartment you share. You observe a very sad, withdrawn appearance and minimal spontaneous social interaction. Lately your roommate has been drinking more than usual on social occasions and this week cancelled a scheduled weekly therapy appointment. You ask if everything is alright, and the reply is "no, not really." "I'm thinking of killing myself, I just can't take it anymore." "How do you think you would do it?" you ask. "I'm not quite sure, I think I have a couple of options here, belts, knives, I'm not sure which way I want to go, but I have to do it soon, maybe by the end of the week. Yes, definitely by the end of the week. All things considered, I think I'll jump out the window. I'm pretty sure the fall would kill me." What risk factors for suicide are you observing in your roommate, what levels of suicide lethality are present, and what should be your first intervention?

7. You are conducting a group for individuals with recently acquired spinal cord injuries that now have paraplegia and need to use a wheelchair for mobility. Adjusting to this abrupt change in their lives has been difficult and group members have developed depression. Several have anger issues as well. While participating in a group, one of the participants says to you "you really have no idea what it's like to have to face using a wheelchair for the rest of your life, when just a month ago I ran my sixth marathon. Running has been my whole life. It was the way I relieved stress and stayed in shape. I guess that's all over now." What type of therapeutic approach should you take? What types of individual and group interventions might benefit this individual?

15

Evaluation and Intervention for Performance in Areas of Occupation

RITA P. FLEMING-CASTALDY

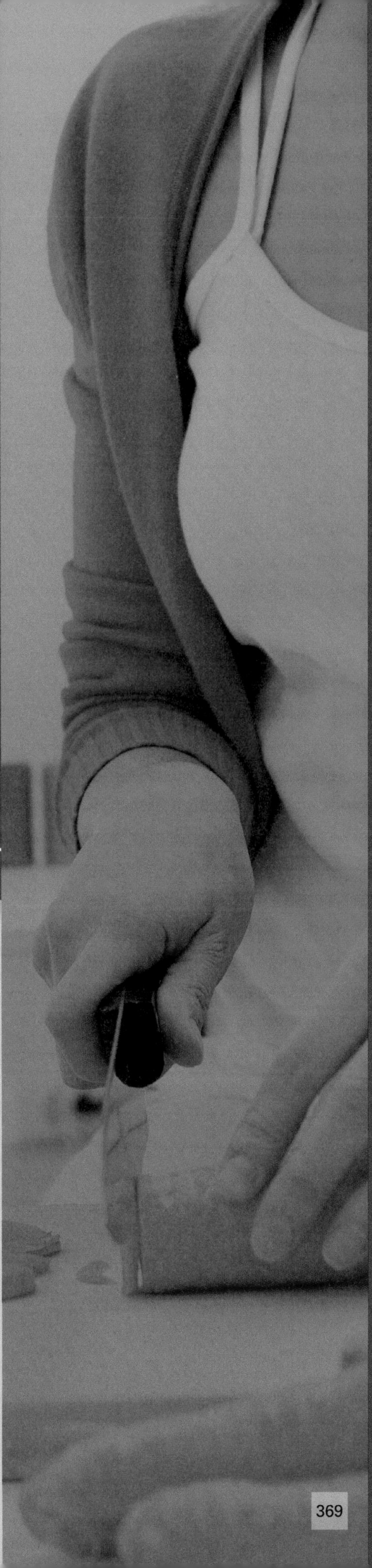

Chapter Outline

Areas of Occupation

Definition

1. "Various life activities in which people, populations, or organizations engage" (AOTA, 2008, p. 631). They include:
   a. Basic activities of daily living (BADL) includes self-care tasks such as grooming, oral hygiene, bathing/showering, toilet hygiene, dressing, eating, functional mobility, and sexual activity. This is also termed "personal" activities of daily living (PADL).
   b. Instrumental activities of daily living (IADL) includes activities that are more complex than BADL and which support community living such as home management tasks (e.g., cleaning, clothing care, shopping, money management, and meal preparation); care of others (e.g., children, pets); and community mobility.
   c. Work includes competitive employment for pay and other productive activities that make a societal contribution such as volunteer work.
   d. Education includes activities needed to participate in a learning environment and fulfill the role of student.
   e. Play and leisure include intrinsically motivated discretionary activities done for personal pleasure, diversion, and entertainment.
   f. Social participation includes activities engaged in as a member of a community, family, and/or peer/friend group.
   g. Rest and sleep include restorative activities which support health and occupational engagement.
2. Refer to Appendix 1 for a complete description of areas of occupation as defined in the AOTA's Practice Framework.

Overall Evaluation Guidelines

1. The focus of OT evaluation must be the individual's ability to perform meaningful occupations that are needed and desired by the individual.
2. Assessments should follow a 'top down' progression of considering the person's areas of occupation first, rather than a 'bottoms up' approach, which focuses on performance skills.
   a. The first step in evaluation is obtaining "an understanding of the client's occupational history and experiences, patterns of daily living, interests, values, and needs" (AOTA, 2008, p. 646).
   b. The desired outcome of evaluation is the identification of the person's occupational performance concerns and difficulties and the establishment of the individual's priorities for performance in areas of occupation.
   c. In the OT Practice Framework, this determination is called the occupational profile.
3. After the completion of a person's occupational profile, the person's client factors, performance skills, patterns, and contexts, and activity demands are assessed to identify specific strengths and limitations that impact on desired and needed occupational performance.
   a. All of the factors that may influence performance in areas of occupation are considered during screening.
      (1) Based on the results of screening, aspects that are determined to warrant further evaluation are specifically assessed.
   b. In certain practice settings (e.g., acute care with a three-day length of stay) and in certain clinical situations (e.g., there are major concerns for a client's safety) this determination of underlying problems may take precedence over the determination of an occupational profile.
   c. To determine these capabilities, the evaluation process should include observation of the person's actual performance of an activity in context.
      (1) If it is pragmatically not possible during the evaluation process for the person to perform the activity in its natural context, an environment that closely simulates the natural one should be provided for the assessment (e.g., an ADL apartment on a rehabilitation unit to simulate the person's home).
   d. In the OT Practice Framework, this part of the evaluation process is called an analysis of occupational performance.
4. Occupational performance assessment tools include interviews, checklists, task performance, rating scales, and standardized instruments.
   a. Subsequent sections in this chapter will outline the major assessment methods and published instruments used for the evaluation of performance in areas of occupation.
      (1) Information on reliability and validity studies conducted on occupational performance assessments will not be included in this chapter.
         (a) There is great variability in the quality and availability of these studies; therefore, the NBCOT exam is unlikely to test this information.
         (b) Readers seeking this information should consult specific assessment manuals.

b. Assessment tools which primarily use an interview format to comprehensively evaluate an individual's occupational functioning (e.g., COPM) and measures that evaluate performance in social participation (e.g., OCAIRS) and the interaction/communication skills needed for socialization (e.g., BAFPE) are described in Chapter 14.
c. Assessments that evaluate functional communication, functional mobility, and community mobility are provided in Chapter 16.
5. Interpretation of occupational performance assessments that are used to determine a person's ability to live independently must be made cautiously due to the self-report and/or simulated nature of certain items and the limited number of items tested in many evaluation tools.
6. Many assessments used to measure occupational performance provide a determination of the person's level of functional performance along a level of assistance continuum (Table 15-1).

Table 15-1

Scales to Measure Functional Performance
TOTAL ASSISTANCE:
The need for 100% assistance by one or more persons to perform all physical activities and/or cognitive assistance to elicit a functional response to an external stimulation.
MAXIMUM ASSISTANCE:
The need for 75% assistance by one person to physically perform any part of a functional activity and/or cognitive assistance to perform gross motor actions in response to direction.
MODERATE ASSISTANCE:
The need for 50% assistance by one person to perform physical activities or provide cognitive assistance to sustain/complete simple, repetitive activities safely.
MINIMUM ASSISTANCE:
The need for 25% assistance by one person for physical activities and/or periodic, cognitive assistance to perform functional activities safely.
STANDBY ASSISTANCE:
The need for supervision by one person for the patient to perform new activity procedures that were adapted by the therapist for safe and effective performance. A patient requires standby assistance when errors and the need for safety precautions are not always anticipated by the patient.
INDEPENDENT STATUS:
No physical or cognitive assistance is required to perform functional activities. Patients at this level are able to implement the selected courses of action, consider potential errors, and anticipate safety hazards in familiar and new situations.

Adapted from Health Care Financing Administration. (1996). *Medicare intermediary manual, Publication 13, Section 3906.4.* Washington, DC: U.S. Government Printing Office, 21–21.

Evaluation Methods and the NBCOT Examination

1. While some institutions and practitioners may develop their own occupational performance assessments to use in practice, the NBCOT examination can only ask questions about published evaluation tools.
2. The NBCOT examination may include a description of evaluation methods and/or the names of specific published assessment tools; therefore, a review of major occupational performance assessments is important for examination preparation.
   a. This can also increase understanding and knowledge of major principles and common approaches in the evaluation of occupational performance assets and deficits.
   b. This can further strengthen the clinical reasoning skills needed to answer examination questions that address the evaluation process.
3. As of the publication of this text, NBCOT has not made public the names of all of the specific assessments that may be on the examination.
   a. The assessments included in this chapter are based on the author's review of NBCOT self-assessment tools, major OT textbooks, and feedback obtained from OT practitioners regarding measures used in practice.

General Intervention Guidelines

1. Intervention should follow a 'top down' progression of considering the person's areas of occupation first rather than a 'bottoms up' approach which focuses initially and/or solely on performance skills and client factors.
   a. The impact of performance skill deficits and client factors on occupational performance is considered after the establishment of individual's desired occupational outcome.
   b. Specific interventions to remediate, alleviate, and/or compensate for the effects of performance skill deficits and client factors on occupational performance are often required.
   c. The focus of remediation interventions for performance skill deficits and client factors must be related to the individual's ability to perform meaningful occupations that are needed and desired by the individual.
2. Interventions for deficits that cannot be remediated should include recommendations for adaptive

strategies and/or adaptive equipment that compensate for the deficits and ease performance in areas of occupation.

a. Strategies that can be generalized to different situations are particularly helpful (e.g., principles of energy conservation).

b. Multiple factors should be considered when recommending adaptive strategies (Table 15-2).

(1) These factors are also relevant to consider when selecting adaptive equipment.

c. Training in adaptive strategies and/or equipment used to enhance performance must consider the person's privacy and dignity.

(1) This is especially critical in interventions for the performance of BADL/PADL.

Table 15-2

Factors to Consider When Recommending Adaptive Strategies
• What is important to the individual about the task?
• Is the strategy viewed as compatible with the particular social context?
• Does the strategy enhance the individual's sense of personal control?
• Does the strategy minimize the effort?
• Does the strategy interfere with social opportunities or diminish the presentation of self?
• Is the recommended strategy temporally realistic given the context?
• Does the strategy provide for safety?

From: McCraig, M. (1994). Self-care management for adults with movement disorders. In C. Christiansen (Ed.), *Ways of living: Self-care strategies for special needs* (p. 261). Bethesda, MD: American Occupational Therapy Association. Reprinted with permission.

Evaluation of Activities of Daily Living

Assessment of Motor and Process Skills (AMPS)

1. Focus: assessment of the effectiveness, efficiency, or safety of a person's ADL task performance, including personal activities of daily living (PADL), instrumental or domestic activities of daily living (IADL), and some leisure activities.
2. Method.
   a. Interview of the individual to determine 3–5 tasks that are relevant to the client and that will be sufficiently challenging.
   b. Selection by the client of 2–3 tasks from those offered by the therapist.
   c. Observation of a person's quality of performance of selected ADL tasks according to standardized task guidelines and client-chosen task options in a person's usual environment or in a closely simulated environment.
   d. Flexibility in task options allows for cultural diversity and individual differences in methods of performing tasks.
   e. Administration of the AMPS requires the therapist to complete a special AMPS training course which includes rater calibration.
3. Materials.
   a. The AMPS manual, which currently contains over 120 standardized task choices, specific task guidelines, and AMPS score sheet.
   b. The AMPS computer scoring program and a pencil.
   c. Materials and tools for each task as selected to be performed by the individual are described in the manual to include everyday items an individual would normally use.
4. Scoring and interpretation.
   a. The rater scores the quality of the individual's 16 motor skills and 20 process abilities on a 4-point ordinal scale of 1 = deficit, 2 = ineffective, 3 = questionable, 4 = competent.
   b. Raw scores are entered into the therapist's AMPS computer scoring program which converts the raw scores into ability measures along the AMPS motor and process skill scales.
   c. Individual's ability measures are adjusted by the AMPS computer program to account for certain test conditions.
      (1) Rater severity based upon calibration of rater during AMPS training.
      (2) Task challenge.
      (3) Skill item difficulty.
   d. Interpretation of scores enables the therapist to determine several functional aspects of performance.
      (1) The nature of the individual's difficulty in task performance.
      (2) The level of task challenges a person can manage.
      (3) The quality of change in ADL performance after intervention.

5. Population: anyone with a developmental age older than two years old with any diagnosis that causes functional limitations in ADL.
   a. The use of the AMPS has been extended to well populations comprised of healthy people.

Barthel Index

1. Focus: measurement of a person's independence in BADL and functional mobility before and after intervention and the level of personal care needed by the individual.
2. It includes 10 items.
   a. Feeding.
   b. Transferring.
   c. Personal grooming.
   d. Toileting.
   e. Control of bowel.
   f. Control of bladder.
   g. Bathing.
   h. Dressing.
   i. Walking on level ground.
   j. Negotiating/climbing stairs.
3. Method: direct observation of task performance, interview of individual and/or caregivers, and/or review of medical records.
4. Materials: score sheet, pencil, and everyday materials for task performance.
5. Scoring and interpretation.
   a. Items are scored according to a weighted system that reflects assisted performance (e.g., the individual receives minimal assistance during toilet transfer).
   b. The maximum score is 100 and reflects an individual's ability to do all 10 tasks independently.
   c. Achievement of a high score on a Barthel does not equate with the ability to live independently, since the Barthel's 10 tasks are limited to basic self-care.
   d. Scores on the Barthel can be used to determine the need for personal assistance (e.g., a home health aide) to perform basic ADL.
6. Population: adults and elders with physical disabilities and/or chronic illnesses, typically used in medical model settings.

Cognitive Performance Test (CPT)

1. Focus: the assessment of six functional ADL tasks that require cognitive processing skills based on Allen's Cognitive Disabilities Model.
   a. Dressing.
   b. Shopping.
   c. Making toast.
   d. Making a phone call.
   e. Washing.
   f. Traveling.
2. Method.
   a. Standardized administration procedures are followed for each task.
   b. Evaluator asks the individual to do each task, providing demonstration, reassurance, cueing, more directions, and/or the addition or elimination of sensory cues, if needed, to facilitate task performance.
3. Materials: specific/common items are delineated for each task.
4. Scoring and interpretation.
   a. Scoring guidelines according to Allen's levels are provided for each task.
   b. Level 1 represents the lowest functional level and Level 6 represents the highest.
   c. Total test scores range from 6 to 36.
   d. Average task performance score can be determined by dividing total test score by 6.
   e. CPT scores are used along with Allen's model to determine a person's capabilities and needs in other ADL tasks and his/her ability to live independently.
5. Population: adults and elders with psychiatric and/or cognitive dysfunction.

FIM System and WeeFIM System

1. Originally called the Functional Independence Measure and Functional Independence Measure for Children.
2. Focus: the assessment of the severity of a disability as determined by what the individual actually does and the amount of assistance needed by the individual to complete each task.
   a. Six performance areas are assessed.
      (1) Self-care: toileting, bowel and bladder management, grooming, bathing, dressing, and eating.
      (2) Sphincter management: bowel and bladder control.
      (3) Mobility: bed/chair/wheelchair, toilet, and tub/shower transfers.
      (4) Locomotion: walking, using stairs, and using a wheelchair.
      (5) Communication: expression and comprehension.
      (6) Social cognition: social interaction, memory, and problem solving.
3. Method: observation of activity performance with or without the assistance of a helper as determined by the person's ability to do the task.
   a. In the WeeFIM, caregiver interview may be used to obtain data.

4. Materials: the FIM (or WeeFIM) manual, score sheets, pencil, common items for ADL tasks. A FIM computer program is available to record and evaluate FIM results.
5. Scoring and interpretation.
   a. Each item on the FIM and WeeFIM for 3–7-year-olds is scored on a 1 to 7 scale graded from dependent to independent and the amount of assistance needed for task performance.
   b. A score of one indicates the person could not be evaluated performing the task or he/she required total assistance in task performance.
   c. Scores of two through five indicate increasing levels of assistance required from a helper for the individual to do the task.
   d. Scores of six or seven indicate that the person is independent in task performance and does not require a helper.
   e. The WeeFIM for children less than 3 year olds is scored on a 1 to 3 scale (1 = rarely, 2 = sometimes, 3 = usually).
   f. Behavioral criteria are provided for each scoring level for all test items.
   g. Documentation of demographics, diagnoses, impairment groups, length of stay, and costs of hospitalization are also included on the FIMs to provide data on the social and economic costs of disability.
   h. Results of the FIM and WeeFIM can provide relevant information about an individual's level of independence and severity of disability.
6. Population.
   a. Adults with disabilities who are not functionally independent for the FIM.
   b. Children from six months to seven years for the WeeFIM.
      (1) All those above age seven with intellectual abilities that are less than those of a typical seven year old can also be assessed with the WeeFIM.

Katz Index of ADL

1. Focus: assessment of level of independent functioning and type of assistance required in six areas of ADL.
   a. Bathing.
   b. Dressing.
   c. Toileting.
   d. Transferring.
   e. Continence.
   f. Feeding.
2. Method: evaluator observes activity performance or interviews the individual about performance.
3. Materials: rating scale, pencil and common task objects if activity is actually performed.
4. Scoring and interpretation.
   a. Evaluator rates each of the six activities as independent, some assistance required, or dependent.
   b. Specific criteria for each rating are provided for each activity.
   c. The individual ratings for the six activities are converted into a global letter score.
      (1) A = independent in all 6 activities.
      (2) B = independent in any 5 activities.
      (3) C = independent in all but bathing and one other activity.
      (4) D = independent in all but bathing, dressing, and one other activity.
      (5) E = independent in all but bathing, dressing, toileting, and one other activity.
      (6) F = independent in all but bathing, dressing, toileting, transfers, and one other activity.
      (7) G = dependent in all activities.
      (8) Other = individual's functional performance cannot be classified in A–G categories.
   d. Scores can be used to evaluate intervention outcomes and prognosis in a broad, general manner.
5. Population: adults and elders with chronic illness.

Kitchen Task Assessment (KTA)

1. Focus: measurement of the judgment, planning, and organizational skills used to perform a simple cooking task.
2. Method.
   a. A pre-test of washing hands is used to determine baseline abilities.
   b. Evaluator instructs and observes the individual in making cooked pudding from a mix.
   c. Large print task instructions are provided for the individual to review if needed.
   d. Evaluator can provide assistance, if needed, to facilitate successful task performance.
3. Materials: Large print task instructions, pudding mix, milk, pan, utensils, dishes, soap, water, and paper towels.
4. Scoring and interpretation.
   a. Scores of 0 = independent, 1 = verbal assistance, 2 = physical assistance, and 3 = totally incapable are rated for six categories of task skills.
      (1) Initiation.
      (2) Organization.
      (3) Performing all steps.
      (4) Proper sequence.
      (5) Judgment and safety.
      (6) Completion of task.
   b. Final scores can range from 0–18 with higher scores indicating increased impairment.

c. Information on performance in this task can be used to develop interventions for individual and adaptation strategies for caregivers.
5. Population: originally developed for adults and elders with senile dementia of the Alzheimer's type (SDAT), but its use has expanded to other populations that have cognitive dysfunction.

Klein-Bell Activities of Daily Living Scale (K-B Scale)

1. Focus: assessment of independent functioning in activities of daily living as evidenced by achievement of 170 items in six areas.
   a. Dressing.
   b. Elimination.
   c. Mobility.
   d. Bathing/hygiene.
   e. Eating.
   f. Emergency telephone communication.
2. Method.
   a. Evaluator observes and scores the individual's performance of each item and the behavioral components of each task.
   b. The use of assistive devices to perform activities is allowed.
3. Materials: manual, ADL scale, score sheet, pencil, everyday items for task performance.
4. Scoring and interpretation.
   a. All 170 items are rated as "achieved" or "failed".
   b. A rating of "achieved" is given if the individual is able to perform the task independently, with or without adaptive equipment.
   c. A rating of "failed" is given if the person requires physical or verbal assistance to perform the task.
   d. Use of this scale can increase caregivers' understanding of the individual's need for assistance.
   e. The detailed behavioral component information is useful for intervention planning and evaluation of intervention outcomes.
      (1) As a result, this measure is often used in research studies.
5. Population: individuals from six months old to the elderly with any diagnosis (physical, psychosocial, cognitive, and/or developmental).

Kohlman Evaluation of Living Skills (KELS)

1. Focus: determination of an individual's knowledge and/or performance of 17 basic living skills needed to live independently in five main areas.
   a. Self-care.
   b. Safety and health.
   c. Money management.
   d. Transportation and telephone.
   e. Work and leisure.
2. Method.
   a. Evaluator provides standard instructions for individual to complete some tasks (e.g., money management).
   b. Evaluator uses standard questions to obtain the individual's self-report regarding performance of other tasks (e.g., leisure pursuits).
   c. Evaluator does not provide additional instructions or feedback during the evaluation.
3. Materials: KELS manual which contains standard test forms, safety pictures, an equipment list for additional common materials, and score sheets.
4. Scoring and interpretation.
   a. A score of "independent" or "needs assistance" is given according to standard scoring criteria established for each of the 17 items.
   b. A "not applicable" or "see note" score is used if warranted (e.g., a person has no need to do monthly bills).
   c. Scores of "independent," "not applicable," and/or "see note" receive a number value of zero.
   d. Scores of "needs assistance" receive a number value of one, except for items in the work/leisure area which receive a number value of ½.
   e. All numerical values for each item are added together for a total score.
      (1) A total score of 5½ or less indicates the presence of skills for independent living.
      (2) A total score of 6 or more indicates the absence of skills needed for independent living.
   f. A separate Community Support Scale can be completed by evaluator to use as a guide to determine the level of assistance the individual may need to live in the community.
   g. KELS scores can provide a general overview of person's functional level and give a baseline for further evaluation and intervention.
5. Population: originally designed for adolescents and adults in acute psychiatric hospitals but its use has expanded to elders and those with a diversity of diagnoses is a variety of settings.

Milwaukee Evaluation of Daily Living Skills (MEDLS)

1. Focus: the assessment of actual or simulated performance of basic living skills needed to function in the individual's expected environment.
   a. Basic communication.
   b. Personal care and hygiene (toileting, brushing teeth).

Chapter 15

c. Medication management.
d. Personal health care (eyeglass care).
e. Time awareness.
f. Eating.
g. Dressing.
h. Safety in the home.
i. Safety in the community.
j. Use of telephone.
k. Transportation.
l. Maintenance of clothing.
m. Use of money.

2. Method.
   a. A screening form is used to determine which of the MEDLS subtests are relevant to the individual and his/her expected environment (e.g., eyeglass care is only relevant to a person who wears eyeglasses, a person who is moving to a group home does not need to do household bills).
   b. Items screened as needing evaluation are then administered according to standardized procedures.
   c. All items have standard instructions and a time limit for task completion.
   d. It is recommended that the evaluator schedule administration of the test items to be during an integral part of the person's normal routine (e.g., personal care, hygiene, and dressing in the morning).
3. Materials: MEDLS manual with screening and reporting test procedures, forms, clothing and safety pictures, and an extensive equipment list of common everyday items. It is recommended that the individual's own supplies be used.
4. Scoring and interpretation.
   a. All items are scored according to standard criteria established for each subtest.
   b. Results from MEDLS can provide comprehensive data on a number of performance-based ADL tasks that are useful for intervention and discharge planning.
5. Population: originally developed for adults (18 or older) who have chronic mental illness (at least a 2-year history) and who have resided, for at least 6 months, in a psychiatric hospital, halfway house, group home, or skilled nursing facility, or who have participated for at least 2 years in an outpatient day treatment program, but its use has expanded to other populations with ADL deficits.

Routine Task Inventory (RTI)

1. Focus: measurement of an individual's level of impairment in activities of daily living according to Allen's model of cognitive disabilities.
   a. Six physical scales in the areas of grooming, dressing, bathing, walking, feeding, and toileting.
   b. Eight instrumental scales in the areas of housekeeping, preparing food, spending money, taking medication, doing laundry, shopping, telephoning, and traveling.
2. Method: three different methods can be used.
   a. Observation of individual's performance and completion of the rating scale for each item by evaluator.
   b. Self-report by the individual if cognitively able to complete RTI questionnaire.
   c. Report of a caregiver familiar with the individual's functional performance through completion of the RTI questionnaire.
3. Materials: RTI questionnaire and a pencil.
4. Scoring and interpretation.
   a. Each item is rated according to behavioral criteria based upon Allen's cognitive levels of 1–6.
   b. Comparisons between scores obtained when more than one evaluation method is used can be helpful in determining similarities and/or discrepancies between the individual's self-awareness of abilities, caregiver's view of performance, and/or evaluator's observance of performance.
   c. Interpretation of evaluation results can be used to design intervention based on Allen's model (refer to Chapter 14).
5. Population: adults and elders with cognitive impairments.

Scoreable Self-Care Evaluation

1. Focus: measurement of functional performance and identification of difficulties in 18 basic living tasks in four main areas.
   a. Personal care.
   b. Housekeeping chores.
   c. Work and leisure.
   d. Financial management.
2. Method.
   a. A Motivational Questionnaire is given to the individual to assess his/her values and beliefs about self-care skills.
   b. Evaluator then administers each task according to standardized instructions.
   c. Individual's performance is observed and scored by the evaluator.
3. Materials: manual, task completion sheets, score sheets, index cards, telephone directory and numbers, and play money.
4. Scoring and interpretation.
   a. The individual's performance is scored based on inability to do the task.

b. Task scores are added to obtain a score for each of the 4 main test areas and then a total score.
c. Interventions can be planned based on observed deficits.
5. Population: adolescents, adults, and elders with psychiatric illnesses in acute hospital settings or living in the community.

Test of Grocery Shopping Skills (TOGSS)

1. Focus: determination of a person's ability to shop for groceries in a grocery store using a grocery list.
   a. Because there are two grocery lists provided in the TOGSS, it can be used as an intervention pre/post-test to measure a person's skill acquisition.
   b. A companion tool called the Knowledge of Grocery Shopping Skills (KOGSS) can be used to assess a person's knowledge of grocery shopping.
2. Method.
   a. The evaluation is completed in the person's natural environment at a community grocery store.
   b. The individual is provided with a grocery list of ten items of specific sizes and asked to locate and select the items at the lowest price.
   c. The therapist observes the person during the performance of this task in the grocery store.
   d. The KOGSS is completed as a self-report.
3. Materials: grocery lists, self-assessment, and score forms.
4. Scoring and interpretation.
   a. A score is obtained based on the person's ability to efficiently and accurately find the correct items at the lowest price. There are three subscale scores.
      (1) Accuracy: the person's ability to find the correct item at the required size and lowest price.
      (2) Time: how long it took the person to find the items.
      (3) Redundancy: the number of aisles the person entered to look for items and how many times a person returned to the same aisle.
      (4) The therapist also uses observation to assess the strategies the person uses to shop (e.g., scanning overhead signs, asking for help, scanning shelves, checking prices).
      (5) The KOGSS is scored to indicate person's knowledge about grocery shopping; higher scores indicate greater knowledge.
5. Population: originally developed for persons with serious mental illness, the TOGSS can be used with persons who have cognitive impairments due to other diagnoses (e.g., TBI, CVA, ID, PDD, dementia) which interfere with community living skills.

Sexual Expression/Activity Evaluation

1. The ADL skill of sexual expression/activity is typically not included on commonly used ADL assessments and it does not have a published OT assessment available for clinical use.
2. The occupational therapist should assess this ADL during routine screenings and interviews, as appropriate.
   a. Determine if sexual expression/activity is valued.
   b. Identify potential obstacles for the attainment and maintenance of safe, satisfying sexual expression/activity.
      (1) Pathophysiological changes related to disease, disability, and/or the aging process.
      (2) Psychological and/or cognitive changes related to disease, disability, and/or the aging process.
         (a) Judgment, impulse control, and decision-making skills must be assessed to ensure safety.
      (3) Limited partner availability due to social demographics and/or sociocultural attitudes.
   c. Determine if a person's knowledge of his/her sexuality is adequate and appropriate for his/her age, developmental level, expected roles, and environmental contexts.
3. If an individual is reticent about discussing his/her sexuality during the OT evaluation, the therapist must respect and accept this preference.
   a. Sexual concerns that are unexpressed during initial OT sessions are often brought forth during later sessions as a therapeutic relationship develops between the individual and his/her occupational therapist.
   b. Sessions focused on intimate self-care issues frequently precipitate questions regarding sexuality.
   c. An atmosphere of continuing permission to discuss sexual expression should be maintained throughout the person's engagement in OT.
4. The potential realities of sexual abuse, assault, and exploitation must be considered during the evaluation of all individuals regardless of age.
   a. Occupational therapists are required by practice acts, protective legislation, and our professional code of ethics to report any suspected incidents of child, adult, or elder abuse or assault to the appropriate agency and/or local law enforcement.

Activities of Daily Living Intervention

Self-Care Intervention

1. Determine whether the self-care activity should be modified to enable individual performance, performance with external assistance, or eliminated.
   a. Activities that are valued, meaningful, and enjoyable to the person and related to desired role performance should be modified for individual performance, with appropriate supports provided as needed (e.g., brushing one's hair using an adapted brush to maintain one's appearance at school/work).
   b. Activities that are difficult to perform and/or are not enjoyable should be eliminated or performed with the assistance of others (e.g., dressing which requires a great deal of exertion that can exhaust an individual; fasteners can be modified or eliminated, assistance can facilitate task performance).
2. Recommend adaptive strategies for self-care task performance (Table 15-2).
3. Provide adaptive equipment to compensate for functional impairments during self-care activity performance.
   a. Toileting and toilet hygiene equipment.
      (1) Grab bars and/or toilet safety frame.
      (2) Bedside (3 in 1) commode or raised toilet seat.
      (3) Bowel training device, bladder control devices.
      (4) Skin inspection mirror.
      (5) Toilet paper holder.
   b. Grooming/oral hygiene adaptive equipment.
      (1) Universal cuff to hold toothbrush, razor, comb, and/or brush.
      (2) Built-up, angled, or long-handled brushes and/or razors.
      (3) Blow-dryer, nail clippers, and nail polish holders.
      (4) Faucet turners.
      (5) Electric toothbrush, floss holders, water pik.
   c. Bathing/showering.
      (1) Grab bars and non-skid mat.
      (2) Tub transfer bench/shower bench.
      (3) Shower commode chair.
      (4) Handheld shower.
      (5) Anti-scald valves and/or faucets.
      (6) Built-up, angled, and/or long-handled bath sponge or bath mitt.
      (7) Soap on a rope, soap dish with suction cup.
      (8) Storage units.
   d. Dressing.
      (1) Reachers, dressing sticks, and pants dressing poles.
      (2) Built-up, angled, or long-handled shoe horn.
      (3) Pull-on clothing, Velcro-type closures, and/or front opening closures for clothing.
      (4) Elastic shoelaces, slip-on shoes.
      (5) Button hook, zipper pull and zipper loop or ring.
      (6) Sock/stocking aid.
   e. Feeding/eating.
      (1) Adapted nipples and bottles for infants.
      (2) Scoop dish or plate guards.
      (3) Non-slip placemat or dycem.
      (4) Built-up, angled, weighted, or long-handled utensils, swivel utensils.
      (5) Rocker knife and/or spork.
      (6) Adapted cups and long or angled straws.
      (7) See Chapter 5 for information on interventions to facilitate development of oral-motor control and feeding skills.
   f. Medication management.
      (1) Easy open, non-child-proof medication bottles.
      (2) Pill organizers, medication minders.
   g. Refer to Table 15-3 for spinal cord injury (SCI) levels and self-care abilities.
4. Recognize the multiple dimensions of a person with a disability and the complexities of many disorders. For example, Friedrich's ataxia is characterized by tremors that may indicate the need for weighted utensils, but muscle strength is also limited so utensils may be too heavy for functional use.
5. Train in safe use of adaptive equipment and assistive technology.
6. Practice to attain proficiency in activity performance at appropriate times and in real environments (e.g., brush teeth in the bathroom in the morning).
7. Provide cues and assistance as needed.
   a. Verbal reminders and prompts.
   b. Nonverbal gestures, written directions, physical prompt to initiate.
   c. Physical hand-over-hand assistance through complete activity movement.
   d. Visual supervision to ensure safety with minimal or no verbal or nonverbal cues.
8. Use thematic and topical groups to develop needed skills (e.g., grooming group, medication management).
9. Teach principles and methods of energy conservation, work simplification, joint protection, and proper body mechanics. Refer to Chapter 11.
10. Educate and train caregivers to provide needed cues, physical assistance, and/or supervision.

Table 15-3

SCI Levels and Self-Care Abilities

C1–C3	Totally dependent in all self-care but can instruct others in preferences for care. Can chew and swallow.
C4	Totally dependent in all self-care but can instruct others in preferences for care. Can drink from a glass with a long straw.
C5	Feeding requires total assist for setup; then independent with equipment. Equipment used may include: • Suspension sling or mobile arm support. • Dorsal wrist splint with universal cuff. • Dycem to prevent slippage of plate. • Scoop dish or plate guard. • Angled utensils. Dressing requires minimal to moderate assistance with upper body dressing. Dependent with lower body dressing. Bathing requires moderate to minimal assistance. Grooming requires assistance with setup; however, with splint and universal cuff can be independent with brushing teeth and combing hair. Independent using electric shaver that fits around the hand.
C6	Feeding: Independent using adaptive equipment which may include • Universal cuff or tenodesis splint. • Rocker knife. • Scoop dish or plate guard • Cup with large handles. Dressing: Independent in lower body dressing performed while in bed. Requires maximal assistance with socks and shoes. Independent with upper body dressing using button hook, zipper pull, velcro fasteners. Bathing: Minimal assistance using hand-held shower, tub bench, and sliding board transfer. Grooming: Independent using tenodesis grasp or splint.
C7	Feeding: Independent Dressing: Independent, but may need button hook. Bathing: independent using hand-held shower, tub bench, and depression transfers. Grooming: Same as C6.
C8–T1	Independent in all self-care; uses tub bench and hand-held shower. Performs depressions transfers. Can transfer from wheelchair to floor and back to chair with standby assist.
T6 to L4	Independent in all self-care.

a. Teach organizational strategies (e.g., place clothing in proper sequence for dressing).

b. Teach activity analysis, gradation, simplification, and adaptation skills (e.g., for a person with Alzheimer's disease, provide multiple small meals to decrease the amount of attention required to eat).

11. Educate the individual with disabilities on personal care attendant training.
    a. Practice methods for directing self-care in the personally desired and acceptable manner.
    b. Provide assertiveness and personal advocacy training.
12. Modify the environment to maximize performance and ensure safety. Refer to Chapter 16.

Sexual Expression/Activity Intervention

1. Occupational therapy intervention is provided to enable satisfying, safe sexual expression/activity regardless of disability, disease, or advanced age.
2. Myths about the sexuality of the aged and individuals with disability or disease processes must be confronted and debunked. Myths include:
   a. They are asexual and have less interest in sexual expression than younger and/or healthier persons.
   b. They are physically unattractive and not desirable as a sexual partner and will be a burden to their partners.
   c. They inherently have poor judgment and cannot make appropriate decisions about their sexuality.
   d. Intercourse with mutual orgasm is the desired and primary means to express oneself sexually.
      (1) Intimate behaviors, such as mutual stimulation, cuddling, oral sex, and/or caressing are not adequate sexual activity.
      (2) Self-stimulation/masturbation is not an appropriate means of sexual expression.
   e. Individuals who live in shared residential settings such as nursing homes, group homes, and assisted living facilities are asexual.
      (1) They should be segregated according to gender.
      (2) Privacy for the individual is not essential and does not need to be respected.

f. Individuals with disabilities and/or elders who desire and/or engage in sexual activity are oversexed and inappropriate.

3. Occupational therapists should use the PLISSIT model as a guide for appropriate interventions.
   a. P = permission which requires the therapist to create an atmosphere which gives the individual permission to raise concerns about his/her sexuality and sexual activity(ies).
      (1) Incorporating sexuality into the OT initial and ongoing evaluation in a matter-of-fact manner is an effective method.
      (2) A therapist who is not comfortable with creating a permissive atmosphere for the discussion of sexuality due to personal, social, cultural, and/or religious reasons must honestly acknowledge this fact to the client and refer him/her immediately to a team member who is comfortable with addressing the individual's concerns.
      (3) It is the team's responsibility to ensure that at least one team member is comfortable with evaluating and intervening with individuals with sexual expression concerns.
      (4) Supervision and continuing professional development activities should be pursued by all to develop this needed comfort.
   b. LI = limited information that is provided by the therapist to ensure that the individual has accurate knowledge about his/her sexual abilities and potentials.
      (1) Facts are shared (e.g., there is sex after disability), and myths are dispelled (see prior section).
   c. SS = specific suggestions that are provided by the therapist to facilitate the individual's pursuit of satisfying sexual expression, either alone or with a partner.
      (1) The individual's (and partner's) goals for sexual expression and activity are identified and strategies for achieving goals are explored.
      (2) Principles of activity analysis, gradation, modification, and simplification are used to facilitate goal attainment.
      (3) Nonmedical methods to manage pain and stiffness (e.g., warm baths) are provided.
      (4) Positioning alternatives and adaptive equipment to facilitate desired sexual expression are suggested.
      (5) Energy conservation methods (e.g., timing sex for when one has the most energy and use of sexual positions that require less energy expenditures) are suggested to those with limited endurance.
      (6) Catheter care, hygiene concerns, and skin care are addressed.
      (7) Referrals to a physician for medical management of pain, impotence or other sexual dysfunctions, and hormonal treatment.
   d. IT = intensive therapy which is indicated when the individual requires intervention for long-standing relationship problems and/or enduring sexual problems.
      (1) These problems are often due to difficulties beyond the onset or presence of a disability.
      (2) Specialized training is required to provide intensive therapy so a referral to the appropriate professional (e.g., marriage counselor, sex therapist) is indicated.
      (3) Occupational therapists can become specialists in this area upon completion of an appropriate professional training program.
4. Methods of intervention can include one-on-one counseling sessions, therapeutic groups, and/or dissemination of printed materials.
5. Interventions for individuals with cognitive impairments (e.g., poor impulse control, limited judgment) are essential to ensure safety and to protect the individual from sexual abuse, assault, and/or exploitation.
   a. Assertiveness training to increase understanding of the right, and develop the ability, to set limits.
   b. Training and practice in physical self-protection techniques.
   c. Role playing to simulate potential scenarios which can challenge the individual's sexual judgment.
   d. Sex education (e.g. menstrual cycle information, prevention of sexually transmitted diseases).
   e. Caregiver and family education.
      (1) Socially inappropriate sexual activity is often difficult for families to understand (e.g., an elder with Alzheimer's disease begins to disrobe in the living room).
         (a) Recognizing that this behavior is indicative of an underlying disease process is important.
         (b) Providing strategies for effectively managing undesirable behaviors is a main OT focus (e.g., eliminate clothing fasteners in the front, divert the person's attention to an activity of interest).

Home Management Intervention

1. Determine the home management expectations and demands of the individual's current and expected environment.
   a. Supportive living environments can range in expectations from requiring that a resident only clean his/her room (e.g., in a group home) to complete management of a home with minimal supervision (e.g., a supported apartment).

b. Independent living environments can also have a range of expectations and demands (e.g., one spouse always does the budget, the other spouse always cooks).

2. Determine whether the home management activity should be modified to enable independent performance, self-directed performance with external assistance, or eliminated.
   a. Activities that are valued, meaningful and enjoyable to the person and related to desired role performance should be modified for individual performance, with appropriate supports provided as needed (e.g., preparing after-school snacks for children).
   b. Activities that are difficult to perform and/or are not enjoyable should be eliminated or performed with the assistance of others (e.g., cleaning a refrigerator can be delegated to another person, or a self-cleaning oven can eliminate a task).
3. Recommend adaptive strategies for home management task performance. Refer to Table 15-2.
4. Provide adaptive equipment to compensate for functional impairments during home management activity performance.
   a. Cleaning.
      (1) Suction bottom bottle and glass brushes.
      (2) Reachers.
      (3) Aerosol can holders.
      (4) Built up, angled, or long-handled sponges, dusters, brooms, mops, dustpans.
      (5) Front-loading washers and dryers.
      (6) Electronic dishwasher, self-cleaning oven, automatic defrosting refrigerator.
   b. Cooking.
      (1) Faucet and knob turners.
      (2) Anti-scald faucets and/or valves.
      (3) Jar openers, bowl holders, and saucepan stabilizers.
      (4) Nonskid pad, placemat, or dycem.
      (5) Cutting board with a stabilizing nail and built-up edges.
      (6) Built-up or angled utensils and rocker knives.
      (7) Adapted timers.
      (8) Electric can opener.
      (9) Lightweight pots, pans, dishware.
      (10) Automatic hot water dispenser and/or hot-pots.
      (11) Strap loops to open refrigerator, cabinets, and oven doors.
      (12) Reachers and step stools.
      (13) Utility cart.
      (14) High kitchen stool.
5. Train in safe use of adaptive equipment and assistive technology.
6. Teach principles and methods of energy conservation, work simplification, joint protection, and proper body mechanics. Refer to Chapter 11.
7. Provide cues and assistance as needed.
   a. Verbal reminders and prompts.
   b. Nonverbal gestures, written directions, physical prompt to initiate.
   c. Physical hand-over-hand assistance through complete activity movement.
   d. Visual supervision to ensure safety with minimal or no verbal or nonverbal cues.
8. Practice to attain proficiency in activity performance at appropriate times and in real environments (e.g., cooking a meal in a kitchen at lunchtime).
9. Recognize and respect personal, sociocultural, and socioeconomic differences (e.g., standards of cleanliness, dietary restrictions, and preferences).
   a. Use equipment that is socioeconomically appropriate (e.g., do not use an oven to teach meal preparation if someone only owns a microwave).
10. Use thematic and topical groups to develop needed skills (e.g., cooking group, money management group).
11. Modify environment to maximize performance and ensure safety. Refer to Chapter 14.
12. Educate and train caregivers to provide needed cues, physical assistance, and/or supervision.
13. Refer to relevant social service programs (e.g., food stamps, home energy assistance program [HEAP]).
14. Refer to the appropriate supportive living environment if independent living is not attainable (e.g., group home, halfway house, supported apartment).

Family Participation Evaluation

Overview

1. There are no specific OT published assessments that deal exclusively with family interaction.
   a. Some commonly used assessments include family participation (e.g., the Role Checklist).
2. The occupational therapist should assess this occupational performance during routine screenings and interviews.
   a. Determine past, current, and anticipated roles, responsibilities, and expectations of family members.

b. Identify potential obstacles for the attainment and maintenance of satisfying family participation.
3. If the family and the therapist do not share a common language, interpreters must be used to ensure the validity of information obtained.
4. The sociocultural background, values, and dynamics of the family must be considered during the evaluation process.
5. Individuals who live in shared residential settings such as nursing homes, group homes, and assisted living facilities and their families should receive intervention to assist with role transitions.
   a. Fellow residents and staff in these settings often assume the roles of surrogate family members.

Parenting/Child Care

1. Determine ability to care for child's physical needs.
2. Determine ability to care for child's emotional needs.
3. Determine knowledge of child's developmental level and its corresponding play and communication level.

Family Participation Intervention

General Intervention Guidelines

1. Collaborate with family on identifying desired goals.
   a. Provide interpreters, if necessary.
2. Determine whether the family activity should be modified to enable independent performance, self-directed performance with external assistance, or eliminated.
   a. Activities that are valued, meaningful, and enjoyable to the person and related to desired role performance should be modified for individual performance, with appropriate supports provided as needed (e.g., reading a bedtime story to children).
   b. Activities that are difficult to perform and/or are not safe should be eliminated or performed with the assistance of others (e.g., bathing a toddler).
3. Methods of intervention can include one-on-one counseling sessions, therapeutic groups, and/or dissemination of printed materials.
4. Design interventions using activities that are meaningful to the individual's role within the family.
5. Use topical and thematic groups to develop effective family participation skills.
   a. Role play to simulate potential scenarios which can challenge the individual's family skills (e.g., assertiveness training, anger management).
   b. Practice effective family communication.
   c. Teach principles and methods of energy conservation, work simplification, joint protection, and proper body mechanics for family activities. Refer to Chapter 11.
   d. Develop parenting skills, if needed.

Intervention for Parenting Activities

1. Teach parent how to care for child's physical needs and physically practice parenting tasks (e.g., placing child into a front pack using proper body mechanics).
2. Instruct parent about normal developmental roles and tasks to ensure expectations of child/children are realistic.
3. Recommend adaptive strategies for home management task performance that are related to parenting (e.g., preparation of child's bag lunch for school). See Table 15-2.
4. Provide adaptive equipment to compensate for functional impairments during parenting tasks.
   a. Adapted drop-side crib, raised and/or adjustable height crib mattress, child-resistant one-handed crib wall release mechanism.
   b. Foam rubber bathing pads for sink, portable plastic tub and/or reclining infant seat placed in tub.
   c. Changing tables at proper height with safety straps and touch fasteners.
   d. Pillow to support breast feeding (which physically is the easiest method to feed an infant).
   e. Lightweight and/or angled bottles.
   f. One-handed swing away release tray on high chair with safety strap.
   g. Food warmer tray.
   h. Pullover clothes, Velcro fasteners for bibs, diaper covers, clothing.
   i. Infant carriers.
5. Baby furniture and equipment should be tested and used on a trial basis to ensure it matches parent's capabilities.

6. The family's socioeconomic status and cost of recommendations must be considered (e.g., premeasured formula and disposable diapers are convenient, energy saving, and expensive options).
7. Recognize and respect personal, sociocultural, and socioeconomic differences within families.
8. Teach the child/children of a parent with a disability self-reliance at a young age.
   a. Arrange tasks so they are accessible to a child (e.g., storage for dishes and glasses next to dishwasher, not in a high cabinet).
   b. Delegate tasks that are achievable for child's/children's developmental level (e.g., even a young child can move clothes from a front-loading washer to a front-loading dryer).
9. Modify the environment to maximize parenting task performance and ensure safety of the parent and child. Refer to Chapter 16.
10. Refer family members to support groups, local and national organizations.
11. Provide caregiver/family education in verbal and written formats in family's language of choice.
12. Be aware of signs of family neglect or abuse.
    a. OTs are required by practice acts, protective legislation, and our professional code of ethics to report any suspected incidents of child, adult, or elder abuse, assault, or exploitation, to the appropriate agency and local law enforcement.

Play/Leisure Evaluation

Activity Index

1. Focus: determination of the individual's perception of the meaning of leisure and the extent the individual participates in leisure activities.
2. Method.
   a. Evaluator provides the individual with the Activity Index Questionnaire.
   b. Instructions are given to indicate the individual's level of participation in each of the 23 listed activities.
   c. The individual is instructed to fill in additional leisure activities of interest in the space provided, if appropriate.
3. Materials: questionnaire and a pencil.
4. Scoring and interpretation.
   a. The individual checks his/her level of interest and participation in each activity along a 4-point scale.
      (1) Don't do/not interested.
      (2) Don't do/would like to do.
      (3) Do at least once a week.
      (4) Do at least 3 times a week.
   b. Interpretation of self-report results can be used to design interventions using activities that are meaningful to the individual and to promote his/her pursuit of preferred activities.
5. Population: developed for elders, aged 65 and over, but has been used with other populations.

Interest Checklist

1. Focus: assessment of a person's level of interest in 80 leisure activities, additional leisure interests, and his/her perspective on how leisure interests and involvement has evolved over time.
   a. A modified Interest Checklist has fewer activities.
2. Method.
   a. The evaluator provides the individual with the 80 item checklist.
   b. Instructions direct the individual to check their level of interest in each activity.
   c. Additional interests can be listed by the individual at the end of the checklist.
   d. Evaluator interviews the individual about his/her life history of leisure interests and pursuits.
3. Materials: checklist and a pencil.
4. Scoring and interpretation.
   a. Individual's level of interest is rated as strong, casual, or no interest.
   b. These scores do not indicate if the person actually pursues the activity.
   c. Interview is not rated; questions can be asked to provide information about activity engagement.
   d. Checklist scores and qualitative data can provide guidance for planning interventions that use meaningful activities and to promote active pursuit of activities of interest.
5. Population: originally developed for adults but it has been used with adolescents to elders.

Leisure Diagnostic Battery (LDB)

1. Focus: measurement of an individual's leisure experience, and motivational and situational issues that influence leisure (e.g., perceived barriers to leisure and knowledge of leisure opportunities).
2. Method.
   a. Evaluator provides the individual with LDB questionnaire and asks the individual to indicate his/her responses on LDB's response sheet.

3. Materials: LDB questionnaire, response sheet, and pencil.
4. Scoring and interpretation.
   a. A 1 to 3 rating scale indicating agreement with statements.
   b. Information can be used to identify individual's knowledge of leisure opportunities, environmental resources and barriers, and leisure characteristics that are motivating and interesting to the person.
5. Population: adults for original LDB. Adapted scales have been developed for children aged 9–14 with no cognitive deficits and for children aged 9–14 with a diagnosis of educable mental retardation.

Leisure Satisfaction Questionnaire

1. Focus: measurement of an individual's perception that leisure pursuits are meeting personal needs in six needs categories.
   a. Psychological.
   b. Educational.
   c. Social.
   d. Relaxation.
   e. Psysiological.
   f. Aesthetic.
2. Method: evaluator gives the individual the questionnaire and asks him/her to respond to each question on a 5-point scale.
3. Materials: questionnaire and a pencil.
4. Scoring and interpretation.
   a. Responses for each question are rated on a 5-point scale with 1 = almost never true and 5 = almost always true.
   b. Information can be used to examine a person's use of leisure time, to discuss needs satisfied by leisure pursuits, and to identify ways leisure can be modified to better meet individual needs.
5. Population: adults and elders.

Meaningfulness of Activity Scale

1. Focus: the measurement of the individual's level of enjoyment, motivational source, perception of competence, and participation in leisure.
2. Method: evaluator provides the individual with a questionnaire and asks the individual to mark his/her responses on the form's rating scale.
3. Materials: questionnaire and a pencil.
4. Scoring and interpretation.
   a. Likert-type scales are used for three subscales.
      (1) Level of activity enjoyment.
      (2) Reason for doing activity.
      (3) Perception of activity competence.
   b. The three subscale scores are totaled to obtain an overall meaningfulness of activity score.
   c. Information can be used to reinforce the pursuit of meaningful leisure and to plan intervention to promote adaptive leisure functioning.
5. Population: adults and elders.

Minnesota Leisure Time Physical Activity Questionnaire

1. Focus: measurement of the energy expended by a person during engagement in leisure activities.
2. Method: evaluator interviews the person using a list of 63 physical activities (excluding work) to determine which activities the individual has performed in the past 12 months.
3. Scoring.
   a. For each activity performed the individual specifies the level of participation for each month.
   b. The evaluator determines whether activity is light, medium, or heavy according to evaluation standards.
   c. A total activity metabolic index and an estimate of average daily caloric expenditures are obtained.
   d. Information can be used to assess pre-morbid physical activity levels and examine their relationship with general health, disease, cardiovascular fitness, weight control.
   e. Intervention plans can be made to increase physical activity to enhance health and fitness and reduce stress.
4. Population: adults.

Play History

1. Focus: assessment of a child's or adolescent's developmental level and the adequacy of his/her play environments.
2. Method: the evaluator conducts a semi-structured interview with the parents or caregivers of the child/adolescent being evaluated.
3. Materials: manual with interview questions.
4. Scoring and interpretation.
   a. Values are assigned to the historical interview information according to manual standards.
   b. Knowledge of a child's/adolescent's play history and play environments can increase understanding of current play behaviors.
5. Population: children and adolescents.

Preschool Play Scale

1. Focus: observation of a child's play behavior within four play dimensions.
   a. Space management.

b. Material management.
c. Imitation.
d. Participation.
2. Method.
a. Observation of a child's free play for 15–30 minute periods.
b. Comparison of observations with expected play behaviors for specific age groups.
3. Materials: child's everyday materials, equipment and toys, play scale, and pencil.
4. Scoring and interpretation.
a. A 'play age' score is derived by comparing observed behaviors to expected age-specific behaviors.
b. Evaluator should have knowledge of play theory and child development and experience in observing play behavior prior to scoring and interpreting evaluation.

Additional Play/Leisure Assessments

1. Developmental assessments (refer to Chapter 5).
2. Activity configurations and temporal adaptation assessments (refer to Chapter 14).
3. Occupational role and occupational performance interviews (refer to Chapter 14).

Play/Leisure Intervention

General Intervention Guidelines

1. Recognize that the acquisition of a disability often results in increased leisure time due to loss of roles.
a. Provide support for losses, refer to support group and/or disability advocacy groups.
b. Renew or adapt old interests.
2. Leisure activities that are valued, meaningful, and enjoyable to the person should be adapted, modified, and/or simplified to facilitate satisfying engagement.
3. Provide assistive technology and adaptive equipment to compensate for functional impairments during leisure activity performance.
a. Universal cuff.
b. Card holders.
c. Book holders and page turners.
d. Writing orthosis, typing aids, weighted pens.
e. Headsticks, mouthsticks.
f. Environmental control unit (ECU) to activate electronic equipment (e.g., CD players, TVs).
g. Adapted computer, keyboard guards, and voice-activated computer.
h. Smart phone applications.
i. Speaker phones.
j. Switches to activate toys that a child with a disability cannot operate by conventional means.
k. Refer to Table 15-4 for a description of SCI levels and play/leisure abilities.
4. Use thematic and topical groups to develop needed skills (e.g., a parenting play group, a retirement planning group).
5. Teach principles and methods of energy conservation, work simplification, joint protection, and proper body mechanics. Refer to Chapter 11.
6. Refer to relevant community and national resources (e.g., senior centers, free concerts, parks, Compeer, Special Olympics).
7. Explore and present internet and web-based opportunities for play and leisure participation (e.g., social networking, chat rooms, gaming sites).

Table 15-4

SCI Levels and Play/Leisure Abilities

C1–C4	Can play computer games, access the Internet and e-mail, and control radios, TVs, and other electronic devices using a mouthstick, head pointer, or voice activation. Can read using a mouthstick, head pointer, or electronic page turner to turn pages. Can paint with a mouthstick or head pointer.
C5	Can independently play computer games, turn pages for reading, play board games, do some crafts, use a speakerphone and access electronic devices, the Internet and e-mail using a splint, universal cuff, and typing splint.
C6 and C7	Can hold a phone, typing stick, and pen using a tenodesis grasp. Can independently do some crafts, turn pages for reading, use a computer, and access electronic devices, the Internet and e-mail using a tenodesis grasp or universal cuff to hold a typing stick. Can play board games and some wheelchair sports.
C8–T1	Can do the most leisure activities due to good functional use of both upper extremities.

Developmental Considerations for Play Interventions

1. Plan play interventions that consider the child's developmental level.
   a. Facilitate active participation in cause and effect learning.
2. Provide opportunities for culturally relevant solitary play and environmental mastery.
3. Facilitate active participation in cause and effect learning.
4. Provide opportunities for play with siblings and/or peers.
5. Provide toys that are safe, durable, and colorful.
6. Provide toys and activities that are visually and auditorally stimulating.

Work Evaluation

Prevocational Assessment Process

1. Screen to identify deficits in occupational performance areas and/or performance components that could impact on work abilities and potential.
2. Determine if the individual is interested in prevocational assessment and intervention.
3. Gather relevant work, educational, social, and medical history information.
4. Identify prevocational interests through the use of interest inventories and/or structured interviews.
5. Assess current level of work-related skills.
   a. Conduct structured observations of an individual performing work tasks in a prevocational group or rehabilitation workshop (formerly called sheltered workshop) or during a job simulation.
      (1) Rating scales or checklists of prevocational skills and behaviors are used.
      (2) Refer to Table 15-5 for a listing of essential behavior skills.
   b. Administer standardized work assessments.
      (1) Aptitude tests to determine individual's strengths and weaknesses in a variety of areas such as verbal and numerical abilities.
      (2) Behavioral and personality tests to determine personality characteristics, attitudes, motivators, and intra- and inter-personal strengths.
      (3) Manual dexterity tests to determine motor coordination skills such as speed and accuracy in performing motor tasks.
6. Determine if individual can return to past employment.
   a. Identify existing abilities and supports.
   b. Identify existing limitations and barriers.
   c. Identify needed reasonable accommodations.
7. Determine if pre-vocational and/or vocational training is indicated.
8. Refer to Table 15-6 for an overview of the prevocational assessment process.

Work Assessment

1. Initial screening and prevocational assessment as described above.
2. Functional capacity evaluation (FCE) which evaluates an individual's capabilities in relation to one of several dimensions.
   a. The physical demands of a job, which is often termed a physical capacity evaluation, to assess the physical demands of a job according to the descriptions provided in the Dictionary of Occupational Titles (DOT) (e.g., the Smith Physical Capacity Evaluation).
   b. The critical demands of a specific job.
   c. The critical demands of an occupational group.
   d. The demands of competitive employment.
3. Work capacity evaluation using real or simulated work activities to assess an individual's ability to return to work (e.g., Valpar Work Samples or BTE).
4. Job site analysis to evaluate its expectations, supports, ergonomics, essential functions of the job, the marginal functions of the job, and the potential reasonable accommodations in accordance with ADA.
   a. See Table 15-7 for assessment guidelines for determining the general ergonomic risks of work tasks and Table 15-8 for assessment guidelines for determining the ergonomic risks of computer work.
   b. Refer to Chapter 4 for ADA information.

Specific Work Assessments

1. EPIC Functional Evaluation System.
   a. Focus: determination of the individual's capacity for lifting, carrying, climbing, industrial pulling and pushing, balance while walking, motor coordination, standing, whole body range of motion, and finger and hand dexterity.
   b. Method: use of the commercially available standardized EPIC six modules.

Table 15-5

Work Behavior Skills

PHYSICAL TOLERANCE & DEMANDS	SENSORY/ PERCEPTION	MOTOR
• Work pace/ rhythm • Standing tolerance • Sitting tolerance • Endurance • Performance with repetition • Muscle strength • Walking • Lifting • Carrying • Pushing • Pulling • Climbing	• Color discrimination • Form perception • Size discrimination • Spatial relationship • Ability to follow visual instruction • Texture discrimination • Digital discrimination • Figure-ground • Form constancy • Visual closure • Parts-to-whole • Shape discrimination • Kinesthesia	• Finger dexterity • Manual dexterity • Coordination: – eye-hand – eye-hand-foot – fine motor – gross motor – bimanual – bilateral • Use of hand tools • ROM: – stooping – kneeling – crouching – crawling – reaching • Balancing
DAILY LIVING SKILLS	**COGNITION**	**AFFECTIVE**
• Self care: – personal hygiene – grooming – dressing – eating/feeding – object manipulation • Mobility – transfers – travel (mode of) – transportation • Communication – with peers – with supervisor – writing – dialing phone – talking on phone – typing	• Numerical ability • Measuring ability • Safety consciousness • Care in handling work and tools • Work quality • Accuracy • Neatness • Attention span • Planning/organization • Ability to follow: – verbal instruction – written instruction • Retention of instruction • Work judgment • Ability to learn new task • Orientation	• Attendance • Punctuality • Response to: – praise – criticism – assistance – frustrating situation • Relationship with – evaluator – co-worker • Work flexibility • Attitude toward work • Behavior in structured setting • Ability to work independently • Initiative (In psychiatry you would also observe for additional pathological behavior.)
• Wayne County Community College, Occupational Therapy Assistant Program		

Reprinted with permission from the Occupational Therapy Assistant Program, Wayne County Community College. 1001 West Fort St. Detroit, Michigan.

Table 15-6

Occupational Therapy Prevocational Assessment Process

Gather Background information

1. Work history, education, and training background
2. Current medications and their side effects
3. History of mental and physical illnesses
4. Factors/stressors influencing symptomatology

Determine Consumer Work Interests and Support Systems

1. Available emotional support persons
2. Cultural/familial influences affecting employment
3. Skills needed for most recent employment
   a. Is that job still available?
   b. Will employer rehire?
   c. Are skills still in place?
   d. Does patient want to return to the job?

Return to Most Recent Employment

1. Identify job stressors
2. Identify accommodations needed to stay employed
3. Identify strategies needed to be practiced to return to work (e.g., relaxation techniques, medication management, cognitive therapy, etc.)
4. Which employment opportunities are considered desired by consumer?
   a. Which skills are needed for identified employment?
   b. What training is needed?
   c. Is a job analysis needed?

Assess Skill Level for Employment Opportunity

1. Determine assessments directly relating to employment tasks
   a. Work tolerance screening
   b. Functional capacity evaluation
   c. Simulated job try-out
   d. Work samples
   e. Standardized assessments for specific job tasks
2. Consider a work behavior assessment
3. Determine job interview skills

Assess for Reasonable Accommodations

Reprinted from Hemphill-Pearson, B. (Ed.). (1999). *Assessments in occupational therapy mental health: An integrative approach*, p. 113, with permission by Slack Incorporated, Thorofare, NJ.

c. Materials: materials to simulate work for each of the six modules.
d. Scoring and interpretation: formal training and certification are required for evaluators.
e. Population: adults.

2. Jacob's Prevocational Assessment (JPVA).
   a. Focus: assessment of work-related skills in fourteen major areas (e.g., cognitive-perceptual skills, motor skills).
   b. Method: individual completes 15 brief tasks (e.g., money management, filing).
   c. Materials: JPVA manual and profile sheet; common items and readily available materials are identified for use.
   d. Scoring and interpretation: evaluator checks off areas that were observed to present difficulty to the individual during task performance on a Profile Sheet. Time for task completion and comments about behavior are also recorded.
   e. Population: adolescents and preadolescents with learning disabilities.

Table 15-7

General Ergonomic Risk Analysis Checklist

Check the box if your answer is "yes" to the question. A "yes" response indicates that an ergonomic risk factor that requires further analysis may be present.

MANUAL MATERIAL HANDLING

- ☐ Is there lifting of loads, tools, or parts?
- ☐ Is there lowering of loads, tools, or parts?
- ☐ Is there overhead reaching for loads, tools, or parts?
- ☐ Is there bending at the waist to handle loads, tools, or parts?
- ☐ Is there twisting at the waist to handle loads, tools or parts?

PHYSICAL ENERGY DEMANDS

- ☐ Do tools and parts weight more than 10 lbs?
- ☐ Is reaching greater than 20 inches?
- ☐ Is bending, stooping, or squatting a primary task activity?
- ☐ Is lifting or lowering loads a primary task activity?
- ☐ Is walking or carrying loads a primary task activity?
- ☐ Is stair or ladder climbing with loads a primary task activity?
- ☐ Is pushing or pulling loads a primary task activity?
- ☐ Is reaching overhead a primary task activity?
- ☐ Do any of the above tasks require five or more complete work cycles to be done within a minute?
- ☐ Do workers complain that rest breaks and fatigue allowances are insufficient?

OTHER MUSCULOSKELETAL DEMANDS

- ☐ Do manual jobs require frequent, repetitive motions?
- ☐ Do work postures require frequent bending of the neck, shoulder, elbow, wrist, or finger joints?
- ☐ For seated work, do reaches for tools and materials exceed 15 inches from the worker's position?
- ☐ Is the worker unable to change his or her position often?
- ☐ Does the work involve forceful, quick, or sudden motions?
- ☐ Does the work involve shock or rapid buildup of forces?
- ☐ Is finger-pinch gripping used?
- ☐ Do job postures involve sustained muscle contraction of any limb?

COMPUTER WORKSTATION

- ☐ Do operators use computer workstations for more than 4 hours a day?
- ☐ Are there complaints of discomfort from those working at these stations?
- ☐ Is the chair or desk nonadjustable?
- ☐ Is the display monitor, keyboard, or document holder nonadjustable?
- ☐ Does lighting cause glare or make the monitor screen hard to read?
- ☐ Is the room temperature too hot or too cold?
- ☐ Is there irritating vibration or noise?

Table 15-7

General Ergonomic Risk Analysis Checklist (*Continued*)

ENVIRONMENT

- ☐ Is the temperature too hot or too cold?
- ☐ Are the worker's hands exposed to temperatures less than 70° F?
- ☐ Is the workplace poorly lit?
- ☐ Is there glare?
- ☐ Is there excessive noise that is annoying, distracting, or producing hearing loss?
- ☐ Is there upper extremity or whole body vibration?
- ☐ Is air circulation too high or too low?

GENERAL WORKPLACE

- ☐ Are walkways uneven, slippery, or obstructed?
- ☐ Is housekeeping poor?
- ☐ Is there inadequate clearance or accessibility for performing tasks?
- ☐ Are stairs cluttered or lacking railings?
- ☐ Is proper footwear worn?

TOOLS

- ☐ Is the handle too small or too large?
- ☐ Does the handle shape cause the operator to bend the wrist in order to use the tool?
- ☐ Is the tool hard to access?
- ☐ Does the tool weigh more than 9 pounds?
- ☐ Does the tool vibrate excessively?
- ☐ Does the tool cause excessive kickback to the operator?
- ☐ Does the tool become too hot or too cold?

GLOVES

- ☐ Do the gloves require the worker to use more force when performing job tasks?
- ☐ Do the gloves provide inadequate protection?
- ☐ Do the gloves present a hazard of catch points on the tool or in the workplace?

ADMINISTRATION

- ☐ Is there little worker control over the work process?
- ☐ Is the task highly repetitive and monotonous?
- ☐ Does the job involve critical tasks with high accountability and little or no tolerance for error?
- ☐ Are work hours and breaks poorly organized?

General ergonomic risk analysis checklist. (From Cohen, A. L., et al. (1997). *Elements of ergonomics programs: A primer based on workplace evaluations of musculoskeletal disorders.* Washington DC: US Government Printing Office.)

3. McCarron-Dial System (MDS).
   a. Focus: assessment of the prevocational, vocational, and educational abilities of individuals with disabilities and/or sociocultural disadvantages in five main areas.
      (1) Cognitive, verbal, and spatial.
      (2) Sensory.
      (3) Motor.
      (4) Emotional.
      (5) Coping, integrative, and adaptive behaviors.
   b. Method.
      (1) A pre-screening interview is conducted and referral information is reviewed.
      (2) Work samples for each of the above five main areas are administered in a structured test setting.
      (3) Systematic observation of the individual in a work or classroom setting is conducted.
   c. Materials.
      (1) The MDS is composed of three large briefcase sized kits which include work samples, answer

Table 15-8

Risk Analysis Checklist for Computer-User Workstations		
"No" responses indicate potential problem areas which should receive further investigation.		
1. Does the workstation ensure proper worker posture, such as		
• horizontal thighs?	☐ Yes	☐ No
• vertical lower legs?	☐ Yes	☐ No
• feet flat on floor or footrest?	☐ Yes	☐ No
• neutral wrists?	☐ Yes	☐ No
2. Does the chair		
• adjust easily?	☐ Yes	☐ No
• have a padded seat with a rounded front?	☐ Yes	☐ No
• have an adjustable backrest?	☐ Yes	☐ No
• provide lumbar support?	☐ Yes	☐ No
• have casters?	☐ Yes	☐ No
3. Are the height and tilt of the work surface on which the keyboard is located adjustable?	☐ Yes	☐ No
4. Is the keyboard detachable?	☐ Yes	☐ No
5. Do keying actions require minimal force?	☐ Yes	☐ No
6. Is there an adjustable document holder?	☐ Yes	☐ No
7. Are arm rests provided where needed?	☐ Yes	☐ No
8. Are glare and reflections avoided?	☐ Yes	☐ No
9. Does the monitor have brightness and contrast controls?	☐ Yes	☐ No
10. Do the operators judge the distance between eyes and work to be satisfactory for their viewing needs?	☐ Yes	☐ No
11. Is there sufficient space for knees and feet?	☐ Yes	☐ No
12. Can the workstation be used for either right- or left-handed activity?	☐ Yes	☐ No
13. Are adequate rest breaks provided for task demands	☐ Yes	☐ No
14. Are high stroke rates avoided by		
• job rotation?	☐ Yes	☐ No
• self-pacing?	☐ Yes	☐ No
• adjusting the job to the skill of the worker?	☐ Yes	☐ No
15. Are employees trained in		
• proper postures?	☐ Yes	☐ No
• proper work methods?	☐ Yes	☐ No
• when and how to adjust their workstations?	☐ Yes	☐ No
• how to seek assistance for their concerns?	☐ Yes	☐ No

Risk analysis checklist for computer-user workstations. (From Cohen, A. L. et al. (1997). *Elements of ergonomics programs: A primer based on workplace evaluations of musculoskeletal disorders.* Washington DC: US Government Printing Office.)

sheets, observation of behavior forms, and reporting forms.

(2) Six established and published assessment tools (e.g., the Peabody and Wechsler tests) are used along with the work samples and behavioral observations.

(3) A computer program to assist with computation and interpretation of data and report documentation is available.

d. Scoring and interpretation.

(1) Each of the six published instruments is scored according to their individual scoring protocol.

(2) Work samples and behavioral observations are scored according to the quantity and quality of performance.

(3) Completion of a minimum three-day workshop to develop administration, scoring, and interpretation skills is required of all purchasers of the MDS.

e. Population: individuals who are aged 16 years or older and who have a neurophysiological and/or neuropsychological impairment.

4. Reading-Free Vocational Interest Inventory.
   a. Focus: identification of vocational areas of interest and/or patterns of interest in a number of vocational areas (e.g., animal care, automotive, housekeeping, clerical work).
   b. Method.
      (1) Evaluator presents a group of three pictures representing unskilled, semi-skilled, and skilled job tasks, and requests that the individual select the picture that represents the job task most preferred.
      (2) This process continues for 55 sets of pictures.
      (3) Literacy is not required as the method uses entirely visual illustrations.
   c. Materials: a manual containing 165 pictures and a scoring profile sheet.
   d. Scoring and interpretation: the individual's selections are converted into a numerical score that represents his/her level of interest (i.e., low, average, high) in the eleven interest areas.
   e. Population: adolescents and adults with learning or developmental disabilities.
5. Smith Physical Capacity Evaluation.
   a. Focus: the individual's performance on 154 items.
   b. Method: performance of real or simulated work tasks based on person's interests.
   c. Materials: equipment and supplies as needed to perform each specific work task.
   d. Population: adults.
6. Testing, Orientation, and Work Evaluation in Rehabilitation (TOWER).
   a. Focus: assessment of the individual's ability to complete specific work samples.
      (1) The TOWER system focuses on 14 job training areas through the provision of 110 work samples.
      (2) Clerical, assembly, and manufacturing jobs are the main focus.
   b. Method.
      (1) Evaluator selects pre-assembled work samples for the individual to complete that are appropriate to the individual's area(s) of interest for job training.
      (2) Work samples progress from simple to complex.
   c. Materials.
      (1) All equipment and items needed to complete each work sample.
      (2) Materials are not standardized but specific guidelines are provided for assembly of work samples.
   d. Scoring and interpretation.
      (1) Individual's performance can be compared to TOWER norms which were obtained for persons with disabilities.
      (2) Interpretation of results of work sample performance can be applied to jobs that relate directly to the work samples.
   e. Population: adults with physical and/or psychiatric disorders.
7. Valpar Component Work Sample (VCWS).
   a. Focus: assessment of groups of skills that are required for specific employment tasks (e.g., clerical) and basic functional capabilities (e.g., upper extremity function, dexterity, visual coordination).
   b. Method: completion of up to 23 work samples that are administered individually except for the cooperative assembly task. Samples can be completed repeatedly as part of an intervention program to improve functional performance.
   c. Materials: each work sample has standardized equipment (e.g., pegboard, tape recorder). Specialized large equipment is required for certain work samples. A manual includes a materials list, administration guidelines, and scoring directions. A separate kit for administration to the visually impaired includes tactile or verbal modifications.
   d. Scoring and interpretation: quality of and time for task performance are scored and converted to a Methods-Time Measurement (MTM) which is an industrial standard with normative data for comparisons. Seventeen worker behavior characteristics (e.g., ability to work with others/alone) are rated on a 5-point scale.
   e. Population: adults with disabilities and adults without disabilities. There is an adapted VCWS for the visually impaired.
8. Vocational Interest Inventory - Revised (VII-R).
   a. Focus: measurement of student interest in eight employment areas for adolescents who are unclear about their vocational interests.
   b. Method: completion of a questionnaire with 112 forced choice statements related to familiar job activities and job titles.
   c. Materials: manual, pencil, and computer-scored test report.
   d. Scoring and interpretation: individual's occupational interests are compared to established norms and a list of interest-compatible college majors are obtained. Information is used for educational and vocational guidance.
   e. Population: high school students.
9. Vocational Interest, Temperament, and Aptitude System (VITAS).
   a. Focus: assessment of vocational interests, temperament, and aptitudes to assist with career guidance and vocational placement.
   b. Method: completion of up to 22 work samples and vocational interest interview. A sixth-grade reading level is needed to complete the VITAS.
   c. Materials: work samples, tools, manual.

d. Scoring and interpretation: time and quality of performance are scored based upon evaluator's observations and compared to established norms.
e. Population: adolescents aged 14 years and older and adults.

10. Worker Role Interview (WRI).
  a. Focus: determination of psychosocial and environmental factors related to an individual's past work experience, job setting, and ability to return to work.
  b. Method: completion of a structured interview.
  c. Materials: manual, rating forms, and a pencil.
  d. Scoring and interpretation: client's responses are scored on a 1–4 rating scale with 1 indicating problems related to a return to work and 4 indicating supports for a return to work.
  e. Population: adults involved in a work-hardening program.

Work Intervention

General Intervention Guidelines

1. Evaluate the work site and adapt the environment and job tasks to enable the individual to perform essential job functions. See Figure 15-1 and Figure 15-2.
  a. Determine feasibility to return to work.
2. Provide assistive devices, adaptive strategies, and equipment to compensate for functional impairments during work activity performance (see Table 15-2).
  a. Smart phone applications.
  b. Adapted computers.
  c. Typing aids.
  d. Universal cuff, tenodesis splint.
  e. Teach principles and methods of energy conservation and work simplification. Refer to Chapter 11.
3. Practice, modify, and instruct in work activities.
4. Provide conditioning exercises and activities.
5. Educate about work safety and injury prevention.
  a. Teach principles and methods of joint protection and proper body mechanics. Refer to Chapter 11.
6. Educate employer regarding reasonable accommodations to enable performance of essential job functions. Refer to Table 15-9 and Chapter 4.

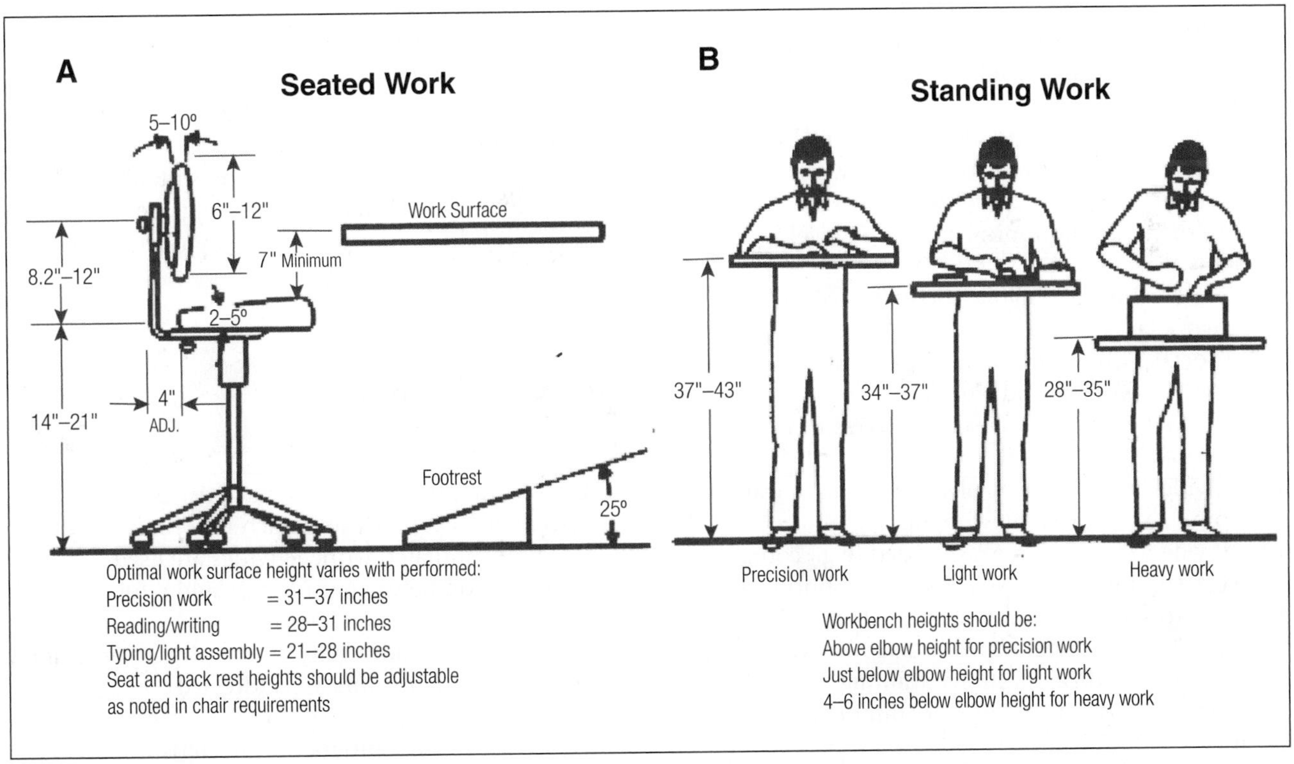

Figure 15-1 **Recommended dimensions of workstations.**
A, Seated work. **B,** Standing work. (From Cohen A. L., et al. (1997). *Elements of ergonomics programs: A primer based on workplace evaluations of musculoskeletal disorders*. Washington DC: US Government Printing Office.)

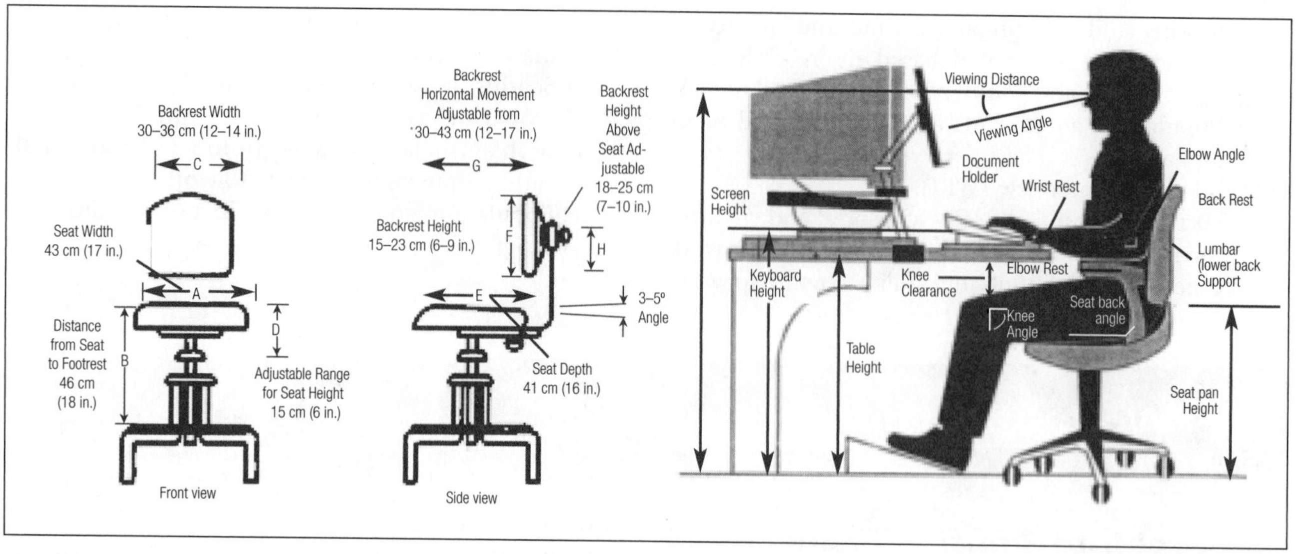

Figure 15-2 Recommended chair characteristics. Dimensions are given using both front and side views for width **(A)**, depth **(E)**, vertical adjustability **(D)**, and angle **(I)** and for backrest width **(C)**, height **(F)**, and vertical **(H)** and horizontal **(G)** adjustability relative to the chair seat. The angle of the backrest should be adjustable horizontally from 12–17 inches (30–43 cm), by either a slide-adjust or a spring, and vertically from 7–10 inches (18–25 cm). The adjustability is needed to provide back support during different types of seated work. The seat should be adjustable within at least a 6-inch (15 cm) range. The height above the floor of the chair seat with this adjustment range will be determined by the workplace, with or without a footrest.

(From Eggleton, E. (Ed.). (1983). *Ergonomic design for people at work,* Vol 1. New York: Van Nostrand Reinhold.) B, Proper seated position for computer user. From Occupational Safety and Health Administration. (1997). *Working safely with video display terminals,* Washington DC: US Government Printing Office, *www.osha.gov. Publications/osha3092.pdf.*)

7. Collaborate with employee assistance programs to obtain additional needed services (e.g., substance abuse counseling).
8. Educate family about work capacities and limitations.
9. Explore alternatives to competitive work if it is not an attainable goal (e.g., volunteer work).
10. Use thematic and topical groups to develop needed skills.
    a. Task skills to enable successful completion of work tasks.
    b. Social skills to facilitate appropriate interactions with coworkers and employer.
    c. Work behaviors to ensure a successful work experience. Refer to Table 15-5.
11. Provide pre-retirement planning to ease transition from competitive employment.
12. Provide follow-up care, as needed (e.g., counseling, work support group, psychosocial clubhouse).
13. Refer to state offices for vocational and educational services for individuals with disabilities for further education and/or vocational training.
14. Interventions for the most common work related injuries.
    a. Cumulative trauma such as carpal tunnel syndrome and low back pain.
        (1) Avoid static positions, repetition, awkward postures, forceful exertions, and vibration.
        (2) Design workplace and work station to be ergonomically correct to prevent further trauma. See Figure 15-1 and Figure 15-2.
    b. Psychosocial and cognitive deficits.
        (1) Engage person in program suitable to functional vocational abilities (e.g., rehabilitation workshop, supportive employment).
        (2) Refer to Table 15-9.

Specific Work Programs

1. Work-hardening program characteristics.
    a. An interdisciplinary approach is used.
    b. Real or simulated work activities are used.
    c. A transition between acute care and return to work is provided.
    d. The issues of productivity, safety, physical tolerance, and worker behaviors are addressed.
    e. CARF accreditation is required.
2. Work conditioning program characteristics.
    a. One discipline is the provider of services.
    b. Real or simulated work activities are used.
    c. A transition between acute care and return to work is provided.

Table 15-9

Reasonable Accommodations for Recurrent Functional Problems Among Persons with Psychiatric Disorders

PERSONAL SELF-EFFICACY
• Reinforce or coach appropriate behaviors. • Test for job skills on the job and avoid self-report of abilities. • Place in job where there is a model to follow or imitate. • Teach self-advocacy skills. • Provide successful job experiences. Use positive feedback. • Begin with close supervision and then cut back slowly as skills are maintained. • Maintain similarity or consistency in work tasks. • Encourage positive self-talk and eliminate negative self-talk.
DURATION OF CONCENTRATION[1]
• Put each work request in writing and leave in "to do" box to avoid interruptions. • Provide ongoing consultation, mediation, problem solving, and conflict resolution. • Provide good working conditions, such as adequate light, smoke-free environment, and reduced noise. • Provide directive commands on a regular basis.
SCREENING OUT ENVIRONMENTAL STIMULI[1]
• Place in a separate office. • Provide opaque room dividers between workstations. • Allow person to work after hours or when others are not around. • Ensure that workstation facilitates work production and organization.
MAINTAINING STAMINA THROUGHOUT THE WORKDAY[1]
• Provide additional breaks or shortened workday. • Allow an extended day to allow for breaks or rest periods. • Avoid work during lunch, such as answering the phone; use of an answering machine instead. • Distribute tasks throughout the day according to energy level. • Job-share with another employee. • Develop work simplification techniques, such as collect all copying to be done at one time or use a wheeled cart to move supplies. • Have a liberal leave policy for health problems, flexible hours, and back-up coverage. • Individualize work agreements. • Verify employees' efficacy regarding their ability to sustain effort or persist with a task. • Teach on-the-job relaxation and stress-reduction techniques.
MANAGING TIME PRESSURE AND DEADLINES[1]
• Maintain structure through a daily time and task schedule using hourly goals. • Provide positive reinforcement when tasks are completed within the expected time lines. • Arrange a separate work area to reduce noise and interruptions. • Screen out unnecessary business.

Table 15-9

Reasonable Accommodations for Recurrent Functional Problems Among Persons with Psychiatric Disorders

INITIATING INTERPERSONAL CONTACT[1]
• Purposely plan orientation to meet and work alongside co-workers. • Allow sufficient time to make good, unhurried contacts. • Make contacts during work, break, and even lunch times, adjusting the conversation to the situation. • When standing, instead of facing each other, try standing at a 90° angle to each other. • Allow the person to work at home. • Have an advocate to advise and support the person. • Communicate honestly. • Plan supervision times and maintain them. • Develop tolerance for and helpful responses to unusual behaviors. • Provide awareness and advocacy training for all workers.
FOCUSING ON MULTIPLE TASKS SIMULTANEOUSLY[1]
• Eliminate the number of simultaneous tasks. • Redistribute tasks among employees with the same responsibilities, so each can do more of one type of job task than a lot of different tasks. • Establish priorities for task completion. • Arrange for all work tasks to be put in writing with due dates or times.
RESPONDING TO NEGATIVE FEEDBACK[1]
• Have employee prepare own work appraisal to compare with supervisor's. • Work together to establish methods employee can use to change negative behavior. • Provide positive reinforcement for observed behavioral change. • Provide on-site crisis intervention and counseling services to develop self-esteem, provide emotional support, and promote comfort with accommodations. • Establish guidelines for feedback.
SYMPTOMS SECONDARY TO PRESCRIBED PSYCHOTROPIC MEDICATIONS[1]
• Provide release time to see psychiatrist or primary physician. • Encourage employee to work with physician to establish a time schedule to take medications that are conducive to work responsibilities. • Provide release time or changes in job tasks that match condition.

[1]From: Mancuso (1990).

From: Crist, P. & V. Stoffel. (1996). The Americans with Disabilities Act of 1990 and employees with mental impairments: Personal efficacy and the environment. In R. P. Cottrell (Ed.), *Perspectives on purposeful activity: Foundation and future of occupational therapy* (pp. 227–228). Bethesda, MD: American Occupational Therapy Association. Reprinted with permission.

d. Flexibility, strength, movement, and endurance are addressed.

e. Accreditation is not a requirement.

3. Ergonomic program characteristics.

a. Prevention is the main focus to fit the work place to the human body.

b. Types of programs.

(1) Ergonomic survey. See Tables 15-7 and 15-8.

(2) Specific job site analysis.

(3) Manager and employee training.

(4) Educational seminars.

(5) Exercise and stretching programs.

Chapter 15

4. Rehabilitation (sheltered) workshops, supported employment programs, transitional employment programs (TEP).
   a. A multidisciplinary or interdisciplinary approach is used.
   b. Real work activities are used.
      (1) Participants are paid at a piece-work rate in rehabilitation (sheltered) workshops.
      (2) Participants are paid at the prevailing competitive wage for positions in TEP and supported employment programs.
   c. Participants are considered as employees with supports provided as needed.
      (1) Job coaches are used.
      (2) Reasonable accommodations are provided. Refer to Table 15-9.
   d. A transition between program participation and competitive employment is provided according to participant's functional level.
   e. Rehabilitation (sheltered) workshops and supported employment can be the final and permanent employment goal for an individual.
   f. Accreditation is not a requirement.
      (1) Rehabilitation (sheltered) workshops, TEPs, and supported employment programs are usually part of an accredited hospital system or a major agency (e.g., TheARC).
5. Discharge criteria from work programs.
   a. Individual exhibits limited potential for improvement.
   b. Individual has declined services.
   c. Individual is non-compliant with the program.
   d. Individual has met program goals.
   e. Individual has returned to work.

Rest and Sleep Evaluation

1. The use of OT assessments which focus on time use and temporal adaptation (e.g., Barth Time Construction, Activities Configuration) can provide helpful information about a person's rest and sleep patterns. See Chapter 14.
2. Rest and sleep are typically not included in commonly used OT published assessments of areas of occupation.
   a. Given the inclusion of rest and sleep in the AOTA Practice Framework and increased research on the importance of rest and sleep to health and occupational performance, this area of occupation is becoming more integrated into OT evaluation and intervention.
3. The occupational therapist should assess this area of occupation during routine screenings and interviews.
   a. Asking a person if he/she feels drowsy during the day is a quick and easy way to screen for problems with rest and sleep.
4. More indepth evaluation should focus on the identification of:
   a. The person's ability to identify the need for restorative rest and sleep.
   b. Typical rest and sleep patterns and routines.
   c. Obstacles to the attainment and maintenance of satisfying rest and sleep.
      (1) Personal issues (e.g., being a "light" sleeper who awakens easily).
      (2) Pathophysiological changes related to disease, disability, and/or the aging process (e.g., chronic pain, unrelenting fatigue).
      (3) Socio-cultural barriers (e.g., need to work a night shift job requires sleeping during daytime hours).
5. Sleep checklists and sleep diaries can be used to obtain detailed information.
6. Persons with chronic and unrelenting insomnia should be referred to a sleep clinic/laboratory for an extensive overnight evaluation.

Rest and Sleep Intervention

1. Intervention must be client-centered, and focused on behavioral and environmental modifications to enable restorative rest and sleep. The therapist should help the person:
   a. Develop a daily pattern of relaxation activities (e.g., meditation, prayers, progressive muscle relaxation. visualization) and pre-sleep routines (e.g., turning off electronic devices, saying goodnight).
      (1) Pre-sleep meals should be consumed at least two hours before sleep is initiated.
   b. Establish healthy and restorative sleep-wake patterns (e.g., going to bed at a consistent time each evening).
   c. Remediate symptoms which hinder rest and sleep (e.g., using energy conservation techniques, effective pain management).
   d. Modify the rest and sleep environment (e.g., playing soothing music to relax, using room darkening shades if daytime sleep is needed due to night shift work, using earplugs and/or 'white noise' machines to block sound).
      (1) Dark, cool, quiet environments are most conducive to sleep.
   e. Implement sleep restriction training.
      (1) Wake up at the same time every day (i.e., no "sleeping in" on weekends).
      (2) Avoid naps until nighttime sleeping improves.
      (3) Limit the bedroom to sleep and sexual activities (i.e., not watching TV or cruising the Internet).
      (4) When sleepy, go to sleep.
      (5) If sleep is not attained, get up and do an activity that is boring until sleepy again.

(6) Allow time for sleep restriction training to work.
   (a) It typically takes two to three weeks for the body to adjust to a new sleep routine.

f. Employ cognitive-behavioral therapy (CBT) strategies to address thought processes which cause anxiety and hinder sleep (e.g., make a list of concerns to address upon awakening and leave them outside the bedroom door). See Chapter 14.

2. A referral to a physician must be completed immediately for persons with (or at risk for) obstructive sleep apnea syndrome (OSAS).
   a. Referrals to physicans are also indicated for persons with conditions which require medical intervention (e.g., restless leg syndrome, narcolepsy, sleep walking, spasticity, pain).

References

Allen, C. K., Earhart, C. A., & Blue, T. (1992). *Occupational therapy treatment goals for the physically and cognitively disabled.* Bethesda, MD: American Occupational Therapy Association.

American Occupational Therapy Association. (2006). *Reference manual of the official documents of the American Occupational Therapy Association,* 11th ed. Bethesda, MD: Author.

American Occupational Therapy Association. (2008). Occupational therapy practice framework: Domain and process, 2nd ed. *American Journal of Occupational Therapy, 62,* 625–688.

American Occupational Therapy Association. (2010). Standards of practice for occupational therapy. *American Journal of Occupational Therapy, 64*(6, Supplement), S106–S110.

AMPS Project International (2013). *Assessment of Motor and Process Skills (AMPS).* Retrieved August 10, 2013 from http://www.innovativeotsolutions.com/content/amps/.

Asher, I. E. (2007). *An annotated index of occupational therapy evaluation tools,* 3rd ed. Bethesda, MD: AOTA Press.

Asrael, W. (1993). The PLISSIT model of sexuality counseling and education. In R.P. Cottrell (Ed.), *Psychosocial occupational therapy: Proactive approaches* (pp. 451–452). Bethesda, MD: American Occupational Therapy.

Backman, C. (1994). Assessment of self-care skills. In C. Christiansen (Ed.), *Ways of living: Self-care strategies for special needs* (pp. 51–75). Bethesda, MD: American Occupational Therapy Association.

Brown, C., Rempfer, M., & Hamera, E. (2009). *The Test of Grocery Shopping Skills (TOGSS).* Bethesda, MD: AOTA Press.

Brown, C., & Stoffel, V. (Eds.). (2011) *Occupational therapy in mental health: A vision for participation.* Philadelphia: F.A. Davis.

Case-Smith, J. (Ed.). (2005). *Occupational therapy for children* 5th ed. St. Louis, MO: Elsevier Mosby.

Christiansen, C. (1994). *Ways of living: Self-care strategies for special needs.* Bethesda, MD: American Occupational Therapy Association.

Clifton, D. (2004, December). Workers' Comp: A plethora of opportunities. *Rehab Management,* 32, 34–36.

Cohen, A., et al. (1997). *Elements of ergonomic programs: A primer based on workplace evaluations of musculoskeletal disorders.* Washington, DC: US Government Printing Office.

Crist, P. A., & Stoffel, V. C. (2005). The Americans with Disabilities Act of 1990 and employees with mental impairments: Personal efficacy and the environment. In R.P. Cottrell (Ed.), *Perspectives for occupation-based practice: Foundation and future of occupational therapy* (pp. 289–299). Bethesda, MD: American Occupational Therapy Association.

Gentry, T., & Loveland, J. (2013, January 21). Sleep: Essential to living life to its fullest. *OT Practice,* 9–14.

Gutman, S., Mortera, M. Hinojosa, J., & Kramer, P. (2007). The issue is: Revision of the occupational therapy Practice Framework *American Journal of Occupational Therapy, 61,*119–126.

Hemphill-Pearson, B. (Ed.). (1999). *Assessments in occupational therapy mental health: An integrative approach.* Thorofare, NJ: Slack.

Hinojosa, J., Kramer, P., & Crist, P. (Eds.) (2005). *Evaluation: Obtaining and interpreting data,* 2nd ed. Bethesda, MD: AOTA Press.

Hussey, S., Sabonis-Chafee, B., & O'Brien, J. (2007). *Introduction to occupational therapy,* 3rd ed. St. Louis, MO: Elsevier Mosby.

Larson, K., Stevens-Ratchford, R. G., Pedretti, L., & Crabtree, J. (1996). ROTE: *The role of occupational therapy with the elderly,* 2nd ed. Bethesda, MD: American Occupational Therapy Association.

Leonardelli, C. (1988). *The Milwaukee Evaluation of Daily Living Skills.* Thorofare, NJ: Slack.

Mosey, A. (1996). *Psychosocial components of occupational therapy.* Philadelphia: Lippincott-Raven.

Moyers, P., & Dale, L. (2007). *The guide to occupational therapy practice.* Bethesda, MD: AOTA Press.

McHugh Pendleton, H., & Schultz-Krohn, W. (Eds.) (2006). *Pedretti's occupational therapy: Practice skills for physical dysfunction,* 6th ed. St. Louis, MO: Mosby.

Schell, B., Gillen, G., & Scaffa, M. (Eds). *Willard and Spackman's occupational therapy,* 12th ed. Philadelphia: Lippincott Williams & Wilkins.

Schultz-Krohn, W., & Pendleton, H. (Eds.) (2006). *Occupational therapy: Practice skills for physical dysfunction,* 6th ed. St. Louis, MO: Elsevier Science/Mosby.

Sladyk, K., Jacobs. K., & MacRae, N. (2010). *Occupational therapy essentials for clinical competence.* Thorofare, NJ: Slack.

Vining-Radomski, M., & Trombly-Latham, C. A. (2007). *Occupational therapy for physical dysfunction,* 6th ed. Baltimore: Williams & Wilkins.

Review Questions

Evaluation and Intervention for Performance in Areas of Occupation

Below are five questions about key content covered in this chapter. These questions are not inclusive of the entirety of content related to evaluation and intervention for performance in areas of occupation that you must know for success on the NBCOT exam. These questions are provided to help you "jump start" the thought processes you will need to apply your studying of content to the answering of exam questions; hence they are not in the NBCOT exam format. Exam items in the NBCOT format which cover the depth and breadth of content you will need to know to pass the NBCOT exam are provided on this text's disc. The answers to the below questions are provided in Appendix 4.

1. The supervisor of a hospital-based occupational therapy department which provides services to persons with medical conditions and physical disabilities is reviewing its guidelines for the evaluation of BADL with newly hired therapists. What assessments should the supervisor identify as core evaluations for all therapists (including entry-level therapists) to include in their "toolbox"? What assessments should the supervisor identify as requiring therapists to complete additional training prior to their use?

2. A person with a C-7 SCI sets a goal to return to work as an accountant. The person expresses concern about the ability to complete a morning self-care routine and job tasks. What will be realistic for the person to expect to be able to do after receiving occupational therapy services to develop self-care and work skills?

3. An occupational therapist seeks to ensure that the BADL of sexual activity is addressed throughout the OT process. Which model can help the therapist achieve this aim? Describe the key points of this model.

4. An occupational therapist provides consultation to a local business which employs people with cognitive limitations due to psychiatric, physical, and intellectual disabilities.What strategies should the therapist share with employers to increase their employees' ability to concentrate, manage time, and focus on multiple tasks at the same time during the work day?

5. During an occupational therapy screening, a client reports feeling tired all of the time. What should the occupational therapist address during evaluation?

16

Mastery of the Environment: Evaluation and Intervention

RITA P. FLEMING-CASTALDY AND COLLEEN McCAUL DeRITIS

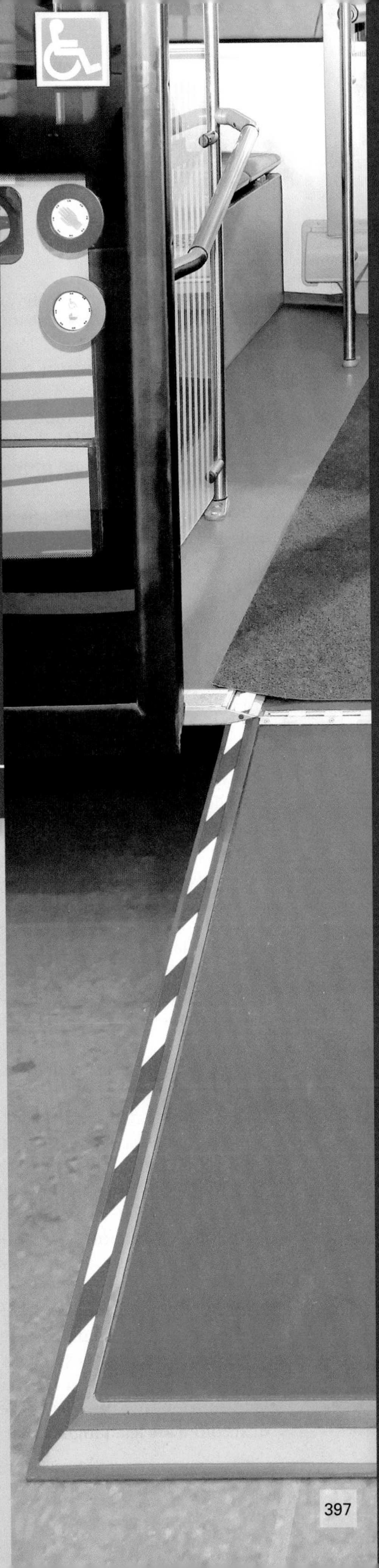

Chapter Outline

General Environmental Considerations

Definition and Major Concepts

1. The environment is "the aggregate of phenomena that surrounds the individual and influences his (her) development and existence" (Mosey, 1996, p. 171).
2. The environment in which a person lives, and the exposure to various settings, influences his or her development and adaptation.
3. The environment can facilitate growth because it allows for adaptation and problem solving strategies to be developed.
4. Conversely, the environment can hinder development and adaptation if it is impoverished or hostile.
5. A person's abilities, skills, limitations, problems, activities, and/or occupations cannot be fully understood without considerations of his/her current and expected environment.
6. Physical/non-human environment.
   a. Everything that is non-human (i.e., buildings, objects, tools, devices, animals, trees).
7. Sensory environment.
   a. Visual: lighting, colors, clutter (i.e., posters all over a wall).
   b. Auditory: loudness of radios, loudspeakers, classroom noise.
   c. Tactile: room temperature, seating textures.
   d. Olfactory: pleasant or offensive odors.
   e. Gustatory: pleasant or offensive tastes.
8. Social-cultural/human environment.
   a. Social roles: "an organized pattern of behavior that is characteristic and expected of the occupant of a defined position in a social system" (Mosey, 1986, p. 64). For example, a student, a parent, a worker.
   b. Social network: "the web of voluntary relationships that make up an individual's social environment" (Mosey, 1996, p. 184).
   c. Cultural aspects: "the social structures, values, norms, and expectations that are accepted and shared by a group of people" (Mosey, 1996, p. 172).
   d. Psychological aspects: environmental characteristics that can effect mood and stress level (e.g., a calming, comfortable, cheerful environment versus a chaotic, uncomfortable, depressing setting).
9. The AOTA practice framework has expanded the description of environment beyond the physical and social environment to include the concept of context.
   a. In the AOTA practice framework, context "refers to a variety of interrelated conditions that are within and surrounding the client. These interrelated contexts often are less tangible than physical and social environments but nonetheless exert a strong influence on performance" (AOTA 2008, p. 642).
   b. Contexts include cultural, personal, temporal, and virtual.
      (1) The "cultural context includes customs, beliefs, activity patterns, behavior standards, and expectations accepted by the society of which the client is a member (AOTA 2008, p. 642).
      (2) The "personal context refers to demographic features of the individual such as age, gender, socioeconomic status, and educational level that are not part of a health condition (AOTA 2008, p. 642).
      (3) The "temporal context includes stages of life, time of year, time of day and duration rhythm of activity, or history" (AOTA 2008, p. 645).
      (4) The virtual context refers to the "environment in which communication occurs by means of airways or computers and an absence of physical contact" (AOTA 2008, p. 645); for example, email, video-conferencing, web-based social networking.

Legislation Related to the Environment

1. Americans with Disabilities Act (ADA): a civil rights law aimed at allowing full participation in society for people with disabilities.
   a. Several sections mandate accessible environments for persons with disabilities.
   b. Included are policies dealing with public service, employment, and public accommodations.
2. Omnibus Budget Reconciliation Act (OBRA): mandates that restraints cannot be used without proper justification, agreement, and documentation.
3. Individuals with Disabilities Education Act (IDEA): mandates that children with disabilities receive education in the least restrictive and most natural environment.
   a. Inclusive models are to be used to enable the child to be taught in a general education classroom.
   b. Education must prepare a child for independent living, employment and social participation.
4. The role of the occupational therapist in environmental assessment and modification has increased with the implementation of the ADA, OBRA and IDEA. (Refer to Chapter 4 for specific information on the ADA, OBRA, and IDEA.)

The Role of the Occupational Therapist

1. Occupational therapists should be familiar with all aspects of a person's environment – living, vocational, and leisure – whether it takes place in a hospital, nursing home, school, or home.
2. Occupational therapists can advocate for and design environments that use principles of universal design to meet the physical, sensory, sociocultural, and psychological needs of the individual.
   a. See Table 16-1.
3. Occupational therapists can help to identify settings and approaches to implement the ADA, OBRA, and IDEA.
4. Occupational therapists can advocate for ADA, OBRA, and IDEA compliance to enable individuals to live independently and with the least restriction possible in their environments of choice.

Table 16-1

Principles of Universal Design
PRINCIPLE 1
Equitable Use: The design is useful and marketable to people with diverse abilities.
Guidelines: **1a.** Provide the same means of use for all users; identical whenever possible; equivalent when not. **1b.** Avoid segregating or stigmatizing any users. **1c.** Provisions for privacy, security, and safety should be equally available to all users. **1d.** Make the design appealing to all users.
PRINCIPLE 2
Flexibility in Use: The design accommodates a wide range of individual preferences and abilities.
Guidelines: **2a.** Provide choice in methods of use. **2b.** Accommodate right- or left-handed access and use. **2c.** Facilitate the user's accuracy and precision. **2d.** Provide adaptability to the user's pace.
PRINCIPLE 3
Simple and Intuitive Use: Use of the design is easy to understand, regardless of the user's experience, knowledge, language skills, or current concentration level.
Guidelines: **3a.** Eliminate unnecessary complexity. **3b.** Be consistent with user expectations and intuition. **3c.** Accommodate a wide range of literacy and language skills. **3d.** Arrange information consistent with its importance **3e.** Provide effective prompting and feedback during and after task completion.
PRINCIPLE 4
Perceptible Information: The design communicates necessary information effectively to the user, regardless of ambient conditions or the user's sensory abilities.
Guidelines: **4a.** Use different modes (pictorial, verbal, tactile) for redundant presentation of essential information. **4b.** Provide adequate contrast between essential information and its surroundings. **4c.** Maximize "legibility" of essential information. **4d.** Differentiate elements in ways that can be described (i.e., make it easy to give instructions or directions). **4e.** Provide compatibility with a variety of techniques or devices used by people with sensory limitations.
PRINCIPLE 5
Tolerance for Error: The design minimizes hazards and the adverse consequences of accidental or unintended actions.
Guidelines: **5a.** Arrange elements to minimize hazards and errors: most used elements, most accessible; hazardous elements eliminated, isolated, or shielded. **5b.** Provide warnings of hazards and errors. **5c.** Provide fail-safe features. **5d.** Discourage unconscious action in tasks that require vigilance.

(Continued)

Table 16-1

Principles of Universal Design (*Continued*)
PRINCIPLE 6
Low Physical Effort: The design can be used efficiently and comfortably and with a minimum of fatigue.
Guidelines: **6a.** Allow user to maintain a neutral body position. **6b.** Use reasonable operating forces. **6c.** Minimize repetitive actions. **6d.** Minimize sustained physical effort.
PRINCIPLE 7
Size and Space for Approach and Use: Appropriate size and space is provided for approach, reach, manipulation, and use regardless of user's body size, posture, or mobility.
Guidelines: **7a.** Provide a clear line of sight to important elements for any seated or standing user. **7b.** Make reach to all components comfortable for any seated or standing user. **7c.** Accommodate variations in hand and grip size. **7d.** Provide adequate space for the use of assistive devices or personal assistance.
From C. Christiansen and K. Matuska. (Eds.). (2004). *Ways of living: Adaptive strategies for special needs,* 3rd ed. (p. 428). Bethesda, MD: American Occupational Therapy Association. Reprinted with permission.

The Role of the Team

1. An occupational therapist is often part of an interdisciplinary team that determines the needs and abilities of an individual with a disability in a specific environment.
2. Basis for team construction.
   a. The facility in which the individual with a disability presently resides and/or participates.
   b. The individual's needs, his or her abilities, and functional status.
   c. Geographical location.
   d. Funding available to the individual with a disability (both individually and through third party payers and/or state offices for individuals with disabilities).
   e. Support available from caregivers.
3. The team should always include the person and caregivers, if any.
4. Professional team members may belong to the Rehabilitation Engineers Society of North America (RESNA) and/or National Registry of Rehabilitation Technology Suppliers (NRRTS).
   a. Both professional organizations help to develop standards and measuring tools to ensure proper design, fabrication, prescription, and delivery of rehabilitation technology.
   b. RESNA offers certification programs for Assistive Technology Professionals (ATPs) Seating and Mobility Specialist (SMSs). Occupational therapists are eligible to acquire these professional certifications.
5. Potential professional team members.
   a. Physician: to authorize and assess services and purchases.
   b. Occupational therapist: refer to prior section.
   c. Physical therapist: to assess mobility difficulties an individual may encounter in the environment.
   d. Speech language pathologist: to assess and recommend augmentative communication aids.
   e. Rehabilitation engineer: to design equipment and to assist with modifications of adaptive equipment.
   f. Computer expert: to assist with the design and provision of efficient technology.
   g. Assistive technology professional (ATP): to analyze consumer needs, help select appropriate assistive technology to meet identified needs, and provide training in the use of the AT.
   h. Seating and mobility specialist (SMS): to evaluate seating, positioning, and mobility needs and make appropriate recommendations.
   i. Rehabilitation counselor: to assess and advise on vocational issues.
   j. Social worker: to assist in obtaining funding.
   k. Psychologist: to assist with adjustment disorders, if indicated.
   l. Nurse: to ensure carry-over of medical care and medication regimes prescribed by the doctor.
   m. Teacher: for children in the school system, to help carry over any modifications within the classroom setting.
   n. Driver trainer: for those who may require training and/or adaptations to drive.

o. Vendor: to provide items requested by therapists and required for the individual to function.
p. Third party payers and/or their respective case manager: to approve and/or provide funding for the individual's needed environmental modifications.

Purposes of Environmental Evaluation and Intervention

1. Identify and prioritize the needs, goals, desires, and problem areas of an individual with a disability within his/her environments.
2. Establish the individual's abilities regarding everyday functional activities within his/her environment.
3. Assess functional use of devices being considered for a particular individual to facilitate mastery of the environment.
4. Identify a device's availability, safety, and cost.
5. Determine a device's location and frequency of use.
6. Determine funding and financial resources for equipment and/or modifications.
   a. It is of questionable ethics and not in the best interest of clients to show them devices or order top of the line equipment that is not covered by their insurance, if they does not have the financial resources to self-pay.
7. Determine environmental constraints.
   a. For example, an individual may be living in a four flight walk-up apartment and have to leave a device locked up in a lobby, opening it up to the risk of vandalism or theft.
8. Assess if the individual with a disability and the device will allow for re-evaluation.
   a. Ensure the device will allow for possible modifications, if upon reassessment of the individual a change in status is found.

Overall Environmental Evaluation

Evaluation of Performance Skills and Client Factors

1. Performance skills and client factors are essential to assess when conducting an environmental evaluation, for they are the fundamental abilities that allow a person to function in his or her environment.
2. There are numerous assessments available for specific performance skills and client factors.
3. A comprehensive evaluation should assess:
   a. Sensory skills (e.g., tactile, pain, visual acuity) to determine if there is an impairment that could influence safety in the manipulation of devices.
   b. Visual-perceptual processing skills (e.g., Minnesota Rate of Manipulation Test, a standardized test to assess visual motor perception) to assess for potential difficulties with computer use.
   c. Musculoskeletal skills (e.g., range of motion, strength, and endurance) to assess if the person will be able to physically use the devices to optimal capability.
   d. Neuromuscular skills (e.g., tone, coordination) to assess the person's ability to utilize all limbs rhythmically in mobility and environmental manipulation.
   e. Cognitive skills (e.g., following directions, memory, and judgment) to assess if a person is aware of limitations and able to follow and recall directions regarding operation of assistive technology and wheelchairs and the safe use of devices.
   f. Psychosocial skills (e.g., social interaction) to assess if an individual with a disability can ask for assistance and obtain needed information from the right person; to assess the individual's ability to give instructions.

Contextual Evaluation

1. Physical considerations.
   a. Arrangement of furniture.
   b. Accessibility of items needed for desired activities and for safety.
   c. Ease of use.
   d. Housing/workplace design.
   e. Neighborhood characteristics.
      (1) Availability and use of transportation.
      (2) Overall accessibility.
2. Sociocultural considerations.
   a. The individual's social network: the relationships between the individual with the disability and others.
   b. Social roles: expectations for role performance of the individual with a disability and others.
   c. Opportunities for socialization.
   d. Sociocultural norms, values, and expectations for independent function.
   e. Community resources available.

Home Evaluation

General Considerations

1. Occupational therapists perform home assessments and make adaptations, modifications, and recommendations to the anticipated dwelling to increase safe, independent functioning.
2. If an individual with a disability is to be discharged to home from a facility, the on-site home evaluation should be done before the discharge date.
3. The person's current status (abilities and limitations) will drive the need for modification.

Overall Characteristics of the Home

1. Type of dwelling: private house, one-family, two-family, apartment, walk-up, elevator access.
2. Protection from weather/environmental changes.
3. Presence and use of a driveway.
4. Level of the dwelling in which the person lives.
5. Entrance to the dwelling: wheelchair access, ramp, level entrance, stairs.
6. Number of entrances that are accessible to the individual.
   a. Some apartment buildings allow residents to use a delivery entrance because it has a ramp.
7. Steps: the number present outside dwelling, inside the dwelling, to the laundry room, and to the mailbox.
8. Railings: the location and number of railings when outside and facing the entrance door; the presence of secure railings for interior stairways.
   a. Interior railings should be mounted 1½″ from the wall to ease grasp.
   b. Exterior railings should be waist high for those who walk; 34″–38″ depending on person's height.
   c. Railings should be 1½″–2″ in diameter with non-skid surfaces.
9. Door sills: identify where they are present, i.e., entrance to dwelling, bedroom doors, bathroom doors, kitchen doorway.
10. Width of elevator doorway.
11. Width of hallway entrance.
12. Width of entrance door(s); measure from open door to frame; not frame to frame.
13. Direction of opening for entrance door(s) and any other doors throughout dwelling which must be opened.
    a. Space to accommodate door swing must be available.
       (1) A minimum of 18″ is needed for those using walkers.
       (2) A minimum of 26″ is needed for those using wheelchairs.
14. Type(s) of door handles: lever handles are more functional than round knobs.
15. Identification of objects which may be obstructing doorways and/or pathways.
16. Presence of pets: they can become obstacles and/or safety concerns to those with low vision, balance problems, and those who require assistive devices.
17. Carpeting: location and type; i.e., wall to wall, throw rugs, height of pile.
18. Electrical cords: placed out of flow of traffic, in good condition or frayed, overloaded or under rugs/carpeting.
19. Presence of a firm chair in the dwelling and its height.
20. Light switches: accessibility from various levels (standing and chair).
21. Telephones: number of phones, their location, and type (i.e., cordless, cell, push button, rotary); emergency numbers by telephone or stored in telephone memory.
22. Presence of working smoke detectors.
23. Presence of space heaters or wood burning stoves/fireplaces.
24. Presence of an emergency call system and an emergency exit plan.

Bedroom Characteristics

1. Bed: size of bed, height from floor to top mattress, type of mattress, wheeled frame or not, position of bed (against the wall or freestanding).
2. Side of the bed from which the individual with a disability enters/exits.
3. Accessibility of clothes and dresser drawers.
4. Sufficient room available for a bedside commode, if needed.

Bathroom Considerations

1. Number of bathrooms in the home.
2. Location of bathroom(s) relative to the bedroom, living room, kitchen, and other living spaces important to the individual.
3. Width of the bathroom doorway.
4. Type of bathing the individual with a disability performs (i.e., bath, shower, sponge bath).
5. Type of shower: separate stall, glass door tub with shower, curtain-enclosed tub with shower.
6. Presence and location of grab bars (the soap dish and towel bar are not grab bars).
   a. If home is rental, landlord's agreement to allow grab bars to be installed if needed.
7. Height of tub, sink, and toilet.
8. Presence of a non-skid mat or skid-free surface in the shower/tub.
9. Presence of a throw rug outside of shower.
10. Availability of a hand-held shower.
11. Presence of anti-scald valves and/or faucets.

Kitchen Considerations

1. Location of meal preparation devices that the individual uses most frequently (i.e., oven, microwave, stove).
2. Presence of a countertop area between the stove and sink, between the stove and refrigerator.
3. Accessibility of food, pots, pans, dishes, and preparation materials.
4. Direction of opening for refrigerator, cabinetry, and/or pantry doors.
5. Presence of a charged fire extinguisher.
6. Presence of anti-scald valves and/or faucets.

Evaluation of Safety

The Safety Assessment of Function and the Environment for Rehabilitation (SAFER)

1. Focus: identifies possible safety concerns in the home environment and assesses if the person is able to respond to safety situations.
2. Method: an interview and observation of a person are conducted in the home. If available, caregiver input is also sought.
   a. During administration, 128 items covering possible safety concerns are addressed.
      (1) These include the living situation, household, kitchen, bathroom, fire hazards, eating, dressing, grooming, medication, mobility, communication, wandering, and memory aids.
      (2) If there is a problem with an item, the therapist applies task analysis and environmental assessment skills to make suggestions which can help the person and/or caregiver deal with the situation.
3. Scoring and interpretation: a form comprised of three columns (i.e., addressed, not applicable, and problem) is used to rate each item.
   a. A percentage score is obtained by multiplying the number of problem items by 100.
   b. Qualitative comments about each item and recommendations to address areas of concern can be provided on the SAFER form.
4. Population: originally designed for psychogeriatric persons, the SAFER can be used with home-residing clients of all ages.

Safety Assessment Scale (SAS)

1. Focus: assesses the potential safety risks of people with dementia who live at home.
2. Method: observation of a person and a caregiver interview are conducted in the home.
   a. A short version of 19 questions is used to screen for safety risks.
   b. A long version of 32 questions is used to make recommendations and plan interventions to decrease safety risks.
3. Scoring and interpretation: a rating scale of always, most of the time, occasionally, or never is used. The results are used to help caregivers diminish safety risks in the home.
4. Population: older adults with cognitive impairments (e.g., dementia) living at home.
   a. The SAS has also been used with community-residing older adults without cognitive impairments.

Fall Prevention and Management

Falls Etiology, Prevalence, and Prognosis

1. The unintentional loss of balance causing one to make unexpected contact with ground or floor.
2. Falls and fall injury are a major public health concern for the elderly.
   a. The facts and figures listed below will not be on the NBCOT examination. These statistics are provided to highlight the reality that the incidence of falls is not rare.
      (1) Consequently, the NBCOT exam will likely include exam items that include scenarios related to falls and fall prevention.
   b. Between 30%–50% of persons over the age of 65 fall each year. Note: percentages may be greater because data is based only upon reported falls.
   c. Women are more at risk for falls than men, due to their increased incidence of osteoporosis; 20% of men aged 65–74 fall, whereas 42% of women of the same age fall.
   d. 24% of falls result in severe soft tissue injury and fractures.
   e. Falls are the sixth-leading cause of death for the elderly; 12% of all deaths for persons aged 65 or older are caused by falls.
   f. Falls are a factor in 40% of admissions to nursing homes.
   g. Within six months of a fall, more than two-thirds of the elderly who have fallen will fall again.
3. Results of falls.
   a. Fractures: most common fracture sites are the pelvis, hip, femur, vertebrae, and humerus head.
   b. Increased caution and fear of falling.
   c. Loss of confidence to function independently.
   d. Decreased engagement in activity and restriction of activities which can result in severe physical deconditioning and deterioration, contributing to the likelihood of reoccurrence.
   e. Increased risk of recurrent falls.

Evaluation of Risk Factors for Falls

1. Intrinsic factors requiring evaluation.
   a. Age related changes in sensory system resulting in reduced sensory capacity.
      (1) Vision.
         (a) Presbyopia (decreased acuity).
         (b) Reduced night vision means that vision in low light situations is also reduced.
         (c) Impaired depth perception.
      (2) Vestibular.
         (a) Vertigo.
         (b) Postural sway combined with vision problems results in a compound risk.
   b. Age related changes in the neuromuscular system.
      (1) Decreased number of neurons results in decreased response time.
      (2) Decreased number of muscle fibers leads to decreased strength and endurance.
      (3) Two manifestations of the combination of the above factors include difficulties in rising from a chair and maintaining gait speed.
   c. Pathological states including congestive heart failure, arrhythmias, hypotension, cerebrovascular disease, Parkinson's disease, arteriosclerosis and atherosclerosis, diabetes mellitus.
   d. Medication side effects and/or polypharmacy.
   e. Delirium and/or dementia.
   f. Anxiety and/or depression.
   g. Prior history of falls.
   h. Fear of falling can lead to decreased mobility and progressive deconditioning, which increase the risk of subsequent falls.
2. Extrinsic factors requiring evaluation.
   a. General.
      (1) Floors: slippery or uneven, presence of throw rugs.
      (2) Toys or other clutter left on floors or stairs.
      (3) Pets under foot.
      (4) High pile carpets.
      (5) Low lying furniture.
      (6) Stairs, excessive steepness, lack of or loose handrails.
      (7) Improper footwear.
      (8) Poor lighting or glare.
      (9) Poor thresholds.
      (10) Extension cords.
      (11) Use of furniture or other unstable objects for support.
      (12) Improper transfer techniques.
      (13) Problems with adaptive equipment or lack of needed equipment.
   b. Bathroom.
      (1) No grab bars.
      (2) Utilization of unstable soap dish or towel bar for support.

(3) Toilet seat too low.
(4) Wet floor surfaces.
(5) Utilization of wet sink surface for support.

c. Kitchen.
(1) Low cabinet doors open.
(2) Step stool without handles.
(3) Chairs pulled out.

d. Bedroom.
(1) Bed too high or too low.
(2) Reaching into closets.

e. Living room.
(1) Wires and/or clutter across floor.
(2) Chairs too high or too low.

Fall Efficacy Scale (FES)

1. Focus: measures a person's fear of falling during nonhazardous activities of daily living (e.g., BADL, meal preparation, functional mobility).
2. Method: the person's level of perceived self-efficacy at avoiding falls is measured by asking how confident the person feels about completing the FES activities without falling.
3. Scoring and interpretation: the person's level of concern about falling during activites is measured on a four point Likert scale with 1 representing not at all concerned to 4 representing very concerned.
4. Population: community-dwelling older adults with or without a history of fear of falling.

Interventions to Prevent Falls

1. Intervention is based upon the determination of the individual's functional problems and the causative factors of falls as identified in evaluation.
2. Eliminate or minimize all fall risk factors; stabilize disease states, manage medication.
3. Improve functional mobility.
   a. Active or resistive muscle strengthening exercises and general conditioning exercises (GCE) to improve or maintain flexibility, strength, endurance, and coordination.
   b. PROM stretching as indicated to increase joint ROM.
   c. Specific coordination training.
   d. Neuromuscular reeducation training.
   e. Balance training.
      (1) Sit and stand positions.
      (2) Static and dynamic.
      (3) Turning, walking, stairs.
   f. Transfer training.
   g. Bed mobility training.
   h. Wheelchair safety training.
   i. Referral to physical therapy for gait/ambulation training.
4. Provide sensory compensation strategies.
5. Modify activities of daily living for safety.
   a. Order appropriate adaptive devices and train in safe use (i.e., reachers, long shoe horn, stocking/sock aid, leg lifter, dressing stick, walker baskets, etc.).
   b. Allow adequate time for activities; instruct in gradual position changes.
6. Teach energy conservation techniques.
7. Communicate with family and caregivers.
8. Modify environment to reduce falls and instability; use environmental checklist.
   a. Ensure adequate lighting.
   b. Use contrasting colors to delineate hazardous areas.
   c. Simplify environment, reduce clutter.
   d. Firmly attach carpet.
   e. Stairs.
      (1) Securely fasten handrails on both sides of stairs.
      (2) Provide light switches at top and bottom.
      (3) Install non-skid secure surface.
   f. Bathrooms.
      (1) Install grab bars located in and out of tubs and shower and near toilets.
      (2) Provide nonskid mats and nightlights.
      (3) Use elevated toilet seat.
   g. Bedrooms.
      (1) Install night lights or light switch within reach of bed.
      (2) Place telephones in an easy to reach position near bed.
      (3) Replace existing mattress with one either thinner or thicker to lower or to raise bed height as needed.
      (4) Arrange furniture for easy maneuverability.
   h. Living areas.
      (1) Ensure couches and chairs are at proper height to get in and out of easily.
      (2) Remove clutter and loose electrical cords.
      (3) Arrange furniture for easy maneuverability.
   i. Kitchen and closet shelves.
      (1) Store items on reachable shelves (between person's eye and hip level).
   j. Outdoors.
      (1) Fix cracked pavement or steps.
      (2) Install stable outside handrail.
9. Provide specific safety guidelines for the individual to follow. Advise them to:
   a. Ask for assistance to transfer or ambulate.
      (1) Not stand up alone; not walk to the bathroom or kitchen alone.

b. Utilize prescribed assistive device(s) to ambulate, especially on any uneven or unfamiliar ground. Keep assistive device near at all times.
c. Use prescribed adaptive equipment.
d. Stand in place before beginning to walk to avoid dizziness from change in position and to regain balance.
e. Do not bend forward.
f. Wear supportive rubber-soled or low heeled shoes.
g. Avoid wearing smooth-soled slippers or only socks, which makes it easier to slip.

10. Provide psychological support and specific interventions to deal with the fear of falling.
    a. Acknowledge the validity of the individual's concerns.
    b. Initiate discussions about risk factors and encourage active problem solving.
    c. Modify activities to be safe and achievable to build confidence.
    d. Provide activities to maintain physical conditioning to decrease risk of fear becoming a reality.
    e. Develop a contingency plan to use in the event of a fall to maintain safety.

Interventions for Occurrence of a Fall

1. Check for fall injury.
   a. Hip fracture: complaints of pain in hip, especially on palpation; external rotation of leg; inability to bear weight on leg; changes in gait or weight bearing status.
   b. Head injury: loss of consciousness, mental confusion.
   c. Spinal cord injury: loss of sensation or voluntary movement.
   d. Cuts, bruises, painful swelling.
2. Check for dizziness that may have preceded the fall.
3. Provide reassurance.
4. Provide first aid, call emergency services if necessary.
5. Do not attempt to lift the individual alone, get help.
6. Solicit witnesses of fall event.
7. Document the incident as per setting's established procedures.
8. Refer the individual to a fall prevention intervention program to prevent reoccurrences.

Modifications for Sensorimotor Deficits

Architectural Barriers

1. Architectural features in the home and the community that make negotiation of space difficult or impossible or require modifications to allow accessibility (e.g., steps, narrow doors).
2. Modifications should be made according to established standards, such as the International Code Council, Inc.
3. Wheelchair dimensions and accessibility needs.
   a. Average wheelchair width is 24″–26″ rim to rim. See Figure 16-1.
      (1) Some doorways and room spaces may be too narrow, limiting clear mobility.
      (2) The minimal clearance width for doorways and halls: 32″ doorway width minimum, with ideal being 36″. See Figure 16-2.
         (a) An additional 26″ is needed beside the door to allow for door swing.
         (b) Doorways can be widened or removed if necessary.
            - Removing doorstops can add ¾″ in width.
            - Replacing existing hinges with offset hinges can add 1½″–2″ in width.
         (c) Doorway saddles can be removed and the floor patched, a wedge can be placed in front of the saddle, or a thin rubber mat can be placed over the saddle.
      (3) Hallways should be 36″ wide. See Figure 16-2.
   b. Average wheelchair length is 42″–43″.
      (1) Adequate turning spaces are needed.
      (2) A 360° wheelchair turning space requires a clearance space of 60″ × 60″. See Figure 16-3.
   c. The maximal height the individual can reach forward from sitting is 48″ and at least 15″ is needed to prevent tipping. See Figure 16-4.
   d. Maximal height for reaching sideways is 48″ and when an obstruction is present is 46″. See Figure 16-5.
   e. The maximal height for countertops should be 31″.
   f. Parking spaces should have an adjacent 4′ aisle to allow wheelchairs to maneuver.
   g. Pathways and walkways should be 48″ wide.
   h. Ramps should be a minimum of 36″ wide and should have a non-skid surface on upper and lower levels.
      (1) The ratio of slope to rise is 1:12 (for every 1″ of vertical rise, 12″ of ramp is required). See Figure 16-6.
      (2) Railings should be between 29″ and 36″ high depending on person's arm reach; 32″ is average.

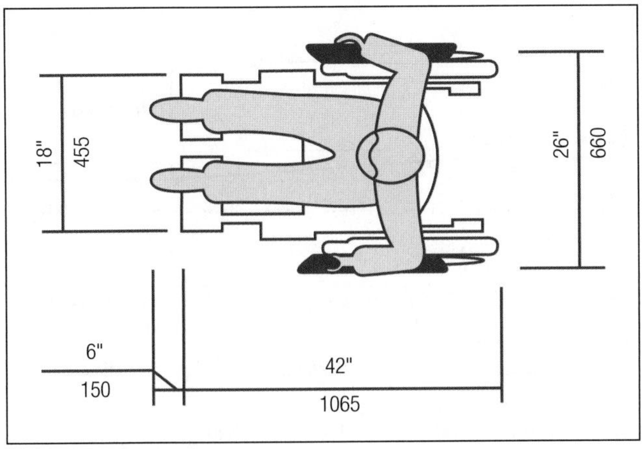

Figure 16-1 **Dimensions of standard adult manual wheelchair.**

Width 24 to 26" from rim to rim. Length: 42 to 43". Height to push handles from floor: 36". Height to seat from floor: 19 to 19.5" (excluding cushion). Height to armrest from floor: 29 to 30". Note: Footrests may extend farther for very large people.

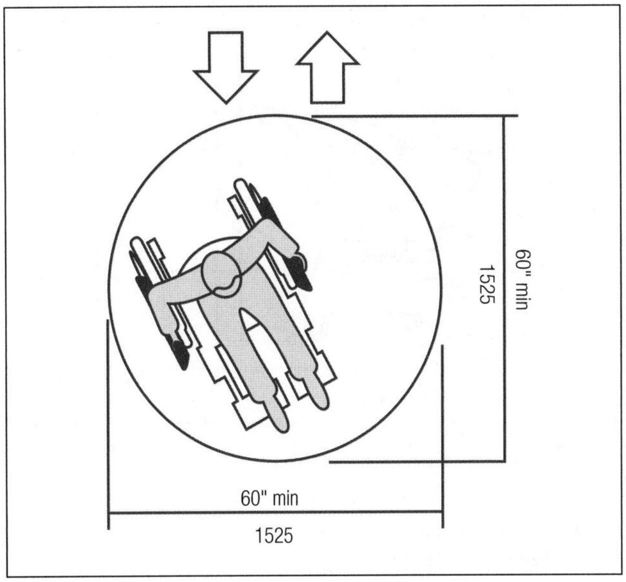

Figure 16-3 **360° wheelchair turning space.**

A 360° turn requires a clear space of 60" by 60". This space enables the individual to turn without scraping the feet or maneuvering multiple times to accomplish a full turn.

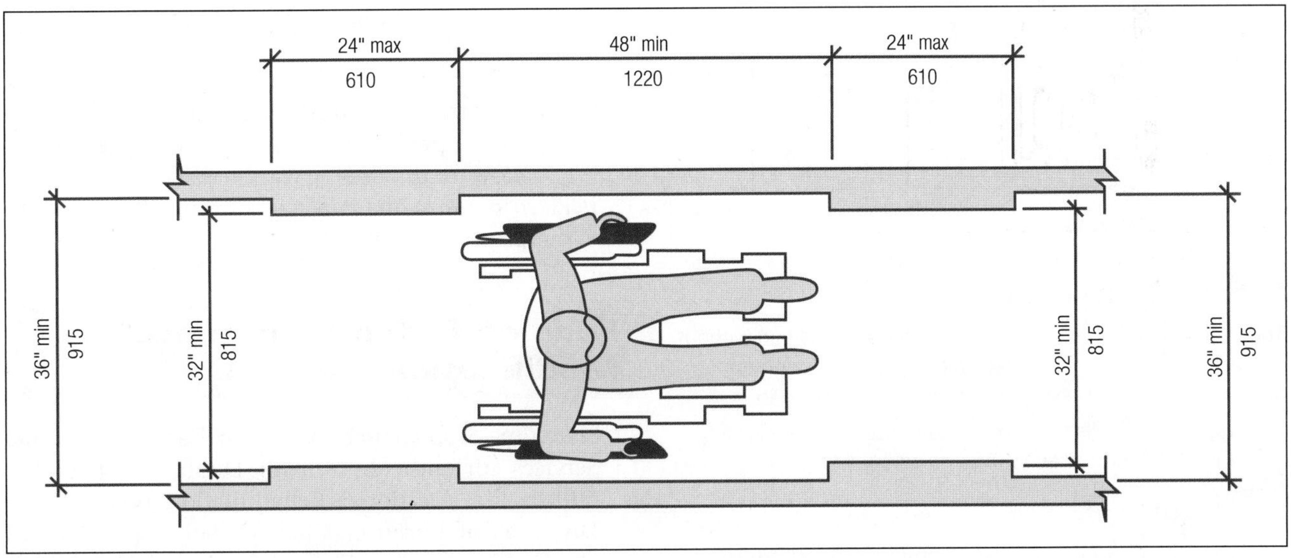

Figure 16-2 **Minimum clear width for doorways and halls.**

A minimum of 32" of doorway width is required; the ideal is 36". Hallways should be a minimum of 36" wide to provide sufficient clearance for wheelchair passage and allow the user to propel the chair without scraping the hands.

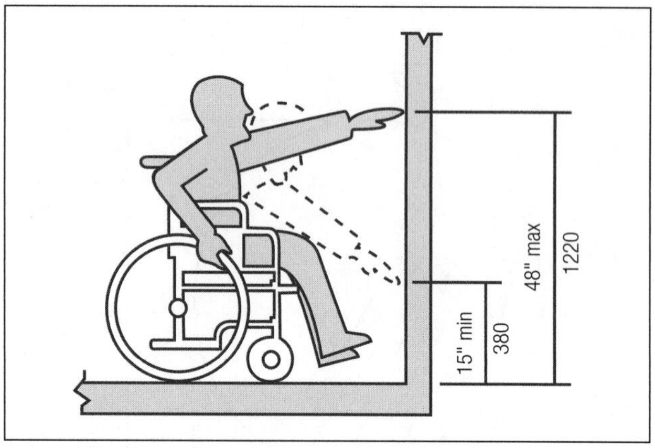

Figure 16-4 **Forward reach.**

The maximal height an individual can reach from a seated position is 48". Height should be at least 15" to prevent the wheelchair from tipping forward.

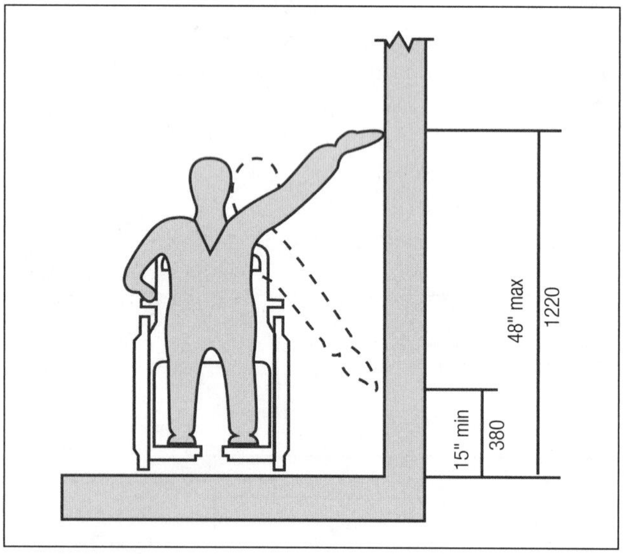

Figure 16-5 **Side reach.**

The maximal height for reaching from the side position without an obstruction is 48". If an obstruction such as a countertop or shelf is present the maximal height for side reach is 46".

(3) Curbs on ramps should be at least 4″ high.

(4) Level platforms must be included in the ramp design.

(a) If the ramp is excessively long, 4′ × 4′ landing(s) are required to allow for rest.

(b) If the person using the ramp has limited upper extremity strength or decreased

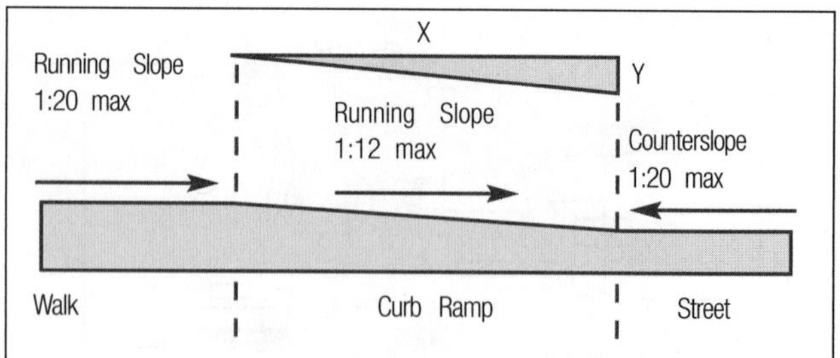

	Maximum rise		Maximum horizontal projection	
Slope	in	mm	ft	m
1:12 to 1:15	30	760	30	9
1:16 to 1:19	30	760	40	12
1:20	30	760	50	15

Figure 16-6 **Slope and rise of ramps.**

This diagram provides the components of a single ramp run and a sample of ramp dimensions. The slope ratio is an important consideration when designing a ramp; slope creates hazardous wheelchair propulsion conditions if it is too steep.

cardiopulmonary capacity, 4′ × 4′ landing(s) are required.

(c) If there is a sharp turn in the direction of the ramp, landing(s) are required for turning space. A 90 degree turn requires a minimum 4′ × 4′ landing; a 180 degree turn requires a minimum 4′ × 8′ landing.

(5) If the ramp leads to a door, there must be a 5′ × 5′ platform before the door that extends at least 12″ (18″ is preferred) along the side of the door to allow for door swing without backing up.

i. Electric porch lifts and stair lifts are alternatives to ramps.

Funding for Environmental Modifications

1. State One-Stop Centers, Vocational and Educational Services for Individuals with Disabilities (VESID), Offices for Vocational Rehabilitation (OVRs), and Divisions of Vocational Rehabilitation (DVRs) will pay for home and work modifications, if the modifications enable a person to go to work or school.
2. Private companies will fund modifications to ensure ADA compliance.
3. Private insurance, Medicare, Medicaid and Worker's Compensation will possibly reimburse for certain devices/adaptations.

Wheelchair Prescription and Assessment

Purposes of Wheelchairs and Wheelchair Seating and Positioning

1. Enable functional mobility with what means the person with a disability has available.
2. Facilitate mastery of the environment.
3. Enable occupational engagement and social participation.
4. Promote functional posture by provision of appropriate back, trunk, and/or leg supports.
5. Facilitate upper limb function which can occur with proper trunk support.
6. Promote comfort during upright ADL.
7. Provide physiological maintenance and tissue protection through prevention of shearing.
8. Promote sensory readiness through provision of proper eye and head position.
9. Decrease progression of deformity through customized seating as needed.
10. Decrease pain through provision of proper support.

General Assessment and Prescription Considerations

1. Assess the ability of the wheelchair to interact/interface with other assistive devices.
2. Determine the individual's medical status, including prognosis (is condition temporary, stable, or progressive?) and functional level/needs.
3. Collaborate with the consumer, caregiver(s), and interdisciplinary team members as identified in prior section of this chapter.

Specific Assessments for Wheelchair Prescription

1. Client factor and performance skill assessments.
   a. Sensory (e.g., sensory loss places the person at risk for the development of decubiti, therefore necessitating a special seat cushion).
   b. Neuromuscular (e.g., the individual's sitting posture can require application of seating and positioning knowledge; poor trunk control requires postural supports).
   c. Musculoskeletal (e.g., physical limitations, such as a compromised respiratory status may impede mobility and require a powered wheelchair prescription).
   d. Cognition (e.g., deficits in cognitive function may impede ability to operate powered devices).
   e. Psychosocial (e.g., the availability of social supports to assist with transferring to transporting a wheelchair).
2. Personal assessment.
   a. Age and developmental status. See subsequent section on developmental considerations.
   b. Nature of disability (i.e., temporary, permanent, stable, or progressive).
   c. Education and work interests and pursuits (e.g., the need for desk arms).
   d. Leisure interests and pursuits (e.g., a special sports chair can enable the individual to pursue past or new interests).
   e. Daily routines and habits.
   f. Goals and desired occupations.
   g. Assistive technology and/or medical equipment used while in the wheelchair (e.g., a communication board, ventilator).
3. Contextual assessments.
   a. Physical environment.
      (1) Areas of travel and wheelchair use.
      (2) Surfaces and terrains that will be traveled on indoors (e.g., floor surfaces) and outdoors (e.g., sidewalks).
   b. Building characteristics of school, work, leisure, and/or worship.
      (1) Doorways.
      (2) Hallways.
      (3) Restrooms.
      (4) Workspace design.
      (5) Parking.
      (6) Other specifics as described in the home evaluation section of this chapter.
4. Wheelchair characteristics considered in assessment.
   a. Transportability/portability.
   b. Ride quality.
   c. Types of wheelchair features available.
      (1) Control mechanism (e.g., type of brakes used, use of anti-tippers).
      (2) Propulsion method (e.g., one arm drive, use of hand rim projections, motorized, use of lower extremities to propel).
      (3) Personalized features (e.g., use of lap tray and/or backpack to hold personal items and/or medical equipment, hard tires instead of pneumatic tires for increased durability for more

active individuals, postural supports for person with poor trunk control).

5. Developmental considerations in assessment.
   a. Transportability to, from, and in school.
   b. Allowance for adjustment when growth changes are experienced.
   c. Allowance for use of adaptive equipment (i.e., computer, augmentative communication).
   d. Facilitation of social acceptance.

Wheelchair Components

1. Armrests.
   a. Fixed: minimal benefit but may be seen in older wheelchairs and/or in rentals.
   b. Detached: helpful for transfers.
   c. Height adjustable: allows for ease in transfers and better support of a lap tray.
   d. Desk arms: allow for moving closer to work surfaces.
   e. Full arms: allow for holding of a lap tray and possibly ease transfers.
   f. Wraparound, space saver arm rests: reduces the overall width of the chair by 1″.
2. Legrests.
   a. Fixed: minimal benefit but may be seen in older wheelchairs and/or in rentals.
   b. Swing-away: allows feet to be placed on the floor to prepare for transfers and for a front approach to wheelchair.
   c. Detachable: allows for a safe path for transfers.
   d. Elevating: allows for edema control and reduction.
3. Footplates.
   a. Fixed: minimal benefit but may be seen in older wheelchairs and/or in rentals.
   b. Swing-away: allows feet to reach floor.
   c. Heel loops: prevent feet from slipping off footrest in a posterior direction.
   d. Ankle straps: prevent slipping off footrest.
4. Tires.
   a. Pneumatic: air-filled, requires maintenance, more cushioned ride, shock absorbent.
   b. Semi-pneumatic: airless foam inserts, less maintenance, good cushioning.
   c. Solid-core rubber: minimal maintenance, tires are mounted on spoked or molded wheels.
5. Casters.
   a. Smaller ones facilitate maneuverability.
   b. Pneumatic and semi-pneumatic types available, but solid-core are best for indoors and smooth surfaces.
   c. Caster locks can be added for increased stability during transfers.
6. Frame.
   a. Fixed: minimal benefit but may be seen in older wheelchairs or sports chairs.
   b. Folding: eases storage and facilitates mobility in community as it can fold to fit in car or van.
   c. Weight: ultra-light, active-duty lightweight, lightweight, standard, and heavy duty frame construction is available.
      (1) The lighter the weight of the chair generally, the greater the ease of use.
      (2) The demands of the individual's expected and desired activities must be considered.
7. Additional attachments.
   a. Anti-tippers to prevent wheelchair from tipping backward or forward.
      (1) Can get caught on doorsills and curbs.
   b. Seatbelts for safety during mobility and functional activities.
      (1) Attach at hip level not waist level.
      (2) Extend across hips and into lap at 45-degree angle.
   c. Harnesses to position a person lacking sufficient trunk control.
   d. Arm troughs to position and support a flaccid upper extremity and prevent edema through elevation.
   e. Lapboards can serve the same purpose as an arm trough, but are also beneficial as a working 'table top' surface.
   f. Head supports allow for improved eye contact, improved communication, and feeding assistance, as the head is kept in a neutral position.
   g. Mobile arm supports allow for use of an upper extremity with proximal weakness to engage in feeding,and other activities.
   h. Brake extensions allow a person with limited range in one upper extremity to independently manipulate the wheelchair's brakes.
   i. Handrim projections ease independent propulsion in persons with weak handgrip.
      (1) These increase the width of the chair and can decrease mobility through narrow doors and/or narrow spaces.
   j. Hillholder devices (also called hillclimber and grade aid devices) allow the wheelchair to move forward but automatically brake when the chair goes backward by engaging a level attached to each wheel.
      (1) Useful for individuals unable to ascend a steep grade (e.g., a long ramp or hill) without a rest.
   k. Seating and positioning systems (refer to subsequent section for details).

Wheelchair Measurement and Considerations

1. General.
   a. The size of a wheelchair should be proportional to the person. See next section for bariatric considerations.
      (1) Standard-sized chairs should be matched to a person whenever possible due to the increased expense of customized chairs.
      (2) Refer to Table 16-2.
   b. Measure on a firm surface, but also observe in a variety of positions to account for tonal influences on posture.
   c. The cushion that will be selected for the individual needs to be considered.
2. Seat width.
   a. Measure the widest point across the hips and thighs to allow for maximal seating space and comfort, and then add 2 inches.
   b. This allows for clearance on the sides to prevent friction/rubbing and to allow the individual to wear heavier material clothing without being cumbersome.
   c. The bariatric client with a pear-shape will have increased gluteal femoral weight distribution.
      (1) Measurement should consider the widest portion of the seated position (e.g., at the forward edge of the seated position).
      (2) Also consider room for weightshifting maneuvers for pressure relief and possible use of lift devices.
3. Seat depth.
   a. Measure both lower extremities (LEs) and take the greatest length; measure from the posterior portion of the buttocks to the popliteal fossa and then subtract 2 inches from this measurement.
   b. This prevents rubbing and potential decubiti to posterior knee region, while also allowing maximal leg swing.
4. Back height.
   a. Measurement is based on the need for postural stability, upper extremity (UE) movements, and potential for independent wheelchair propulsion.
   b. Take measurement from seat surface (including the cushion) upward to one of the following depending on the person's trunk control, activity level, strength, and size.
      (1) Mid-back under scapula: 1–2 inches below.
      (2) Mid-scapula or axilla.
      (3) Top of the shoulder.
   c. Lower back height can increase functional mobility as in sports chairs.
      (1) Lower back height can increase back strain.
   d. Higher back height may be needed if poor trunk stability.
      (1) If back height of chair is extended, potential problems must be recognized.
         (a) Added back height may prevent the individual from locking onto the push handle for stabilization and/or weight shifting.
         (b) Added back height may increase difficulty of fitting chair into car or van.
5. Seat height.
   a. Knees and ankles should be positioned at 90 degrees; measure from distal thigh to heel.
   b. Footrests should have 2″ clearance from the floor, so cushion selected will affect this measurement.
   c. Standard height: 19.5″.
   d. Hemi-height: 17.5″.
   e. Super-low: 14.5″.
6. Armrest height.
   a. Shoulders should be neutral; arms hanging at the sides; elbow flexed to 90 degrees.
   b. Measure under each elbow to cushioned seating surface.
   c. Armrests that are too low will encourage leaning forward.
   d. Armrests that are too high will cause shoulder elevation.

Table 16-2

Standard Dimensions for Wheelchairs

CHAIR STYLE	SEAT WIDTH	SEAT DEPTH	SEAT HEIGHT
Adult	18″	16″	20″
Narrow Adult	16″	16″	20″
Slim Adult	14″	16″	20″
Hemi/low Seat			17.5″
Junior	16″	16″	18.5″
Child	14″	11.5″	18.75″
Tiny Tot	12″	11.5″	19.5″

Types of Wheelchairs

1. Refer to Table 16-3 for descriptions of general types of wheelchairs and indications/contraindications for use.
2. Specialized wheelchairs.
   a. Reclining back: indicated for individuals who are unable to independently maintain an upright sitting position.

Chapter 16

Table 16-3

Types of Wheelchairs

ATTENDANT PROPELLED	MANUAL WHEELCHAIR	POWERED MOBILITY
Description	**Description**	**Description**
• Pushed by another • Usually is manual wheelchair • Can be a full-size chair or a stroller type chair (e.g., airplane aisle transit chairs)	• Rigid or folding frames • Various frames and weights • Lightweight chair: 25–40 pounds • Standard: > 50 pounds without seating • Amputee frame: axle can be moved posteriorly for increased stability and accommodate for change in gravity center • Hemi-chair: use non-affected upper extremity and/or lower extremity • One-arm drive • Gurneys: for prone position	• Power-base typically independent of seating system • Diverse 4 wheel designs and 3 wheel scooters • Add-on power units to manual chairs • Battery operated: - deep cycle lead acid - wet cell - sealed cell • Method of operation: - micro-switch - proportional joystick - sip and puff - sensing system - body part to be used
Indications/Benefits	**Indications/Benefits**	**Indications/Benefits**
• Brief or chronic disability prevents the ability to self-propel • Transport in the community • When powered mobility cannot be used or is being repaired • Fit and comfort considered for all involved	• Can independently propel and brake using upper extremities • May use quick release wheels (easier for cars) • Can be easily tilted to go up and down curbs.	• Cannot use hands or feet • Energy expenditure limitations • Arthritic upper extremities • Prone to repetitive stress injury • Neuromuscular injury: to prevent associated reactions • Can change seat height or tilt • Sturdy and useful indoors and outdoors.
Limitations	**Limitations**	**Limitations**
• Dependent on another person	• Standard weight is heavy when considering adding seating system	• Large and heavy to transport • Difficult to maneuver in small places • Cannot be tilted over curbs • May need to use lifts

Based upon Dudgeon, B. & Deitz, J. (2008).

b. Tilt-in-space: indicated for pressure relief or for an individual with severe extensor spasms that may throw him or her out of the chair; entire seat and back tilt back to maintain a normal seat to back angle.
c. One arm-drive, hemi-chair, amputee frame, and powered chairs as outlined in Table 16-3.
d. Recreational: designed with large thick inner tube type tires and large front casters for all terrain use including sand, mud, snow, and off-road surfaces.
e. Sports: specially designed for racing, cycling, basketball, and other competitive sports; typically ultra lightweight.
f. Stander: designed to enable a person to independently change seat height and/or elevate to a standing position.
g. Stair-climbing: designed to navigate stairs while balancing on two wheels using sensors and gyroscopes.
h. Bariatric wheelchair: heavy-duty, extra-wide wheelchair designed to assist mobility for individuals who are obese. See following section.

Bariatric Wheelchairs and Prescription Considerations[1]

1. Wheelchair users who are obese must be prescribed wheelchairs that are rated for their obesity category.
   a. Selection based on patient characteristics, safety, and function.
2. The bariatric client has a center of body mass that is positioned several inches forward in comparison with the non-obese person.
   a. In order to ensure wheelchair stability, the rear axle is displaced forward in comparison with the standard wheelchair.
      (1) This forward position allows for a more efficient arm push (full arm stroke with less wrist extension).

[1]This section and the section on bariatric considerations for wheelchair measurement were contributed by Susan O'Sullivan.

3. Bariatric wheelchair can be ordered with special adaptations.
   a. Hard tires versus pneumatic tires for increased durability.
   b. Adjustable backrest to accommodate excessive posterior bulk.
   c. Reclining wheelchair to accommodate excessive anterior bulk, cardiorespiratory compromise (e.g., orthostatic hypotension).
   d. Power application attached to a heavy duty wheelchair to accommodate excessive fatigue.

Wheelchair Mobility Training

1. Assess cognitive and physical capabilities to determine the individual's ability to learn and use a wheelchair independently.
   a. Include personal care attendants and caregivers in training, as needed.
2. Determine goals for community mobility.
3. Check wheelchair and seating system for fit and needed adjustments.
4. Instruct in proper sitting posture.
5. Instruct in pressure relief (i.e., push ups, weight shifts leaning to one side, then the other).
   a. Provide time schedule for weight shifts.
6. Instruct in the purpose and use of additional devices used with the wheelchair (i.e., cushion, lap board).
7. Instruct in wheelchair propulsion (e.g., manual, joystick, head control, sip and puff).
   a. Use of wheelchair gloves to ease propulsion and protect hands.
   b. Compensation techniques (e.g., use of feet to assist for propulsion when upper extremity is affected).
8. Instruct in safety concerns when operating a mobility device.
   a. Need to set/release locks.
   b. Use of swing-away legrests and removable armrests with transferring.
   c. Caution when using powered wheelchair.
   d. Safe ways to fall from a wheelchair and to return to wheelchair from the ground, if possible.
9. Instruct in how to manipulate basic parts of the wheelchair and break them down to ease transport (e.g., removal of parts to ease storage in a car trunk).
10. Instruct in how to maneuver wheelchair throughout the community.
    a. Practice in natural interior and exterior environments is essential.
       (1) Traverse over different surfaces (e.g., carpeted, asphalt, uneven).
       (2) Ascend and descend inclines.
       (3) Negotiate lips and curbs; how to "pop a wheelie".
       (4) Negotiate obstacles (e.g., garbage cans on streets, chairs in restaurants).
       (5) Use car and stair lifts.
11. Train in how to transfer from wheelchair to diverse surfaces. See section on transfer training.
12. Instruct in basic maintenance of wheelchair parts.
13. Developmental considerations.
    a. Teach children early to foster independence with wheelchair mobility in their environment.
    b. Discourage use of strollers that prevent child from independent propulsion.

Chapter 16

Seating and Positioning Systems

Definition

1. The primary unit that properly positions and correctly aligns the trunk and extremities.

Goals

1. Enhance posture.
2. Provide stability, control, and comfort.
3. Promote proximal stability.
4. Allow for pressure distribution and support.
5. Decrease the risk of muscle contracture, deformity, and decubiti.
6. Increase sitting tolerance and energy level.
7. Allow visual readiness and use of the upper extremities during activities.
8. Increase function and enable participation.

Assessment Considerations

1. It is crucial to distinguish between flexible deformity (i.e., where the occupational therapist can manually correct the position), and fixed abnormal postures and deformities (i.e., where changes cannot occur).
2. The pelvis should be evaluated first, and then LEs, trunk, UEs, head and neck, and feet as stability is required prior to mobility and proximal control allows for better distal function.

Basic Styles of Seating

1. Linear.
   a. Flat, non-contoured.
   b. Custom or factory-ordered.
   c. Firm, rigid seating.
   d. Good for active individuals, those who perform independent transfers, and/or those with minimal musculoskeletal involvement.
2. Contoured and/or custom-contoured.
   a. Ergonomically supports the individual.
   b. Provides excellent support.
   c. Enhances postural alignment.
   d. Decreases abnormal posturing.
   e. Provides pressure relief.
   f. May be difficult for independent transfers if decreased UE muscle strength.
   g. Good for individuals with moderate to severe central nervous system dysfunction or neurological disease.

Major Styles and Accessories of Seating Systems

1. Solid wood insert prevents hammock effect; provides solid base of support.
2. Solid seat prevents hammock effect; provides stable base of support; easy to remove.
3. Lumbar back support helps to give proper lumbar curve.
4. Foam cushions (of various densities) can enhance sitting posture and comfort.
5. Contoured foam cushion enhances pelvic and LE alignment.
6. Pressure relief cushions.
   a. Fluid.
      (1) Facilitates pelvic and LE alignment.
      (2) Provides pressure relief without changing support.
      (3) Good for individuals who need increased stability.
   b. Air.
      (1) Minimal postural support offered.
      (2) Provides pressure relief.
      (3) Good trunk control is needed.
7. Wedge cushions or antithrust seats have a front that is higher than the back to prevent the individual from sliding out of their seat.
8. Pelvic guides inserted on the interior sides of the wheelchair at hip level keep hips stable.
9. Lateral supports extend up the side of the chair to just below person's armpits to provide trunk support.

Pediatric Seating and Positioning Systems

1. Purposes.
   a. Accommodate for contractures and deformities.
   b. Enable function in home, school, and community settings.
   c. Facilitate eye contact and parent/teacher/sibling/peer interactions.
   d. Attain general positioning goals as previously stated.
2. Types.
   a. Usually custom molded created systems.
   b. Standers provide weight bearing experience which maintains hips, knees, ankles and trunk in optimal position, facilitate formation of acetabulum and long bone development, and aid in bowel and bladder function.
      (1) Prone standers decrease effect of tonic labyrinthine reflex (TLR).
      (2) Supine standers provide more support posteriorly.
   c. Sidelyers decrease effects of TLR and put hands in visual field.
   d. Triwall construction for infants and toddlers.
   e. Abductor pads at hips decrease scissoring extensor pattern.

Mobility and Mobility Aids

Overview

1. Functional mobility involves "moving from one position or place to another (during performance of everyday activities), such as in-bed mobility, wheelchair mobility, and transfers (e.g., wheelchair, bed, car, tub, toilet, tub/shower, chair, floor). Includes functional ambulation and transporting objects" (AOTA, 2008, p. 631).
2. Functional mobility is needed to perform ADL, IADL, work, education, leisure, and social participation tasks and activities.
3. Evaluation includes a full client factor and performance skill assessment to determine potential ability to perform mobility (including sensation, perceptual, neuromuscular, musculoskeletal, cognitive, and psychosocial areas).

Functional Mobility Aids

1. Ambulation aids.
   a. Orthotic devices (sometimes referred to as braces) are used to prevent contractures and provide stability to joints involved.
      (1) AFO: ankle-foot orthosis.
      (2) KAFO: knee-ankle-foot orthosis.
      (3) HKAFO: hip-knee-ankle-foot orthosis.
   b. Canes.
      (1) Straight: one leg.
      (2) Wide-based quad cane (WBQC): one shaft is connected to a four-pronged base to increase stability when a person is not able to balance on a straight cane.
      (3) Narrow-based quad cane (NBQC): same premise as WBQC, but prongs are situated closer together for a client who may not require as much support.
   c. Walkers.
      (1) Standard: requires the person to have fair balance and the ability to lift device with upper extremities to advance.
      (2) Hemi-walker: for those who do not have the ability to use two hands.
      (3) Side-stepper: a walker situated on a non-affected side of a person.
      (4) Rolling walker: for those who cannot lift a standard walker due to upper extremity weakness or impaired balance.
      (5) Three-wheeled walker: large pneumatic wheels, hand brakes, and a fold-down seat for those who need increased stability and/or fatigue easily.
      (6) Walker bags, trays and baskets are used to assist in transporting personal items.
   d. Crutches.
      (1) Standard: situated in person's axillary region to allow ambulation.
      (2) Platform: forearms are neutral and are supported and hands are in neutral position.
      (3) Lofstrand: proximal arm has closure around it instead of support in axillary region.
   e. Slings provide support to an upper extremity which may have fractured and prevent poor handling of flaccid upper extremity.
2. Wheelchairs and wheelchair training: see information previously provided in this chapter.
3. Scooters provide mobility to those who are not able to ambulate for distances.
4. Sliding boards allow independent transfers from different surfaces for those who are not able to stand-pivot.
5. Upper extremity mobility aids for task performance (e.g., mobile arm support).

Bed Mobility

1. Rolling, bridging, sidelying, supine, and sitting.
2. Some diagnoses require special positioning in bed to:
   a. Maintain alignment of vulnerable joints.
   b. Provide variation in postures.
   c. Decrease the effect of pathological reflex activity.
   d. Provide variations in ranges of motion.
   e. Provide stretch to muscles prone to contracture.
   f. Increase comfort.
   g. Include supine as well as right and left side positioning.
3. Specific mobility/positioning techniques.
   a. Status-post total hip replacement.
      (1) May not be permitted to roll on the non-operated side. This may result in internal rotation of the operated hip, which may cause dislocation.
      (2) May require use of abductor pillow between lower extremities to prevent adduction of the operated hip.
   b. Status-post CVA.
      (1) May need education regarding proper positioning of upper extremity to increase awareness, minimize pain, decrease swelling, and promote normalization of tone.
      (2) May also require use of pillows between knees while in sidelying to increase comfort and promote proper positioning.
   c. Status-post amputation of the lower extremity.
      (1) May require training regarding use of pillows to prevent edema in the lower extremity.
      (2) May also need training on how to provide passive stretching to residual limb while in bed to prevent shortening or contracture, which would make prosthetic training difficult and painful.
4. Bed mobility aids.
   a. Hospital beds, usually with bedrails and elevating head and foot surfaces to increase safety and comfort.
      (1) Bedrails can assist with rolling, positioning for sleep, and assuming to a short-legged seated position.
   b. Overhead trapeze frame,attached to bed to assist with rolling over and assuming to a long-legged seated position.
   c. Rope ladders to assist in pulling to a seated position.
   d. Hoyer lift/trans-aid, a hammock device that is attached to either hydraulic or manual lift systems to transfer individuals who are dependent.
   e. Bedpans and urinals to decrease need to leave bed.

Transfers

Purpose

1. To move from one surface to another safely and effectively with (dependent) or without (independent) the assistance of others.

Transfer Considerations

1. Assess and identify an individual's assets and deficits, especially cognitive and physical abilities.
2. The occupational therapist should be aware of his or her own limitations to avoid personal or consumer injury.
3. Use of proper body mechanics should be strictly enforced.
   a. Use broad base of support.
   b. The therapist must know where his/her center of gravity is at all times.
   c. Individual to be transferred should be lifted with the therapist using his/her lower extremities to lift and not his/her back.
4. Perform wheelchair transfers safely.
   a. Clear areas involved in transfers of any clutter.
   b. Ask for help or standby assist if questioning ability to transfer safely.
   c. Use transfer belts if needed.
   d. Stabilize/lock brakes.
   e. Swing away legrests and flip up footplates.
   f. Remove armrest if individual is unable to assist, is too heavy to bring to a standing position, or if the individual has a weight bearing precaution.
5. Allow for variability of individuals and environment.
   a. Adjust transfer methods according to the individual's strengths and limitations regarding performance components/skills and client factors.
   b. Be aware of different floor/ground surfaces.
   c. Be aware of the increased risk of personal injury when transferring a bariatric client.
      (1) Use good body mechanics, obtain adequate assistance during transfers, and use mechanical lifts.
6. Train in transfers to and from a variety of different surfaces (i.e., bed, wheelchair, chair, toilet, tub, and/or car).

Transfer Types

1. Stand-pivot: individual stands and turns to transfer surface.
2. Pop-over or seated sitting: a full stand position is not required and is used for those with decreased endurance and/or weight-bearing precautions.
3. Sliding (transfer) board for those who are not able to stand to transfer (i.e., individuals with spinal cord injuries or amputations).
   a. Board is placed under individual's gluteal region during a weight shift, while the other end of board is placed on surface being transferred to.
   b. Individual then uses upper extremities to push buttocks up and "slide" over to transfer surface.
   c. If the individual uses a tenodesis grasp or splint for functional activities, the person should weight bear on clenched fists with wrists extended.
4. Dependent: caregiver is required to fully perform the transfer.
5. Mechanical lift: use of ceiling lift, track lift, Hoyer lift or trans-aid.
6. Use of adaptive or mobility devices.
   a. Bed transfer aids.
      (1) Trapeze.
      (2) Bedrail.
   b. Bath transfer aids.
      (1) Grab bars.
      (2) Active-aid commode, a commode with small wheels to allow transfer to bathroom and shower stall when otherwise not possible.
      (3) Bedside or 3-in-1 commode.
      (4) Ambulatory devices (i.e., canes, walkers).
      (5) Wheelchairs (i.e., removable arms, swing arms, leg rests).
7. Chair lifts: chairs with power control to allow elevation from surface for individuals who may otherwise not be able to transfer independently.

Assistive Technology Devices (ATDs)/Electronic Aids to Daily Living (EADLs)

Assistive Technology Devices (ATDs)

1. Definition: "...any piece of equipment or product... used to increase, maintain, and improve functional capabilities of individuals with disabilities..." (Bain, 1998, p. 466).
2. An expansion of adaptive equipment.
3. Assistive devices for the environment may be considered "high tech" or "low tech."
   a. High tech: costly devices that may require custom ordering and may require specific training to use (e.g., environmental control units [ECUs], augmentative and alternative communication [AAC] devices, computers).
   b. Low tech: inexpensive household and/or catalog items that are readily available for use, (e.g., jar opener, shoehorn, and sock aid).
   c. Some components of high tech devices (e.g., ECUs) can be fabricated in a cost-effective manner using inexpensive commercially available microswitch technology (e.g., simple switches to turn on and off lights, appliances, and other electronic equipment).

Electronic Aids to Daily Living (EADLs)

1. Definition: EADLs were formerly known as environmental control units (ECUs) and are a "...means to purposefully manipulate and interact with the environment by alternately accessing one or more electrical devices via switch, voice activation, remote control, computer interface..." (Bain, 1998, p. 469).
2. Purposes.
   a. Enable control of devices within the environment.
   b. Compensate for functional limitations and maximize functional abilities.
   c. Increase independence in home, school, work, and other environments.
   d. Conserve energy during home management and work tasks.
3. Uses.
   a. Turn on/off lights, control appliances, open and close doors/drapes.
   b. Allow use of phones and office machinery.
   c. Summon assistance.
4. Considerations in device selection.
   a. Input method: selection requires knowledge of the distance of throughput/transmission.
   b. Output method.
   c. Portability.
   d. Safety.
   e. Reliability.
   f. Durability.
   g. Assembly ease.
   h. Operation ease.
   i. Maintenance schedule.
   j. Current and future affordability.
5. Types of EADL technology.
   a. Phones: large number pads, automatic dialing phones, speaker-phones, amplifiers, videophones, smart phone applications.
   b. Monitoring systems allow for communication between areas.
   c. Personal emergency response system (PERS): enables a client to summon help by the push of a button or the vocalization of a command.
   d. Electronically controlled door openers and closers.
   e. Computers enable individuals with disabilities to more fully participate in social, leisure, work, and productive activities. They:
      (1) Facilitate performance of multiple functional tasks (e.g., banking, shopping).
      (2) Allow for communication and socialization through e-mail and Internet support groups.
      (3) Provide the means for productive work via telecommuting.
      (4) Have alternative access modes that can compensate for a diversity of disabilities. Adaptations can include:
         (a) Eye gaze for individuals with severe mobility and speech impairments (e.g., individuals with amyotrophic lateral sclerosis).
         (b) Voice activation for individuals with severe mobility impairments with functional speech (e.g., upper extremity contractures).
         (c) Programmable keyboards that allow for customized overlays (e.g., enlarged letters and numbers for persons with low vision; graphics and symbols for individuals with cognitive impairments).
         (d) Expanded keyboards that provide large keys for persons with visual-motor deficits.
         (e) Key guards for persons with limited motor accuracy and control (e.g., individuals with ataxia).

(f) Contracted keyboards that provide smaller keys in a constrained space for persons with limited range of motion and functional motor control (e.g., individuals with arthritis).
(g) Light-touch keyboard activation systems for persons with decreased strength and/or mobility (e.g., individuals with muscular dystrophy).
(h) Delayed touch keyboard activation systems for persons with poor motor control (e.g., individuals with athetoid movements).
(i) Chorded keyboards that consist of a few keys which generate standard characters by pressing various combinations of keys for persons with one-handed use (e.g., individuals with hemiplegia).
(j) Tongue-touch keypad (TTK) imbedded in an orthotic device for persons with severe motor deficits and good tongue control.

f. Augmentative alternative communication (AAC): methods of communication that do not require speech. Need to consider:
(1) Speed at which message is conveyed.
(2) Portability: easy to use in a variety of environmental settings.
(3) Accessibility: ability of individual to independently operate.
(4) Dependability: quality, durability, and warranty/service record.
(5) Independence of user.
(6) Vocabulary flexibility.
(7) Time for repairs and maintenance.
(8) Types range from simple communication boards or albums with a limited number of pictures to complex portable computer systems with extensive language capacity.

Evaluation and Intervention

1. Evaluation focus.
a. Identify the activities the individual wants to engage in and the occupational roles the person wants to pursue.
b. Determine the person's values about the use of AT.
c. Assess the individual's abilities and deficits, including client factors and performance skills.
(1) Stability of positioning and seating must be assessed as this will affect ability to use device.
(2) The anatomic site at which the person demonstrates purposeful controlled movement must be determined as this will influence device's control site (e.g., device activated by shoulder, head, elbow, hand, tongue, or eye movements).
(a) If no physical interaction with an input is possible, the ability to use speech to use voice recognition AT should be assessed.
d. Determine the environments in which the device will be used and when it will be used.
e. Identify potential assistive technology devices.
(1) Consider input method; how the device will be activated (e.g., infrared, sonic, electric, or radio frequency switches) and by what action (e.g., voice recognition, eye gazing, using a joystick, head pointer, mouthstick, or tongue).
(2) Consider the processing method; how the device will process the information from the input method.
(3) Consider the output method; results are needed (response from input occurs).
(4) Consider the feedback method; ensures the device is being used in the right way (could be auditory, visual, or proprioceptive).

2. Intervention principles.
a. Select and use several devices on a trial basis to determine what serves the individual's needs best.
b. Determine the specific device, after reviewing and incorporating all of the team members' information.
c. Keep devices as simple as possible.
d. If device is stationary, ensure that it is positioned to enable ease of access.
e. Provide multiple training sessions.

3. Documentation.
a. Document the evaluation process.
b. Document recommended ATD(s) selected and the rationale for each item for reimbursement justification.
(1) Based on individual's needs and goals.
(2) Based on functional status, abilities, and limitations.
(3) Based on school/work/leisure status and needs.
(4) Justify cost-effectiveness of recommended equipment.

4. Re-evaluation guidelines.
a. Assess for change in status of the individual with a disability.
b. Determine efficiency and efficacy of use of assistive devices.
c. Check parts of the device for durability.

Additional Considerations for ATDs and EADLs

1. The appliances and electrical cords to be used with ATDs and EADLs must be determined.
2. Charging instructions must be followed, as some have strict schedules.

3. The technological and computer abilities of an individual with a disability should be determined.
4. Surge protectors must be used to avoid blown circuits.
5. Back-up systems for electrical high-tech devices should be established. ✓
6. Instruction must be provided to the individual to ensure carry-over when OT and/or other supports are not present. ✓
7. Warranty information should be obtained and the consumer educated about these terms and conditions.

Funding for ATDs and EADLs

1. State Vocational and Educational Services for Individuals with Disabilities (VESID), Offices for Vocational Rehabilitation (OVRs), and Divisions of Vocational Rehabilitation (DVRs) will pay for ATDs and EADLs, if they enable a person to go to work or school.
2. Private companies may fund ATDs and EADLs to ensure ADA compliance.
3. Private insurance, Medicare, Medicaid and Worker's Compensation mayreimburse for certain devices.

Community Mobility

Overview

1. Community mobility is the ability to move around one's community to engage in desired occupations and pursue meaningful activities.
2. Community mobility includes the ability to access and use public and/or private transportation systems; i.e., buses, subways, trains, taxi cabs or other community-based transportation systems.
 a. Transportation systems specifically developed to meet the community mobility needs of persons with disabilities are typically called "paratransit."
3. Community mobility also includes the ability to drive, walk, and/or bicycle.

Driver Rehabilitation

1. Driving is defined as an instrumental activity of living.
2. Purposes.
 a. Provide mobility within one's community.
 b. Allow for autonomy for self-directed activity pursuit.
 c. Enable engagement in life roles including vocational, social, and familial role activities.
3. Physical, cognitive, psychiatric, and developmental disabilities can affect the ability to drive safely and effectively.
4. Driver rehabilitation requires extensive on-the-road training and behind the wheel driving in a diversity of driving environments.
 a. Knowledge of general state driving regulations and statutes specifically related to individuals with disabilities must be acquired prior to initiating a driver rehabilitation program. ✱

 b. An occupational therapist who performs on-the-road driver training must become a state licensed driving instructor.
 c. Occupational therapists who practice driver rehabilitation should become certified driving rehabilitation specialists.

Evaluation of Driver Ability

1. Clinical screening of performance skills, prerequisite abilities, and client factors.
 a. Visual-perceptual: intact acuity, night vision, contrast sensitivity, peripheral field, scanning, spatial relations, and depth perception are needed to access essential visual input and to accurately interpret the driving environment.
 (1) Color recognition is not a state mandated requirement as color blindness can be readily compensated for while driving.
 b. Cognitive-perceptual: intact orientation, alertness, memory, ability to shift attention, problem solving, response time, topographical orientation, sign recognition, and knowledge of "rules of the road" are required to drive safely and appropriately for different driving conditions, and to anticipate the actions of other drivers on the road and the consequences of one's own actions.
 c. Motor: adequate range of motion, strength, endurance, and response time are needed for basic vehicle control including accurate steering to remain in lane and make turns, and for smooth acceleration and braking.
 d. Psychosocial: the presence of impulsive and/or agitated behaviors, and/or psychiatric symptoms such as, suicidal intentions, delusions, and hallucinations can affect an individual's ability to drive safely.

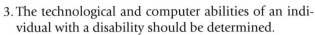

e. Side-effects of medications can affect motor performance, alertness, attention, judgment, and reaction time.
f. Past driving experiences (which can range from none, to poor, to competent) can influence the individual's potential to drive with a disability.
g. Occupational therapists can perform clinical screenings for all of the above factors that can affect driving without additional specialized training.
(1) If screening identifies areas requiring further evaluation, the occupational therapist should refer the individual to a driving rehabilitation specialist.

2. On-the-road evaluation: there are two levels of driving that must be considered when evaluating a person's abilities when they are behind the wheel and actually driving. These are:
a. Operation: the ability to steer, brake, and turn.
b. Tactical: the ability to respond to changes in road conditions and traffic/driving risks.
3. The ergonomics of driving should also be assessed to increase safety and prevent discomfort. Considerations include:
a. Seat position in relation to visibility of car's endpoints.
b. Positioning of seatbelt and shoulder restraint.
c. Access to foot pedals and/or steering column controls.
d. Airbag clearance of 12 inches between the person and the steering wheel in case of airbag deployment.
4. The person's ability to manage automotive emergencies (e.g., a breakdown) and obtain assistance should also be assessed.

Interventions for Driver Rehabilitation

1. Adaptive driving equipment can be prescribed for individuals with specific limitations.
a. Hand controls can replace accelerators and brake foot pedals.
b. Steering knobs for one-handed steering control can include a:
(1) Standard round spinning knob for a person with one intact upper extremity.
(2) Ring to accommodate a prosthesis.
(3) Tri-pin or cuff to accommodate absent or weak grasp.
c. Pedal extensions can be added if feet do not reach standard foot pedals.
d. Zero effort or reduced effort steering can accommodate for decreased range, strength, and endurance.
e. Steering wheel positioning adjustments can place the steering wheel in atypical positions to allow for access.
2. If, and when, a person is determined to be unsafe or unable to drive, alternatives to maintain community mobility must be explored and implemented (i.e., public transportation, walking).
a. Support must be provided to the individual to deal with this loss and its ramifications on the person's daily life.
b. Interventions to ensure safety as a public transit user and pedestrian are required.

Funding for Driver Rehabilitation

1. State Vocational and Educational Services for Individuals with Disabilities (VESID), Offices for Vocational Rehabilitation (OVRs), and Divisions of Vocational Rehabilitation (DVRs) will pay for driver rehabilitation if it will enable a person to go to work or school.
2. Private insurance, Medicare, Medicaid, and Worker's Compensation may reimburse for certain driver rehabilitation devices/adaptations.

Environmental Modifications for Cognitive and Sensory Deficits

General Interventions

1. The environment needs to be familiar, consistent, and predictable.
a. Provide structure in the environment to increase orientation to time, place, person, and situation.
b. Remove clutter to decrease extraneous stimuli when an individual is easily distracted or has limited vision.
c. Provide visual reminders or tactile cues to decrease confusion, increase awareness, and facilitate independence (e.g., written directions, Braille labels).
d. Keep things in the same place for consistency and ease.
2. Use contrasting colors to discriminate background from foreground or figures from background.
3. Use restraint reduction techniques if a person is confused, agitated, and/or a wanderer.

4. Educate consumer, caregiver, and family.
   a. Train caregivers for persons with memory and/or sensory impairments on effective communication techniques.
   b. Facilitate carry-over of intervention techniques in the modified environment.
   c. Increase awareness of potential resources available to the individual and his/her family.
   d. Increase awareness of his/her rights to access these resources.
5. Monitor changes and adjustment after a disability to assess carry-over of information.
6. Make home modifications to ensure safety as needed.
   a. Remove potential hazards such as cleaning solutions, medications, sharp objects, matches, stove knobs, and firearms if a person is confused or forgetful.
   b. Follow modifications identified earlier in this chapter for the prevention of falls.
   c. Refer to Chapter 5 for additional modifications for sensory loss.
7. Provide a personal emergency system and train in its use.

Restraint Reduction

1. Assessment of behaviors that result in agitation, restlessness, and/or wandering.
   a. Pain, physical discomfort.
   b. Hunger, thirst, need for toileting.
   c. Loneliness, fear.
   d. Boredom.
   e. Unfamiliar environment.
2. Intervention to address contributing factors/correct underlying problems.
   a. Referral to physician for medical evaluation/pain management.
   b. Proper positioning.
   c. Provision of snacks, unbreakable water bottles, or other appropriate safe source of nourishment and hydration.
   d. Adequate and client-directed toileting routine.
   e. Active listening; attention to underlying feelings and expressed concerns to promote trust.
   f. Family, peer, and/or pastoral visits.
   g. Animal-assisted or pet therapy.
   h. Social and leisure activities.
   i. Exercise and/or other outlets for restless, anxious behavior.
   j. Night-time activities.
   k. Eliminate loudspeaker and other extraneous noise; provide soothing background music.
   l. Inclusion of familiar and favorite objects in person's living space to personalize it.
   m. Provide a structured home-like environment with a set routine to promote sense of safety and security.
3. Interventions to address agitation and/or wandering incidents.
   a. Approach from person's front at his/her eye level.
   b. Communicate calmly with the use of simple statements/instructions.
   c. Distract with an activity or topic of interest to the person.
   d. Re-direct back to desired location.
   e. Engage in an activity of interest or diversion.
   f. Camouflage doors, exits, and elevators with full-length mirrors, stop or no-crossing signs, wallpaper, and/or vertical blinds.
   g. Put tape on floors or planters to mark end of hall.
   h. Install locks or Velcro doors.
   i. Use door alarms, personal alarms, or monitoring devices.
   j. Make contained areas interesting and safe.
   k. Rearrange furniture to deter wandering.
   l. Provide a variety of comfortable seating and furniture including broad-based rockers and footstools.

References

American National Standards Institute. (1992). *Accessible and usable buildings and facilities*. New York: Author.

American Occupational Therapy Association. (2010). Driving and community mobility. *American Journal of Occupational Therapy, 64*(6, Supplement), S112–S124.

American Occupational Therapy Association. (2008). Occupational therapy practice framework: Domain and process, 2nd ed. *American Journal of Occupational Therapy, 62*, 625–688.

American Occupational Therapy Association. (2010). Specialized knowledge and skills in technology and environmental interventions for occupational therapy practice. *American Journal of Occupational Therapy, 64*(6, Supplement), S44–S56.

Bain, B. (1998). Assistive technology. In G. Gillen & A. Burkhardt (Eds.), *Stroke rehabilitation: A function based approach* (pp. 465–478). St. Louis, MO: Mosby.

Bain, B., & Leger, D. (1997). *Assistive technology: An interdisciplinary approach.* New York: Churchill Livingstone.

Bolding, D., Adler, C., Tipton-Burton, M., & Lillie, S. (2007). Mobility. In H. McHugh Pendleton & W. Schultz-Krohn

Chapter 16

(Eds.), *Pedretti's occupational therapy: Practice skills for physical dysfunction*, 6th ed. (pp. 195–247.). St. Louis, MO: Mosby.
Buning, M. E. (2008). High-technology adaptations to compensate for disability. In M.V. Radomski & C.A. Trombly Latham (Eds.), *Occupational therapy for physical dysfunction*, 6th ed. (pp. 510–541). Philadelphia: Lippincott Williams & Wilkins.
Case-Smith, J. (Ed.). (2005). *Occupational therapy for children*, 5th ed. St. Louis, MO: Elsevier Mosby.
Dudgeon, B., & Deitz , J. C. (2008). Wheelchair selection. In M. V. Radomski & C. A. Trombly Latham (Eds.), *Occupational therapy for physical dysfunction*, 6th ed. (pp. 487–509). Baltimore: Williams & Wilkins.
Foti, D., & Kanazawa, L. (2006). Activities of daily living. In H. McHugh Pendleton & W. Schultz-Krohn (Eds.). *Pedretti's occupational therapy: Practice skills for physical dysfunction*, 6th ed. (pp. 146–194). St. Louis, MO: Mosby.
Gourley, M. (2002, March 25). Driver rehabilitation. *OT Practice*, 15–20.
Johann, C. (1998). Seating and wheeled mobility prescription. In G. Gillen & A. Burkhardt (Eds.), *Stroke rehabilitation: A function based approach* (pp. 437–451). St. Louis, MO: Mosby.
Kane, L., & Buckley, K. (1998). Functional mobility. In G. Gillen & A. Burkhardt (Eds.), *Stroke rehabilitation: A function based approach* (pp. 305–242). St. Louis, MO: Mosby.
Lange, M. L. (2001, July 2). Alternative keyboards. *OT Practice*, 19–20.
Lange, M. L. (2001, Aug. 6). EADLs and aging clients. *OT Practice*, 16–18.
Lange, M. L. (2001, Aug. 6). EADLs in the school setting. *OT Practice*, 17–18.
Larson, K., Stevens-Ratchford, Pedretti, L., & Crabtree, J. (1996). *ROTE: The role of occupational therapy with the elderly*, 2nd ed. Bethesda, MD: American Occupational Therapy Association.
Mosey, A. C. (1996). *Psychosocial components of occupational therapy*. New York: Raven Press.
Moyers, P., & Dale, L. (2007). *The guide to occupational therapy practice*. Bethesda, MD: American Occupational Therapy Association.
Oliver, R., Blathwayt, J., Brackley, C., & Tamaki, T. (1993). Development of the Safety Assessment of Function and the Environment for Rehabilitation (SAFER) tool. *Canadian Journal of Occupational Therapy, 60*, 70–82.
O'Toole, M. (Ed.). (1997). *Miller-Keane encyclopedia and dictionary of medicine, nursing, and allied health*, 6th ed. Philadelphia: W. B. Saunders.
Pedretti, L. (1990). Activities of daily living. In L. Pedretti & B. Zoltan (Eds.), *Occupational therapy: Practice skills for physical dysfunction*, 3rd ed. (pp. 230–271). St. Louis, MO: Mosby.
Peterson, E. W., & Murphy, S. (2002). Fear of falling: Part II - Assessment and intervention. *Home and Community Health Special Interest Section Quarterly, 9*(1),1, 2, 4.
Pierce, S. L. (2008). Restoring mobility. In M.V. Radomski & C.A. Trombly Latham (Eds.), *Occupational therapy for physical dysfunction*, 6th ed. (pp. 817–853). Philadelphia: Lippincott Williams & Wilkins.
Radomski, M. V. (2008). Assessing context: Personal, social, and cultural. In M.V. Radomski & C.A Trombly Latham (Eds.), *Occupational therapy for physical dysfunction*, 6th ed. (pp. 284–309). Philadelphia: Lippincott Williams & Wilkins.
Rigby, P., Lowe M., & Stewart, D. (2008). Assessing environment, home, community, and workplace access. In M.V. Radomski & C.A. Trombly Latham (Eds.). *Occupational therapy for physical dysfunction*, 6th ed. (pp. 310–337). Philadelphia: Lippincott Williams & Wilkins.
Sabata, D. B., Shamberg, S., & Williams, M. (2008). Optimizing access to home, community, and work environments. In M. V. Radomski & C. A. Trombly Latham (Eds.). *Occupational therapy for physical dysfunction*, 6th ed. (pp. 951–973). Philadelphia: Lippincott Williams & Wilkins.
Salerno, C. (1998). Home evaluation and modification. In G. Gillen & A. Burkhardt (Eds.). *Stroke rehabilitation: A function based approach* (pp. 452–464). St. Louis, MO: Mosby.
Schell, B., Gillen, G., & Scaffa, M. (Eds). (2013). *Willard and Spackman's occupational therapy*, 12th ed. Philadelphia: Lippincott Williams & Wilkins
Sladyk, K., Jacobs. K., & MacRae, N. (2010). *Occupational therapy essentials for clinical competence*. Thorofare, NJ: Slack.
Spencer, E. (1998). Functional restoration: Preliminary concepts and planning. In H. Hopkins & H. Smith (Eds.). *Willard and Spackman's occupational therapy*, 7th ed. (pp. 435–460). Philadelphia: Lippincott Company.
Stav, W., Pierce, S., Wheatley, C., & Schold Davis, E. (2005). Driving and community mobility. *American Journal of Occupational Therapy 59*, 666–670.
Tinetti, M. E., Richman, D., & Powell, L. (1990). Falls efficacy as a measure of fear of falling. *Journal of Gerontology, 45*(6), 239–243.
Walls, B. S. (1999, December 6). A dangerous secret: I had a fall. *OT Practice*, 12–16.
West Virginia Research and Training Center. (1990). *ADA - The Americans with Disabilities Act of 1990 PL 101–336, Volume I - The Law*. Dunbar, WV: Author.
Wheatley, C. J. (2001, July 16). Shifting into drive: Evaluating potential drivers with disabilities. *OT Practice*, 12–15.

Review Questions

Mastery of the Environment: Evaluation and Intervention

Below are five questions about key content covered in this chapter. These questions are not inclusive of the entirety of content on occupational therapy evaluation and intervention related to mastery of the environment that you must know for success on the NBCOT exam. These questions are provided to help you "jump start" the thought processes you will need to apply your studying of content to the answering of exam questions; hence they are not in the NBCOT exam format. Exam items in the NBCOT format which cover the depth and breadth of content you will need to know to pass the NBCOT exam are provided on this text's disc. The answers to the below questions are provided in Appendix 4.

1. An occupational therapist provides consultation services to a group of religious organizations who want to improve the accessibility of the entrances to their buildings. All entrances currently have stairs. What should the occupational therapist recommend to allow access for persons who use mobility aides (e.g., walkers and canes) and wheelchairs?

2. An occupational therapist provides a weekly home safety group to members of a senior center. What strategies should the therapist recommend the group members use inside and outside their homes to prevent falls?

3. A client is status-post posterolateral hip replacement surgery. What recommendations should the therapist make for bed mobility?

4. A school-based occupational therapist provides recommendations for alternative access modes to computers to compensate for a diversity of disabilities and maximize students' independence in the school environment. What adaptations can the therapist recommend? Explain their use.

5. An occupational therapist begins employment at a new skilled nursing facility (SNF). To ensure compliance with OBRA and reduce the use of restraints in the facility, what policies and procedures should the therapist have the SNF administrators implement?

EPILOGUE

Professional Development After Initial Certification

RITA P. FLEMING-CASTALDY

Successfully passing the NBCOT® examination for the occupational therapist enables you to meet an essential criterion for initial certification as an occupational therapist. The regulatory boards of all 50 states in the United States (US), the District of Columbia, and the US territories of Guam and Puerto Rico require a passing NBCOT® examination score to legally practice as an occupational therapist in their resepective jurisdictions. Passing the NBCOT® examination also enables you to use the designation of registered (OTR®) if you choose to participate in the NBCOT® certification program. Thus, your success on this high-stakes examination can mark the beginning of a rewarding and fulfilling professional career. This concept of beginning is a critical one for you to embrace. While the pursuit of the goal to become an occupational therapist may end with professional licensure and/or NBCOT® certification, it is at this point that the life-long process of being a professional has just begun.

> Being a member of a profession requires an ongoing commitment to the attainment and maintenance of excellence. Competent occupational therapists value this pursuit of excellence and are personally responsible for this professional development. . . . The benefits of a life-long commitment to one's professional development are numerous. Increased personal pride and satisfaction in one's work; improved health care services for consumers and their families; enhanced professional image among policy makers, reimbursers, administrators, and the multidisciplinary team; and the prevention of burnout and professional stagnation are all viable outcomes of the continual pursuit of professional excellence (Cottrell, 2000, p.465).

Numerous professional development resources are available to facilitate your growth from entry-level novice to master practitioner. Clinical supervision, peer support, networking, professional associations, mentorships, self-study, inservices, workshops, conferences, and post-professional education can all be used to attain and maintain professional mastery and excellence. The advent of the technological era has increased the availability and decreased the cost of many professional development activities through the use of e-mail, chat rooms, and distance learning. I strongly urge you to take advantage of both high-tech (e.g., video conferencing) and low-tech (e.g., brainstorming with a colleague over a practice dilemma) learning opportunities early and often in your professional life. I also highly recommend that you become an active member in the American Occupational Therapy Association and your state association (and/or the local district in a large state). These actions will immediately provide you with access to a network of OT practitioners and leaders in the field who are proactive forces for professional advancement and role models for excellence. Moreover, the AOTA website at www.aota.org has countless resources available to members to ensure they provide evidence-based and occupation-based practice. See Appendix 3 for State Association contact information.

As Yerxa (1985) noted, an authentic professional is one who recognizes his/her responsibility to be a life-long student. I wish you well at the beginning of this journey, the journey to learn and pursue an authentic occupational therapy career. I can think of no better way to practice or live.

References

American Occupational Therapy Association Continuing Competency Task Force (1999). *Professional development for continuing competency*. Bethesda, MD: AOTA.

Cottrell, R. P. (2000). Professional development: The attainment, maintenance and promotion of excellence. In R. P. Cottrell (Ed.), *Proactive approaches in psychosocial occupational therapy*, (pp. 465–468). Thorofare, NJ: Slack.

Yerxa, E. (1966). Authentic occupational therapy. *American Journal of Occupational Therapy, 21*, 1–9.

APPENDIX 1

The Practice Framework

Areas of Occupation

Various kinds of life activities in which people, populations, or organizations engage, including ADL, IADL, rest and sleep, education, work, play, leisure, and social participation.

Activities of Daily Living (ADL)—activities that are oriented toward taking care of one's own body (adapted from Rogers & Holm, 1994, pp. 181–202). ADL also is referred to as *basic activities of daily living (BADLs)* and *personal activities of daily living (PADLs)*. These activities are "fundamental to living in a social world; they enable basic survival and well-being" (Christiansen & Hammecker, 2001, p. 156).

- **Bathing, showering**—Obtaining and using supplies; soaping, rinsing, and drying body parts; maintaining bathing position; and transferring to and from bathing positions.
- **Bowel and bladder management**—Includes completing intentional control of bowel movements and urinary bladder and, if necessary, using equipment or agents for bladder control (Uniform Data System for Medical Rehabilitation, 1996, pp. III-20, III-24).
- **Dressing**—Selecting clothing and accessories appropriate to time of day, weather, and occasion; obtaining clothing from storage area; dressing and undressing in a sequential fashion; fastening and adjusting clothing and shoes; and applying and removing personal devices, prostheses, or orthoses.
- **Eating**—"The ability to keep and manipulate food or fluid in the mouth and swallow it; *eating* and *swallowing* are often used interchangeably" (AOTA, 2007b).
- **Feeding**—"The process of setting up, arranging, and bringing food [or fluid] from the plate or cup to the mouth; sometimes called self-feeding" (AOTA, 2007b).
- **Functional mobility**—Moving from one position or place to another [during performance of everyday activities], such as in-bed mobility, wheelchair mobility, and transfers (e.g., wheelchair, bed, car, tub, toilet, tub/shower, chair, floor). Includes functional ambulation and transporting objects.
- **Personal device care**—Using, cleaning, and maintaining personal care items, such as hearing aids, contact lenses, glasses, orthotics, prosthetics, adaptive equipment, and contraceptive and sexual devices.
- **Personal hygiene and grooming**—Obtaining and using supplies; removing body hair (e.g., use of razors, tweezers, lotions); applying and removing cosmetics; washing, drying, combing, styling, brushing, and trimming hair, caring for nails (hands and feet); caring for skin, ears, eyes, and nose; applying deodorant; cleaning mouth; brushing and flossing teeth; or removing, cleaning, and reinserting dental orthotics and prosthetics.

- **Sexual activity**—Engagement in activities that result in sexual satisfaction.
- **Toilet hygiene**—Obtaining and using supplies; clothing management; maintaining toileting position; transferring to and from toileting position; cleaning body; and caring for menstrual and continence needs (including catheters, colostomies, and suppository management).

Instrumental Activities of Daily Living (IADLs)—Activities to support daily life within the home and community that often require more complex interactions than self-care used in ADL.

- **Care of others (including selecting and supervising caregivers)**—Arranging, supervising, or providing the care for others.
- **Care of pets**—Arranging, supervising, or providing the care for pets and service animals.
- **Child rearing**—Providing the care and supervision to support the developmental needs of a child.
- **Communication management**—Sending, receiving, and interpreting information using a variety of systems and equipment, including writing tools, telephones, typewriters, audiovisual recorders, computers, communication boards, call lights, emergency systems, Braille writers, telecommunication devices for the deaf, augmentative communication systems, and personal digital assistants.
- **Community mobility**—Moving around in the community and using public or private transportation, such as driving, walking, bicycling, or accessing and riding in buses, taxi cabs, or other transportation systems.
- **Financial management**—Using fiscal resources, including alternate methods of financial transaction and planning and using finances with long-term and short-term goals.
- **Health management and maintenance**—Developing, managing, and maintaining routines for health and wellness promotion, such as physical fitness, nutrition, decreasing health risk behaviors, and medication routines.
- **Home establishment and management**—Obtaining and maintaining personal and household possessions and environment (e.g., home, yard, garden, appliances, vehicles), including maintaining and repairing personal possessions (clothing and household items) and knowing how to seek help or whom to contact.
- **Meal preparation and cleanup**—Planning, preparing, and serving well-balanced, nutritional meals and cleaning up food and utensils after meals.
- **Religious observance**— Participation in religion, "an organized system of beliefs, practices, rituals, and symbols designed to facilitate closeness to the sacred or transcendent" (Moreira-Almeida & Koenig, 2006, p. 844).
- **Safety and emergency maintenance**—Knowing and performing preventive procedures to maintain a safe environment as well as recognizing sudden, unexpected hazardous situations and initialing emergency action to reduce the threat to health and safety.
- **Shopping**—Preparing shopping lists (grocery and other); selecting, purchasing, and transporting items; selecting method of payment; and completing money transactions.

Rest and Sleep—Includes activities related to obtaining restorative rest and sleep that supports healthy active engagement in other areas of occupation.

- **Rest**—Quiet and effortless actions that interrupt physical and mental activity resulting in a relaxed state (Nurit & Michel, 2003, p. 227). Includes identifying the need to relax; reducing involvement in taxing physical, mental or social activities; and engaging in relaxation or other endeavors that restore energy, calm, and renewed interest in engagement.
- **Sleep**—A series of activities resulting in going to sleep, staying asleep, and ensuring health and safety through participation in sleep involving engagement with the physical and social environments.
- **Sleep preparation**—(1) Engaging in routines that prepare the self for a comfortable rest, such as grooming and undressing, reading or listening to music to fall asleep, saying goodnight to others, and meditation or prayers; determining the time of day and length of time desired for sleeping or the time needed to wake; and establishing sleep patterns that support growth and health (patterns are often personally and culturally determined). (2) Preparing the physical environment for periods of unconsciousness, such as making the bed or space on which to sleep; ensuring warmth/coolness and protection; setting an alarm clock; securing the home, such as locking doors or closing windows or curtains; and turning off electronics or lights.
- **Sleep participation**—Taking care of personal need for sleep such as cessation of activities to ensure onset of sleep, napping, dreaming, sustaining a sleep state without disruption, and nighttime care of toileting needs or hydration. Negotiating the needs and requirements of others within the social environment, interacting with those sharing the sleep space such as children or partners, providing nighttime care giving such as breastfeeding, and monitoring the comfort and safety of others such as the family while sleeping.

Education—Includes activities needed for learning and participating in the environment.

- **Formal educational participation**—Including the categories of academic (e.g., math, reading, working on a degree), nonacademic (e.g., recess, lunchroom, hallway), extracurricular (e.g., sports, band, cheerleading, dances), and vocational (pre-vocational and vocational) participation.
- **Informal personal educational needs or interests exploration (beyond formal education)**—Identifying topics and methods for obtaining topic-related information or skills
- **Informal personal education participation**—Participating in classes, programs, and activities that provide instruction/training in identified areas of interest.

Work—Includes activities needed for engaging in remunerative employment or volunteer activities (Mosey, 1996, p. 341).

- **Employment interests and pursuits**—Identifying and selecting work opportunities based on assets, limitations, likes, and dislikes relative to work (adapted from Mosey, 1996 p. 342).
- **Employment seeking and acquisition**—Identifying and recruiting for job opportunities; completing, submitting, and reviewing appropriate application materials; preparing for interviews; participating in interviews and following up afterward; discussing job benefits; and finalizing negotiations.
- **Job performance**—Job performance including work skills and patterns; time management; relationships with co-workers, managers, and customers; creation, production, and distribution of products and services; initiation, sustainment, and completion of work; and compliance with work norms and procedures.
- **Retirement preparation and adjustment**—Determining aptitudes, developing interests and skills, and selecting appropriate avocational pursuits.
- **Volunteer exploration**—Determining community causes, organizations, or opportunities for unpaid "work" in relationship to personal skills, interests, location, and time available.
- **Volunteer participation**—Performing unpaid "work" activities for the benefit of identified selected causes, organizations, or facilities.

Play—"Any spontaneous or organized activity that provides enjoyment, entertainment, amusement, or diversion" (Parham & Fazio, 1997, p. 252).

- **Play exploration**—Identifying appropriate play activities, which can include exploration play, practice play, pretend play, games with rules, constructive play, and symbolic play (adapted from Bergen, 1986, pp. 64–65).
- **Play participation**—Participating in play; maintaining a balance of play with other areas of occupation; and obtaining, using, and maintaining toys, equipment, and supplies appropriately.

Leisure—"A nonobligatory activity that is intrinsically motivated and engaged in during discretionary item, that is, time not committed to obligatory occupations such as work, self-care, or sleep" (Parham & Fazio, 1997, p. 250).

- **Leisure exploration**—identifying interests, skills opportunities, and appropriate leisure activities.
- **Leisure participation**—Planning and participating in appropriate leisure activities; maintaining a balance of leisure activities with other areas of occupation; and obtaining, using, and maintaining equipment and supplies as appropriate.

Social Participation—"Organized patterns of behavior that are characteristic and expected of an individual or a given position within a social system" (Mosey, 1996, p. 340).

- **Community**—Engaging in activities that result in successful interaction at the community level (i.e., neighborhood, organizations, work, school).
- **Family**—Engaging in "[activities that result in] successful interaction in specific required and/or desired familial roles" (Mosey, 1996, p. 340).
- **Peer, friend**—Engaging in activities at different levels of intimacy, including engaging in desired sexual activity.

From *Occupational therapy practice framework: Domain and process,* 2nd ed. (pp.631–633). Copyright by the American Occupational Therapy Association, Inc. Reprinted with permission.

Note. Some of the terms used in this table are from, or adapted from, the rescinded *Uniform Terminology for Occupational Therapy*—Third Edition (AOTA, 1994, pp. 1047–1054).

Client Factors	
Client factors include (1) values, beliefs, and spirituality; (2) body functions; and (3) body structures that reside within the client and may affect performance in areas of occupation.	
VALUES, BELIEFS, AND SPIRITUALITY	
CATEGORY AND DEFINITION	**EXAMPLES**
Values: Principles, standards, or qualities considered worthwhile or desirable by the client who holds them.	**Person** 1. Honesty with self and with others. 2. Personal religious convictions. 3. Commitment to family. **Organization** 1. Obligation to serve the community. 2. Fairness. **Population** 1. Freedom of speech. 2. Equal opportunities for all. 3. Tolerance toward others.
Beliefs: Cognitive content held as true.	**Person** 1. He or she is powerless to influence others. 2. Hard work pays off. **Organization** 1. Profits are more important than people. 2. Achieving the mission of providing service can effect positive change in the world. **Population** 1. People can influence government by voting. 2. Accessibility is a right, not a privilege.
Spiritual: The "personal quest for understanding answers to ultimate questions about life, about meaning, and the sacred" (Moyers & Dale, 2007, p, 28).	**Person** 1. Daily search for purpose and meaning in one's life. 2. Guiding actions from a sense of value beyond the personal acquisition of wealth or fame. **Organization and Population** (See "Person" examples related to individuals within an organization and population.)
BODY FUNCTIONS: "[t]he physiological functions of body systems (including psychological functions)" (WHO, 2001, p. 10). The "Body Functions" section of the table below is organized according to the classifications of the International Classification of Functioning, Disability, and Health (ICF) classifications. For fuller descriptions and definitions, refer to WHO (2001).	
CATEGORIES	**BODY FUNCTIONS COMMONLY CONSIDERED BY OCCUPATIONAL THERAPY PRACTITIONERS (Not intended to be all-inclusive list)**
Mental functions (affective, cognitive, perceptual)	
■ **Specific mental functions**	**Specific mental functions**
• Higher-level cognitive	Judgement, concept formation, metacognition, cognitive flexibility, insight, attention, awareness
• Attention	Sustained, selective, and divided attention
• Memory	Short-term, long-term, and working memory
• Perception	Discrimination of sensations (e.g., auditory, tactile, visual, olfactory, gusfatory, vestibular-proprioception), including multi-sensory processing, sensory memory, spatial, and temporal relationships (Calvert, Spence, & Stein, 2004)

Mental functions (affective, cognitive, perceptual) (continued)	
■ **Specific mental functions**	**Specific mental functions**
• Thought	Recognition, categorization, generalization, awareness of reality, logical/coherent thought, and appropriate thought content
• Mental functions of sequencing complex movement	Execution of learned movement patterns
• Emotional	Coping and behavioral regulation (Scheil, Cohn, & Crepeau, 2008)
• Experience of self and time	Body image, self-concept, self-esteem
■ **Global mental functions**	**Global mental functions**
• Consciousness	Level of arousal, level of consciousness
• Orientation	Orientation to person, place, time, self, and others
• Temperament of personality	Emotional stablity
• Energy and drive	Motivation, impulse control, and appetite
• Sleep (physiological process)	
Sensory functions and pain	**Sensory functions and pain**
• Seeing and related functions, including visual acuity, visual stability, visual field functions	Detection/registration, modulation, and integration of sensations from the body and environment Visual awareness of environment at various distances
• Hearing functions	Tolerance of ambient sounds; awareness of location and distance of sounds such as an approaching car
• Vestibular functions	Sensation of securely moving against gravity
• Taste functions	Association of taste
• Smell functions	Association of smell
• Proprioceptive functions	Awareness of body position and space
• Touch functions	Comfort with the feeling of being touched by others or touching various textures such as food
• Pain (e.g., diffuse, dull, sharp, phantom)	Localizing pain
• Temperature and pressure	Thermal awareness
Neuromusculoskeletal and movement-related functions	**Neuromusculoskeletal and movement-related functions**
■ **Functions of joints and bones**	
• Joint mobility	Joint range of motion
• Joint stability	Postural alignment (this refers to the physiological stability of the joint related to its structural integrity as compared to the motor skill of aligning the body while moving in relation to task objects)
• Muscle power	Strength
• Muscle tone	Degree of muscle tone (e.g., flaccidity, spasticity, fluctuation)
• Muscle endurance	Endurance
• Involuntary movements reactions	Stretch, asymmetrical tonic neck, symmetrical tonic neck Righting and supporting Eye-hand/foot coordination, bilateral integration, crossing the midline, fine- and gross-motor control, and oculomotor (e.g., saccades, pursuits, accommodation, binocularity) Walking patterns and impairment such as asymmetric gait, stiff gait (Note: Gait patterns are considered in relation to how they affect ability to engage in occupations in daily life activities.)
Cardiovascular, hematological, immunological, and respiratory system function	**Cardiovascular, hematological, immunological, and respiratory system function**
• Cardiovascular system function	Blood pressure functions (hypertension, hypotension, postural hypotension), and heart rate
• Hematological and immunological system function • Respiratory system function	(Note: Occupational therapy practitioners have knowledge of these body functions and understand broadly the interaction that occurs between these functions to support health and participation in life through engagement in occupation. Some therapists may specialize in evaluating and intervening with a specific function as it is related to supporting performance and engagement in occupations and activities targeted for intervention.)
• Additional functions and sensations of the cardiovascular and respiratory systems	Rate, rhythm, and depth of respiration Physical endurance, aerobic capacity, stamina, and fatigability

(Continued)

Voice and speech functions • Voice functions • Fluency and rhythm • Alternative vocalization functions **Digestive, metabolic, and endocrine system function** • Digestive system function • Metabolic system and endocrine system function **Genitourinary and reproductive functions** • Urinary functions • Genital and reproductive functions	(Note: Occupational therapy practitioners have knowledge of these body functions and understand broadly the interaction that occurs between these functions to support health and participation in life through engagement in occupation. Some therapists may specialize in evaluating and intervening with a specific function, such as incontinence and pelvic floor disorders, as it is related to supporting performance and engagement in occupations and activities targeted for intervention.)
Skin and related-structure functions • Skin functions • Hair and nail functions	**Skin and related-structure functions** Protective functions of the skin—presence or absence of wounds, cuts, or abrasions Repair function of the skin—wound healing (Note: Occupational therapy practitioners have knowledge of these body functions and understand broadly the interaction that occurs between these functions to support health and participation in life through engagement in occupation. Some therapists may specialize in evaluating and intervening with a specific function, as it is related to supporting performance and engagement in occupations and activities targeted for intervention.)
BODY STRUCTURES: "*Body structures* are "anatomical parts of the body, such as organs, limbs, and their components [that support body function]" (WHO, 2001, p. 10). The "Body Structures" section of the table below is organized according to the ICF classifications. For fuller descriptions and definitions, refer to WHO (2001).	
CATEGORIES	**BODY FUNCTIONS COMMONLY CONSIDERED BY Occupational Therapy Practitioners (Not intended to be all-inclusive list)**
Structure of the nervous system **Eyes, ear, and related structures** **Structures involved in voice and speech** **Structures of the cardiovascular, immunological, and respiratory systems** **Structures related to the digestive, metabolic, and endocrine systems** **Structures related to the genitourinary and reproductive systems** **Structures related to movement** **Skin and related structures**	(Note: Occupational therapy practitioners have knowledge of these body functions and understand broadly the interaction that occurs between these functions to support health and participation in life through engagement in occupation. Some therapists may specialize in evaluating and intervening with a specific function, as it is related to supporting performance and engagement in occupations and activities targeted for intervention.)

Note. Some data adapted from the ICF (WHO, 2001).

From *Occupational therapy practice framework: Domain and process*, 2nd ed. (pp. 634–638). Copyright by the American Occupational Therapy Association, Inc. Reprinted with permission.

Performance Skills

Performance skills are the abilities clients demonstrate in the actions they perform.

SKILL	DEFINITION	EXAMPLES
Motor and praxis skills	*Motor:* actions or behaviors a client uses to move and physically interact with tasks, objects, contexts, and environments (adapted from Fisher, 2006). Includes planning, sequencing, and executing new and novel movements. *Praxis*: skilled purposeful movements (Heilman & Rothl, 1993). Ability to carry out sequential motor acts as part of an overall plan rather than individual acts (Liepmann 1920). Ability to carry our learned motor activity, including following through on a verbal command, visual-spatial construction, ocular and oral-motor skills, imitation of a person or an object, and sequencing actions (Ayres, 1985; Filey, 2001). Organization of temporal sequences of actions within the spatial context, which form meaningful occupations (Blanche & Parham, 2002).	• *Bending and reaching* for a toy or tool in a storage bin • *Pacing* tempo of movements to clean the room • *Coordinating* the body movements to complete a job task • *Maintaining balance* while walking on an uneven surface or while showering • *Anticipating or adjusting posture and body position* in response to environmental circumstances, such as obstacles • *Manipulating keys* or lock to open the door

Sensory-perceptual skills	Actions or behaviors a client uses to locate, identify, and respond to sensations and to select, interpret, associate, organize, and remember sensory events based on discriminating experiences through a variety of sensations that include visual, auditory, proprioceptive, tactile, olfactory, gustatory, and vestibular	• *Positioning the body* in the exact location of a safe jump • *Hearing and locating* the voice of your child in a crowd • *Visually* determining the correct size of a storage container for leftover soup • *Locating* keys by touch from many objects in a pocket or purse (i.e., stereognosis) • *Timing the appropriate moment* to cross the street safely by determining one's own position and speed relative to the speed of traffic • *Discerning* distinct flavors within foods or beverages
Emotional regulation skills	Actions or behaviors a client uses to identify, manage, and express feelings while engaging in activities or interacting with others	• *Responding* to the feelings of others by acknowledgement or showing support • *Persisting* in a task despite frustrations • *Controlling* anger toward others and reducing aggressive acts • *Recovering* from a hurt or disappointment without lashing out at others
Cognitive skills	Actions or behaviors a client uses to plan and manage the performance of an activity	• *Judging* the importance or appropriateness of clothes for the circumstance • *Selecting* tools and supplies needed to clean the bathroom • *Sequencing* tasks needed for a school project • *Organizing* activities within the time required to meet a deadline • *Prioritizing* steps and *identifying* solutions to access transportation • *Creating* different activities with friends that are fun, novel, and enjoyable • *Multitasking*—doing more than one thing at a time, necessary for tasks such as work, driving, and household management
Communication and social skills	Actions or behaviors a person uses to comminicate and interact with others in an interactive environment (Fisher, 2006)	• *Looking* where someone else is pointing or gazing • *Gesturing* to emphasize intentions • *Maintaining* acceptable physical space during conversation • *Initating and answering* questions with relevant information • *Taking turns* during an interchange with another person verbally and physically • *Acknowledging* another peron's perspective during an interchange

From *Occupational therapy practice framework: Domain and process*, 2nd ed. (pp. 640–641). Copyright by the American Occupational Therapy Association, Inc. Reprinted with permission.

APPENDIX 2

Selected Prefixes and Suffixes

A working knowledge of the components of medical terminology can often help decipher the meaning of an unknown word. This can assist in question analysis and the selection of the best answer. Remember, Latin is not a dying language, it is alive and well in the language of health care. This Appendix does not list all medical terms that may be on the examination, but it does provide many foundational components of medical terminology. For a complete and exhaustive presentation of medical terminology, the reader is referred to this Appendix's reference.

a-	without
ab-	away from
abdomin/o	abdomen
acous/o	hearing
acr/o	extremity or topmost
-acusis	hearing condition
ad-	.to, toward, or near
aden/o	gland
adip/o	fat
adren/o	adrenal gland
aer/o	air or gas
-algia	pain
alveol/o	alveolus (air sac)
ambi-	both
an-	without
angi/o	vessel
ankyl/o	crooked or stiff
ante-	before
anti-	against or opposed to
-arche	beginning
arteri/o	artery
arthr/o	joint
articul/o	joint
-ase	enzyme
-asthenia	weakness
ather/o	fat
-ation	process
audi/o	hearing
aur/i	ear
bi-	two or both
-blast	germ or bud
blast/o	germ or bud
brachi/o	arm
brady-	slow
bronch/o	bronchus (airway)
bucc/o	cheek
carcin/o	cancer
cardi/o	heart
celi/o	abdomen
cephal/o	head
cerebell/o	cerebellum (little brain)
cerebr/o	brain
cervic/o	neck or cervix
chondr/o	cartilage
chrom/o	color
circum-	around
con-	together or with
contra-	against or opposed to

cost/o	rib
crani/o	skull
cutane/o	skin
cyan/o	blue
cyst/o	bladder or sac
dacry/o	.tear
dactyl/o	digit (finger or toe)
de-	from, down, or not
derm/o	skin
-desis	binding
dextr/o	right, or on the right side
dia-	across or through
diaphor/o	profuse sweat
dips/o	thirst
dis-	separate from or apart
-dynia	pain
dys-	painful, difficult, or faulty
ec-	out or away
-ectasis	expansion or dilation
ecto-	outside
-ectomy	excision (removal)
-emesis	vomiting
-emia	blood condition
en-	within
encephal/o	brain
endo-	within
epi-	upon
erythr/o	red
esthesi/o	sensation
eu-	good or normal
ex-	out or away
exo-	outside
extra-	outside
fasci/o	fascia (a band)
fibr/o	fiber
gangli/o	ganglion (knot)
gastr/o	stomach
-gen	origin or production
glomerul/o	glomerulus (little ball)
gloss/o	.tongue
glott/o	opening
gluc/o	sugar
glyc/o	sugar
gnos/o	knowing
-gram	record
-graph	instrument for recording
-graphy	process of recording
hem/o	blood
hemat/o	blood
hemi-	half
hepat/o	liver
hepatic/o	liver
herni/o	hernia
hidr/o	sweat

hist/o	tissue
histi/o	tissue
hydr/o	water
hyper-	above or excessive
hypo-	below or deficient
-ia	condition of
-iasis	formation of or presence of
-iatrics	treatment
-iatry	treatment
-icle	small
immun/o	safe
infra-	below or under
inter-	between
intra-	within
-ism	condition of
iso-	equal, like
-itis	inflammation
-ium	structure or tissue
kyph/o	humped
lacrim/o	tear
lapar/o	abdomen
lei/o	smooth
lip/o	fat
lob/o	lobe (a portion)
lord/o	bent
lumb/o	loin (lower back)
lymph/o	clear fluid
-lysis	breaking down or dissolution
macr/o	large or long
-malacia	softening
meat/o	opening
-megaly	enlargement
meso-	middle
meta-	beyond, after, or change
-meter	instrument for measuring
-metry	process of measuring
micro-	small
mono-	one
morph/o	form
multi-	many
muscul/o	muscle
myel/o	bone marrow or spinal cord
myring/o	eardrum
narc/o	stupor
nas/o	nose
nat/i	birth
necr/o	death
neo-	new
nephr/o	kidney
neur/o	nerve
ocul/o	eye
-oid	resembling
-ole	small
olig/o	few or deficient
-oma	tumor

ophthalm/o	eye
opt/o	eye
or/o	mouth
orth/o	straight, normal, or correct
-osis	condition or increase
oste/o	bone
ot/o	ear
pachy-	thick
pan-	all
para-	alongside of or abnormal
-paresis	slight paralysis
path/o	disease
pector/o	chest
ped/o	child or foot
pelv/i	hip bone
pelv/o	hip bone
-penia	abnormal reduction
per-	through
peri-	around
phag/o	eat or swallow
phas/o	speech
-phil	attraction for
-philia	attraction for
phleb/o	vein
phob/o	exaggerated fear or sensitivity
phon/o	voice or speech
phot/o	light
phren/o	diaphragm (also mind)
plas/o	formation
-plasty	surgical repair or reconstruction
-plegia	paralysis
pleur/o	pleura
-pnea	breathing
pneum/o	air or lung
pod/o	foot
-poiesis	formation
poly-	many
post-	after or behind
pre-	before
presby/o	old age
pro-	before
-ptosis	falling or downward displacement
pulmon/o	lung
quadr/i	four
re-	again or back
reticul/o	a net
retro-	backward or behind
rhabd/o	rod shaped or striated (skeletal)
-rrhage	to burst forth
-rrhexis	rupture
sarc/o	flesh
scler/o	hard or sclera
scoli/o	twisted
semi	half
sinistr/o	left, or on the left side
somat/o	body
somn/o	sleep
son/o	sound
-spasm	involuntary contraction
sphygm/o	pulse
spin/o	spine (thorn)
spir/o	breathing
spondyl/o	vertebra
squam/o	scale
-stasis	stop or stand
steat/o	fat
sten/o	narrow
stere/o	three dimensional or solid
stern/o	sternum (breastbone)
steth/o	chest
stomat/o	mouth
-stomy	creation of an opening
sub-	below or under
super-	above or excessive
supra-	above or excessive
sym-	together or with
syn-	together or with
tachy-	fast
tax/o	order or coordination
ten/o	tendon (to stretch)
thorac/o	chest
thromb/o	clot
-tomy	incision
ton/o	tone or tension
top/o	place
tox/o	poison
trache/o	trachea (windpipe)
trans-	across or through
tri-	three
-tripsy	crushing
troph/o	nourishment or development
-ula, -ule	small
ultra-	beyond or excessive
uni-	one
ur/o	urine
varic/o	swollen or twistedvein
vas/o	vessel
vertebr/o	vertebra
vesic/o	bladder or sac
xanth/o	yellow
xer/o	dry
-y	condition or process of

References

Willis, M. C. (1996). *Medical terminology: The language of healthcare*. Philadelphia: Williams & Wilkins.

APPENDIX 3

State Occupational Therapy Regulatory Board and State OT Association Contact Information

ALABAMA
Type of Regulation: Licensure

Regulatory Authority Contact:
Alabama State Board of Occupational Therapy
64 N. Union Street, Suite 734
Montgomery, AL 36130-4510
Phone: 334-353-4466
Email: info@ot.alabama.gov
Website: www.ot.alabama.gov

State Association Contact:
Alabama Occupational Therapy Association (ALOTA)
P.O. Box 55764
Birmingham, AL 35255
Website: www.alota.org

ALASKA
Type of Regulation: Licensure

Regulatory Authority Contact:
Alaska State PT & OT Board
Division of Corporations, Business, & Professional Licensing
333 Willoughby Avenue, 9th Floor
Juneau, AK 99811-1770
Phone: 907-465-2580
Website: http://www.commerce.state.ak.us/occ/pphy.htm

State Association Contact:
Alaska Occupational Therapy Association (AKOTA)
3705 Arctic Blvd.
PMB 1616
Anchorage, AK 99503
Website: http://www.akota.org

ARIZONA
Type of Regulation: Licensure

Regulatory Authority Contact:
Arizona Board of Occupational Therapy Examiners
5060 North 19th Avenue, Suite 216
4205 N. 7th Avenue, Suite 305
Phoenix, AZ 85013
Phone: 602-589-8352
Website: http://www.occupationaltherapyboard.az.gov/

State Association Contact:
Arizona Occupational Therapy Association (ArizOTA)
P.O. Box 5214
Peoria, AZ 85385
Phone: 623-937-0920
Email: admin@arizota.org
Website: arizota.org

ARKANSAS
Type of Regulation: Licensure

Regulatory Authority Contact:
Arkansas State Occupational Therapy Examining Committee
1401 West Capitol Avenue, Suite 340
Little Rock, AR 72201-2936
Phone: 501-296-1802
Website: www.armedicalboard.org

State Association Contact:
Arkansas Occupational Therapy Association (AROTA)
P.O. Box 10674
Conway, AR 72034
Email: office@arota.org
Website: www.arota.org

CALIFORNIA
Type of Regulation: Licensure - OT, Certification - OTA

Regulatory Authority Contact:
California Board of Occupational Therapy
2005 Evergreen Street, Suite 2050
Sacramento, CA 95815
Phone: 916-263-2294
Website: http://www.bot.ca.gov/

State Association Contact:
Occupational Therapy Association of California (OTAC)
P.O. Box 276567
Sacramento, CA 95827-6567
Phone: 916-567-7000
Email: info@otaconline.org
Website: www.otaconline.org

COLORADO
Type of Regulation: Registration (Does not regulate OTAs)

Regulatory Authority Contact:
Division of Professions and Occupations
Department of Regulatory Agencies
1560 Broadway, Suite 110
Denver, CO 80202
Phone: 303-894-7855, 800-886-7675
Website: www.dora.state.co.us/occupational-therapists

State Association Contact:
OT Association of Colorado
P.O. Box 632136
Littleton, CO 80163
Email: support@otacco.org
Website: www.otacco.org

CONNECTICUT
Type of Regulation: Licensure

Regulatory Authority Contact:
Department of Public Health Occupational Therapy Licensure
410 Capital Avenue
P.O. Box 340308
Hartford, CT 06134
Phone: 860-509-8000
Website: http://www.ct.gov/dph/cwp/view.asp?a=3121&q=389442

State Association Contact:
Connecticut Occupational Therapy Association (ConnOTA)
370 Prospect Street
Wethersfield, CT 06109
Phone: 860-257-1371
Email: info@connOTA.org
Website: http://www.connota.org/

DELAWARE
Type of Regulation: Licensure

Regulatory Authority Contact:
Department of Administrative Services Professional Regulation
Division of Professional Regulation
861 Silver Lake Blvd., Suite 203
Dover, DE 19904
Phone: 302-744-4500
Website: http://dpr.delaware.gov/

State Association Contact:
Delaware Occupational Therapy Association (DOTA)
Phone: 302-456-1962
Website: http://www.dotaonline.org/

DISTRICT OF COLUMBIA
Type of Regulation: Licensure

Regulatory Authority Contact:
District of Columbia Board of Occupational Therapy
899 North Capitol Street NE
Washington, DC 20002
Phone: 877-672-2174
Website: http://doh.dc.gov/service/occupational-therapy-licensing

District of Columbia Association Contact:
330 13th Street, SE
Washington, DC 20003
Phone: 202-806-7614

FLORIDA
Type of Regulation: Licensure

Regulatory Authority Contact:
Florida Board of Occupational Therapy Practice
4052 Bald Cypress Way, Bin # C05
Tallahassee, FL 32399-3255
Phone: 850-245-4373
Email: MQA_OccupationalTherapy@doh.state.fl.us
Website: http://www.doh.state.fl.us/mqa/occupational/index.html

State Association Contact:
Florida Occupational Therapy Association (FOTA)
P.O. Box 1459
Englewood, FL 34295
Phone: 954-840-FOTA (3682)
Website: http:// www.flota.org

GEORGIA
Type of Regulation: Licensure

Regulatory Authority Contact:
Georgia State Board of Occupational Therapy
237 Coliseum Drive
Macon, GA 31217
Phone: 478-207-2440
Website: http://www.sos.state.ga.us/plb/ot

State Association Contact:
Georgia Occupational Therapy Association (GOTA)
1260 Winchester Parkway, Suite 205
Smyrna, GA 30080
Phone: 770-435-5910
Website: http://www.gaota.com

HAWAII
Type of Regulation: Licensure (Does not regulate OTAs)

Regulatory Authority Contact:
Hawaii Professional & Vocational Licensing Division
DCCA/PVL-Occupational Therapist Program
P.O. Box 3469
Honolulu, HI 6801
Phone: 808-586-2701
Website: http://hawaii.gov/dccal/pvl/programs/occupational/

State Association Contact:
Occupational Therapy Association of Hawaii (OTAH)
1360 S.Beretania St, Suite 301
Honolulu, HI 96814
Phone: 808-544-3336
Email: OTAssociationofHawaii@gmail.com
Website: http://www.otah-hawaii.com

IDAHO
Type of Regulation: Licensure

Regulatory Authority Contact:
Idaho Occupational Therapy Board
Idaho State Board of Medicine
P.O. Box 83720
Boise, ID 83720-0058
Phone: 208-327-7000
Email: info@bom.idaho.gov
Website: http://www.bom.state.id.us

State Association Contact:
Idaho Occupational Therapy Association (IOTA)
P.O. Box 7364
Boise, ID 83707
Phone: 208-388-4682
Email: info@id-ota.com
Website: http://www.id-ota.com/

ILLINOIS
Type of Regulation: Licensure

Regulatory Authority Contact:
Illinois Occupational Therapy Board (ILOTA)
320 West Washington
Springfield, IL 62786
Phone: 217-782-8556
Email: mkim.scoh@illinois.gov
Website: http://www.ilota.org/licensure-in-illinois

State Association Contact:
Illinois Occupational Therapy Association (ILOTA)
7234 West North Avenue, Suite 409
Elmwood Park, IL 60707
Phone: 708-452-7640
Website: http://ilota.org

INDIANA
Type of Regulation: Certification

Regulatory Authority Contact:
Indiana Occupational Therapy Committee
P.O. Box 4520
Lisle, IN 60532
Phone: 708-452-7640
Email: office@ilota.org
Website: http://www.in.gov/hpb/boards/otc/

State Association Contact:
Indiana Occupational Therapy Association (IOTA)
P.O. Box 47803
Indianapolis, IN 46247
Phone: 866-653-7429
Email: info@inota.com
Website: http://www.inota.com

IOWA

Type of Regulation: Licensure

Regulatory Authority Contact:
Iowa Board of PT and OT Examiners
Professional Licensure
Office Lucas State Office Bldg., 5th Floor
321 East 12th Street
Des Moines, IA 50319
Phone: 515-281-0254
Website: http://www.idph.state.ia.us/licensure/

State Association Contact:
Iowa Occupational Therapy Association (IOTA)
P.O. Box 57221
Des Moines, IA 50317
Phone: 515-720-7346
Website: http://www.iowaot.org

KANSAS

Type of Regulation: Registration

Regulatory Authority Contact:
Kansas State Board of Healing Arts
800 SW Jackson Lower Level, Suite A
Topeka, KS 66602
Phone: 785-296-7413
Website: http://www.ksbha.org/

State Association Contact:
Kansas Occupational Therapy Association (KOTA)
825 S. Kansas Avenue, Suite 500
Topeka, KS 66612-1253
Phone: 785-232-8044
Toll Free: 877-904-0529
Website: http://www.kotaonline.org/

KENTUCKY

Type of Regulation: Licensure

Regulatory Authority Contact:
Kentucky Board of Licensure for Occupational Therapy
911 Leawood Drive
Frankfort, KY 40601
Phone: 502-564-3296 ext 226
Email: Jennifer.Hutcherson@ky.gov
Website: http://bot.ky.gov/Pages/default.aspx

State Association Contact:
Kentucky Occupational Therapy Association (KOTA)
P.O. Box 5531
Louisville, KY 40255
Phone: 1-888-987-KOTA (5682)
Email: kotaweb@kotaweb.org
Website: http://www.kotaweb.org/

LOUISIANA

Type of Regulation: Licensure

Regulatory Authority Contact:
Louisiana State Board of Medical Examiners
State Board of Medical Examiners
630 Camp Street
New Orleans, LA 70130
Phone: 504-568-6820
Website: http://www.lsbme.louisiana.gov/

State Association Contact:
Louisiana Occupational Therapy Association (LOTA)
P.O. Box 14806
Baton Rouge, LA 70898
Phone: 225-291-2806
Website: http://www.lota.org/

MAINE

Type of Regulation: Licensure

Regulatory Authority Contact:
Maine Board of Occupational Therapy Practice
Dept. of Prof. & Financial Regulation
35 State House Station
Augusta, ME 04333-0035
Phone: 207-624-8603
Website: http://www.state.me.us/pfr/olr/categories/cat28.htm

State Association Contact:
Maine Occupational Therapy Association (MEOTA)
Phone: 207-453-5172
Website: http://www.meota.org/

MARYLAND

Type of Regulation: Licensure

Regulatory Authority Contact:
Maryland Board of Occupational Therapy Practice
201 West Preston Street
Baltimore, MD 21201
Phone: 410-767-6500
Email: mdotboard@dhmh.state.md.us
Website: http://dhmh.maryland.gov/botp/SitePages/Home.aspx

State Association Contact:
Maryland Occupational Therapy Association
P.O. Box 2742
Columbia, MD 21045
Phone: 1-888-290-2662
Email: email.mota@gmail.com
Website: http://www.mota.memberlodge.org/

MASSACHUSETTS
Type of Regulation: Licensure

Regulatory Authority Contact:
Massachusetts Board of Registration Allied Health Professions
Division of Professional Licensure
1000 Washington Street, Suite 710
Boston, MA 02118-6100
Phone: 617-727-3074
617-727-1944
Website: www.mass.gov/dpl

State Association Contact:
Massachusetts Occupational Therapy Association (MAOTA)
57 Madison Road
Waltham, MA 02453-6718
Phone: 781-647-5556
Email: info@maot.org
Website: http://www.maot.org/

MICHIGAN
Type of Regulation: Licensure

Regulatory Authority Contact:
Michigan Board of Occupational Therapy
Department of Community Health Bureau of Health Professions
P.O. Box 30004
Lansing, MI 48909
Phone: 517-373-1820
Website: http://www.michigan.gov/mdch/0,1607,7-132-27417_27529_27545---,00.html

State Association Contact:
Michigan Occupational Therapy Association (MiOTA)
124 W. Allegan, Suite 1900
Lansing, MI 48933
Phone: 517-267-3918
Email: office@miota.org
Website: http://www.mi-ota.com/

MINNESOTA
Type of Regulation: Licensure

Regulatory Authority Contact:
Minnesota Department of Health OT/OTA Licensing Advisory Council
MDH/HOP, OTP Licensing Advisory Council
P.O. Box 64975
St. Paul, MN 55164-0975
Phone: 651-201-5000
Website: http://www.health.state.mn.us/divs/hpsc/hop/otp/index.html

State Association Contact:
Minnesota Occupational Therapy Association (MOTA)
1000 Westgate Drive, Suite 252
St. Paul, MN 55114
Phone: 651-290-7498
Website: http://www.motafunctionfirst.org/

MISSISSIPPI
Type of Regulation: Licensure

Regulatory Authority Contact:
MSDH Professional Licensure Division
P.O. Box 1700
Jackson, MS 39215-1700
Phone: 601-364-7360
Website: www.msdh.state.ms.us

State Association Contact:
Mississippi Occupational Therapy Association (MSOTA)
P.O. Box 13706
Jackson, MS 39236
Phone: 601-956-4105
Website: http://www.angelfire.com/ms/msota/

MISSOURI
Type of Regulation: Licensure

Regulatory Authority Contact:
Missouri State Board of Occupational Therapy
3605 Missouri Blvd.
P.O. Box 1335
Jefferson City, MO 65102-1335
Phone: 573-751-0877
Email: ot@pr.mo.gov
Website: http://pr.mo.gov/

State Association Contact:
Missouri Occupational Therapy Association (MOTA)
360 S. Missouri Blvd.
Jefferson City, MO 65102
Phone: 636-441-4146
Email: motamoweb@gmail.com
Website: http://www.motamo.net/index.htm

MONTANA
Type of Regulation: Licensure

Regulatory Authority Contact:
Montana Board of Occupational Therapy Practice
Department of Labor and Industry
P.O. Box 200513
301 South Park, 4th Floor
Helena, MT 59620
Phone: 406-841-2385
Website: http://www.discoveringmontana.com/dli/otp

State Association Contact:
Montana Occupational Therapy Association (MOTA)
Phone: 406-855-5894
Email: admin@mtota.org
Website: http://www.mtota.org/

NEBRASKA
Type of Regulation: Licensure

Regulatory Authority Contact:
Nebraska Board of Occupational Therapy Practice
Credentialing Division,
301 Centennial Mall South, 3rd Floor
P.O. Box 94986
Lincoln, NE 68509-4986
Phone: (402) 471-2115
Website: www.hhs.state.ne.us/crl/profindex1.htm

State Association Contact:
Nebraska Occupational Therapy Association (NOTA)
P.O. Box 31594
Omaha, NE 68131-0594
Email: notassistant@gmail.com
Website: http://www.notaonline.org/

NEW HAMPSHIRE
Type of Regulation: Licensure

Regulatory Authority Contact:
Occupational Therapy Governing Board
2 Industrial Park Drive
Concord, NH 03301
Phone: 603-271-8389
Email: traci.e.weber@nh.gov
Website: http://www.nh.gov/alliedhealth/boards/occupationaltherapy/index.htm

State Association Contact:
New Hampshire Occupational Therapy Association (NHOTA)
P.O. Box 4232
Concord, NH 03302-4232
Phone: 603-225-9290
Email: office@nhota.org
Website: http://www.nhota.org/

NEW JERSEY
Type of Regulation: Licensure

Regulatory Authority Contact:
NJ Occupational Therapy Advisory Council
P.O. Box 45037
Newark, NJ 07101
Phone: 973-504-6570
Website: www.state.nj.us/lps/ca/medical/occuptherapy.htm

State Association Contact:
New Jersey Occupational Therapy Association (NJOTA)
P.O. Box 401
Summit, NJ 07902
Phone: 732-968-5038
Website: http://www.njota.org/

NEW MEXICO
Type of Regulation: Licensure

Regulatory Authority Contact:
NM Board of Examiners for Occupational Therapy
P.O. Box 25101
Santa Fe, NM 87505
Phone: 505-476-4940
Email: occupationaltherapy@state.nm.us
Website: http://www.rld.state.nm.us/boards/Occupational_Therapy.aspx

State Association Contact:
New Mexico Occupational Therapy Association (NMOTA)
Phone: 603-225-9290
Website: http://www.nmota.org/

NEW YORK
Type of Regulation: Licensure—OT, Registration—OTA

Regulatory Authority Contact:
New York State Board for Occupational Therapy
89 Washington Avenue
Albany, NY 12234
Phone: 518-474-3817 ext. 270
Email: opunit3@mail.nysed.gov
Website: http://www.op.nysed.gov/prof/ot/otlic.htm

State Association Contact:
New York Occupational Therapy Association (NYOTA)
119 Washington Avenue, 2nd Floor
Albany, NY 12210
Phone: 518-462-3717
Website: http://www.nysota.org/

NORTH CAROLINA
Type of Regulation: Licensure

Regulatory Authority Contact:
North Carolina Board of Occupational Therapy
P.O. Box 2280
Raleigh, NC 27602
Phone: 919-832-1380
Email: administrator@ncbot.org
Website: http://www.ncbot.org/

State Association Contact:
North Carolina Occupational Therapy Association (NCOTA)
P.O. Box 20432
Raleigh, NC 27619
Phone: 919-785-9700
Website: http://www.ncota.org

NORTH DAKOTA
Type of Regulation: Licensure

Regulatory Authority Contact:
North Dakota State Board of OT Practice
P.O. Box 4005
Bismarck, ND 58502-4005
Phone: 701-250-0847
Website: http://www.ndotboard.com

State Association Contact:
North Dakota Occupational Therapy Association (NDOTA)
P.O. Box 14118
Grand Forks, ND 585208-4118
Website: http://www.ndota.com

OHIO
Type of Regulation: Licensure

Regulatory Authority Contact:
Ohio Occupational Therapy, Physical Therapy and Athletic Trainers Board
77 South High Street, 16th Floor
Columbus, OH 43215-6108
Phone: 614-466-3774
Email: board@otptat.ohio.gov
Website: www.otptat.ohio.gov

State Association Contact:
Ohio Occupational Therapy Association (OOTA)
P.O. Box 693
Canal Winchester, OH 43110-0693
Phone: 614-920-9445
Email: webmaster@oota.org
Website: http://www.oota.org/

OKLAHOMA
Type of Regulation: Licensure

Regulatory Authority Contact:
Oklahoma State Board of Medical Licensure and Supervision
P.O. Box 18256
Oklahoma City, OK 73154-0256
Phone: 405-962-1400
Website: www.okmedicalboard.org

State Association Contact:
Oklahoma Occupational Therapy Association (OOTA)
P.O. Box 2602
Oklahoma City, OK 73101-2602
Phone: 405-205-3942
Website: http://www.okota.org/

OREGON
Type of Regulation: Licensure

Regulatory Authority Contact:
Oregon Occupational Therapy Licensing Board
800 NE Oregon Street, Suite 407
Portland, OR 97232
Phone: 971-673-0198
Email: Felicia.M.Holgate@state.or.us
Website: http://www.otlb.state.or.us

State Association Contact:
Occupational Therapy Association of Oregon (OTAO)
P.O. Box 7133
Aloha, OR 97007
Email: otao@otao.com
Website: http://www.otao.com

PENNSYLVANIA
Type of Regulation: Licensure

Regulatory Authority Contact:
Pennsylvania State Board of Occupational Therapy Education and Licensure
P.O. Box 2649
Harrisburg, PA 17105-2649
Phone: 717-783-1389
Email: ST-OCCUPATIONAL@pa.gov
Website: http://www.dos.state.pa.us/therapy

State Association Contact:
Pennsylvania Occupational Therapy Association (POTA)
610 Freedom Business Center, Suite 110
King of Prussia, PA 19406
Phone: 1-800-UR1POTA
Email: help@pota.org
Website: http://www.pota.org/

RHODE ISLAND
Type of Regulation: Licensure

Regulatory Authority Contact:
Rhode Island Board of Occupational Therapy Practice Health Professions Regulation
Cannon Building 3 Capital Hill, Room 104
Providence, RI 02908
Phone: 401-222-2828
Email: jmichel.martineau@health,ri.gov
Website: http://www.health.ri.gov/hsr/professions/occ_therap.php

State Association Contact:
Rhode Island Occupational Therapy Association (RIOTA)
P.O. Box 8585
Warwick, RI 02888-0599
Phone: 401-484-5207
Email: riota@ritoa.org
Website: http://www.riota.org/

SOUTH CAROLINA
Type of Regulation: Licensure

Regulatory Authority Contact:
South Carolina Board of Occupational Therapy
110 Centerview Drive
P.O. Box 11329
Columbia, SC 29211
Phone: 803-896-4683
Email: contactllr@llr.sc.gov
Website: http://www.llr.state.sc.us/POL/OccupationalTherapy/

State Association Contact:
South Carolina Occupational Therapy Association (SCOTA)
401 Pittsdowne Road
Columbia, SC 29210
Phone: 888-647-2682
Website: http://www.scota.net/

SOUTH DAKOTA
Type of Regulation: Licensure

Regulatory Authority Contact:
South Dakota Occupational Therapy Committee
101 N. Main Ave, Suite 301
Sioux Falls, SD 57104
Phone: 605-367-7781
Website: http://www.state.sd.us/dcr/medical/ot.htm

State Association Contact:
South Dakota Occupational Therapy Association (SDOTA)
P.O. Box 1120
Aberdeen, SD 57402
Phone: 605-215-2659
Email: SDOTA@msn.com
Website: http://www.sdota.org

TENNESSEE
Type of Regulation: Licensure

Regulatory Authority Contact:
Tennessee Board of Occupational Therapy & Physical Therapy Examiners
665 Mainstream Drive, 2nd Floor
Nashville, TN 37243
Phone: 615-741-3807
Email: tn.health@tn.gov
Website: http://health.state.tn.us/boards/ot/

State Association Contact:
Tennessee Occupational Therapy Association (TOTA)
P.O. Box 198126
Nashville, TN 37219
Phone: 615-425-5310
Email: joyce@tnota.org
Website: http://www.tnota.org

TEXAS
Type of Regulation: Licensure

Regulatory Authority Contact:
Texas Executive Council of PT & OT Examiners
333 Guadalupe Street #2-510
Austin, TX 78701-3942
Phone: 512-305-6900
Email: info@ptot.texas.gov
Website: http://www.ecptote.state.tx.us/ot/

State Association Contact:
Texas Occupational Therapy Association (TOTA)
1106 Clayton Lane, Suite 516W
Austin, TX 78723
Phone: 512-454-8682
Website: http://www.tota.org

UTAH
Type of Regulation: Licensure

Regulatory Authority Contact:
Utah Occupational Therapy Board
P.O. Box 146741
Salt Lake City, UT 84114-6741
Phone: 801-530-6628
Email: doplweb@utah.gov
Website: www.dopl.utah.gov

State Association Contact:
Utah Occupational Therapy Association (UOTA)
P.O. Box 58412
Salt Lake City, Utah 84158-0412
Phone: 800-748-4063
Website: http://www.utahotassociation.org/

VERMONT
Type of Regulation: Licensure (Does not regulate OTAs)

Regulatory Authority Contact:
Vermont Occupational Therapy Advisors
89 Main Street, 3rd Floor
Montpelier, VT 05620-3402
Phone: 802-828-1505
Website: http://www.vtprofessionals.org/opr1/o_therapists/

State Association Contact:
Vermont Occupational Therapy Association (VOTA)
P.O. Box 5567
Essex Junction, VT 05453-5567
Phone: 802-264-9671
Website: http://vermontot.blogspot.com/

VIRGINIA
Type of Regulation: Licensure

Regulatory Authority Contact:
Virginia Advisory Board on Occupational Therapy
Perimeter Center
9960 Maryland Drive, Suite 300
Henrico, VA 23233-1463
Phone: 804-367-4600
Website: http://www.dhp.virginia.gov/Medicine/advisory/ot/

State Association Contact:
Virginia Occupational Therapy Association (VOTA)
3720 Parchment Circle
Richmond, VA 23229
Email: office@vaota.org
Website: http://www.vaota.org/

WASHINGTON
Type of Regulation: Licensure

Regulatory Authority Contact:
Washington Occupational Therapy Practice Board
P.O. Box 1099
Olympia, WA 98507-1099
Phone: 360-236-4700
Email: hsqa.csc@doh.wa.gov
Website: http://www.doh.wa.gov/LicensesPermitsandCertificates/ProfessionsNewReneworUpdate/OccupationalTherapist.aspx

State Association Contact:
Washington Occupational Therapy Association (WOTA)
23607 Hwy 99, Suite 2C
Edmonds, WA 98092
Phone: 425-778-6162
Website: http://www.wota.org/

WEST VIRGINIA
Type of Regulation: Licensure

Regulatory Authority Contact:
West Virginia Board of Occupational Therapy
WVBOT - 3041 University Avenue
2nd Floor, Suite 6
Morgantown, WV 26505
Phone: 304-285-3150
Email: help@wvbot.org
Website: http://www.wvbot.org/

State Association Contact:
West Virginia Occupational Therapy Association (WVOTA)
1840 Oakridge Drive
Charleston, WV 25311
Website: http://www.wvota.org/

WISCONSIN
Type of Regulation: Licensure

Regulatory Authority Contact:
Bureau of Health Professions Department of Regulation and Licensing
OT Affiliated Credentialing Board
P.O. Box 8935
Madison, WI 53708-8935
Phone: 608-266-2112
Email: dsps@wisconsin.gov
Website: http://drl.wi.gov/prof/occt/def.htm

State Association Contact:
Wisconsin Occupational Therapy Association (WOTA)
122 E. Olin Avenue, Suite 165
Madison, WI 53713
Phone: 608-287-1606
Email: wota@wota.net
Website: http://www.wota.net/

WYOMING
Type of Regulation: Licensure

Regulatory Authority Contact:
Wyoming Board of Occupational Therapy
6101 Yellowstone Road, Suite 510
Cheyenne, WY 82002
Phone: 307-777-7764
Email: Vickie.spires@wyo.gov
Website: http://ot.state.wy.us/

State Association Contact:
Wyoming Occupational Therapy Association (WYOTA)
201 E. 2nd Street, Suite 18
Casper, WY 86201
Phone: 307-215-3894
Email: Cheryl@centralwyomingtherapy.com
Website: http://www.wyota.org/

APPENDIX 4

Review Questions and Answers

Chapter 3 Review Questions

The Process of Occupational Therapy

1. An occupational therapist is preparing to evaluate a client. What contextual considerations should the therapist take into account when determining the assessments that will be appropriate to use with the client?

The therapist should consider the environmental contexts of the practice setting in which the assessment will be conducted (e.g., the length of stay, the setting's primary focus, legislative guidelines and restrictions, and the facility's resources of space, equipment, and supplies). In addition, the physical and sociocultural contexts of the client's current and expected environment (e.g., roles, values, norms, supports) should be taken into account by the therapist. The temporal context of the client and his/her disability (e.g., the client's chronological and developmental age, anticipated duration of disability, and stage of illness) should also be considered when determining which assessment tools are best to use during an evaluation.

2. An occupational therapist owns and operates a pre-school facility for children with developmental, intellectual, and physical disabilities. When should the therapist instruct the facility staff members to use standard precautions? What policies and procedures should the therapist implement for the use of standard precautions in this practice setting?

Standard precautions are infection prevention practices that are applied at *all* times when working with *all* persons in *all* practice settings. They include standards for hand hygiene and the use of gloves, gown, mask, eye protection, or face shield (depending on the anticipated exposure). There are also standards for handling and caring for equipment or items in a practice setting to prevent transmission of infectious agents. The application of standard precautions during service delivery is determined by the nature of the interactions with clients and the extent of anticipated blood, body fluid, or pathogen exposure. In a pediatric pre-school setting, the therapist should ensure that all staff members consistently adhere to hand hygiene and respiratory hygiene/cough etiquette standards. Signs should be posted in the facility with instructions to persons with symptoms of a respiratory infection to cover their mouths/noses when coughing or sneezing, use and dispose of tissues, and perform hand hygiene after hands have been in contact with respiratory secretions. The facility should provide tissues and no-touch receptacles (e.g., foot pedal-operated lid or open, plastic-lined waste baskets) for disposal of tissues. Resources and instructions for performing hand hygiene should be conveniently located throughout the facility. Policies and procedures for routine and targeted cleaning and disinfecting of the facility's environmental surfaces and toys used by the children must be established. Toys selected for use with the children during evaluation and intervention must be ones that can be easily cleaned and disinfected (e.g., hard plastic building blocks, not furry stuffed animals). Toys that are mouthed must be immediately cleaned, disinfected and then rinsed with water after use. After cleaning and disinfection, toys should be stored in a designated labeled container which identifies them as clean and ready for use. Large stationary toys (e.g., climbing equipment) must be cleaned and disinfected at least weekly and whenever visibly soiled.

3. An occupational therapist provides services in a community-based setting which offers individual and group interventions. What factors should the therapist consider when determining if it is best to use an individual intervention versus a group intervention with a client?

The level of the client's cognitive, physical, and interpersonal skills should be considered to determine if an individual or a group intervention is best to use with a client. Clients with lower capabilities and a greater need for attention and structure from the occupational therapist due to body structure and functional impairments will benefit from an individualized approach. The client's need for privacy and/or greater control over the environment also support the use of an individual intervention. Individualized interventions are indicated if the activity demands, performance skills, and performance patterns of an intervention are complex. Most important, if the client exhibits inappropriate and/or dangerous behaviors, group interventions are not appropriate. Group interventions are indicated when the intervention focus is on the development of interpersonal skills and the ability to engage socially with others. Group interventions provide the opportunity to receive feedback from people experiencing similar conditions, learn from them, place one's own condition into perspective, and become motivated by peer role models. Groups are also indicated when an intervention goal is to develop behaviors that are needed for successful performance in shared occupations (e.g., work, study, and leisure groups).

4. An occupational therapist working in a long-term care facility co-leads a discharge planning group with a social worker. What are the advantages to this co-leadership? What issues may arise to impede effective co-leadership that the therapist should be prepared to address?

Co-leadership enables each leader to share his/her professional knowledge and skills and use their unique professional expertise to assume different leadership roles and tasks. Both leaders can provide and obtain mutual support to each other, share their observations, and model effective behaviors. Issues that may arise and must be dealt to ensure effective co-leadership include the splitting by group member(s) of one leader against the other, excessive competition among co-leaders, and unequal responsibilities resulting in an unbalanced work load among co-leaders.

5. An occupational therapist provides services to a group of parents of infants and toddlers. Each parent recently incurred a disability. The therapist plans to use a thematic and a topical group with the clients to address goals related to their parental role. What would be appropriate foci and relevant activities for these groups?

The purpose of a thematic group is to assist members in acquiring the knowledge, skills, and/or attitudes needed to perform a specific activity. Because the clients in this group are parents who each recently incurred a disability, this group should focus on the improvement of members' ability to engage in desired parenting activities outside of group by teaching and practicing these activities within group (e.g., how to perform childcare activities using adaptive equipment and compensatory strategies; how to transfer to and from a wheelchair to the floor to enable play with a toddler). In a thematic group, simulated, clearly defined, structured activities are used for group members to practice and learn needed skills within the group (e.g., using a doll to practice diapering an infant from a wheelchair or by using a one-handed technique).

The purpose of a topical group is to discuss specific activities that members are engaged in outside of group to enable them to engage in the activities in a more effective, need-satisfying manner. Because the clients are already parents, this group would be considered a concurrent topical group. In this group, discussion would include members' current or anticipated fears and problems about parenting with a disability, potential solutions for dealing with these concerns, and coping mechanisms for increasing personal self-efficacy as a parent. The therapist would facilitate a focused group discussion on parenting activities, help members problem-solve, give feedback and support, and reinforce skill acquisition.

Chapter 4 Review Questions

Professional Standards and Responsibilities

1. You are working in a skilled nursing facility. An administrator asks you to actively treat a new resident who is very frail with multiple medical complications. Upon admission, you had evaluated the resident and determined that the resident would not be able to tolerate occupational therapy services. During the evaluation, the resident had stated that chronic pain made all activities very difficult. Pain relief and rest were the only things the resident identified as personally desired. How should you respond to the administrator's request? Which principles of the AOTA Code of Ethics should you use to guide your response? Explain how these principles relate to this situation.

You must refuse to place the person on an active occupational therapy intervention program because doing so would violate the ethical principles of beneficence, nonmaleficence, autonomy, and procedural justice. The ethical principle of beneficence requires you to demonstrate your concern for the resident's well-being and safety. The resident has chronic pain which compromises health and well-being; thus, pain relief must be a priority. The ethical principle of nonmaleficence requires you to avoid doing anything that can harm or injure a person. You must use your professional judgment and avoid compromising the resident's rights or health. This arbitrary administrative directive to place the resident on an active intervention program must be confronted. The administrator's request does not consider the person's current status and can cause harm. This request also violates the ethical principle of autonomy which requires you to respect the right of the individual to self-determination and the person's right to refuse occupational therapy services. The resident has stated that pain relief and rest were the only things personally desired. According to the ethical principle of procedural justice, you must know and apply our profession's Code and Ethics to the work setting and share them with employers when indicated to make sure that they are aware of your ethical obligations. Providing occupational therapy services to a person who is frail and too ill to participate in therapy would violate all of the above ethical principles; therefore, the administrator must be informed that you will not do this.

2. A large regional health care system provides occupational therapy services across the continuum of care. Settings in which occupational therapy services are provided include an acute care hospital, an outpatient clinic, a subacute rehabilitation unit, a skilled nursing facility (SNF), a palliative care unit, and a home health agency. All settings employ occupational therapists and occupational therapy assistants. What factors should be considered when determining the level of supervision that the occupational therapist should provide to the occupational therapy assistant? What is a key determinant for deciding if an occupational therapy assistant (OTA) can ethically be given more responsibility?

The degree, amount, and pattern of supervision required in each setting will depend on the OTA's knowledge and skills (e.g., the OTA has completed advanced training in splinting); the complexities of client needs (e.g., the presence of co-morbidities) and caseload characteristics and demands (e.g., focused primarily on one diagnostic category and a core intervention approach such as training clients in hip precautions pre-and post-hip replacement surgery). An OTA providing services to an acutely ill person with rapidly changing status on the inpatient unit will require a closer occupational therapist/OTA partnership than an OTA providing services to a more stable client in a long-term care setting. State laws, licensure requirements, and other regulatory mandates must also be considered when determining the level of OTA supervision required. Ethically, the OT supervisor must ensure that the type, amount, and pattern of supervision match the supervisee's level of role performance. An OTA can be given more responsibility by the occupational therapist after the OTA establishes service competency. Service competency is the ability to use a specified intervention in a safe, effective, and reliable manner. Before assigning greater responsibilities to the OTA, the occupational therapist must determine that the OTA can perform a procedure in a manner that obtains the same results as the therapist would have obtained. OTAs who establish service competency do not become independent; they continue to work under the occupational therapist's supervision.

3. An occupational therapist is opening a private practice. What procedures should the therapist implement to ensure full compliance with the Health Insurance and Portability Accountability Act (HIPAA)?

The therapist needs to set standards and establish safeguards to ensure the privacy and security of health care records. Procedures must be established for informing all clients of the practice's privacy policies and obtaining clients' written acknowledgement that they received this information. Guidelines for staff members to follow if there are difficulties obtaining signed assent are needed. All staff must be advised that prior to discussing a client's status with another person, they must obtain the person's permission. Guidelines for staff members to follow if there are questions about the client's ability to give permission are needed (e.g., a client is at risk of harming self due to lack of judgment; consultation with a specialist is essential to ensure quality of care). Staff must be advised that all information used or disclosed about a person's status must be limited to the minimum needed for the immediate purpose. The therapist must set procedures to ensure patient confidentiality in oral, written, and electronic forms of communication (e.g., all conversations with clients should be conducted in private areas and in low tones; sign-in sheets should only ask for clients' names; computer monitors should have privacy screens; emails should be protected by encrypted passwords).

4. You are beginning a new job as an occupational therapist for a Medicare-certified home health agency. Most of your clients will have limited independence or be dependent in basic activities of daily living. What are key Medicare guidelines for home-based occupational therapy you must consider when working with these individuals and their caregivers?

Home-based occupational therapy (OT) services for medical, physical, cognitive, and psychiatric conditions are covered if the individual is under a physician's care and needed intermittent skilled nursing care, physical therapy (PT), or speech therapy (ST) before OT began. OT services can continue after the person's need for skilled nursing, PT, or ST has ended. Services must be provided under a plan of care that was established by a physician. Care plans must be reviewed regularly by the physician. The person must be considered home-bound to receive home care services. Medicare has specific criteria for determining if a person is homebound. To be considered homebound, the person is "confined" to the home and not able to easily leave the home due to a need to use an ambulatory device, the assistance of others, or special transportation. If the person leaves the home, it requires considerable effort that is taxing to the person. The person may leave his/her home for medical appointments (e.g., kidney dialysis) and non-medical short-term and infrequent appointments/events (e.g., attendance at religious services). If the person receives adult day care services, he or she can still receive OT services in the home. Rental or purchase expenses for durable medical equipment (DME) are covered if prescribed by a physician. The DME must be considered necessary and reasonable to treat an illness or injury or to improve functioning. It must be used in the person's home and be able to withstand repeated use. To be reimbursable, the DME must be primarily and customarily used for a medical purpose (e.g., a wheelchair or walker). DME will not be reimbursed if it is useful to a person in the absence of injury or illness (e.g., self-help items such as bathtub grab bars, and raised toilet seats).

5. You are developing a new driver rehabilitation program. What are important issues for you to consider as you develop your budget and fiscal management plan?

When developing a new program it is important to make realistic revenue and volume projections. You should complete a break-even analysis to determine the volume of services you will need to provide to obtain sufficient revenue to equal the costs of operating the program. You will need to plan for short and long-term program needs. This includes budgeting for capital expenses (i.e., typically any item or action above a fixed amount such as a driver simulator) and operating expenses. Operating expenses include direct expenses costs related to OT service provision (i.e., salaries and benefits, office supplies, and treatment equipment) and indirect expenses (i.e., utilities, housekeeping, and marketing). Because the amount of services you provide will increase as your program grows, it will be important to determine which expenses are fixed and which are variable. Fixed expenses will remain at the same level (e.g., rent), while variable expenses will change in direct proportion to the amount of services provided (e.g., computer paper and ink).

Chapter 5 Review Questions

Human Development Across the Lifespan: Pediatric Through Geriatric Considerations for Occupational Therapy Practice

1. You are part of an intra-professional screening team to determine children's readiness for kindergarten. A 5-year-old child whom you are evaluating has performed at or above level on every aspect of the screening and has not demonstrated any fine motor, visual motor, or gross motor delays. The child has no cognitive deficits. The child performed well on the Beery-Buktenica Developmental Test of Visual-Motor Integration. Given the child's performance so far, which of Erhardt's developmental levels of prewriting skills would you expect the child to use for writing tasks? Explain your answer.

Your evaluation indicated that the child is functioning at an age-appropriate developmental level; thus, the child would be expected to use a developmentally appropriate grasp for writing tasks. Given that the child is five years old, the child would be expected to use a dynamic tripod posture for writing tasks. The dynamic tripod posture is observed in children ages 4 ½ to 6 years.

2. A typically developing child with no developmental delays independently creates a building made of blocks from a mental image. Identify the child's age range and describe the skills the child would use during this play activity.

A child aged 3 to 4 years would have the fine motor, balance and coordination skills needed to build a structure using blocks and the cognitive ability to build a structure from a mental image. This activity requires the child to recognize color and shape. The child must organize the blocks by size and shape to produce a three-dimensional block structure based on a mental image.

3. A 15-year-old has a group of friends who have recently become involved in experimenting with drugs, alcohol and other risky behaviors. The teen is torn between wanting to remain friends with this group and not wanting to join them in these behaviors. The teen decides to join another group of teens who are engaged in a competitive soccer league in order to meet and become connected to a new group of friends. According to Erikson's eight stages of man, what stage of development is the teenager undergoing? Describe the characteristics of this stage.

According to Erikson, there are eight stages of man and each stage includes a critical personal-social crisis. When the crisis is resolved by the individual, the individual gains a sense of mastery and acquires a personality quality. Erikson identifies the crisis of the teenage years as self-identity versus role diffusion. During this stage, the teenager is challenged to make choices about adult roles. The resolution of this identity crisis provides the teenager with a sense of fidelity and an integrated sense of belonging to and being a member of society.

4. A 16-month-old toddler is brought to occupational therapy for an evaluation. The parents are concerned with the frequency of the toddler's falls, which result in bangs to the head. The child demonstrates delayed motor skills. You notice that the toddler has not yet integrated primitive reflexes. Which primary primitive reflex is most likely absent in this toddler? Explain its relevance to the toddler's health status, safety and its impact on occupational performance.

The toddler likely does not have a protective extension reflex. Protective extension occurs in response to a challenge to an individual's balance and it involves arm extension in the direction of the fall, protecting the head from injury. The forward protective extension reflex develops at 6–9 months, protective extension sideward develops at 7 months, and backward protective extension develops at 9–10 months. This reflex persists upon development. Absence of the protective extension reflex is indicative of a neurological condition or a potential disease process. The absence of the protective extension reflex is a safety concern and may require environmental adaptations and the use of a protective helmet to allow the child to safely participate in gross motor play activities to promote normal growth and development.

5. You provide wellness and prevention services to older adults who attend a community-based senior center. What strategies to slow, reverse and/or compensate for age-related changes to their muscular, skeletal and neurological systems can you share with these older adults?

You can advise the older adults on ways to improve their general health (e.g., stop smoking, exercise regularly) and maintain an adequate nutritional intake (e.g., if budget is limited, use community-based food programs to supplement diet). You should stress that active engagement in functional activities and activity programs can be used to increase their levels of physical activity. Strength training can be used to increase or maintain muscle strength required for functional activity while flexibility and range of motion exercises can be used to increase range of motion. The older adults should be advised to gradually increase the intensity of their physical activity to avoid injury. They should plan and include adequate warm-ups and cool downs and appropriate pacing and rest periods in their routine.

Weight-bearing (gravity-loading) exercises (e.g., walking, stair climbing, all activities performed in standing) can decrease bone loss. You can advise the older adults to allow for increased reaction and movement times to improve accuracy of movements and to avoid long sequences of movements to allow for memory limitations. You can provide safety education to reduce fall risk.

Chapter 6 Review Questions

Musculoskeletal System Disorders

1. You provide post-operative occupational therapy for clients who have undergone tendon repair surgery. You receive a referral for a client diagnosed with a Zone 1 extensor tendon repair. What is this diagnosis typically termed? According to established protocol, what is your diagnostic-specific intervention for the first six weeks? What are the overall goals for tendon repair surgeries that you will use to guide your intervention?

A Zone 1 extensor tendon repair is commonly referred to as a "mallet finger." Standard protocol for extensor tendon repairs at Zone 1 is to immobilize for 6 weeks, 24 hours a day, 7 days a week (except for the performance of skin checks). General occupational therapy goals for tendon repairs are to increase tendon excursion, improve strength at repair site, increase joint ROM, prevent adhesions and facilitate resumption of meaningful roles, occupations and activities.

2. A client incurred a right Colles' fracture. One week ago, the client's cast was removed. You have worked with this client since the initial evaluation and during several intervention sessions. When arriving for the current therapy session, the client is tearful and holding the right arm in a protected position. The client reports that severe pain developed over the weekend in the wrist, hand and shoulder and that it has not gone away. The right hand is swollen and skin is shiny. On a pain scale of 0–10, the client reports a 10+. The client describes an inability (over the past 2 days) to complete exercises and basic self-care activities due to the pain. What do you suspect is causing the client's increase in symptoms? How would you address the client's new presenting symptoms?

This client is presenting symptoms that are typical of complex regional pain syndrome (CRPS), which may follow a trauma such as a Colles' fracture. CRPS symptoms include swelling, shiny skin, pain beyond what is expected for a Colles' fracture, and difficulty using the extremity during ADL. The physician should be contacted and symptoms described. Occupational therapy intervention for CRPS include modalities to decrease pain, edema management (e.g., elevation, manual edema mobilization, compression glove), AROM to involved joints to avoid joint contractures and muscle atrophy, ADL to encourage pain-free active use, stress loading (e.g., weight-bearing and joint distraction activities, including scrubbing and carrying activities), splinting to prevent contractures and self-management to enable the ability to engage in occupation-based activities. Interventions to avoid or to proceed with caution include passive range of motion, passive stretching, joint mobilization, dynamic splinting, and casting.

3. A client is referred to you with a diagnosis of (R) de Quervain's. The client's major complaint is pain when lifting (e.g., the client's newborn child, grocery bags). Pain is reported as 8/10. What findings will you expect upon formal evaluation? What interventions should you implement?

De Quervain's is a tenosynovitis of the first dorsal compartment of the extensor tendons. It is characterized by pain and swelling over the radial styloid and a positive Finkelstein's Test. A forearm-based thumb splint should be fabricated to place the tendons at rest until pain decreases. The client should be instructed in ways to modify lifting and other activities without causing further trauma to the extensor tendons. Ice massage over the radial wrist and gentle AROM of wrist and thumb to prevent stiffness can be used.

4. You receive a referral for a client with a third-degree burn to the hand which includes a prescription for a splint. What is the optimal anti-deformity position you should use to guide your splint construction? Explain your reasoning.

When splinting a person with a burn to the hand, you should position the wrist in 20°–30° extension (increases MCP flexion via tenodesis), MCP joints in 70° flexion (places the collateral ligaments in a lengthened position), IP joints in extension (prevents contracture of the volar plates) and thumb abducted and extended (preserves the first web space).

5. You receive a referral for a person with a diagnosis of carpal tunnel syndrome (CTS). What conservative treatment methods are indicated for this diagnosis?

A splint that positions the wrist in neutral should be provided to the client and the client should be advised to wear the splint at night and during the day when performing repetitive activity. Median nerve gliding exercises and differential tendon gliding exercises should be used. The client should be taught how to modify activities to prevent compression of the median nerve and avoid activities with extreme positions of wrist flexion, wrist flexion with repetitive finger flexion and wrist flexion with a static grip.

6. A child with a diagnosis of osteogenesis imperfecta receives occupational therapy services. What should be the primary foci of occupational therapy intervention? Describe how safety precautions should be integrated into the treatment of a child with osteogenesis imperfecta.

A primary focus of occupational therapy in treating a child with osteogenesis imperfecta is the education of family members, caregivers and educators about proper handling and positioning techniques to use with the child to avoid fractures. As the child grows, interventions must focus on revising these precautions and teaching family members and caregivers to adapt to the demands and environmental challenges encountered by the child (e.g., playground play). The occupational therapist should also reinforce the importance of nutrition for bone health and weight control. Occupational therapy interventions should focus on weight-bearing activities to facilitate bone growth and activities to increase muscle strength. The occupational therapist should also provide school-related activities and environmental modifications to enable participation. Throughout all interventions, precautions to avoid fractures must be followed. For instance, the occupational therapist may fabricate or order special equipment for the child to safely participate in playground or gym activities or design splints to enable the completion of desktop school activities.

Chapter 7 Review Questions

Neurological System Disorders

1. You will be evaluating two persons who have survived strokes. One incurred a left MCA stroke and one incurred a right MCA stroke. What symptoms might each patient present during his/her respective evaluation session?

The person with a left MCA may exhibit right-sided sensory and motor loss, aphasia, apraxia and right visual field loss. The person with a right MCA may exhibit left-sided sensory and motor loss, unilateral neglect, spatial dysfunction and left visual field loss.

2. You are working on a spinal cord unit. You are about to evaluate a client who has an injury classified as ASIA A. The injury is at the C5 level. What is the expected sensory and motor status of your client?

Complete loss of sensation and motor function below the lesion. No sensory or motor function is preserved in the sacral segments.

3. You have just completed your first evaluation session with a client that sustained a TBI 2 weeks ago. Your findings include that the patient was alert and in a heightened state of activity (easily overstimulated) and attempting to pull out the IV and feeding tube. The patient could not remember directions, exhibiting poor short-term memory. The patient screamed out for no reason several times during the session and was observed to be aggressive (e.g., attempting to hit you and the nurse). The patient required maximum assist for BADL. Your facility requires you to document each TBI patient's Rancho Level of Cognitive Function. What is the appropriate level for you to record?

The behaviors described are indicative of Level IV: Confused and Agitated. Rancho Levels I–III present with very low levels of arousal and require total assistance for BADL. Persons at these levels do not respond or respond inconsistently to stimuli. Persons at Rancho Levels V and higher do not demonstrate agitation, they are not aggressive and their ability to participate in ADL continues to improve.

4. During an occupational therapy evaluation of a toddler, you observe that the child tends to sit or lay as placed, without moving. The parent reports that the child shows interest in toys, but never seems to reach out to them or handle them. The child is reported to be a "picky eater" who shows no interest in self-feeding. When you attempt to approach or make eye contact, the child cries. Based on this information, how would you describe the child's disorder to the parent?

This child exhibits signs of sensory modulation disorder, specifically sensory avoidance behaviors. These sensory avoidance behaviors were evidenced in the child's avoidance of movement, avoidance of touching and handling toys or foods, avoidance of eye contact and non-response to being approached.

5. You are working with a child who suddenly has a series of seizures that occur in rapid succession and are prolonged. When the parents are contacted, they report that they ran out of the child's medicine the day before. What type of seizure do these symptoms represent? How should you have responded to in this situation?

The child incurred status epilepticus, which can be triggered by an abrupt disruption of the child's medications. Procedures in responding to status epilepticus include remaining calm and having someone call for immediate medical attention (although rare, sudden death can occur in status epilepticus). You should have removed dangerous objects from the area and protected the child from harm, without interfering with the child's movement. If the child was standing or sitting in a chair, you should have gently guided the child to the floor.

Chapter 8 Review Questions

Cardiovascular and Pulmonary System Disorders

1. An adult with a diagnosis of left ventricular failure congestive heart failure (CHF) has been referred to occupational therapy for Phase I cardiac rehabilitation during an acute hospitalization. What are the primary goals of inpatient cardiac rehabilitation? What symptoms of CHF does the occupational therapist need to be aware of that might manifest during therapeutic activities?

A primary focus of Phase I cardiac rehabilitation is patient and family education about the disease process and recovery. This includes teaching energy conservation and work simplification techniques and the connection between MET levels and activity. Interventions should also focus on improving the person's ability to carry out BADL, including mobility with low-level out of bed functional activities. Decreasing the patient's anxiety around activity performance and support for smoking cessation and dietary modification are also primary goals for Phase I cardiac rehabilitation. The ultimate goal of this phase is to discharge the patient to home and outpatient cardiac rehabilitation. During therapeutic activities, the therapist must be aware that the patient may experience tachycardia, fatigue with activity or mobility, decreased endurance to sustain activity, and/or dyspnea.

2. What are the clinical indications that may lead an occupational therapist to stop an activity during a cardiac rehabilitation intervention session? How does the occupational therapist monitor the patient during activity for signs/symptoms of distress?

Indications that the patient is experiencing an adverse response to treatment include a rise in diastolic blood pressure (BP) greater than or equal to 110 mmHg, a decrease in systolic BP greater than 10 mmHg, significant ventricular or atrial dysrhythmias, second- or third-degree heart block, and signs/symptoms of exercise intolerance including angina and/or marked dyspnea. To monitor a patient for signs/symptoms of distress during activities, the therapist should keep track of the person's vital signs. Vital signs are an important and reliable indicator of activity tolerance and response to treatment. These include heart rate, blood pressure, respiratory rate, and O_2 and CO_2 levels. In addition to monitoring vital signs, the occupational therapist should seek feedback from the patient using angina and dyspnea rating scales, intermittent claudication rating scale, and the BORG Scale for Rating Perceived Exertion.

3. An older adult status-post myocardial infarction (S/P MI) has been referred to occupational therapy for Phase II outpatient cardiac rehabilitation. The client is able to carry out all basic ADL independently and has fair tolerance for activities that require standing and overhead movements. The client lives with a spouse and identifies being a partner, home maintainer, and gardener as primary roles. The client would like to be able to resume role-related activities. The occupational therapy prescription calls for activities beginning at MET level 3 and increasing to MET level 5 according to the patient's activity tolerance. Taking into consideration the therapy prescription, the patient's current status, desired occupational roles, and activity preferences, which treatment approaches and activities should the occupational therapist include in intervention?

The occupational therapist should include energy conservation and work simplification techniques and IADL activities in treatment to address the patient's preferences and goals. Beginning with activities at MET level 3-4, the occupational therapist could include making a bed, sweeping, mopping, and gardening. As the patient tolerates these activities, the therapy program would be upgraded to MET level 4-5 activities including changing bed linens, weeding and raking the garden. A discussion about resuming sexual activity is also appropriate at this level.

4. You have been asked to consult with a teacher to discuss precautions for a student who has a diagnosis of cystic fibrosis. What precautions should you discuss with the teacher? Provide a rationale for your recommendations.

You should inform the teacher about the student's need for adequate nutrition and hydration. Nutrition and hydration are important for managing mucous production. You should advise the teacher to create an inclusive environment to promote social participation and safe participation in physical activities. You should instruct the teacher in energy conservation techniques the student can use during activities. These techniques are required to help the child work toward participating in a full school day. During physical activity, the child should be actively monitored for signs of fatigue and dehydration which may lead to cardiac and respiratory problems.

5. You are completing an evaluation on a 20-month-old toddler who was diagnosed with Bronchopulmonary Dysplasia (BPD) shortly after birth. What are the typical deficits resulting from BPD that the child may exhibit during the occupational evaluation? Provide an explanation for your answers.

Delays may be observed in all areas of development including gross motor, fine motor, visual motor, cognitive and social-emotional development The toddler may present with hypotonia and exhibit fatigue and a low tolerance for physical activity. Poor autonomic and sensory state regulation and poor vision may be evident. Extended time on respirators and artificial ventilation can affect vision and visual motor development and state regulation. Central nervous system problems can lead to contribute to global developmental delays. Malabsorption problems can lead to brittle bones and also to cognitive delays. Because children with BPD experience dependence on technology and lengthy hospitalizations, some children also experience attachment disorders, which may impact social-emotional development and social participation.

Chapter 9 Review Questions

Gastrointestinal, Renal-Genitourinary, Endocrine, Immunological, and Integumentary Systems Disorders

1. You work with clients who have dysphagia and swallowing disorders to develop their feeding skills. What would you do if a client chokes and cannot clear his/her airway during the activity?

If the person gasps for breath, but has a partial or complete airway obstruction, you should clear the obstruction and raise the bolus that has been aspirated. You can use the Heimlich maneuver as long as the person is awake and responsive. If the person loses consciousness, basic life support procedures are used to continue to try to reestablish the airway.

2. If clients have a colostomy or a stoma due to surgery to their bowel, must they have intact fine motor functioning to learn to manage their stoma independently? What can an occupational therapy practitioner do to work with clients to develop their ability to manage their stoma care independently?

It is best for clients with a colostomy or a stoma to have intact fine motor functioning to manage their stoma care. However, they can be taught to compensate using adaptive devices and techniques (e.g., the use of spring clasps verses twist valves). Self-care aspects of stoma care must be addressed for persons with decreased fine motor skills (e.g., individuals with peripheral neuropathy secondary to chemotherapy treatment). The occupational therapist can determine why a person has fine motor impairments. The therapist can plan a course of therapy to improve the person's fine motor ability. If abilities cannot be improved, the therapist can determine the types of adaptations that could be used to substitute for lost functional mobility and train the person in their use.

3. What intervention options are useful for someone who has bladder urgency with stress urinary incontinence and a diagnosis of non-insulin dependent diabetes mellitus?

Intervention might include using Kegel exercises to strengthen the pelvic floor and timed routines for emptying the bladder before it is full enough to cause spillage. Lifestyle adjustments to use incontinence supporting garments for a socially acceptable solution and to decrease public attention to the incontinence are also effective. Medications may be used when the physician feels the client can tolerate the side effects of drug therapy support. Electric stimulation may be used, if the client fits the parameters of recovery for the condition. For example, if the nerve damage is permanent from neuropathy, exercises may not be a useful strategy, since the muscles would not get the enervation needed to effect a change.

4. You are treating an adult client with a diagnosis of scleroderma and colon cancer who was referred to occupational therapy because soft tissue/connective tissue changes are affecting hand function. Would it be appropriate to have a restorative goal for evolving contractures? Describe your rationale.

Yes, it can still be beneficial to try to prevent progression of the contractures using stretching, splinting and scar management principles. By teaching the person to stretch and giving him or her supplies to assist the scar management, he or she can be taught to preserve hand function over time.

5. You work in a community that has people living and working in it who have spinal cord injuries. A primary care doctor refers clients to you who have reddening of skin in their sacral regions. What could you do to work with these clients to improve their skin integrity and prevent decubiti?

You can educate them about conditions that predispose an individual to the formation of decubitus ulcers. These include immobility or altered mobility, weight loss, edema, incontinence, sensory deficiencies, circulatory abnormalities, dehydration, inadequate nutrition, obesity, pathological conditions/multiple comorbidities, and/or changes in skin condition due to aging. You can use principles of lifestyle redesign, habit formation, and/or habit change to plan an individual course of action for behavioral change and improved self-care patterns. If there is presence of substance abuse, cognitive deficits, and/or psychological impairments which can jeopardize the individual's ability to understand and complete the required daily ulcer prevention regimen, you can alter the form of education so that a caregiver can assist with the care plan.

Chapter 10 Review Questions

Psychiatric and Cognitive Disorders

1. You are asked to provide consultation services for an individual who lives in a group home. The resident has become dehydrated and inconsistent in taking oral medications. You interview the resident about his/her daily habits and routines and learn that the resident will not drink the tap water in the group home. The resident states "The water is poisoned. They are trying to poison me. If I drink the water I will die." Identify the psychiatric symptom that is preventing this person from drinking the water. Describe an intervention approach you would use to help the resident hydrate and take prescribed medications. Explain the importance of this person staying hydrated and taking prescribed medications.

This person has a delusion. The best intervention strategy would be to ask the resident if he/she will agree to drink fruit juice or sealed bottles of water which he/she can independently open. Telling the person that the water is not being poisoned would not be an option as one must not argue with or try to refute a delusion, which by definition is a fixed, unshakeable, false belief. Working with the person to ensure consistent hydration is important because dehydration threatens the person's physical health. It is important for the resident to take prescribed medications because it stabilizes the person sufficiently so he/she can live in a less restrictive setting and participate in life within the group home and the community. To increase medication compliance, you can provide external structure and consistency by involving and encouraging the support of caregivers in the group home, establishing a set routine for taking medication (e.g., at a specific time of day such as right before the evening news or after a meal), using medication containers marked with the day of the week, and using calendars or daily checklists. Depending on the type of medication, the use of long acting injections may prove useful in facilitating medication compliance.

2. Upon evaluation of an adolescent you find that the teen has great difficulty reading the various nonverbal behaviors of others (e.g., eye contact, facial expression, gestures and body language) that are needed to regulate social interactions. The adolescent has not been able to develop relationships with a peer group. The teen is preoccupied and intensely interested in World War II, its history, battles, and generals and talks about nothing else. The teen's bedroom is filled with World War II memorabilia and books about the war. This adolescent's cognitive, language and communication skills, and ADL development has been age-appropriate; however the teen has not developed age-appropriate social interaction skills. Based on this information, what diagnosis is most reflective of this teen's functional status? What intervention goals would be helpful to work on with this adolescent?

This adolescent's described behaviors are most reflective of a diagnosis of Asperger's disorder. The teen has difficulty with social interaction, restricted interests and behaviors, adequate language skills, and misses the social interaction cues that others provide. These behaviors impair the adolescent's establishment of peer interactions and relationships. The teen's ADL, cognitive, language, and communication skills are reported as age appropriate, which is often the case for individuals with Asperger's. Intervention goals include increasing social interaction skills. Interventions can include the use of groups. Involvement in extracurricular activities, clubs, and sports may also broaden the adolescent's interests. Depending on the individual, addressing any milestone developmental delays may be necessary to improve age-appropriate interactions, such as impairment in sensorimotor skills. Additional intervention goals may include vocational readiness and community participation. Interventions for adolescents should also include family involvement.

3. You are conducting an evaluation of a 16-month-old toddler. The parent reports that the toddler has frequent tantrums with no clear precipitant. The parent thinks these behaviors may be the result of the toddler's frustration due to language delays. When unable to reach a toy, the toddler pulled the parent's hand toward the toy without pointing. The toddler also did not point to pictures in books. When playing with blocks or cars, the toddler lined them up, but did not spontaneously manipulate or move them. The toddler exhibited a rigid and limited repertoire of play and interaction skills. What diagnosis is most consistent with the toddler's presenting behaviors? Explain your rationale.

The toddler's behaviors are indicative of Autism/ Autism Spectrum Disorder (ASD). Children with Autism/ASD typically have limited communication skills and language. Because pointing to express interest and/or fulfill a need is a primary means of communication, the toddler's non-use of the pointing gesture suggests a lower level of communication skills. This also is indicative of the lack of inferred sharing that is commonly seen in children with ASD. The tantrums reported by the parent may indicate sensory induced behavioral responses that are also common in ASD. The limited and rigid repertoire of play behaviors (as exhibited in the lining up of objects) is also consistent with the play of children with Autism Spectrum Disorder.

4. You are a home health therapist providing services to an elderly client. The client's caregiver reports that the client is having trouble remembering things, sustaining attention, and making decisions. The caregiver reports the client seems mentally confused and asks whether the symptoms are indicative of dementia. As a therapist, you know that there are possible reversible causes of mental confusion. What are the reversible causes of mental confusion that you should consider during your intervention and inform the caregiver to consider for further evaluation?

When working with a client who appears mentally confused, you should always consider the possible reversible causes for mental confusion. These can include sensory changes and problems caused by age-related losses in hearing, vision, and/or touch and sensory overload or deprivation. The client's need for a hearing aid or glasses (and if these prostheses are available and working properly) should also be considered. The client's environment should be assessed because it may lack cues to aid orientation (i.e., clocks and calendars). Other causes for mental confusion that you should consider and inform the caregiver about are depression and drug use or misuse (i.e., drug interactions, medication side effects, poly-medication/the combination of prescription and over-the-counter drugs). Urinary tract infections, viral or bacterial infections, pneumonia or gallbladder disease are often causes of mental confusion in geriatric patients so these need to be ruled out. Metabolic problems such as liver or kidney disease, thyroid disorders, dehydration and poorly controlled diabetes may also present as mental confusion and need to be further assessed by a physician.

5. You observe that a very thin client in your outpatient partial hospital program has been losing weight. The individual has no medical problems. The physician supervising the program states the client is well below the normal weight for age and height. The client participates in cooking groups with peers, but will not eat whatever is prepared other than salad without dressing. When encouraged to try other foods, the client says "I don't want to get fat, and I already need to lose a few pounds." You are concerned that the individual has anorexia nervosa. What signs of this eating disorder are being exhibited? What additional symptoms would you expect to see that would indicate this diagnosis?

The client refuses to maintain a body weight that is normal for age and height and has a fear of gaining weight and becoming fat, even though underweight. There is a disturbance in the way this individual perceives or experiences personal weight and appearance. Other symptoms of this disorder include the undue influence of body weight or shape on self-evaluation and denial of the seriousness of the current low body weight, even if the person were to be hospitalized or seriously ill. If the client is a postmenarchical female, amenorrhea may occur.

Chapter 11 Review Questions

Biomechanical Approaches: Evaluation and Intervention

1. You work in a practice setting which serves many clients with musculoskeletal disorders. The majority of clients have decreased ROM. What are the different types of ROM you should consider during assessment? How should you document your evaluation and its results?

When assessing ROM, you should consider functional ROM, which is the ROM needed to perform functional movements (e.g., reach to top of head to brush hair, reach to the small of the back to tuck a shirt into pants); active ROM (AROM), which is the movement produced by one's own muscle; passive ROM (PROM), which is movement produced by an external force; and active assistive ROM (AAROM), movement produced by one's own muscles and assisted by an external force. When recording ROM measurements, you should always record the starting position and ending position (e.g., 0°–150°) and not use negatives. You can use the terms within functional limits (WFL) to denote that the client's ROM is functional (e.g., can don socks) and within normal limits (WNL) to denote ROM which achieves established ranges (e.g., shoulder flexion 0°–180°).

2. A new client is admitted into an intensive care unit with a diagnosis of a spinal cord injury. The physician requests an evaluation to aide in determining the level of injury. How would you perform a light touch sensory test? How does this method of testing differ from the procedures used during sensory testing for other major diagnostic categories?

When determining sensation of a client diagnosed with a spinal cord injury, the test stimulus (i.e., cotton ball) is presented proximal to distal following dermatomes (beginning at cervical level and moving distal). Following the dermatome pattern will provide you with information about the client's status at each sensory level. When completing sensory testing for neurological disorders, you assess according to dermatome patterns. Peripheral nerve injuries are tested distal to proximal following peripheral nerves.

3. An adult client is having difficulty performing daily activities due to decreased ROM and pain in both shoulders. You decide to treat the client with preparatory interventions followed by an occupation-based intervention. What interventions can you use to increase ROM and decrease pain?

Applying heat and performing gentle passive ROM on the client's shoulders are preparatory interventions. The application of heat prior to stretch can increase extensibility. Manual stretching within the individual's tolerance and contract/relax and hold/relax are additional preparatory methods which can increase ROM. Working with the client to perform activities which require shoulder movements to engage in desired occupational roles (e.g., completing hair care, placing groceries on upper cabinet shelves) would be an appropriate occupation-based intervention.

4. You provide consultation services to a Center for Independent Living which serves persons with a diversity of disabilities. You are scheduled to conduct an educational session on energy conservation and work simplification. What key principles and methods should you be sure to include in your presentation?

You should advise presentation participants to plan short rest periods (e.g., 5–10 minutes) during their daily routine and to schedule daily tasks which alternate between and balance heavy and light work tasks. Tasks that are non-essential and/or those that are beyond personal capacity can be eliminated. To decrease extraneous work, tasks can be combined. Prior to initiating a task, all necessary items and equipment should be gathered. The use of a utility cart, a bucket, walker bag, and/or backpack can be used to carry all items needed in one trip to avoid multiple trips. The participants should be advised to sit to work at a table or use a high stool for counter-top work and to use lightweight equipment, tools, and utensils. Cabinets can be organized so that items are easy to reach and in convenient locations. The sliding of items across counter-tops is preferable to lifting them. Adaptive equipment (e.g., reachers) can be used to avoid bending and stooping and electrical appliances (e.g., mixers) can be used to decrease personal effort. Because intermittent rest during an activity is more effective than resting after exhaustion has occurred, participants should be advised to rest before they experience fatigue.

5. Your client is diagnosed with rotator cuff tendonitis and is experiencing severe pain. The physician has ordered the use of transcutaneous electrical nerve stimulator (TENS), gentle ROM, and below shoulder level ADL. During your evaluation, you review the client's past medical history. You learn that the person has a history of cardiac issues that required the implantation of a pacemaker. Which of the prescribed interventions will you use with this client? What are additional interventions you can use with this client to decrease pain and prepare the person for occupation-based interventions?

Gentle ROM and below shoulder level ADL are appropriate interventions to use with this client. The use of TENs is contraindicated and should not be used with this client. TENS can interfere with the electrical current of the defibrillator. Additional preparatory methods to decrease pain include cryotherapy and superficial heat therapy.

6. Your client is status post a below knee amputation. You assess the strength of the client's triceps in preparation for transfer training. The results of the MMT reveal that the client can take moderate resistance and then break. What muscle grade would you document the client possesses?

A client who can extend against gravity and take moderate resistance has a 4/5 (good) muscle strength.

Chapter 12 Review Questions

Neurological Approaches: Evaluation and Intervention

1. What level of motor control must be present for a person to be a candidate for CIMT?

The person must exhibit at least partial control of the wrist and hand, 20° of extension of the wrist and 10° of extension of each finger or 10° extension of the wrist, 10° abduction of the thumb, and 10° extension of any two other digits or able to lift a wash rag off a table top using any type of prehension and then release it.

2. What is the correct procedure to evaluate the severity of spasticity in a muscle or group of muscles?

Spasticity is evaluated by the elicitation of velocity-dependent stretch reflexes. The limb is quickly stretched in a direction opposite the pull of the muscle group being tested.

3. What is the purpose of applying a static orthosis (splint) to an affected body part?

Utilized for external support, prevention of motion, stretching of contractures, aligning joints for healing, resting joints, or reducing pain.

4. You are working with a client with hemiplegia after a brain tumor resection. The client is learning to transfer using a tub bench for the first time. Thus, the person is at the cognitive stage of learning. According to principles of motor learning, what types of interventions would be appropriate to teach this transfer skill at this stage of learning?

Examples of appropriate types of interventions include having the client demonstrate ideal performance of the task to establish a reference of correctness, verbalize the task components and requirements, point out similarities to other learned tasks (e.g., a toilet transfer), direct attention to critical task elements (e.g., lock brakes for safety, judge height of the tub), use blocked practice (i.e. repeated practice of the transfer), encourage the use of mental practice, use manual guidance to assist as appropriate (e.g., guiding legs over and into the tub), break the tasks down to component parts (e.g., wheelchair alignment and management, sit to stand).

5. You receive a referral for occupational therapy services for a toddler. The parents report that the toddler dislikes changes to daily routines, meeting strangers, and being touched. During your evaluation, you observe that the toddler does not like to move or explore unfamiliar objects and toys. Upon analysis of evaluation results, you determine that the toddler is over-responsive to sensory stimuli and avoids all sensory experiences. According to the principles of Ayres Sensory Integration® approach, what types of sensory stimuli should you introduce during interventions with this toddler and how should you structure your initial intervention sessions? Explain your rationale.

You should introduce controlled sensory activities that simultaneously combine vestibular and proprioceptive stimuli. It would be best to begin with the toddler in the prone position and provide slow linear movement combined with joint compression and deep firm touch pressure. You should observe, monitor and adjust stimuli that influence modulation. You should be alert to the toddler's behavioral responses and assess these during treatment and up to a few hours following treatment. Slow linear movement combined with firm deep touch and pressure resistance is less threatening than light touch. When combined these inputs have an integrative effect.

Chapter 13 Review Questions

Cognitive-Perceptual Approaches: Evaluation and Intervention

1. You are observing a client with apraxia eat breakfast. What behaviors would you most likely observe?

   You may see problems with tool use, such as stirring coffee with a knife or eating cereal with a fork. You would observe difficulty with the sequencing of the steps of the task, such as eating cereal without first pouring the milk into it. In severe cases, the person will not perform the task at all. He or she will stare blankly at the breakfast tray as the concept of the task of eating breakfast will have been completely lost.

2. Your client presents with unilateral spatial neglect and poor awareness. The client has a supportive partner. What environmental modifications will be useful to maximize performance and safety indoors?

   Place perceptual anchors (e.g., brightly colored objects or strips of colored tape) in the places where the person usually engages in occupation. Place necessary grooming objects on the left side of the sink. Reorganize closets and dressers so that needed items are biased to the left. Place cell phones or safety alert systems in the person's right shirt pocket.

3. What are examples of activities you can use to evaluate components of attention?

   Activities which require vigilance (e.g., reading or listening to the news) can be used to assess sustained attention. Engaging the client in two tasks (e.g., as making tea and toast) can determine divided attention skills. Engaging the client in activities in an environment that is stimulating (e.g., a cafeteria or playground) can determine selective attention abilities.

4. Your client has left-sided body neglect. Describe the behaviors would you expect to see during the person's morning self-care routine.

   You may observe the person spending more time combing the right side of his/her hair as compared to the left. The person may not shave or only partially shave the left side of the face or legs. He or she may not engage the left arm in the task despite having the physical capacity.

5. You are working in acute care with a person with low arousal after a head trauma. Describe approaches and activities that would be useful to include during interventions with this person.

   The use of sensory stimulating activities would be beneficial. Examples include washing the face and upper body with a cold wash cloth, using a loud and direct voice when cuing, providing visually stimulating objects, turning all lights on, opening bedroom curtains, sitting the person up to provide vestibular input, and playing music.

Chapter 14 Review Questions

Psychosocial Approaches: Evaluation and Intervention

1. What are key general postulates for change that are used in cognitive behavioral therapy (CBT) to guide the intervention process? How can these be applied throughout the occupational therapy process?

According to CBT, dysfunctional thought processes produce or lead to the development of mental health symptoms and can result in psychological dysfunction and/or psychiatric disorders. Negative thoughts, which are considered a dysfunctional process in CBT, function as a sustaining factor for illnesses such as depression. CBT proposes that altering a person's cognition can improve psychological health. In occupational therapy, a practitioner can help the person alter dysfunctional thoughts and cognitive processes by addressing them through the use of CBT interventions. For example, using work sheets in psychoeducational groups or individual sessions can assist clients in looking at their perceptions of their problems, situations and/or feelings. CBT interventions are also used to help clients make changes that can lead to improved emotional health.

2. Identify three evaluation tools that can be used to assess an individual's cognitive level according to the Cognitive Disabilities model. Describe a practice situation in which each evaluation would be most effectively used.

The Allen Cognitive Level Screen-5 (ACLS-5) is a structured task that allows the therapist to observe the individual performing three increasingly complex leather lacing stitches. Based on these observations, the therapist makes determinations about that person's cognitive skill level. Guidelines are available for designing other tasks that will also elicit the component skills of each level. (See this chapter's evaluation section.) In practice, the ACLS-5 can be used in any setting where the practitioner's observations lead him or her to believe that the client is experiencing cognitive dysfunction. The ACLS-5 can be effectively used, in conjunction with other evaluations, to assist in intervention and discharge planning. Clinical settings where adult individuals present with a traumatic brain injury (TBI), CVA, or mental health disorders are among the various settings where this evaluation can be used. For example, veterans hospitals would be a current setting that may use the ACLS-5 because many returning soldiers present with TBIs.

The Routine Task Inventory (RTI) gathers data about the individual's ADL performance from an informed caregiver. See Chapter 15. Therapists practicing in home health may use the information obtained from this evaluation to improve a patient's ADL performance by providing activity adaptations and making home modifications as indicated. Based on the RTI results, the therapist can also provide patient and family education to enhance occupational performance and ease caregiver burden.

The Cognitive Performance Test (CPT) was designed to assess the functional performance of individuals with Alzheimer's disease. The focus is on the identification of the effects that particular deficits have on the performance of ADL. This test can be used in any clinical situation where individuals present with the symptoms of Alzheimer's disease. The CPT can screen and identify for low level cognitive ability to refine the results of the occupational therapy evaluation.

3. Describe five current intervention approaches that use sensory models to guide treatment and how they can be effectively applied in occupational therapy practice.

The use of "Snoezelen" multi-sensory environments can be effective in calming or alerting individuals with psychiatric illness, autism, pervasive developmental disorders, and dementia. Such rooms can be used with an individual or with a group depending upon intervention goals and objectives. The use of therapeutic weighted blankets, dolls, and stuffed animals can also be used as a modality to assist in self-soothing and as an alternative to the use of restraints in inpatient mental health settings, skilled nursing facilities, and/ or any setting where individuals could benefit from interventions to decrease agitation. "Comfort Rooms" are increasingly used as an alternative to restraints in mental health settings. Occupational therapists' unique knowledge in creating comfort rooms based on sensory principles can be very useful in increasing the efficacy of these rooms, particularly in acute, inpatient psychiatric settings.

Occupational therapists can also use a psycho-education approach along with sensory models during intervention. For example, after the administration of an evaluation such as the Adolescent and Adult Sensory Profile, the therapist can use worksheets in a group to help clients identify their reactions to sensory input and learn adaptive ways of coping with their sensory issues. Sensory diets including alerting/calming stimuli and heavy work patterns can be provided in any setting by occupational therapists and individualized to the specific sensory needs of the client. By helping clients learn how to use their sensory diets whenever sensory processing issues arise, occupational therapists can extend the effective use of occupational therapy interventions throughout the day.

4. Describe interventions that can effectively help individuals experiencing hallucinations and/or delusions manage their symptoms during an occupational therapy group.

Therapists can create an environment free of the distractions that trigger hallucinatory and/or delusionary thoughts and interfere with the performance of a reality-based activity for the individual. Therapists can use highly structured simple, concrete and tangible activities that hold the individual's attention (e.g., craft projects or meal preparation tasks) to provide reality-based experiences. These activities can be used to successfully redirect persons experiencing hallucinations and/or delusions and help move their focus away from the internal stimuli they are experiencing to refocus on their task. When a person is observed experiencing a hallucination or expressing a delusion, the therapist can intervene with verbalizations about what the client is doing with respect to the activity and facilitate reality-based thinking and actions. A good clinical example is when clients work in a greenhouse which provides the opportunity to engage in simple concrete tasks such as planting, pruning, and watering. Their participation in reality-based activities, the setting's consistent structure, and the therapist's positive feedback can effectively help clients manage their psychotic symptoms.

5. The RADAR approach is used to screen for and respond to domestic abuse. How would an occupational therapist apply this approach?

R = Routinely ask. During evaluation sessions, the therapist should routinely ask appropriate questions to screen for abuse. Inquiring about potential abuse when interviewing all clients can be the first step in intervention because this acknowledges that abuse is not an acceptable secret.

A = Affirm and ask. Acknowledge and support the person who discloses abuse at anytime throughout the OT process. Ask direct questions of all clients to determine risk (e.g., Do you feel safe with your partner? Are you afraid when he/she comes home?).

D = Document objective findings whenever anything that may be indicative of abuse is observed (e.g., the person has multiple bruises) and record client statements in quotes (e.g., "I am scared to go home"). This information can establish useful clinical evidence.

A = Assess and address the person's safety (i.e., Has abuse become more violent? Are there weapons in the home?). This can help determine the urgency for action by the therapist to help the person remain safe.

R = Review options and referrals. As needed, refer the person to domestic violence hotlines, domestic violence shelters, and/or safe houses which have staff trained in family violence and safety planning. This is an essential and ethical step in preventing further domestic violence experiences. Therapists should always have the contact information for these resources readily available. The public display of these resources in occupational therapy practice settings can also diminish the silence which enshrouds domestic violence.

6. You are watching television with your roommate in the eighth-floor apartment you share. You observe a very sad, withdrawn appearance and minimal spontaneous social interaction. Lately your roommate has been drinking more than usual on social occasions and this week cancelled a scheduled weekly therapy appointment. You ask if everything is alright, and the reply is "no, not really." "I'm thinking of killing myself, I just can't take it anymore." "How do you think you would do it?" you ask. "I'm not quite sure, I think I have a couple of options here, belts, knives, I'm not sure which way I want to go, but I have to do it soon, maybe by the end of the week. Yes, definitely by the end of the week. All things considered, I think I'll jump out the window. I'm pretty sure the fall would kill me." What risk factors for suicide are you observing in your roommate, what levels of suicide lethality are present, and what should be your first intervention?

The risk factors for suicide based on this scenario is a sad affect, limited interaction or social isolation and withdrawal, a mental health history, increased alcohol use, and a verbalized suicidal statement, which must be taken seriously. The roommate has suicidal ideation and a plan and intent, which presents a great potential risk for attempting suicide. Assessing this situation, your first plan of action is to stay with and not allow your roommate to be alone at any moment. You should encourage your roommate to go to the emergency room, call the doctor or therapist, and/or call the National Suicide Hotline 1-800-273-TALK (8255). If those interventions are ineffective and it cannot be done without leaving the individual alone, you should call 911.

7. You are conducting a group for individuals with recently acquired spinal cord injuries that now have paraplegia and need to use a wheelchair for mobility. Adjusting to this abrupt change in their lives has been difficult and group members have developed depression. Several have anger issues as well. While participating in a group, one of the participants says to you "you really have no idea what it's like to have to face using a wheelchair for the rest of your life, when just a month ago I ran my sixth marathon. Running has been my whole life. It was the way I relieved stress and stayed in shape. I guess that's all over now." What type of therapeutic approach should you take? What types of individual and group interventions might benefit this individual?

   In this case, validation of this person's feelings is indicated by making statements such as "I can only imagine what you are going through. I respect your perspective on your experience. I know and accept that this is a hard adjustment, not being able to run, or walk for that matter, and on top of that you need to use a wheelchair. I can understand why you are concerned about how to manage stress and stay active." This acknowledges the person's loss issues and may establish rapport and trust as you do not attempt to assume to know how the person feels. In providing a client-centered approach, you would next ask the group member to identify personal treatment goals. You would then provide individual or group interventions based on this feedback. Appropriate interventions would include addressing the person's wish to be involved in running and athletics and providing psychoeducational groups for anger management and the development of adaptive coping skills. Thematic or patient and family education to address lifestyle changes and resultant depression and to develop a plan for recovery are also appropriate.

Chapter 15 Review Questions

Evaluation and Intervention for Performance in Areas of Occupation

1. The supervisor of a hospital-based occupational therapy department which provides services to persons with medical conditions and physical disabilities is reviewing its guidelines for the evaluation of BADL with newly hired therapists. What assessments should the supervisor identify as core evaluations for all therapists (including entry-level therapists) to include in their "toolbox"? What assessments should the supervisor identify as requiring therapists to complete additional training prior to their use?

Core BADL evaluations for all therapists to include in their "toolbox" include the Barthel Index, Katz Index of ADL, and the Klein-Bell Activities of Daily Living Scale (K-B Scale). BADL assessments that require additional training beyond entry-level occupational therapy education are the Assessment of Motor and Process Skills (AMPS) and the FIM System (originally called the Functional Independence Measure).

2. A person with a C-7 SCI sets a goal to return to work as an accountant. The person expresses concern over the ability to complete a morning self-care routine and job tasks. What will be realistic for the person to expect to be able to do after receiving occupational therapy services to develop self-care and work skills?

At C-7, the person can use a tenodesis grasp or splint to perform many tasks. Thus, the person can expect to be independent in feeding, grooming, and dressing. A button hook may be used, if needed. The person will be able to transfer independently using depression transfers. For bathing, a handheld shower head and a tub bench are needed. At work, the person will be able to independently hold a phone, typing stick, and pen using a tenodesis grasp or splint. Thus, the person can expect to be able to independently complete work tasks requiring the use of a calculator, computer, and telephone.

3. An occupational therapist seeks to ensure that the BADL of sexual activity is addressed throughout the OT process. Which model can help the therapist achieve this aim? Describe the key points of this model.

The occupational therapist can use the PLISSIT model as a guide to address sexual activity throughout the OT process. In this model, the "P" stands for "permission" which requires the therapist to create an atmosphere which gives the individual permission to raise concerns about his/her sexuality and sexual activity(ies). This can be accomplished by incorporating sexuality into the OT initial and ongoing evaluation in a matter-of-fact manner. "LI" represents "limited information" which the the therapist can provide to ensure that the individual has accurate knowledge about his/her sexual abilities and potentials. The therapist can share facts (e.g., there is sex after disability) and dispel myths (e.g., people with disabilities are asexual). "S" stands for "specific suggestions" that the therapist can provide to facilitate the individual's pursuit of satisfying sexual activities, either alone or with a partner. These can include strategies for achieving clients' goals for sexual expression (e.g., energy conservation methods, the use of nonmedical methods to manage pain and stiffness, positioning alternatives and adaptive equipment, and applying principles of activity analysis, gradation, modification, and simplification to sexual activities). In this model, "IT" represents "intensive therapy" which is indicated when the individual requires intervention for long-standing relationship problems and/or enduring sexual problems. The application of this part of the PLISSIT model requires specialized training, so the therapist would complete a referral to the appropriate professional (e.g., marriage counselor, sex therapist) if indicated.

4. An occupational therapist provides consultation to a local business which employs people with cognitive limitations due to psychiatric, physical, and intellectual disabilities. What strategies should the therapist share with employers to increase their employees' ability to manage time, concentrate, and focus on multiple tasks at the same time during the work day?

To help the employees manage time, the employer can provide directive commands on a regular basis and maintain structure through a daily time and task schedule using hourly goals. The provision of positive reinforcement when tasks are completed within the expected time lines is also helpful. To improve employees' concentration and management of multiple tasks, the employer can put each work request in writing and leave it in a "to do" box to avoid interrupting the employees' work in progress. The provision of good working conditions (e.g., adequate light, reduced noise, a separate work area to reduce noise and interruptions) can also help employees concentrate. The number of tasks that need to be completed simultaneously can be decreased or eliminated and priorities for task completion can be established. All work tasks can be put in writing with due dates or times identified. Tasks among employees with the same responsibilities can be redistributed, so that each can do more of one type of job task than a lot of different tasks.

5. During an occupational therapy screening, a client reports feeling tired all of the time. What should the occupational therapist be sure to address during evaluation?

The therapist should assess the person's ability to identify the need for restorative rest and sleep, his/her typical rest and sleep patterns and routines, and obstacles to the attainment and maintenance of satisfying rest and sleep. In addition, personal issues (e.g., being a "light" sleeper who awakens easily), pathophysiological changes related to disease, disability, and/or the aging process (e.g., chronic pain, unrelenting fatigue), and socio-cultural barriers (e.g., night shift job work) should be considered. The therapist can use sleep checklists and sleep diaries to obtain detailed information.

Chapter 16 Review Questions

Mastery of the Environment: Evaluation and Intervention

1. An occupational therapist provides consultation services to a group of religious organizations who want to improve the accessibility of the entrances to their buildings. All entrances currently have stairs. What should the occupational therapist recommend to allow access for persons who use mobility aides (e.g., walkers and canes) and wheelchairs?

The therapist should recommend the installation of railings on the stairs and ramps as an alternative to the stairs. The exterior railings should be placed at 36″. This is the average of the recommended 34″–38″ waist height for those who walk (variance depends on people's height). The railings should be $1^1/_2$″–2″ in diameter with non-skid surfaces. The ramps should be built with a ratio of slope to rise of 1:12. The ramps should be a minimum of 36″ wide with a non-skid surface. Ramp railings should be at the average of 32″ high. If possible two railings (one lower and one higher) should be provided to allow for differences in people's arm reach. Curbs on the ramps should be at least 4″ high. Level platforms should be included in the ramp design. If the ramp is excessively long, 4′ × 4′ landing(s) are needed to allow for rest. If a sharp turn is needed in the direction of the ramp, a landing for turning space is needed. A 90° turn will require a minimum 4′ × 4′ landing; a 180° turn will require a minimum 4′ × 8′ landing. At the top of the ramp, a 5′ × 5′ platform is needed before the door to allow for persons in a wheelchair to swing the door without backing up. Electronic opening doors are optimal. If these are not feasible, doors should be able to be opened with a closed fist via the use of lever handles or push bars. Objects which may obstruct entrance ways should be removed (e.g., planters, garbage cans).

2. An occupational therapist provides a weekly home safety group to members of a senior center. What strategies should the therapist recommend the group members use inside and outside their homes to prevent falls?

The therapist should recommend that the members ensure that their living spaces have adequate lighting with no loose electrical cords, minimal clutter, firmly attached carpet, and furniture arranged for easy maneuverability. For homes with stairs, the therapist should recommend that members make sure that there are stair handrails securely fastened on both sides of the stairs. There should be light switches at the top and bottom of the stairs and the stairs should be covered by a non-skid secure surface. In the bathrooms, members should have grab bars located in and out of tubs and shower stalls and near toilets. The use of nonskid mats, nightlights, and an elevated toilet seat are also effective in decreasing fall risk. Good recommendations for the therapist to make to prevent falls in the bedroom are the installation of night lights or light switches within reach of the bed, the placement of telephones in an easy to reach position near the bed, and the use of a mattress which is at a height that makes it easy to get in and out of bed. In the members' living areas, the therapist should advise the members to be sure their couches and chairs are at proper height to get in and out of easily. To decrease fall risk in the kitchen, the therapist should advise members to store items on reachable shelves (i.e., between the person's eye and hip level). Outside the home, members should be sure that cracked pavement or steps are fixed and stable handrails are installed if there are steps.

3. A client is status-post posterolateral hip replacement surgery. What recommendations should the therapist make for bed mobility?

The therapist should advise the person to not roll on the non-operated side because this may result in internal rotation of the operated hip, which may cause dislocation. An abductor pillow between the lower extremities can be used to prevent adduction of the operated hip. The therapist should recommend that the person does not flex the hip beyond 90° or internally rotate or pivot at the hip. The therapist should teach the person to transfer by keeping operated the hip in slight abduction and extended out in front.

4. A school-based occupational therapist provides recommendations for alternative access modes to computers to compensate for a diversity of disabilities and maximize students' independence in the school environment. What adaptations can the therapist recommend? Explain their use.

The therapist can recommend programmable keyboards that allow for customized overlays (e.g., enlarged letters and numbers for students with low vision; graphics and symbols for students with cognitive impairments). Key guards and expanded keyboards that provide large keys can be helpful for students with limited motor accuracy and control (e.g., students with ataxia). Contracted keyboards that provide smaller keys in a constrained space can be useful for students with limited range of motion and functional motor control (e.g., students with arthritis) and light-touch keyboard activation systems can be useful for students with decreased strength and/or mobility (e.g., students with muscular dystrophy). The therapist can recommend delayed touch keyboard activation systems for students with poor motor control (e.g., students with athetoid movements) and chorded keyboards (which consist of a few keys which generate standard characters by pressing various combinations of keys) for students who use only one hand (e.g., students with hemiplegia). Finally, eye gaze and voice activated computers can be useful for students with severe mobility impairments (e.g., upper extremity contractures).

5. An occupational therapist begins employment at a new skilled nursing facility (SNF). To ensure compliance with OBRA and reduce the use of restraints in the facility, what policies and procedures should the therapist have the SNF administrators implement?

All staff should be aware of the conditions and situations that can contribute to agitated, restless, and/or wandering behaviors. These include pain, physical discomfort, hunger, thirst, need for toileting, loneliness, fear, boredom, and an unfamiliar environment. Staff should be trained in the provision of interventions which can effectively address these contributing factors and correct underlying problems without the use of restraints. These can include active listening, attention to underlying feelings and expressed concerns to promote trust, a medical evaluation for pain management, proper positioning, an adequate and client-directed toileting routine, and the provision of snacks, unbreakable water bottles, or other appropriate safe source of nourishment and hydration. Family, peer, and/or pastoral visits; animal-assisted or pet therapy; and social, leisure, and physical activities can also be helpful in decreasing agitated, restless, and/or wandering behaviors. Activities should be provided at night as well as in the day. Loudspeaker and other extraneous noise should be eliminated and replaced with soft soothing background music. All resident rooms should include familiar and favorite objects to personalize them. A structured home-like environment with a set routine should be provided to promote a sense of safety and security. Contained areas should be interesting and safe. Furniture should be arranged to deter wandering with a variety of comfortable seating and furniture provided including broad-based rockers and footstools.

Guidelines for Effective Use of the Computer-Based Examinations

The computer disk included with this text has three exams designed to simulate the NBCOT exam. We strongly advise that you do *NOT* take a simulated exam until after you have reviewed the content of this text. Taking an exam before you have studied the information that will be tested on the NBCOT exam will only reinforce all you do not know. In contrast, taking your first exam after you have studied will provide more specific feedback on your strengths and weaknesses. This information can be then used to develop a targeted study plan and acquire mastery of the knowledge you need to pass the NBCOT exam.

Like the NBCOT exam, each exam on the disc begins with three simulation test (ST) items followed by 170 multiple choice (MC) items. This replication of the NBCOT format enables you to simulate the NBCOT exam experience. Therefore, we advise you to complete each of the TherapyEd exams during a four-hour period with any breaks you take included in the total time. This will allow you to practice your timing for your actual NBCOT exam. As discussed in Chapter 1, we recommend you spend 10–12 minutes to complete each of the three ST problems for a total of 30–36 minutes for this exam section. This will give you approximately 3 ½ hours to complete the 170 MC items.

Because the exam clock stops when you complete and exit the ST section, you can take a brief break. Before you begin the MC section, the NBCOT exam offers a short (about 10–15 minutes) tutorial about the MC section that does not count toward the exam administration time. Once you begin the MC section, the exam clock keeps running until you exit the exam. Thus, the tutorial break is a good time to pause and congratulate yourself on the successful completion of the ST section and re-focus your thoughts on the most effective ways to answer MC items. If you need to take a brief break during your completion of the MC section, do so; sometimes a short break can help restore energy and focus. Do not, however, add this time to your four-hour simulated exam session. During both the ST and MC sections, the exam clock keeps running and does not stop until you exit each exam section.

Upon completing each TherapyEd computer-based exam, you will receive an analysis of your exam performance. This detailed analysis will identify which items you answered incorrectly. Extensive rationales for correct and incorrect answers are provided in this text section. ***DO NOT*** read these rationales until after you have completed the exam in its computerized format. The computer analysis of your performance on the MC items will also give you an indication of your strengths and weaknesses according to the content categories and critical reasoning strategies listed after this introduction. To ensure you obtain a complete picture of your content knowledge, you should supplement the computer analysis of your performance on the MC items with a personal review of the content category designations that are provided in this text section for each of the ST item answer choices.

After reviewing the answer rationales for the ST and MC exam items, the computerized analysis of your performance in the specific content areas, and your self-assessment of the Simulation test content categories, you should revise your study plan. To help you know what to study, the content categories are labeled in accordance with this text's chapter titles. You should also reflect on the feedback provided on your critical reasoning strategies. If the analysis of your exam performance identifies difficulty with a specific area of reasoning, review the self-assessment questions and the exam preparation guidelines provided in Table 5 in Chapter 2.

After implementing your revised study plan and using effective exam preparation strategies, complete the second computer-based exam. Use your next exam performance analysis to further revise your study plan. After implementing this revised study plan, take the third exam. Use the feedback provided on this exam to further revise your study plan and implement your final exam preparations before your NBCOT exam.

If you realize the feedback provided indicates you are particularly weak in one content area (e.g., pediatric practice), the computer program will allow you to "design" a content-specific exam of MC items. Using this feature can help you further assess the efficacy of your study plan. Additional guidelines for effective examination preparation are provided in Chapter 2 of this text. The feedback provided for some of the ST item answers may be more extensive than the feedback on your NBCOT exam. We provide additional information in our feedback because our focus is on preparing you for exam success and these feedback boxes provide effective "teachable moments."

It is important to understand your performance on these practice exams is *not* predictive of your future performance on the NBCOT exam. Many students who successfully pass the NBCOT exam have reported less than perfect scores on the TherapyEd exams. Remember, the items on these practice tests are *purposefully* designed to assist you in developing, critiquing, and revising your study plan so you are well prepared for the NBCOT exam. Therefore, if your scores on these exams are less than you anticipated you should critically review the rationales for the answers, as well as the computerized content analysis of your performance on the MC items and the content category designations for the ST items.

If the items you are getting wrong are scattered over a number of content areas and your errors tend to be made on the more complex and/or harder questions, it is likely that you will do well on the exam *if* you understand the item rationales upon reviewing them. If your wrong answers are clustered in a major content area, you should revise your study plan to be sure you develop the foundational knowledge of this area before you take your examination. Similarly, if most of your wrong answers indicate the persistence of a test-taking personality that is not effective for exam success (e.g., changing your answers without a good reason, reading into the question), you should practice the behavioral management strategies identified in Table 2-4 of this text before taking your exam. As previously noted, if the analysis of your exam performance identifies difficulty with a specific area of reasoning, review the self-assessment questions and the exam preparation guidelines provided in Table 5 in Chapter 2.

We believe engaging in this extensive (and at times challenging) preparation based on your simulated exam performance is far better than being under-prepared for the high-stakes NBCOT exam. Students consistently report the time they spend taking the TherapyEd exams, reviewing the answer rationales, and revising their study plans is well worth the effort when they successfully pass the NBCOT exam on their first attempt.

Content Categories

C1 Human Development and Aging
C2 The Process of Occupational Therapy
C3 Musculoskeletal System Disorders and Biomechanical Approaches
C4 Neurological System and Neurological Approaches
C5 Cardiopulmonary, Gastrointestinal, Renal-genitourinary, Immunological, Endocrine, and Integumentary System Disorders and Evaluation and Intervention Approaches
C6 Psychiatric Disorders and Psychosocial Approaches
C7 Cognitive-perceptual Disorders and Approaches
C8 Evaluation and Intervention for Performance in Areas of Occupation and Environmental Mastery
C9 Professional Standards and Responsibilities

CRITICAL REASONING STRATEGIES

Inductive Reasoning

Inference

Analysis

Deductive Reasoning

Evaluation

Examination A

Simulation Test Item A.I.

Opening Scene:

An adult with chronic obstructive pulmonary disease (COPD) is admitted to a rehabilitation facility after a brief hospital stay for stabilization. The patient is deconditioned and fatigues easily. Prior to hospitalization, the patient lived with a spouse and worked full-time as a home inspector. The occupational therapist receives a physician order for evaluation and treatment.

Section A

The occupational therapist is preparing to evaluate the patient to determine functional abilities and premorbid status. The patient uses two liters of oxygen and complains of shortness of breath during most activities. Which approaches should the occupational therapist include during the evaluation process? Choose all that apply.

1. C5 Provide education and information about smoking cessation.

Feedback: The patient becomes irritated and exclaims, "I don't smoke!"

Outcome and Rationale: Not all patients develop COPD from smoking. The background information provided did not indicate that the patient smoked. The therapist should not automatically assume that smoking is a contributing factor for a patient's COPD. It is important to remember that this section of the ST item is about evaluation, not intervention. It is inappropriate to provide interventions without an evaluation. A better approach that would be consistent with the evaluation stage of the OT process would be to determine past habits and routines that contributed to the patient's condition. This information can then be used to determine appropriate intervention approaches. Moreover, this choice created patient distress. This action would not be reimbursable since it is not an evaluation and is not relevant to the patient's status or based on any reported information about the patient's lifestyle. Consequently, the selection of this option would result in a loss of points.

2. C2 Interview the patient about everyday routine and habits at home.

Feedback: The patient reports independent performance of all BADL and home maintenance tasks prior to hospitalization.

Outcome and Rationale: Determining the patient's prior routine and level of functioning is a pivotal aspect of the evaluation process. This approach can provide the basis for effective intervention planning and implementation to promote the patient's return to his/her prior living situation and prior level of independence. This choice has a positive impact and therefore would result in receiving points.

3. C3 Administer manual muscle test to determine current level of strength.

Feedback: The patient demonstrates weakness in bilateral upper extremities, with level 4 of 5 strength in the shoulders and 4 of 5 strength in the elbows and hands.

Outcome and Rationale: Manual muscle testing is an important part of the evaluation process to determine functional abilities that relate directly to ADL skills. This provides the basis for intervention planning and implementation to improve strength and endurance in functional skills. This choice has a positive impact and would result in receiving points.

4. C8 Demonstrate the use of a reacher, dressing stick, and sock aide to promote ADL independence.

Feedback: The patient thanks the therapist for this demonstration.

Outcome and Rationale: While the demonstration of adaptive equipment may be informative to this patient, it is premature at this time. It is important to remember that this section of the ST item is about evaluation, not intervention. It is inappropriate to provide interventions without an evaluation. A therapist should not demonstrate adaptive devices until after a comprehensive ADL evaluation has been completed to determine if the equipment is needed. Based on the evaluation results, the therapist can then recommend and demonstrate equipment. Recommending equipment without an evaluation also incurs an unjustified expense. Since this action was premature, its selection reflects poor understanding of the OT process and it is fiscally unsound. Therefore, the selection of this action is negative and it would result in a loss of points.

5. C5 Assess ability to persist in activity by having the patient walk on a treadmill until fatigued.

Feedback: The patient complains of extreme fatigue and dizziness during the activity. The patient stops and is very short of breath.

Outcome and Rationale: The goal of pulmonary rehabilitation is to build tolerance to activity over time as functional abilities improve. Assessing the patient's ability to perform an activity such as treadmill walking is too much for a patient who has just been discharged from a hospital. This activity is likely to invoke shortness of breath and reduced oxygen capacity, which leads to dizziness. The evaluation should first determine all of the patient's capabilities and limitations prior to implementing an activity that tests pulmonary capacity. This choice has a negative impact on the patient and an entry-level practitioner should know that this is contraindicated for this patient at this stage of the therapy process. Consequently, it would result in a loss of points.

6. C5 Use pulseoximeter to determine oxygen levels at rest and with activity.

Feedback: Pulse oximetry readings indicate 92% at rest and 87% with seated activities.

Outcome and Rationale: Pulse oximetry is an important part of the pulmonary rehabilitation process. The therapist must monitor saturation levels both while at rest and during functional activities. The oximeter is left on the patient while engaging in activities to monitor the trends and changes. It should not be used for "spot checks" as this provides an incomplete picture of the patient's saturation changes with activity. This choice has a positive impact and would result in receiving points.

7. C8 Administer a career exploration questionnaire.

Feedback: The patient reports satisfaction with current job and refuses to complete the questionnaire.

Outcome and Rationale: There is no information provided in this scenario to indicate that the patient needs to explore careers; therefore, this action is premature. The patient has the ability to improve functional abilities and potentially return to his/her existing job. A vocational evaluation is typically initiated later in the therapy process after ADL and IADL skills have improved. Career exploration would only be sought if the patient is unable to return to his/her previous vocation or states a desire for a career change. This action does not move the patient forward in the therapy process, but it did not harm the patient to receive the questionnaire. Therefore, this selection is neutral and would not result in receiving or losing points.

8. C8 Assess performance in basic ADL skills.

Feedback: The patient requires minimal assistance for bathing and dressing the lower body and set-up and rest periods for upper body care and grooming.

Outcome and Rationale: Performing a basic ADL evaluation is an important aspect of the evaluation process in order to determine the patient's limitations and functional abilities. With this information, effective intervention planning can be designed and relevant intervention approaches implemented to promote functional recovery to the baseline level at home. This is a positive choice and would result in receiving points.

9. C5 Increase oxygen intake to 3 liters during periods of shortness of breath.

Feedback: The head nurse asks the therapist why oxygen was increased without a physician's order.

Outcome and Rationale: An occupational therapist is not allowed to make changes in a patient's level of oxygen intake without standing orders by the physician in charge of the patient's care. Changes in oxygen intake (either by increasing or decreasing levels) can have detrimental effects on the patient's well-being, which is why a physician must approve all changes. This choice has a negative impact and would result in the loss of points.

Section B

Evaluation results reveal that the patient is deconditioned with deficits in upper body strength, endurance, and basic ADL. The patient's goals are to return home at the pre-morbid level, which includes no oxygen use and full-time employment as a home inspector. This job requires climbing on ladders, bending, squatting, and standing for up to 20 minutes at a time. In initiating intervention, which activities should the OT use? Choose all that apply.

1. C5 Incorporate pursed-lip strategies into basic ADL.

Feedback: The patient states feeling less short of breath when completing ADL.

Outcome and Rationale: Pursed-lip breathing techniques are an important facet of pulmonary rehabilitation. With these techniques, the patient focuses on breathing patterns and maximizing use of the diaphragm when inhaling, rather than accessory muscles around the shoulder girdle. This maximizes oxygen saturation and reduces stress on the cardiovascular system during stressful activities. This selection is beneficial for the patient and therefore would result in receiving points.

2. C5 Provide informative brochures about the symptoms and progression of COPD.

Feedback: The patient thanks the therapist for the information.

Outcome and Rationale: Having accurate information about the disease process is beneficial to patients. However, it is likely that the patient has already received this information since the COPD diagnosis is a long-standing one (present prior to hospitalization) and the patient was just hospitalized for a recent exacerbation of symptoms. This action does not harm the patient but does it not move the patient forward in the therapy process. Therefore, this selection is neutral and would not result in a deduction or the awarding of points.

3. C3 Implement training in ways to simplify work-related activities to maximize endurance.

Feedback: The patient learns new work simplification techniques that can be applied to the job of home inspector.

Outcome and Rationale: Work simplification techniques are an important part of a pulmonary rehabilitation program. Here, the patient learns how to maximize endurance through pacing. These techniques can also include the use of adaptive equipment to ease performance in strenuous activities. This approach is an effective intervention that would have a positive impact on the patient's progress. Its selection would result in the awarding of points.

4. C5 Practice climbs up and down a ladder to simulate work activity.

Feedback: The patient complains of severe dyspnea and dizziness while engaging in this activity.

Outcome and Rationale: While work simulation tasks are a positive approach for this patient, it is too soon in the intervention process to engage in such an activity. This activity requires a high amount of strength and endurance and is not appropriate for a person in the initial stages of intervention. It could also result in a fall due to the patient's deconditioned status. It would be more beneficial to simulate basic work tasks in a seated or static standing position to build endurance over time until higher demand tasks can be tolerated. This choice is not safe and it has a negative impact on the patient. Consequently, its selection would result in the loss of points.

5. C5 Educate in stress management techniques.

Feedback: The patient learns new stress management techniques that have a positive impact on pulmonary status.

Outcome and Rationale: Stress management techniques are beneficial for the majority of patients with COPD as stress can negatively impact one's cardiovascular status. The American Association of Cardiovascular and Pulmonary

Rehabilitation (AACPR) establishes standards for pulmonary rehabilitation practice, which include the implementation of stress management and relaxation techniques by occupational therapists. Patients with high levels of stress can experience breathlessness and panic, which causes shortness of breath. Stress management reduces these episodes. This action is a positive and effective intervention and would result in receiving points.

6. C3 Perform meal preparation in standing without breaks to simulate activity performance in the home.

Feedback: The patient reports being too fatigued to continue after five minutes of standing.

Outcome and Rationale: This technique goes against energy conservation guidelines, which encourage a person to maximize his/her available energy while engaging in functional tasks and to rest when fatigued in order to replenish energy to persist in the task. Pushing a patient to persist beyond the point of fatigue is harmful. It leads to dyspnea and potential dizziness, which is counterproductive. The selection of this approach would result in a loss of points.

7. C5 Practice the Valsalva maneuver during strengthening activities in order to maximize strength.

Feedback: The patient complains of extreme dizziness, breathes heavily, and places head down on the table.

Outcome and Rationale: The Valsalva maneuver is a technique where a patient 'bears down' or holds his/her breath while engaging in strenuous activity in order to gain more power. This is taxing on the lungs, creates shortness of breath, and stresses the cardiovascular system by initially elevating blood pressure. It is contraindicated in patients with cardiovascular conditions, such as COPD and coronary artery bypass graft (CABG). The patient should only be encouraged to breathe through strenuous activity which includes exhaling through the concentric phase of a contraction (such as lifting) and inhaling with eccentric contraction (lowering). Selection of this technique (Valsalva maneuver) is a negative action and would result in a loss of points.

8. C5 Use free weights and ergometer exercises to improve upper body strength.

Feedback: The patient builds upper body strength and learns to pace self through these exercises.

Outcome and Rationale: Strengthening activities for patients with COPD should include approaches such as free weights, arm ergometer (a flywheel moved by a pedaling action of the arms), and elastic bands, which all help to build strength. The therapist should encourage the patient to pace him/herself during these activities and to rest when feeling short of breath. Guidelines to indicate the need to rest is when the patient can no longer say a complete sentence during a strengthening activity without mild difficulty. Pulse oximetry levels should be monitored during strengthening. This action is a positive selection and would result in the awarding of points.

Section C

The patient has demonstrated functional gains in deficit areas and the rehabilitation team is planning for the patient's discharge home. The patient independently completes basic and instrumental ADL but requires extra time for task completion. The patient has been weaned off oxygen, but continues to complain of shortness of breath with chaotic breathing when anxious. The patient states difficulty sleeping at night and is fearful about suffocation when lying flat, though nursing staff report no saturation changes when lying flat. Which of the following choices are most beneficial in preparation for the patient's discharge to home? Check all that apply.

1. C5 Instruct the patient to engage in hyperventilation strategies when experiencing shortness of breath to increase oxygen saturation.

Feedback: The patient complains of light-headedness and states not feeling better.

Outcome and Rationale: Hyperventilation, also known as over-breathing, is a rapid breathing pattern where the patient inhales and exhales quickly. This type of breathing pattern should not be encouraged as it does not promote the required controlled breathing for the condition of COPD. This approach only adds to shortness of breath and chaotic breathing pattern, which should be discouraged. This is a negative approach and its selection would result in a loss of points.

2. C2 Refer the patient to a psychologist to address anxiety issues.

Feedback: The patient appreciates the suggestion, but feels this is not needed.

Outcome and Rationale: A referral can provide help for the patient's anxiety, but it does not directly address the patient's pre-discharge preparation needs, which is the primary focus of this section. This option does not move the patient forward in the therapy process but it does not create harm. Therefore, this selection is neutral and would not result in a deduction or the awarding of points.

3. C8 Provide a wedge cushion for use in bed to elevate the head at night.

Feedback: The patient uses the new cushion and reports less anxiety about sleeping at night.

Outcome and Rationale: The use of a wedge cushion provides elevation of the head at night, which is a cost-effective solution that will help the patient to sleep better and lessen anxiety. This is a positive approach which will result in the awarding of points.

4. C8 Conduct a home evaluation to ensure safety and independence in home tasks.

Feedback: The patient is able to transfer and retrieve items from high and low locations independently. The patient requires safety cues and reminders of breathing strategies.

Outcome and Rationale: A home evaluation is an important aspect of the discharge planning process to ensure the patient is safe in the home and can perform all required tasks independently. It can also help determine the need for services in the home and identify indications for adaptive equipment. This is a positive action and its selection would result in the awarding of points.

5. C9 Contact a home care agency for delivery of a hospital bed to the home.

Feedback: The home care agency states that the patient does not meet the criteria of medical necessity for a hospital bed. Insurance reimbursement is denied.

Outcome and Rationale: A hospital bed is considered durable medical equipment (DME) and requires medical necessity for reimbursement by most insurance carriers. Guidelines that indicate medical necessity can include a diagnosis that requires the use of a hospital bed (such as congestive heart failure or pulmonary disease where the bed must be elevated higher than 30°, pressure sores, or the need for traction equipment attached to a hospital bed) and the requirement for positioning that cannot be accomplished in a standard bed. Though the patient has a pulmonary disease, the patient does not require elevation of the head beyond 30° since saturation levels do not change when lying flat. The patient's shortness of breath is related to anxiousness, not medical necessity. Anxiety is not a reimbursable condition for a hospital bed. Therefore, this recommendation can create financial harm and its selection demonstrates a lack of knowledge about established reimbursement standards for DME. Consequently, its selection would result in a loss of points.

6. C6 Recommend participation in a local pulmonary diseases support group.

Feedback: The patient contacts the support group coordinator.

Outcome and Rationale: The patient can benefit from a support group to discuss feelings and coping related to the disease process. With the patient's reported anxiousness, a support group can be an ideal place to work through this issue. This is a positive action and its selection would result in the awarding of points.

7. C5 Teach the patient diaphragmatic breathing exercises to complete at home.

Feedback: The patient implements the exercises.

Outcome and Rationale: Diaphragmatic breathing exercises are an important aspect of the rehabilitation process which should be carried through upon return to home. These exercises promote controlled breathing with maximizing use of the diaphragm, rather than accessory muscles for breathing. This is an effective intervention which contributes to a positive patient outcome; therefore, its selection would result in the awarding of points.

8. C8 Recommend the patient visit a vocational rehabilitation agency for career exploration.

Feedback: The patient questions this recommendation stating no desire for a different job and happiness with current job.

Outcome and Rationale: The patient indicated during the evaluation phase the desire to return to the job that is currently held, therefore career exploration is unnecessary. This would only be necessary if the patient indicated a desire to do so and the condition and inability to perform required job tasks warranted a career change. This recommendation did not harm the patient nor did it move the patient forward in the therapy process. Therefore this selection is neutral and would not result in a change of points.

Simulation Test Item A.II.

Opening Scene:

An occupational therapist working as a private practitioner receives a referral from a primary care physician to evaluate a 92-year-old individual. The physician reports that the individual is exhibiting symptoms of dementia non-Alzheimer's type which are indicative of Stage 4 on Reisburg's Stages of Dementia Scale. The client recently moved into a family member's two-story home.

Section A

The occupational therapist meets with the client and family caregiver in their home. Which evaluation approaches should the occupational therapist use in this situation? Choose all effective evaluation approaches.

1. C2 Ask the family caregiver to explain the reasons for seeking a physician's referral for an OT evaluation of the family member.

Feedback: The family caregiver reports that the client is distractible, forgetful, and easily confused when performing previously familiar activities.

Outcome and Rationale: Asking the caregiver for input can be very helpful toward building rapport. This is a primary goal for an occupational therapist's initial visit to a client's home. The information provided by the caregiver is consistent with the behavioral indicators of Stage 4 on Reisburg's Stages for Dementia Scale. Although this action can lead to the building of rapport, it is not an evaluation approach that will provide any information to the therapist. Therefore, its selection would be considered neutral. No points would be awarded or deducted for this choice.

2. C1 Assess the client's balance.

Feedback: The client's static balance is good, dynamic is balance is poor.

Outcome and Rationale: At 92 years of age, this client can be expected to have musculoskeletal and sensory system changes due to the aging process. These typically result in slower movements, delayed reaction times, decreased functional mobility, poor balance, decreased vision, and disorganized postural responses. All of these factors can contribute to an increased risk for falls. An accurate assessment of risk for falls must include an evaluation of balance. Adequate balance skills are a necessary component/prerequisite for many functional activities (e.g., dressing, bathing). Therefore, balance should be an assessment priority. Obtaining information about the client's static and dynamic balance is a good outcome; therefore points would be awarded for this selection.

3. C1 Assess the client's functional mobility by having the client independently ascend the home's interior stairway.

Feedback: The client unsteadily walks up the stairs, stops halfway, and sways backwards.

Outcome and Rationale: As noted above, this 92-year-old client can be expected to have age-related sensori-motor losses which put him/her at an increased risk for falls. Having the client ascend the stairs without first completing an assessment of balance and functional mobility places the client at great risk. The selection of this action reflects poor judgment and would result in the deduction of points.

4. C8 Assess the client's IADL using the Kohlman Evaluation of Daily Living Skills.

Feedback: Client becomes confused and cannot engage in the evaluation process.

Outcome and Rationale: The Kohlman Evaluation of Daily Living Skills (KELS) determines an individual's knowledge and/or performance of 17 basic living skills needed to live independently in five main areas. These areas include self-care, safety and health, money management, transportation and telephone use and work and leisure. Many of these tests would not be appropriate for a person who is at Stage 4 of Reisburg's Stages for Dementia Scale. Moreover, the administration of the KELS requires the individual to complete some tasks using written forms (e.g., money management) or to respond to the therapist's questions to obtain the individual's self-report regarding the performance of other tasks (e.g., leisure pursuits). These abilities are beyond this client's capabilities. At Stage 4 of Reisburg's Stages for Dementia Scale, the person has difficulty with word finding and cannot follow written cues. The selection of this evaluation reflects a poor understanding of the client's current functional level. Consequently, points would be deducted for this choice.

5. C8 Interview the caregiver using the Routine Task Inventory.

Feedback: Caregiver reports that the client is able to perform simple routine ADL independently.

Outcome and Rationale: The Routine Task Inventory (RTI) measures an individual's level of impairment in activities of daily living according to Allen's model of cognitive levels. This is an appropriate practice model to use with persons with dementia. The RTI includes six physical scales in the areas of grooming, dressing, bathing, walking, feeding, and toileting and eight instrumental scales in the areas of housekeeping, preparing food, spending money, taking medication, doing laundry, shopping, telephoning, and traveling. It can be completed through observation of an individual's performance and completion of the rating scale for each item by the evaluator; self-report by the individual if cognitively able to complete RTI questionnaire; and/or report of a caregiver familiar with the individual's functional performance through completion of the RTI questionnaire. This is an appropriate measure to use to evaluate the client's functional abilities and the information obtained will be helpful toward designing a relevant intervention plan for this client. Consequently, this selection would result in the awarding of points.

6. C8 Observe the client's performance using the Routine Task Inventory.

Feedback: The therapist observes that client is able to perform simple routine ADL independently.

Outcome and Rationale: As noted above, the RTI measures an individual's level of impairment in activities of daily living according to Allen's model of cognitive levels. This model is appropriate to use to guide evaluation and intervention for persons with dementia. The RTI is an appropriate measure to use to evaluate the client's functional abilities. Directly observing the client's ability to perform ADL can provide information that can help design a relevant intervention plan for this client. Consequently, this selection would result in the awarding of points.

7. C8 Assess the home for potential environmental factors that can contribute to falls.

Feedback: Potential fall hazards are identified.

Outcome and Rationale: As noted previously in the above rationales for selections 2 and 3, this client can be expected to have an increased risk for falls. Therefore, the evaluation of environmental factors that may contribute to falls is essential to ensure the client's safety. These environmental risk factors can include, but are not limited to, slippery or uneven floor surfaces, the presence of throw rugs, high pile carpets, low lying furniture, lack of or loose stairway handrails, and poor lighting or glare. Identifying potential fall hazards in the home will help the occupational therapist make appropriate recommendations for modifying the environment to reduce the risk of falls. This is a good outcome and points would be awarded for this selection.

Section B

The occupational therapist determines that the individual is experiencing sensori-motor losses that are consistent with the aging process. The therapist provides recommendations to the family caregiver on how to effectively manage the sensori-motor and cognitive deficits of the client to ensure safety in the home and facilitate the completion of daily activities. Which should the occupational therapist recommend to the family caregiver? Choose all recommendations that would effectively apply to this client and this situation.

1. C8 Use similar toned colors in the environment and during activities to decrease distractions.

Feedback: The caregiver modifies the client's living space and activity characteristics to be monotone.

Outcome and Rationale: The use of similar toned colors is not helpful for persons with sensory deficits because these do not provide the necessary visual contrast needed to enhance visual discrimination. This can decrease the person's ability to complete basic tasks (e.g., feeding becomes difficult when white foods such as potatoes or cauliflower are placed on a white plate). Safety can also be compromised when there is not a clear visual distinction between walls, floors, and steps. This is a negative outcome and the selection of this action would result in the deduction of points. High contrast colors enable the individual with visual deficits to see items more clearly in his/her environment and their use would be a more appropriate and effective recommendation.

2. C8 Vary the characteristics of the environment and activities on a daily basis to maintain the client's interest and attention.

Feedback: The caregiver changes the characteristics of the client's living space and activities each day.

Outcome and Rationale: Persons with dementia are able to function best in environments that are familiar and consistent. In addition, the completion of activities that are simple and repetitive are indicated for a person at Stage 4 of Reisburg's Stages for Dementia. Varying the environment and activities on a daily basis would increase the client's confusion and not support the adaptive use of any of the client's remaining functional capacities. This is contraindicated and the selection of this outcome would result in the deduction of points.

3. C6 Contact the local chapter of the Alzheimer's disease and Related Disorders Association to receive support.

Feedback: The caregiver calls this local chapter and schedules an appointment.

Outcome and Rationale: The ability to obtain support from a well-established association is important to prevent caregiver burden. While this is a good outcome, it does not directly address this section's focus on providing direct interventions and/or concrete recommendations to help the caregiver effectively manage the sensori-motor and cognitive deficits of the client to ensure safety in the home and facilitate the completion of daily activities. Consequently, this action would be considered neutral and no points would be awarded or deducted for its selection.

4. C6 Speak loudly and provide a comprehensive orientation to the activity being performed.

Feedback: The caregiver speaks loudly and gives a comprehensive orientation to activities.

Outcome and Rationale: Speaking loudly can frighten or confuse a person with cognitive impairments. Providing a comprehensive orientation is contraindicated for persons at Stage 4 of Reisburg's Stages for Dementia. At this level, the person can follow simple verbal and demonstrated cues that are provided throughout an activity. The client in this situation could not be expected to remember a comprehensive orientation to an activity; therefore, he/she would not be able to successfully engage in or complete the activity. This is a negative outcome which would likely increase both the client's and the caregiver's level of frustration. Consequently, points would be deducted for the selection of this action.

5. C6 Speak slowly and validate statements made by the client.

Feedback: The caregiver speaks slowly and validates statements made by the client.

Outcome and Rationale: Speaking slowly to allow time for processing and the validation of statements has proven to enhance the performance and carry-over of skills in persons with cognitive impairments. This approach is consistent with the client's current functional level and its use would likely enable the client to successfully engage in activities. This is a good outcome and points would be awarded for this selection.

6. C6 Provide consistent reality orientation.

Feedback: The caregiver consistently reminds the client of the date, time, where the client is, and who is present.

Outcome and Rationale: Reality orientation is not an effective approach for a person with dementia. Orienting the person who is forgetful or confused due to an irreversible cognitive impairment to time, place, person and situation does not improve functional capabilities. Doing this on a consistent basis would only highlight the client's deficits and could likely lead to increased caregiver stress. Moreover, reality orientation provides no guidance to help the caregiver effectively engage the client in activities. This selection does not provide a recommendation relevant to the client's functional level and it reflects a lack of awareness of effective intervention strategies for persons with dementia. Consequently, points would be deducted for the selection of this action.

7. C8 Remove clutter to decrease extraneous stimuli.

Feedback: The caregiver removes clutter from the client's living space.

Outcome and Rationale: Decreasing environmental stimulation by eliminating clutter can help an individual with cognitive and sensory impairments maintain his/her concentration and attention. This is a positive outcome and points would be awarded for this selection.

8. C8 Move the client to an assisted living setting with a dementia care unit.

Feedback: The caregiver declines this recommendation and describes being grateful to be able to care for the client in his/her home.

Outcome and Rationale: This recommendation does not address the stated question focus of providing recommendations to ensure the client's safety in the home and facilitate his/her completion of daily activities. However, it does not cause any harm; therefore, it would be considered a neutral action and points would not be awarded or deducted for its selection.

9. C8 Install light switches at the top and bottom of the stairway.

Feedback: The caregiver installs the light switches.

Outcome and Rationale: With normal aging there is decreased visual acuity (presbyopia), reduced night vision, and impaired depth perception. These deficits can make ascending and descending stairs dangerous. To decrease the risk of falls, it is advisable to install light switches at both ends of a stairway so that the stairs can be easily illuminated. This is a good outcome and points would be awarded for the selection of this action.

Section C

During a subsequent home visit, the family caregiver expresses concern over the client's wandering behavior during the night. The caregiver is afraid the client will leave the house while everyone is asleep, placing the client in a dangerous situation. The caregiver is also concerned that the client becomes restless in the early evening prior to dinner. What should the occupational therapist tell the caregiver to do to manage these behaviors? Choose all recommendations that could effectively deal with this situation.

1. C8 Use full-length mirrors or wallpaper to camouflage exit doorways.

Feedback: The caregiver camouflages the exit doorways.

Outcome and Rationale: Camouflaging the doorways is often an effective intervention to decrease wandering behavior in individuals with dementia or other cognitive deficits. One cannot open a door if one does not see a door. This is a good outcome and points would be awarded for the selection of this action.

2. C8 Provide the client with a pre-dinner snack to eat while watching a video of a favorite musical.

Feedback: The caregiver provides the client with a snack which the client eats while watching the video.

Outcome and Rationale: Restless behavior can increase in the early evening hours due to hunger and the increased environmental stimulation that occurs in a household when everyone returns home in the evening. Providing a snack can help ameliorate hunger, decreasing the effect of this stressor. Watching a video of a favorite musical can provide appropriate sensory stimulation and positive reminiscent feelings. This is a good outcome and points would be awarded for the selection of this action.

3. C8 Install a deadbolt lock on the client's bedroom door.

Feedback: The caregiver installs a deadbolt lock.

Outcome and Rationale: The installation of a deadbolt lock on the person's bedroom door is very dangerous for it can prevent timely rescue in the event of a fire or accident. This is a negative outcome and the selection of this action would result in the deduction of points. There are many intervention options to recommend to decrease wandering (i.e., the use of personal alarms, camouflaged doors, and/or diversional activities, and/or the rearrangement of furniture) that would be much safer to recommend the caregiver employ.

4. C8 Install bed guard rails to ensure that the client remains in bed at night.

Feedback: The caregiver installs bed guard rails.

Outcome and Rationale: The use of bed guard rails can be dangerous as the client may attempt to climb over the rails and fall. This is a negative outcome and the selection of this action would result in the deduction of points.

5. C1 Provide the client with an aerobic exercise video to follow along with the exercises and expend excess energy.

Feedback: The client falls while attempting to follow along with the exercises.

Outcome and Rationale: Exercising to a video can provide a positive sensorimotor outlet; however, this activity would need to be closely supervised due to the motor deficits that can occur as a result of dementia. In addition, the normal aging process can compromise one's balance and equilibrium reactions. This selection resulted in a negative outcome; therefore it would result in the deduction of points.

6. C6 Encourage the client to participate in meal preparation by tearing lettuce into small pieces for a salad.

Feedback: The client successfully completes the task.

Outcome and Rationale: At Stage 4 of Reisburg's Stages of Dementia, a person can perform simple repetitive tasks independently. Being engaged in an activity that is familiar uses the client's remaining capabilities. This is a good outcome and points would be awarded for the selection of this action.

7. C9 Consult with the home care case manager for an assessment for skilled nursing facility placement.

Feedback: The caregiver declines this recommendation and describes being grateful to be able to care for the client in his/her home.

Outcome and Rationale: This recommendation was premature since the client just moved into the caregiver's home and the caregiver is actively seeking the expertise of the occupational therapist to enable the client to remain in the home. However, this recommendation does not likely cause harm; therefore it would be considered neutral. No points would be awarded or deducted for its selection.

Section D

The caregiver reports that the client repeats the same questions and tells the same stories about the "old days" throughout the day. Extended family members and friends visit consistently but express difficulty with these behaviors. The family caregiver expresses fear to the occupational therapist that these visits will cease if they are not made "easier." Which activities and/or approaches are most effective for the therapist to recommend that the caregiver suggest to the client's visitors? Choose all effective recommendations.

1. C6 Engage in many different activities to keep the client interested.

Feedback: Visitors introduce many diverse activities to the client, but the client cannot attend to them.

Outcome and Rationale: The provision of many different activities can be confusing and over-stimulating for a person with cognitive deficits. At Stage 4 of Reisburg's Stages for Dementia, consistency and repetition are indicated, not diversity and variety. This recommendation is contraindicated at this person's stage of dementia and its selection would result in the deduction of points.

2. C6 Reminiscence about shared memories.

Feedback: Visitors reminiscence with the client and the client shares favorite memories.

Outcome and Rationale: Reminiscence is an effective approach to use with a person with mid-stage dementia. At this stage, long-term, remote memory is intact and in this situation the caregiver reports that the client consistently tells stories about the past. Reminiscence enables the client to review past life experiences with his/her visitors which promotes the use of intact long-term memory. This is a positive outcome so points would be awarded for this selection.

3. C6 Play a matching card game that includes pictures of the client's past interests.

Feedback: The client cannot match the cards but the pictures prompt the client to tell a story.

Outcome and Rationale: Immediate memory is required for successful participation in a matching card game. Individuals with mid-stage dementia typically have poor immediate memory so the client's difficulty with this game can be anticipated. However, the use of pictures of past interests was a good suggestion as these pictures can (and did) trigger memories that lead to client telling a story. Since reminiscence is a good strategy to use with clients with dementia, the client's inability to complete the game is balanced by the prompt the pictures provided. This can be considered a neutral outcome and no points would be deducted or awarded for the selection of this recommendation.

4. C6 Watch a DVD of a classic film.

Feedback: The client ignores the movie and wanders into the kitchen.

Outcome and Rationale: Watching a film is a passive activity. A movie requires attention over an extended period of time which is difficult for a person with mid-stage dementia. The recommendation of this activity demonstrates a poor use of activity analysis skills for determining an appropriate activity for a person with cognitive deficits. This selection also does not provide any strategies to enable the visitors to effectively engage the client in an activity, which is what the caregiver explicitly requested. Since this recommendation does not address the caregiver's stated need nor provide the client with an opportunity to use his/her remaining capabilities, the outcome is poor. Consequently, this action would result in a deduction of points.

5. C6 Ask the client to share more information about the client's favorite stories.

Feedback: Visitors and the client chat about the client's favorite stories.

Outcome and Rationale: In this situation, the caregiver reports that the client consistently tells stories about the past; therefore, engaging the client in conversation about his/her favorite stories is an appropriate social activity. This reminiscence can effectively promote the use of the client's intact long-term memory. This is a positive outcome so points would be awarded for this selection.

6. C6 Reinforce reality by orienting the client to time, place, person and situation.

Feedback: Visitors question the client about the date, time, place, and what is occurring.

Outcome and Rationale: Reality orientation is not effective with persons who have mid-stage dementia. This client's memory deficits, confusion, and distractibility would result in his/her responses being inaccurate and/or incomplete. This lack of success can highlight the client's deficits and make it even more difficult for the visitors. Selecting this option demonstrates a poor understanding of the functional effects of dementia and can be detrimental to the client and his/her visitors as they both can become frustrated with the client's inability to correctly respond to the posed questions. Frustration on the part of the client can result in agitated behavior. Moreover, the family caregiver had sought the therapist's input to make visits "easier." If the visitors feel frustrated with their inability to successfully engage the client, the likelihood of attaining this goal is very poor. This is a negative outcome and the selection of this action would result in the deduction of points.

7. C6 Play a board game to use remaining cognitive abilities.

Feedback: Visitors begin playing a board game with the client but the client is unable to follow the game rules or its progress.

Outcome and Rationale: Due to the client's memory deficits, confusion, and distractibility, playing a board game is an activity that is beyond the client's capabilities. The effective use of activity analysis is an important skill of the entry-level occupational therapist. Selecting this option demonstrates poor activity analysis skills and can be detrimental to the client and his/her visitors as they both can become frustrated with the client's inability to successfully engage in the recommended activity. Frustration on the part of the client can result in agitated behavior. Moreover, the family caregiver had sought the therapist's input to make visits "easier." If the visitors feel frustrated with their inability to successfully engage the client, the likelihood of attaining this goal is very poor. This is a negative outcome and would result in the deduction of points.

8. C6 Review photo albums containing pictures of people the client knew in the past.

Feedback: Visitors look at pictures with the client of people the client previously knew.

Outcome and Rationale: Reviewing old photos can facilitate positive remote memories for the client to share with the visitors. This can serve as a precipitant to meaningful conversation about familiar people and favorite activities. This is a positive outcome so points would be awarded for this selection.

Simulation Test Item A.III.

Opening Scene:

A 17-year-old student with Asperger's syndrome begins the senior year at a public high school. The student consistently attends classes and demonstrates adequate performance in the school's technical training program, which began during the student's junior year. The school's Individualized Education Plan (IEP) planning team has scheduled a meeting with the student and family to collaborate on goals and update the student's IEP for the senior year.

Section A

The occupational therapist prepares to revise the occupational therapy service component of the IEP to present at the IEP meeting. Which of the following should the therapist do to ensure that the recommendations made for occupational therapy are appropriate to the student's current status? Choose all of the approaches that apply.

1. C4 Administer the Sensory Profile.

Feedback: The student's scores indicate no differences between the student's identified responses and typical performance.

Outcome and Rationale: The Sensory Profile (SP) has three versions for different age ranges; i.e. infants/toddlers, children aged 3–10 and adolescents/adults aged 11–65 years. The pediatric versions of the Sensory Profile use a caregiver questionnaire to obtain caregiver's judgment and observations of a child's sensory processing, modulation, and behavioral and emotional responses in each sensory system. The Adolescent/Adult SP allows clients to identify their personal behavioral responses and develop strategies for enhanced participation through the completion of a questionnaire which measures the individual's reactions to daily sensory experiences. Cut-off scores indicate typical performance and probable, definite, and significant differences. Differences indicate which sensory system is hindering performance. In this case, there was no information provided in the scenario to indicate the need for the evaluation of the student's sensory system. According to the OT process, evaluations are selected based upon screening information; therefore, the selection of this action reflects a lack of understanding of standard evaluation procedures. In addition, this evaluation does not provide any information to add to the team's knowledge about the student's current status or to help update the transition plan. As a result, it is a waste of the therapist's and student's time. Consequently, the selection of this option would be considered negative and points would be deducted for its selection.

2. C6 Administer the Coping Inventory.

Feedback: Results show the client scores low average in all areas of coping behaviors.

Outcome and Rationale: The Coping Inventory assesses coping skills, habits, and behaviors to cope with self and with the environment in three areas: productive, active, and flexible, for those aged 15 years and older. This is an appropriate evaluation for a student who will be transitioning to life after high school and points would be awarded for its selection.

3. C8 Re-administer the School Function Assessment previously completed at the end of the student's junior year.

Feedback: The results of the SFA show student's functional performance has not changed since the evaluation's prior administration.

Outcome and Rationale: The School Function Assessment (SFA) assesses and monitors functional performance to promote participation in the school environment. While it does not measure academic performance, the SFA assesses the student's level of performance in school-related tasks and the type of support needed for successful performance. The SFA was administered at the end of the student's junior year and the information obtained was likely used to place the student in the correct school environment for the senior year. At this point, the student is doing well in the current program so a re- assessment would not be required at this time. The administration of this evaluation in the senior year would be indicated if the student was reported to be having difficulty with school-related tasks (e.g., a decline in-class participation). According to the OT process, evaluations are selected based upon screening information; therefore, the selection of this action reflects a lack of understanding of standard evaluation procedures. In addition, this evaluation did not provide any new information to add to the team's knowledge about the student's current status or to help update the transition plan. As a result, it is a waste of the therapist's and student's time. Consequently, the selection of this option would be considered negative and points would be deducted for its selection.

4. C6 Recommend weekly occupational therapy groups to develop behavioral management skills.

Feedback: The IEP team leader notes that all disciplines must complete their evaluations prior to making an intervention recommendation.

Outcome and Rationale: According to the OT process, the occupational therapist must first complete all evaluations prior to making a recommendation for intervention. In a school-based setting, the therapist should also meet with the interdisciplinary team to discuss evaluation results and review all service options, prior to recommending an intervention. Based upon this shared information, the therapist would then establish goals and develop the OT intervention plan. There is a possibility that OT intervention to develop behavioral management skills may be needed for a student with the diagnosis of Asperger's, but this determination is dependent on each student's needs and the other services offered at the school. The selection of this option represents a lack of understanding of the OT process and school-based practice. Therefore, it would result in a deduction of points.

5. C2 Interview the student to determine aptitudes, interests, and preferences to establish self-determined goals.

Feedback: The student discusses plans to go to a local technical training institute upon graduation but is uncertain about which field to pursue.

Outcome and Rationale: The interview provides essential information about the student's personal goals, an essential component in planning for secondary transition. In addition, the IDEA requires active student participation in the composition, revision, and implementation of a transition plan for post-secondary school life. This plan should prepare the student for adult life including community participation, independent living, post-secondary education, and/or employment. This plan must be based on the student's active input and the student must be invited to all IEP meetings that discuss his/her transition plan to allow for self-advocacy and self-determination. Consequently, interviewing the student to acquire a personal perspective is a positive action and would result in the awarding of points.

6. C8 Refer the client to the state vocational rehabilitation services.

Feedback: The referral is declined with the explanation that it is premature.

Outcome and Rationale: The student shows adequate performance in the high school technical training program to date. Consequently the student is likely to be a good candidate for a referral to the state vocational rehabilitation (VR) services. Although VR services are typically not available until age 18 and/or upon high school graduation, a referral can be initiated while an individual is still in high school. Pre-vocational interventions can be coordinated in the school setting to develop the skills needed to make the student's use of VR services more effective.

However at this point in the provided scenario, a complete OT evaluation and an IEP team plan would need to be completed to determine the student's appropriateness as a candidate for VR services. While this referral was premature, it did not cause any harm. Consequently, the selection of this option would be considered neutral and no points would be awarded nor deducted for its selection.

7. C6 Administer the Childhood Autism Rating Scale (CARS).

Feedback: The therapist's supervisor states that the student does not meet the criteria for the CARS.

Outcome and Rationale: Although the student has a diagnosis of Asperger's, which is an autism spectrum disorder, the CARs is not an appropriate assessment for the therapist to administer. The CARS determines the severity of autism (i.e., mild, moderate or severe) in children over 2 years of age. It is a diagnostic tool that distinguishes children with autism from children with developmental delays who do not have autism. This is a highly inappropriate evaluation for a teenager with Asperger's. Consequently, its selection reflects a lack of knowledge about basic pediatric diagnostic assessments and would result in the deduction of points.

8. C4 Provide the student with a sensory diet.

Feedback: The IEP team, student, and family question the appropriateness of this intervention.

Outcome and Rationale: Individuals with Asperger's tend to demonstrate limitations in social, communication, and cognitive skills, along with gross motor incoordination. If there were concerns about the student's sensory processing, the therapist must first evaluate the student (e.g., using the Adolescent/Adult SP) prior to providing the student with a sensory diet. Implementing an intervention prior to the completion of an evaluation is poor practice and represents an inadequate understanding of the OT process. Consequently, the selection of this action would result in the deduction of points.

9. C6 Administer the Social Interaction Scale (SIS) of the Bay Area Functional Performance Evaluation (BAFPE).

Feedback: The student complies with social norms. The student exhibits limited interaction skills in 1:1 and group settings and reports discomfort in social situations.

Outcome and Rationale: The SIS of the BAFPE assesses a person's general ability to relate appropriately to other people within the environment through observations of the individual in up to five situations (i.e., one to one, mealtime, unstructured group, structured activity group, structured verbal group). The SIS also has an optional self-report social interaction questionnaire. Since this evaluation can be conducted during the school day by the therapist's direct observations of the student or by the therapist obtaining input from the student's teachers or other school personnel, it is appropriate to the setting. In addition, if time or setting constraints preclude the evaluation of the student's behavior in all five social situations, the scoring can be adjusted. Obtaining information based on direct observations along with the student's self-report provides useful information to the IEP team. Consequently, the selection of this action would be awarded points.

Section B

The occupational therapy evaluation reveals that the student shows low average coping skills and difficulty initiating and maintaining group and one-on-one social interactions. The student complies with social norms but expresses discomfort in social situations. At the IEP meeting, the team members concur that the student's present class placement adequately meets academic needs. Team members report that the student exhibits good technical drawing skills, the ability to initiate and complete classroom tasks with minimal verbal direction, and minimal gross motor incoordination. The student's and family's goals are for the student to study at a technical training institute upon graduation. Which actions are most effective for the therapist to recommend for inclusion in the IEP to enable goal attainment? Choose all actions that are appropriate.

1. C2 Participation in a parallel task group to develop attention and concentration skills.

Feedback: The student independently initiates and completes tasks with limited interaction with peers.

Outcome and Rationale: A parallel group is the first developmental group level. It is indicated for persons who have great difficulty in social situations. The purpose of a parallel group is to develop members' basic level of awareness, trust, and comfort with others in the group by having them perform individual tasks in the presence of others. Parallel groups require minimal verbal or non-verbal interaction with others since interactions are not needed for the successful completion of members' individual tasks. In this case, the student is reported to be appropriately placed in classes with no difficulties reported. Therefore, one can clinically reason that parallel social interaction skills are intact since these abilities are required for adequate classroom performance. As a result, placement in this group level is too low for this student. This selection reflects a lack of knowledge about basic group interventions and it would result in the deduction of points.

2. C8 Participation in the school's pre-vocational program.

Feedback: The student consistently participates in the group. Task and social skills are strengthened and essential work habits are developed.

Outcome and Rationale: The purpose of a pre-vocational program is to develop an individual's task skills, social interaction skills, and work habits that are prerequisite to work (e.g., independent task initiation and completion, decision making and problem solving, appropriate response to supervision, constructive interactions with co-workers, punctuality, and consistent attendance). This is an appropriate intervention program for this student. By participating in this group, the student's current level of task and social skills can be built on to develop abilities that are required in a vocational program (such as the technology training institute that the student desires to attend post-high school). In addition, the prevocational program can help the student develop work habits that are needed for success in future employment. This is a positive outcome and the selection of this action would result in the awarding of points.

3. C8 Tours of community-based employment settings.

Feedback: The student asks why job site visits are necessary.

Outcome and Rationale: It is premature at this point to have the student visiting employment settings. The high school program should enhance and hone the student's skills for future success in the post-secondary technical training program. Employment observation tours could be included in the school's pre-vocational program to further explore the student's vocational interests and identify sites that may meet future employment goals. Although this action is not indicated at this time, it does not cause harm. Therefore points would neither be deducted nor awarded for its selection.

4. C8 Inclusion in the school basic life skills preparation class.

Feedback: The teacher states that the student demonstrates no deficits in basic activities of daily living.

Outcome and Rationale: A basic life skills class addresses basic activities of daily living (BADL) such as dressing, feeding, and hygiene for students who are unable to complete these tasks due to severe cognitive limitations. The skills noted in the OT evaluation indicate a higher cognitive level and greater functional skills than those that would indicate a need for membership in this group. The student is performing well in the technical training program with no problems noted by the IEP team to indicate deficits in BADL. The selection of this action indicates inadequate understanding of the student's functional abilities and poor analysis of the student's intervention needs. As a result, it would result in the deduction of points.

5. C8 Referral to a vocational workshop.

Feedback: The IEP team, student, and family question the appropriateness of this referral.

Outcome and Rationale: The student's functional level is higher than the functional level appropriate for a vocational (previously called sheltered) workshop. Participants in vocational workshops typically have significant cognitive deficits and intellectual disorders that limit their ability to participate in unstructured work environments. The work tasks performed at a vocational workshop are typically highly structured, repetitive, concrete tasks that require minimal technical skills (e.g., assembly work paid at a piece-work rate). The selection of this action demonstrates poor knowledge about a basic vocational program and a poor grasp of the student's current functional level. Consequently, its selection would result in the deduction of points.

6. C2 Participation in an OT communication skills group at the project group level.

Feedback: The student develops the ability to interact more comfortably with peers.

Rationale and Outcome: A communication skills group is an appropriate intervention for a person who has limited social interaction skills. A project group is a type of developmental group. The purpose of a developmental group is to teach the social interaction skills needed for group participation in a sequential manner. It provides relevant group structure and activities along a continuum that is consistent with how interaction skills develop normally. A project group focuses on developing the ability to perform a shared, short-term activity with another member in a comfortable, cooperative manner and facilitating interactions beyond those that the activity requires. It also focuses on helping members be able to give and seek assistance. This group level is consistent with the client's reported poor group and 1:1 interaction skills and it is an appropriate intervention to develop the skills needed to pursue the student's post-secondary education goal. As a result, the selection of this option would result in the awarding of points.

Section C

During the fall semester, the student consistently attends an occupational therapy communication skills group and meets the established goals to initiate and maintain one-on-one and group interactions with minimal verbal prompts. The student also attends the school's technical pre-vocational class. At midpoint in the school year, the teacher requests that the occupational therapist complete objective evaluations of the student's skills relevant to stated vocational interests. This information will be used in a pre-graduation referral to the state vocational rehabilitation (VR) services. The student and family plan to seek funding from VR to pay the student's tuition at the technical training institute as a commuter student. As a result, the student will need to independently travel to the program site. Which of the following evaluation and/or intervention actions should the therapist take to facilitate attainment of the VR referral and post-graduation plans? Choose all that apply.

1. C1 Administer the Bruininks-Oseretsky Test of Motor Proficiency.

Feedback: The student scores within normal limits (WNL) on fine motor and manual coordination and minimal limitations on body coordination, strength, and agility.

Outcome and Rationale: The Bruininks-Oseretsky Test of Motor Proficiency assesses persons aged 4–21 with clinical validity tests for persons with Asperger's. It is a standardized test that assesses and provides information on fine motor coordination, manual coordination, body coordination, and strength and agility A total motor composite score consisting of these four motor areas is provided. The administration of this evaluation will provide objective information on the student's specific motor skills that will be needed for successful participation in a post-secondary technical training program. The evaluation results can be useful for the completion of the referral to the state VR services and the admission application to the post-secondary technical training program. The evaluation results can also provide information on the student's strengths that can be supported and areas of difficulty or deficits that can be addressed by the IEP team during the student's last year of high school. In this case, the evaluation identified functional abilities in fine motor and manual coordination. These skills are essential to the ability to complete technical work tasks and can support the student's application for VR funding to attend the technical training institute. The evaluation results indicated that the student has minimal limitations in body coordination, strength, and agility. However, these skills are not essential for the student's identified post-secondary plan. The acquisition of specific information about the student's motor strengths and limitations is a positive outcome as it will help the IEP team and student revise the IEP plan as needed and complete accurate referrals to meet the student's goals. This is a positive outcome and would result in the awarding of points.

2. C1 Administer the Erhardt Developmental Prehension Assessment (EDPA).

Feedback: The student does not demonstrate any deficits in the hand components evaluated by this measure.

Outcome and Rationale: The Erhardt Developmental Prehension Assessment assesses prehensile development by observing 341 test components which are categorized according to involuntary arm hand patterns, voluntary movements of approach, and prewriting skills. This observational checklist is used to evaluate children with moderate to severe hand and upper extremity impairments related to neurodevelopmental disorders (e.g., CP, TBI.). The selection of this evaluation represents poor knowledge of developmental assessments and a lack of understanding of this student's functional status. The administration of the EDPA would not provide any results that would be valid for pre-vocational and vocational planning for this student. Consequently, its selection would result in the deduction of points.

3. C6 Discharge the student from the OT communication skills group.

Feedback: The student does not develop social skills beyond current abilities.

Outcome and Rationale: Although the student has met the goals of initiating and maintaining one-on-one and group interactions with minimal verbal prompts, the student still has social skill needs that can be addressed through continued participation in this group. Independent social interaction skills are essential for success in the technical training institute program that the student will be pursuing post-graduation and in the future work setting. Consequently, the continuation of the student's participation in this group would be appropriate. Discharge from the communication skills group would be contraindicated as it would prevent the student from developing essential interaction skills needed to achieve post-high school goals. Consequently, the selection of this action would result in the deduction of points.

4. C8 Modify the student's OT program to include participation in the thematic travel skills group.

Feedback: The student develops the ability to independently travel on public transportation.

Outcome and Rationale: Thematic groups are structured to assist members in acquiring the knowledge, skills, and/or attitudes needed to perform a specific activity, in this case the ability to travel independently (i.e., the ability to read a public transportation schedule, ask for directions/information from transit personnel as needed, pay for transit fees, etc.). In thematic groups, learning is facilitated by practicing and experiencing needed behaviors in a real-world setting. Activity gradation and reinforcement of appropriate behaviors are provided to develop needed skills. In addition, thematic groups enable members to discuss their thoughts and feelings about the group's activity (e.g., increased anxiety when the bus is crowded, preferences to not use public transportation and a desire to learn to drive). This group is an appropriate intervention that can help the student develop the skills needed to attain post-secondary goals. Therefore, the selection of this action would result in the awarding of points.

5. C8 Administer a vocational interest inventory.

Feedback: The student identifies interests in drawing, working with animals, and clerical/technical work in a low-stress environment.

Outcome and Rationale: A vocational interest inventory can provide relevant information about the student's areas of interest and/or patterns of interest in a number of vocational areas (e.g., the Reading-Free Vocational Interest Inventory enables the participant to identify interests in categories such as animal care, automotive, housekeeping, and clerical work). This evaluation can provide essential information to help the IEP team implement an effective pre-vocational program for the remainder of the school year and more effectively direct post-secondary plans in the referral to vocational rehabilitation services. This is a positive outcome and points would be awarded for its selection.

6. C8 Refer the student to a public driver training program.

Feedback: The student and family disagree about the appropriateness of this referral.

Outcome and Rationale: The occupational therapist should consult with the student and family prior to making a referral to a program that can have an impact on the family's finances (i.e., the cost of driving lessons, the expense of a car and its maintenance and insurance). In addition, the family's values and opinions about the occupational pursuits of their minor child must be considered. Prior to a referral to a driver training program the therapist should ensure that a driver evaluation is completed. A driver evaluation assesses the person's performance skills, prerequisite abilities, and client factors, (e.g., reaction time and reflexes). It also includes an evaluation of a person's ability to operate a motor vehicle (e.g., the ability to steer, brake, and turn) through the use of a driver simulator and then through the completion of an on-road evaluation. The on-road evaluation also includes the assessment of the person's tactical driving abilities (e.g., the ability to respond to changes in road conditions and traffic/driving risks). Referring the student to a driver training program prior to the completion of an evaluation of the student's skills represents a poor understanding of the OT process. Most importantly, this action can be unsafe since public driving programs do not typically provide driver assessments to persons with disabilities. Therefore, the selection of this action would result in the deduction of points.

7. C9 Recommend a physical therapy evaluation of coordination.

Feedback: The physical therapist responds that the student does not meet the criteria for school–based physical therapy.

Outcome and Rationale: There is nothing in the provided case scenario information to indicate the need for a physical therapy evaluation. While this is not an appropriate referral, it did not cause harm; therefore, it is considered a neutral action. Points would neither be deducted nor awarded for the selection of this action.

Section D

The student develops the requisite skills in the pre-vocational program but remains unsure of a specific vocational interest. The student advances to the high school's vocational transition program. This program includes a class at the technical training institute that the student hopes to attend post-high school and visits to potential work sites of interest to the student. In the weekly occupational therapy social skills group, the student has attained previous goals and has established a new goal to initiate workplace communication with minimal verbal prompts. The student has also achieved an established goal in the travel training group and can now independently use public transportation. Which actions should the occupational therapist take to prepare the student to transition from the school system to post-secondary life? Choose all actions that apply.

1. C8 Recommend a referral to a transitional employment program.

Feedback: The team advises that this referral is premature.

Outcome and Rationale: A transitional employment program (TEP) provides training in a specific job. TEPs are generally time limited (3–6 months) with discharge to competitive employment, supportive employment, or rehabilitation workshops. The student has not identified a specific vocational interest but has identified a desire to complete post-secondary education at a technical training institute. As a result, this referral recommendation is inappropriate for this student. However, a recommendation does not waste resources or cause harm; therefore, this option would be considered neutral. Points would neither be awarded nor deducted for its selection.

2. C8 Develop a list of needed accommodations for the vocational transition program teachers with the IEP team.

Feedback: The team develops a list of needed accommodations.

Outcome and Rationale: The occupational therapist can provide essential information that can help the IEP transition team develop accommodations for the student to successfully participate in the school-based vocational transition program. For example, placing supplies on the desk, providing complex multi-step directions in a written format and presenting information in a clear and direct manner are accommodations that can enable independent task completion. This success can facilitate the student's transition from the school system to the technical training institute. Collaborating with the team (e.g., teachers, psychologist, and other members) can ensure a comprehensive list. This is a positive outcome and the selection of this action would result in the awarding of points.

3. C9 Ask the student's teachers to provide objective information about the student's skills for the discharge report.

Feedback: The teachers share various data on the student's skills with some variability noted in different classroom settings.

Outcome and Rationale: Teachers can provide relevant information about the student's skills based on anecdotal knowledge and objective assessments. This information can help the team compose an accurate discharge summary but it does not include any action that moves the student forward in attaining post-secondary goals. Consequently, this action would be considered neutral and points would neither be awarded nor deducted for its selection.

4. C8 Develop an OT goal for the student to present information about the local public transportation system to the vocational transition program class.

Feedback: The student attains this goal and presents the information to classmates with minimal verbal prompts.

Outcome and Rationale: This is a good goal that requires the student to acquire knowledge about the local public transportation system. Working to attain this goal can concurrently and effectively address the student's goal to develop workplace interaction skills. This is a positive outcome and the selection of this action would result in the awarding of points.

5. C2 Observe the student's behaviors during the vocational transition program classes.

Feedback: The therapist observes the student's abilities to relate to peers and to teachers, and to complete tasks during several classes.

Outcome and Rationale: Observation of a student's behavior can provide relevant information, but it is not the most efficient use of the therapist's time. Teachers who spend direct time with the student can provide this observational data. Although this is not an effective choice for preparing the student for post-secondary life, it does not cause harm. Consequently, this action would be considered neutral and points would neither be awarded nor deducted for its selection.

6. C6 Implement role playing activities in the communication skills group based on student's concerns about workplace interactions.

Feedback: The student engages in the role-plays and develops desired interaction skills.

Outcome and Rationale: The student has done well in the communication skills group so designing group activities relevant to the student's new goal is most appropriate. Role-playing is an effective intervention for the development of social interaction skills. Basing role-play scenarios on the student's expressed concerns will be most effective for developing the skills needed to socially interact in the workplace. This is a positive outcome and points would be awarded for its selection.

Multiple Choice Test Items A1–A170

A1 C8 ✓

An elder with peripheral neuropathies resulting from the chronic effects of diabetes expresses concern over the ability to have a satisfying sexual relationship with a partner. Which is the most beneficial recommendation for the occupational therapist to make to the elder?

Answer Choices:
A. Experiment with different positions during sexual expression activities. ⟶ *for neuromuscular/ortho deficits*
B. Focus on intact senses and areas of intact sensation. ✗
C. Schedule sexual expression activities after rest periods. → *fatigue; MS*
D. Advise the elder to accept decreased abilities in sexual expression as a normal part of aging.

Correct Answer: B.

Rationale:
Peripheral neuropathies result in sensory loss; therefore, focusing on intact senses and intact areas of sensation can help the elder and his/her partner achieve satisfying methods for sexual expression. Experimenting with different positions during sexual expression activities is an effective recommendation for individuals with neuromuscular or musculoskeletal deficits. Scheduling sexual expression activities after rest periods is effective for persons who experience fatigue that limits activity (e.g., multiple sclerosis). While the effects of aging may decrease some abilities in sexual expression, the desire to engage in sexual expression does not necessarily diminish with age. Sexual desire and interest in pursuing sexual expression activities is deeply personal and highly individualized. Advising the elder to accept decreased abilities in sexual expression as a normal part of aging reflects an ageist bias. Moreover, in this situation the elder has expressed concerns which should be directly addressed by the therapist. See Chapter 15 for evaluation and intervention guidelines related to sexuality.

Type of Reasoning: Inductive
This question requires one to determine the best recommendation for a person according to the current deficits and diagnosis. This requires inductive reasoning skill, where clinical judgment is paramount in arriving at a correct conclusion. For this situation the therapist should recommend focusing on intact senses and areas of intact sensation. If answered incorrectly, review sexual expression guidelines for individuals with disabilities or chronic impairments.

A2 C8 ✓

An individual with amyotrophic lateral sclerosis requires the use of an environmental control unit (ECU) to access electrical devices and a personal emergency response system. The individual lives alone and self-directs personal care attendants to perform personal activities of daily living. During instruction to the individual on the capabilities and use of the ECU, which is most important for the occupational therapist to discuss with the client?

Answer Choices:
A. The ECU's back-up power source and charging instructions.
B. Additional assistive technology available.
C. Augmentative alternative communication options.) important but not most
D. Funding for assistive technology.

Correct Answer: A.

Rationale:
Back-up systems for electronic devices must be specified, especially if the device is used to access emergency assistance. Batteries used as back-up systems often have very strict schedules for charging (e.g., water cell batteries must be regularly checked for adequate water levels). Information about additional assistive technology, augmentative alternative communication, and funding can be helpful but they are not the most important area for consumer education in this case.

Type of Reasoning: Inferential
One must determine the most important information to provide for a patient about an ECU, given an understanding of the patient's diagnosis. This requires inferential reasoning skill, where one must infer or draw conclusions about a best course of action. In this situation, the therapist should provide information about a back-up power source and charging instructions as the device may be used to access emergency assistance. If answered incorrectly, review information on ECUs and patient training.

A3 C1 ✓

A nine-year-old child identifies the assembly of a model as the most desired play activity. The occupational therapist determines that the child would have difficulty completing the selected model. Which action is most effective for the therapist to take during the next intervention session?

Answer Choices:
A. Allow the child to work on the model and provide maximum assistance as the child completes the project. X
B. Explore with the child why completing the model is desired by the child and provide alternative project choices. X → too young
C. Break the project down into accomplishable segments and instruct the child to complete one segment at a time.
D. Explain to the child several reasons why the selected model is not the best choice for the child and provide alternative project choices. → too young

Correct Answer: C.

Rationale:
The child is in the concrete operational phase of cognitive development according to Piaget. It is best to give specific information with clear guidelines at this age. Allowing someone to do a project or activity that he/she cannot accomplish is inappropriate. The occupational therapist can use his/her activity analysis skills to break the model down into achievable steps which allow the child to successfully engage in the activity of interest. The exploration of motivation and the rational explanation of a decision require higher cognitive abilities that are consistent with Piaget's formal operational period, from age 11 through the teen years.

Type of Reasoning: Inductive
Clinical knowledge and judgment are the most important skills needed for answering this question, which is an inductive reasoning skill. An understanding of the cognitive development of a six-year-old is important in choosing the best solution. In this case, breaking the project down into segments the child can complete and telling the child to complete one segment at a time is the best action. Review cognitive development guidelines, especially the concrete operational phase if answered incorrectly.

A4 C1

A child with myelomeningocele meets the short-term goals of achieving functional gross grasp and lateral pinch. After several additional weeks of occupational therapy, the child does not meet the goals of demonstrating pincer grasp and three jaw chuck. Consequently, the therapist modifies the child's intervention plan. Which intervention is best to include in the revised plan?

Answer Choices:
A. Splint the index finger in 30° PIP flexion and 30° DIP flexion to achieve pincer grasp. X won't help; may worsen
B. Increase strength of lateral pinch as a basis to develop pincer grasp and three jaw chuck. X not coordination
C. Teach the child to use gross grasp and lateral pinch for functional activities. ☆ can use for funct act.
D. Teach the child to use ulnar grasp for functional activities.

Correct Answer: C.

Rationale:
The child can use gross grasp and lateral pinch to do most functional activities including buttoning, zipping, and playing. Splinting in the manner described will not increase pincer grasp and may actually impede development of pincer grasp. Increasing strength of lateral pinch does not contribute to the coordination needed for pincer grasp and three jaw chuck. Even though gross grasp precedes ulnar grasp, the latter is not as functional as lateral pinch for fine motor skills.

Type of Reasoning: Inductive
One must determine a best course of action utilizing clinical judgment and knowledge of the child's developmental level. This requires inductive reasoning skill in order to determine how to best modify the treatment plan. For this situation, teaching the child to use gross grasp and lateral pinch in functional activities is the best modification to the treatment plan in order to achieve pincer grasp and three jaw chuck. If answered incorrectly, review the developmental stages of grasp.

A5 C6

An individual attends an outpatient parenting skills group. The person has a history of serious recurrent depression and is taking Nardil. The client complains of recurrent headaches and difficulty focusing during the day (e.g., when helping children with their homework). Which action is best for the occupational therapist to make in response to the client's expressed concerns?

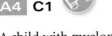

Answer Choices:
A. Instruct the client in stress reduction techniques.
B. Ask the group for suggestions on how to deal with the parenting stress of homework.
C. Suggest that the individual consult with a nurse practitioner for headache relief strategies.
D. Tell the client you will be notifying the psychiatrist of these complaints.

Correct Answer: D.

Rationale:
Nardil is a monoamine oxidase inhibitor (MAOI). It has serious side effects when a person eats foods that contain the amino acid tyramine. Tyramine increases blood pressure and may lead to stroke or other cardiovascular reactions. Headache and heart palpitations are the first sign of a problem. This must be considered a serious medical situation and the physician must be contacted. To assume that the headaches are stress-related is dangerous. Suggesting that the person contact a nurse practitioner does not guarantee follow through. The individual needs to collaborate with the psychiatrist to determine if an MAOI is the best medication, given its restrictions. Chapter 10 in this text provides these restrictions.

Type of Reasoning: Evaluative
One must weigh the possible courses of action and then make a value judgment about the best course to take. This requires evaluative reasoning skill, which often utilizes guiding principles of action in order to arrive at a correct conclusion. In this case, because the patient is describing potentially serious side effects of the medication, the therapist must notify the person's psychiatrist. Questions of this nature can be challenging. Essential to arriving at a correct conclusion is concern for the person's well-being and safety.

A6 C8

A religious congregation obtained private funding to build a ramp so that members with disabilities can attend services. The entrance to the congregation's building has six steps with a rise of 7 inches each. Which is best for the occupational therapist hired by the congregation to recommend for construction of this ramp?

Answer Choices:
A. 42 feet long.
B. 48 feet long.
C. 42 feet long with a 4′ × 4′ landing at the ramp's midpoint.
D. 48 feet long with a 4′ × 4′ landing at the ramp's midpoint.

Correct Answer: C.

Rationale:
A ramp should provide one foot of slope for every inch of rise. Six steps that have a rise of 7 inches results in a total rise of 42 inches. A 42-foot ramp may be too long for some individuals to independently access. Therefore, a landing at the ramp's midpoint would be best to allow the opportunity to safely take a rest break.

Type of Reasoning: Deductive
One must recall the guidelines for ramp construction in order to choose a correct solution. This is factual knowledge, which is a deductive reasoning skill. For this scenario, construction of the ramp should be 42 feet long with a 4′ × 4′ landing at the ramp midpoint. If answered incorrectly, review ramp construction guidelines of the International Code Council's accessibility standards.

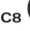

A7 C3 ✓

A child with juvenile rheumatoid arthritis wears bilateral night resting splints with wrists in 0° of extension, MPs and IPs flexed, ulnar deviation of 10°, and thumbs in opposition. The child complains of pain in the wrists upon awakening. No redness is noted upon removing splints. ROM measurements show ulnar deviation of 5°. Which action should the occupational therapist take in response to this complaint and these observations?

Answer Choices:

A. Modify the splints at the wrist. ✗

B. Pad the ulnar aspect on the inside of the splints.

C. Discontinue the splints and monitor the status of pain for two weeks.

D. Construct volar cock-up splints for use during the day.

Correct Answer: A.

Rationale:

The splints should be adjusted by use of heat to accommodate to the current position of ulnar deviation. Padding is frequently used to attempt to modify the position of a splint, but it does not correctly allow distribution of pressure. Discontinuing the splints will serve to increase deformities and pain. The child might benefit from day splints, but this does not address the issue of splints causing pain and being set at an incorrect angle for the child's ulnar deviation measurement.

Type of Reasoning: Evaluative

One must evaluate the symptoms provided and then determine a best course of action based upon this information. This utilizes evaluative reasoning skill, where the value of the information should guide one's thinking and action in clinical situations. In this case, the most appropriate action would be to modify the night splints at the wrist.

Exam A

A8 C9

A 15-year-old with asymptomatic HIV attends an outpatient clinic. The occupational therapy protocol for patients diagnosed with HIV includes presentation of information on safe sex. The adolescent's parents refuse to allow this information to be presented to their child. Which is the best action for the therapist to take in response to this situation?

Answer Choices:

A. Ask the patient's opinion and act on the patient's refusal or consent.

B. Document that the parents refuse the intervention for their child. ✗ → parent's choice w/ children

C. Refer the family to the social worker for counseling.

D. Have the parents sign a waiver that they refused the intervention for their child.

Correct Answer: B.

Rationale:

The therapist should document that the information was refused. Parents are the teenager's legal guardians and have a right to refuse treatment for him/her. If this refusal constitutes a life-threatening situation, a facility can take legal action on behalf of the child. This situation is not considered life-threatening. Although teenagers will often make important personal decisions, including ones about their sexual behavior, legally, parents can make decisions about their children until they are 18 years old. The information about the parents' refusal should be documented to ensure that other team members do not violate the parents' rights. This also protects the setting from potential liability. Asking the teen-aged patient his/her opinion is irrelevant for the therapist could not act on the patient's wishes if they defied the parents' stated wishes about the course and scope of treatment. The therapist may refer the case to the social worker or bring the issue up in a team meeting, but this team collaboration about a difficult issue does not preclude the need to accurately document what has occurred. The parents do not have to sign a waiver to refuse treatment options.

Type of Reasoning: Evaluative

One must weigh the possible courses of action and then make a value judgment about the best course to take. This requires evaluative reasoning skill, which often utilizes guiding principles of action in order to arrive at a correct conclusion. For this case, because the patient is a minor and the decision does not involve a life-threatening situation, the therapist should document the parent's refusal to allow discussion of the information during occupational therapy intervention.

A9 C4

An individual who has Parkinson's disease presents with poor trunk rotation during ambulation and while performing activities of daily living. According to neurophysiologic frames of reference, which is the most effective therapeutic intervention for the occupational therapist to use with this person?

Answer Choices:

A. Facilitation of trunk rotation using neurodevelopmental handling techniques. X
B. Slow rolling with the person supine with knees and hips flexed.
C. Engagement in activities of daily living using diagonal patterns. PNF
D. Provision of a rolling walker to compensate for limited rotation and enhance mobility. X

Correct Answer: C.

Rationale:

The person is presenting with poor trunk rotation during ADL and functional mobility. This is typical in individuals with Parkinson's disease. According to neurophysiologic frames of reference, the most appropriate approach is to use a technique to facilitate rotation during activity performance. PNF diagonals are the best choice because many activities (e.g., loading/unloading the dishwasher, putting away groceries) can be performed using diagonal patterns. NDT handling techniques and the Rood technique of slow rolling may facilitate rotation; however, they do not incorporate functional activities. Therefore, they are not the best choice. The provision of a rolling walker is a compensatory approach and does not directly address the effects of poor rotation on the person's performance of activities of daily living.

Type of Reasoning: Inferential

One must determine the most appropriate intervention approach, given knowledge of the presenting diagnosis, neurophysiologic frames of reference, and incorporation of functional activity. This requires inferential reasoning skill, where one must infer or draw conclusions about a best course of action. In this situation, the therapist should choose ADL activities incorporating diagonal patterns. Review information on intervention approaches for Parkinson's disease and PNF intervention techniques. Answering this question correctly requires integration of this knowledge.

A10 C9

An individual who had a CVA one year ago continues to demonstrate unilateral neglect. The individual drives daily to therapy despite several suggestions from the occupational therapist to discontinue this activity. The therapist has determined that the client is an unsafe driver. Which is the best action for the therapist to take in response to this situation?

Answer Choices:

A. Report the individual to the department of motor vehicles.
B. Suggest that the individual attends a driver training program.
C. Report the information to the physician.
D. Tell the individual's family that the client is at risk for injuring self and others while driving.

Correct Answer: C.

Rationale:

The therapist must report the information to the physician, who is responsible to take action on the individual's ability to drive. The driver's license agency addresses the issues of administration of licenses. The agency does not address cognitive evaluation or remedial issues concerning driving. A driver training program is a good suggestion to help the person improve skills but it does not address the unsafe driver on the road. The option to inform the family can be presented in the context of the skills that OT addresses, such as unilateral neglect. However, it does not address the safety issue.

Type of Reasoning: Evaluative

One must weigh the merits of each of the four possible courses of action in order to determine the best response to the situation. This necessitates evaluative reasoning skill, where guiding principles of action are paramount in arriving at a correct conclusion. In this situation it is best to report the information to the physician. If answered incorrectly, review driver re-education guidelines and reporting potentially unsafe driving.

A11 C7

Following a left CVA, an individual receives OT services at a sub-acute rehabilitation facility. The patient's personal goal is to be independent in dressing. The patient demonstrates decreased memory, poor sequencing skills, and ideational apraxia. Which of the following is most effective for the therapist to provide when teaching one-handed dressing techniques to this patient?

Answer Choices:

A. Step-by-step verbal instructions.
B. Sequenced photographs of the steps in dressing.
C. Physical prompts to initiate the steps in dressing.
D. A full length mirror for the client to observe self-dressing performance.

Correct Answer: C.

Rationale:

Ideational apraxia is the breakdown in the knowledge of what is to be done and how to perform specific activities. This means that one cannot perform a task either spontaneously or upon request. However, the sensorimotor aspects needed to perform the activity can be intact. Providing physical prompts to initiate dressing may be a sufficient cue for the individual to begin and then complete the task. Providing verbal instructions or sequenced photographs will not address the fundamental deficit of ideational apraxia and therefore will not enhance performance. Observing one's self dressing in front of a mirror results in a view opposite of actual performance. This can increase confusion, especially with apraxia.

Type of Reasoning: Inductive

One must utilize clinical knowledge and judgment to determine the best approach for teaching one-handed dressing techniques, given the patient's symptoms. In this case, because the patient has ideational apraxia, it is best to provide physical prompts to initiate dressing tasks. If answered incorrectly, review ideational apraxia symptoms and ADL intervention guidelines.

A12 **C8**

An elementary school teacher has been recently diagnosed with multiple sclerosis (MS). Which adaptation is best for the occupational therapist to recommend the teacher use to accommodate for the effects of MS on classroom teaching?

Answer Choices:

A. Large print written material to compensate for visual impairments.
B. A daily list of tasks to compensate for cognitive deficits.
C. A motorized scooter to compensate for decreased endurance.
D. A high stool to compensate for lower extremity weakness.

Correct Answer: D.

Rationale:

Lower extremity muscle weakness is common in the early stages of MS. Using a high stool will provide the teacher with an alternative to standing while maintaining visibility to the entire classroom. In addition, the use of a stool can help minimize the effects of fatigue which is often common in all stages of MS. Visual impairments, cognitive deficits, and/or decreased endurance are not common in the early stages of MS.

Type of Reasoning: Inferential

One must determine the most appropriate recommendation for an individual, given knowledge of the presenting diagnosis. This requires inferential reasoning skill, where one must infer or draw conclusions about a best course of action. In this situation, the therapist should recommend a high stool to compensate for lower extremity weakness, given an understanding that lower extremity muscle weakness is common in the early stages of MS. Review symptoms of early stage MS if answered incorrectly.

A13 **C2**

An occupational therapist conducts an initial home visit to a family with a premature infant who, at four months and 5 lbs., has just been sent home. The child has multiple disabilities. Which is the best primary goal for the therapist to work on with the family during this first session?

Answer Choices:

A. Communicate effectively to develop a therapeutic relationship with the family.
B. Teach the family proper body mechanics for lifting the child.
C. Teach the family assertiveness training to develop advocacy skills.
D. Determine whether adaptive aids or positioning equipment is needed.

Correct Answer: A.

Rationale:

During the first visit, it is essential that the therapist practice effective communication and work on developing a therapeutic relationship with the family. Since the child has multiple disabilities, the occupational therapist will need to work closely and frequently with the family to address their child's needs over an extended period of time. The other choices can be addressed when, and if the need evolves. In addition, one cannot assume that the family will need assertiveness training.

Type of Reasoning: Inferential

One must determine the most likely intervention approach for a child on an initial home visit. This requires inferential reasoning skill, where one must draw conclusions based on the information presented. In this situation, practicing effective communication and developing a therapeutic relationship is the primary goal. If answered incorrectly, review guidelines for family centered practice and home health care of premature infants.

A14 C7

A three-year-old child with left spastic hemiplegia due to cerebral palsy is evaluated for early intervention services. During the evaluation the occupational therapist observes behaviors that seem to indicate the presence of visual deficits. Based on these observations, which action should the occupational therapist take?

Answer Choices:

A. Completion a motor-free visual perceptual assessment.
B. Completion a developmental vision assessment.
C. Refer the child to an optician.
D. Refer the child to an optometrist.

Correct Answer: D.

Rationale:
Prior to conducting a visual perceptual evaluation, an anatomical visual assessment to determine visual acuity is required. Optometrists are the professionals who are qualified to perform eye examinations to determine visual acuity, level of visual impairments, and damage to or disease in the visual system.

Type of Reasoning: Evaluative
One must weigh the possible courses of action and then make a value judgment about the best course to take. This requires evaluative reasoning skill, which often utilizes guiding principles of action in order to arrive at a correct conclusion. For this case, because the child demonstrates visual deficits, the therapist should refer the child to an optometrist.

A15 C3

An occupational therapist constructs a splint for a person who incurred full thickness facial and anterior neck burns. In which position should the therapist splint the neck?

Answer Choices:

A. Neutral.
B. 15° flexion.
C. 15° lateral flexion.
D. 15° hyperextension.

Correct Answer: A.

Rationale:
The neck should be splinted in neutral. A major focus of acute burn care is proper positioning to maintain involved areas in anti-deformity positions. The anti-deformity position for the neck is neutral. The other positions are contraindicated. A full thickness burn involves the epidermis and dermis, hair follicles, sweat glands, and nerve endings. Skin grafting is required and healing time can take months. Post-operative occupational therapy care following skin grafts involves the wearing of a splint at all times.

Type of Reasoning: Deductive
This question requires recall of guidelines and principles, which is factual knowledge. Deductive reasoning skills are utilized whenever one must recall facts to solve clinical problems. In this situation, the therapist should splint the patient in neutral. Review splinting guidelines for anterior neck and facial burns if answered incorrectly.

Exam A

A16 C9

An occupational therapist reviews the use of the occupational therapy department's resources to determine medical necessity and cost efficiency. Which service management task is the therapist performing?

Answer Choices:
A. Utilization review. ~~A~~ ✗
B. Retrospective peer review.
C. Total quality management.
D. Risk management.

Correct Answer: A.

Rationale:
Utilization review is a plan to review the use of resources within a facility to determine medical necessity and cost efficiency. It is often a component of a continuous quality improvement (CQI) or a performance assessment and improvement (PAI) system. Total quality management is the creation of an organizational culture that enables all employees to contribute to an environment of continuous improvement. Risk management is a process that identifies, evaluates and takes corrective action against risk; and plans, organizes and controls the activities and resources of OT services to decrease actual or potential losses. Retrospective review involves the auditing of medical records by third-party payers to ensure appropriate care was rendered. Peer review is a system in which the quality of work by a group of health professionals is reviewed by their peers.

Type of Reasoning: Deductive
One must recall the definition of a utilization review for this question. This requires deductive reasoning skill, where factual knowledge is vital in choosing the correct solution. Utilization review is defined as a plan to review the use of resources in a facility, which should be reviewed if answered incorrectly.

A17 C1

A six-year-old has thumb weakness, noted mostly in poor ability to perform thumb opposition. During evaluation, which activity will the therapist most likely observe the child having difficulty performing?

Answer Choices:
A. Holding a penny on the ulnar side of the hand while moving a nickel from the palm to the tips of the thumb and the index finger. — translation
B. Rotating a pencil 180°. ✗
C. Sliding the fingers up and down a pencil while holding the pencil in a tripod grasp. — shift
D. Moving a ring from pad-to-pad pinch position to the palm.

Correct Answer: B.

Rationale:
Rotating a pencil describes simple rotation of 180°. Complex rotation is 360 degrees. The child with poor thumb opposition has the most difficulty performing this skill of all of the in-hand manipulation skills. The penny example describes translation with stabilization. Sliding the fingers along the pencil is shift. Moving a ring describes translation without stabilization.

Type of Reasoning: Inferential
One must link the child's symptoms to the activities presented in order to determine which activity would pose the most challenge. This requires inferential reasoning, where one must mentally picture the activities occurring and then determine which one uses the most thumb opposition to complete the activity. In this case the rotation of a pencil 180° uses the most thumb opposition.

Multiple Choice Scenario Item A.I.

Questions A18 to A22 are based on the following information.

A private practice comprised of five occupational therapists provides home-based services to a variety of adult clients in a two-county area. They are expanding their practice to include home-based services in another county. In addition, this private practice has recently been awarded the early intervention service provider contract for all three counties. The practitioners plan to hire three entry-level occupational therapists and two occupational therapy assistants (OTAs) to fill the service needs of their growing practice. The OTAs have extensive experience in home-based service provision. The private practitioners plan to provide all of their new employees with a comprehensive orientation program and the shadowing of an experienced therapist for two weeks.

A18 C9

To ensure the provision of best practice, the new entry-level occupational therapists will be provided with supervision of their caseloads. At what level should this supervision be provided?

Answer Choices:
A. Routine.
B. General.
C. Close.
D. Minimal.

Correct Answer: C.

Rationale:
It is recommended that entry-level occupational therapists receive close supervision, that is, daily, direct contact for patient care. Intermediate-level occupational therapists can receive routine supervision, every two weeks, to general supervision, at least monthly. Advanced practitioners need minimal supervision, on an as-needed basis, for patient care.

Type of Reasoning: Deductive
This question requires one to recall factual guidelines pertaining to supervision of occupational therapists, which is a deductive reasoning skill. The question essentially tests whether one recalls the recommendations for supervision of entry-level occupational therapists. In this situation, the entry-level occupational therapists should receive close supervision with their own caseloads. If answered incorrectly, review standards of practice guidelines related to supervision of occupational therapists.

A19 C9

The private practitioners pay for their newly hired occupational therapists' registration for an advanced course on pediatric assessment. Which is the most important outcome of attending this course for the occupational therapists?

Answer Choices:
A. Fulfillment of continuing education requirements for independent credentialing agencies.
B. Keeping up-to-date on current trends in occupational therapy.
C. Networking with other pediatric professionals.
D. Improvement of their professional skills and competence.

Correct Answer: D.

Rationale:
The most important goal of continuing professional education is to improve skills and develop competence for service delivery. Networking opportunities, keeping up-to-date with trends and the fulfilment of external credentialing requirements are all a benefit of participation in continued education. However, these are not the primary aim of professional development activities. The most important objective is to improve service delivery skills and competencies.

Type of Reasoning: Inferential
One must determine the benefits of an advanced assessment course in order to determine the most important goal of the program. This requires inferential reasoning, where one must draw conclusions based on the information provided. In this situation, an advanced handling course would improve professional skills and competence. If answered incorrectly, review benefits of continuing education and professional development activities.

A20 C9

The supervising occupational therapists meet to plan the workload of the recently hired OTAs. Which is an appropriate task for them to assign to the OTAs?

Answer Choices:
A. The in-home evaluation of the adult clients' instrumental activities of daily living.
B. The determination of long-term goals to include in the adult clients' occupational therapy home care intervention plan.
C. The design of home-based sensory integration protocols for infants and toddlers with sensory processing disorders.
D. The administration and interpretation of the Hawaii Early Learning Profile (HELP) to infants and toddlers.

Correct Answer: A.

Rationale:
An OTA can complete IADL evaluations under the supervision of an occupational therapist. The interpretation of the evaluation results and the determination of goals are the responsibility of the occupational therapist. The design of sensory integration protocols and the completion and interpretation of evaluations cannot be completed by an OTA. An OTA can contribute to these processes but cannot independently complete them.

Type of Reasoning: Inferential
This question requires one to recall the standards of practice for the OTA. Inferential reasoning skills are utilized as the test taker must determine, based on knowledge of practice guidelines, what is likely to be true. For this situation an OTA can complete an evaluation of instrumental activities of daily living. If answered incorrectly, review information on standards of practice for the OTA.

A21 C9

The private practitioners meet with their accountant to plan fiscally for their expanded practice. How would the accountant classify the fees that the practice receives from their early intervention contract?

Answer Choices:
A. Accounts payable.
B. Capital assets.
C. Productivity standards.
D. Accounts receivable.

Correct Answer: D.

Rationale:

Accounts receivable are the payments received by a program, setting, or institution for services rendered. They are the assets in a budget. Accounts payable are the payments that are due for purchases by or services rendered to a program, setting, or institution. They are the debts in a budget. Capital assets are improvements or purchases that cost more than a set amount (often $500.00 or $1000.00) and that are expected to last more than a year (e.g., a new ADL kitchen, computer equipment). Productivity standards establish the amount of direct care and reimbursable services each therapist must provide each day.

Type of Reasoning: Analytical

This question provides a description of a service and the test taker must determine the definition of such a service. This is an analytical reasoning skill, as questions of this nature often ask one to analyze descriptors in order to determine a definition. In this situation the description is that of accounts receivable, which should be reviewed if answered incorrectly.

A22 C9

The accountant asks the private practitioners to present their budget for anticipated direct expenses of their growing practice. Which is the most appropriate item to include in this budget request?

Answer Choices:

A. The rent and utilities of the practice's primary office.
B. An integrated computer system for paperless documentation by all staff.
C. Staff vacation and sick time.
D. Supplies of items used in in-home therapy sessions.

Correct Answer: C.

Rationale:

Direct expenses include costs related to OT service provision such as salaries and benefits. Vacation and sick time are benefits that must be budgeted. An integrated computer system will cost a substantial amount of money which renders it a capital expense. As noted above, capital expenses are any item above a fixed amount. Capital items are separated from other expenses due to their depreciation in value and potential tax credits that may be available for purchases and/or investments. Supplies are considered a variable expense since this expense will change in direct proportion to the amount of services provided. Rent is a fixed expense. Utilities are indirect expenses.

Type of Reasoning: Inferential

One must infer or draw conclusions about a likely course of action, given the information presented. This is an inferential reasoning skill, where knowledge of an approach, such as describing direct expenses of a new program, is essential to choosing a correct solution. In this case, the therapist should include staff vacation and sick time. Review fiscal management terms if answered incorrectly.

A23 C8

A young adult with a diagnosis of schizophrenia, paranoid type is scheduled to be discharged from an inpatient setting to a halfway house and psychosocial clubhouse. The occupational therapist is assisting the team with the discharge plan. Which is the most important information for the therapist to provide to the team about this person?

Answer Choices:

A. The person's instrumental ADL skills.

B. The possible effects of medication on the person's performance.

C. The person's vocational potential.

D. The person's social interaction skills.

Correct Answer: A.

Rationale:

Knowledge of the person's level of skills for the performance of IADL is essential for the occupational therapist to share with the team. This can provide the halfway house staff with information that can be used to determine the level of structure and support this person may need to make a successful transition. In a halfway house, residents are typically responsible for the maintenance of their rooms and personal items (e.g., laundry). They are also expected to contribute to the maintenance of the entire household (e.g., cleaning and cooking). Successful adjustment to the halfway house will require the performance of instrumental ADL, whether independently or with assistance. In addition, the IADL of community mobility will be needed to travel from the halfway house to the clubhouse. The occupational therapist is the only member of the team who is able to assess the specifics of the individual's functioning in these areas. While OT input in the other areas identified in the answer choices can be helpful, it is not as essential as the individual's IADL status. Nursing can provide information on the functional effects of medications. All team members can provide information on social skills. The individual's vocational potential can be assessed at the clubhouse because an inherent component of the clubhouse model is vocational services.

Type of Reasoning: Inductive

This question requires one to determine the most important information to provide to the discharge planning team. This requires inductive reasoning skill, where clinical judgment is paramount in arriving at a correct conclusion. For this situation the therapist should provide information about the person's instrumental ADL skills, since the person will be transitioning to a halfway house. If answered incorrectly, review discharge planning guidelines for persons in inpatient settings and the expectations of community-based settings. Answering this question correctly requires the integration of this knowledge.

A24 C3

Following the performance of a home exercise program prescribed one week ago, an individual with bilateral upper extremity muscle weakness reports experiencing pain in both shoulders and elbows. The pain is consistent for up to eight hours. The individual's occupational therapist is on vacation for two weeks and a recently hired entry-level therapist has been assigned to cover the vacationing therapist's caseload. Which is the most appropriate action for the covering therapist to take in response to this individual's reporting symptoms?

Answer Choices:

A. Stop exercising completely until the primary therapist returns and can re-evaluate the person's status.

B. Reduce the intensity of exercise by 50% and reassess the person during the next intervention session.

C. Continue with the current exercise program to develop tolerance.

D. Advise the individual to take a pain relief medication 30 minutes prior to exercising.

Correct Answer: B.

Rationale:
A decrease in the exercise by 50% allows for the continuation of the treatment regime and addresses the individual's complaints of excessive pain. The person needs to maintain the exercise program in order to address range of motion deficits and muscle weakness, however the intensity is causing excessive pain. The 50% decrease reduces the regime intensity and still allows the person to exercise. Further modification of the home program can occur at the next intervention session, if needed. An abrupt cessation of the exercise program may cause joint stiffness and is not necessary. The continuation of the current regimen is contraindicated due to the longevity of residual pain reported by the person. There is potential for harm to the affected joints if pain is not respected and the current exercise regimen is continued. Ingestion of pain medication 30 minutes prior to exercising will not address post-exercise pain.

Type of Reasoning: Evaluative
This question requires a value judgment in a therapeutic situation, which is an evaluative reasoning skill. In this situation, because the treating therapist is on vacation, the covering therapist should recommend a reduction in the home program by 50% and then reassess at the next treatment session. This solution allows the individual to continue the therapeutic exercises, while addressing the individual's pain.

A25 C8

A child with spinal muscle atrophy can no longer reach beyond 90° of shoulder abduction and 90° of shoulder flexion. The parents state that the child can no longer don or doff a T-shirt. Which is the best approach for the occupational therapist to recommend the child use for dressing?

Answer Choices:
A. Place the T-shirt directly on the child's lap, have the child don the arms first, then don the head of the T-shirt.
B. Have the child learn to don and doff front-opening shirts instead of T-shirts.
C. Have the child support the elbows on a table at chest height to don the T-shirt over arms, then don over head.
D. Have the child sit with the trunk well-supported, lean to the right and don the right arm, repeat to the left, and then don the head of the T-shirt.

Correct Answer: C.

Rationale:
Spinal muscle atrophy is a progressive disorder and the therapist needs to prepare the child and family for progressive loss of skills. The best technique, as shoulder ROM decreases, is to use a table for support to don arms then over the head.

Type of Reasoning: Inductive
This question requires one to consider the best approach for completing the ADL task, given an understanding of the diagnosis and limitations. This requires inductive reasoning skill, where the test taker must utilize clinical judgment based on knowledge of the diagnosis to arrive at a correct conclusion. If answered incorrectly, review information on spinal muscle atrophy and on activity analysis. A correct answer requires you to analyze the activity adaptations provided to find the one that best matches the child's capabilities.

Exam A

A26 C4

An individual recovering from a CVA has received extensive motor learning intervention. The client can now transfer a learned motor skill to different contexts. The client also demonstrates the ability to successfully motor problem solve during activities in different contexts. In documenting the client's progress, which stage of motor learning is most accurate for the occupational therapist to document the individual has achieved?

Answer Choices:

A. Skill acquisition.
B. Skill retention.
C. Practice context.
D. Generalized context stage.

Correct Answer: B.

Rationale:

During the skill retention stage of motor learning, the individual can successfully retain the motor skill and transfer its application and use to a diversity of contexts. In these different settings and situations the person must modify his/her timing, sequencing, posture, and many other neuromotor component skills. These modifications and adjustments reflect successful motor problem solving abilities. During the skill acquisition stage of motor learning, the individual will make frequent errors and motor performance is inconsistent and inefficient. Although practice, context, and generalization are important motor learning concepts, they are not considered stages of motor learning.

Type of Reasoning: Analytical

This question provides a description of a functional stage of motor learning and the test taker must determine the appropriate stage that the patient is functioning within. This is an analytical reasoning skill, as questions of this nature often ask one to analyze a group of functional skills in order to determine a level of performance. In this situation the functional level is that of the skill retention stage of motor learning. Review motor learning stages, especially skill retention if answered incorrectly.

A27 C8

An occupational therapist provides consultation services to members of a town chamber of commerce who have expressed interest in improving their businesses' accessibility. Which is the minimum door width that the occupational therapist should recommend to the chamber members as accessible and not requiring modification?

Answer Choices:

A. 28 inches.
B. 32 inches.
C. 30 inches.
D. 34 inches.

Correct Answer: B.

Rationale:

The minimum clearance width for doorways to allow for wheelchair access is 32 inches. Measurements less than 32 inches must be modified. Measurements equal to or greater than 32 inches are acceptable.

Type of Reasoning: Deductive

One must recall the minimum clearance width for doorways in order to arrive at a correct conclusion. This requires deductive reasoning skill, where factual knowledge is essential to choosing the correct solution. Thirty-two inches is the minimum clearance for door widths in this situation. Review accessibility guidelines, especially door width measurements if answered incorrectly.

A28 C2

A client expresses an interest in playing a computer game with another group member during a leisure skills group. The occupational therapist reviews the client's cognitive evaluation and agrees that the game is a good choice for the client's cognitive level. After 15 minutes of engaging in the computer game, the client rubs both eyes, looks around, and reports trouble focusing. Which should the therapist do in response to these observations and client statements?

Answer Choices:
A. Provide verbal encouragement for the client to complete the game before taking a break.✗
B. Suggest the client and the other member play a different video game that is easier for the client.✗
C. Discontinue the session and advise the client to select a different leisure activity to do with the other member.✗
D. Suggest the client and the other member talk about the game's progress in between completing their turns.✗

Correct Answer: D.

Rationale:
The client appears to be experiencing visual strain which can be caused by staring at a computer screen without a break. Consequently, the best choice is to decrease the visual strain by providing periodic brief breaks from looking intently at the screen. Having the clients talk between taking turns will facilitate them looking at each other rather than the computer screen. Providing verbal encouragement and suggesting a new game that is easier does not address the visual fatigue/strain issue. There is no need to discontinue the session at this point. Ending the session would be inappropriate because it would not enable the therapist to use the client's experience to teach ways to effectively manage discomfort and successfully engage in activities of interest. This could leave the client with a feeling of failure and contribute to a low self-esteem, which would be counterproductive to leisure skill development.

Type of Reasoning: Inductive
This question requires clinical judgment to determine a best course of action, which is an inductive reasoning skill. For this situation, the behavior exhibited by the client indicates that a decrease in visual stimuli is warranted; therefore the client should talk about the game's progress with the other member in between completing turns. If answered incorrectly, review information on visual fatigue in computer use.

A29 C9

A 19-year-old with diagnoses of dysthymic disorder and narcissistic personality disorder attends a vocational rehabilitation program. When the client arrives for the work adjustment group, the therapist notes that the client demonstrates an unsteady gait and slurred speech. The client's breath smells of alcohol. Which is the best action for the therapist to take in response to these observations?

Answer Choices:
A. Follow program procedures to arrange for transportation to bring the client home.✗
B. Introduce the topic of alcohol's effect on work performance as the focus of the scheduled group session.
C. Have the client meet with the social worker to discuss treatment options for potential alcohol abuse.
D. Contact the client's parents to pick the client up to bring the client home.

Correct Answer: A.

Rationale:
The person is showing signs of being under the influence of alcohol. It is not appropriate at this time to use the group or an individual session to discuss the observed behaviors and/or potential treatment needs. In the client's current state, he/she is impaired and cannot fully participate in this discussion. The client is a 19-year-old adult so there is no need to contact the client's parents.

Type of Reasoning: Evaluative

This question requires professional judgment based on guiding principles, which is an evaluative reasoning skill. Because the person is showing signs of being under the influence of alcohol, the therapist should arrange for transportation back to the client's home. Questions such as these are challenging to answer as clear cut answers may not be readily available. Essential to choosing the correct conclusion is to do what is in the best interest of the individual.

A30 C5

A toddler with spastic quadriplegic cerebral palsy demonstrates a consistent gag reflex. Which technique should the occupational therapist use to help inhibit this reflex?

Answer Choices:

A. Move a spoon from side to side on the tongue.
B. Walk a spoon down the tongue, going from proximal to distal with even pressure.
C. Press a spoon down firmly on the center of the tongue.
D. Stroke the tongue in a circular motion with a firm object.

Correct Answer: C.

Rationale:

The best approach to decrease a gag reflex is to press down firmly on the center of the tongue and to apply pressure from distal to proximal. Lateral and circular movements can facilitate the gag reflex.

Type of Reasoning: Deductive

This question requires recall of guidelines for feeding children with spastic cerebral palsy, which is factual knowledge. Deductive reasoning skills are utilized whenever one must recall facts to solve clinical problems. In this situation, the therapist can inhibit the gag reflex by pressing down firmly on the center of the tongue. Review feeding guidelines for children with a persistent gag reflex if answered incorrectly.

A31 C4

A child with a tactile defensive sensory modulation disorder attends a private early intervention clinic. The occupational therapist collaborates with the child's parents to develop strategies and guidelines to help the child handle the symptoms of this disorder at home. Which is the best recommendation for the therapist to make to the parents?

Answer Choices:

A. Avoid the use of swings and other moving equipment during play activities.
B. Encourage the use of swings and other moving equipment during play activities.
C. Soften the child's clothing by repeated laundering and remove clothing tags.
D. Provide a variety of textures in the clothing the child wears.

Correct Answer: C.

Rationale:

Children with tactile defensive sensory modulation disorder find stiff clothing, textured clothing, and clothing tags aversive. The use or avoidance of, swings and other moving play equipment is indicated for vestibular processing disorders.

Type of Reasoning: Inductive

This question requires one to determine the most appropriate recommendation for a child with tactile defensiveness. This requires inductive reasoning skill, where clinical judgment is paramount in arriving at a correct conclusion. For this situation, given knowledge of tactile defensive behaviors, the therapist should recommend softening clothing and removing clothing tags. If answered incorrectly, review intervention guidelines for children with tactile defensive behaviors.

A32 C9

A newly hired OTA is instructed by the director of rehabilitation to supervise two hospital volunteers as they learn how to assist patients in safely completing bed to wheelchair transfers. The OTA informs the supervising occupational therapist of the director's request. Which is the first action the occupational therapist should take in response to this request?

Answer Choices:

A. Advise the OTA to comply with the request.
B. Advise the OTA to refuse the request.
C. Observe the OTA to assess service competence in transfer training.
D. Explain to the director of rehabilitation why the request is inappropriate.

Correct Answer: D.

Rationale:

Volunteers are not trained health care professionals and they cannot perform transfers with patients. Therefore, the OTA cannot comply with the director's request to supervise volunteers in performing transfers. The occupational therapist is responsible for the practice of the OTA he/she supervises; therefore, he/she must inform the director of rehabilitation of the inappropriateness of this request. While it is appropriate for the OTA to decline the director's request, it is most important that the rationale for this denial be explained by the OT supervisor in order to prevent future inappropriate requests of the OTA.

Type of Reasoning: Evaluative

One must weigh the possible courses of action and then make a value judgment about the best course to take. This requires evaluative reasoning skill, which often utilizes guiding principles of action in order to arrive at a correct conclusion. For this case, because the request to supervise volunteers in transfer training is an inappropriate request, the OT supervisor should speak to the director to explain why the request is inappropriate. Review guidelines for supervision of personnel if answered incorrectly.

A33 C8

A single parent is hospitalized for an exacerbation of schizophrenia. Actively psychotic upon admission, the client has been stabilized on medication. The client is currently not demonstrating hallucinations or delusions. Residual deficits include several negative symptoms and decreased cognitive skills. At the team meeting, the psychiatrist decides to discharge the client within 48 hours. The client lives with his/her elementary-school aged children. Which is the best recommendation for the occupational therapist to make during this team meeting?

Answer Choices:

A. An extension of hospitalization to further evaluate cognitive skills.
B. A family meeting to discuss the need for the children to assume home management tasks.
C. A home visit to assess the client's safety skills within the home environment.
D. A referral to social services to explore foster care for the children.

Correct Answer: C.

Rationale:
A home visit is necessary to determine the individual's ability to safely carry out home management and parenting responsibilities. The therapist should recommend a home visit to determine if the physician's recommendation is appropriate and/or if home-based services are needed. It is not necessary to extend the hospital stay to evaluate cognitive skills. It is most effective to evaluate cognitive skills in the home setting where the individual will be carrying out occupational tasks. While children can help with home management tasks, they should not fully assume these responsibilities. There is no information in the scenario to indicate that the children need foster care.

Type of Reasoning: Inductive
One must determine a best course of action for this patient, which requires inductive reasoning skill. For this patient, to ensure safety in the home, a home visit is ideal prior to discharge. The home visit can help determine if discharge is appropriate. Recommendations can then be made to extend treatment and/or provide concrete supports to enhance the patient's functional abilities. If answered incorrectly, review principles of discharge planning and the symptoms of schizophrenia. Answering this question correctly requires the integration of this knowledge.

A34 C5

An individual recovering from hip replacement surgery prepares for discharge home. The client has a secondary diagnosis of gastric esophageal reflux disease (GERD). Which is the best bed position for the occupational therapist to recommend to this client?

Answer Choices:
A. Supine with elevation of the shoulders and head.
B. Sidelying with the neck in neutral.
C. Sidelying with elevation of the shoulders and head.
D. Supine with elevation of the hips.

Correct Answer: A.

Rationale:
In GERD, the lower esophageal sphincter (which acts as a valve between the esophagus and stomach) becomes weak or relaxes when it should not. This results in the stomach contents rising up into the esophagus. Elevation of the head above the stomach when the person is reclined may decrease the upward retropulsion of the bolus from the stomach. The other positions are not effective for an individual with GERD and they are contraindicated for a person recovering from hip surgery.

Type of Reasoning: Inferential
One must infer or draw conclusions about a likely course of action, given the information presented. This is an inferential reasoning skill, where knowledge of a therapeutic approach, such as the appropriate bed positioning in this situation, is essential to choosing a correct solution. In this case, the therapist should recommend a supine position with elevation of the shoulders and head. Review the bed positioning for individuals with GERD if answered incorrectly.

A35 C3

An occupational therapist designs a dynamic splint for an individual recovering from tendon repair. At which angle should the therapist position the outrigger?

Answer Choices:

A. 45° to the joint.
B. 90° to the joint.
C. 60° to the joint.
D. 110° to the joint.

Correct Answer: B.

Rationale:

90° is the appropriate angle of pull for it provides the most effective application of force. The application of a perpendicular force prevents unwanted traction on the joint and shearing stress. As the person's condition improves and mobility increases, the therapist must adjust the outrigger to maintain the 90° angle of pull.

Type of Reasoning: Deductive

One must recall the guidelines for dynamic splinting and angle of pull. This is factual knowledge, which is a deductive reasoning skill. 90° is the appropriate angle of pull for this situation. If answered incorrectly, review guidelines for dynamic splinting, especially the angle of pull after tendon repair.

A36 C8

The transition plan for a high school senior with developmental delay includes a referral to a vocational rehabilitation (sheltered) workshop job setting. The student has set a goal to live independent of family. Which is the best living environment for the occupational therapist to recommend for this student?

Answer Choices:

A. An apartment in a subsidized housing project.
B. A group home with case managers available on-call.
C. A supported apartment with a roommate.
D. A group home with daily on-site supervision.

Correct Answer: D.

Rationale:

A person with developmental disabilities who meets the referral criteria for a vocational rehabilitation (formerly called sheltered) workshop will typically have cognitive deficits that require structure and supervision to successfully and safely complete tasks. A group home with on-site staff would provide this type of support. In addition, since this student has lived with family for all of his/her life, it is likely that he/she will need training to develop instrumental activities of daily living skills (IADL). Upon the attainment of IADL skills in the group home and vocational skills in the vocational rehabilitation (sheltered) workshop, the person may be able to progress to a higher level of independence in work and home management. The person would have to first develop IADL skills to live more independently in a housing project apartment, unsupervised group home, or supported apartment.

Type of Reasoning: Inferential

This question requires clinical judgment in order to determine the best living environment for an individual with developmental delay. This requires inductive reasoning skill, where knowledge of the diagnosis and ability to live independently are paramount in arriving at a correct conclusion. For this situation, the therapist should recommend a group home with daily on-site supervision. If answered incorrectly, review community living options for individuals with developmental disabilities.

A37 C1

The parents of a two-year-old child with bilateral congenital upper extremity amputations express concern to the homecare occupational therapist about their child's complete disinterest in toilet training. At which point should the occupational therapist advise the parents to begin toilet training?

Answer Choices:

A. When the child indicates discomfort with being wet or soiled.
B. Immediately, because toileting is a developmentally appropriate task.
C. When the child is three years old, as this is the typical developmental age for toilet training.
D. By placing the child on a "potty" chair for five minutes per hour each day.

Correct Answer: A.

Rationale:

The first toileting skill developed is the child's recognition of being wet or soiled as uncomfortable. All children develop differently and typical developmental time tables include a range of ages for skill development. In addition, these ranges can vary for children with congenital disabilities.

Type of Reasoning: Deductive

One must recall the developmental guidelines for children in toilet training. This is factual knowledge, which is a deductive reasoning skill. In this situation, the therapist should advise the parents to begin toilet training when the child indicates discomfort with being wet or soiled. If answered incorrectly, review toilet training guidelines for children.

A38 C3

A school-aged child who is right-hand dominant complains of numbness and tingling after writing for more than 15 minutes. A neurological exam shows no reason for the numbness and tingling. Which action would be most beneficial for the occupational therapist to recommend to the child?

Answer Choices:

A. Use a pencil held in a universal cuff to complete writing activities.
B. Elevate the right upper extremity at night and whenever possible during the day.
C. Stretch the right upper extremity every 15-20 minutes during writing activities.
D. Use a custom-molded pencil grip made of splinting material when writing.

Correct Answer: C.

Rationale:

The neurological exam is negative. The best choice is to educate the child in active ROM and stretching of the upper extremity to increase circulation and to attempt to prevent numbness and tingling. The universal cuff and custom-molded grip are adaptations that do not address treatment of numbness and tingling. Elevation can reduce edema; however, edema is not a symptom here.

Type of Reasoning: Inductive

One must determine the reason for the child's symptoms in order to determine the best recommendation for the child to alleviate the symptoms. This requires inductive reasoning skill, where clinical judgment and diagnostic thinking are central to choosing a best solution. In this situation, stretching the right upper extremity every 15-20 minutes during writing is the best recommendation to increase circulation and prevent symptoms. Review intervention approaches for paresthesia if answered incorrectly.

A39 C9

An occupational therapist leads a transitional planning group for high school students with conduct disorders. The school fire alarm goes off five minutes before the group's scheduled termination. There have been six false alarms during the past three days at the school. Several of the students laugh and say, "There it goes again." Which is the occupational therapist's best response to this situation?

Answer Choices:

A. Call the school's main office to determine the validity of this alarm.
B. Escort the students to the nearest fire exit.
C. Conclude the group with a discussion about the implications of false alarms.
D. Escort the students back to their homeroom classrooms to await directions.

Correct Answer: B.

Rationale:
All alarms must be taken seriously to ensure safety. In the event of an actual fire, any delay can be deadly. All the other choices are incorrect for they place students at potential risk.

Type of Reasoning: Evaluative
This question requires a value judgment in an emergency situation, which is an evaluative reasoning skill. In this type of situation, the safest procedure should be followed, which is to escort the students to the nearest fire exit. Questions that inquire about a course of action in a potential emergency often require the test taker to respond in the safest, most effective manner possible.

A40 C2

A clubhouse program hires an occupational therapist as a consultant. The clubhouse board of directors requests that the OT consultant focus on the development of evening and weekend leisure activities. Which recommendations should the therapist make for the selection and completion of the group activities?

Answer Choices:

A. Activities to be selected and completed by clubhouse members according to guidelines provided by the therapist. → too direct
B. Activities to be selected by the therapist with written instructions provided to the group attendees for activity completion.
C. Activities to be selected by clubhouse members with activity completion led by the clubhouse members.
D. Activities to be selected by the therapist and completed by the clubhouse members after demonstration by the therapist.

Correct Answer: C.

Rationale:
Clubhouse programs utilize a consumer empowerment model that emphasizes the active involvement of all participants in the decision-making and implementation processes of the clubhouse. The other choices are too directive for this model.

Type of Reasoning: Inferential
One must infer or draw conclusions about a likely course of action, given the information presented. This is an inferential reasoning skill, where knowledge of a therapeutic approach, such as the recommendations for activities in a clubhouse setting, is essential to choosing a correct solution. In this case, the therapist should allow the members to select and lead the activities, given the clubhouse setting. Review therapeutic group approaches and practice standards for clubhouse programs if answered incorrectly.

A41 C4

A two-year-old child is placed in foster care due to child abuse and neglect. The child was frequently beaten and locked in a dark closet. The child is fearful and suffering from sensory deprivation. Which sensory input is best for the occupational therapist to recommend the foster parents provide for the child?

Answer Choices:
A. Slow rocking.
B. Fast rocking.
C. Bright lights.
D. Upbeat music.

Correct Answer: A.

Rationale:
Intervention for sensory deprivation should begin with slow linear movements such as slow rocking. The other options can lead to sensory overload due to the severity of the child's sensory deprivation.

Type of Reasoning: Inductive
One must utilize clinical knowledge and judgment to determine the recommendation that best addresses the child's deficit. This requires inductive reasoning skill. In this case, the occupational therapist should recommend slow rocking. If answered incorrectly, review intervention guidelines for sensory deprivation.

A42 C8

An occupational therapist advises the parent of an 18-month-old with developmental delays on techniques to facilitate feeding. The child has a reflexive bite. Which utensil is most beneficial for the therapist to recommend the parent use when feeding the child?

Answer Choices:
A. A deep-bowled soup spoon.
B. A narrow shallow coated spoon.
C. A traditional teaspoon.
D. A plastic spork.

Correct Answer: B.

Rationale:
The use of a narrow shallow coated spoon will help the food slide off. Deeper spoons or a spork will make it more difficult for the food to slide off, which would not be indicated for a child with a reflexive bite. In addition, the prong edges of the spork may hurt the child as he/she bites.

Type of Reasoning: Inferential
One must have knowledge of reflexive bite in children in order to choose the best feeding utensil. This is an inferential reasoning skill where knowledge of the diagnosis coupled with an understanding of the benefits of each of the utensils is essential to arriving at a correct conclusion. In this situation the therapist should suggest a narrow shallow plastic spoon. If answered incorrectly, review guidelines for issuing utensils for children with reflexive bite.

A43 **C8**

During a wheelchair evaluation, an individual with limited functional mobility expresses concern about the ability to continue volunteer work at a local church. The church's doorways are 31 inches wide. The client knows (from a recent home remodeling project) that 32 inches is the minimum width recommended for wheelchair access. Which recommendation should the occupational therapist make to the client to most effectively address the client's concerns and functional mobility needs?

Answer Choices:
A. Have the church widen its doorways to comply with ADA requirements.
B. Order a wheelchair with wraparound armrests. ✗
C. Have the client explore alternative volunteer activities in accessible locations. ✗
D. Order a customized narrow adult wheelchair. ✗

Correct Answer: B.

Rationale:
Wraparound armrests (also called space saver armrests) reduce the overall width of a wheelchair by one inch. A customized chair can be very expensive. The case does not indicate the individual's measurements, so it is not possible to ascertain if a narrow wheelchair would actually fit the person. Religious organizations are exempt from ADA accessibility requirements. The individual does not need to explore alternative volunteer experiences since valued established activities can continue with an appropriate wheelchair.

Type of Reasoning: Inductive
Clinical knowledge and judgment are the most important skills needed for answering this question, which requires inductive reasoning skill. Knowledge of available mobility equipment to remedy the issue of a narrow doorway is paramount to arrive at a correct conclusion. In this case, the most appropriate recommendation is to order a wheelchair with wraparound armrests, which should be reviewed if answered incorrectly.

 A44 **C9**

An occupational therapist provides home-based services to a person recovering from a recent CVA. The individual lives alone and receives home care Medicare Part A benefits. The therapist arrives at the client's house at the scheduled session time, but there is no response to the knocking on the door. A neighbor reports seeing the client leave with a friend. Which is the best action for the therapist to take in response to this situation?

Answer Choices:
A. Document that no one answered the door and that the appointment will be rescheduled. ✗
B. Call the nurse case manager to report the missed appointment and the need to reschedule. ✗
C. Document that no one was home and that the appointment will be rescheduled. ✗
D. Document that the client is engaged in community mobility activities and should be evaluated for discharge. —best not to jeopardize homebound status

Correct Answer: A.

Rationale:
Documentation must state that no one answered the door. This is factually correct and allows the individual to continue to receive home care service reimbursement from Medicare. To receive Medicare home care reimbursement, an individual must be homebound which means he/she can only leave home according to specific criteria. See Chapter 4 for these criteria. The client may have left for a reason that would meet these criteria. It is best not to document any behaviors that may jeopardize a person's homebound status. It is not necessary to notify the nurse case manager about a missed appointment. The therapist can speak directly to the individual. One missed appointment is not a basis for discharge.

Type of Reasoning: Evaluative
One must weigh the possible courses of action and then make a value judgment about the best course to take. This requires evaluative reasoning skill, which often utilizes guiding principles of action in order to arrive at a correct conclusion. For this case, the therapist should document that the patient did not answer the door and that the appointment will be rescheduled. Review Medicare guidelines for homebound status if answered incorrectly.

A45 C6

A client with a diagnosis of paranoid schizophrenia is participating in an initial evaluation session at a psychiatric day treatment program. Halfway through the completion of an activities configuration, the client states the referral to this day program is inappropriate and unnecessary because it was made by an incompetent psychiatrist. The client becomes visibly upset and loud when talking about the unfounded referral and the psychiatrist's incompetence. Which is the best initial action for the occupational therapist to take in response to the client's statements?

Answer Choices:
A. End the evaluation session and tell the client to call to re-schedule when feeling better. ✗
B. Assure the client of the referring psychiatrist's competence and advise the client to discuss concerns with the doctor. ✗
C. Acknowledge that the client appears upset and ask if the client is able to focus on the remaining evaluation. ✗
D. Contact the day program's chief psychiatrist to report the client's stated concerns about the referring psychiatrist's competence. ✗

Correct Answer: C.

Rationale:
A simple acknowledgement of the individual's concerns can validate his/her feelings in a non-threatening manner without validating potentially delusional thought content. Asking the person in a calm business-like manner if he/she can return to the task at hand can diffuse the situation. If the client states he/she is not able to regain focus, the therapist can then provide the needed support. Immediately ending the evaluation does not deal with the issue of potentially escalating behavior and does not provide the individual with the opportunity to engage in a therapeutic relationship. Continuing the evaluation can allow concrete opportunities for support and reality testing. Assuring the client of the doctor's competence could contribute to further escalation if the client's concerns are based on a delusional thought process, which is unshaken by external explanations. There is no need to report the client's concerns for there is no concrete evidence of physician incompetence at this time. The therapist should relay the client's expressed concerns at the next team meeting.

Type of Reasoning: Evaluative
One must weigh the possible courses of action and then make a value judgment about the best course to take. This requires evaluative reasoning skill, which often utilizes guiding principles of action in order to arrive at a correct conclusion. In this case, the client is upset and his/her feelings appear to be escalating. To address potential agitation and prevent escalation, the therapist should acknowledge the client's feelings and try to redirect him/her to the task at hand. Review redirection strategies for clients with escalating behavior if answered incorrectly.

A46 C3

An occupational therapist measures the active range of motion of an individual's index finger. The measurements are MCP 0-45, PIP 10-60, and DIP 10-40. Which is most accurate for the therapist to document as the finger's total active motion (TAM)?

Answer Choices:

A. 62.5°.
B. 125.0°.
C. 72.5°.
D. 145.0°.

Correct Answer: B.

Rationale:
To obtain the TAM measurement, the extension deficits are added and then subtracted from the flexion measurement total. In this scenario, the extension deficits total 20°. The flexion measurements total 145°. 145 minus 20 equals 125.0°.

Type of Reasoning: Deductive
This question requires recall of guidelines and principles, which is factual knowledge. Deductive reasoning skills are utilized whenever one must recall facts to solve clinical problems. In this situation, the TAM is 125°, which is calculated by subtracting the extension deficits from the flexion measurement total. Review TAM guidelines if answered incorrectly.

A47 C9

The family of an individual being admitted to a rehabilitation center offers the occupational therapist a cash gift. The therapist refuses the money but the family continues to insist that the therapist take the cash gift. After thanking the family for their generous gesture, which is the therapist's best response?

Answer Choices:

A. Donate the money to the hospital.
B. Donate the money to charity.
C. Use the money to purchase an item for the OT department.
D. Decline the gift.

Correct Answer: D.

Rationale:
In accordance with the OT Code of Ethics, OT practitioners should not enter into transactions that could be interpreted as financially exploitive. Accepting a substantial cash gift would bring into question the ethical issue of financial gain; therefore, declining the gift is the best response. In certain circumstances, it could be appropriate to suggest a donation to the department or facility (e.g., if the family is determined to concretize their gratitude). In some cultures, it is appropriate to offer tokens of appreciation to staff. It might be considered rude and offensive to some persons to refuse a small gift. Some facilities may alter their policies about accepting gifts in these cases.

Type of Reasoning: Evaluative
This question requires one to weigh the merits of the four possible choices and determine the most ethical response to the situation. In keeping with the OT Code of Ethics the therapist should refuse the gift. Citing hospital policy can depersonalize this response and decrease the possibility of insulting the family. Ethical questions often require evaluative reasoning skill, as there is not always a clear cut or simple answer to the situation.

Exam A

A48　C9

An individual who successfully completed an inpatient drug rehabilitation program returns to the setting to thank staff members for their assistance with recovery. The individual offers to share personal insights and experiences with the members of the OT values clarification group scheduled for the next hour. After thanking the individual, which is the best response for the occupational therapist to make in response to this offer?

Answer Choices:
A. Welcome the individual as a guest to the group to share personal perspectives on recovery and inspire group members.
B. Inform the individual that former clients cannot visit the group due to the need to maintain member confidentiality. ✗
C. Ask the individual to prepare a presentation on how values clarification aided in recovery for the next scheduled group session.
D. Tell the individual that the therapist will discuss this offer with the group and afterwards inform the individual regarding the group decision.

Correct Answer: B.

Rationale:
Confidentiality of all members of a group on an inpatient unit must be preserved at all times. Even if the therapist discussed the possibility of a guest speaker with members and the members verbally agreed to this visit, the therapist could not be certain that all members are in complete agreement. More reticent members may be hesitant to voice their opposition to a visit. The therapist is professionally responsible to maintain confidentiality.

Type of Reasoning: Evaluative
This question requires a value judgment in an ethical situation, which is an evaluative reasoning skill. In this situation, it is paramount to protect patient confidentiality; therefore the therapist must decline the person's visit to the group. Judgment in this situation relies on the OT Code of Ethics, which includes the principle of confidentiality. Review the OT Code of Ethics, if answered incorrectly.

A49　C1

A 21-month-old child with severe spastic quadriplegia is evaluated by an occupational therapist. The therapist determines that the child is cognitively intact, exhibiting age-appropriate cognitive skills despite major sensorimotor deficits. The therapist recommends a play activity to enhance these cognitive abilities and provide the child with a fun and pleasurable experience. Which is the best object for the therapist to recommend?

Answer Choices:
A. A multi-colored mobile of objects of interest placed over the child's stroller. ✗
B. A mechanical toy with a chin controlled on/off switch. ✗
C. A shape sorter with foam squares, triangles, and circles. ✗
D. A battery controlled hammock swing. ✗

Correct Answer: B.

Rationale:
At 21 months, a child is cognitively able to operate and control mechanical toys. The chin controlled switch will enable this child to self-direct his/her play despite the spastic quadriplegia. A mobile is cognitively too low for this child's ability. It is a passive activity that would not provide active engagement of the child. The ability to identify and sort shapes does occur at 21 months, but the use of a shape sorter requires motor abilities beyond this child's capacity.

Type of Reasoning: Inductive
This question requires one to determine the most appropriate object for enhancing cognitive abilities of this child. This requires inductive reasoning skill, where clinical judgment is paramount in arriving at a correct conclusion. For this situation, a mechanical toy with a chin controlled on/off switch is most appropriate. If answered incorrectly, review developmental levels of cognition and play and treatment guidelines for small children with spastic quadriplegia. The integration of this knowledge is required to answer this question correctly.

A50 C4

An individual recovering from a traumatic brain injury is assessed to be at Level VI of the Rancho Level of Cognitive Functioning Scale. Which should the occupational therapist use to implement treatment?

Answer Choices:
A. Sensory stimulation activities such as moving to music.
B. Repetitive self-care tasks such as brushing hair.
C. Community re-entry activities such as taking a bus.
D. Simple meal preparation tasks such as making a sandwich.

Correct Answer: D.

Rationale:
At Level VI the individual is appropriate and goal-directed but can become confused. Cues are required. Community re-entry activities are too high-level for an individual at Level VI. They are more appropriate for Level VII and VIII. Sensory stimulation activities such as moving to music would be appropriate for Level III. Repetitive self-care tasks would be appropriate for Level V.

Type of Reasoning: Inductive
One must utilize clinical knowledge and judgment to determine the approach that provides appropriate therapeutic challenge for a patient at Level VI. In this case, the therapist should implement treatment by having the individual prepare a simple meal, such as a sandwich. If answered incorrectly, review treatment guidelines for patients at Level VI on the Rancho Level of Cognitive Functioning Scale.

A51 C8

An individual with hemiplegia has inadequate ankle dorsiflexion on the affected side. Which of the following equipment is best for the occupational therapist to recommend the person use to compensate for this deficit and facilitate safe and effective ambulation?

Answer Choices:
A. An ankle-foot orthosis (AFO).
B. A wide-based quad cane (WBQC).
C. A narrow-based quad cane (NBQC).
D. A knee-ankle-foot orthosis (KAFO).

Correct Answer: A.

Rationale:
An AFO will provide the needed stability to the ankle joint to enable safe and effective ambulation. In this case, the knee is not involved so a KAFO is not indicated. A WBQC and a NBQC would be indicated for an individual with poor balance. Although canes can be very helpful ambulation aids, the concern in this case was to provide equipment to compensate for the lack of ankle dorsiflexion.

Type of Reasoning: Analytical
This question provides a description of a functional device and the test taker must determine the best device to address the patient's deficits. This is an analytical reasoning skill, as questions of this nature often ask one to analyze descriptors or equipment to determine the best match for a patient's deficit(s). In this situation an AFO is the best recommendation. Review guidelines for use of AFOs if answered incorrectly.

A52 C6

The parent of two elementary school-aged children receives home care hospice services due to metastasized bone cancer. The client is in pain and has poor endurance and decreased muscle strength. The client requires moderate assistance with self-care and dressing. Which is the best intervention for the occupational therapist to incorporate into sessions with this parent?

Answer Choices:
A. Training in energy conservation techniques for self-care and dressing. ✗
B. Training in joint protection techniques for self-care and dressing. ✗
C. Using biofeedback to reduce the client's pain.
D. Exploring play activities for the parent to do with the children. ✗

Correct Answer: D.

Rationale:
A major focus of hospice care is to maintain the individual's control over his/her life while enabling engagement in meaningful activities that are related to the person's valued roles. Although the person is dying, he/she is still a parent and will likely enjoy playing with his/her children when they are not in school. There are many play activities suitable for elementary school-aged children that can be completed by a person with decreased endurance and muscle strength. In addition, research has found that diversional activities can decrease the intensity of an individual's pain experience. There is no indication of a need to train the client in techniques for self-care or dressing. The client currently is in pain and requires moderate assistance due to functional deficits. It is likely that the client will continue to need this assistance due to the fact that his/her cancer is at the terminal stage. Even with training in energy conservation or joint protection, the individual would still need assistance with these tasks due to the effects of advanced cancer. Biofeedback is not effective in managing pain that results from metastasized bone cancer.

Type of Reasoning: Inductive
One must utilize clinical knowledge and judgment to determine the intervention approach that best incorporates control over the patient's life. In this case, because the patient is a parent of school-aged children, the therapist should incorporate play activities to do with the children after school. Review principles of hospice care and intervention approaches for patients with terminal illness if answered incorrectly.

A53 C8

An occupational therapist working in a school has been asked to recommend technological devices for a student with severe spastic quadriplegia and dysarthria. Which action should the therapist take prior to recommending specific equipment?

Answer Choices:
A. Determine access capabilities in collaboration with the speech language pathologist ✗
B. Identify funding source(s) in collaboration with the social worker. ✗
C. Obtain family support in collaboration with the psychologist. ✗
D. Determine intervention goals in collaboration with the student. ✗

Correct Answer: D.

Rationale:
Establishing the goals of technological interventions in collaboration with the student is essential to ensure that all equipment recommendations are meaningful and relevant to the student's unique needs and desired goals. For example, technology can facilitate interpersonal communication, functional mobility, engagement in leisure activities, and/or the completion of schoolwork. Determining access capabilities is an important step to take after the goal of the device is established. Funding for a device would be provided by the school in accordance with IDEA. While obtaining family support is always important and is required by IDEA, the occupational therapist must be able to explain the need and rationale for the recommended equipment to effectively obtain this support.

Type of Reasoning: Inductive
This question requires one to determine the best approach for recommending assistive technology. This requires inductive reasoning skill, where clinical judgment is paramount in arriving at a correct conclusion. For this situation, the occupational therapist should determine the intervention goals in order to ensure that the equipment recommendations are relevant to what the student needs and wants. If answered incorrectly, review assessment guidelines for assistive technology.

A54 C8

A patient with a complete injury of the spinal cord at the C5 level completed inpatient rehabilitation which concentrated on increasing independence in activities of daily living. In the discharge documentation, which is most likely for the occupational therapist to state the client is able to do?

Answer Choices:
A. Button buttons using a button hook. 67+
B. Use mobile arm supports for feeding. ✗
C. Tie shoes using thick shoelaces. — C8
D. Brush teeth using a tenodesis splint. C6

Correct Answer: B.

Rationale:
Mobile arm supports are likely to be able to be used by a person with a C5 level of injury. The ability to complete grooming tasks using a tenodesis splint and buttoning with a button hook are likely skills for a person with a SCI at the C6 level. A person with a C8 level of SCI would likely be able to tie shoes.

Type of Reasoning: Inferential
One must match the patient's level of injury to the expected functional outcome in order to arrive at a correct conclusion. This requires inferential reasoning, where one must draw conclusions based on the information presented. If answered incorrectly, review expected functional outcomes in dressing skills for patients with C6 injury.

A55 C4

An individual presents with intention tremor, dysmetria, decreased equilibrium and nystagmus caused by a cerebellar lesion. The person expresses difficulty with routine tasks. Which intervention is best for the occupational therapist to provide?

Answer Choices:

A. A cone and pegboard activity with wrist weights to control tremors.

B. Quick stretch to lateral trunk muscles during a functional activity.

C. A power wheelchair to prevent falls during routine activities.

D. Upper extremity weight bearing during self-care activities at a sink.

Correct Answer: D.

Rationale:

The treatment goals for persons with cerebellar dysfunction are focused on strengthening proximal muscles, improving postural responses, and increasing stability. Weight bearing of the upper extremities can increase shoulder girdle stability. A cone and pegboard activity does not describe a functional activity and would not generalize to activities of daily living. This activity is also very difficult to complete with dysmetria and intention tremor. Quick stretch is not an intervention method. It is a method to assess spasticity. It is applied in a direction opposite the pull of the muscle group being tested and then graded utilizing a "minimal/moderate/severe" rating scale. A power wheelchair is not indicated in this scenario nor would a power wheelchair help the person perform routine tasks with intention tremors and dysmetria.

Type of Reasoning: Inductive

Clinical knowledge and judgment are the most important skills needed for answering this question, which requires inductive reasoning skill. Knowledge of the diagnosis, its presenting symptoms, and the most appropriate clinical outcomes is essential to choose the best solution. In this case, the therapist should provide upper extremity weight bearing during self-care routine at the sink. Review the functional impact of cerebellar lesions and intervention approaches for persons with motor disturbances if answered incorrectly. The integration of this knowledge is required to determine a correct answer.

A56 C3

A middle school-aged child with osteogenesis imperfecta reports feelings of low self-esteem, social isolation, boredom, and lethargy. The occupational therapist collaborates with the child to identify resources for after-school leisure activities to promote socialization and community participation. Which of the following activities is best for the therapist to explore with the child?

Answer Choices:

A. Team sports.

B. Therapeutic horseback riding.

C. Scouting programs.

D. Computer clubs.

Correct Answer: D.

Rationale:

Osteogenesis imperfecta results in brittle bones that fracture easily. Fracture prevention through activity restrictions is a primary focus. This can result in social isolation, decreased self-efficacy, and depression. Exploring different computer clubs can provide the child with a number of age-appropriate viable options for leisure activities that the child can successfully pursue after school without risking fractures. The other options involve more physically-based activities that would be difficult for the child to safely pursue. These activities would highlight what the child is unable to do, rather than his/her abilities. This would be contraindicated in the treatment of depression. In computer clubs, physical abilities are not needed, for any physical deficit can be readily compensated for with adaptations and modifications.

Type of Reasoning: Inferential

One must determine the most appropriate activity recommendation, given knowledge of the presenting diagnosis. This requires inferential reasoning skill, where one must infer or draw conclusions about a best course of action. In this situation, the therapist should recommend that the child join a computer club. If answered incorrectly, review symptoms of osteogenesis imperfecta and developmentally appropriate leisure activities. The integration of this knowledge is required to answer this question correctly.

A57 C9

An occupational therapist interviews an OTA for a position at a high school for gay and lesbian youth. The position involves the provision of transitional vocational programming and life skills training. The OTA uses a wheelchair for mobility and has dysarthric speech. Which of the following is most relevant for the occupational therapist to ask the OTA about during the interview?

Answer Choices:

A. Verbal group leadership skills.
B. Sexual orientation.
C. Personal beliefs about homosexuality.
D. Accommodations needed due to the evident disabilities.

Correct Answer: A.

Rationale:

The other questions are in violation of civil rights legislation and the ADA. One can ask an applicant about his/her ability to perform essential job tasks. Vocational programming and life skills training is most often done in group settings; therefore inquiring about the applicant's verbal group leadership skills is appropriate and legal. It is up to the applicant to declare a disability and to request any reasonable accommodations needed to perform essential job tasks. An interviewer cannot directly question an individual about his/her disability nor needed accommodations.

Type of Reasoning: Deductive

This question requires recall of guidelines and protocols, which is a deductive reasoning skill. Having an understanding of the ADA, the test taker should conclude that the only question that can be asked in this situation is the OTA's verbal group leadership skills. Review ADA regulations related to job interviewing if answered incorrectly.

A58 C8

A nine-year-old girl with the diagnosis of cystic fibrosis is hospitalized in a small rural hospital. Currently, there are no other children in the hospital and the hospital does not have a pediatric play area. The head nurse asks the occupational therapist to suggest appropriate play activities that hospital volunteers can provide for the child. Which is the most age appropriate activity for the therapist to suggest?

Answer Choices:

A. Dressing paper dolls.
B. Coloring in coloring books.
C. Playing card games.
D. Cutting and pasting pictures onto cards.

Correct Answer: C.

Rationale:
Children aged 7–12 are developmentally able to participate in games with rules, competition, and social interaction. The other activities reflect creative play that is developed between ages the ages of 4 and 7. In addition, they are solitary activities and do not afford opportunities for competitive fun and socialization. Hospitalization can be lonely and frightening so having volunteers play with the child can be psychologically beneficial, as well as developmentally appropriate.

Type of Reasoning: Inferential
One must determine the most appropriate play activities for a child, given knowledge of the child's age and developmental ability. This requires inferential reasoning skill, where one must infer or draw conclusions about a best course of action. In this situation, the therapist should suggest playing card games. Review information on play activities for nine-year-old children if answered incorrectly.

A59 C4

After evaluating a client with right-sided weakness and decreased motor control an occupational therapist decides to use interventions based on the proprioceptive neuromuscular facilitation (PNF) approach. When applying PNF principles, which of the following actions should the therapist have the client do during an intervention session to increase use of the right upper extremity and hand?

Answer Choices:
A. Reach overhead with the right hand to retrieve a dish out of a higher cabinet and set it down on the countertop in front.
B. Reach to the right side to retrieve an item out of refrigerator at hip height and place it into the left hand to set it on the countertop to the left.
C. Use both hands together to pour juice out of a heavy pitcher into a glass on a countertop.
D. Take items out of a dishwasher on the right side and reach across the body to place them in the upper cabinet on the opposite side.

Correct Answer: D.

Rationale:
PNF (proprioceptive neuromuscular facilitation) is a technique which involves use of diagonal patterns of movement and involves rotational trunk movement. Using the right upper extremity to reach down to one side to take items out of a dishwasher and reaching across one's body (trunk rotation) to place these items into a higher cabinet on the opposite side of body creates this diagonal pattern and encourages use of the affected side to increase motor control and volitional movement. The other answer choices do not include activities which require diagonal movements of the upper extremity or trunk rotation. Thus, they are not consistent with a PNF approach.

Type of Reasoning: Inductive
This case requires the test taker to first recall PNF principles and then determine the approach that will best facilitate improved functioning given the deficits. This necessitates inductive reasoning skill, where clinical judgment is paramount in arriving at a correct conclusion. In this situation, the therapist should have the patient take items out of a dishwasher on the right side and then place the items above and to the left side. If answered incorrectly, review PNF principles and assumptions.

A60 C8

A teenage girl with juvenile rheumatoid arthritis (JRA) identifies a goal of applying her own makeup. Which adaptation is most beneficial for the therapist to recommend?

Answer Choices:

A. Silver ring splints to hold makeup applicators.
B. Enlarged soft foam handles on makeup applicators.
C. Long thin handles on makeup applicators.
D. A universal cuff to hold makeup applicators.

Correct Answer: B.

Rationale:

Enlarged soft foam handles will facilitate independent grasp and increase independence in makeup application. Silver ring splints are not designed to hold objects. They are used on individual fingers to prevent boutonniere deformities which can contribute to improved functional grasp. However, there is no mention of the presence of boutonniere deformities in this item's scenario. Long thin handles would increase the difficulty of holding applicators. A universal cuff is an adaptation for a person with no ability to grasp. It is not indicated in this case.

Type of Reasoning: Inductive

Clinical knowledge and judgment are the most important skills needed for answering this question, which requires inductive reasoning skill. Knowledge of the diagnosis and most appropriate recommendations for the functional activity is essential in order to choose the best solution. In this case, the therapist should recommend enlarged soft foam handles on the makeup applicators. Review self-care adaptations and adaptive devices for persons with rheumatoid arthritis if answered incorrectly.

A61 C9

An occupational therapist conducts a satisfaction survey to evaluate the quality of OT services in an outpatient program. The questionnaire developed by the therapist asks respondents to rate their responses to quality statements according to a 4-point Likert scale of agreement. Which statement best reflects an adequate measure of satisfaction?

Answer Choices:

A. "The amount of time devoted to stress management was adequate."
B. "Setting my own goals was important to me."
C. "My experience in occupational therapy helped me."
D. "The OT staff was respectful and fair to me."

Correct Answer: A.

Rationale:

The response "The amount of time devoted to stress management was adequate" is the most helpful for those listed because it provides concrete information to evaluate service quality and improve service provision. Statements that reflect the personal value of an item to an individual, or that are vague and non-measurable do not measure satisfaction with the services delivered. As a result, they do not meet the measurement requirements of a satisfaction survey.

Type of Reasoning: Analytical

This question requires one to determine which statement is the best reflection of one's level of satisfaction with a service. This requires analytical reasoning skill, where the test taker must determine the meaning of the phrases and interpret their inherent characteristics as it relates to measuring quality. In this situation, the phrase asking about the adequacy of the amount of time devoted to stress management best reflects a measure of satisfaction.

A62 C6

An occupational therapist working on an acute psychiatric inpatient unit conducts a series of groups for clients newly admitted to the unit. Which group leadership style is most effective for the therapist to assume when leading these groups?

Answer Choices:
A. Advisory.
B. Facilitative.
C. Laissez-faire.
D. Directive.

Correct Answer: D.

Rationale:
Directive leadership involves the provision of structure, clear directions, and immediate and consistent feedback. These qualities are needed in a group whose members are acutely ill with psychiatric disorders. The other choices do not provide the structure or organization needed for individuals whose symptoms often include decreased attention span, distractibility, poor social skills, and/or thought disorders.

Type of Reasoning: Inductive
Clinical knowledge and judgment are the most important skills needed for answering this question, which requires inductive reasoning skill. Knowledge of the leadership styles and the most effective style in leading groups of newly admitted clients is essential to arriving at a correct conclusion. In this case, the most effective style is directive leadership, which should be reviewed if answered incorrectly.

Multiple Choice Scenario Item A.II.

Questions A63 to A66 are based on the following information.

An individual with degenerative joint disease (DJD) incurred an injury to the right hand. The client is referred to occupational therapy due to complaints of severe pain, stiffness, and extreme temperature changes in the hand. The occupational therapy referral states that the person has pitting edema and blotchy, shiny skin. Based on a screening, the occupational therapist determines that the client's presenting symptoms are consistent with the diagnosis of complex regional pain syndrome (CRPS) Type I.

A63 C3

The occupational therapist evaluates the client's pain by asking the client which movements or activities elicit pain. Which of the following is the therapist assessing?

Answer Choices:
A. The quality of pain.
B. The location of pain.
C. The intensity of pain.
D. The triggers of pain.

Correct Answer: D.

Rationale:
Pain triggers are those activities and/or movements that result in pain. The quality of pain is determined by asking the person to describe the pain; common descriptors are sharp, throbbing, burning, tender, and shooting. The intensity of pain is measured by pain scales; a 0 to 10 scale is most commonly used. The location of pain is determined by having the person describe or point to the location.

Type of Reasoning: Analytical
This question provides a description of a functional activity and the test taker must determine the likely definition of such an activity. This is an analytical reasoning skill, as questions of this nature often ask one to analyze descriptors of functional skills to determine the overall skill involved. In this situation the activity is assessing pain triggers, which should be reviewed if answered incorrectly.

A64 C3

The occupational therapist completes the pain evaluation. What additional evaluation methods should the therapist use to assess this client?

Answer Choices:
A. Vigormeter.
B. Dynamometer.
C. Volumeter.
D. Sphygmomanometer.

Correct Answer: C.

Rationale:
One of the client's major presenting problems is edema. The volumeter is an assessment tool that objectively measures edema based on the displacement law of physics. A dynamometer, vigormeter, and sphygmomanometer are tools that can be used to measure grip strength. An evaluation using these measures would be contraindicated at this time due to the client's presenting complaints of severe pain and stiffness.

Type of Reasoning: Inferential
One must have knowledge of all the assessment tools described and reasons for administration in order to arrive at a correct conclusion. This is an inferential reasoning skill where knowledge of clinical guidelines and judgment based on facts are utilized to reach conclusions. If answered incorrectly, review volumeter assessment guidelines.

A65 C3

The occupational therapist plans intervention to address the client's goals to engage in meaningful occupations. Which physical agent modality (PAM) should the occupational therapist use in preparation for functional activity?

Answer Choices:
A. Transcutaneous electrical nerve stimulator (TENS).
B. Contrast baths.
C. Whirlpool.
D. None; PAMs are contraindicated for this diagnosis.

Correct Answer: B.

Rationale:
CRPS Type I is a vasomotor dysfunction. The use of contrast baths facilitates the opening and closing of the vascular and lymphatic vessels and is the preferred modality for CRPS. Initially, treatment of CRPS focuses on the reduction of pain and edema and then progresses to functional movement. Techniques to address pain and edema are a priority and should be used gently and as tolerated. Contrast baths are the gentlest PAM intervention listed. Other options include cold packs, retrograde massage, Coban wraps, and desensitization. TENS may be too painful to implement initially. Whirlpools are typically used to clean and debride wounds and are not indicated in this case.

Type of Reasoning: Inferential
One must link the individual's diagnosis to the treatment approaches provided in order to determine which treatment approach would most effectively address the individual's deficits. This requires inferential reasoning, where one must draw conclusions about the potential treatment outcomes. In this case the therapist should use contrast baths to appropriately address deficits. Review treatment approaches for CRPS Type I if answered incorrectly.

A66 C3

Which is the most appropriate activity for the occupational therapist to recommend for the person to complete at home?

Answer Choices:
A. Doing light craft work.
B. Playing a table-top game.
C. Performing relaxation exercises.
D. Manually washing a car.

Correct Answer: D.

Rationale:
Manually washing a car involves scrubbing and the carrying of buckets of water which are stress loading activities. Stress loading is a recommended intervention for CRPS, Type I (formerly known as reflex sympathetic dystrophy or RSD). Light crafts, table-top games, and/or visualization relaxation exercises can be meaningful and relevant to the person, but they do not provide any weight bearing. Therefore, these activities are not indicated as an intervention approach for this disorder.

Type of Reasoning: Inferential
This question requires the test taker to recall characteristics of CRPS Type I and then match this to a home program that most effectively addresses the patient's symptoms. In this situation, manually washing a car would provide the best approach to address the symptoms, which allows for stress loading activity. If answered incorrectly, review intervention guidelines for CRPS, especially Type I.

A67 C8

An individual with advanced Huntington's chorea is newly admitted to a skilled nursing facility. The resident weighs 280 pounds and cannot independently transfer. What is the best recommendation for the occupational therapist to make to the resident's direct care staff to ensure a safe transfer?

Answer Choices:
A. A mechanical lift transfer.
B. A two-person lift transfer.
C. A stand pivot transfer.
D. An assisted sliding board transfer.

Correct Answer: A.

Rationale:
A mechanical lift transfer is the safest for both the resident and the staff. The other transfers require motor and cognitive abilities that are beyond the capacity of an individual with advanced Huntington's chorea. Huntington's chorea, an autosomal dominant neuromuscular disease, is characterized by choreiform movements, progressive intellectual deterioration, and psychiatric disturbances. The individual's movement disorder combined with potential confused and/or agitated behaviors requires the use of a mechanical lift for safe and efficient transfers.

Type of Reasoning: Inductive
This question requires one to determine the best recommendation for an individual, given an understanding of the diagnosis and limitations. This requires inductive reasoning skill, where clinical judgment is paramount in arriving at a correct conclusion. For this situation, the therapist should recommend a mechanical lift transfer for the safety of the resident and staff. If answered incorrectly, review guidelines for mechanical lift transfers and the information about the sequelae of Huntington's chorea. The integration of this knowledge is needed to determine the correct answer.

A68 C9

The staff of an acute inpatient medical unit consists of an occupational therapist and an entry-level occupational therapy assistant (OTA). The admission rate has increased and the occupational therapist is having difficulty completing evaluations in a timely manner. Which is the best action for the therapist to take in response to these practice realities?

Answer Choices:
A. Evaluate patients screened by nursing staff as appropriate for occupational therapy.
B. Plan intervention based on the physical therapy evaluation.
C. Train the OTA to independently complete the evaluation process.
D. Redesign the program to allow more time for evaluation.

Correct Answer: D.

Rationale:
Since the lengths of stay on acute care units are very short, it is most important to complete assessments that can help with prioritizing interventions and planning discharge. Effective interventions cannot be implemented and relevant discharge plans cannot be made without the benefit of an evaluation. Interventions must be continued after discharge so it is essential to identify a person's functional status to ensure a proper recommendation for aftercare. The occupational therapist can redesign the program to include evaluation methods that are more efficient. The occupational therapist can also redesign the program to include supervision of the OTA in the completion of structured standardized evaluations, and the implementation of the intervention plan. While nursing staff can refer clients to occupational therapy, only occupational therapy practitioners can screen for occupational therapy. The physical therapy evaluation can be informative but its usefulness for planning OT interventions is limited. Only OT practitioners can complete an OT evaluation. OTAs can contribute to the evaluation process with the supervision of an occupational therapist, but they cannot independently carry out the evaluation process.

Type of Reasoning: Evaluative
This question requires professional judgment based on guiding principles, which is an evaluative reasoning skill. Because the therapist is having difficulty completing evaluations in a timely manner, he/she should redesign the OT program to allow more time for evaluation. This way the therapist can complete evaluations more efficiently.

A69 C4

An occupational therapist receives a referral to construct a splint for an individual with Erb's palsy. Which orthosis would be most effective for this condition?

Answer Choices:
A. A flail arm splint.
B. An elbow lock splint.
C. A figure-of-eight splint.
D. A deltoid sling.

Exam A

Correct Answer: B.

Rationale:
Erb's palsy results from injury to the fifth and sixth brachial plexus roots. The resulting clinical picture is that the arm hangs limp with the shoulder rotated inward due to atrophy and paralysis in the biceps, deltoid, brachialis, and brachioradialis muscles. This significantly limits functional movement. The elbow lock splint stabilizes the elbow to enable the individual to position the hand closer to or away from his/her body for functional use. A flail arm splint is recommended for a brachial plexus injury of C5-T1 resulting in whole upper extremity involvement. It provides the needed stability at both the shoulder and elbow for functional positioning of the hand. A figure-of-eight splint is used for a combined median ulnar nerve injury and to prevent MP hyperextension. A deltoid sling is used for upper extremity muscle weakness.

Type of Reasoning: Inferential
One must first determine the benefits and indications of each of the orthoses above in order to determine the orthosis that best addresses the patient's condition. This requires inferential reasoning, where one must draw conclusions based on the information provided. In this situation, an elbow lock splint is the ideal orthosis for Erb's palsy. If answered incorrectly, review Erb's palsy and appropriate orthoses.

A70 C7

Following medical treatment for a brain tumor, a client is referred to OT home care services for a functional evaluation. During the initial interview, the client reports difficulty locating desired items. For example, at lunchtime the client could not find a can of soup in the pantry. Based upon this self-report, which functional ability should the occupational therapist evaluate?

Answer Choices:
A. Visual scanning.
B. Visual acuity.
C. Spatial relations.
D. Topographical orientation.

Correct Answer: A.

Rationale:
Visual scanning is the ability to systematically observe and locate items in the environment. Visual acuity is the clarity of both near and far. Spatial relations is the ability to relate objects to each other (i.e., above/below). Topographical orientation is the ability to find one's way in space.

Type of Reasoning: Analytical
This question provides symptoms and the test taker must determine the likely cause for them. This is an analytical reasoning skill, as questions of this nature often ask one to analyze a group of symptoms in order to determine a diagnosis. In this situation the symptoms indicate visual scanning deficits, which should be reviewed if answered incorrectly.

A71 C9

A patient has been discharged from a rehabilitation facility six months ago. A staff therapist who works at the facility sees the former patient and the senior therapist who treated the patient in a dating situation. The senior therapist confirms involvement in a personal relationship with the former patient. Which is the staff therapist's best response to this situation?

Answer Choices:
A. Report the therapist to the NBCOT.
B. Advise the facility director.
C. Do nothing.
D. Report the therapist to the OT supervisor.

Correct Answer: C.

Rationale:
A health care practitioner can date a former but not a current patient. This is no evidence that they dated while the person was a patient. The therapist is doing nothing wrong and there is no need to take any action.

Type of Reasoning: Evaluative
This question requires a value judgment in an ethical situation, which is an evaluative reasoning skill. In this situation, there is only evidence of a relationship between the therapist and patient after the patient was discharged, therefore no action needs to be taken. Ethical situations such as these often rely upon the OT Code of Ethics to provide guiding principles of action. Because there is no harm involved in dating a former patient, the therapist's actions do not constitute harm. Review the AOTA Code of Ethics if answered incorrectly.

A72 C4

An adult is hospitalized in the recovery phase of Guillain-Barré syndrome. The patient complains of tingling, aching and weakness in both hands, causing difficulty in grasping grooming supplies. The patient requests relief from the hand symptoms. Which action should the occupational therapist take to address the patient's concerns?

Answer Choices:
A. Provide soft tissue massage to both hands prior to grooming activities.
B. Apply hot packs to both hands and complete stretching exercises prior to grooming activities.
C. Refer the client to a neurologist for follow-up of possible condition regression.
D. Educate the patient about sensory deficits and related adaptive ADL strategies.

Correct Answer: D.

Rationale:
Guillain-Barré (GBS) is characterized by ascending motor weakness in the limbs, usually beginning in the hands and feet. Paresthesias and pain are also a common occurrence. The best approach to this patient is to educate the patient about the sensory deficits that are common to the condition and provide adaptive strategies for ADL so the patient is successful. Soft tissue massage will not remedy the aching in the hands as the inflammation of the peripheral nerves must decrease for this to resolve. Hot packs are contraindicated in this situation due to the potential for burns from altered sensation. Referral to a neurologist is not needed as the symptoms are typical of the syndrome.

Type of Reasoning: Inductive
This question requires the test taker to understand the nature of the course of Guillain-Barré syndrome in order to determine the best approach to address the patient's concerns. In this case, because the patient's symptoms will require time to improve, the therapist should educate the patient about the sensory deficits and adaptive ADL strategies. If answered incorrectly, review information on the recovery phase of Guillain-Barré syndrome, especially sensory deficits of the hands.

A73 C2

A child with attention deficit with hyperactivity disorder (ADHD) and conduct disorder attends an after-school program that utilizes sensory-integrative and behavioral management approaches to achieve intervention goals. Snacks are provided and occasionally used as rewards. A parent insists that a child not be given any foods containing sugar. Which is the occupational therapist's best response to this request?

Answer Choices:

A. Discontinue providing sugary snacks but continue their use as rewards in the behavioral management program.
B. Provide the parent with recent research that refutes the link between sugar and problem behaviors.
C. Discontinue providing sugary snacks for the child to comply with the parent's request.
D. Inform the parent that the therapist will discuss the issue with the program's administrator to determine the best course of action.

Correct Answer: C.

Rationale:

The parent's request must be respected and honored. While a therapist may provide a parent with research information related to a child's condition, it is not the therapist's role to attempt to prove the parent wrong in his/her beliefs. The therapist can directly address the issue with the parent and does not need to discuss the issue with the administrator prior to responding. Behavioral rewards and appropriate snacks that do not contain sugar can be used in the program. The use of non-sugar items can also be beneficial for children at risk with a secondary diagnosis of diabetes or other medical conditions.

Type of Reasoning: Evaluative

One must weigh the possible courses of action and then make a value judgment about the best course to take. This requires evaluative reasoning skill, which often utilizes guiding principles of action in order to arrive at a correct conclusion. In this case, because the parent has requested no food containing sugar, the therapist should comply with the parent's request.

A74 C2

An individual with myasthenia gravis is being discharged home after a hospitalization for the treatment of pneumonia. The person's spouse has expressed concern about caregiving responsibilities and the client's ability to function in the home. Which is the most beneficial recommendation for the occupational therapist to make to address the spouse's concerns and the client's needs?

Answer Choices:

A. The extension of client's length of stay to allow for caregiver training
B. The extension of client's length of stay to provide intervention to develop ADL skills
C. A referral for the client to an adult day care program to relieve caregiver stress and to develop functional skills.
D. A referral to a home care agency for a functional evaluation and home assessment.

Correct Answer: D.

Rationale:

A functional evaluation in the client's home and an assessment of the home environment is the best choice listed to provide accurate information about the client's functional status and caregiver needs. This information will enable the home care team to collaborate with the family to develop an appropriate intervention plan to address their identified needs. An extension of length of stay is very difficult to justify because the individual was hospitalized for the medical treatment of pneumonia. Once this illness is effectively treated, discharge must occur. In addition, it is more effective to provide caregiver and ADL training in the person's home environment. A referral to adult day care may be determined based on the home care therapist's evaluation.

Type of Reasoning: Inferential

One must determine the most appropriate recommendation for this patient, given the caregiver's stated concerns. This requires inferential reasoning skill, where one must draw conclusions based upon presented evidence. In this situation, referral to a home care agency for a functional evaluation and home assessment is the most appropriate recommendation. Review home care services for individuals with disabilities and the functional impact of myasthenia gravis if answered incorrectly. The integration of this knowledge is needed to determine the best answer.

A75 C9

An occupational therapist becomes aware of the practice of a colleague who teaches an energy conservation class to persons with arthritis. This colleague has been sending the names of class participants to a vendor who sells adaptive equipment. Which action is best for the occupational therapist to take in response to the situation?

Answer Choices:

A. Ignore the situation for it does not harm anyone. ✗
B. Speak to the therapist privately and tell him/her this action is unethical. ☆
C. Advise the therapist to disclose this practice and if he/she refuses report the therapist to the state regulatory board.
D. Report the therapist's unethical behavior to the state regulatory board. ✗

Correct Answer: B.

Rationale:

This occupational therapist should talk directly to the colleague to allow the person to self-correct his/her behavior by ending this practice. Ignoring the situation is incorrect for it allows an unethical practice to continue. Advising the therapist to disclose this practice makes the assumption that this practice will continue. Reporting the therapist to the state regulatory board is over-reactive at this time and would result in little action for these boards only regulate issues of potential harm and/or fraud. Providing a vendor with the names of potential clients may be of questionable ethics, but it is not illegal or dangerous.

Type of Reasoning: Evaluative

This question requires a value judgment in an ethical situation, which is an evaluative reasoning skill. Ethical situations such as these often rely upon the OT Code of Ethics to provide guiding principles of action. In this situation, the best course of action is to speak to the therapist privately and inform the therapist that the actions are unethical.

A76 C8

An occupational therapist providing home-based occupational therapy services implements a bed positioning plan for a person recovering from a cerebral vascular accident. The person is receiving care from family members and personal care assistants employed by a home care agency. Which action should the therapist take to ensure the accurate implementation of this plan by the client's caregivers?

Answer Choices:

A. Provide verbal step-by-step directions of the desired positions to the client's caregivers. ✗
B. Post written step-by-step directions of the desired positions on the wall by the client's bed. ✗
C. Post pictures of the desired positions next to the headboard of the client's bed. ✗
D. Require each caregiver to demonstrate the replication of the desired positions.
⤷ unlikely all could come in

Correct Answer: C.

Rationale:
A visual representation of the exact positions desired can decrease any misinterpretations of a written description. Placing this picture by the bed's headboard will ensure that it is visible to all caregivers. It is the most effective method provided to ensure compliance. Providing verbal step-by-step directions for positioning is reliant on the caregiver's memory which can be incomplete or faulty. Posting written step-by-step directions is reliant on the initiation of all caregivers to read the documented procedures and on the caregivers' accurate interpretation of the written word. These methods may also assume a knowledge base (e.g., 30° of shoulder abduction) that is beyond the level of some of the client's caregivers. Requiring caregivers to demonstrate replication of the positions can be helpful but it is highly unlikely that the therapist would be able to access every personal care assistant who will be providing direct care to this client. In addition, home care agencies often use on-call per diem staff that would not be available to participate in a demonstration session.

Type of Reasoning: Inductive
This question requires one to determine the best approach for implementing a bed positioning plan. This requires inductive reasoning skill, where clinical judgment is paramount in arriving at a correct conclusion. For this situation, posting a picture of the person in the desired bed position next to the person's bed's headboard is best to ensure effective carryover. Review caregiver training guidelines if answered incorrectly.

A77 C6

A young adult with a 10-year history of bulimia nervosa participates in an outpatient vocational exploration group and completes a vocational interest inventory. This evaluation identifies four possible areas for a career. Which career choice is best for the occupational therapist to advise the client to explore further?

Answer Choices:
A. Web designer.
B. Dietitian.
C. Athletic trainer.
D. Fashion designer.

Correct Answer: A.

Rationale:
Persons with eating disorders have inaccurate and distorted body images and their self-evaluation is unduly influenced by their body shape and weight. There is a strong preoccupation with food and exercise activities may be pursued excessively in order to decrease weight. Consequently, web design would be the best choice for vocational exploration of the four listed because it offers many options that do not focus on food, exercise, or personal appearance. While a dietitian's job focuses on the science of food and provides education about nutrition, this constant contact with food might be difficult a person with a long history of an eating disorder. An athletic trainer is involved with exercise on a daily basis which might contribute to over-exercise and prove stressful for the client. Fashion design lends itself to a constant emphasis on body image and consistent contact with thin women in the fashion industry. This would also be contraindicated.

Type of Reasoning: Inductive
This question requires one to determine which career choices would best avoid triggers associated with bulimia nervosa. Having an understanding of the disorder, one should realize that a web designer is the only career choice that does not primarily focus on food, body image, or exercise, which are all triggers for bulimia. Inductive reasoning skill is utilized for this question, as one must use clinical judgment to determine a best course of action. If answered incorrectly, review symptoms of bulimia and the behavioral characteristics of eating disorders.

A78 C6

An occupational therapist develops a task group for the newly admitted patients of a psychiatric inpatient unit of a busy city hospital. The therapist considers several activities to use for the group's first session. Which activity is best for the therapist to present to the group members?

Answer Choices:
A. Planning a weekend pizza party for the patients and their visitors.
B. Decorating styrofoam cups and planting cuttings in them.
C. Publishing a weekly newsletter about city attractions for patients on the unit.
D. Painting a large mural to cover one wall of the day room.

Correct Answer: B.

Rationale:
Decorating cups and planting cuttings is a simple, concrete, and safe task, which can be structured to ensure successful completion by individuals with acute psychiatric disorders who have been newly admitted to an acute psychiatric hospital. In addition, individuals on an acute unit have a short length of stay and require activities that can be completed in one session. The other choices require multiple sessions, which are not realistic on an inpatient unit.

Type of Reasoning: Inferential
One must determine the most appropriate activity for an initial group session, given knowledge of the treatment setting. This requires inferential reasoning skill, where one must infer or draw conclusions about a best course of action. In this situation, the therapist should choose decorating styrofoam cups and planning cuttings in them as a first activity. If answered incorrectly, review group activities for inpatient psychiatric settings.

A79 C3

An individual is evaluated for a repetitive stress disorder. The individual complains of numbness and tingling of the thumb, index, middle, and radial half of the ring finger and aching pain in the proximal forearm. The client states that these symptoms are not evident at night. The occupational therapist notes a positive Tinel's sign. Which site should the therapist document as the location of this sign for this client?

Answer Choices:
A. The wrist. → CTS
B. The Guyon's canal. → GC syndrome
C. The elbow. → cubital tunnel syndrome
D. The forearm. → pronator teres

Correct Answer: D.

Rationale:
The presenting signs described in this case scenario indicate pronator teres syndrome. A positive Tinel's sign at the forearm is consistent with this syndrome which is a medial nerve compression between the two heads of the pronator teres. Symptoms are similar to carpal tunnel syndrome (CTS) except there is aching pain in the forearm and no night symptoms. A person with CTS has paresthesias occurring at night, does not have pain in the forearm, and has a positive Tinel's sign at the wrist. A positive Tinel's sign that is noted at the Guyon's canal indicates Guyon's canal syndrome which is a compression of the ulnar nerve with sensorimotor symptoms reflecting ulnar nerve distribution. A positive Tinel's sign at the elbow is indicative of cubital tunnel syndrome. This is an ulnar nerve compression at the elbow that has the symptoms of numbness and tingling along the ulnar aspect of the forearm and hand, and pain at the elbow with extreme elbow flexion.

Type of Reasoning: Analytical
This question provides symptoms and the test taker must determine the likely cause for them in order to determine the location of the positive Tinel's sign. This is an analytical reasoning skill, as questions of this nature often ask one to analyze a group of symptoms in order to determine a diagnosis and draw a correct conclusion. In this situation the symptoms indicate pronator teres syndrome and the positive Tinel's sign would be located in the forearm, which should be reviewed if answered incorrectly.

A80 C3

A client with a right below-elbow amputation begins prosthetic training with a body-powered myoelectric prosthesis. The occupational therapist collaborates with the client to begin training in the use of the terminal device to grasp and release objects. Which elbow position is best for the therapist to place the client's elbow in during grasp and release activities?

Answer Choices:
A. Flexed at 90° with neutral degrees of pronation/supination.
B. Flexed at 90° and pronated 60°.
C. Flexed at 120° and with neutral degrees of pronation/supination.
D. Flexed at 90° and supinated 60°.

Correct Answer: A.

Rationale:
The elbow flexed at 90° with neutral degrees of pronation/supination is the easiest position in which to begin grasp and release activities. It is also the most functional and natural. The other positions are more difficult positions and can be attempted after achievement of the mentioned position, if needed.

Type of Reasoning: Inductive
This question requires that test taker to determine the best initial grasp and release position for a patient beginning below-elbow amputation prosthetic training. This requires clinical judgment and knowledge of prosthetic training in order to choose the best solution. In this case, the position of 90° of flexion with neutral degrees of pronation/supination is the best initial grasp and release position.

A81 C1

During an early intervention planning meeting, an occupational therapist explains the results of a play assessment to the parents of an 18-month-old toddler with multiple developmental disabilities. The child has been assessed as delayed by 6–8 months in all developmental parameters. Which intervention approach is most effective for the therapist to recommend using first to develop the toddler's play skills?

Answer Choices:
A. The use of toys that encourage creative and imaginative play.
B. The use of toys that are visually and auditorily stimulating.
C. Participation in a small parallel play group with other toddlers. → too young
D. Engagement in activities that use sensorimotor skills prerequisite to play.

1 year developmentally

Correct Answer: B.

Rationale:

Providing toys that are visually and auditorily stimulating will help engage the child in the intervention process. As the child explores the sensory properties and characteristics of these toys, he/she will engage in activities that will facilitate developmentally appropriate play. Through this process, the child will develop sensorimotor and cognitive skills. Many toys that provide visual and auditory stimulation also provide opportunities to explore relationships between actions and objects (e.g., striking a colorful keyboard to produce music). The exploration of relationships between actions and consequences is typical of the cognitive development of a 9–12 month-old, which is this child's developmental age. Creative play occurs developmentally at 4–7 years, so this option is not developmentally appropriate for this child. Placing a toddler with the developmental age of a 10–12 month-old into a parallel play group is not age appropriate. Engaging the child in activities that use sensorimotor skills prerequisite to play would not achieve the stated aim of developing play skills. It is more effective to directly use play activities during intervention to develop play skills.

Type of Reasoning: Inferential

One must infer or draw conclusions about a likely course of action, given the information presented. This is an inferential reasoning skill, where knowledge of a therapeutic approach is essential in choosing a correct solution. In this case, the therapist should recommend initiating intervention with toys that are visually and auditorily stimulating, given the child's diagnosis and delays. If answered incorrectly, review intervention approaches for small children with developmental disabilities.

A82 C1

A two-year-old child receives home care early intervention services. The occupational therapy intervention plan includes a goal to develop the child's pincer grasp. Which is the most appropriate activity for the occupational therapist to work on with the child during an intervention session?

Answer Choices:

A. Finger-feeding of O-shaped cereal.
B. Picking up marbles.
C. Drawing with jumbo crayons.
D. Stacking one-inch cubes.

Correct Answer: A.

Rationale:

Picking up O-shaped cereal to finger-feed will facilitate the use a pincer grasp. While picking up marbles also uses a pincer grasp, this activity presents a potential choking hazard, as two-year-olds frequently put items they pick up into their mouths. Drawing with a jumbo crayon uses a gross grasp. Stacking cubes uses a radial digital grasp.

Type of Reasoning: Inductive

Clinical knowledge and judgment are the most important skills needed for answering this question, which requires inductive reasoning skill. Knowledge of the development of pincer grasp and effective strategies to facilitate it are essential to choosing the best solution. In this case, the therapist should recommend finger-feeding O-shaped cereal. Review the developmental sequence of grasp and the characteristics of different grasp patterns if answered incorrectly.

A83 C2

An occupational therapist works with an individual with chest and upper extremity burns. During the intervention session, the client expresses vague fears about personal safety at home and asks the therapist to advocate for an extension in the discharge date. According to the medical record, the client had incurred the burns during a cooking accident. Which is the therapist's best initial response to the client's stated concerns?

Answer Choices:

A. Encourage the client to speak to the social worker about discharge plans.
B. Assure the client that pre-discharge fears are normal and expected.
C. Document the client's concerns and recommend an extension of the length of stay.
D. Invite the client to expand upon the nature of these concerns.

Correct Answer: D.

Rationale:

The occupational therapist needs more information to determine the basis for the client's fears and evaluate for appropriate interventions. Referring the client to the social worker can be helpful, but it will not address his/her concerns at this moment. A delay may result in the client deciding that his/her concerns are not worth mentioning. Many clients find it difficult to express fears so it is important to respond immediately when they do. This is of particular importance in cases of domestic violence, which this case (and any case) can have as a contributing and complicating factor. In addition, the client's fears may be functionally based and the therapist can address these immediately in the current intervention session. Assurance that fears are normal and expected does not address the issue at hand. A request to extend a client's length of stay requires a documented need for inpatient services. Client's stated concerns about home safety are not sufficient justification for a length of stay extension.

Type of Reasoning: Evaluative

This question requires professional judgment based on guiding principles, which is an evaluative reasoning skill. Because the therapist cannot determine the source of the patient's fears, the therapist should ask for the patient to elaborate on the nature of his/her concerns. This way the therapist can determine the most appropriate course of action based on further information. Without further information, clinical decision making is subject to being inaccurate or incomplete.

A84 C6

The occupational therapist employed at a day treatment center for clients with psychiatric disorders is conducting a leisure planning group. The members of the group decide to take a day trip to the local sculpture garden. Which side effect of psychotropic medications is most important for the therapist to discuss preventative precautions for with the group?

Answer Choices:

A. Orthostatic hypotension.
B. Akathisia.
C. Photosensitivity.
D. Tremors.

Correct Answer: C.

Rationale:

Photosensitivity results in severe sunburn which can occur during an outdoor trip. The other answer choices identify potential side effects of medications but they are not exacerbated by being outside.

Type of Reasoning: Deductive

This question requires the test taker to recall the common precautions for clients using psychotropic medications in order to arrive at a correct conclusion. This requires deductive reasoning skill, where the recall of facts is utilized to draw a correct conclusion. In this situation, the most important precaution to discuss is photosensitivity. Review psychotropic medication side effects and preventative precautions for clients taking psychotropic medications if answered incorrectly.

A85 C4

A child with mild spastic diplegia wants to participate in neighborhood activities with peers. The family's main goal for the child is to ride a bicycle. Which bicycle is best for the occupational therapist to recommend?

Answer Choices:

A. A hand-propelled bicycle with hand brakes.
B. A foot-propelled bicycle with hand brakes.
C. A foot-propelled bicycle with foot brakes.
D. An adapted tricycle with foot brakes.

Correct Answer: B.

Rationale:

Mild spastic diplegic cerebral palsy is characterized by mild lower extremity involvement and minimal to no upper extremity involvement. The use of legs to propel the bicycle increases lower extremity strength while encouraging lower extremity dissociation. Hand brakes are best for safety because the child usually has better control of the upper extremities than the lower extremities. Hand propulsion is not the best option since a bicycle will provide an excellent opportunity to develop lower extremity strengthening and dissociation. An adapted tricycle would be more suitable for a child with more involvement and less control of lower and upper extremities.

Type of Reasoning: Inductive

This question requires one to determine the benefits and potential outcomes of providing each of the four possible recommendations for a child with mild spastic diplegia. Questions of this nature require clinical judgment, which is an inductive reasoning skill. In this situation, a foot-propelled bicycle with hand brakes is the best recommendation, given the child's diagnosis. If answered incorrectly, review information on diplegic cerebral palsy.

A86 C9

An occupational therapist receives a referral from a physician that outlines a specific course of treatment. Following the evaluation of the person, the therapist believes that a different course of treatment would be more beneficial. Which course of action is best for the therapist to take?

Answer Choices:

A. Contact the physician and discuss the alternative treatment.
B. Provide the prescribed treatment on a three to four-week trial.
C. Combine the prescribed treatment with the therapist's preferred treatment.
D. Provide the treatment the therapist believes would be more beneficial for the person.

Correct Answer: A.

Rationale:

This action enables the occupational therapist to share his/her professional expertise with the physician in a collaborative manner. The other choices do not do this.

Type of Reasoning: Evaluative
This question requires professional judgment based on guiding principles, which is an evaluative reasoning skill. Questions of this nature often require the test taker to determine a best course of action. The goal of arriving at a correct conclusion is to determine what solution will best meet the needs of the recipient of services. Because the therapist believes a different course of treatment would be more beneficial, the occupational therapist should contact the physician to discuss the alternative treatment.

A87 C8

A woman with a complete spinal cord injury at the C-5 level has given birth to her first child. The client seeks suggestions on methods to facilitate independent and safe parenting. Which of the following is most beneficial for the occupational therapist to recommend the mother use to help her independently feed her child?

Answer Choices:
A. A pillow to support the mother's arms during breast feeding.
B. Bottles with pre-measured formula.
C. Bottles that have molded easy to grip shapes.
D. A sling to support the infant's head during breast feeding.

Correct Answer: A.

Rationale:
Providing support of the mother's upper extremities will enable her to independently breast feed her child. Breast feeding is physically the easiest method for feeding an infant and it is the healthiest for the infant. The individual with a C-5 spinal cord injury has sufficient upper extremity function to be able to support the infant's head without the use of a sling, especially since the mother's arms will be supported by a pillow to decrease fatigue. Pre-measured formula is not indicated in this case. The individual would need a splint or other piece of adaptive equipment to hold a baby's bottle.

Type of Reasoning: Inductive
Clinical knowledge and judgment are the most important skills needed for answering this question, which requires inductive reasoning skill. Knowledge of the diagnosis and most appropriate courses of action is essential to choose the best solution. In this case, a pillow to support the mother's arms is the best recommendation to enable independent breast feeding. Review child care adaptations for individuals with disabilities if answered incorrectly.

A88 C4

During a classroom screening, an 8-year-old is observed holding a pencil with a tight grip. The student appears to rely heavily on visual cues to assist during both fine and gross motor tasks. During gross motor activities, the student moves in an uncoordinated manner. The occupational therapist uses a sensory integrative frame of reference to interpret evaluation data. Which impairment should the therapist document as needing further evaluation?

Answer Choices:
A. Vestibular processing dysfunction.
B. Proprioceptive system dysfunction.
C. Hyporesponsive tactile system.
D. Hyperresponsive tactile system.

Correct Answer: B.

Rationale:
The tight pencil grip, incoordination, and the use of visual cues could indicate proprioceptive deficits that require further evaluation. Vision is often used to compensate for proprioceptive deficits. An evaluation is needed to determine the nature of these deficits. Hyperresponsivity/over-responsivity to tactile stimuli would be demonstrated by tactile defensiveness, (e.g., irritation and discomfort from a variety from textures such as clothing, sand, grass, glue, water, paint, and/or food). Hyporesponsiveness/under-responsivity to tactile stimuli would be demonstrated by diminished sensory registration and responsiveness. The student would not respond to normal levels of tactile input and would seek disproportionate amounts of stimuli to gain environmental information (e.g., excessive touching of people and objects). Behaviors that would indicate the need to further evaluate vestibular processing could include hyper- or hypo-responsiveness to movement and gravitational insecurity.

Type of Reasoning: Analytical
This question provides symptoms and the test taker must determine the likely cause for them. This is an analytical reasoning skill, as questions of this nature often ask one to analyze a group of symptoms in order to determine the impairment. In this situation the symptoms indicate a need to further evaluate the proprioceptive system. Review the sensory integrative frame of reference and sensory processing disorders, especially of the proprioceptive system, if answered incorrectly.

A89 C2

An individual with borderline personality disorder is admitted to the hospital following a suicide attempt. After attending an occupational therapy orientation group, the patient tells the occupational therapist, "You are the only therapist who has ever been really helpful." The patient asks to meet with the therapist privately on a regular basis instead of the assigned primary individual therapist. Which action is best for the therapist to take in response to the patient's request?

Answer Choices:
A. Refer the patient to the assigned primary individual therapist.
B. Agree to meet with the patient since a positive therapeutic connection has been expressed.
C. Tell the patient that an occupational therapist provides only occupation-based group treatment.
D. Explain that this type of manipulative behavior is not acceptable.

Correct Answer: A.

Rationale:
The patient must be referred to the primary individual therapist assigned to his/her case. Although the patient has responded favorably to the initial occupational therapy group session, this does not preclude the patient's need for individual therapy. On inpatient psychiatric units, occupational therapy practitioners often serve as primary individual therapists in addition to their group therapist role. However, the assignment of caseloads is not (and cannot be) based upon patients' requests. Labeling the individual's behavior as manipulative is judgmental and can be considered antagonistic.

Type of Reasoning: Evaluative
This question requires professional judgment based on guiding principles, which is an evaluative reasoning skill. For this situation, the therapist should refer the person to her primary individual therapist for individual therapy. If answered incorrectly, review individual versus group therapy guidelines for inpatient psychiatric settings.

A90 C6

An occupational therapist plans a task-oriented activity group for adolescent girls recently diagnosed with anorexia nervosa. Which is the best activity for the therapist to include in the initial session of this group?

Answer Choices:
A. Making cards to send to veterans in a local hospital.
B. Baking cookies for the residents in a homeless shelter.
C. Performing low impact aerobic exercises.
D. Composing lyrics and melody for a group song.

Correct Answer: D.

Rationale:
A task-oriented group utilizes a psychodynamic approach to increase participants' understanding of their needs, values, ideas, feelings, and behaviors. Activities are selected and designed to facilitate self-expression and the exploration of feelings, thoughts, and behaviors. Composing a song is a self-expressive activity that allows each member to contribute his/her thoughts and feelings. It is an activity that can be stopped to discuss behaviors, feelings, and issues that arise during the group. The other activity choices do not provide this self-expression opportunity. In addition, baking and exercising are not the best initial activities for a person with eating disorders.

Type of Reasoning: Inductive
Clinical knowledge and judgment are the most important skills needed for answering this question, which requires inductive reasoning skill. Knowledge of the diagnosis and most appropriate activities for a task-oriented group are essential to arriving at a correct conclusion. In this case, the most appropriate initial activity is composing lyrics and melody for a group song. If answered incorrectly review task-oriented activities for adolescents with anorexia nervosa.

A91 C1

An occupational therapist completes an early intervention screening of an 8-month-old child. The results indicate that the child is able to sit independently by propping forward on both arms. Which is the best action for the occupational therapist to complete next?

Answer Choices:
A. Evaluate the child's sensorimotor skills using a standardized evaluation. ✓
B. Inform the parents that the child exhibits typical behavior. ✗
C. Develop goals to improve sitting balance. ✗
D. Provide play activities to develop sitting balance. ✗

Correct Answer: A.

Rationale:
The screening indicated a sensorimotor delay, which requires further evaluation. Sitting with arms propped forward is typical of a 5–6 month-old. At 8 months, a child typically sits without support; therefore, further evaluation of the child's sensorimotor status is indicated. The therapist cannot set goals or prescribe activities prior to the completion of a full evaluation.

Type of Reasoning: Inferential
One must determine the most likely next course of action for a child, given the diagnosis and functional ability described. This requires inferential reasoning skill, where one must draw conclusions based on the information presented. In this situation, the next step after screening would be to complete a sensorimotor evaluation since the child is demonstrating a sensorimotor delay. Review motor development of infants, especially 6–8 month range, if answered incorrectly.

A92 C9

An entry-level occupational therapist is hired to work on an acute psychiatric unit. The occupational therapy supervisor orients the therapist to hospital policies and procedures. Which are the most important policies and procedures for the supervisor to include in the initial orientation session?

Answer Choices:

A. Crisis intervention.
B. Reimbursement.
C. Employee benefits.
D. Group program scheduling.

Correct Answer: A.

Rationale:

Crises can occur at any time in any acute facility. All employees must immediately learn the policies and procedures for dealing with crises to ensure the safety of patients and staff. Reimbursement issues and group program scheduling can be reviewed during regular supervisory sessions. These issues are not immediate concerns. Employee benefits are the responsibility of the personnel/human resources department.

Type of Reasoning: Evaluative

One must weigh the possible courses of action and then make a judgment about which focus is the most immediate need. This requires evaluative reasoning skill, which often requires one to make value judgments. In this case, the supervisor should initially discuss crisis intervention policies and procedure as they are the most critical to know in an acute psychiatric setting. The other policies and procedures are important but they are not immediate concerns. Review policies and procedures guidelines for acute psychiatric practice settings if answered incorrectly.

A93 C7

An occupational therapist evaluates a client using the Allen Cognitive Level (ACL) Screen. The client successfully completes three running stitches. Which step should the therapist take next?

Answer Choices:

A. Demonstrate the whip stitch and ask the client to imitate this and complete three stitches.
B. Demonstrate the single cordovan stitch and ask the client to imitate this and complete three stitches.
C. Demonstrate the double cordovan stitch and ask the client to imitate this and complete three stitches.
D. Document that the person demonstrates a cognitive level consistent with Level 3 of the Cognitive Disabilities model.

Correct Answer: A.

Rationale:

According to the Allen Cognitive Level (ACL) Screen, after the completion of three running stitches the person should move on to the next step in the screening process, which is the completion of three whip stitches. After the completion of three whip stitches, the therapist then demonstrates the single cordovan stitch. The double cordovan stitch is not used in the ACL Screen. The documentation of a person's cognitive level should be completed after the person has had the opportunity to perform all components of the evaluation.

Type of Reasoning: Deductive

This question requires the test taker to recall the procedural steps in administering the Allen Cognitive Level (ACL) Screen. This is factual information, which is a deductive reasoning skill. For this scenario, after a client completes three running stitches, the therapist should instruct the client to complete the next step, which is three whip stitches. If answered incorrectly, review the procedures for the ACL Screen.

A94 C8

During an occupational therapy session, a veteran recovering from bilateral traumatic lower extremity amputations expresses several concerns about having a changed body and questions its sexual appeal. Which response is best for the therapist to take in response to client's concerns?

Answer Choices:
A. Refer the client to the primary care physician.
B. Ask open-ended questions to explore the concerns further.
C. Reassure the client that the concerns are a normal part of the recovery process.
D. Explain that positioning can compensate for changes in functional mobility.

Correct Answer: B.

Rationale:
Sexuality and sexual expression are within occupational therapy's domain of concern; therefore, there is no need to refer the person to the physician. The therapist should immediately recognize the validity of the individual's concerns and provide the client with the opportunity to discuss these concerns further. Providing reassurance does not deal with the concerns at the moment. Discussing positioning alternatives can occur after the person's concerns have been identified.

Type of Reasoning: Evaluative
One must weigh the possible courses of action and then make a judgment about the best course to take. This requires evaluative reasoning skill, which often utilizes principles of action in order to arrive at a correct conclusion. For this case, because the patient has expressed concerns about sexual appeal after traumatic amputations, the therapist should ask open-ended questions to explore the concerns further.

A95 C6

An older adult who is recovering from a cerebral vascular accident attends occupational therapy two times per day. The intervention environment is highly structured and not over-stimulating, yet the occupational therapist observes that the client's mood often changes abruptly. Within one session, the client will laugh and then become tearful with no apparent precipitant. Which is most accurate for the occupational therapist to document the client is exhibiting in the client's daily progress note?

Answer Choices:
A. Early Alzheimer's disease.
B. Anhedonia.
C. A response to auditory hallucinations.
D. Emotional lability.

Correct Answer: D.

Rationale:
Emotional lability describes abrupt changes in mood without external precipitants. It is often observed in persons recovering from CVAs. Anhedonia is the inability to experience pleasure. There is no information in the case that would substantiate a conclusion that the individual is developing Alzheimer's disease or is responding to the internal stimulation of hallucinations.

Type of Reasoning: Analytical
This question provides symptoms and the test taker must determine the likely cause for them. This is an analytical reasoning skill, as questions of this nature often ask one to analyze a group of symptoms in order to determine a diagnosis. In this situation the symptoms indicate emotional lability, which should be reviewed if answered incorrectly.

A96 C9

A large general hospital in an urban area initiates several quality improvement committees that include occupational therapists. Which of the following does participation in these committees provide to the occupational therapists?

Answer Choices:

A. The ability to develop personal performance skills.
B. The capability to enhance leadership skills.
C. The power to promote occupational therapy services.
D. The opportunity to improve overall service delivery.

Correct Answer: D.

Rationale:

Quality improvement (QI) involves a prospective analysis of specific services to improve service quality and meet the needs of a population. The QI approach is designed to use a team effort to empower employees to improve service quality. Participants may develop skills while working on the committee, but personal performance and leadership development are not the goals of QI. Participating in a QI committee can provide opportunities for the occupational therapists to informally promote occupational therapy services, but this is not the purpose of a QI committee.

Type of Reasoning: Deductive

This question requires one to recall factual guidelines of a QI program. This is a deductive reasoning skill, where concrete knowledge is utilized to draw a correct conclusion. In this situation, a QI committee would focus on improving overall service delivery. If answered incorrectly, review guidelines for QI programs.

A97 C8

An adolescent student with Duchenne muscular dystrophy and depression is being evaluated for a power wheelchair. Which is the most important area to be considered during the occupational therapy evaluation of the student to determine the student's readiness for the wheelchair?

Answer Choices:

A. Level of interest.
B. Fine motor skills.
C. Cognitive skills.
D. Postural control.

Correct Answer: C.

Rationale:

Cognitive skills include alertness, spatial operations, judgment, decision making and problem solving, which can be affected by depression. Since these abilities are needed for the safe operation of a power wheelchair, it is essential that the occupational therapist assesses the student's cognitive level. An individual's level of interest can help engage him/her in mobility training but it is not the most important area to assess. Fine motor skills and postural control are likely absent due to the progression of Duchenne muscular dystrophy. Wheelchair adaptations can compensate for decreased fine motor skills and poor postural control.

Type of Reasoning: Inferential

One must determine the critical skills needing to be assessed prior to providing a power wheelchair. This requires inferential reasoning, where one must infer or draw conclusions based on the information provided. In this situation, the student should be assessed for cognitive skills as this is the most important element in determining the safe and appropriate use of the device. If answered incorrectly, review power wheelchair prescription guidelines.

A98 C5

An individual incurred a spinal cord injury at the C-5 level. During an occupational therapy session focused on developing the ability to feed independently using adaptive equipment, the occupational therapist notes that the client is flushed and sweating excessively. The client requests that the session end early due to a pounding headache. Which action is best for the occupational therapist to take first in response to this situation?

Answer Choices:

A. End the session and call the transporter to return the client to the client's room.
B. Empty the client's filled catheter bag and maintain the client's upright position.
C. Return the individual to the unit and report symptoms to the head nurse.
D. Stop the session and recline the individual in the wheelchair for a rest break.

Correct Answer: B

Rationale:

The client's symptoms are indicative of autonomic dysreflexia. This is an extreme rise in blood pressure caused by a noxious stimulus. This complication is deemed a medical emergency that must be treated immediately by quickly removing the noxious stimulus that caused the problem. Common stimuli are blocked catheters or sitting on sharp objects. Other symptoms of autonomic dysreflexia include profuse sweating and a pounding headache. The other choices do not deal with this medical emergency in an appropriate or timely manner. The patient should remain in an upright position to help manage the rise in blood pressure.

Type of Reasoning: Evaluative

One must weigh the possible courses of action and then make a value judgment about the best course to take. This requires evaluative reasoning skill, where an understanding of what the symptoms indicate is pivotal in arriving at a correct conclusion. In this case, the symptoms indicate autonomic dysreflexia and the therapist's first action should be to empty the filled catheter bag to remove the noxious stimulus causing the dangerous rise in blood pressure. If answered incorrectly, review symptoms and management of autonomic dysreflexia.

A99 C2

An occupational therapist and an OTA co-lead a work adjustment group. One member has become progressively more dependent on the OTA for directions, praise, and input throughout the group activities. Which action should the group leaders initially take in response to these behaviors?

Answer Choices:

A. Schedule several individual sessions with the OTA and group member to examine the issues of dependency and transference.
B. Inform the attending psychiatrist that the group member is exhibiting signs of dependency and transference.
C. Have the OTA work with the person during group sessions to develop independence in task completion.
D. Have another therapist co-lead the group with the occupational therapist and reassign the OTA to another group.

Correct Answer: C.

Rationale:

This question addresses therapeutic use of self and effective group process. The best answer is to utilize the group situation and have the OTA function as a change agent during the group's activities. It is not necessary to devote individual sessions to this issue. Notifying the psychiatrist is not necessary as these behaviors are not indicative of a need for a modification in the person's medication regimen and does not address the potential of modifying behavior through the group process. Removing the OTA is not a good choice because it does not provide the member a chance to work through these issues and develop needed skills. This also does not give an opportunity for the member to benefit from the therapeutic use of self by the OTA.

Type of Reasoning: Evaluative
One must determine a best course of action, based upon the four possible choices. This requires evaluating the choices and determining which one best meets the needs of all parties involved. In this case, having the OTA work with the person during group sessions to develop independence best meets the needs of the individual and effectively uses the skills of the OTA. Questions that require one to weigh the merits of situations and determine a best course of action often require evaluative reasoning skills.

A100 C1

The parents of an 8-month-old child bring their child to a free community health developmental screening program. The occupational therapist evaluates the oral motor development of the child and determines that the child's development is within normal limits. When documenting this determination, which is most likely for the therapist to state the child demonstrates?

Answer Choices:
A. Rotary chewing. ✗ 12 mths
B. Diagonal jaw movements. ✗ 7mths
C. Effective mastication. ✓ 9 mths
D. Cup drinking with a firm jaw. ✗ 12 mths

Correct Answer: B.

Rationale:
Diagonal jaw movements can develop as early as 7 months and would be evident by 8 months. Effective mastication typically develops at 9 months. Cup drinking with a firm jaw and rotary chewing are typical for a child at 12 months.

Type of Reasoning: Deductive
One must recall the developmental guidelines for 8-month-old children in oral motor skills. This is factual knowledge, which is a deductive reasoning skill. The child's demonstration of diagonal jaw movement indicates development within normal limits. If answered incorrectly, review developmental milestones of infants in oral motor skills.

A101 C9

An elder diagnosed with dementia, Alzheimer's type was recently admitted to a skilled nursing facility (SNF). The OTA working with the resident reports to the occupational therapist that during the morning care session, the OTA observed bruises on the resident's back and upper arms. Which action is best for the occupational therapist to initially take?

Answer Choices:
A. Talk to the resident to obtain more information.
B. Follow facility procedures for investigating resident safety. ✗
C. Contact the resident's family to obtain more information.
D. Contact the state office for adult protective services.

Correct Answer: B.

Rationale:
Whenever there are concerns for a client's safety and well-being facility procedures for investigating the situation must be followed. Talking to the resident may not enable the occupational therapist to obtain accurate information due to the person's diagnosis of dementia. At this point there is no need to contact the family. An internal investigation would determine if the family could provide helpful information or if they should be contacted by a professional who is trained in abuse investigation. The source of the bruises needs to be determined before any other action is taken. Contacting state authorities may be premature, for there may be a reasonable explanation for the bruises. Further investigation into the situation by the appropriate facility personnel according to established institutional policies is indicated. All health care facilities have clear guidelines for investigating and reporting potential abuse.

Type of Reasoning: Evaluative
One must weigh the possible courses of action and then make a value judgment about the best course to take. This requires evaluative reasoning skill, which often utilizes guiding principles of action in order to arrive at a correct conclusion. In this case, the occupational therapist follows facility procedures for investigating resident safety. If answered incorrectly, review guidelines for investigating potential abuse in older adults.

A102 C6

An occupational therapist assesses a retired carpenter and war veteran who was recently admitted to an acute psychiatric unit due to an exacerbation of post-traumatic stress disorder. The individual is observed to initiate interactions with others during structured tasks but is withdrawn when not engaged in a task. Which activity is best for the therapist to recommend to the individual?

Answer Choices:
A. Writing thoughts and feelings in a daily journal.
B. Engaging in meditation when alone in a hospital room.
C. Assisting another patient with a woodworking project.
D. Writing about personal experiences in the unit's newspaper.

Correct Answer: C.

Rationale:
Assisting someone with a woodworking project uses the patient's carpentry skills and facilitates the curative factor of altruism. Completing a shared project will provide the individual with an opportunity for socialization. Self-expressive activities and meditation can be very helpful to many individuals. However, they can be extremely stressful for someone who is experiencing an exacerbation of post-traumatic stress disorder. This disorder is characterized by flashbacks or the reliving of very traumatic events. Focusing on these thoughts and feelings are contraindicated in an acute episode.

Type of Reasoning: Inductive
Clinical knowledge and judgment are the most important skills needed for answering this question, which requires inductive reasoning. Knowledge of the diagnosis and most appropriate clinical outcomes is essential to choose the best solution. In this case, the therapist should recommend assisting another patient with a woodworking project.

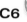

A103 C8

Upon evaluating a client for a wheelchair, the occupational therapist determines that a standard narrow adult chair would be suitable for the individual. Which dimensions most accurately identify this chair?

Answer Choices:

A. 18" wide × 18" deep × 20" high.
B. 16" wide × 16" deep × 20" high.
C. 16" wide × 16" deep × 18.5" high.
D. 14" wide × 16" deep × 18.5" high.

Correct Answer: B.

Rationale:

These are the standard dimensions for a narrow adult chair. The other choices do not identify measurements consistent with standard adult wheelchairs. These measurements would reflect a customized chair. A regular adult chair has dimensions of 18" wide × 16" deep × 20" high. A slim adult standard chair has dimensions of 14" wide × 16" deep × 20" high and a junior standard chair has dimensions of 16" wide by 16" deep by 18.5" high.

Type of Reasoning: Deductive

This question requires recall of guidelines and principles, which is factual knowledge. Deductive reasoning skills are utilized whenever one must recall facts to solve novel problems. In this situation, the dimensions of a standard adult narrow wheelchair are 16" wide × 16" deep × 20" high. Review dimensions of adult wheelchairs, especially narrow chairs if answered incorrectly.

A104 C9

An adult is referred to occupational therapy for treatment of chronic back pain that hinders the satisfactory performance of home maintenance tasks. The occupational therapists in the department have little experience with back pain, while the physical therapists in the rehabilitation department have extensive experience in this area. Which action is the best choice for the occupational therapist to take in response to this situation?

Answer Choices:

A. Refer the patient to physical therapy.
B. Co-treat the person with a physical therapist.
C. Give the patient the option to work in occupational or physical therapy.
D. Review a video on treatment of back pain.

Correct Answer: B.

Rationale:

This is an opportunity to improve the therapist's skills by collaborating with a team member. The primary focus of physical therapy is different than that of occupational therapy; consequently, co-treating the individual allows each discipline to contribute its unique expertise to address the person's pain. Referring the person to physical therapy would not allow the person to benefit from the occupational therapist's activity analysis, activity adaptation, and environmental modification knowledge and skills which can be very helpful for the pain-free performance of home management tasks. The decision as to the form of therapy that can best meet a person's needs should be made by professional staff, not by the person. A review of a video is not the best method for developing the knowledge and skills needed to provide individualized intervention. Working with an experienced therapist to provide treatment is an excellent opportunity for individualization of intervention and is the best answer.

Type of Reasoning: Evaluative
One must weigh the possible courses of action and then make a value judgment about the best course to take. This requires evaluative reasoning skills, which often utilize guiding principles of action in order to arrive at a correct conclusion. In this situation, the occupational therapist should co-treat the person since this would allow the therapist to receive ongoing input from the experienced physical therapist. This choice allows an opportunity to improve the occupational; therapist's knowledge and skill in back rehabilitation.

A105 C7

A six-year-old child with difficulties in figure-ground perception is being discharged from occupational therapy services. In the discharge plan, which should the therapist recommend for this child?

Answer Choices:
A. Use a different solid-colored folder to hold materials for each class subject.
B. Use a toothbrush and comb that are the same colors as the counter.
C. Wear clothing with bold colors and loud patterns.
D. Place all school books and handouts on the desk while completing homework.

Correct Answer: A.

Rationale:
Using a different solid-colored folder to hold class materials for each subject (e.g., blue is for math, red is for social studies, green is for science) can help the child more easily find desired class work. Contrasting colors facilitate performance by accommodating for the figure-ground difficulties. Monotone colors can make it more difficult to find grooming items. Loud, bright prints can make it more difficult to find armholes and don shirts. Working on a desk that is cluttered can make it more difficult to find needed work.

Type of Reasoning: Inferential
One must link the child's deficit to the activities presented in order to determine which activity would best address figure-ground perception after discharge. This requires inferential reasoning, where one must mentally picture the activities occurring and then determine which one uses the most figure-ground perception. In this case, the use of colored folders to organize schoolwork is the most likely recommendation from the therapist. If answered incorrectly review figure-ground perception deficits.

A106 C4

An occupational therapist is working with a child presenting with sensory-seeking behaviors and under reactivity to touch and movement. The child has an unusually high activity level, inability to self-calm, motor impulsivity, and frequent touching and handling of items in the environment. Using Ayres classic sensory integrative (SI) approach which would be most effective for the therapist to use with this child to facilitate an adaptive response?

Answer Choices:
A. A pre-determined schedule of sensory activities designed by the occupational therapist.
B. The child's passive participation in a variety of vestibular and proprioceptive experiences.
C. Use of a sensory void environment to promote self-regulation.
D. Individualized therapeutic activities based on the interests of the child.

Correct Answer: D.

Rationale:
Classic Ayres SI treatment is based on the principles of inner drive and active involvement of the child. Individualizing the activities used in therapy based on the child's interests is consistent with these principles; the use of a pre-determined schedule of activities designed by the occupational therapist is not. According to Ayres, sensory systems are impacted by a sensory rich environment and the balance between structure and freedom in regards to activity and participation. The occupational therapist is constantly vigilant to ensure that the interaction between the child and the therapist promotes the "just right" challenge. Passive participation and a sensory void environment do not provide the opportunity for the child to engage in this process.

Type of Reasoning: Inductive
One must utilize clinical judgment and knowledge of therapeutic guidelines in order to determine the most effective approach for a child with sensory seeking behaviors. This requires inductive reasoning skill. For this case, the therapist should provide individualized therapy based on the interests of the child. If answered incorrectly, review the sensory integration frame of reference and therapeutic approaches for sensory-seeking behaviors.

A107 C2

A non-English speaking individual with a recent left-sided CVA comes to occupational therapy for the first evaluation session. The assigned therapist cannot communicate verbally with the person. Which action is best for the therapist to take first?

Answer Choices:
A. Perform a screening to determine the specific areas to evaluate.
B. Seek out a translator to assist with the evaluation.
C. Communicate with the individual using non-verbal communication.
D. Evaluate the individual according to established protocols.

Correct Answer: B.

Rationale:
The best choice to ensure that the individual's desires are included in each step of the occupational therapy process is to seek out a translator to help the therapist communicate directly and verbally with the person during the evaluation. This action is consistent with Principle 3: Autonomy of the OT Code of Ethics. Without a translator, the individual is not autonomously able to participate in the screening or evaluation process. According to this principle, the therapist must "take appropriate steps to facilitate meaningful communication and comprehension in cases in which the recipient of service, student, or research participant has limited ability to communicate (e.g., aphasia or differences in language, literacy, culture)" (AOTA, 2010, p. S21). Non-verbal communication does not transcend a language barrier for abstract concepts such as incorporating the individual's needs, values, and goals into the occupational therapy process.

Type of Reasoning: Evaluative
This question requires one to determine the best course of action that considers the needs of the person and most effectively facilitates delivery of services. Questions that ask the test-taker to use judgment to determine a best course of action often utilize evaluative reasoning skills. In this situation, and in keeping with the OT Code of Ethics, the therapist should seek out a translator.

A108 C6

Which is the most effective approach for an occupational therapist to use when giving directions for a task to an individual with schizophrenia who is experiencing auditory hallucinations?

Answer Choices:

A. Written directions for making vanilla pudding.
B. Verbal step-by-step directions for making a leather link belt.
C. General verbal directions for the completion of a group collage.
D. Demonstration of steps during a swing dance class.

Correct Answer: A.

Rationale:

When designing activities for an individual with psychotic symptoms, the therapist must consider the activity components and how best to present the activity. Written directions with a structured, expected outcome are best to reinforce reality and to provide concrete feedback for the person experiencing hallucinations. Verbal directions are hardest to follow for a person who is experiencing auditory hallucinations. Working near others with some interaction can help to decrease auditory hallucinations, but an unstructured open-ended group project like a collage may be too vague and ambiguous. Demonstration can be an excellent way to provide directions. However, the increased auditory input of background music and the additional tactile stimulation of being touched by others while dancing may contribute to hallucinations due to increased sensory input. The quick movements of swing dancing may be contraindicated if the person is experiencing certain medication side effects, such as orthostatic hypotension.

Type of Reasoning: Inductive

This question requires one to assess the needs of the client based upon his/her diagnosis and knowledge of the symptoms of schizophrenia. This necessitates clinical judgment in determining a best course of action, which is an inductive reasoning skill. For this case, the therapist should choose structured activities with written directions to best ensure success and minimize the impact of auditory hallucinations. Review therapeutic approaches for patients with schizophrenia and auditory hallucinations.

A109 C3

As the result of a trauma 10 months ago, a 13-year-old incurred a unilateral below-elbow amputation. Due to a recent growth spurt, the adolescent is being re-evaluated for a new prosthesis. During the evaluation, the adolescent angrily tells the occupational therapist that a prosthesis is "annoying to have to wear every day." The adolescent reports not liking "the claw" and as a result often takes off the current prosthesis. However, the adolescent acknowledges that the prosthesis is "needed sometimes" to perform desired bilateral activities. Which action is best for the therapist to take in response to this adolescent's statements?

Answer Choices:

A. Refer the adolescent to the child psychologist to deal with adjustment to disability.
B. Work on developing unilateral skills for completion of meaningful activities.
C. Refer the adolescent to a prosthetist for a prosthesis with a cosmetic hand.
D. Recommend the adolescent attend a teen amputee support group.

Correct Answer: B.

Rationale:
Most individuals with unilateral below elbow amputations are able to achieve functional independence in desired activities using their intact UE for skilled task functions with their residual limb serving as a stabilizer. A prosthesis can readily become unnecessary as a person develops unilateral skills and can then be viewed as more of an annoyance than a facilitator. The adolescent's response is a normal response and does not indicate a need for a referral to a psychologist or a support group. A cosmetic prosthesis requires more muscle function to operate and it does not enhance functional abilities. The adolescent currently expresses the need to occasionally use the prosthesis to perform desired activities so a cosmetic device would not be helpful. The new prosthesis can be used for bilateral activities when needed and desired by the adolescent.

Type of Reasoning: Evaluative
One must weigh the possible courses of action and then make a value judgment about the best course to take. This requires evaluative reasoning skill, which often utilizes guiding principles of action in order to arrive at a correct conclusion. In this case, because the patient has indicated annoyance with wearing the prosthesis and frequent removal, the therapist should work on developing unilateral skills for completion of meaningful activities.

A110 C2

An occupational therapist conducts an after-school transition skills group with adolescents with a diversity of disabilities. One of the student's behaviors is very different than in prior groups (e.g., difficulty focusing when typically serving as the group initiator, making statements that are irrelevant to the topic at hand). The therapist smells a strong alcohol scent on the student's breath. Which action should the therapist take in response to this situation?

Answer Choices:
A. Directly ask the student if the student has been drinking.
B. Initiate a group discussion about the effects of substance abuse on occupational performance.
C. Proceed with the group and report suspicions of alcohol use at the next transition planning team meeting.
D. Call for a school aide to escort the student to the school's on-site health care facility.

Correct Answer: D.

Rationale:
The occupational therapist must ensure the student's safety. The medical staff of the school's on-site health care facility can evaluate the student to determine the cause of the student's atypical behavior and alcohol-smelling breath. These symptoms can be the result of alcohol use or an indication of ketoacidosis. In either case, it is best for the student to receive a medical evaluation and the corresponding care. The other options do not address the student's need for a medical evaluation and they can be disruptive to the group process for the other group participants.

Type of Reasoning: Evaluative
This judgment question requires one to determine what will not only address the situation at hand, but protect the student from future harm. The test taker must choose the answer that addresses the situation immediately and with the professionals who hold ultimate responsibility for the patient. Evaluation questions are challenging in that one must evaluate the merits of each statement and conclude what will result in the best possible outcome. Review first aid procedures and symptoms of ketoacidosis if answered incorrectly.

A111 C6

An occupational therapist uses behavior modification techniques to help shape the behavioral responses of students with behavioral disorders. Which action is most consistent with this intervention approach?

Answer Choices:
A. Provide frequent positive reinforcement for all desired behaviors.
B. Reprimand the students every time an undesirable behavior occurs.
C. Allow each student enough time for self-correction of the behavior.
D. Encourage the teaching staff to tell the students which behaviors are correct and incorrect.

Correct Answer: A.

Rationale:
Behavioral modification is best achieved through use of positive reinforcements for all desired behaviors. Negative behaviors should be ignored. Self-correction is not a form of behavior modification.

Type of Reasoning: Deductive
For this question the test taker utilizes knowledge and recall of behavioral modification techniques to choose the correct answer. This necessitates the factual recall of guidelines, which is a deductive reasoning skill. For this scenario, the therapist should provide frequent positive reinforcement for all desired behaviors, which is aligned with behavioral modification guidelines. Review behavioral modification guidelines if answered incorrectly.

A112 C4

During a home visit, a client who had incurred a CVA reports difficulty finding objects during BADL and IADL. The client reports that the directions family members provide (e.g., look on the refrigerator's door, look in the medicine cabinet) are not helpful. Which cognitive perceptual ability should the occupational therapist further evaluate?

Answer Choices:
A. Stereognosis.
B. Organization.
C. Spatial relations.
D. Visual closure.

Correct Answer: D.

Rationale:
This behavior may be evidence of difficulties with visual closure since the person may not be able to find an item if it is in its incomplete form (i.e., covered partially by other objects in the refrigerator or cabinet). The other options describe cognitive-perceptual deficits with different manifestations. Stereognosis is the ability to recognize objects by touch alone. Organization is the ability to structure thoughts and actions. Spatial relations are the ability to relate objects in relationship to each other or the self (e.g., up/down, front/back, under/over).

Type of Reasoning: Analytical
This question provides a description of a functional deficit and the test taker must determine the likely cause for this deficit. This requires analysis of symptoms, which is an analytical reasoning skill. In this case, the client is reporting difficulties with visual closure. If answered incorrectly, review signs and symptoms of visual closure dysfunction.

A113 **C1**

An occupational therapist is treating an eight-month-old child with mild developmental delay. The child exhibits normal cognitive development. The child has developed adequate static sitting balance but has poor dynamic sitting balance. The therapist implements intervention by positioning the child and having the child find a toy that is covered with a cloth. Which positioning and toy placement are most beneficial for the therapist to use with this child?

Answer Choices:

A. Sit the child between the therapist's extended legs and alternate placing the covered toy to the child's right and left side.

B. Sit the child in a child seat and alternate placing the covered toy to the child's right and left side.

C. Lay the child in a prone position and place the covered toy in front of the child.

D. Lay the child in on the right side and place the covered toy to the left of the child.

Correct Answer: A.

Rationale:

Having the child sit between the therapist's extended legs can enable the therapist to easily provide postural support for the child as needed. Placing the covered toy to the right and then left of the seated child will facilitate the child's sideward protective extension response. Sideward protective extension in sitting is a functional, protective reaction that typically occurs at 7 months and persists in normal development. Sideward protective extension is a key component to the development of dynamic sitting balance as it protects the child from a fall. This reaction also supports the body for unilateral use of the opposite arm. Sitting the child in a child seat would provide too much support and would not provide the child with the "just-right" challenge to develop dynamic sitting. Laying the child in a prone position and placing the covered toy in front of the child would help facilitate a prone on elbows position. If the child has begun to sit, this position would have already been mastered so this intervention is not needed. Laying the child in on the right side and placing the covered toy to the left of the child would facilitate rolling. If the child has begun to sit, rolling would have already been mastered so this intervention is not needed.

Type of Reasoning: Inferential

One must recall the developmental milestones of infants and infer the best choice for positioning in order to choose the correct solution. For this child, who just achieved static sitting balance, positioning that provides postural support during dynamic sitting activity with facilitation of the protective extensive response is most beneficial because this skill is essential for dynamic sitting. If answered incorrectly, review the motor developmental milestones of infants.

A114 **C8**

A child with moderate spastic cerebral palsy works on ambulation with a walker in physical therapy. The occupational therapy evaluation reveals problems in lower extremity dressing, transitional skills, self-feeding, and grasp and release skills. To facilitate the attainment of the child's ambulation goal, which activity is best for the occupational therapist to include in OT intervention session?

Answer Choices:

A. Rolling in and out of prone and supine while on a mat, with minimal hands-on facilitation.

B. Donning and doffing shoes and socks in bench sitting with one leg externally rotated and placed on the opposite knee.

C. Self-feeding with elbows supported on a cut-out table at waist height, using a spoon with a built-up handle.

D. Practicing grasp and release of small objects while wearing bilateral soft splints to support a more functional hand position.

Correct Answer: B.

Rationale:
Dressing the lower extremities in bench sitting encourages dynamic trunk balance, lower extremity external rotation, and dissociation. This activity is the best one listed to address the skills needed for ambulation while meeting OT goals related to performance in areas of occupation. The use of elbows to stabilize the upper extremity for feeding does not address dynamic balance and focuses more on fine motor control and coordination. Practicing the grasp and release of small objects while wearing soft splints might help improve the child's ability to grasp the walker handles but this activity does not directly address the child's ambulation goal, which is the stated focus of the question.

Type of Reasoning: Inductive
This question requires one to utilize clinical judgment to determine what activities would best address the child's goal of ambulation, which is an inductive reasoning skill. From all the activities listed, donning and doffing shoes and socks best facilitates the precursory skills needed for ambulation. If answered incorrectly, review information on the components of functional ambulation and apply your activity analysis skills to the answer choices.

A115 C9

A co-worker in the therapy department complains excessively during working hours of personal problems. The co-worker does not respond to colleagues' statements that this is disruptive to their work. Which action is best for the occupational therapist to take in response to this situation?

Answer Choices:
A. Call the employee assistance program for the co-worker.
B. Talk with the co-worker using a client-centered approach.
C. Tactfully and firmly redirect the co-worker to work issues.
D. Inform the department supervisor of the situation.

Correct Answer: D.

Rationale:
The supervisor should be informed of the situation because the employee's personal problems are entering the workplace, which is not in the best interests of the employee, the other staff, or the facility. This situation falls in the area of the supervisor's responsibility. A therapist should not call the employee assistance program or counseling service for a co-worker. The decision for taking these actions is the co-worker's choice. Co-workers are not responsible to and should not treat fellow employees. Tactfully redirecting the co-worker is a common technique to avoid being drawn into the problems of others, but it will not address the problem in the department.

Type of Reasoning: Evaluative
One must make a decision based on ethical guidelines and value judgment, which is an evaluative reasoning skill. In this situation, the therapist should inform the supervisor of the issue, as it is in the best interests of everyone involved. Questions of this nature can be challenging to answer as a simple solution is not often found and clear cut guidelines are not always at hand to refer to in situations such as these.

A116 C1

A five-year-old is referred to occupational therapy. Upon the completion of a standardized test evaluation, the occupational therapist determines that the child demonstrates age-appropriate cognitive and fine motor skills. Which activity would the child be able to complete at this developmental level?

Answer Choices:
A. Cutting long thin strips with scissors.
B. Holding and snipping with scissors.
C. Cutting simple figure shapes with scissors.
D. Opening and closing scissors in a controlled fashion.

Correct Answer: C.

Rationale:
Cutting simple figure shapes is a four to six year-old cognitive and fine motor skill. Cutting strips is a three to four-year-old skill. Holding and snipping with scissors and opening and closing scissors in a controlled fashion are 2–3 year old skills.

Type of Reasoning: Deductive
This question requires one to recall factual knowledge, which is a deductive reasoning skill. The question necessitates one to recall the developmental skills of a four-year-old. In this situation, cutting simple figure shapes is a four-year-old skill. If answered incorrectly, review the developmental sequence of scissor skills.

A117 C8

An occupational therapist provides recommendations for play activities that a parent with a complete spinal cord injury at the C-7 level can do with children, aged eight, and ten. Which is the best adapted activity for the therapist to recommend?

Answer Choices:
A. An arts and crafts project using a mouthstick brush to paint.
B. A woodworking project using a universal cuff to hold tools.
C. A board game using a tenodesis grasp to move game pieces.
D. A computer game using a typing stick to keyboard.

Correct Answer: C.

Rationale:
An individual with a C-7 SCI has a tenodesis grasp that can be effective for picking up and releasing game pieces. The other activity adaptations are appropriate for individuals with higher spinal cord injuries.

Type of Reasoning: Inductive
One must utilize clinical knowledge and judgment to determine the most appropriate activity for a patient with C7 injury. In this case, a board game using a tenodesis grasp to move game pieces is most appropriate given the person's level of injury. If answered incorrectly, review functional abilities and intact musculature for persons with C7 injury.

A118 C6

An individual recently lost significant functional abilities due to post-polio syndrome. The occupational therapist works with the individual to develop compensation skills for performing daily tasks. During a meal preparation session, the person angrily throws all of the adaptive equipment onto the floor. At the next team meeting, which defense mechanism should the therapist report the individual appears to be demonstrating?

Answer Choices:
A. Acting out.
B. Passive-aggressive behavior.
C. Reaction formation.
D. Displacement.

Correct Answer: D.

Rationale:
Displacement occurs when an individual redirects an emotion from one "object" (in this case, the anger over the progression of the disease) to another "object" (i.e., the adaptive equipment). Acting out is a term used to describe behaviors that violate societal norms (e.g., sexually provocative behavior, physically assaultive behavior). Passive-aggressive behavior is characterized by indirect or unassertive aggression (e.g., being chronically late when meeting someone you had an argument with years ago). Reaction formation is the switching of an unacceptable impulse into its opposite (e.g., hugging someone you would like to hit).

Type of Reasoning: Analytical
This question provides a description of a behavior and the test taker must draw conclusions about what the behavior indicates. This is an analytical reasoning skill, as questions of this nature often ask one to analyze descriptors and symptoms in order to determine a diagnosis or draw a conclusion. In this situation the behavior indicates displacement. Review defense mechanisms if answered incorrectly.

A119 C5

An occupational therapist works with a patient with diabetes and a below-knee (BK) amputation to learn how to effectively perform home management tasks while wearing a BK prosthesis. When taking laundry from a front-loading washer and placing it into a top-loading dryer, the patient reports feeling weak, dizzy, and somewhat nauseous. The occupational therapist notices that the patient is sweating profusely and is unsteady when standing. Which is the best immediate course of action for the therapist to take in response to the patient's complaints and these observations?

Answer Choices:
A. Return the person to the unit of care due to an insulin reaction. X
B. Administer orange juice for developing hypoglycemia. ☆
C. Call a nurse to administer an insulin injection for developing hyperglycemia.
D. Have the patient sit down until the orthostatic hypotension resolves. X

Correct Answer: B.

Rationale:
Hypoglycemia, abnormally low blood glucose, results from too much insulin (insulin reaction). It requires accurate assessment of symptoms and prompt intervention. Having the patient sit down and ingest an oral sugar (e.g., orange juice) is the best immediate action for the therapist to take. Once the patient is stabilized, the physician should be notified. Profuse sweating and nausea do not usually accompany orthostatic hypotension.

Type of Reasoning: Inductive

The test taker must determine first what the cause is for the patient's symptoms and then what is the appropriate course of action. Questions such as these utilize one's clinical judgment and diagnostic thinking, which is an inductive reasoning skill. One should recognize that these symptoms are indicative of hypoglycemia and require immediate administration of sugar to relieve symptoms. Review first aid guidelines for hypoglycemia if answered incorrectly.

A120 C4

A child with spastic quadriplegic cerebral palsy has increased tone and flexor synergies in both upper extremities. The child receives Botox injections into both biceps. In designing play activities to use during intervention, which is most important for the occupational therapist to include as an activity performance characteristic?

Answer Choices:

A. Reaching overhead and to both sides in supine.
B. Bilateral upper extremity weight-bearing in sitting and in prone.
C. Grasp and release of objects in supported sitting.
D. Transitions into and out of sitting, supine, and prone.

Correct Answer: B.

Rationale:

The theory supporting the use of Botox injections is that the Botox lessens spasticity for three to six months to allow for the strengthening of the opposing non-spastic muscles. In this case, the child has flexor spasticity so relaxation of the biceps to allow strengthening of the triceps is indicated. Therefore, the most important focus of intervention is weight-bearing of the upper extremities since this can strengthen the triceps muscles. Reaching overhead and grasp and release are helpful in refining gross and fine motor skills, respectively; but these activities would not be effective in achieving the post-Botox injection aim of strengthening the triceps. Although the performance of transitions in sitting and supine involves upper extremity weight-bearing, a child with spastic quadriplegia would probably not be able to do this activity.

Type of Reasoning: Inferential

One must determine the most important activity to include in the intervention plan for a child with spastic quadriplegic cerebral palsy who just received Botox injections into the biceps. This requires inferential reasoning skill, where the test taker must determine the best course of action based on the information provided. In this case the plan of care should include bilateral upper extremity weight-bearing in sitting and in prone.

A121 C9

A person recovering from hip replacement surgery wants to begin meal preparation. The client refuses to use the walker that was ordered by the physician. The physician is unavailable for consultation. Which is the best initial action for the occupational therapist to take in response to this situation?

Answer Choices:

A. Work on meal preparation activities with the client sitting at a table.
B. Work on meal preparation activities with the client standing without the walker.
C. Delay working on meal preparation activities until the physician can be contacted.
D. Tell the client the walker must be used until the physician changes the order.

Correct Answer: A.

Rationale:
There are many meal preparation activities that can be done while seated so there is no need to delay meal preparation activities. The therapist should not conduct the session without the prescribed walker or ambulatory aid until a written or verbal order is received. This is not negotiable as the client's safety is the paramount concern. Telling the client that the walker must be used violates the client's rights to self-determination.

Type of Reasoning: Evaluative
One must make a judgment call based on values and ethical principles, which is an evaluative reasoning skill. Situations such as these are challenging as one must weigh the interests of all the parties involved. The only solution that considers the safety and needs of the client is to work on meal preparation activities with the client sitting at the table. Review safety guidelines for clients with total hip arthroplasty if answered incorrectly.

A122 C6

The occupational therapist administers the Allen Cognitive Level (ACL) Screen to an individual. During this evaluation, the most complex behavior the individual can perform is to do the three running stitches, imitating the therapist's example. Based upon these results, the therapist selects an activity to use for intervention that is consistent with the individual's functional level. According to the Cognitive Disabilities model, which activity is best for the therapist to use when implementing intervention with this patient?

Answer Choices:
A. Exercises that require the imitation of another's posture. too low (2)
B. Sorting laundry by matching the colors of clothing items. (4)
C. Sanding wooden bookends. (3)
D. Planning a three-course meal. (5)

Correct Answer: C.

Rationale:
According to the rating criteria of the ACL, the ability to imitate the running stitch indicates level 3 of cognitive performance. According to Allen's Cognitive Disability model, people at level 3 can use their hands to manipulate objects and they are able to perform a limited number of simple tasks that are repetitive. Sanding wood is an activity that is consistent with level 3 of the Allen Cognitive Levels. In addition, sanding bookends will result in the completion of a tangible object that has functional use which can facilitate the person's feelings of self-efficacy. According to the Cognitive Disabilities model, the imitation of postures is a level 2 skill, so exercises that require postural imitation would be too low for this individual. Sorting laundry by matching clothing colors is a level 4 skill. Planning a three-course meal would require the level 5 skills of problem solving. This is too high of a level for this person.

Type of Reasoning: Inferential
This question requires one to first determine the level of ACL functioning according to the description provided (completing a running stitch following an example) and then match this to the listed activity that is also characteristic of this level of functioning. This requires knowledge of the Cognitive Disability model as well as functional abilities within each level. In this situation, the characteristics are associated with level 3 ACL functioning. In this case, sanding wooden blocks is an ideal approach, as it provides a repetitive task within the capabilities of this individual. If answered incorrectly, review the Allen Cognitive Levels and characteristics of level 3 functioning.

A123 C9

A skilled nursing facility (SNF) wants to provide an activities program to meet the needs of each resident. The occupational therapy supervisor has been asked to write a job description for the position of an activities program director and delineate the qualifications needed for that position. Which should the occupational therapist recommend for this position?

Answer Choices:

A. An OTA who receives general supervision from an occupational therapist.
B. An OTA who receives close supervision from an occupational therapist.
C. An OTA who receives routine supervision from an occupational therapist.
D. An OTA who does not require the supervision of an occupational therapist.

Correct Answer: D.

Rationale:
According to AOTA standards of practice and Medicare guidelines, an OTA who works strictly as an activities program director is not providing occupational therapy. While OTAs who work as activities program directors likely use their OT knowledge (e.g., the impact of client factors on activity performance) and skills (e.g., activity analysis, adaptation, and gradation) in this position; they are not providing OT services. Rather they are providing directorship to the SNF's activity program. Therefore, they do not require the supervision of an occupational therapist.

Type of Reasoning: Deductive
One must recall the supervisory guidelines for OTAs in the role of activities program director. This is factual knowledge, which is a deductive reasoning skill. Because OTAs can perform duties as an activities director without supervision, no supervision from an occupational therapist is required. If answered incorrectly, review supervisory guidelines for OTAs and Medicare guidelines for activity program director positions in SNFs.

A124 C2

An occupational therapist works with adolescents who have been victims of child abuse. Treatment can be carried out in groups or on an individual basis. Which of the following would indicate to the therapist that intervention should be provided to an adolescent on an individual basis rather than in a group?

Answer Choices:

A. The adolescent wants more socialization experiences.
B. The adolescent could benefit from feedback from peers.
C. The adolescent desires greater control over the environment.
D. The adolescent needs an opportunity to gain situational perspective.

Correct Answer: C.

Rationale:
The person who wants to have more control over the environment would benefit from working on an individual basis. Groups are unpredictable and effective group process requires trust and the sharing of control among all members. This may be difficult for an adolescent who has survived child abuse and is understandably seeking personal control. Someone who wants increased socialization would benefit from group interventions. A group is also the best intervention format to obtain peer feedback and to put one's own personal situation into perspective.

Type of Reasoning: Inferential
One must determine the benefits of individual therapy for adolescents who are survivors of abuse in order to arrive at a correct conclusion. This requires inferential reasoning, where one must draw conclusions based on the information provided. In this situation, if the client requires greater control over the environment, individual therapy is best, as a group situation can be unpredictable. If answered incorrectly, review the benefits of individual therapy versus group therapy and the characteristics of victims of abuse. Integration of this knowledge is required for a correct answer.

A125 C3

A house painter is referred to occupational therapy after a re-occurrence of rotator cuff tendinitis. The physician prescribes a conservative intervention approach. Which recommendation is best for the occupational therapist to make to the individual?

Answer Choices:
A. Continue performing above shoulder activities to build rotator cuff strength.
B. Use an extension handle in the paint roller when painting ceilings.
C. Sleep with the shoulder extended and adducted.
D. Sleep with the shoulder fully flexed and adducted.

Correct Answer: C.

Rationale:
Sleeping with the shoulder extended and adducted is an acceptable position for this condition. Above shoulder activities and positions are contraindicated for persons with rotator cuff injuries. Even with an extended roller handle the individual would still be performing above shoulder activities while painting.

Type of Reasoning: Inductive
One must utilize clinical knowledge and judgment to determine the most appropriate recommendation. In this case, sleeping with the shoulder extended and adducted is the most appropriate recommendation out of the choices provided. If answered incorrectly, review activity guidelines and positioning recommendations for patients with rotator cuff tendinitis.

A126 C4

An occupational therapist implements intervention in a preschool program for children with tactile defensiveness. In the prior intervention session, the children had responded favorably when the therapist had rolled a large ball over their bodies as they lay supine on a mat. Which intervention method should the therapist use next?

Answer Choices:
A. Roll the large ball with increased pressure across the children's bodies.
B. Bounce the ball across the children's bodies.
C. Have the children jump into a pool filled with small balls.
D. Roll the large ball, as in the prior session, with the children prone.

Correct Answer: A.

Rationale:
Increasing pressure on the ball is the next gradation of the activity that has been reported to be successful. Children with tactile defensiveness respond well to firm pressure. Jumping into a pool with small balls is too large of a progression to make from comfort with a ball rolling over one's body for children who have tactile defensiveness. Bouncing a ball across their bodies can be frightening and it does not provide the desired deep pressure input. Changing the children's position from supine to prone does not provide an activity gradation related to intervention for tactile defensiveness.

Type of Reasoning: Inferential
One must have knowledge of tactile defensiveness in children and gradation of sensory activity in order to choose the next most appropriate gradation of activity. This is an inferential reasoning skill where knowledge of the diagnosis and progression of activity is pivotal to choosing the correct solution. If answered incorrectly, review sensory activities for children with tactile defensiveness, especially activities that provide deep pressure.

A127 C8

The parent of a newborn infant has bilateral shoulder weakness and is referred to occupational therapy for training in energy conservation techniques for the performance of parenting and home management tasks. Which adaptation(s) is/are most effective for the occupational therapist to recommend the parent use?

Answer Choices:
A. A top-loading washer and dryer for clothing care.
B. A steamer, steamer basket, and/or crock pot for meal preparation.
C. A front pack carrier for holding the infant.
D. Cloth diapers and the use of a weekly diaper care service.

Correct Answer: B.

Rationale:
A steamer, steamer basket, and crock pot eliminate the need to move and lift heavy pans and pots; tasks which require intact bilateral upper extremity strength. A top-loading washer and dryer require more work than front-loading machines. The extra lifting required for top-loading appliances would be difficult with shoulder weakness. A front pack infant carrier has straps which cross the shoulders so this would be contraindicated in this case. The child's weight in the carrier could contribute to shoulder strain. While a weekly diaper service can provide clean diapers each week, cloth diapers require additional care (i.e., rinsing) which can consume the client's time and energy. Lifting the week's load of wet diapers to bring to the door and picking up the week's allotment of clean diapers can be difficult with shoulder weakness.

Type of Reasoning: Inductive
This question requires one to review all of the potential recommendations and determine which one is most aligned with conserving energy, given the patient's limitations. For this situation, use of a steamer, steamer basket or crock pot to prepare meals will best conserve energy. Inductive reasoning skills are utilized as clinical judgment is paramount in choosing the best solution. Review energy conservation strategies for home management tasks if answered incorrectly.

A128 C9

A 14-year-old with spastic quadriplegia cerebral palsy and mild intellectual disability begins high school. The occupational therapist determines that the adolescent's academic needs are being adequately addressed by the use of the equipment and strategies that the adolescent had acquired during the middle school years. Which recommendation is best for the therapist to make to the individualized education planning team?

Answer Choices:
A. Adaptation of the middle school strategies and equipment to the adolescent's high school classes.
B. The development of a transition plan with the adolescent for a desired post-school life.
C. The development of peer relationships through engagement in extracurricular activities.
D. A referral to the local center for independent living for community-based activities.

Correct Answer: B.

Rationale:
The IEP must include transitional planning to help a student identify desired post-school goals and develop a plan for achieving these goals for adult life. This plan must begin at 14 (or younger if indicated) with transition services implemented at 16 (or younger if indicated). In the exam item scenario it states that the strategies and equipment acquired during middle school are effective. There is no indication that adaptations are needed. Having used these strategies and equipment during middle school, an adolescent with mild intellectual disability would be able to use these in high school without additional intervention. There is no information in the scenario to indicate that the adolescent requires intervention to develop peer relationships or engage in community-based activities.

Type of Reasoning: Inferential
One must infer or draw conclusions about a likely course of action, given the information presented. This is an inferential reasoning skill, where knowledge of a therapeutic approach, such as the recommendations for a teenager with spastic quadriplegic CP and mild intellectual disability, is essential to choosing a correct solution. In this case, the therapist should recommend a transition plan for post-school life. Review recommendations for post-school transition planning for students with disabilities if answered incorrectly.

A129 C5

An occupational therapist provides services to a homeless shelter which includes residents who are HIV positive. The therapist conducts several activity groups. Which should the therapist do while working with this population?

Answer Choices:
A. Wash hands before and after each group session.
B. Always wear latex gloves during groups.
C. Wear latex gloves when handling food.
D. Implement transmission-based precautions.

Correct Answer: A.

Rationale:
Health professionals should use standard precautions at all times, regardless of clients' diagnoses. Washing hands is a basic precautionary step all individuals should take to prevent the spread of infections and diseases (even in their own homes). The diagnosis of HIV is irrelevant to the question's correct answer for HIV is transmitted only through the exchange of body fluids. See Chapter 9. Wearing gloves while handling food is a health department regulation but it only addresses sessions involving food. One must still wash one's hands before and after glove use. In addition, due to potential latex allergies, health care environments must be latex-free. Transmission-based precautions are used when the route(s) of transmission is (are) not completely interrupted using standard precautions alone. For some diseases that have multiple routes of transmission (e.g., SARS), more than one transmission-based precaution category may be used. Transmission-based precautions have three categories: contact precautions, droplet precautions, and airborne precautions. None of these are indicated for HIV. See Chapter 3 for comprehensive information about standard and transmission-based precautions

Type of Reasoning: Deductive
This question requires recall of guidelines and principles, which is factual knowledge. Deductive reasoning skills are utilized whenever one must recall facts to solve everyday problems. In this situation, the therapist should follow standard precautions, which includes washing hands before and after each session. Review standard precautions if answered incorrectly.

A130 C6

A client with chronic depression and a spouse attend a discharge meeting with the occupational therapist following the client's six-week hospitalization for a major depressive episode. They state that they have few activities in common and spend little time together. The client retired two months ago and the spouse continues to work full time. Which of the following should the therapist encourage this couple to do first to address this concern?

Answer Choices:

A. Immediately participate in one activity together.
B. Become involved in their own individualized activities during the day.
C. Explore activities enjoyed together and alone.
D. Delay planning activities until the depression is totally resolved.

Correct Answer: C.

Rationale:

Assistance with an exploration of activities is a priority given the client's recent hospitalization for depression. The client's life has changed significantly with the loss of the worker role due to retirement and the resultant change in the amount of time spent alone. It will be important for the client to explore activities enjoyed alone so that retirement and time separated from his/her spouse will be enjoyable and meaningful. Exploring activities that the couple enjoy together will assist both in the maintenance of their relationship and in the establishment of a new activities pattern. Immediate participation in one activity together is premature for there has been no determination of shared interests. While involvement in their own individualized activities during the day may be helpful, this also must be done after their involvement in treatment planning and activity selection. A delay in planning activities until the depression is totally resolved is contraindicated. The client has chronic depression and needs treatment now.

Type of Reasoning: Inferential

One must infer or draw conclusions about a likely course of action, given the information presented. This is an inferential reasoning skill, where knowledge of a therapeutic approach is essential to choosing a correct solution. In this case, the therapist should begin with an exploration of activities that the individual and the spouse have enjoyed together and alone. Review meaningful activities and activity exploration for individuals with depression if answered incorrectly.

A131 C3

Two months ago a child received full thickness circumferential burns of both upper extremities. The child shows progressively decreasing ROM of the right elbow with a 25° loss to date with a stiff endpoint. The child complains of increased pain in the elbow. Which action should the occupational therapist take first in response to this change in status?

Answer Choices:

A. Begin use of a continuous passive motion device.
B. Apply heat prior to active ROM.
C. Contact the child's physician.
D. Splint the child's elbows in static splints.

Correct Answer: C.

Rationale:

The child shows probable symptoms of heterotopic ossification, a calcium deposit that may occur in or near a joint after burns. Circumferential burns are most susceptible to this condition. Symptoms include decreased joint excursion, a stiff endpoint, and increased pain. The best action is to call the physician. Aggressive passive ROM, especially to increase range, is contraindicated in treatment of this condition. The physician must determine the intervention. Heat may be contraindicated at this time. Splinting may be contraindicated in the treatment of heterotopic ossification.

Type of Reasoning: Analytical
This question asks the test taker to first determine the diagnosis and then determine a course of action based on this knowledge. Analytical reasoning is used whenever one must determine a diagnosis from a set of symptoms. If answered incorrectly, review symptoms of heterotopic ossification.

A132 C2

An occupational therapist conducts a communication skills group in a wellness program for a large accounting company. In this mature level group, what should the therapist do?

Answer Choices:
A. Help to develop the group norms.
B. Participate as a member.
C. Actively resolve group conflicts.
D. Maintain a leader role.

Correct Answer: B.

Rationale:
In a mature group, the therapist participates at the level of a member and does not serve as group leader except in special circumstances such as a member becoming destructive to the group process. The members decide formally and informally the group norms. The therapist does not usually participate in conflict resolution except to facilitate the members' participation in extreme situations, such as deadlocked conflicts. The therapist functions in a variety of task, maintenance, or egocentric roles as needed to show members how these roles function in the group.

Type of Reasoning: Deductive
This question essentially asks what the role is of an occupational therapist conducting a mature level group. Questions inquiring about guidelines or definitions test deductive reasoning skill, which is a more factual type of reasoning. For this question, an occupational therapist conducting a mature level group acts as a group participant. If answered incorrectly review group levels and the role of the group leader in facilitating groups.

A133 C2

When performing a chart audit for an on-site accreditation visit, an occupational therapist realizes that a date of service was documented wrong. Which actions are best for the therapist to take?

Answer Choices:
A. Use whiteout to remove the incorrect date, write the correct date of service, and then initial and date the correction.
B. Write the correct date over the incorrect date and then write the rehabilitation department director's initials.
C. Put a single line through the incorrect date, write the correct date of service, and then initial and date the correction.
D. Meet with the rehabilitation department director to discuss the need to correct this documentation.

Correct Answer: C.

Rationale:
Medical charts are legal documents that cannot be altered without accountability. Therefore, the error found must be acknowledged with the date of correction and the initials of the person making the correction. According to established guidelines for documentation, charting errors should be corrected by drawing a single line through the error and initialing and dating the chart. The permanent removal of an error by using whiteout is not acceptable nor is it acceptable to place another practitioner's initials on documentation. There is no need for the therapist to meet with the rehabilitation department director to discuss this situation. The therapist can make the needed correction according to established documentation standards.

Exam A

Type of Reasoning: Evaluative
This question requires one to evaluate the merits of the four possible solutions in order to determine which response is consistent with documentation standards of practice. Evaluative reasoning skills are utilized whenever one must make a judgment about a best course of action. In this type of situation, drawing a single line through the incorrect information with initials and then making and dating the correction is consistent with established guidelines for OT documentation, which should be reviewed if answered incorrectly.

A134 C3

A patient incurred a traumatic upper extremity amputation. During pre-prosthetic treatment, the occupational therapist molds the contours of the residual limb to shape it in preparation for a prosthesis. Which method is most effective for the occupational therapist to use?

Answer Choices:
A. Wrapping.
B. Percussion.
C. Shrinking.
D. Massage.

Correct Answer: A.

Rationale:
Wrapping by applying an elastic bandage to the residual limb in a figure-of-eight pattern will reduce the volume of the residual limb and shape it for a prosthesis. Shrinking is the result of wrapping. Percussion and massage are used to desensitize a residual limb.

Type of Reasoning: Analytical
This question provides a description of an intervention method and the test taker must determine the likely definition of the described method. This is an analytical reasoning skill, as questions of this nature often ask one to analyze a descriptor to determine the specific method being defined. In this situation the intervention method is that of residual limb wrapping, which should be reviewed if answered incorrectly.

A135 C6

An individual receives treatment for major depression on an inpatient psychiatric unit. The patient has received an electroconvulsive treatment (ECT) treatment at 8 am. At 2 pm, the patient walks into the occupational therapy department stating a desire to participate in the leisure skills group. Which is the occupational therapist's best response?

Answer Choices:
A. Encourage the client to select one of three structured leisure activities to complete.
B. Call nursing staff to escort the client back to the client's room so that the client can rest.
C. Commend the client's motivation but remind the client that rest is recommended for 24 hours after ECT.
D. Have the client complete a leisure history questionnaire to enable individualized treatment.

Correct Answer: A.

Rationale:
Six hours after ECT, the individual is capable of engaging in a structured task. Giving the individual a choice of activities to complete increases the likelihood that the person will be interested in the task selected. There is no need to return the client to his/her room and 24 hours of rest is not necessary after an ECT. However, there is some temporary memory loss after an ECT so it would not be appropriate to give the individual an activity that requires memory to complete.

Type of Reasoning: Inductive

This question requires one to determine the best response to a patient who had ECT treatment six hours ago. This requires inductive reasoning skill, where clinical judgment is paramount in arriving at a correct conclusion. For this situation, the test taker should recall the guidelines for activity after ECT treatment. Six hours after treatment the individual can engage in a structured task; therefore, the therapist should encourage the individual to engage in such a task. If answered incorrectly, review guidelines for OT intervention post ECT.

A136 C2

An occupational therapist designs an activity group program for twelve adults with multiple physical disabilities and/or illnesses who attend a day hospital family respite program. Which method is most effective for the therapist to use to determine the members' needs upon which to base the program?

Answer Choices:

A. Interview family caregivers.
B. Interview each member.
C. Interview day hospital staff.
D. Research the program's population characteristics.

Correct Answer: B.

Rationale:

Interviewing each member allows the therapist to assess members' assets, limitations, interests and roles. This information can be used to identify commonalities among members upon which meaningful activities can be developed. People are more likely to engage in activities that are related to their interests and roles and are at a level appropriate to their assets and limitations. Interviewing others will provide information about their perspectives but one cannot assume that these perceptions are valid representations of member concerns. Research on population characteristics is too broad for planning a relevant and meaningful activity program for a discrete group of people.

Type of Reasoning: Inductive

This question requires one to determine the best approach for determining group members' needs. This requires inductive reasoning skill, where clinical judgment is paramount in arriving at a correct conclusion. For this situation, the therapist should interview the group members to determine their needs. If answered incorrectly, review group program planning, especially needs assessment.

A137 C8

An occupational therapist leads a work group at a vocational rehabilitation program for persons with traumatic brain injuries. One member begins to make sexually suggestive comments to other group members. The therapist redirects the client to the work in progress but the member continues to make sexually suggestive statements. Which is the therapist's best initial response to this situation?

Answer Choices:

A. Explain to the client that such statements are not tolerated at work and call security to have the client removed from the group.
B. Explain to the client that such statements are not tolerated at work and the client must stop or leave the group.
C. End the group before the situation escalates and reschedule the group to meet without the disruptive client.
D. Set the client up at a different work station so the client is not in contact with other group members and cannot disrupt the group's work.

Correct Answer: B.

Rationale:
This response reinforces the norms of a work environment and gives the individual the opportunity to practice making a decision about the most appropriate course of action. An important aspect of vocational rehabilitation for persons with traumatic brain injuries is the development of appropriate social interaction skills. Ending the group, removing the client from the group, or decreasing contact with others does not address the client's need to develop appropriate interaction skills for work. In addition, the role of the therapist in a vocational rehabilitation program is to act as a work supervisor, enforcing the realities of a work situation. Inappropriate sexual remarks are not tolerated in a work setting. If the client cannot comply with work norms in a vocational program, he/she may need to be referred to a pre-vocational program for basic social skills and work habit training. These basic skills are not the focus of vocational rehabilitation.

Type of Reasoning: Evaluative
One must weigh the possible courses of action and then make a value judgment about the best course to take. This requires evaluative reasoning skill, which often utilizes guiding principles of action in order to arrive at a correct conclusion. In this case, the therapist should explain that the client's statements are not tolerated and he/she must either stop or leave the group. Refer to group leadership guidelines and reinforcement of group norms if answered incorrectly.

A138 C3

A carpenter recovering from injuries incurred during a fall from a ladder has decreased strength in the triceps, bilaterally. The most recent manual muscle test indicated that the triceps muscle strength is 3. The occupational therapist provides the individual with a tabletop wood project to complete. To develop triceps muscle strength, how should the therapist position the tabletop when the person sands the project?

Answer Choices:
A. At a 45° incline angled so that the individual's hands are above the elbows when the elbows are flexed.
B. At the individual's waist height so that the individual's hands and elbows are on the same plane when the elbows flex.
C. At the individual's chest height so that the individual's hands and elbows are on the same plane when the elbows flex.
D. At a 45° incline angled so that the individual's hands are below the elbows when the elbows are flexed.

Correct Answer: A.

Rationale:
This position requires the triceps to perform movement against gravity, which is possible at a muscle strength of 3 (fair). The sanding activity will provide slight resistance, which is the next level of muscle strength (3+, fair plus). Sanding wood placed on a table at waist or chest height, or inclined so that the hand is below the elbow when it is flexed, uses gravity-eliminated or gravity-assisted positions. These positions are too low of an activity for a person with fair muscle strength who can perform complete range of motion against gravity and they will not increase strength.

Type of Reasoning: Inductive
One must utilize clinical knowledge and judgment to determine the exercise approach that provides gravity-resisted movement. This requires inductive reasoning skill. In this case, the tabletop should be at a 45° inclined angle so the hands are above the elbows when the elbows are flexed. If answered incorrectly, review activity analysis principles and strengthening guidelines. The integration of this knowledge is needed to determine the correct answer.

A139 C1

An occupational therapist provides home-based early intervention evaluations. A referral for an 18-month-old child notes that the child is able to finger feed effectively but is not able to use a spoon or suck from a straw. The occupational therapist puts together supplies to bring to the child's home and plans activities to use during the developmental evaluation. Which developmental age is most important for the therapist to consider when selecting objects and activities to bring to the evaluation session?

Answer Choices:
A. 6–9 months.
B. 9–12 months.
C. 12–18 months.
D. 18–20 months.

Correct Answer: B.

Rationale:
The referral notes abilities that are typical of the age of 9–12 months. Therefore, the therapist would begin the assessment by using activities that are at the child's developmental age as reflected in the referral. If the child's performance in certain parameters is more or less advanced than this developmental age, the therapist can adjust the evaluation accordingly. However, initially the therapist would begin evaluation at the developmental age consistent with the referral. Since the child cannot use a spoon or a straw, activities that are typical of the developmental ages of 12–18 months and 18–20 months may be too difficult for the child. Spoon use typically develops at 12–18 months. Straw use typically develops at about 18 months. Since the child's finger feeding is noted to be effective, activities that are typical at 6–9 months would be too low developmentally for the child.

Type of Reasoning: Inductive
Clinical knowledge and judgment are the most important skills needed for answering this question, which requires inductive reasoning skill. Knowledge of the child's developmental age and most important activities to bring to the evaluation is essential to choose the best solution. In this case, the therapist should bring objects and activities for the developmental age of 9–12 months. If answered incorrectly, review developmental milestones for feeding in infants.

A140 C4

An occupational therapist is instructing a patient who had a left CVA on how to lock the brakes on a wheelchair. The patient is right-handed and the right upper extremity has partial paralysis. Based on motor learning theory, which is the best intervention approach for the therapist to use when instructing the person to lock the right brake?

Answer Choices:
A. Practice with the left hand first and then with the right.
B. Show the person how to use an extension brake.
C. Practice the locking motions with both hands simultaneously.
D. Have the patient use the left hand to assist the right hand.

Correct Answer: A.

Rationale:
Approaches based on motor learning theory acknowledge the importance of practice and repetition. When the patient practices with the left hand first and then the right, transfer of learning is promoted. Adapting the wheelchair to have an extension brake and then showing the person how to use the brake is a method used in a compensatory model of intervention. Using the left hand to assist the right hand is also a compensatory approach. These actions negate the person's ability to practice and acquire the skill, a core component of motor learning theory. Practicing with both hands simultaneously is more challenging than practicing with one hand at a time.

Type of Reasoning: Analytical

In this scenario, the test taker must identify the therapeutic approach to teaching an individual how to lock the wheelchair that follows the principles of motor learning theory. This requires analysis of the different approaches in order to determine the one approach that meets motor learning theory guidelines. For this situation, practicing with the left hand first, followed by the right hand is most aligned with this theory. Review motor learning theory guidelines if answered incorrectly.

A141 C2

An occupational therapist develops a protocol for a topical group to be implemented on an acute inpatient unit for individuals recovering from substance abuse. Which intervention focus is best for the occupational therapist to identify for this topical group?

Answer Choices:

A. The improvement of self-esteem.
B. The development of coping skills.
C. The identification of leisure pursuits.
D. The practice of assertive behaviors.

Correct Answer: C.

Rationale:

A topical group is a verbal discussion group focused on a specific activity engaged in outside of the group. Identifying leisure activities that can be pursued in a substance-free environment is a relevant focus for individuals on an inpatient unit who need to plan concretely for discharge. Recovery from substance abuse is long-term. Having non-substance-related leisure activity ideas to pursue upon discharge can aid in this recovery process. Improving self-esteem, developing coping skills, and practicing assertive behaviors are very broad and not related to a specific activity. Topical groups are activity focused.

Type of Reasoning: Inductive

One must utilize clinical knowledge and judgment to determine the most appropriate intervention goal for this topical group. In this case, a goal of identifying leisure pursuits is most appropriate as it is activity focused. If answered incorrectly, review the characteristics of topical groups and the goals of inpatient substance abuse intervention. Integration of this information is required to correctly answer this question.

A142 C3

An adult incurred severe lacerations to the extrinsic flexor tendons in Zone V of the hand. The tendons were surgically repaired and have healed. The surgeon's most recent orders have upgraded the patient to active ROM without restrictions. The occupational therapist is preparing for discharge and performs a final evaluation, which reveals limitations inactive finger flexion 10–20° of full active ROM in the MCP, PIP and DIP joints of all fingers. The therapist collaborates with the patient to prepare a home program. Which intervention is most important for the therapist to include in this program?

Answer Choices:

A. Use of a resting splint.
B. Tendon gliding exercises.
C. Weight-bearing activities.
D. Home management tasks.

Correct Answer: B.

Rationale:
Tendon gliding exercises help to prevent adhesions of the tendons in the healing process. Initially after tendon repair, a resting splint would be used for 23 hours and removed only for bathing and gentle active ROM. At the point of discharge from therapy, the patient should be pursuing more active movement. A volar splint for day use that allows active finger and thumb use may be prescribed based on the client's needs. Weight-bearing activities help to strengthen the upper extremity, but lacks focus on the location of injury—the flexor tendons of the hand. The focus after tendon trauma or surgery is prevention of adhesions with tendon gliding exercises and avoidance of heavy work to prevent tearing or re-injury. Home management tasks do not specifically address ROM to the flexor tendons to prevent tendon adhesions and losses in ROM.

Type of Reasoning: Analytical
One must analyze the evaluation findings and match this to the most appropriate home exercise program, which requires analytical reasoning skill. In this case, the findings indicate that the patient would benefit most from a home program that incorporates tendon gliding exercises to prevent adhesions of the tendons. If answered incorrectly, review exercise guidelines for hand tendons post laceration.

A143 C8

A child with moderate Klumpke's paralysis on the right side wants to cut meat. The child holds the fork with the right hand and the knife in the left hand, and practices with therapy putty. To begin cutting, which is the best way to configure the therapy putty?

Answer Choices:
A. Flattened and placed directly on the table.
B. Rolled and placed on a plate on the table.
C. Flattened on a plate that rests on a non-skid mat.
D. Flattened and placed on a plate on the table.

Correct Answer: A.

Rationale:
Klumpke's palsy is a brachial plexus injury affecting C8 and T1. Placing the therapy putty on the table is the first step in learning to cut meat. Here the putty is stabilized and the child practices and refines technique. The second gradation in the activity is to put the putty on a plate on a non-skid surface. The third gradation is to put the flattened putty on a plate without the non-skid surface. The fourth gradation is to make the putty thicker and harder to cut by rolling it up. Additional gradations can include using harder grades of putty. Having the child work on cutting different textured real foods is also an appropriate intervention approach.

Type of Reasoning: Inductive
This question requires one to determine the best approach for learning cutting skills using a knife. This requires inductive reasoning skill, where clinical judgment is paramount in arriving at a correct conclusion. In this situation, placing the therapy putty flattened on a table is the best way to learn how to cut meat.

A144 **C7**

During an occupational therapy intervention session, a client with a left CVA demonstrates extinction to the right and a tendency to ignore items on the right side. When documenting this behavior what should the therapist report?

Answer Choices:
A. Agnosia.
B. Unilateral inattention.
C. Poor right/left discrimination.
D. Poor visual scanning.

Correct Answer: B.

Rationale:
Unilateral inattention is when the individual neglects the side of the body contralateral to the CVA site and the environment on that side. The other options describe cognitive-perceptual deficits with different manifestations. Agnosia can be the inability to identify body parts. Right/left discrimination is the differentiation of one side of the body from the other. Visual scanning is the engagement and disengagement of visual attention as the eye moves its focus from one object to another.

Type of Reasoning: Analytical
This question provides symptoms and the test taker must determine the likely cause for them. This is an analytical reasoning skill, as questions of this nature often ask one to analyze a group of symptoms in order to determine a diagnosis. In this situation the symptoms indicate unilateral inattention, which should be reviewed if answered incorrectly.

A145 **C3**

An individual with post-polio syndrome receives an occupational therapy re-evaluation of functional status. How should the therapist initiate sensory testing with this client?

Answer Choices:
A. Demonstrate the test with the individual's vision occluded.
B. Proceed proximal to distal.
C. Demonstrate the test with the client's vision not occluded.
D. Proceed distal to proximal.

Correct Answer: C.

Rationale:
Sensory testing must begin with a demonstration of the test with the client being able to visually observe the demonstration. If the client's vision is impaired, the therapist must verbally explain each step of the demonstration to ensure that the individual understands the testing process. After this demonstration is complete, the testing proceeds with vision occluded. Sensory testing for individuals with spinal cord injuries proceeds from proximal to distal. Sensory testing for individuals with peripheral nerve injuries proceed from distal to proximal.

Type of Reasoning: Deductive
One must recall the testing guidelines for sensory testing in order to arrive at a correct conclusion. This requires deductive reasoning skill, where factual knowledge is essential to choosing the correct solution. In this case, all sensory testing must begin with demonstration of the test that the patient can visualize. Review guidelines for administration of sensory testing if answered incorrectly.

A146 C4

An occupational therapist is working with a preschool student who was born with congenital Cytomegalovirus (CMV) infection. As a result, the child has difficulty seeing. The child enjoys playing with classmates but has difficulty when the play activity is highly dependent on vision. Which of the following actions is best for the therapist to recommend for improving the child's play experiences with classmates?

Answer Choices:

A. Train a personal assistant to provide verbal cues during play activities.
B. Have the child read books in Braille aloud to the classmates.
C. Train a classmate to guide the child during play activities.
D. Incorporate three-dimensional objects into play activities.

Correct Answer: D.

Rationale:

The use of three-dimensional objects during play can enable the child to use intact tactile skills. Strengthening the use of other senses (i.e., touch, hearing, smell, and taste) is an effective intervention to compensate for low vision. Strengthening the sense of touch cannot only enhance play with limited vision, but it can also improve the child's ability to learn. Children depend on touch for learning about the world including the qualities of temperature, texture, shape, softness, sharpness, elasticity, and resilience. Incorporating three dimensional objects into play activities can help a child with low vision participate through touch while not having to rely on others for information. Having 1:1 assistance from an aide or a classmate are not practical or effective options when the goal is to improve the child's play experiences with peers. Typically, pre-schoolers do not have someone help them play with each other. Reading books in Braille aloud does not have components of active play and would not provide developmentally appropriate pre-school learning opportunities.

Type of Reasoning: Inductive

This item requires the test taker to determine a best course of action for a child with CMV infection with visual impairment. This requires inductive reasoning skill, where clinical judgment is used to reach a conclusion. For this case, considering the child's deficit, the therapist should incorporate three-dimensional objects into play activities. If answered incorrectly, review principles of activity analysis and interventions for low vision. The integration of this knowledge is required to determine the therapeutic activity which would be most effective for a child with visual impairments.

A147 C1

Upon screening, an eight-month-old child demonstrates a positive downward parachute reflex. Which action should the occupational therapist take next in response to this observed behavior?

Answer Choices:

A. Document that the child exhibits normal reflex development.
B. Document that the child exhibits a developmental delay.
C. Evaluate the protective extension downward reflex.
D. Evaluate the standing tilting reflex.

Correct Answer: A.

Rationale:

A downward parachute reflex is normal from four months and persists throughout one's lifetime unless neurological damage occurs. It is also called the protective extension downward reflex. The onset of the standing tilting reflex is from 12–21 months so an evaluation of this reflex is premature.

Type of Reasoning: Evaluative
One must weigh the possible courses of action and then make a value judgment about the best course to take. This requires evaluative reasoning skill, which often utilizes guiding principles of action in order to arrive at a correct conclusion. For this case, because the child is displaying normal reflex development, the therapist should document this finding as normal. Review downward parachute reflex and age of integration if answered incorrectly.

A148 C3

The occupational therapist wishes to compare the results of an evaluation of lateral pinch to the norms. Which is the best positioning for the therapist to place the individual in when using the pinch meter?

Answer Choices:
A. Forearm in neutral and the pinch meter placed on the DIP joint.
B. Forearm in neutral and the pinch meter placed on the middle phalanx.
C. Forearm in pronation and the pinch meter placed on the DIP joint.
D. Forearm in pronation and the pinch meter placed on the middle phalanx.

Correct Answer: B.

Rationale:
Norms for lateral pinch have been established with the forearm in neutral and the pinch meter placed on the middle phalanx. The other described positions do not match the normed position.

Type of Reasoning: Deductive
This question requires recall of guidelines and principles, which is factual knowledge. Deductive reasoning skills are utilized whenever one must recall facts to solve clinical problems. In this situation, the therapist should place the forearm in neutral and the pinch meter on the middle phalanx. Review pinch strength testing procedures if answered incorrectly.

A149 C4

An elementary school-aged child is referred to occupational therapy by a pediatrician. The pediatrician has ruled out attention deficit disorder and notes that the child demonstrates poor school performance and unexplained clumsiness. The occupational therapist screens the child and determines that the child is a candidate for a sensory processing evaluation. Which skills are most likely to have been observed to be intact during the screening and needing no further evaluation?

Answer Choices:
A. Fine motor coordination.
B. Sequencing motor tasks.
C. Initiation of activities.
D. Ocular pursuits.

Correct Answer: A.

Rationale:
Poor fine motor coordination may occur along with a sensory processing problem, but it is not one of the criteria for sensory processing disorders. Impairments in the other skills listed are typical of sensory processing disorder. The presence of these presenting signs and symptoms would indicate that a child would benefit from assessment of sensory processing. Depending on the results, treatment based on sensory integrative principles may be indicated.

Type of Reasoning: Inferential
One must determine the likely deficits of a child with sensory processing disorder. This requires inferential reasoning, where one must draw conclusions based on the information provided. In this situation, fine motor coordination deficits are likely to be present with sensory integrative dysfunction. If answered incorrectly, review characteristics of sensory integrative deficits.

A150 C4

A seven-year-old with complete spina bifida at the T10 level attends outpatient OT weekly. The child's parent reports that the child is losing bladder control. Upon re-evaluating the child, the occupational therapist notes that the child shows a minimal decrease in strength of bilateral lower and upper extremities and an increase in the equinovarus position of the feet. The therapist contacts the physician to report that the child's change in status may indicate which of the following?

Answer Choices:
A. Shunt malformation.
B. A recent growth spurt.
C. Arnold-Chiari formation.
D. Tethered cord.

Correct Answer: D.

Rationale:
Tethered cord is noted by all of the symptoms listed. The spinal cord of the child with spina bifida is sometimes attached to the spinal column and becomes taut as the child grows. The child requires a surgical release of the tethered cord. Shunt malformation is marked by intermittent headaches, shortened attention span, increased paralysis, decreased upper extremity strength, noticeable decrease in school performance, and increased irritability. Young children often demonstrate increased head size, nausea, and vomiting. The tethered cord presents whether the child has an even rate of growth or goes through a recent growth spurt. Arnold-Chiari formation occurs in the process of development and involves the part of the lower portion of the brain slipping or being pushed through the foramen ovale.

Type of Reasoning: Analytical
One must recall the signs and symptoms of tethered cord. Questions that provide a group of symptoms and the test taker must determine the cause requires analytical reasoning skill. In this case the symptoms indicate tethered cord with spina bifida, which should be reviewed if answered incorrectly.

A151 C9

An occupational therapy assistant (OTA) recently attended a two-day splinting workshop. The OTA asks the supervising occupational therapist for a caseload that includes more clients that require splinting interventions. Which action is best for the occupational therapist to take in response to this request?

Answer Choices:
A. Decline the request because splinting is an advanced practice skill.
B. Ask the OTA to give a splinting in-service to demonstrate acquired knowledge.
C. Establish the OTA's service competency in splinting.
D. Distribute the department's caseload to meet the OTA's request.

Correct Answer: C.

Rationale:
The establishment of service competency is required before the OTA takes on a new task. This ensures that the OTA will achieve the same intervention outcome as the occupational therapist. If service competency is established, splinting is not considered an advanced skill. Providing an in-service can demonstrate knowledge but it does not provide adequate information about the OTA's intervention abilities. Service competency must be established prior to revising the OTA's caseload.

Type of Reasoning: Inductive
This question requires one to determine the best approach for responding to the OTA's request. This requires inductive reasoning skill, where clinical judgment is paramount in arriving at a correct conclusion. For this situation, the occupational therapist should first establish that the OTA is competent to perform the delivery of splinting services. Review service competency and supervisory guidelines if answered incorrectly.

A152 C8

An occupational therapist works with the new foster parent of a two-year-old child diagnosed with major developmental delays and severe hypotonia. The therapist advises the foster parent to position the head in midline during feeding. Which additional positioning recommendations for feeding are best for this child?

Answer Choices:
A. Sitting with hips and knees at 90° flexion, neck in neutral.
B. Sitting with hips and knees at 90° flexion, neck in extension.
C. Semi-reclined with neck in neutral.
D. Semi-reclined with neck in extension.

Correct Answer: C.

Rationale:
This semi-reclined position can be easily maintained with the use of a commercially available child seat and it allows for correct postural alignment during the feeding activity. The support of positioning equipment is needed due to the child's severe hypotonia which prevents the child from independently maintaining a sitting position. Although it is possible to design equipment to support a seated position, the child's severe hypotonia would require equipment that is over-restrictive (e.g., a chest restraint). Feeding in a semi-reclined position is the least restrictive and most comfortable option for the child. It is not safe to feed anyone with neck in extension for this can result in choking.

Type of Reasoning: Inductive
One must utilize clinical knowledge and judgment to determine the best position for feeding the child, given knowledge of the diagnosis. In this case, positioning the child semi-reclined with the neck in neutral is the best position for feeding. If answered incorrectly, review positioning guidelines for children with hypotonia and for feeding. Integration of this knowledge is required to answer this question correctly.

A153 C7

During an intervention session focused on developing home management skills, a client made a grocery list. The client grouped needed items together to make shopping easier and listed eggs separately from all of the other items. When explaining how the list was composed, the client stated, "Eggs break, they should be on top." Which of the following is the most accurate for the occupational therapist to report that the client's approach to this task represents?

Answer Choices:
A. Diminished insight.
B. Concreteness.
C. Anosognosia.
D. Poor sequencing.

Correct Answer: B.

Rationale:
The statement reflects concrete thinking which is concerned with the actual properties of things and the realities of situations, rather than abstract properties or situational potentialities. In this situation, it is a functional strength. Insight is an awareness and understanding of oneself and behavior. Anosognosia is unawareness or denial of deficits. Sequencing is the ability to determine the proper ordering of steps in a task.

Type of Reasoning: Analytical
This question provides a description of a behavior and the test taker must determine the definition of the behavior displayed. This requires analytical reasoning skill where one must analyze the behavior in order to correctly determine the appropriate behavioral characteristic. In this situation, the behavior indicates concrete thinking. Review concrete thinking behaviors if answered incorrectly.

A154 C8

A client with a traumatic below-elbow amputation of the dominant right arm has participated in occupational therapy for prosthetic training. The therapist prepares a discharge plan that incorporates recommendations to facilitate independence in meal preparation and feeding. Which method is best for the therapist to recommend the client use to cut meat?

Answer Choices:
A. Hold a regular knife in the terminal device and hold a regular fork in the left hand.
B. Hold a knife with a built-up handle in the terminal device and hold the plate with the left hand.
C. Use a one-handed technique with a rocker knife in the left hand and hold the plate with the terminal device.
D. Hold a regular fork in the terminal device and hold a regular knife in the left hand.

Correct Answer: D.

Rationale:
Holding a regular fork in the terminal device and the knife in the hand is the best and safest option for using the prosthesis to cut meat. It is also the method most people use to cut food so it will facilitate the person's resumption of typical activities. OT training should include safe options for use of the prosthesis as well as one-handed techniques for use without the prosthesis. The use of the knife in the terminal device is not as safe and secure as holding the knife in the hand. Holding the plate with the hand or prosthesis is not consistent with typical performance of this activity and may be considered by some to not reflect the best manners for eating. Therapists should teach typical, socially acceptable methods for performing activities, including appropriate table manners, as much as possible. Therefore, learning to cut meat without holding the plate with either the hand or the prosthesis is best.

Type of Reasoning: Inductive
This question requires one to use clinical judgment in order to arrive at a reasonable conclusion about a best course of action during prosthetic training. This necessitates inductive reasoning skill. For this case, the therapist should recommend that the client hold a regular fork in the terminal device and hold a regular knife in the left hand. If answered incorrectly, review upper extremity prosthetic training guidelines, especially feeding skills.

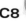

A155 C6

An occupational therapist working for a partial hospital program arranges the seats for a topical group. The room is small and there are eight people in the group. Two of the members have been diagnosed with schizophrenia, paranoid type. Which is the best arrangement of the room for this group composition?

Answer Choices:

A. Eight chairs placed around a table, with no assigned seats and the therapist at the front of the room.
B. Nine chairs placed in a circle, with assigned seats and the therapist between the two persons with schizophrenia.
C. Two semi-circles of four chairs facing the therapist, with the two patients with schizophrenia, in the front row.
D. Nine chairs placed in a circle, with no assigned seats for the patients or therapist.

Correct Answer: D.

Rationale:
In groups, members are typically more comfortable if they are allowed to sit where they wish. Providing individuals with this choice is respectful and supportive of their autonomy. This can facilitate the development of trust and group cohesion. These issues are important in a partial hospital program because patients are actively engaged in their recovery from an acute illness or an exacerbation of a persistent illness. Assigning seats and/or having the therapist in front of the group mimic a school-type setting. This can be perceived as infantilizing, authoritarian, and/or threatening. This type of atmosphere would be contra-indicated for individuals with schizophrenia, paranoid type.

Type of Reasoning: Inductive
One must utilize clinical knowledge and judgment to determine the best arrangement of the room that meets the needs of the group members. This requires inductive reasoning skill. In this case, nine chairs should be placed in a circle with no assigned seats. If answered incorrectly, review group facilitation guidelines.

A156 C7

A client exhibits residual difficulties in a variety of perceptual skills. Which procedure should the therapist include in the evaluation of the client's proprioception?

Answer Choices:

A. The therapist positions one extremity and asks the patient to duplicate the position with the contralateral extremity.
B. The therapist moves one extremity and asks the patient to duplicate the movement with the contralateral extremity.
C. The therapist demonstrates the desired position and asks the person to replicate the position in mirror fashion.
D. The therapist shows the client a picture of a position and asks the client to replicate the position with each extremity.

Correct Answer: A.

Rationale:
Proprioception or position sense is evaluated by having a person duplicate a position in which an extremity has been previously placed. Proprioception is not evaluated by replicating a demonstrated position or the picture of a position. The evaluation of movement is kinesthesia, not proprioception.

Type of Reasoning: Deductive

This question requires one to recall how to conduct an evaluation of proprioception. This is factual recall of knowledge, which is a deductive reasoning skill. The correct way to conduct this test is to have the therapist position the involved extremity and asks the patient to duplicate the position with the contralateral extremity. If answered incorrectly, review testing guidelines for proprioception.

A157 C2

An occupational therapist implements a transitional program for a high school student with a history of numerous school-related failures. Which is the most important principle of intervention for the therapist to use with this student?

Answer Choices:

A. Utilize activities that are typically at the developmental level of a middle school student to ensure successful completion.
B. Grade an activity of interest into achievable steps to facilitate successful completion.
C. Introduce several activities during each session and change them frequently to decrease boredom.
D. Terminate the activity during a treatment session when there is difficulty with activity completion to eliminate frustration.

Correct Answer: B.

Rationale:

Grading an activity to be presented in achievable steps is the most appropriate intervention principle for a person with a history of diminished success experiences. Employing activities appropriate for a younger child and terminating the activity will not address the teen's need for transitional services. Introducing several activities during one session can be overwhelming and decrease the ability to work in a focused manner on the attainment of transition goals.

Type of Reasoning: Inductive

Clinical knowledge and judgment are the most important skills needed for answering this question, which requires inductive reasoning skill. Knowledge of the person's limitations and most appropriate interventions to foster success is essential to choosing the correct solution. In this case, the most appropriate principle of intervention planning is to grade the activity of interest into achievable steps to ensure successful completion. Review intervention planning guidelines for teens in transitional programs if answered incorrectly.

A158 C9

An elementary school-aged child incurred burns, lacerations, and a femur fracture in a motor vehicle accident and was hospitalized for three weeks. During outpatient occupational therapy sessions, the parent expresses concern that the child has begun wetting the bed daily. Which professional is most relevant for the occupational therapist to advise the parent to contact?

Answer Choices:

A. A rehabilitation nurse to develop a bladder control program.
B. A child life therapist for intervention for developmental delays.
C. A psychiatric occupational therapist for behavior management strategies.
D. A clinical social worker to explore potential regression issues.

Correct Answer: D.

Rationale:
The child has no reported developmental delay and the injuries he/she incurred would not have likely affected the renal-genitourinary system. If there had been internal organ complications as a result of the accident, these would have been treated in the hospital prior to discharge. Therefore, the development of bedwetting is likely a symptom of regression. Regression is a common reaction to trauma. A social worker can provide supportive counseling for the regressive behaviors. Behavior management is typically indicated for acting-out and aggressive behaviors and there is nothing in the provided scenario to indicate that the child's bedwetting is intentional.

Type of Reasoning: Inductive
This question requires one to recall the practice parameters of each of the professionals listed and reason the exact nature of the problem, which is an inductive reasoning skill. For this situation, a clinical social worker would best address the problem, as the issue is regression. Regression issues are best handled by a clinical social worker.

Multiple Choice Scenario Item A.III.

Questions A159 to A163 are based on the following information.

A single parent of two children, a four-year-old and a six-year-old, is referred to occupational therapy services in a rehabilitation center. The client had a brain tumor removed one month ago. The referral states that the client has residual cognitive-perceptual deficits. Screening indicates that the client's sensori-motor abilities are within functional limits.

A159 C7

The occupational therapist administers a standardized cognitive-perceptual assessment to the client. The client demonstrates difficulty performing the first two tasks of the evaluation. Which is the most appropriate action for the therapist to take?

Answer Choices:
A. Continue the evaluation and provide verbal cues during task performance.
B. Continue the evaluation and model each evaluation task.
C. Continue the evaluation according to the established administration protocol. A
D. Discontinue the evaluation to avoid frustrating the client.

Correct Answer: C.

Rationale:
A standardized assessment must be administered according to its established protocol to be reliable. Providing additional verbal cues or modeling would compromise the reliability of the assessment tool. Discontinuing the evaluation would not enable the therapist to obtain needed information about the person's cognitive-perceptual status. Since most cognitive-perceptual assessments measure several skills, one cannot assume that poor performance on the first two tasks will mean poor performance on the other tasks.

Type of Reasoning: Deductive
This question requires recall of guidelines, which is factual knowledge. Deductive reasoning skills are utilized whenever one must rely on facts to solve problems. In this situation, because the therapist is administering a standardized assessment, the established protocol must be followed. Review guidelines for administering standardized assessments if answered incorrectly.

A160 C7

During the evaluation, the occupational therapist observes that the client has difficulty dealing with increasing amounts of stimuli. This is observed in all modalities. Based on this observation, which cognitive perceptual dysfunction does the therapist record as present when reporting the client's evaluation results?

Answer Choices:

A. Inability to abstract.
B. Poor organizational skills.
C. Poor semantic memory.
D. Generalized attention deficit.

Correct Answer: D.

Rationale:

Attention requires the ability to focus on a specific stimulus without being distracted by external or internal stimuli. The other options describe deficits with different manifestations. The ability to abstract requires the person to see relationships between concepts, ideas, and events. Organization is the ability to structure thoughts and actions. Semantic memory is the general knowledge shared by groups of people, such as social norms.

Type of Reasoning: Analytical

This question provides a group of symptoms and the test taker must determine the cause. This requires analytical reasoning skill where one must analyze the symptoms in order to correctly determine a diagnosis. In this situation, the symptoms indicate generalized attention deficit. Review symptoms of generalized attention deficit disorder, and other cognitive-perceptual deficits, especially related to CVA if answered incorrectly.

A161 C7

The occupational therapist uses a neurofunctional approach to remediate the client's cognitive dysfunction. Which is most appropriate for the occupational therapist to include in the intervention program?

Answer Choices:

A. Functional activities in their real contexts.
B. Client education on strategies to remediate deficits.
C. Tabletop activities to practice remediation strategies.
D. Computer games to develop performance component skills.

Correct Answer: A.

Rationale:

A neurofunctional approach emphasizes functional activity performance in the actual environment. The other options reflect a transfer of training approach.

Type of Reasoning: Deductive

One must recall factual knowledge of the neurofunctional approach to rehabilitation in order to choose the correct solution. This is a deductive reasoning skill. A typical neurofunctional approach emphasizes functional activity performance in a real-life context. If answered incorrectly, review guidelines for providing treatment under a neurofunctional approach.

A162 C7

During an intervention session using a transfer of training approach, the occupational therapist gives the client a list of items commonly found in a closet and asks the client to separate the items into grooming and dressing items. Which skill is the occupational therapist working on?

Answer Choices:
A. Categorization.
B. Sequencing.
C. Problem solving.
D. Memory.

Correct Answer: A.

Rationale:
Separating items into two groups requires placing them into a category. Sequencing involves the planning, organization and implementation of the steps of a task in an appropriate order. Problem solving requires the recognition and definition of a problem and the selection and implementation of a plan. Memory is the registration, integration, recall, and retrieval of information.

Type of Reasoning: Analytical
A descriptor of an activity is provided and the test taker must determine what these guidelines indicate, which is an analytical reasoning skill One should determine that the description of this sorting activity most closely represents categorization. If answered incorrectly, review cognitive retraining guidelines.

A163 C7

The occupational therapist re-evaluates the client prior to discharge from the rehabilitation center. The client exhibits residual cognitive deficits in problem solving. To develop requisite problem solving skills for independent functioning at home, which ability should the occupational therapist work on with the client during OT intervention?

Answer Choices:
A. Performing routine morning self-care.
B. Making a shopping list of grocery staples.
C. Washing the family's laundry.
D. Reading a bedtime story to the client's children.

Correct Answer: C.

Rationale:
Problem solving is the ability to recognize and define a problem, identify alternative plans for solving the problem, select a plan, organize steps in the plan, implement the plan, and evaluate the plan's outcome. Doing laundry can present a number of potential problems that must be solved (i.e., stain removal, appropriate care for different textured and/or colored fabrics). The other task choices are more structured and have less of a problem-solving component.

Type of Reasoning: Inferential

One must infer or draw conclusions about the likely intervention approach needed at home, given the information presented. This is an inferential reasoning skill, where knowledge of a therapeutic skill, such as problem solving in this situation, is essential in choosing a correct solution. In this case, the person will mostly likely require intervention for developing independence in laundry skills. If answered incorrectly, review problem solving skills after brain injury and instrumental ADL. The integration of this knowledge is required to answer to this question correctly.

A164 C1

An elderly person has lost significant functional vision over the last four years and complains of blurred vision and difficulty reading. The patient frequently mistakes images directly in front, especially in bright light. When walking across a room, the patient is able to locate items in the environment using peripheral vision when items are located on both sides. Based on these findings, which visual deficit should the occupational report the client is exhibiting?

Answer Choices:

A. Glaucoma.
B. Presbyopia
C. Hemianopsia.
D. Cataracts.

Correct Answer: D.

Rationale:

Cataracts are a clouding of the lens which results in a gradual loss of vision. Central vision is lost first, then peripheral. There are increased problems with glare and a general darkening of vision with loss of acuity and distortion. Glaucoma produces the reverse symptoms: loss of peripheral vision is first (tunnel vision), then central, progressing to total blindness. Presbyopia is a visual loss in middle and older ages that is characterized by an inability to focus properly and blurred images. Hemianopsia is field defect in both eyes that often occurs following CVA.

Type of Reasoning: Analytical

In this question, symptoms are presented and one must make a determination of the most likely diagnosis. These types of questions require analysis of the meaning of information presented, which is an analytical reasoning skill. For this situation, the symptoms are indicative of cataracts. Refer to information on visual deficits associated with aging if answered incorrectly.

A165 C9

The director of an occupational therapy driver rehabilitation program must determine if the program is meeting its objectives. Which of the following is most important for the director to measure during the evaluation of the program outcomes?

Answer Choices:

A. Participants' satisfaction with program services.
B. Family members' satisfaction with program services.
C. The effect of program participation on participants' automobile insurance premiums.
D. The percentage of participants who successfully return to driving.

Correct Answer: D.

Rationale:
The desired outcome of a driver rehabilitation program is to enable participants to be able to safely and independently drive. Therefore, the most relevant outcome measure is the determination of the percentage of participants who successfully return to driving after participation in the program. While consumer satisfaction is important it does not provide a measure of program outcomes. A positive result of being a safe driver can be decreased automobile insurance rates. However, it would be impossible to determine if any reduction was a direct result of participation in the program since there are many factors that can affect insurance rates (e.g., credit scores, geographic location, number of drivers on a plan, type of coverage, etc.).

Type of Reasoning: Inferential
This question requires the test taker to determine the most important outcome to measure for a driver rehabilitation program. This requires one to infer or draw a reasonable conclusion for what would have the most benefit, which is an inferential reasoning skill. In this case, measuring the percentage of participants who successfully return to driving would be the most important measure. If answered incorrectly, review driver rehabilitation program guidelines and outcomes.

A166 C5

An individual with an incomplete C6 spinal cord injury has a secondary diagnosis of thromboangiitis obliterans. The occupational therapist conducts a pre-discharge home evaluation of the client's rented apartment. Which is the most important area for the therapist to assess?

Answer Choices:
A. The apartment's electrical capacity for an environmental control unit.
B. The apartment's electrical capacity for an emergency call system.
C. The apartment's water temperature.
D. The landlord's willingness to modify the bathroom.

Correct Answer: C.

Rationale:
Thromboangiitis obliterans, also known as Buerger's disease, results in diminished temperature sense, paresthesias, pain, and cold extremities. It is most common in young men who smoke. Poor or absent temperature sense can place a person at serious risk for scalding burns. If the apartment's water temperature is higher than 102°F, an anti-scalding faucet and/or valve must be installed. An individual with a C6 SCI is independent in many tasks and does not require an environmental control unit to access the environment. A special emergency call system is also not needed because this person can independently access a telephone to call 911 with minimal modifications (i.e., large push buttons, speaker phone). Structural bathroom modifications are not needed. A person with a C6 SCI can bathe with minimal assistance using a tub bench, a sliding board transfer, and a handheld shower. None of these modifications would require a landlord's permission.

Type of Reasoning: Inductive
One must utilize clinical knowledge and judgment to determine the most important area for assessment. In this case, the therapist should assess the apartment's water temperature to prevent scalding burns from hot water. If answered incorrectly, review home evaluation skills for patients with cervical spinal cord injuries, especially diminished sensation.

A167 C7

An occupational therapist receives a referral to evaluate an individual's executive functioning following a mild cerebral vascular accident. Which are the most relevant foci for this evaluation?

Answer Choices:

A. The person's attention and memory.
B. The person's job interests and efficacy.
C. The person's spatial relations and praxis.
D. The person's initiation and planning.

Correct Answer: D.

Rationale:
Executive functions are higher level cognitive abilities that are needed to perform unstructured multi-step activities and role tasks. The four main components of executive functioning are volition, planning, purposeful action, and effective performance. Attention and memory are considered primary cognitive capacities that are prerequisite to higher-level cognitive abilities. The other choices do not relate to cognitive functioning.

Type of Reasoning: Inferential
One must infer or draw conclusions about a likely course of action, given the information presented. This is an inferential reasoning skill, where knowledge of a therapeutic approach, such as executive functioning in this situation, is essential to choosing a correct solution. In this case, the therapist would most likely assess the person's initiation and planning. Review executive functions if answered incorrectly.

A168 C4

An occupational therapist is evaluating a child with developmental delay characterized by hypotonicity. According to the Rood approach, which is the first stability pattern that the therapist should facilitate during intervention?

Answer Choices:

A. Roll over.
B. Quadruped.
C. Neck co-contraction.
D. Prone on elbows.

Correct Answer: C.

Rationale:
According to Rood, motor development follows a sequence termed 'ontogenic motor patterns' that includes eight different patterns in sequence (i.e., supine withdrawal, rollover, prone extension, neck co-contraction, prone on elbows, quadruped, standing). In this model, neck co-contraction is the first stability pattern because it requires simultaneous activation or contraction of the neck flexors and extensors. Neck co-contraction is essential for head control. Roll over is an early mobility pattern and occurs when the arm and leg on the same side of the body flex as the trunk rotates. It is utilized to elicit lateral trunk responses. The positions of prone on elbows and quadruped are stability patterns that develop after neck co-contraction. The prone on elbows position provides trunk and proximal limb stability. The quadruped position develops limb and trunk co-contraction.

Type of Reasoning: Deductive
This question requires recall of guidelines and principles, which is factual knowledge. Deductive reasoning skills are utilized whenever one must recall facts to solve clinical problems. In this situation, the therapist should facilitate neck co-contraction in this child. Review Rood's sequence of motor development in children if answered incorrectly.

A169 C3

A person recovering from skin grafting due to full thickness burns is prescribed splints to immobilize the grafted areas in anti-deformity positions. Which splint wearing schedule is best to include in the splinting protocol for the first 72 hours post-surgery?

Answer Choices:
A. One hour on, with 10 minutes off.
B. Four hours on, with 20 minutes off.
C. Eight hours on, with 30 minutes off.
D. On at all times, except for dressing changes.

Correct Answer: D.

Rationale:
The usual post-operative splinting schedule for persons who have undergone skin grafting is to keep the splint on at all times, except during dressing changes. The duration of this period of immobilization can vary according to surgeon's recommendations and the burn center's protocol. The average period of immobilization is reported as five to ten days.

Type of Reasoning: Deductive
One must recall the guidelines for splinting after skin grafting with burns in order to arrive at a correct conclusion. This requires deductive reasoning skill, where factual knowledge is essential to choosing the correct solution. In this situation, the splint should be worn at all times, except for dressing changes. Review splinting after burns, especially skin grafting if answered incorrectly.

A170 C4

A child with tactile defensiveness is receiving intervention from an occupational therapist using a sensory integrative approach. Which method is most effective for the therapist to use when introducing tactile stimuli to the child?

Answer Choices:
A. Provide deep touch and firm pressure where the child can see the stimuli.
B. Apply the stimuli in the direction opposite of hair growth with vision occluded.
C. Apply light touch across the face and abdomen with vision occluded.
D. Provide light brushing across the palmar surfaces of the extremities with the child watching.

Correct Answer: A.

Rationale:
Deep touch and firm pressure help to decrease tactile defensiveness. To decrease defensiveness, the child needs to see the stimuli. The self application of stimuli can also increase toleration. Light touch, brushing across the face and abdomen, and application of stimuli in the direction opposite of hair growth are all averse to a person with tactile defensiveness. Stimuli should be applied in the direction of hair growth for this is less averse.

Type of Reasoning: Inductive
This question requires one to determine the most appropriate method for introducing tactile stimuli. This requires inductive reasoning skill, where clinical judgment is paramount in arriving at a correct conclusion. For this situation, the therapist should provide deep touch and firm pressure where the child can see the stimuli. If answered incorrectly, review tactile approaches for sensory integration intervention.

Exam B

Examination B

Simulation Test Item B.I.

Opening Scene:

An unemployed medical professional is referred to a partial hospitalization program after a four day hospitalization. This adult client has recently experienced a severe episode of major depression with panic disorder. The client was alcohol dependent until seven years ago but has been in full remission for six years. The client lives with an employed spouse and an unemployed adult child. The family members complain that the client leaves clutter all over the house and does not do much to help the family. The physician anticipates that the client, now moderately depressed, will become increasingly less symptomatic as antidepressant medication is titrated to adequate dose over the next eight weeks. The plan is to help the client participate in meaningful desired family and community roles.

Section A

The occupational therapist meets with the client and family members to complete the partial hospitalization evaluation process. The client's appearance is disheveled. The client expresses anger that family members think mental illness is a character flaw and its resulting limitations are personal choices. Based on the available information, which evaluation approaches are best for the occupational therapist to use? Choose all approaches that can contribute to effective intervention planning.

1. C2 With the client's consent, interview the client's family to learn about their understanding of the impact of depression on the client's occupational performance.

Feedback: The client's spouse reports frustration with client's inability to engage in activities. The client's child is critical of the client's "laziness."

Outcome and Rationale: Obtaining the perspectives of family members can provide helpful insights to family communication patterns and family role expectations. This information combined with observation of the family's dynamics can contribute to an understanding about how the family views the impact of a biological brain disorder on performance. This knowledge can help the client and therapist set realistic goals that are meaningful to the client's family role expectations. It is important to remember that the discussion of a client's illness with family members can only be done with the client's consent. Since the client's permission was obtained, this is an acceptable action in this case. In addition, this action provided the therapist and client with helpful information. As a result, this is a positive action and its selection would result in the awarding of points.

2. C8 Administer the Occupational Performance History Interview (OPHI) to compare past and present function.

Feedback: The client's responses are vague and guarded when discussing the present. The client declines to discuss the past.

Outcome and Rationale: This assessment asks the client to describe previous functioning and compare it to the present. While this can be a relevant evaluation of a person who is stabilized and engaged in a long-term treatment program, it is not the best evaluation for someone who has just been discharged from an acute psychiatric hospital. The client's past level of functioning was likely much better than his/her current abilities to engage in occupations. At the present time, the client is unemployed as a medical professional. It is likely that the client cannot return to work in the near future due to presenting symptoms and residual deficits. Asking a person who is in a vulnerable state to talk about past performance capabilities that are currently not intact will likely increase a sense of hopelessness and helplessness. This is not a good outcome for a person who has been recently hospitalized for severe depression and who currently requires partial hospitalization services due to moderate depression. The selection of this option reflects a lack of understanding of the recovery process. As a result, it is negative and its selection would result in the deduction of points.

3. C6 Assess the client's self-esteem.

Feedback: The client reports feeling worthless, helpless and ashamed to be a family burden.

Outcome and Rationale: It is not necessary to ask a person with moderate depression who is recovering from a severe episode of depression about his/her self-esteem. Poor self-esteem is a major symptom of this health condition. This line of inquiry reminds the client how bad he/she feels, which can cause harm to a person who has just been hospitalized. The selection of this option reflects a lack of understanding of depression and its symptoms. As a result, it is negative and its selection would result in the deduction of points.

4. C6 Ask the client to describe key symptoms that influence the ability to rest, work and complete home management tasks.

Feedback: The client explains that fatigue and irritability increase and ability to attend and concentrate decrease when depressive symptoms are present.

Outcome and Rationale: A person with a chronic biologic brain disorder (such as depression) needs to learn to accommodate and adapt to fluctuating symptoms. It is important to help this client determine the early warning signs for depressive episodes so that he/she can develop strategies to effectively manage symptoms. This increased knowledge can also be used to help the client identify which activities to engage in and those to avoid. Activity gradations and modifications can then be developed to maximize occupational performance during symptomatic time periods. The selection of this option provided the therapist and client with helpful information. As a result, this is a positive action and its selection would result in the awarding of points.

5. C7 Evaluate the client's cognitive skills and the impact of activity demands on performance by having the client purchase five items from a list in the partial hospital consumer-run store.

Feedback: The therapist observes that the client has difficulty with initiation, attention and organization. Activity performance worsens with auditory stimuli and social demands.

Outcome and Rationale: Depression can affect cognitive skills and the ability to perform home management tasks, such as shopping. Environmental factors, activity demands and the structure of an activity can make performance easier or more difficult. Evaluating cognitive skills and the impact of activity demands on performance is a 'real-world' environment greatly enhances the contextual validity of the evaluation. Acquiring knowledge about the client's abilities and limitations can help the therapist and client develop an intervention plan to build on capabilities, develop needed skills, design adaptive strategies and/or modify the environment to maximize occupational performance. As a result, this is a positive action and its selection would result in the awarding of points.

6. C7 Provide the client with a notebook to record a daily schedule.

Feedback: The client records daily activities and events.

Outcome and Rationale: Recording one's daily schedule can be a helpful organizational tool for a person with cognitive deficits. However, it is not an evaluation approach that will provide information to effectively assist with intervention planning. A daily journal that is reviewed after a week or two and is expanded to include questions that are typically included in an activities configuration evaluation (e.g., Do you do this activity because you want to? Do you do this activity because you want to need to? Do others require you to do this activity), could provide helpful information for intervention planning. However, merely listing what happened in a day does not facilitate reflection on interests, goals, activity demands or performance. While this option does not contribute to intervention planning, it does not harm the client. Therefore, this action is considered neutral. No points would be awarded or deducted for its selection.

Section B

The therapist determines that the client can link fatigue, irritability and the ability to concentrate to mood states. The client has difficulty with initiation, attention and organization. Activity performance worsens with auditory stimuli and social demands. Family stress contributes to the client's anxiety, helplessness, low self-esteem and shame. As medication is adjusted, the client's symptoms are likely to fluctuate until a baseline of optimal function is reached. Which intervention approaches are most effective at this time to help the client manage symptoms and participate in meaningful family and community roles? Choose all that apply.

1. C6 Provide training in effective strategies the client can use to help counter negative thinking.

Feedback: The client develops the ability to react to negative thinking in an adaptive manner.

Outcome and Rationale: Since negative thinking cannot be ignored; it is a symptom that has to be managed. Learning to manage symptoms is an important aspect of recovery from mental illness. There are numerous techniques based on the principles of cognitive-behavioral therapy (CBT) that the client can learn to use to effective counter his/her negative thoughts. The provision of training in these strategies is a positive action and its selection would result in the awarding of points.

2. C6 Collaborate with the client to determine resources to help family members learn about depression and its biological foundation.

Feedback: The client identifies internet sites for mental health support groups and movies about people living with depression to share with family members.

Outcome and Rationale: This approach to family education fosters self-advocacy, puts the client in a leadership role within the family, and strengthens the client's support system. As the client's family members learn more about the biological foundations of depression, it is likely that they will be more understanding of the client's illness. As they explore the internet sites for mental health support groups (e.g., National Alliance for Mentally Ill [NAMI]), it is likely that they will become more supportive of the client's recovery. These outcomes can help decrease the client's anxiety, helplessness and shame and increase the client's self-esteem. These are positive outcomes; therefore, the selection of this action would result in the awarding of points.

3. C6 Refer the client to a local volunteer agency so the client can find ways to help others to build self-esteem.

Feedback: The client is overwhelmed by this referral and feels demoralized about not being able to do what used to be easy.

Outcome and Rationale: Though volunteering in an area of interest can be beneficial to a person recovering from mental illness, this recommendation is premature in this case. Volunteering would be too difficult for this client at this time. The client has not yet been stabilized on medications and presents active depressive symptoms. The client reports fatigue, irritability, anxiety, helplessness and low self-esteem. The client has difficulty with initiation, attention and organization. Activity performance worsens with auditory stimuli and social demands. Volunteering typically requires sufficient self-management, cognitive and social skills to respond effectively to multiple activity demands. The client has not yet engaged in treatment to develop these requisite skills. The selection of this option reflects a lack of understanding of depression and the recovery process. As a result, it is negative and its selection would result in the deduction of points.

4. C6 Collaborate with the client to set up a weekly schedule that includes a balance in activity demands to enable desired role performance.

Feedback: The client reports feeling less overwhelmed with a schedule that respects symptoms and also builds capabilities for engaging in desired activities.

Outcome and Rationale: A weekly schedule that balances activity demands can effectively support successful role performance. Collaborating with the client to develop this schedule would allow the therapist to teach the client how to "chunk" related activities together to increase efficiency. The therapist can also teach the client how to break down an activity into reasonable sub-tasks to more effectively manage activity demands. Learning these skills can facilitate successful engagement in desired role activities. The process of setting up a weekly schedule for activity performance can also help strengthen the client's capacity to set realistic expectations. This is important for people with depression who often continue to compare a present loss of function to what they were able to do when not depressed. Learning to set a new baseline for performance can reduce the stressors that contribute to feelings of worthlessness. All of the potential outcomes of this selected action are positive; therefore, its selection would result in the awarding of points.

5. C6 Encourage the client to attend a support group to maintain sobriety.

O

Feedback: The client regularly attends support group meetings.

Outcome and Rationale: Obtaining support to maintain sobriety is an important part of this client's recovery. Support groups, such as Alcoholics Anonymous, can help the client sustain self-management of his/her co-morbid alcohol dependence and continued abstinence. However, encouraging the client to attend a peer support group is not an active occupational therapy intervention. While this does not move the person forward in the OT process, it is inherently supportive. Consequently, this action is neutral and its selection would have no point ramifications.

6. C8 Establish a routine with the client to include food shopping and paying the family's bills so that the client can resume an active home maintainer role.

X

Feedback: The client has trouble following this routine and does not shop for food or pay bills.

Outcome and Rationale: This intervention focus is more appropriate for a person with mild depression. When introduced to a person with moderate depression immediately after discharge from a hospitalization (which was precipitated by a severe episode of a major depression), it is can be anticipated that the client will have difficulty with the completion of these activities. Due to the complex activity demands of bill paying and shopping, it is likely that the client's symptoms will increase rather than decrease as a result of this action. The client has not yet been stabilized on medications and presents active depressive symptoms. The client has difficulty with initiation, attention and organization. These skills are essential for the successful completion of bill paying and food shopping. Bill paying and food shopping also requires the executive functions of planning, problem-solving and making decisions; all of these are compromised by depression. The client has not yet engaged in treatment to develop the requisite skills needed for the successful assumption of these home management activities. In addition, the client's activity performance is known to worsen with auditory stimuli and social demands. As a result, shopping for food in a supermarket would overwhelm this client at this point in his/her recovery process. The selection of this option reflects a lack of understanding of depression and the recovery process. As a result, it is negative would result in the deduction of points.

7. C6 Engage the client in a communication skills group to increase assertiveness skills.

✓

Feedback: The client develops assertive communication skills and talks with family members about the effect of their criticism.

Outcome and Rationale: The ability to communicate in an assertive manner is helpful to this client since it was reported that the client is angry at family members' lack of understanding about his/her mental illness. Developing assertive communication skills can help the client explain his/her mood symptoms and their effect on occupational performance to family members. Learning to interact with others in an assertive manner is a skill that will benefit the client at this level of depression in all occupational roles. These are positive outcomes; therefore the selection of this action would result in the awarding of points.

Section C

The client actively participates in an occupational therapy intervention program to facilitate effective self-management of major depression and develop the requisite skills for successful occupational role performance. The client can now identify the effect of depression on functioning and is improving at evaluating the physical, social, emotional and cognitive demands of desired activities. However, the client has difficulty structuring activities to meet desired goals and often sets unrealistic expectations. The client's inability to successfully complete desired tasks exacerbates the client's symptoms. The therapist seeks evidence for interventions to help the client successfully grade and/or modify activity engagement according to activity demands. Which evidence is relevant for the therapist to use as a basis for modification of the client's intervention plan? Choose all that apply.

1. C9 A single subject case study describing the course of occupational intervention for a client with depression.

Feedback: The subject of the study provides personal insights but shares only a few of the client's life circumstances and goals.

Outcome and Rationale: Case studies are descriptive and/or explanatory. They do not provide evidence to support the efficacy of an intervention. Case studies have a low level of evidence since there are no controls for factors that may affect the results. While the findings of a single case study can be helpful in understanding the lived experience of a person, they cannot be generalized to the experiences of others. As a result, this action will provide limited information to use as a basis for the modification of the client's intervention plan. However, the therapist may gain some insights about occupational therapy intervention from the perspective of a person with depression that can help with the therapeutic relationship. Consequently, this action is neutral and no points would be awarded or deducted for its selection.

2. C9 A comparative study of the reported self-esteem of persons with depression versus those with schizophrenia.

Feedback: Both groups report low self-esteem. The group with depression does not anticipate anything will improve.

Outcome and Rationale: Gaining knowledge about the reported similarities and differences in self-esteem among persons with two different psychiatric diagnoses will not provide information to help modify the intervention plan. This intervention plan's stated focus is to help the client learn how to successfully grade and/or modify activities according to activity demands. Acquiring information about self-esteem will not inform this intervention modification in any meaningful way. The selection of this option reflects a lack of understanding of this section's focus and relevant research. As a result this action is negative and points would be deducted for its selection.

3. C9 A longitudinal study of people with depression who are able to work.

Feedback: Specific factors that contribute to the ability to work are identified.

Outcome and Rationale: The focus of this section is the identification of evidence to modify the intervention plan to help the client successfully grade and/or modify activity engagement according to activity demands. The client will need to actively engage in this modified intervention plan prior to considering the resumption of a worker role. When the client develops the desired skills identified as the focus of this current intervention plan modification, the therapist can then modify the intervention program to include work-related goals. Since this client is currently not at the level of returning to work, the information provided by this study is irrelevant to the modification of the client's intervention plan at this time. The selection of this action reflects a poor understanding of the client's current status and the scenario's stated focus. As a result it is negative and points would be deducted for its selection.

4. C9 A systemic review of studies which examined the efficacy of intervention programs focused on the development of skills for activity engagement and role participation.

Feedback: The therapist learns about effective interventions for the development of skills for activity engagement and role participation.

Outcome and Rationale: A systemic review is an exhaustive summary of the literature that is focused on a specific research question. A systemic review identifies, selects, critiques and synthesizes all high quality research evidence relevant to the proposed area of inquiry. Systematic reviews of high-quality randomized controlled trials (RCTs) are essential for evidence-based practice. RCT studies, which test a set of related research hypotheses, have high internal validity because the RCTs have controlled for non-intervention factors that may affect the results of each study. The therapist's use of a systemic review to guide modifications to an intervention plan is an excellent example of evidence-based practice. Therefore, the selection of this option reflects a good understanding of the levels of evidence and the focus of this section. As a result, this action is positive and its selection would result in the awarding of points.

5. C9 A randomized control trial (RCT) study which tested the hypothesis that people with depression who use a day planner will manage a routine better than people who do not use a planner.

Feedback: The therapist learns that participants who used day planners were significantly more successful in maintaining a routine.

Outcome and Rationale: Randomized control trial (RCT) studies provide the highest level of evidence. Because a RCT study has controlled for non-intervention factors, it has high internal validity. A RCT that is well-designed can provide strong evidence that research participants' outcomes were the result of having received or not received an intervention (in this case the use of a day planner). The selection of this option reflects a good understanding of the levels of evidence and the focus of this section. As a result, this action is positive and its selection would result in the awarding of points.

6. C9 Web-based blogs describing the outcomes of experimental approaches for persons with depression.

Feedback: Multiple and conflicting opinions about the effective treatment of depression are presented.

Outcome and Rationale: Web-based blogs are not reliable sources of information. Frequently, these are developed and maintained by persons who are promoting specific viewpoints which typically do not have established evidence. In addition, this option stated that the information to be obtained was about experimental approaches. It would be unethical for the therapist to plan intervention based on methods that are not supported by a sound scientific and/or theoretical base. This can cause harm. As a result, this action is negative and its selection would result in the deduction of points.

Simulation Test Item B.II.

Opening Scene:

After a blast-related injury, a military logistics coordinator begins an extensive inpatient rehabilitation program. The client has been diagnosed with polytrauma, including a traumatic brain injury (TBI), left below and right above knee amputations, and right wrist disarticulation. The client is left hand dominant. The client underwent surgical revisions of residual limbs two weeks ago and now wears residual limb shrinkers.

Section A

The client is brought to occupational therapy for an initial evaluation. Upon review of the client's chart, the therapist learns that the client's TBI has been assessed to be at Level VIII of the Rancho Level of Cognitive Functioning Scale. The client's pain in the residual limb revision areas is reported to be level 5 on a 1–10 numerical scale. Which of the following should the therapist initiate or perform at this point? Choose all approaches that apply.

1. C3 Determine the time frame for prosthetic molding and fitting.

X

Feedback: The therapist discusses the prosthetic process with the client.

Outcome and Rationale: This action is premature. The time frame for the fitting and molding of a prosthesis is based upon the medical team's assessment of the adequacy of the client's wound healing and the efficacy of the pre-prosthetic treatment program. Even in optimal circumstances, healing can take several weeks or months before prosthetic fitting and molding can begin. In blast-related injuries, this can take longer. The selection of this action reflects a lack of foundational knowledge about post-amputation care and pre-prosthetic evaluation and intervention priorities. Moreover, this action reflects a poor understanding of the respective role responsibilities of medical team members by overstepping the role responsibilities of the occupational therapist. The occupational therapist should not solely discuss the prosthetic process with a patient. As a result, the selection of this action would result in the deduction of points.

2. C8 Administer a vocational interest inventory.

Feedback: Results show that the client has a tendency to prefer work similar to the logistics coordination job.

Outcome and Rationale: While the assessment of a client's vocational interests can provide useful information to develop an occupational therapy intervention plan, the administration of this evaluation is premature in this situation. This client has just incurred poly-trauma and will be undergoing substantial rehabilitation for multiple amputations and TBI. The client's vocational interests may change when he/she has both progressed in skill development and established strengths and limitations post-rehabilitation. Consequently, it would be more appropriate to administer a vocational interest inventory during the pre-discharge planning stage of the client's rehabilitation. Although this action was premature, it did not cause harm. Consequently, points would neither be deducted nor awarded for its selection.

3. C8 Administer the Barthel Index.

Feedback: The client is independent in feeding, grooming and control of bowel and bladder. The client is dependent in bathing, toileting, dressing and transferring and reports difficulty in cutting meat.

Outcome and Rationale: The Barthel Index measures a person's independence in basic activities of daily living (BADL) before and after intervention and the level of personal care needed by the individual. The administration of this measure includes direct observation of task performance, interview of an individual and/or caregivers and/or review of medical records. The administration of this evaluation provides the therapist with relevant information about the client's baseline BADL. This information can be used to develop a relevant client-centered intervention plan. This is a positive outcome and the selection of this action would result in the awarding of points.

4. C8 Initiate an assessment for a customized one-arm drive wheelchair. ✗

Feedback: The rehabilitation team questions the appropriateness of this evaluation at this time.

Outcome and Rationale: Customized wheelchairs are not prescribed until a client has attained his/her maximal potential in rehabilitation. In this case, the client has recently incurred poly-trauma and has just begun a rehabilitation program. The client will be undergoing months of rehabilitation for multiple amputations. During this rehabilitation stay, the client can use the rehabilitation center's wheelchair mobility resources. As the client progresses beyond this initial phase of rehabilitation more specific information about the client's mobility needs and goals can be determined. It can be expected that the client will make functional mobility gains during the course of rehabilitation. The client may develop sufficient ambulation skills using bilateral lower extremity prostheses and decide not to use a wheelchair at all. Conversely, the client may develop complications in the residual limbs that compromise the ability to achieve independent ambulation with prostheses and may have to use a wheelchair all the time. The client may also decide to use prostheses for ambulation in the community and a wheelchair for prosthetic rest times while at home. The client's need for a one-arm drive wheelchair will depend on the outcomes of the upper-extremity rehabilitation program. Since the nature of the client's wheelchair needs cannot be accurately determined at this time, the selection of this action reflects a lack of foundational knowledge about the rehabilitation process for a person with multiple amputations and pre-prosthetic evaluation and intervention priorities. As a result, the selection of this action would result in the deduction of points.

5. C7 Administer the Contextual Memory Test.

Feedback: The client demonstrates minimal difficulties in memory retention and recall. The client reports moderate difficulty focusing on the test and remembering the complex daily rehabilitation schedule.

Outcome and Rationale: The Contextual Memory Test is a good tool for the evaluation of memory and concentration in a person with a TBI. This assessment can provide relevant information about the person's assets and limitations and awareness of deficits. At a Level VIII on the Rancho Level of Cognitive Functioning, the client will have intact past and recent memory but will require assistive devices to recall more complex information (e.g., schedules with multiple appointments, lengthy "to do" lists). These evaluation results can be used to develop a relevant intervention plan. This is a positive outcome and points would be awarded for the selection of this outcome.

6. C2 Interview the client to determine pre-prosthetic rehabilitation program goals.

Feedback: The client wants to learn to walk using prostheses but "can't be bothered" with learning to use an upper extremity prosthesis.

Outcome and Rationale: The determination of a client's goals is a major focus of an initial evaluation. This action is consistent with the OT process and provides important information that helps the occupational therapist design a client-directed intervention plan. Many individuals with unilateral upper extremity amputations, who have a residual limb of sufficient length to serve as a stabilizer and/or assist during bilateral activities, choose not to use a prosthesis. Knowing the client's preference will enable the occupational therapist to focus intervention on the development of abilities to perform desired tasks without an upper extremity prosthesis. These skills can be beneficial to the client even if the client changes his/her mind and decides that he/she would like to use an upper extremity prosthesis because there may be times when the prosthesis is not available (e.g., when being repaired). Since this evaluation provided relevant information that progresses the person through the OT process, it is a positive outcome. Consequently, points would be awarded for the selection of this action.

7. C3 Measure the upper extremity residual limb length, circumference and sensitivity. ✓

Feedback: The therapist records the residual limb measurements and determines that it is hypersensitive.

Outcome and Rationale: The measurement of the length and circumference of a residual limb is a fundamental component of a post-amputation evaluation. These measurements are taken frequently and consistently in the same location to help determine when the client can be fitted for a prosthesis. At this early stage in the client's rehabilitation, this data is essential to obtain even if a client has expressed no desire for a prosthesis. A client's perspective may change over time and it is important to know when circumference measurements have stabilized to allow for the casting of a limb. Evaluating a residual limb's sensitivity is also important to determine if desensitization techniques are needed to prepare a limb for a prosthesis and/or functional use. The evaluations included in this action provided the therapist with meaningful information that can be used to plan a relevant treatment plan. As a result, it selection would result in the awarding of points.

8. C3 Administer a visual analog pain intensity scale. O

Feedback: The client marks current pain level on the midpoint of this scale.

Outcome and Rationale: A visual analog scale is comprised of a line that has an endpoint of mild pain and an endpoint of severe pain. The client is asked to indicate the intensity of his/her pain by bisecting the line. In this case, the client reports that the intensity of pain is at the scale's midpoint which is consistent with the information obtained during chart review. Since the client has just been admitted, it would be reasonable to expect that the administration of a measure which is equivalent to the one that was administered upon admission would provide similar results. While the administration of this assessment does not provide the therapist with any new information, it does not cause harm. Consequently, this action would be considered neutral and points would neither be deducted nor awarded for its selection. A more appropriate pain measure to use during the initial OT evaluation would be one that obtained information beyond a numerical rating; for example, a description of the client's subjective pain experience.

Section B

Evaluation results indicate that the client is independent in feeding and grooming. The client is dependent in bathing, toileting, dressing and transferring and has difficulty cutting meat. The client has minimal difficulties in memory retention and recall and moderate difficulties in concentration and remembering a daily schedule. The client meets with the therapist to determine intervention goals. The client wants to be independent in the performance of ADL using the residual limb without a prosthesis; however, the limb is painful and very sensitive. Which should the therapist include in the OT intervention program to address these deficits and attain the client's goals? Choose all that apply.

1. C3 Implement an exercise program to strengthen muscles that will enable the effective use of an UE prosthesis. X

Feedback: The client questions why these exercises are focusing on the use of a prosthesis.

Outcome and Rationale: The development of strength is an important clinical outcome for a person with an UE amputation, regardless as to whether the person will use a prosthesis or not to complete functional tasks. If the client decides to use a prosthesis, strength will be required to operate the prosthesis during task performance. If the client decides not to use a prosthesis, UE strength will enable the client to effectively use the residual limb during occupational performance. However, in this action choice the therapist is focusing on exercises for the use of a prosthesis. This is not appropriate in this case since the client has stated a decision not to use an UE prosthesis. The therapist should have implemented the strengthening program with an emphasis on functional task performance without a prosthesis. Although the client may change his/her mind in the future about prosthetic use, implementing an exercise program with a goal that is counter to the client's expressed desired outcome is inappropriate. This action does not demonstrate good interactive reasoning skills as it is likely that the client will become frustrated or annoyed with the therapist's pursuit of a goal that is not consistent with his/her stated wishes. This can impede the client's progress. Consequently, this action would be considered negative and points would be deducted for its selection.

2. C7 Refer the client to the rehabilitation unit's daily current events group.

Feedback: The client joins the group and actively participates.

Outcome and Rationale: A current events group can help the client strengthen concentration and memory. Group participation is appropriate for a person at Level VIII of the Rancho scale. Individuals at this level can respond appropriately to social interactions with minimal assistance, although frustration tolerance may be low. They can recognize when their interactions are not appropriate and take corrective actions with minimal assistance. The current events group leader can assess the client's interaction skills and provide the structure and support the client may need to maximize social functioning. In addition, this group participation can help effectively integrate the client into the rehabilitation unit as it provides an opportunity to develop rapport with other group members and become socially involved on the unit. These are all positive outcomes. Consequently, points would be awarded for the selection of this action.

3. C8 Teach the client to direct personal care aides during the performance of self-care activities.

Feedback: The client self-directs all personal care aides.

Outcome and Rationale: The ability to self-direct personal care aides is an essential skill when a person is dependent in self-care performance. However, it is an action that does not address the client's stated goal to be independent in the performance of ADL using the residual limb without a prosthesis. If the client is not able to attain the goal of independent ADL performance, the ability to self-direct personal care aides is a vital skill that can empower the client to live an independent self-determined life. While this action does not directly address the client's needs or progress towards the client's stated goal, it is an action that can help make the client's current care more self-determined. Consequently, it would be considered a neutral selection and points would neither be awarded nor deducted for this selection.

4. C7 Provide the client with daily check-off logs to record pain levels and concentration status.

Feedback: The client consistently uses the logs and notes a trend in increased pain, inattention, and irritability in the early afternoon.

Outcome and Rationale: The completion and analysis of logs of pain, concentration, and other physiological factors and behavioral elements can be helpful to identify personal trends. This information can be used to modify pain management interventions and cognitive remediation treatment approaches based on the client's individualized needs. For this approach to be effective, the logs should be personalized for each client. In this case, a check-off list format is most helpful since it will decrease the amount of time that the client will need to use the residual limb to stabilize the paper. A narrative log format may be too frustrating for the client who is just beginning rehabilitation. The brief check-off sheet format will also be helpful to this client since he/she has moderate difficulties in concentration. This action is appropriate to the client's current status and it provides an intervention that will help the client progress in the rehabilitation program. Consequently, its selection would result in the awarding of points.

5. C6 Teach the client to incorporate deep breathing into a daily routine.

Feedback: The client learns the techniques and incorporates them into a daily routine during periods of frustration, inattention, and pain.

Outcome and Rationale: Deep breathing can be an effective pain management technique that can also help improve concentration. In addition, it is a technique that can help address frustration and feeling overwhelmed and tense; emotions that typically arise post-traumatically during intensive rehabilitation. This technique can be taught to most clients and it is free of contra-indications. Deep breathing can be a helpful initial technique during the ongoing process of re-evaluating a client's status and revising intervention. As more is learned about the client's response to this basic technique, more focused specific pain management and cognitive remediation strategies can be provided. Deep breathing can also prove to be one of many helpful strategies that the client can use on a long-term basis to manage the adjustment to a life with multiple amputations and a TBI. This is a positive outcome and the selection of this action would result in the awarding of points.

6. C3 Teach the client to protectively wrap the residual limb with an elastic bandage in a circular manner.

Feedback: The client reports that pain and hypersensitivity have increased greatly.

Outcome and Rationale: Wrapping a residual limb with an elastic bandage in a circular manner is a major contraindication in amputee care. This action would cause a tourniquet effect and dangerously restrict the limb's circulation. The wrapping of a residual limb should be done in a figure-of-eight diagonal pattern going from a distal to proximal direction with greater pressure applied at the distal end of the limb. The therapist should treat the client's pain and hypersensitivity with established intervention methods. Pain management techniques can include relaxation techniques, alternative exercise programs (e.g., aquatics, Tai Chi), and physical agent modalities. Methods of desensitization can include the application of diverse textures to the limb, massage, and tapping. The selection of this action represents a serious lack of basic knowledge about interventions for amputations. It is a harmful action that would result in the deduction of points for its selection.

7. C8 Train the client in the use of adaptive strategies and/or equipment to perform BADL.

Feedback: The client develops the ability to independently perform BADL.

Outcome and Rationale: There are many techniques that the client can learn to independently perform BADL. The client can learn to use the dominant LUE to perform unilateral tasks using adaptive equipment such as a rocker knife to cut meat. Instruction on the use of the residual RUE as a stabilizer and/or assist during task performance can also be very effective (e.g., stabilizing clothing to enable the fastening of closures) in attaining independence in BADL. This is a positive outcome and the selection of this action would be awarded points.

Section C

The client has progressed well in rehabilitation. The client demonstrates independence in all BADL and transfers with and without LE prostheses. Physical therapy reports that the client's ambulation with bilateral prostheses is within functional limits. Memory and concentration are consistently in the lower ranges of normal limits, with short periods of difficulty during complex, challenging tasks. The client has incorporated strategies for memory, concentration and behavioral management into a daily routine. Short outbursts of frustration occur less than once a week and the client demonstrates the ability to recover quickly. The client's pain had decreased to a 2 on the pain intensity scale. The client is scheduled to be discharged from the inpatient rehabilitation center in three weeks to live alone in a private home. Which should the occupational therapist include in the client's pre-discharge program and discharge plan to prepare the client for discharge? Choose all interventions and/or recommendations that apply.

1. C8 Refer the client to the rehabilitation center's vocational rehabilitation program.

Feedback: The client is accepted into the program and begins extensive vocational rehabilitation with the goal to return to previous job.

Outcome and Rationale: The referral to the vocational rehabilitation program is appropriate to the client's current status. Vocational rehabilitation departments in long-term rehabilitation centers typically provide extensive services including the administration of a work capacity evaluation which is critical for determining the person's ability to return to work. Services also include instruction and practice in real and simulated work tasks, with and without modifications. The client can begin this program as an inpatient and continue participation as an outpatient. Upon completion of the center's vocational rehabilitation program the client can begin competitive employment or seek additional vocational training and/or education. A referral to the state vocational rehabilitation services for economic support of the client's vocational goals can also be made by the rehabilitation center's staff based on the client's objective performance in their program. This is a positive outcome and points would be awarded for its selection.

2. C8 Recommend the client participate in the community mobility group. ✓

Feedback: The client learns how to ambulate with prostheses on varying terrain and in diverse environments.

Outcome and Rationale: Although the PT report states that the client's ambulation is WFL, the surfaces in a rehabilitation center are typically flat and even. In contrast, surfaces in the community are typically uneven with variations in grade and multiple potential obstacles and hazards. Consequently, applying the ambulation skills acquired during PT to the community environment is essential for a successful transition to community living. This action is very relevant to this case and its selection would be awarded points.

3. C8 Refer the client to the area home care agency for an evaluation for a personal care assistant (PCA). ✗

Feedback: The agency intake supervisor determines that the client does not meet the criteria for a PCA.

Outcome and Rationale: A PCA is indicated when a person is dependent in BADL. This client is independent in BADL so this referral is inappropriate. This action represents a lack of understanding of the role of the PCA and is a waste of the client's and home care agency intake supervisor's time. Consequently, points would be deducted for its selection.

4. C8 Administer the Leisure Diagnostic Battery. ✓

Feedback: The client identifies outdoor leisure activities as motivating. The client wants to resume skiing and hunting, but has limited knowledge of accessible community leisure opportunities.

Outcome and Rationale: The Leisure Diagnostic Battery measures an individual's leisure experience and motivational and situational issues that influence leisure (e.g., perceived barriers to leisure and knowledge of leisure opportunities). This is an appropriate evaluation that provides relevant information to assist the occupational therapist and rehabilitation team in making discharge recommendations relevant to the client's leisure interests (e.g., an adaptive ski program, a local rifle range). This is a positive outcome and points would be awarded for the selection of this action.

5. C8 Administer the Katz Index of ADL to determine home management skills. ✗

Feedback: The client scores independent in all six areas on the Katz.

Outcome and Rationale: It is most appropriate to evaluate the client's ability to perform home management skills and other IADL since the client will be living alone in his/her own home post-discharge. Based upon the results of this evaluation, the occupational therapist can plan interventions that can enable the client to develop the desired skills in IADL. However, the Katz will not provide this essential information. The Katz assesses a person's level of independent functioning and type of assistance required in six areas of BADL. It does not assess any IADL Consequently, it is an inappropriate evaluation for determining the client's home management skills and points would be deducted for the selection of this action.

6. C8 Encourage the client to locate supportive community resources. ✓

Feedback: The client identifies several community resources that may be available for support.

Outcome and Rationale: The identification of community resources to support independent living and community participation can be helpful to a client's post-discharge adjustment. However, as stated this recommendation is vague and not directly related to the client's goals or interests. It would be more effective to work with the client on identifying specific community participation goals and concerns prior to seeking external supports. These supports can include outpatient services offered by the rehabilitation center, public and private agencies, centers for independent living, and disability rights groups. Although this recommendation is not optimal, it does not cause harm; therefore it would be considered a neutral action. Points would neither be deducted nor awarded for its selection.

7. C8 Recommend an assessment for an ambulatory device to be used during lower extremity prosthetic "down time." ✓

Feedback: The client is evaluated for a wheelchair that can be independently propelled.

Outcome and Rationale: A wheelchair is often a valuable resource for the client with bilateral LE prostheses. It can provide independent mobility during prosthetic downtime (e.g., during repairs) and for long distances or over rough terrain. Crutches and/or a walker can also be used as an ambulatory aid in these situations by clients with a unilateral prosthesis. This action will enable the client to have functional mobility even when the prostheses are unavailable or ineffective. This is a good outcome and points would be awarded for this action.

Simulation Test Item B.III.

Opening Scene:

An adult with Type II diabetes, peripheral neuropathy of the hands and feet, and retinopathy receives services in an inpatient rehabilitation setting due to persistent difficulties with medication management and IADL tasks at home. The client lives alone in a one-story home and reports a recent fall while reaching into a high cabinet. The client is referred to occupational therapy for evaluation and intervention.

Section A

The occupational therapist begins the evaluation process with an interview and history. The client describes personal responsibilities for meal preparation, medication management, and light housekeeping tasks at home. The client has assistance with cleaning, laundry and grocery shopping. The client no longer drives due to significant vision deficits in both eyes. Which assessments are most important for the occupational therapist to implement to determine the client's deficits? Choose all that apply.

1. C2 A stair negotiation evaluation.

Feedback: The client attempts the stairs, stops and states a fear of falling.

Outcome and Rationale: Evaluating stair negotiation is premature. The therapist must first determine the client's level of pain, mobility and visual skills first before attempting a higher level task. Completing a client factor evaluation first will help the therapist identify deficits that could impact the ability to safely negotiate stairs. Without completion of the client factor evaluation, the therapist can place the patient at risk for harm. Consequently, this selection would result in the deduction of points.

2. C8 A leisure interests inventory.

Feedback: The client identifies being interested in listening to the radio and books on tape.

Outcome and Rationale: While the identification of leisure interests can be an important component of a client-centered evaluation, leisure pursuits have not been identified as an area of concern in this scenario. Thus, leisure exploration is not a high priority for an initial evaluation. This choice does not cause harm nor does it move the person forward in the evaluation process; therefore, it would be considered a neutral selection and points would neither be awarded nor deducted for its selection.

3. C3 The Semmes Weinstein monofilament test.

Feedback: Evaluation results reveal moderate sensory deficits of light touch in both hands.

Outcome and Rationale: Monofilament testing is very valuable in this situation as it helps the therapist to determine deficits in light touch related to the peripheral neuropathy. Through this evaluation, the therapist can identify whether the patient will have difficulty with manipulation of objects or be at risk for injury secondary to sensory impairments in the hand, such as impairments in detection of temperature or pain. This is a positive outcome so points would be awarded for this selection.

4. C3 Active and passive ROM assessment of the upper extremities.

Feedback: The client moves both arms though full passive range. Active ROM shows deficits in flexion and abduction to 1/4 of the end range bilaterally.

Outcome and Rationale: Active ROM evaluation can provide valuable information about the patient's ability to tolerate motion, potential for pain and ultimately to engage in everyday tasks using his/her available range to complete ADL tasks. Without completion of this evaluation, the therapist will not be effective in developing an intervention plan that addresses the patient's needs related to his/her deficits. This is a positive outcome so points would be awarded for this selection.

5. C3 A subjective pain assessment.

Feedback: The client reports burning and tingling in both hands and rates this pain at a level of 5 out of 10.

Outcome and Rationale: A subjective pain assessment can provide valuable information about the patient's potential pain, especially as it relates to a chronic condition. A subjective pain assessment addresses sources of pain, remedies that reduce pain, duration of pain and qualitative aspects of pain. The therapist can then use this information to assist the patient in the safe completion of ADL tasks. This is a positive outcome so points would be awarded for this selection.

6. C8 A kitchen mobility evaluation with the use of a standard cane. ✗

Feedback: The client is very unsteady using a cane and stumbles during ambulation. The therapist must intervene to prevent a fall.

Outcome and Rationale: The therapist needs to finish the client factor evaluation before asking a patient to ambulate in the kitchen. If the therapist finishes the evaluation first, then the client's ability to ambulate will be determined. To do so beforehand places the client at risk. Consequently, this selection would result in the deduction of points.

7. C8 Issue adaptive kitchen devices for meal preparation tasks, such as a suction cutting board and rocker knife for chopping tasks. ◯

Feedback: The client expresses disinterest in these devices since the progression of the retinopathy and neuropathy has limited meal preparation to simple meals.

Outcome and Rationale: Adaptive devices should be issued after the evaluation. It is not a harmful action, but it would be more beneficial to wait and determine after a complete evaluation that these devices are needed and provide appropriate training in its use. Otherwise unnecessary training and purchase of this equipment may result. This choice does not cause harm nor does it move the person forward in the evaluation process; therefore, it would be considered a neutral selection and points would neither be awarded nor deducted for its selection.

8. C3 Thermal testing of both hands.

Feedback: Testing reveals the client has moderate impairments in the detection of hot and cold temperatures in both hands.

Outcome and Rationale: Thermal testing is an important evaluation with clients who have peripheral neuropathy. Testing can provide valuable information about the potential risk of injury from extreme temperatures, such as the ability to distinguish threatening cold when outside or conversely threatening heat, especially when bathing and cooking. This is a positive outcome so points would be awarded for this selection.

9. C9 Visual acuity evaluation with use of an eye chart. ✗

Feedback: The client questions this testing since an ophthalmologist recently conducted a vision test.

Outcome and Rationale: Visual acuity testing is outside the scope of practice for occupational therapists. Visual acuity is important information to have, but it must come from a professional trained in acuity testing. Conducting this testing without proper training can cause financial harm (not reimbursable) and physical harm (if the client is improperly assessed as having a level of acuity that is incorrect). The therapist must defer this test to a qualified professional, such as an optometrist or ophthalmologist. Consequently, this selection would result in the deduction of points.

Section B

Evaluation results reveal that the patient has mild pain in both hands. The client has difficulty reading moderate-sized print. The client is moderately impaired in detection of light touch and hot/cold sensations. ROM in both extremities is limited to within ¼ of the end range in shoulder flexion and abduction. The client requires contact guard for ambulation with a cane. Strength is rated good in the shoulders. The client wants to return home to resume all previous activities. In implementing the intervention plan, which activities are most beneficial to include? Choose all activities that are appropriate to this situation.

1. C3 Apply cold packs to both hands for relief of pain. X

Feedback: The patient complains that the cold increases pain and numbness in the hands.

Outcome and Rationale: Cold is contraindicated in this situation as diabetic neuropathy results in decreased vascular circulation. Cold negatively impacts vascular circulation and can cause pain and numbness of the affected areas. Gentle heat is an appropriate alternative to promote pain relief and tissue elasticity. Consequently, this selection would result in the deduction of points.

2. C8 Provide adaptive training for medication management. ✓

Feedback: The patient demonstrates increased independence in managing medications using the adaptive methods.

Outcome and Rationale: Because the client has impaired vision, medication management is pivotal to safely manage medications upon return home. Adaptive training such as relabeling bottles with larger print, adding color to the tops of bottles to make them distinctive or the use of a large print medication holder are all ways to improve success in managing medication for people with impaired vision. This is a positive outcome so points would be awarded for this selection.

3. C3 Use high-grade joint mobilization of both shoulders to increase ROM. X

Feedback: The client complains of joint pain during the technique and asks the therapist to stop.

Outcome and Rationale: High-grade joint mobilization is not indicated in patients with diabetes. This technique provides too much stress on the joints and the limitations in ROM of the shoulders do not indicate that this technique is warranted. Gentle stretching exercises are safer and likely to result in improved tissue elasticity for greater ROM. Consequently, this selection would result in the deduction of points.

4. C8 Simulate completion of shopping tasks with education on proper body positioning. O

Feedback: The client does not understand why shopping is being emphasized since all personal shopping is done with assistance.

Outcome and Rationale: Previous information indicated that the client had assistance with shopping. It is important to focus intervention efforts toward the functional improvement in all IADL tasks that the client must complete at home. This approach is not the most effective because it does not address required IADL skills. This choice does not cause harm nor does it move the person forward in the intervention process. Therefore, it would be considered a neutral selection and points would neither be awarded nor deducted for its selection.

5. C3 Provide high resistance exercises to build shoulder strength. X

Feedback: The client yells out in pain when performing the exercises.

Outcome and Rationale: High resistance activities are not appropriate for this client. Resistance should begin at a lower level and build up over time and tolerance increases. This approach will be too stressful on the joints and could cause pain. Consequently, this selection would result in the deduction of points.

6. C8 Train the client in the use of adaptive equipment for meal preparation tasks. ✓

Feedback: The client expresses increased confidence in preparing meals using the stovetop and oven.

Outcome and Rationale: Because the client previously prepared meals and has impairments in touch and temperature sensation, adaptive equipment for meal preparation will be beneficial to improve safety and IADL functioning. The goal is to prevent injury and promote independence in meal preparation tasks, compensating or adapting for deficits related to the neuropathy and retinopathy. This is a positive outcome so points would be awarded for this selection.

7. C3 Train the client in energy conservation techniques for the performance of IADL. ✓

Feedback: The client implements the techniques and demonstrates improved energy during IADL performance.

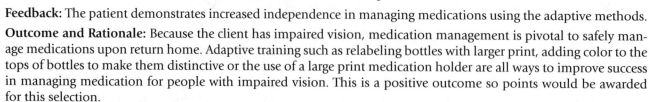

Outcome and Rationale: Energy conservation is very beneficial for persons with chronic diseases. Fatigue is common in people who are recently admitted to inpatient settings. Energy conservation training emphasizes appropriate pacing

of activities to prevent undue exhaustion. Tying this to the performance of IADL is beneficial, as the client is responsible for certain IADL upon return to home. This is a positive outcome so points would be awarded for this selection.

8. C8 Re-train in skills needed for successful driving.

Feedback: The client states a fear of driving because remaining vision is too poor to drive safely.

Outcome and Rationale: Information previously provided stated that the client had difficulty reading moderate-sized print and received assistance for shopping. These are indications that the client did not recently drive and does not have the needed vision in order to engage in safe driving. Consequently, this selection would result in the deduction of points.

9. C8 Train the client in fall prevention and safe reaching during retrieval of common items.

Feedback: The client states less fear of falling and increased safety during retrieval.

Outcome and Rationale: Fall prevention is important in all persons who wish to return home. Retrieval of items is a daily task that has the potential to result in a fall for those with impaired mobility. Due to the client's history of a fall while reaching into a high cabinet, fall prevention training and learning the safe retrieval of items is pivotal. This is a positive outcome so points would be awarded for this selection.

10. C9 Ask the client to invite family members to an educational session about the impact of the client's disease process on independence.

Feedback: The client prefers that family members not be invited or informed.

Outcome and Rationale: The scenario information that has been presented thus far has not indicated family involvement. While family education can be important in certain cases, nothing in the exam item indicates that the client wants family involved or has family that is involved. Because the client declined the action, no harm has been created. Since this choice does not cause harm nor does it move the person forward in the intervention process, it would be considered a neutral selection and points would neither be awarded nor deducted for its selection.

Section C

The client has been progressing in both occupational and physical therapy, however the occupational therapist notices that safety is a concern during the performance of IADL. For example, the client often bumps into objects in the pathway, stumbles during ambulation and knocks the handles of pots and pans on the stove. Which of the following should the therapist include in a modified intervention plan? Choose all actions that would effectively address this situation.

1. C8 Cessation of meal preparation using a stove and emphasize training in microwave meal preparation.

Feedback: The client questions why meal preparation cannot include the use a stove since independent stove use has been previously acquired.

Outcome and Rationale: There is no reason to withdraw use of a stove for meal preparation. The bumping of handles on the stove indicates visual perceptual impairments, which can be improved through compensatory training strategies. The client has stated a desire to resume all previous activities so the cessation of meal preparation using the stove will frustrate the client. Consequently, this selection would result in the deduction of points.

2. C8 Low vision training during mobility tasks.

Feedback: The client states that the training is increasing confidence and decreasing fear during mobility.

Outcome and Rationale: Low vision training is very important, as the current deficits indicate that the client's low vision is part of the problem at hand. As part of this training, clients learn techniques to maximize their visual ability through specific strategies in order to be independent and safe in ADL and IADL. It may also include the use of optical aids during functional tasks. Low vision training is a pivotal intervention prior to discharge to the community. This is a positive outcome so points would be awarded for this selection.

3. C7 Cognitive training tasks including judgment and reasoning skills. X

Feedback: The client shows no impairments during the cognitive training tasks.

Outcome and Rationale: None of the identified current deficits are indicative of cognitive problems. The most common deficits are low vision and peripheral neuropathy in the feet, which are affecting sensation during mobility. If cognitive impairments were a factor, the client would demonstrate additional deficits that are not present in the scenario, such as poor ability to reason through ADL and IADL tasks, ongoing safety issues with decreased carryover and decreased ability to understand the consequences of decisions made. This approach causes financial harm, as it is a waste of time and resources and could affect the client's reimbursement for services. Consequently, this selection would result in the deduction of points.

4. C8 Downgrade the client's assistive device from a cane to a rolling walker. O

Feedback: The client reports working on developing the ability to walk with a cane in physical therapy.

Outcome and Rationale: Because physical therapy is involved in treatment, the occupational therapist should first consult with the physical therapist before changing assistive devices. Collaboration is important before making changes that affect other disciplines involved in care. In this case, changing to a walker will provide more support, so it is not harmful. But it does create confusion for the client on which device to use. This choice does not cause harm nor does it move the person forward in the intervention process. Therefore, it would be considered a neutral selection and points would neither be awarded nor deducted for its selection.

5. C9 Collaboration with physical therapy regarding mobility and safety. ✓

Feedback: The physical therapist believes that vision and fearfulness are key factors in the client's current difficulties.

Outcome and Rationale: When deficits impact more than just the domain of concern of occupational therapy practice, the occupational therapist should collaborate with the other disciplines to ensure effective carryover of changes in the intervention plan. In this case, because the deficits are impacting mobility and ambulation, the physical therapist should definitely be consulted before making any changes to the intervention plan, so care is coordinated. This is a positive outcome so points would be awarded for this selection.

6. C8 Training in compensatory strategies related to vision during ADL and IADL. ✓

Feedback: Less difficulty is noted when the client completes ADL and IADL.

Outcome and Rationale: Because vision is one of this client's primary issues, compensatory strategies are pivotal to independent functioning in ADL and IADL. The client can learn how to compensate for deficits to prevent losses of balance, injury and fatigue during ADL and IADL. This will lead to improved performance upon discharge where the client may have to complete these tasks independently. This is a positive outcome so points would be awarded for this selection.

7. C9 Referral to physician for possible diagnosis of vestibular disorder. X

Feedback: The physician contacts the therapist and states frustration with the unnecessary referral.

Outcome and Rationale: This is a misinterpretation of the current deficits by the therapist. Vestibular issues are not likely given the diagnosis. The fact that the client has low vision and diabetic neuropathy should cause one to conclude that the vision and lack of sensation in the feet are contributing to the deficits. In this case, financial harm is done, as it has cost the client money for the visit and the physician his or her time. Consequently, this selection would result in the deduction of points.

Section D

The client has actively participated in occupational therapy and physical therapy for two weeks. The client's deficits have improved to a level that supports returning home to live alone. The client's primary concern is being safe and preventing injury from a fall. The occupational therapist accompanies the client on a home evaluation prior to discharge. Which areas of home functioning should the therapist evaluate? Choose all that apply.

1. C8 The use of a wheelchair for safe in-home mobility.

Feedback: The client does not understand why a wheelchair is needed.

Outcome and Rationale: This client should not be downgraded to wheelchair mobility. This will result in a loss of LE strength and flexibility over time which can lead to a risk for falls. The client's concerns about falling are important, but downgrading to a wheelchair is a drastic measure. A better option would be training is safe mobility in the home using the client's current assistive device. If further concerns are noted, a recommendation for in-home therapy or outpatient therapy is appropriate. This option reflects a poor understanding of the client's current status; consequently, this selection would result in the deduction of points.

2. C8 Independence in operating kitchen appliances.

Feedback: The client demonstrates the ability to turn stove knobs, open the refrigerator and use the dishwasher.

Outcome and Rationale: This is an important area to assess. Since the client previously stated the need to prepare meals at home and has practiced meal preparation throughout the rehabilitation stay, it is very important to follow up in the home environment and ensure the client can operate appliances safely. This task directly addresses the client's priorities of safety and fall prevention. This is a positive outcome so points would be awarded for this selection.

3. C8 Rearrange cupboard items so food items are closer to the stove.

Feedback: The client cannot find food items because the previous arrangement was in place for years.

Outcome and Rationale: Rearranging items for people with visual impairments should only be done when absolutely necessary because it is harder to locate and identify the rearranged items. This selection reflects a lack of understanding of a basic compensation strategy used by persons with visual impairments; therefore, it would result in the deduction of points.

4. C8 Rearrange cupboard items so pots and pans are stored below the oven.

Feedback: The client becomes unsteady when reaching down for a pan.

Outcome and Rationale: Placing pots and pans at a low location below an oven can increase the risk of falls due to excessive bending. It could also lead to burns if the client uses the stove to steady him/herself during cooking to bend and retrieve. Consequently, this selection would result in the deduction of points.

5. C8 Ability to transport clothes to laundry room in basement.

Feedback: The client is irritated, stating, "I already told you someone helps me with my laundry."

Outcome and Rationale: The therapist was previously informed by the client during the initial evaluation that he/she has assistance with laundry skills. Laundry was not addressed on the intervention plan in the previous section, so it is not fitting to address it now. This has resulted in irritation by the client and loss of confidence in the therapist's knowledge and skills by the client. Consequently, this selection would result in the deduction of points.

6. C8 Recommend the removal of all carpeted surfaces in the home to decrease risk of falls.

Feedback: The client does not think removing the carpet is going to prevent a fall and declines the recommendation.

Outcome and Rationale: Removal of carpeting may or may not lessen the likelihood of a fall. More needs to be done to prevent a fall than just removing carpeting. It is important to note that the recommendation was not to remove throw rugs, which is a good recommendation. It was to remove all carpet, which is burdensome and does not guarantee to prevent falls. In this case, the client declined the recommendation so no harm was done. This choice does not cause harm nor does it move the person forward in the intervention process; therefore, it would be considered a neutral selection and points would neither be awarded nor deducted for its selection.

7. C8 Ability to lock and unlock all the outside doors in the home.

Feedback: The client thanks the therapist for addressing personal safety.

Outcome and Rationale: This is an important safety feature for all persons who live in the community, especially if they live alone. The client must be able to secure his/her home and be able to exit safely in case of an emergency, such as a fire. If the client has difficulty with the operation of locks due to the peripheral neuropathy, modifications can be made, both with devices purchased commercially or custom-made by the therapist. This is a positive outcome so points would be awarded for this selection.

Multiple Choice Test Items B1–B170

B1 C6

An occupational therapist provides consultation services to a psychogeriatric unit for individuals with mid-stage dementia. In designing the activity program, which groups are best for the occupational therapist to include?

Answer Choices:
A. Reality orientation.
B. Sensory stimulation.
C. Reminiscence.
D. Coping skills.

Correct Answer: C.

Rationale:
Reminiscence groups are designed to review past life experiences to promote use of intact long-term memory. Current memory is not required for successful participation in reminiscence groups. Individuals with mid-stage dementia typically have poor recent memory but good long-term memory. Reality orientation typically involves activities that require remembering the current day, date, time, season and activity sequence. Individuals with mid-stage dementia have current memory deficits that would preclude their ability to successfully participate in reality orientation activities. This lack of success can highlight deficits and increase frustration. Sensory stimulation activities are indicated for individuals with later stage dementia who are at risk for sensory deprivation. Coping skills groups use activities to problem solve, apply and critique alternative solutions that can be used to effectively manage potential life stressors/problems. These activities require cognitive abilities that are beyond the capacity of a person with mid-stage dementia.

Type of Reasoning: Inferential
One must determine the most likely intervention approach for a group of individuals, given the treatment setting provided. This requires inferential reasoning skill, where one must draw conclusions based on the information presented. In this situation, the therapist should suggest that groups emphasize reminiscence. If answered incorrectly, review group treatment activities for older adults with dementia.

B2 C4

The parents of a five-year-old with attention deficit with hyperactivity disorder (ADHD) express difficulty managing the child's aggressive behavior towards older siblings. Which is the most effective strategy for the occupational therapist to recommend to the parents?

Answer Choices:
A. Allow the child to vent aggressive feelings on a stuffed animal or doll.
B. Redirect the child's energy into acceptable and safe play activities.
C. Provide consistent punishment for aggressive behavior.
D. Send the child to stay with a family member or close friend for an extended "time-out."

Correct Answer: B.

Rationale:
Redirecting the child's energy to activities can be an effective management of the child's aggressive behavior. It would also be appropriate to have the parents observe and record the precipitants to these behaviors to determine potential environmental modifications. This is not an option provided. Allowing the child to vent aggression onto a stuffed animal or doll would not provide the structure the child needs to learn appropriate, safe behaviors. Also, aggressive behaviors are not always coupled with aggressive feelings. Sometimes the hyperactivity of a child simply asserts itself in socially unacceptable ways, such as when a child pushes a sibling very hard in an effort to get the sibling to play "chase." Punishing the child or removing the child from the family does not address the child's needs. Taking punitive actions towards the child can increase feelings of resentment and promote a decrease in feelings of self-worth, which are typically already low in children with ADHD, which can fuel aggressive behavior.

Type of Reasoning: Inductive
This question requires one to determine the most appropriate recommendation for a child with ADHD. This requires inductive reasoning skill, where clinical judgment is paramount in arriving at a correct conclusion. For this situation, the therapist should recommend redirecting the child's energy into acceptable and safe play activities. If answered incorrectly, review treatment guidelines for children with ADHD, especially behavior management techniques.

B3 C3

An individual with rheumatoid arthritis has developed several boutonniere deformities. Which of the following is the most accurate description for the occupational therapist to include in documentation of the individual's presenting signs?

Answer Choices:
A. Hyperextension of the PIP joint and flexion of the DIP joint.
B. Ulnar deviation and subluxation of the MCP joints.
C. Flexion of the PIP joint and hyperextension of the DIP joint. ✓
D. Heberden's nodes at the DIP joints and Bouchard's nodes at the PIP joints.

Correct Answer: C.

Rationale:
A boutonniere deformity occurs when there is hyperextension of the DIP joint with flexion of the PIP joint. A swan neck deformity is evident when there is hyperextension of the PIP joint and flexion of the DIP joint. Ulnar deviation and subluxation of the MCP joints are additional deformities that can result from rheumatoid arthritis. Herberden's nodes and Bouchard's nodes are types of bone spurs that can result from osteoarthritis.

Type of Reasoning: Inferential
One must link the individual's diagnosis to the signs presented in order to determine which presenting signs are most representative of boutonniere deformities. This requires inferential reasoning, where one must draw conclusions about the likely presentation of a diagnosis. In this case the diagnosis would present with flexion of the PIP joint and hyperextension of the DIP joint.

B4 C5

An occupational therapist receives a referral to provide home-based services to an elder adult who lives alone in a fourth floor walk-up apartment. Upon entering the apartment, the therapist notes the sweltering heat. The apartment has no fans or air conditioners. The client's skin is hot, dry and red, and breathing is labored. The therapist offers the client a glass of water and places ice compresses on the arterial pressure points to help with cooling. Which is the most important action for the therapist to take next?

Answer Choices:

A. Cancel the intervention session and call for an ambulance to provide emergency medical services. ✓
B. Proceed with the planned intervention session and include documentation about client's environmental conditions in the intervention report.
C. Contact the home health agency's case manager to report the client's environmental conditions and then proceed with the planned intervention session.
D. Cancel the intervention session and advise the client to speak to a doctor on how to best address the impact of hot weather on personal health.

Correct Answer: A.

Rationale:
The client is exhibiting signs of heat stroke. The elderly are particularly at risk for heat-induced illnesses. Extended periods of intense heat can be life threatening to the elderly and must be treated as a medical emergency. While lowering the client's body temperature with ice on the arterial pressure points is an appropriate first-aid intervention, it is not sufficient to deal with this serious situation. Immediate medical care is required.

Type of Reasoning: Evaluative
This question requires one to weigh the courses of action presented and determine the approach that will most effectively address the client's needs. This requires evaluative reasoning skill. In this case, because the patient's symptoms indicate a life-threatening situation, the therapist should cancel the evaluation and call for an ambulance. If answered incorrectly, review symptoms of heat stroke and first aid approaches for heat stroke.

B5 C9

An occupational therapist observes an OTA having difficulty transferring a client with athetoid movements from a mat to a wheelchair. Before the therapist can cross the room to help with the transfer, the OTA slides with the client to the floor. The therapist assists the OTA in safely returning the client to the wheelchair. They assess that the client appears to be unharmed and return the client to the unit for a medical evaluation. Which action should the therapist take next?

Answer Choices:

A. Counsel the OTA on the need to ask for assistance with difficult transfers.
B. Require the OTA to attend a transfer training inservice.
C. Document the OTA's unsafe actions in the personnel record.
D. Complete an occurrence report according to facility standards. ✓

Correct Answer: D.

Rationale:
Immediately after an incident occurs, the therapist must complete documentation according to the setting's standards. Counseling an OTA to ask for assistance and requiring attendance at a workshop can be appropriate aspects of risk management but they are not the first steps. In addition, there is no information provided to clearly identify that the OTA was acting unsafely. There are transfer situations that unexpectedly become beyond a practitioner's ability to successfully complete. During those situations, the practitioner should guide the patient to the floor in a controlled manner. This is often done by using one's own body to support the patient and can give the appearance of "sliding." More information is needed to determine if the OTA's actions were actually unsafe.

Type of Reasoning: Inductive
This question requires one to determine the best course of action. This requires inductive reasoning skill, where clinical judgment is paramount in arriving at a correct conclusion. For this situation, after returning the client to the unit for a medical evaluation, the therapist should complete an occurrence report according to the facility standards. If answered incorrectly, review guidelines for completing facility incidence reports.

B6 C4

A teenager with spinal muscle atrophy shows decreased trunk balance and strength. Upper extremity strength and ROM are unchanged from the last evaluation. Which is the best recommendation for the occupational therapist to make?

Answer Choices:
A. A re-evaluation of the client be completed. ✓
B. The client be referred to an orthotist for a soft spinal support. ✗
C. The client be measured for a power wheelchair. ✗
D. A trunk strengthening program be initiated with the client.

Correct Answer: A.

Rationale:
The most important action to take after noticing a change in the functional status of a person with a progressive condition is to re-evaluate. Based on the results of the evaluation, interventions can be planned. These interventions can include orthotics, adaptive equipment, powered mobility, compensation techniques and/or a strengthening program; only the results of a re-evaluation can appropriately determine intervention needs. The physician determines the need for a soft or plastic spinal support, often called a TLSO, thoracolumbosacral orthosis. These are usually used to prevent an increase in, or to maintain, the scoliosis curve. Supports often tend to decrease trunk balance by providing fewer opportunities for trunk mobility. A power wheelchair might be indicated for a person with spinal muscle atrophy. However, indications for a prescription of a power wheelchair are decreased strength and endurance to propel a manual wheelchair, not poor trunk balance.

Type of Reasoning: Inferential
One must determine the recommendation that would best address the adolescent's needs. Re-evaluation of the adolescent's capabilities and limitations is the best approach in order to determine if the decreases in trunk balance and strength will necessitate modifications to the intervention program. If answered incorrectly, review evaluation and intervention planning guidelines for patients with spinal muscle atrophy.

B7 C2

An occupational therapist consults with a home care agency interested in starting a falls prevention program. Which should the occupational therapist do first?

Answer Choices:
A. Review available evaluation protocols.
B. Review available screening tools. ✓
C. Create a new screening tool.
D. Design an evaluation protocol.

Correct Answer: B.

Rationale:
The home care agency's population will need to be screened to determine who would benefit from a falls prevention program. Therefore, the occupational therapist should review available tools to determine the one most suitable for the agency's population. Creating a new screening tool is not cost-effective because there may be several tools readily available that meet the program's needs. One must screen a population prior to reviewing or designing an evaluation protocol. After screening methods are established, the occupational therapist can focus on an evaluation protocol.

Type of Reasoning: Inductive
This question requires one to determine the best initial step for developing a fall prevention program for a specific population. This requires inductive reasoning skill, where clinical judgment is paramount in arriving at a correct conclusion. In this situation, reviewing available screening tools is the best initial action.

B8 C1

A four month-old with arthrogryposis remains in position when placed and shows little spontaneous movement. The occupational therapist implements intervention to work on rolling. Which positional changes should the therapist include in the intervention session?

Answer Choices:
A. Prone to supine.
B. Supine to side-lying. ✓
C. Prone to side-lying.
D. Supine to prone.

Correct Answer: B.

Rationale:
When children exhibit developmental delay, the occupational therapist should begin intervention by working on the first skill that typically occurs. Developmentally, rolling from supine to side-lying starts first. Rolling from prone to supine is the next stage and the other options occur later.

Type of Reasoning: Deductive
One must recall the developmental guidelines in mobility for infants. This is factual knowledge, which is a deductive reasoning skill. Supine to side-lying is the first skill to develop, therefore the therapist should initiate mobility with this skill first. If answered incorrectly, review developmental milestones of infants for gross motor skills.

B9 C5

An occupational therapist designs a dining rehabilitation program in a long-term care facility. The occupational therapist instructs paraprofessional staff in proper feeding techniques. Which point is most important for the therapist to include in this staff training?

Answer Choices:
A. Meals should occur in a homelike environment with staff conversing with the elders being fed. ✓
B. Individuals with swallowing difficulties should be fed in a group so that staff can remind them to swallow at the beginning of each meal.
C. Placing three fingertips on the throat and pressing firmly will stimulate a swallow response.
D. The head should be tilted slightly backward during feeding to facilitate an assisted swallow.

Correct Answer: A.

Rationale:
Proper feeding techniques include a <u>facilitative environment.</u> Dining in a homelike setting with staff who are attentive to the elders' needs and interests during feeding/mealtimes will facilitate eating and socialization during the activity. Grouping individuals with swallowing difficulties diminishes the individualized approach that is essential to quality long-term care. In addition, reminding people to swallow does not effectively deal with the reasons for their swallowing difficulties. If an individual does forget to swallow food, he/she must be reminded/cued throughout the meal to prevent aspiration/choking. Reminding/cueing only at the beginning of a meal is not sufficient. Placing three fingertips on the throat and pressing firmly does not stimulate a swallow response. Tilting the head back may facilitate aspiration and is contraindicated.

Type of Reasoning: Inferential
One must determine the most important feeding instruction to provide to staff, given knowledge of the clinical setting and feeding guidelines. This requires inferential reasoning skill, where one must infer or draw conclusions about a best course of action. In this situation, the therapist should inform staff of the importance of meals occurring in a homelike environment with staff conversing with the elders being fed. Review feeding guidelines in long-term care settings if answered incorrectly.

B10 C3

Following nerve injury repair surgery, an individual is evaluated for sensory return. Which measurement tool is best for the occupational therapist to use to assess for the return of vibration?

Answer Choices:
A. A tuning fork. ✓
B. Nylon filament.
C. A disk-criminator.
D. The ninhydrin test.

Correct Answer: A.

Rationale:
Tuning forks are used to test for the sense of vibration. Nylon filaments are used to assess for cutaneous pressure thresholds. A disk-criminator or caliper is used to test for two point discrimination. A ninhydrin test is a test of the ability to sweat.

Type of Reasoning: Analytical
This question provides a description of a various evaluation tools and the test taker must determine the tool that most appropriately measures sense of vibration. This is an analytical reasoning skill, as questions of this nature often ask one to analyze several choices to determine the appropriate one to perform the specified task at hand. In this situation, measurement of sense of vibration is conducted with a tuning fork.

B11 C1

During a group session at an adult day care program an older adult consistently complains that everyone is mumbling. After the group, which action should the occupational therapist take in response to these statements?

Answer Choices:
A. Notify the client's primary care physician that the person exhibited evidence of paranoia.
B. Collaborate with the program director to remove groups from the client's program plan.
C. Document objective data about the complaints in the person's chart.
D. Notify the primary care physician that the person may need an audiological evaluation. ✓

Correct Answer: D.

Rationale:
It is common for older adults to experience hearing loss. The individual's report that people are mumbling is indicative of a potential hearing loss that warrants further evaluation. Interpreting the person's report as indicative of paranoia is subjective. Modifying the person's program plan to not include groups and documenting the individual's complaints does not deal directly with the issue at hand.

Type of Reasoning: Inductive
One must utilize clinical knowledge and judgment to determine the most appropriate action to take, given the individual's complaint. This requires inductive reasoning skill. In this case, the individual's complaint warrants notifying the physician that an audiological evaluation may be needed. If answered incorrectly, review symptoms of hearing loss in adults.

B12 C9

The occupational therapist completes an intake interview for a work hardening program. As the individual is leaving, the person gives the therapist a hug and expresses much gratitude. The individual then tries to kiss the therapist on the lips. Which action is best for the therapist to take in response to this situation?

Answer Choices:
A. Forcibly push the individual away while telling the person that the behavior is inappropriate and unacceptable.
B. Say nothing but decline the person's admission to the work hardening program based upon the person's inappropriate behavior.
C. State that the individual's behavior oversteps professional boundaries and makes the therapist uncomfortable.
D. Tell the person the behavior is inappropriate and unacceptable and decline the person's admission to the program.

Correct Answer: C.

Rationale:
Informing the person of the boundaries of the client-therapist relationship is the appropriate action. There is no need to admonish the individual or decline the person's admission to the program. Some individuals are more demonstrative with their affections than others and the person may be showing gratitude in a manner that in his/her view is socially and culturally appropriate. The therapist can respond simply by stating that this expression of affection is outside the scope of their professional relationship.

Type of Reasoning: Evaluative
This question requires a value judgment in an ethical situation, which is an evaluative reasoning skill. In this situation, the therapist's most appropriate action is to state that the behavior is outside professional boundaries and makes the therapist uncomfortable. Ethical situations such as these often rely upon the OT Code of Ethics to provide guiding principles of action. Because the behavior is outside of the acceptable realm of the therapist/client relationship, the therapist is appropriate in stating the boundaries.

B13 **C4**

A person with a traumatic brain injury is assessed to score a 6 on the Glasgow Coma Scale. Which should the occupational therapist use to initiate intervention with this person?

Answer Choices:
A. Demonstrated directions.
B. Sensory stimulation. ✓
C. Verbal cues.
D. Hand-over-hand assistance.

Correct Answer: B.

Rationale:
A score of 6 on the Glasgow Coma Scale is just one level above a completely non-responsive coma. As a result, a person at this level has severe deficits. The person can open his/her eyes in response to pain and make incomprehensible sounds; therefore, intervention begins at the sensory stimulation level. The other choices are at levels that are too high for this individual.

Type of Reasoning: Inferential
One must determine the most likely intervention approach for a person, given the diagnosis provided and level of functioning. This requires inferential reasoning skill, where one must draw conclusions based on the information presented. In this situation, the therapist should begin with sensory stimulation, given the score of 6 on the Glasgow Coma Scale (GCS). If answered incorrectly, review intervention activities for individuals with TBI.

B14 **C5**

An occupational therapist working in an outpatient cardiac rehabilitation center develops an intervention plan for an individual who has entered the convalescence stage of cardiac recovery. Which activities should the therapist recommend be included in this intervention plan? *Stage 2 4-5mets*

Answer Choices:
A. Weeding a garden and doing low impact aerobics.
B. Putting away groceries and keyboarding.
C. Washing dishes and playing tabletop board games.
D. Carrying groceries upstairs and playing basketball.

Correct Answer: A.

Rationale:
Outpatient rehabilitation and the convalescence stage of recovery is Phase 2 of cardiac rehabilitation. At this point, activities should begin at a 4–5 MET level and progress to higher MET levels. Weeding a garden and doing low impact aerobics are at this level. Putting away groceries, keyboarding, washing dishes and playing tabletop board games are at a 1.0–2.5 MET level. These activities are appropriate for an individual in Phase I of cardiac rehabilitation. Carrying groceries upstairs and playing basketball are at a 6.0–10 MET level. These activities are not appropriate for a person just beginning Phase 2 of cardiac rehabilitation; however, they may be appropriate as the person progresses in the program.

Type of Reasoning: Deductive
One must recall the guidelines for MET level activity for patients in Phase 2 of cardiac rehabilitation. This is factual knowledge, which is a deductive reasoning skill. For this situation, the intervention plan would include weeding a garden and doing low impact aerobics. Review Phase 2 activity guidelines and MET levels if answered incorrectly.

B15 C8

An individual recovering from an exacerbation of multiple sclerosis is referred by a primary care physician to an outpatient occupational therapy clinic. The referral requests that the occupational therapist complete a functional capacity evaluation. Which is the most likely reason for this referral?

Answer Choices:

A. Determination of cognitive level.
B. Determination of disability status.
C. Assessment of instrumental activities of daily living.
D. Assessment of return-to-work capabilities. ✓

Correct Answer: D.

Rationale:

A functional capacity evaluation (FCE) evaluates an individual's capabilities for the physical demands of a specific job or for a group of occupations. It does not assess the other areas of concern identified.

Type of Reasoning: Inferential

One must determine the benefits of a functional capacity evaluation in order to arrive at a correct conclusion. In this situation, referral for a functional capacity evaluation is most appropriate for assessment of return-to-work capabilities. If answered incorrectly, review guidelines for administration of a functional capacity evaluation.

B16 C2

To develop social interaction skills, an occupational therapist implements a group program for students with Asperger's syndrome. Which group is best for the therapist to include in this program?

Answer Choices:

A. A directive group.
B. A topical group.
C. A developmental group. ✓
D. A task-oriented group.

Correct Answer: C.

Rationale:

A developmental group's focus is to teach the social interaction skills needed for group participation in a sequential manner. It provides relevant group structure and activities along a continuum that is consistent with how interaction skills typically develop. Asperger's syndrome is a pervasive developmental disorder. Individuals with Asperger's often have normal intelligence but significant deficits in social interaction skills. A directive group uses a highly structured 5-step approach to help low functioning patients (e.g., persons with dementia or serious and persistent mental disorders) develop basic skills. This group is too low functioning for students with Asperger's. A topical group is a discussion group that focuses on activities performed outside of the group (e.g., vocational planning). A task-oriented group's focus is to increase members' awareness of their values, ideas and feelings as revealed through group activity. This emphasis on intra-psychic functioning would be inappropriate for individuals with Asperger's syndrome.

Type of Reasoning: Inductive

This question requires the test taker to determine the best group focus for students with Asperger's syndrome and the need to focus on social interaction skills. This requires clinical judgment and knowledge of Asperger's syndrome symptoms in order to arrive at a correct conclusion, which is an inductive reasoning skill. In this case, the therapist should use a developmental group focus. If answered incorrectly, review the foci of different groups (especially developmental groups) and the social interaction needs of individuals with Asperger's syndrome. The integration of this knowledge is required to determine the correct answer.

B17 **C6**

A home-care occupational therapist plans intervention for an individual with agoraphobia with panic attacks. The occupational therapist plans to use a cognitive-behavioral approach. Which approach is most effective for the therapist to use during intervention?

Answer Choices:
A. A token reward system.
B. Behavioral extinction.
C. Sensorimotor tasks.
D. Systematic desensitization. ✓

Correct Answer: D.

Rationale:
Systematic desensitization is a cognitive-behavioral technique that introduces graded levels of the anxiety-producing stimuli. As the person responds to these stimuli, cognitive reframing of the situation and relaxation techniques are used to decrease anxiety. The introduction of graded levels of the stimuli combined with reframing and relaxation continues until the stimuli no longer produce an anxiety response. A token reward system involves the granting of tokens as a reward for desired behaviors. Behavioral extinction is a technique used to decrease undesirable behaviors by ignoring them and reinforcing desirable behaviors. These are not effective techniques for agoraphobia because the person's anxiety must be directly treated. Sensorimotor tasks are not a cognitive-behavioral approach and would not be indicated in this case.

Type of Reasoning: Inferential
One must infer or draw conclusions about a likely course of action, given the information presented. This is an inferential reasoning skill, where knowledge of a therapeutic approach, such as the cognitive-behavioral approach in this situation, is essential to choosing a correct solution. In this case, the therapist should choose systematic desensitization. Review the cognitive-behavioral approach, especially systematic desensitization if answered incorrectly.

B18 **C9**

A non-English speaking family attends a discharge planning session. The assigned occupational therapist does not share the language of the family. Which action should the therapist take first?

Answer Choices:
A. Make a referral for a home-care therapist to visit the family to provide in-home education.
B. Obtain a translator to communicate with the family during the session. ✓
C. Attempt to communicate with the family through non-verbal communication.
D. Consult with the case manager to develop a discharge plan.

Correct Answer: B.

Rationale:
The best choice to ensure the family involvement in the discharge planning process is to seek out a way to communicate directly and verbally with the family via a translator. The family is not included in these processes without a translator. Nonverbal communication does not transcend a language barrier for abstract concepts such as incorporating the individual's needs, values and goals of treatment. There is no need for the therapist to consult with a case manager if the therapist has already been assigned this case. The therapist can independently get a translator to help communicate with the family. In addition, the occupational therapist should not develop a discharge plan without the family's input.

Type of Reasoning: Evaluative
This question requires one to determine the best course of action that considers the needs of the family and most effectively facilitates delivery of services. Questions that ask the test-taker to use judgment to determine a best course of action often utilize evaluative reasoning skills. In this situation, and in keeping with the AOTA Code of Ethics, the therapist should seek out a translator. Review cultural competency guidelines, including providing translation services.

B19 **C1**

The parents of an infant born at 32 weeks gestation are about to take the baby home after four weeks in the neonatal intensive care nursery. Which is most important for the occupational therapist to instruct the parents to avoid?

Answer Choices:
A. Placing the infant in the prone position for sleeping. ✓
B. Placing the infant in the supine position for sleeping.
C. Using an infant swing with a head support for calming.
D. Presenting toys in the mid-line with the infant in the prone position for playing.

Correct Answer: A.

Rationale:
The infant should be encouraged to sleep in supine to prevent Sudden Infant Death Syndrome (SIDS). An infant swing can provide slow, rhythmic vestibular input that can be calming to infants. A swing can also provide visual stimulation and proper alignment in supported sitting. Toys should be presented in mid-line with the infant in the prone position. This positioning provides the infant with visual stimulation and the opportunity to develop play, social and cognitive skills. This "tummy-time" also facilitates head control and prevents a flattened head that can occur when a child sleeps in supine.

Type of Reasoning: Inferential
One must determine the contraindications for activity in premature infants. This requires inferential reasoning, where one must determine a most important course of action. In this situation, the discharge plan should include instruction to avoid sleeping in prone to avoid SIDS. If answered incorrectly, review positioning guidelines for infants and SIDS.

B20 **C4**

Following an acute hospitalization for the medical management of a CVA, an individual receives home-based occupational therapy services. The occupational therapist is working on dressing skills with the patient. During one session, the therapist has the individual dress in the bedroom and during the next session the therapist has the client dress in the bathroom. During the following session, the therapist has the client don and doff a sweater and coat in the living room. Which motor learning technique is the therapist using?

Answer Choices:
A. Variable activities.
B. Variable conditions. ✓
C. Repetition.
D. Generalization.

Correct Answer: B.

Rationale:
Variable conditions involve the practice and performance of skills in various contexts to improve the transfer of learning and retention of skills. Variable activities is a contrived term. Dressing during three different sessions is not repetitive. Varying the performance and practice context can facilitate the ability to generalize a skill but generalization is not a treatment technique; rather it is a desired outcome of intervention.

Type of Reasoning: Inferential
One must link the functional activity to the appropriate motor learning technique. This requires inferential reasoning, where one must infer or draw conclusions based on the evidence presented. In this case the technique described is that of variable conditions. If answered incorrectly, review motor learning theory and the application of variable conditions.

B21 C2

An occupational therapist provides bedside BADL training to a patient recovering from multiple injuries incurred during a motor vehicle accident. The patient's children arrive for a visit and ask the therapist to let them look at their parent's chart while they wait outside the room for the session to conclude. Which response is best for the therapist to make in response to this request?

Answer Choices:
A. Tell the family members that they must have the permission of their parent before they can look at the chart.
B. Commend the family members for their interest in their parent's status and give them the chart to read.
C. Tell the family members they cannot see the chart because they could misinterpret the information.
D. Tell the family members to go ask the unit's charge nurse for permission to look at the chart.

Correct Answer: A.

Rationale:
According to the Health Insurance and Portability Accountability Act (HIPAA), the therapist must obtain the person's permission prior to sharing any information about the person's status with family members or significant others. HIPAA does allow providers to use their clinical judgment to determine whether to discuss the person's case with others if the person cannot give permission or objects. Documentation for this decision is essential (e.g., person is at risk of harming self due to lack of judgment; consultation with a specialist is essential to ensure quality of care). All information used or disclosed about a person's status must be limited to the minimum needed for the immediate purpose. There is no need for the therapist to advise the family members to speak to the charge nurse. The therapist can directly inform the family of the HIPAA guidelines.

Type of Reasoning: Evaluative
One must weigh the courses of action presented and determine which approach will result in the most effective outcome and follow federal guidelines for protecting patient privacy. This is an evaluative reasoning skill. For this situation, having knowledge of HIPAA guidelines, the therapist should tell the family members that they must have the permission of their parent before they can look at the chart. Review HIPAA guidelines for protecting patient privacy if answered incorrectly.

B22 C4

An occupational therapist provides intervention for an individual with a swallowing disorder. To elicit a swallow reflex, the occupational therapist provides sensory input to the inferior faucial arches. Which should the therapist use to provide this intervention?

Answer Choices:
A. A tongue depressor.
B. A moistened cotton swab.
C. A chilled dental examination mirror. ✓
D. A warmed metal teaspoon.

Correct Answer: C.

Rationale:
The use of cold stimulation of the inferior faucial arches via a chilled dental examination mirror will elicit a swallow reflex. The others will not.

Type of Reasoning: Inferential
One must determine the guidelines for eliciting a swallow reflex and then determine which of the listed devices is aligned with the stimulation of this reflex. This requires inferential reasoning skill. In this situation, a chilled dental examination mirror is ideal. If answered incorrectly, review elicitation of the swallow reflex.

B23 C1

A child with a diagnosis of traumatic brain injury (TBI) is evaluated by an occupational therapist. The child presents with extension of both upper extremities and flexion of both lower extremities following a stimulus of neck extension. When interpreting this observation, which statement is most accurate for the therapist to document?

Answer Choices:
A. The presence of + ATNR, which is "abnormal" and has reappeared after the TBI.
B. The presence of a + STNR, which is "normal" and not affected by the TBI.
C. The presence of a + ATNR, which is "normal" and not affected by the TBI.
D. The presence of a + STNR, which is "abnormal" and has reappeared after the TBI. ✓

Correct Answer: D.

Rationale:
STNR is facilitated by flexion of the neck followed by extension of the neck. The response is that flexion of the neck results in bilateral UE flexion with bilateral LE extension. Neck extension results in bilateral UE extension with bilateral LE flexion. Positive reactions are normal up to four to six months of age. Positive reactions after six months of age are indicative of delayed reflexive maturation or pathology.

Type of Reasoning: Analytical
This question provides symptoms and the test taker must determine the likely cause for them. This is an analytical reasoning skill, as questions of this nature often ask one to analyze a group of symptoms in order to determine a diagnosis. In this situation, the symptoms indicate + STNR, an abnormal reflexive response that has reappeared after the TBI. Review the STNR if answered incorrectly.

B24 C6

An individual with moderate intellectual disability moves into a group home. An initial goal established for this resident is the development of socially acceptable table manners. The occupational therapist uses a behavior modification approach to achieve this goal. Which intervention technique is best for the therapist to include in the design of the group home dining experience?

Answer Choices:
A. Negative reinforcement for socially inappropriate behaviors.
B. Clear explanations of behaviors expected during dining.
C. Clear explanations about the effects of inappropriate behaviors on others.
D. Rewards for socially appropriate behaviors. ✓

Correct Answer: D.

Rationale:
A behavior modification program provides positive reinforcement for desired behaviors. Negative reinforcement for undesirable behaviors is not the preferred approach, because it focuses on deficits rather than skill development. While it is important to provide a person with clear explanations of behaviors, this would not be the most effective approach for the development of concrete specific skills in a behavior modification program. In addition, since the person has moderate intellectual disability, the individual's ability to understand these expectations or the effect of the behaviors on others may be limited due to deficits in abstract thinking.

Type of Reasoning: Inferential
One must have knowledge of intellectual disabilities and behavior modification guidelines in order to arrive at a correct conclusion. This is an inferential reasoning skill where knowledge of clinical guidelines and judgment based on facts are utilized to reach conclusions. In this situation, the therapist should provide rewards for socially appropriate behaviors. If answered incorrectly, review behavior modification principles.

B25 C9

A toddler with severe congenital anomalies and an irreparable cleft palate has a do not resuscitate (DNR) order. While being fitted for a molded seat for a wheelchair, the child stops breathing and turns blue. The entry-level occupational therapist determines that the child has a brachial pulse. Which of the following is the first action the therapist should take in response to this situation?

Answer Choices:
A. Inform the physician about the situation and the child's DNR order.
B. Call the supervising occupational therapist to discuss the best response.
C. Implement the facility's emergency procedure. ✓
D. Perform obstructed airway maneuver and monitor heart rate for five minutes.

Correct Answer: C.

Rationale:
The child is not breathing and the therapist should initiate the facility's plan for medical emergencies and cardiac codes. It is not the decision of the therapist to withhold treatment or to provide intervention. The medical team that responds to emergency procedures must make the decision about the best action to take in a DNR situation. It would be desirable to inform the physician, but the current situation requires emergency attention. The therapist can call the supervising occupational therapist to advise of the event and discuss the necessary follow-up after dealing with the event, but this is not the first action. Even a minute delay is too long to wait to notify the emergency team.

Type of Reasoning: Evaluative
This question requires one to make a value judgment about a best course of action, given the information presented. This necessitates evaluative reasoning where one must weigh the merits of the possible course of action in order to make a sound decision. For this situation, the therapist should implement the facility's emergency procedure. If answered incorrectly, review emergency management guidelines, especially DNR orders.

B26 C8

A seven-year-old child with spina bifida at the C-7 level receives home-based occupational therapy services. Which ability is most relevant for the occupational therapist to focus on during intervention?

Answer Choices:
A. Dressing the lower body. ✓
B. Dressing the upper body.
C. Brushing teeth.
D. Playing tabletop games.

Correct Answer: A.

Rationale:
An individual with a spinal cord lesion at C-7 has difficulty dressing the lower extremities. At seven, a child is typically independent in dressing; therefore, an intervention to increase the ability to dress the lower body is age appropriate. An individual with a C-7 lesion is independent in upper extremity dressing, personal grooming and tabletop activities; thus, no intervention is warranted.

Type of Reasoning: Inferential
One must determine the most likely intervention approach for a child, given the diagnosis provided. This requires inferential reasoning skill, where one must draw conclusions based on the information presented. In this situation, dressing the lower body is the likely intervention. If answered incorrectly, review levels of spinal cord injury and their corresponding functional abilities. Understanding how these capabilities would impact on the ADL of children with cervical spina bifida is required to correctly answer this question.

B27 C9

An OT administrator is designing a patient satisfaction questionnaire to be administered upon discharge from the OT program. The administrator designs the questionnaire so that individuals will indicate their level of agreement with a series of statements by circling a number with 1 = very dissatisfied, 2 = dissatisfied, 3 = neutral, 4 = satisfied and 5 = very satisfied. Which method of data collection is the administrator using?

Answer Choices:
A. Gutman scale rank ordering.
B. A Likert scale. ✓
C. Retrospective data.
D. A semantic differential.

Correct Answer: B.

Rationale:
Likert scales have respondents indicate their level of agreement according to a scale, usually with 5 points. Gutman scale rank ordering is a method in which a respondent places a number along side a list of items, indicating their order of importance. Retrospective data is data collected in the past. Semantic differential is a point scale with opposing adjectives at two extremes, measuring affective meaning.

Type of Reasoning: Deductive
One must recall the different types of data collection methods in order to arrive at a correct conclusion. This is factual knowledge, which is a deductive reasoning skill. The described scale is characteristic of a Likert scale, which should be reviewed if answered incorrectly.

B28 C8

A ten-year-old with congenital anomalies wears bilateral ankle-foot orthoses. The parents want the child to be able to don and doff shoes independently, but the child cannot tie shoes. Which is the best footwear recommendation for the therapist to make for the child to wear?

Answer Choices:
A. Leather slip-on loafers.
B. Slip-on tennis shoes with no laces.
C. Running shoes with Velcro shoe closures.
D. Hi-rise sneakers with sliding adapters on the laces.

Correct Answer: C.

Rationale:
Running shoes are the best option for use with ankle-foot-orthoses (AFOs) and Velcro closures will help the child to be independent until tying is learned. Leather slip-on loafers will not correctly support the ankle-foot orthoses (AFOs). Slip-on tennis shoes that do not have laces do not have adequate support in the upper part of the foot to maintain the AFOs. The sliding adapters are a good option to replace the laces, but the hi-rise sneakers will not likely allow for placement of the AFOs on the feet.

Type of Reasoning: Inductive
Clinical knowledge and judgment are the most important skills needed for answering this question, which requires inductive reasoning skill. Knowledge of the diagnosis and most appropriate clinical outcomes is key to choosing the best solution. In this case, shoes with Velcro closures are best as it helps facilitate independence while providing the needed support when wearing AFOs. If answered incorrectly, review footwear adaptations to facilitate independence in fastening and tying.

B29 C4

A patient who is status-post left frontal lobe ischemia has difficulty bearing weight through the right lower extremity during reaching activities (e.g., standing at a sink during morning self-care routine). The occupational therapist implements a Motor Re-Learning Program (MRP). Which is the best intervention for the therapist to provide according to this approach?

Answer Choices:
A. Therapeutic handling to affect the central nervous system.
B. A stool to sit on during reaching activities.
C. Joint compression to the right lower extremity during reaching activities.
D. Verbal and visual feedback while practicing reaching.

Correct Answer: D.

Rationale:
A MRP approach provides verbal and visual feedback to give a person the input needed to make postural and limb adjustments. Therapeutic handling to affect the central nervous system is consistent with a neurodevelopmental therapy approach. Providing a stool to sit on during reaching activities can be used for safety purposes. This is consistent with a compensatory approach. Joint compression is a technique used for sensory modulation disorders (e.g., tactile defensiveness, hypersensitivity/over-responsivity; and hyposensitivity/under-responsivity and sensory seeking).

Type of Reasoning: Deductive
One must recall the guidelines of a Motor Re-Learning Program in order to arrive at a correct conclusion. This is factual knowledge, which is a deductive reasoning skill. For this situation the most appropriate intervention is verbal and visual feedback while practicing reaching. If answered incorrectly, review Motor Re-Learning Program guidelines.

B30 C9

A new outpatient mental health facility offering occupational therapy services opens in a community of 100,000. The occupational therapy director of an established outpatient program is concerned that the new program will affect service delivery. Which action is best for the director of the established program to take in response to this potential competition?

Answer Choices:
A. Wait for the new facility to implement services and develop services in the areas not covered by that facility.
B. Offer the same services that the new facility offers and advertise a competitive price.
C. Conduct a program evaluation and develop a marketing plan based on the results.
D. Design an intensive marketing campaign to local consumers and third party payers.

Correct Answer: C.

Rationale:
The best approach is to conduct a program evaluation to identify the strengths and limitations of the existing program and then develop a promotional plan that highlights the program's strongest aspects. The results of a program evaluation can also be used to address the limitations of the existing program to help it provide services that are reflective of best practice. The development of new services and the offering of services similar to the new facility's services would require a needs assessment to determine the necessity of services. Prior to beginning a marketing campaign, one should first evaluate a program to determine its most marketable aspects.

Type of Reasoning: Inductive
This question requires one to utilize clinical judgment in order to determine a best course of action. In this situation, the therapist should conduct a program evaluation and develop a marketing plan based on those results. Inductive reasoning skill often requires one to predict what is likely to occur, given a current situation. Therefore, in answering this question, one should predict that a program evaluation would result in the most benefit.

B31 C8

An individual with obsessive-compulsive personality disorder participates in a vocational program. The client asks the occupational therapist to speak to the supervisor of the transitional employment program (TEP). The client is concerned that compulsive behaviors are interfering with job performance and may result in the loss of a new TEP placement. Which is the therapist's best response to these expressed concerns?

Answer Choices:
A. Instruct the client to speak directly to the TEP supervisor about the right to receive reasonable accommodations.
B. Schedule a re-evaluation of the client's work behaviors and skills.
C. Assure the client that it is natural to have initial difficulties at a new job.
D. Schedule an appointment with the client and the TEP supervisor.

Correct Answer: D.

Rationale:
Meeting with the individual and the supervisor will enable the therapist to provide support for the individual's concerns. The therapist can also facilitate a dialogue about the specific difficulties the individual is experiencing from both the employee and employer perspective. This will help the therapist analyze the situation and can provide a basis for making recommendations for accommodations, if needed. Instructing the individual to speak directly to the work supervisor ignores the request for the therapist's input. In addition, knowing one's rights for reasonable accommodations as provided by the Americans with Disabilities Act (ADA) does not equate to knowing what accommodations will help with work performance. A complete evaluation of the essential functions of the job and the person's skills and abilities must be completed prior to determining the nature of accommodations. Re-evaluating the individual's work behaviors and skills does not address the individual's stated concerns. In addition, TEP placements are typically made after an extensive evaluation process. This information would be readily available for the therapist to review, if needed. While it is natural to have initial difficulties and concerns when one begins a new job, reassuring the person of this reality does not address the individual's request for the occupational therapist's support.

Type of Reasoning: Evaluative
This question requires professional judgment based on guiding principles, which is an evaluative reasoning skill. For this situation, the therapist should schedule an appointment with the supervisor and the individual in order to analyze the situation and make any needed recommendations. Review transitional employment guidelines and fostering success in individuals if answered incorrectly.

B32 C6

In an acute inpatient psychiatric facility, an occupational therapist designs a therapeutic activity group for individuals with poor orientation to reality. Which is the best activity choice for the therapist to provide in this group?

Answer Choices:
A. A discussion of the effects of hospitalization on occupational roles. ✗
B. The assembly of wooden toys for a children's unit. ✓
C. Guided imagery for stress management. ✗
D. Structured verbalizations of personal assets and limitations. ✗

Correct Answer: B.

Rationale:
On an acute inpatient psychiatric unit, activities should be structured, easily completed in one session and provide a concrete result to reinforce reality. Wooden toy kits meet these criteria and donating them to the children's unit facilitates Yalom's curative factor of altruism. Discussions and verbal activities are abstract and would be difficult for persons with poor orientation to reality. They also involve personal issues that require time to process feelings, adequate verbal skills, and adequate level of insight. This time is not available in a setting with a short length of stay. Guided imagery can be difficult for a disoriented person to focus on and can be frightening to an acutely ill person. Unstructured types of activities can actually increase symptoms and reinforce poor reality orientation.

Type of Reasoning: Inductive
One must determine which activity best meets the needs of persons who are acutely ill and disoriented. This requires inductive reasoning skill, where the test taker must utilize clinical judgment to determine a best course of action. In this situation, assembly of wooden toys for a children's unit is the best choice for individuals with poor orientation to reality as it provides structured activity that is easily completed in one session. If answered incorrectly, review Mosey's taxonomy of groups and recommended therapeutic activities for acutely ill individuals in inpatient psychiatric settings.

B33 C1

An occupational therapy professional education program provides an after-school play program for normally developing children to help students understand typical development. The students observe a child who is beginning to use blunt scissors to snip paper. The child opens and closes the scissors and moves them in a controlled forward motion, but the child cannot cut circles or figure shapes. At which age are these behaviors typical?

Answer Choices:
A. 2 years-old.
B. 3 years-old. ✓
C. 4 years-old.
D. 5 years-old.

Correct Answer: B.

Rationale:
The described activities are typical of 3-year-old children. The behaviors described in this scenario are too advanced for 2 year-old children. While older children can perform the described activities, they typically are cutting circles at $3\frac{1}{2}$–$4\frac{1}{2}$ years and cutting simple figure shapes at 4–6 years.

Type of Reasoning: Deductive
One must recall developmental motor milestones of children in order to arrive at a correct conclusion for this question. This necessitates the recall of factual guidelines, which is a deductive reasoning skill. For this scenario, the behaviors described are typical of 3-year-old children. Review motor skills and developmental milestones of children, especially skills of 3-year-olds, if answered incorrectly.

B34 C9

An adult who incurred a severe traumatic brain injury (TBI) is entering the second week of care at a long-term TBI rehabilitation center. The patient's family visit regularly and frequently asks multiple questions of the treatment team. A team and family conference is planned to address family concerns. Which is the most important information for the team to share with the family?

Answer Choices:
A. Realistic and clear information about the individual's current status and care plan. ✓
B. Each team member's expert opinion about the expected prognosis and discharge recommendations.
C. Reimbursement information about each professional service to assist in determining treatment choices.
D. Community resources that are available to support the family and provide respite care.

Correct Answer: A.

Rationale:
The family needs to understand the individual's current status and what is being done in treatment to facilitate recovery. This information can help the family support the team's care plan. Since the individual has only been in rehabilitation for two weeks, it is not possible for the team to know the prognosis or discharge plan. Reimbursement is always pertinent to the provision of care, but it is not the primary basis for determining interventions. Providing the family with support is always important; however, community-based support programs are focused on individuals with TBI who have completed the acute rehabilitation phase. Most (if not all) TBI rehabilitation centers offer on-site support programs for families, which would be more relevant to this family's current needs. Respite services may or may not be needed by the family, depending upon the individual's level of recovery, which cannot be determined at this point.

Type of Reasoning: Inferential
One must determine the benefits of providing the information described in order to determine which information would be most important. This requires inferential reasoning, where one must draw conclusions of the benefits to the family based on the information provided. In this situation, providing realistic and clear information about the individual's current status and care plan is most important. Review the purposes of family conference meetings and the guidelines for client-centered care if answered incorrectly.

B35 C3

An occupational therapist supervises a Level II Fieldwork student regarding the evaluation procedures of a work hardening program. The therapist explains that some individuals attending the program magnify their symptoms to retain benefits; therefore the validity of some evaluation measures may be compromised. Which assessment tool does the therapist identify as providing the most valid results?

Answer Choices:
A. A volumeter.
B. A dynamometer (all five positions).
C. A standardized pegboard test.
D. A total active motion (TAM) evaluation.

Correct Answer: A.

Rationale:
The volumeter is the only true objective assessment tool that occupational therapists utilize for it is based on the displacement law of physics. It is the only tool that a person cannot manipulate.

Type of Reasoning: Inferential
One must have knowledge of all the assessment tools described and proper administration in order to arrive at a correct conclusion. This is an inferential reasoning skill where knowledge of clinical guidelines and judgment based on facts are utilized to reach conclusions. In this case, the only assessment that cannot be manipulated is volumeter measurements. If answered incorrectly, review volumeter assessment guidelines.

B36 C9

Two occupational therapy assistants (OTAs) working for a school district are assigned to two different schools. One school has a supervising occupational therapist, the other school does not. The OTA without a supervising therapist expresses concern to the OTA who is supervised about the lack of supervision. Which is the best response for the supervised OTA to take in response to this situation?

Answer Choices:
A. Report the situation to the OT supervisor.
B. Share information acquired during supervisory sessions with the unsupervised OTA.
C. Advise the unsupervised OTA to contact the state regulatory board.
D. Report the situation to the school district's administration.

Correct Answer: A.

Rationale:
The first step is for the OTA to discuss the situation with his/her supervisor since all of the concerned parties work in the same school district. The OT supervisor would then be the appropriate person to further explore the situation and find a solution with his/her supervisor. There is no need at this point to go beyond the OT supervisor's level. While it can be beneficial to share information gained during supervisory sessions, this process is no substitute for supervision.

Type of Reasoning: Evaluative

One must weigh the possible courses of action and then make a value judgment about the best course of action to take. This requires evaluative reasoning skill, which often utilizes guiding principles of action in order to arrive at a correct conclusion. In this case, because the OTA is concerned about the lack of supervision, the OTA should report the situation to the OT supervisor.

B37 C2

A single parent of two school-aged children is employed as a truck driver working the 11 pm–7 am shift. The client was hospitalized for depression following the sudden death of the client's spouse one year ago. The deceased spouse's primary role had been home maintainer. The client was re-hospitalized this past weekend for an exacerbation of depression. Which skills are most relevant for the occupational therapist to evaluate?

Answer Choices:

A. Interpersonal.
B. Self-management.
C. Cognitive.
D. Leisure.

Correct Answer: B.

Rationale:

This individual has experienced major role disruptions, including the loss of a spousal role and the assumption of the home maintainer role. These major life changes require significant self-management skills. The evaluation of interpersonal skills and cognitive skills are not indicated in this case for there is no information in the scenario identifying deficits in these areas. Leisure is an area of occupation, not a performance skill.

Type of Reasoning: Inferential

One must infer or draw conclusions about a likely course of action, given the information presented. This is an inferential reasoning skill, where knowledge of a therapeutic approach, such as evaluation of performance skills is essential to choosing a correct solution. In this case, the therapist should evaluate self-management skills. Review evaluation of performance skills in persons with depression if answered incorrectly.

B38 C5

An individual with a body mass index (BMI) of 35 is joining a community-based wellness program conducted by an occupational therapist. When formulating an individualized wellness plan, which condition should the occupational therapist take into consideration as an increased risk for this person?

Answer Choices:

A. Hypothermia during exertion.
B. Hyperthermia during exertion.
C. Rapid weight loss during the initial weeks.
D. Increased anxiety and depression.

Correct Answer: B.

Rationale:

A patient with a body mass index of 35 is considered obese and is at increased risk of hyperthermia during exertion. Weight loss will occur after the person actively engages in a wellness program that includes lifestyle redesign, a nutritional diet and exercise over an extended period of time, not just in the initial weeks. An individualized wellness program should decrease anxiety and depression, not increase them.

Type of Reasoning: Inferential
This question requires one to infer a patient's risk factors based on the diagnosis provided. This is an inferential reasoning skill, as one must determine what may be true of a patient, although one cannot be 100% certain. In this case, the patient is likely to have hyperthermia during exertion. If answered incorrectly, review risk factors for patients with obesity.

B39 C9

The supervisor of an acute inpatient unit requests that a recently hired entry-level therapist write summaries of several evaluation sessions that were completed by another therapist. The evaluating therapist had to leave work unexpectedly due to a medical emergency and is not expected to return to work. Which is the best response for the therapist to make in response to this request?

Answer Choices:
A. Comply with the supervisor's request but ask for the supervisor to co-sign the notes.
B. Request time to complete an independent evaluation of each individual previously evaluated.
C. Report the supervisor's request to the facility's administration.
D. Suggest that the therapist's evaluation results be documented by the supervisor.

Correct Answer: D.

Rationale:
It is not appropriate for a peer to document results of an evaluation session in which he/she did not participate. It is acceptable for a supervisor to provide documentation based upon staff's input, as long as the documentation reports that it is based upon the work of a given staff member. The supervisor must provide an accurate record of the situation (i.e., evaluation completed by therapist X found that. . .). In an acute inpatient setting, there is insufficient time to complete another evaluation. The entry-level therapist should communicate directly with his/her supervisor. There is nothing to report to the administration at this time.

Type of Reasoning: Evaluative
This question requires professional judgment based on guiding principles, which is an evaluative reasoning skill. In this situation, the therapist's most appropriate response is to suggest that the therapist's evaluation results be documented by the supervisor. Accuracy in record keeping is important in this situation and should be used as the guiding principle in finding the best solution to this situation.

B40 C8

An individual prepares for discharge home following rehabilitation for a left CVA. Residual difficulties include fair dynamic balance, decreased upper extremity (UE) strength and poor dexterity. The individual's stated priority is to be able to ambulate safely to the senior center located in the client's apartment building. Which ambulatory aid would be most effective for the occupational therapist to recommend to this client?

Answer Choices:
A. A hemi-walker.
B. A rolling walker.
C. A side-stepper walker.
D. A standard walker.

Correct Answer: B.

Rationale:
A rolling walker is indicated for a person who cannot lift a standard walker due to impaired balance or upper extremity weakness. A hemi-walker and side-stepper are indicated for individuals who do not have use of both hands. This individual has poor dexterity in the affected UE, but only gross grasp is needed to hold a walker.

Type of Reasoning: Inferential
One must determine the most appropriate ambulatory aid, given knowledge of the presenting symptoms and limitations. This requires inferential reasoning skill, where one must infer or draw conclusions about a best course of action. In this situation, the therapist should recommend a rolling walker. Review guidelines for use of a rolling walker and other ambulatory aids if answered incorrectly.

B41 C3

An individual with rheumatoid arthritis (RA) is currently in a stage of remission. During this inactive chronic phase of this disease, the occupational therapist works with the client to maintain range of motion (ROM) and muscle strength. Which of the following is most effective for the therapist to recommend the client include in a daily home exercise program?

Answer Choices:
A. Passive ROM.
B. Active ROM.
C. Isotonics.
D. Progressive resistance.

Correct Answer: B.

Rationale:
Activities that use active ROM are indicated for the treatment of RA both in its acute and chronic phases. Passive ROM is generally contraindicated for persons with RA. If a person is unable to perform AROM, gentle passive ROM may be used with caution. Progressive resistance is also contraindicated in the treatment of RA. The use of isotonic exercises for individuals with RA is somewhat controversial. If isotonics are considered for an intervention, the occupational therapist must establish that the individual's joints are stable and would benefit from isotonic exercises without jeopardizing other joints. The individual's response to these exercises must be monitored; therefore, isotonics are not appropriate for an unmonitored home care program.

Type of Reasoning: Inductive
One must utilize clinical judgment in order to determine the best exercise approach for a patient with RA. Questions that require one to use knowledge of a diagnosis, coupled with therapeutic approaches often require inductive reasoning skill. For this situation, active ROM is indicated in both acute and chronic phases of RA. If answered incorrectly, review exercise guidelines for patients with RA.

B42 C9

An occupational therapist employed in a pediatric clinic participates in an initial performance appraisal. The supervisor identifies the area needing improvement as handling skills in working with children with various types of cerebral palsy. Which is the most effective way for the occupational therapist to improve handling skills?

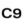

Answer Choices:
A. Observe an experienced occupational or physical therapist use handling techniques.
B. Complete an evidence-based practice literature review on the use of handling techniques for children with cerebral palsy.
C. Participate in an advanced level experiential course on handling techniques. ✓
D. Participate in a teleconference on handling techniques for children with cerebral palsy.

Correct Answer: C.

Rationale:
Participating in an advanced handling skills course provides opportunities to learn and practice these techniques. It would also provide opportunities to interact with other therapists and benefit from visual and kinesthetic learning. Observing a skilled therapist is helpful but does not offer the opportunity to develop hands-on skills. A literature review and a teleconference can cover a variety of information about best practices and handling techniques for children with cerebral palsy. However, these offer little opportunity to learn handling skills, which is a hands-on competence rather than knowledge-based.

Type of Reasoning: Inferential
The test taker must draw conclusions about the best way to improve skills in the use of handling techniques with children who have cerebral palsy. The key to arriving at a correct conclusion is determining the best way to acquire knowledge and skill in a technique that requires hands-on skills. In this situation, participating in an advanced practice course on handling techniques will provide the most hands-on opportunity to learn the skills. If answered incorrectly, review approaches to improve therapeutic techniques and competency.

Multiple Choice Scenario Item B.I.

Questions B43 to B47 are based on the following information.

An adult who incurred a traumatic brain injury three months ago is referred to a home care agency to receive OT services. The client's referral states that cognition is at Level VII of the Rancho Los Amigos scale and that grasp and shoulder mobility are limited. During the initial interview, the client reports being frustrated by the inability to independently engage in the previously enjoyed and personally meaningful activity of cooking. The client reports frequently losing place when reading recipes and an inability to "find" things in the kitchen.

B43 C7

Upon evaluation, the client exhibits difficulty with the letter cancellation task. Which visual deficit should the occupational therapist document as present?

Answer Choices:
A. Imagery.
B. Scanning. ✓
C. Cognition.
D. Memory.

Correct Answer: B.

Rationale:
The behaviors described relate to the ability to scan. Visual imagery is the process of making a mental picture of information so that it can be remembered. Visual cognition is the ability to mentally manipulate visual information and integrate it with other sensory information. Visual memory is the retrieval and recall of information that has been stored and encoded.

Type of Reasoning: Analytical
This question provides symptoms of a deficit and the test taker must determine what these symptoms indicate. This requires analytical reasoning skill, where one must consider all of the pieces of information provided and draw conclusions about what that means as a whole. In this situation, the symptoms indicate deficits in visual scanning ability. If answered incorrectly, review the definitions of visual perceptual skills and the symptoms of visual perceptual deficits.

B44 C7

During meal preparation tasks the client ignores items on the left side of the counter. The therapist decides to use a compensatory functional approach to improve the client's performance. Which is the most appropriate method for the therapist to use during intervention to develop meal preparation skills?

Answer Choices:
A. Encourage bilateral activities.
B. Place all items on the right side of the counter.
C. Practice scanning activities.
D. Place a brightly colored placemat on the left side of the counter.

Correct Answer: D.

Rationale:
The placemat provides an external cue which the person can be taught to scan for during meal preparation. This anchoring technique is a basic compensatory functional approach. Encouraging bilateral activities and placing all items on the right side of the counter would not address the client's performance deficit. Using practice of scanning activities is a transfer of training approach which assumes that remediation of the cause of the presenting symptom will result in increased functional skills.

Type of Reasoning: Inferential
This question requires one to draw conclusions and make certain assumptions about clinical situations based on evidence, which is an inferential reasoning skill. For this scenario, placing a brightly colored placemat on the left side of the counter utilizes a compensatory functional approach to address the person's deficit. If answered incorrectly, review information on cognitive-perceptual intervention strategies.

B45 C7

The client responds well to the compensatory approach when performing countertop meal preparation tasks. The therapist decides to use a dynamic interactional approach as the theoretical foundation for cognitive perceptual intervention for other meal preparation activities. During a session to train the client in scanning strategies, the client accurately finds two items in a refrigerator. Which is the therapist's most appropriate initial response to the client's task success?

Answer Choices:
A. Praise the client for successful task completion.
B. Ask the client to now find three items in the refrigerator.
C. Ask the client how he/she knows that the items are correct.
D. Ask the client to now find two items in the pantry.

Correct Answer: C.

Rationale:

A fundamental technique in the dynamic interactional approach is awareness questioning to help the individual identify successes, detect errors, estimate task difficulty and predict outcomes. The person's processing abilities and the use of self monitoring techniques are used to facilitate learning for different tasks and/or environments. Praising the individual provides positive feedback but it does not develop the desired self-awareness of abilities that is a foundation of this approach. Adding more items to scan and a new environment (for example, the pantry) to scan are approaches that would be used after the person developed awareness of the strategies that led to success in the initial activity.

Type of Reasoning: Inferential

One must have knowledge of the dynamic interactional approach and typical strategies in order to arrive at a correct conclusion. This is an inferential reasoning skill where knowledge of clinical guidelines and judgment based on facts are utilized to reach conclusions. In this situation, the therapist should ask the person how he/she knows that the items are correct. If answered incorrectly, review the dynamic interactional approach and intervention strategies.

B46 C4

During an intervention session focused on the development of grasp and shoulder mobility, the occupational therapist asks the client to move numerous identical one pound cans of vegetables from the counter top to the cabinet shelf above the counter. According to contemporary motor learning approaches, which type of practice has the therapist designed this activity to provide to the client?

Answer Choices:

A. Random practice.
B. Blocked practice.
C. Planned practice.
D. Contextual practice.

Correct Answer: B.

Rationale:

Blocked practice involves repeated performance of the same motor skill. Since the cans are identical and weigh the same, lifting each can requires the same motor skill. If the cans were of different sizes, shapes and/or weights then different motor skills would be required for task performance. This would be an example of random practice which involves the performance of several tasks in random order to encourage the re-formulation of the solution to the presented motor problem. Planned practice and contextual practice are contrived terms.

Type of Reasoning: Analytical

This question requires one to analyze the information provided and determine the best descriptor for this functional activity. This requires analytical reasoning skill, where one must weigh all of the information provided in order to arrive at a correct conclusion. For this situation, the activity presented is that of blocked practice. Review guidelines for motor practice, especially blocked practice if answered incorrectly.

B47 C8

The client is attending a vocational rehabilitation program three days a week but is frequently late due to difficulties with getting ready in the morning. The client asks the home-care therapist for suggestions to address this problem. Which is the most appropriate action for the occupational therapist to take in response to the client's request?

Answer Choices:

A. Advocate that the vocational program provide the client with a flexible start time.

B. Develop a visual chart with the client, depicting the necessary sequence of his morning activities. ✓

C. Advise the client to call the vocational program to tell staff when running late.

D. Advise the client to wake up one hour earlier on vocational rehabilitation program days.

Correct Answer: B.

Rationale:

Individuals at Rancho Los Amigos Level VII have cognitive abilities that are automatic-appropriate. They are able to initiate and attend to highly familiar tasks (e.g., BADL) in a distraction-free environment, but have shallow recall of what has been completed. Creating a visual chart of the necessary sequence of routine morning activities will provide the person with a tool that he/she can use each morning to check off ADL task ✓ completion. This visual cueing device can also help the client refocus if he/she gets distracted. Increasing the time available in the morning to do the daily routine is not needed. The client does not have any sensorimotor deficits that require extended time for ADL performance. In addition, having extra time can increase the potential for distractions and can decrease focus. While it is polite to call when one is going to be late, this action is not addressing the client's need to develop an organized effective routine. Changing the vocational rehabilitation program schedule is also inappropriate for this reason.

Type of Reasoning: Inductive

One must utilize clinical knowledge and judgment to determine the most appropriate action to address an individual's unique challenge. This requires inductive reasoning skill. In this case, the occupational therapist should develop a visual chart with the individual, depicting the sequence of morning activities. If answered incorrectly, review scales and activities for the different cognitive levels, especially activity completion for individuals at Level VII.

B48 **C8**

An occupational therapist is conducting a community transportation group with individuals attending a traumatic brain injury day treatment program in an urban area. Which should the group do first?

Answer Choices:

A. Read a subway or bus map.

B. Take a subway or bus as a group.

C. Determine a destination. ✓

D. Purchase a subway or bus fare card.

Correct Answer: C.

Rationale:

The first step is to determine a desired destination. Then the group would need to decide the mode of transportation that would be used to reach the desired destination. Map reading skills would be used to determine the specific bus and/or subway route(s) to take to arrive at the desired destination. Purchasing a fare card and taking the subway or bus as a group comes after planning a route.

Type of Reasoning: Inferential

One must infer or draw conclusions about the ideal first step in a functional task. After reviewing all of the possible choices, one must determine that one step must come before all the others in order to have a successful outcome. For this situation, determining a destination must come first in order for the remaining steps to be executed effectively. If answered incorrectly, review principles of activity analysis.

B49 C9

The administrator of a large rehabilitation hospital reviews the occupational therapy staffing schedules. The administrator determines that of the 12 full-time therapists, six work full-time in the inpatient department, two work full-time in the outpatient department, two divide their hours equally between the inpatient and outpatient department, and two divide their hours equally between administrative/managerial work and direct care provision on the inpatient unit. Which is most accurate staffing for the administrator to document for the occupational therapy inpatient department in the annual report?

Answer Choices:

A. Twelve full-time equivalent employees.
B. Ten full-time equivalent employees.
C. Eight full-time equivalent employees.
D. Six full-time equivalent employees.

Correct Answer: C.

Rationale:
A full-time equivalent (FTE) is the amount of work time assigned to one full-time staff member in a year. In this scenario, two employees have part-time inpatient responsibilities, so they would each be considered 0.5 FTE and two employees only devote half of their hours to direct care, so they would also each be considered 0.5 FTE. Since $0.5 \times 4 = 2$, and there are six staff members with full-time inpatient responsibilities, the total of FTEs would be eight.

Type of Reasoning: Deductive
This question requires recall of guidelines, which is factual knowledge. Deductive reasoning skills are utilized whenever one must recall facts to solve clinical problems. In this situation, the FTE in the inpatient department is eight. Review clinical management guidelines, including calculations of FTE employees if answered incorrectly.

B50 C5

A person recovering from a cerebral vascular accident has left-sided weakness and dysphagia. Which of the following is the most effective direct intervention approach to help the person successfully swallow ingested food?

Answer Choices:

A. Provide pureed, thick liquids.
B. Provide thermal stimulation to the inferior faucial arches.
C. Tilt the person's head back and towards the left side.
D. Provide small, warm boluses.

Correct Answer: D.

Rationale:
Direct intervention for oral motor control involves techniques that utilize a bolus. These techniques can involve modification of bolus amount, consistency and temperature. Providing thermal stimulation to the inferior faucial arches using a chilled dental examination mirror can elicit a swallow response; however, this is considered an indirect treatment method. Tilting the head back is contraindicated because it increases choking risk.

Type of Reasoning: Inferential
One must infer or draw conclusions about a likely course of action, given the information presented. This is an inferential reasoning skill, where knowledge of a therapeutic approach, such as the direct intervention to swallow food in this situation, is essential to choosing a correct solution. In this case, the therapist should provide small, warm boluses. Review direct and indirect interventions for persons with oral motor disorders if answered incorrectly.

B51 **C8**

An individual cannot independently get from a supine position to a sitting position. The person has good scapular, shoulder and elbow muscle strength. Which of the following should the occupational therapist recommend as most effective for the client to use to improve bed mobility?

Answer Choices:
A. A leg lifter.
B. A bed rail assist.
C. A log roll technique.
D. A rope ladder.

Correct Answer: D.

Rationale:
A rope ladder or bed loops enable the individual to loop the arm(s) into the first "rung"/loop, and then into the next "rung"/loop, and so on until he/she has achieved a sitting position. The other options do not assist with independently moving from supine to sitting. A leg lifter is used to lift a leg that cannot move independently. A bed rail assist is used to help with rising from sitting to standing. A log roll technique can be used to help a person go from supine to sitting but this technique requires the assistance of another person. It is indicated for an individual who cannot use the rope ladder technique.

Type of Reasoning: Inductive
This question requires one to determine the most appropriate device to improve bed mobility in supine to sit. This requires inductive reasoning skill, where clinical judgment is paramount in arriving at a correct conclusion. For this situation, the therapist should recommend a rope ladder. If answered incorrectly, review adaptive devices for bed mobility, especially rope ladders.

B52 **C6**

An adult diagnosed with bipolar disorder has been taking lithium for five years. Prior to a weekly occupational therapy vocational planning group, the client reports noticeable functional changes since the last group session. In describing these changes, the client reports symptoms that may be indicative of a possible lithium overdose. With the client's permission, the therapist contacts the psychiatrist to describe the client's concerns. Which symptom would the therapist most likely report as indicative of this problem?

Answer Choices:
A. Reduction in mood swing.
B. Gross hand tremors.
C. Decreased velocity of speech.
D. Fine hand tremors.

Correct Answer: B.

Rationale:
Gross hand tremors are a sign of a possible lithium overdose and should be reported to the physician immediately. Reduction of mood swings and decreased speech velocity are desired effects of taking lithium to decrease mania. Symptoms of mania include increased activity and speech level, feelings of euphoria and expansiveness. Fine hand tremors are a common side effect of lithium and can be controlled by taking the medication propranolol. They usually do not represent an overdose of the medication.

Type of Reasoning: Analytical
This question requires one to recall the likely symptoms of an overdose of lithium. This requires analyzing the four possible symptoms and determining which symptom best coincides with lithium overdose. In this case, the likely symptom is gross hand tremors. If answered incorrectly, review information on the desired effects of lithium and the symptoms of lithium overdose.

B53 C2

A school-based occupational therapist is teaching orientation and mobility skills to an adolescent with a degenerative visual disorder. Which is the most effective motivational technique for the therapist to use with this student?

Answer Choices:

A. Provide concrete structure and frequent feedback to ensure accurate orientation and safe functional mobility.
B. Keep sessions short to allow time for emotional adjustment to orientation and mobility challenges.
C. Treat the student as an adult and incorporate the student's orientation and mobility goals into intervention sessions.
D. Limit anxiety by practicing the techniques in a quiet and self-contained environment; e.g., an empty classroom.

Correct Answer: C.

Rationale:
Adolescents prefer to be treated as adults. The most important (and most effective) motivational technique is to incorporate the student's goals into the intervention sessions. Too much structure will limit the student's trial and error learning which is vital to learning and retaining orientation and functional mobility skills. The length of intervention sessions should be determined by the student's established goals, the methods identified to attain these goals and the student's progress towards goal attainment. Throughout the orientation and mobility training sessions, the occupational therapist can incorporate the therapeutic use of self to help the student emotionally adjust to the challenges of the situation and effectively deal with any anxiety he/she may be experiencing. Using a quiet self-contained environment can be a helpful intervention approach when first introducing orientation and mobility techniques but it is not a motivational strategy.

Type of Reasoning: Inductive
This question requires one to utilize clinical judgment to reach a sound conclusion, which is an inductive reasoning skill. For this question, the test taker must consider the age of the individual in order to determine the best motivational techniques. In this case, treating the patient as an adult and incorporating the patient's goals into the plan of care is best.

B54 C6

An occupational therapist working in a skilled nursing facility conducts an inservice on validation therapy for the recently hired staff of a new psychogeriatric unit. Which fundamental principle of validation therapy is important for the therapist to include in this presentation?

Answer Choices:

A. Listen to the words an individual uses to ascertain the person's underlying message.
B. Provide highly structured, activities to refocus the individual on reality.
C. Provide unstructured activities to facilitate the expression of feelings.
D. Listen to the words an individual uses and provide reality orientation for invalid statements.

Correct Answer: A.

Rationale:
Validation therapy is an approach to working with individuals with dementia founded on the principle that the unspoken messages an individual conveys in his/her speech are more important than the actual content of the speech. Individuals with dementia often make statements that are not based in reality. For example, an individual introduces a daughter as his/her mother. In validation therapy, the factual aspects of this familial relationship are irrelevant and do not need to be addressed at all. However, the underlying message that this relationship is valued and important is worthy of comment. The use of structured or unstructured activities is not a component of validation therapy. The focus of validation therapy is to facilitate communication with persons with dementia in a caring, respectful and empathetic manner.

Type of Reasoning: Inferential
This question requires one to determine the primary principle of validation therapy. This requires inferential reasoning skill, where one must infer or draw conclusions about a likely guideline or principle. In this case, the therapist should advise staff to listen to the words an individual uses to ascertain the person's underlying message. If answered incorrectly, review validation therapy principles and guidelines.

B55 **C4**

An occupational therapist conducts an intervention session with a client recovering from a CVA to develop transfer skills. The client has a co-morbidity of epilepsy. As the client stands to complete a transfer from the wheelchair to the bed, the client reports feeling sensations that are indicative of an aura. Which is the best immediate action for the therapist to take in response to this situation?

Answer Choices:
A. Provide reassurance and ask for guidance from the physician.
B. Return the client to a seated position in the wheelchair until the sensations pass.
C. End the session so the client can rest.
D. Guide the person into a sidelying position on the bed. ✓

Correct Answer: D.

Rationale:
An aura is the brief warning stage before the tonic phase of an epileptic seizure. During an aura, changes in tactile, gustatory, olfactory or other sensations are experienced (e.g., numbness, unexplained smells). After this brief stage, a tonic-clonic seizure will occur. The tonic phase includes a loss of consciousness, stiffening of the body, heavy and irregular breathing, drooling, skin pallor and occasional bladder and bowel incontinence for a few seconds before the clonic phase begins. The clonic phase includes alternating rigidity and relaxation of muscles. Since a person could fall and harm him/herself during a seizure, the therapist must immediately ensure the client's safety. Therefore, the best action for the therapist to take is to place the person in sidelying on the bed. If there are bed rails these should be raised. This will prevent the client from falling or choking. Providing reassurance, having the client remain seated, and ending the session does not effectively deal with the immediate need to provide interventions for the impending seizure. The therapist does not need (nor should wait for) the input of the physician.

Type of Reasoning: Evaluative
This question requires the test taker to weigh the merits of the four courses of action presented and then determine the action that most effectively addresses the needs of the client. This requires evaluative reasoning skill. For this situation, the therapist should guide the person into a side-lying position on the bed. Review first aid guidelines for clients with seizure disorders if answered incorrectly.

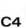

B56 **C9**

An occupational therapist is scheduled to give a one-hour presentation to a support group of parents of infants with a diversity of developmental disabilities. Which of the following is the most important focus of the therapist's presentation?

Answer Choices:

A. Demonstration of infant positioning techniques.
B. Discussion of typical areas of concern addressed by OT practitioners.
C. Demonstration of different types of developmental assessments.
D. Discussion of the Individual Family Service Plan (IFSP).

Correct Answer: B.

Rationale:

An overview of the domain of concern addressed by OT for infants with developmental disabilities is the most appropriate topic for a one-hour presentation to an audience with diverse needs. Demonstration of infant positioning techniques and developmental assessments can be informative, but these techniques and assessments must be tailored to the individual child. A discussion about the IFSP can also be informative, but this information should be provided by the family's early intervention service provider.

Type of Reasoning: Evaluative

One must weigh the possible courses of action and then make a value judgment about the best course to take. This requires evaluative reasoning skill, which often utilizes guiding principles of action in order to arrive at a correct conclusion. In this case, given the audience the therapist is speaking to and the range of diagnoses of the infants, the therapist should discuss typical areas of concern addressed by OT practitioners.

B57 **C2**

Several adolescents with behavior problems attend a school-based after-school program. They work at an egocentric-cooperative level in a group dealing with issues related to school performance and peer pressure. Which of the following would be most likely for the occupational therapist to observe the participants doing in the group?

Answer Choices:

A. Actively taking on roles such as energizer, coordinator or opinion giver.
B. Focusing on the group tasks rather than the feelings of the participants.
C. Making decisions with minimal to no supervision from the group leader.
D. Performing group skills consistent with the developmental level of 15 to 18 years of age.

Correct Answer: B.

Rationale:

The egocentric-cooperative group tends to focus on the tasks to be completed with little attention devoted to the feelings of the participants. At this level, members do not actively assume diverse group roles. A mature group would require little or no supervision and performs at the 15- to 18-year-old developmental level. An egocentric-cooperative group performs at the five to seven year developmental level.

Type of Reasoning: Deductive

One must recall the typical manifestations of clients who function at an egocentric-cooperative level in order to arrive at a correct conclusion. This requires deductive reasoning skill, where recall of guidelines and protocols are utilized to choose the best response. In this situation, the group members are most likely to focus on the group tasks rather than the feelings of the members. If answered incorrectly, review egocentric-cooperative level group guidelines and functional level of group participants.

B58 **C1**

An occupational therapist leads a social skills group for children aged 10–12 with conduct disorders. One of the children complains that the group activity is stupid and boring. Which is the most effective response for the occupational therapist to provide in response to this complaint?

Answer Choices:
A. Encourage the child to complete the activity with the group. ✓
B. Allow the child to leave the group since uninterested.
C. Allow the child to suggest a different group activity.
D. Tell the child the complaint will be discussed at the next family meeting.

Correct Answer: A.

Rationale:
Children between the ages of 10 and 12 are typically at the developmental age of cooperative play which emerges at age 7. During this stage of development, children participate in games and learn to play according to rules in a cooperative manner. Encouraging the child to complete the activity with the group provides the child with the opportunity to develop age-appropriate social skills. Children with conduct disorders often show disregard for others and tend to violate rules; therefore, completing a planned activity with others is particularly relevant. Allowing the child to alter the group's in-progress activity does not address these issues. There is no need for the child to leave the group or for the behavior to be discussed at a family meeting.

Type of Reasoning: Inductive
This question requires one to determine the most appropriate response to a child with conduct disorder. This requires inductive reasoning skill, where clinical judgment is paramount in arriving at a correct conclusion. For this situation, the occupational therapist should encourage the child to complete the activity with the group. If answered incorrectly, review the diagnostic criteria of conduct disorders and the typical developmental sequence of play. Integration of this knowledge is required for a correct answer.

B59 **C3**

The occupational therapist plans intervention for a client with a recent diagnosis of complex regional pain syndrome (CRPS) Type I. Which intervention approach is most effective to use to reduce pain and increase function?

Answer Choices:
A. Hot packs.
B. Biofeedback. ✓
C. Paraffin.
D. Passive range of motion.

Correct Answer: B.

Rationale:
CRPS Type I is a vasomotor dysfunction which causes extreme hypersensitivity to touch, edema, intense burning pain and dramatic temperature and color changes to the affected limb. Goals of treatment include reducing pain and edema, promoting normal positioning and increasing function. Biofeedback is a technique where electrodes are used to measure muscle responses and stress levels. The goal is to train the individual to release tension, which can reduce pain and prepare the individual for increased tolerance to range of motion and functional movement. Hot packs and paraffin can be too painful to tolerate in the initial stages and are contraindicated if the affected limb demonstrates elevated temperature. Passive range of motion is usually not tolerated during the initial stages of the syndrome due to the severe pain and hypersensitivity to touch.

Type of Reasoning: Inferential
One must link the individual's diagnosis to the treatment approaches provided in order to determine which treatment approach would most effectively address the individual's deficits. This requires inferential reasoning, where one must draw conclusions about the potential treatment outcomes. In this case the occupational therapist should use biofeedback to reduce pain and promote tolerance to activity. Review treatment approaches for CRPS Type I if answered incorrectly.

B60 C8

Several newly homeless veterans with a variety of mental health diagnoses attend an occupational therapy community re-entry group conducted in a community-based shelter. Which should be the primary focus of the initial group session?

Answer Choices:
A. Development of home management skills such as meal preparation.
B. Determination of financial assets and money management skills.
C. Identification of local resources such as soup kitchens and thrift stores.
D. Exploration of vocational interests and employment possibilities.

Correct Answer: C.

Rationale:
Locating basic resources is the most essential survival skill listed for people who have recently become homeless. Initial sessions at a homeless shelter would likely focus on basic survival and personal self-care skills prior to focusing on vocational interests, employment opportunities or instrumental activities of daily living (IADL) such as meal preparation and money management skills. Subsequent sessions may focus on the development of IADL and vocational skills.

Type of Reasoning: Inductive
One must consider the needs of the group and benefits of each of the four possible courses of action. This necessitates inductive reasoning skill, where the test taker must use clinical judgment to determine the merits of each of the four choices, based on client needs. In this case, location of resources is the most beneficial topic, as it is focused on meeting the essential survival skills of this group. If answered incorrectly, review guidelines for working with homeless individuals and appropriate community resources.

B61 C4

An occupational therapist provides home-based services to a homemaker who incurred a right CVA eight months ago. The individual and the therapist have chosen to focus on kitchen activities during the intervention session. The therapist has the client stand in front of the counter with an open dishwasher to the left. The therapist asks the client to put the clean dishes into an open overhead cabinet to the right of the client. By setting up the activity in this manner, which proprioceptive neuromuscular facilitation (PNF) technique is the therapist using?

Answer Choices:
A. Heavy work/mobility superimposed on stability.
B. Reciprocal inhibition/innervation.
C. Diagonal patterns of D2 flexion/extension.
D. Diagonal patterns of D1 flexion/extension.

Correct Answer: D.

Rationale:
In this example, the D1 flexion pattern moves the person's left upper extremity "up and away" as the person grasps the dishes from the dishwasher on the left and puts them away in the cabinet above the counter to the right. Heavy work and reciprocal inhibition/innervation are techniques used in the Rood approach. In heavy work (also termed "mobility superimposed on stability"), proximal muscles contract and move and the distal segments are fixed. According to the Rood approach, reciprocal inhibition/innervation is an early mobility pattern that is primarily a reflex governed by spinal and supraspinal centers. D2 is the PNF extension diagonal which moves the UE "down and in."

Type of Reasoning: Analytical
For this question, a description of a functional activity is provided and the test taker must determine the functional activity that is being performed. This requires analytical reasoning skill, as questions of this nature often ask one to analyze descriptors of functional tasks to determine the overall skill involved. In this situation the activity being performed is that of D1 flexion/extension. Review PNF patterns, especially D1 if answered incorrectly.

B62 C7

An occupational therapist conducts a sensory evaluation of an individual recovering from a left cerebral vascular accident. The individual has right hemiplegia and expressive aphasia. During the evaluation of stereognosis, which should the therapist have the client use to identify responses to the testing stimuli?

Answer Choices:
A. Pictures of the objects.
B. A set of identical objects.
C. Cards with "one" and "two" printed on them.
D. Cards with "yes" and "no" printed on them.

Correct Answer: B.

Rationale:
Stereognosis is the ability to identify objects through touch and cognition. Having an identical set of objects from which the individual can select an object that matches the test stimulus will enable a person with expressive aphasia to participate in the evaluation. The person can point to the object to indicate his/her response Cards with "one" and "two" printed on them would be relevant assists for the evaluation of two point discrimination. Cards with "yes" and "no" printed on them would be relevant assists for the evaluation of light touch. Presenting the person with pictures to indicate his/her response requires the ability to generalize the object to its symbolic representation. This ability may be compromised in an individual with a CVA. It is more accurate to have exact matches of the objects used during the evaluation for this will not require the interpretation of pictures.

Type of Reasoning: Deductive
This question requires recall of testing guidelines based on factual knowledge. This is a deductive reasoning skill, where recall of facts is essential to arriving at a correct conclusion. In this scenario, the only appropriate method for identifying the response to a stimulus in stereognosis testing is to use a set of identical objects. Review guidelines for stereognosis testing for patients with expressive aphasia if answered incorrectly.

B63 C8

A young adult with a T9–10 spinal cord injury wishes to engage in sports activities. Which wheelchair features are best for the occupational therapist to recommend to this client?

Answer Choices:
A. A heavy-duty foldable frame with a high back.
B. An ultra-light foldable frame with a high back.
C. An ultra-light rigid frame with a low back. ✓
D. A heavy-duty rigid frame with a low back.

Correct Answer: C.

Rationale:
Sports competition wheelchairs are usually made with rigid construction and very strong lightweight materials. A folding wheelchair does not provide the stability needed for competition sports. A low seat back enhances the user's upper body/arm movements. A higher seat back is indicated for patients with decreased trunk control (not a factor in this example). At T9–10 this patient has partial innervation of the abdominals (innervated T6–12) and full innervation of the upper extremities.

Type of Reasoning: Inductive
One must utilize diagnostic reasoning and clinical judgment to determine the best type of wheelchair for a patient with T10 paraplegia who wishes to participate in sports. This requires inductive reasoning skill. In this case, the therapist should recommend an ultra-light rigid frame with a low back. Review wheelchair prescription guidelines if answered incorrectly.

B64 C9

An entry-level occupational therapy assistant (OTA) recently hired for an outpatient rehabilitation clinic requires supervision during the direct supervisor's scheduled vacations. To maximize departmental efficacy, who should provide supervision to the OTA?

Answer Choices:
A. The rehabilitation clinic's administrator.
B. An OTA with experience.
C. An occupational therapist. ✓
D. An OTA with advanced credentialing.

Correct Answer: C.

Rationale:
Only an occupational therapist can supervise OTAs. The other choices do not meet this criterion.

Type of Reasoning: Deductive
One must recall the supervisory guidelines for OTAs in rehabilitation settings. This is factual knowledge, which is a deductive reasoning skill. Because entry-level OTAs require direct supervision from an occupational therapist, another occupational therapist is required to supervise in the supervisor's absence. If answered incorrectly, review supervisory guidelines for OTAs.

B65 C5

A child with developmental delay has poor oral motor control. Which should the occupational therapist do to facilitate lip closure?

Answer Choices:

A. Give pressure with the index finger under the jaw.
B. Place food on a spoon and firmly place the spoon on the back part of the tongue.
C. Place the thumbs on the lateral ends of the mandibles.
D. Give a slight upward sweep of the index finger from the lower jaw to the lower lip. ✓

Correct Answer: D.

Rationale:

Providing a slight upward sweep of the index finger from the lower jaw to the lower lip can facilitate lip closure. Pressing down on the space between the nose and upper lip is also facilitative for lip closure. Placing pressure with the index finger under the jaw and placing each thumb on the lateral end of the mandibles facilitates jaw closure. Placing food on a spoon and firmly placing the spoon on the back part of the tongue can facilitate the gag reflex.

Type of Reasoning: Inferential

One must determine the most likely intervention approach for a child, given the diagnosis provided and skill described. This requires inferential reasoning skill, where one must draw conclusions based on the information presented. In this situation, the therapist would give a slight upward sweep of the index finger from the lower jaw to the lower lip to facilitate lip closure. If answered incorrectly, review oral motor control techniques for children.

B66 C4

A client recovering from a left CVA demonstrates increased flexor tone in the dominant right upper extremity while trying to re-learn to write with the left hand. Which of the following is most accurate for the therapist to state the client is exhibiting when documenting this observation?

Answer Choices:

A. An associated reaction. ✓
B. A crossed flexion reaction. ✗
C. A tonic labyrinthine reflex.
D. An asymmetrical tonic neck reflex.

Correct Answer: A.

Rationale:

Providing resisted voluntary movements to the unaffected limb facilitates an associated reaction in the affected limb. A tonic labyrinthine response results from changes in the orientation of the head, leading to bilateral flexor or extensor posturing of the arms/legs. The asymmetrical tonic neck reflex response is facilitated by rotation of the head, and results in limb extension on the face side, and limb flexion on the skull side. Crossed flexion reaction is a made up term.

Type of Reasoning: Analytical

This question requires the test taker to determine the functional deficit of the patient, which is an analytical reasoning skill. Questions of this nature often call upon the test taker to determine a deficit based on a functional description. Based on this information, the symptoms of the person indicate the deficit of associated reaction, which should be reviewed if answered incorrectly.

B67 C8

A person with scleroderma has limited upper extremity ROM. Coordination is within functional limits. The occupational therapist assesses the individual's computer inputting capabilities and provides a recommendation to improve efficacy. Which adaptation would be most effective for this person?

Answer Choices:
A. An expanded keyboard.
B. A concept keyboard.
C. A key guard.
D. A contracted keyboard. ✓

Correct Answer: D.

Rationale:
A contracted keyboard decreases the ROM required to strike the keys. It is indicated for someone with limited ROM; however, due to smaller key size coordination must be functional. An expanded keyboard requires increased ROM to strike the keys. A key guard is an overlay on the keyboard used for individuals with poor coordination who frequently miss or overshoot keys. A concept keyboard is used for individuals with cognitive impairments. It replaces the keyboard letters and numbers with pictures, symbols or words to represent the concepts that are needed by a software program.

Type of Reasoning: Inductive
One must utilize clinical knowledge and judgment to determine the keyboard adaptation that is most appropriate for the individual, given the diagnosis and limitations. In this case, a contracted keyboard is most appropriate. If answered incorrectly, review modifications for increasing computer accessibility and indications for issuing a contracted keyboard.

B68 C9

An individual is referred by a physician to an outpatient occupational therapy program for an evaluation. The person's insurance company does not cover outpatient OT services. Which action is best for the therapist to take in response to this situation?

Answer Choices:
A. Follow the physician's order and let the person pay the bill when it is received.
B. Refuse to accept the referral and advise the person to seek additional insurance coverage.
C. Explain the limitation of the insurance coverage and let the person decide whether to complete the evaluation. ✓
D. Request that the program's billing department submit a bill using a code that is covered by the insurance company.

Correct Answer: C.

Rationale:
This provides the individual with accurate information and enables him/her to make an informed choice. Following the physician's order and letting the person pay the bill when it is received does not allow for informed consent. Refusing to accept the referral is unethical. Requesting that the program's billing department submit a bill using a code that is covered by the insurance company is unethical and illegal.

Type of Reasoning: Evaluative
One must weigh the possible courses of action and then make a value judgment about the best course to take. This requires evaluative reasoning skill, which often utilizes guiding principles of action in order to arrive at a correct conclusion. For this case, because the patient does not have coverage for outpatient OT services, the therapist should explain the limitation of the insurance coverage and let the person decide whether to complete the evaluation.

B69 C4

An elementary school-aged child with Duchenne's muscular dystrophy receives occupational therapy services. The family establishes a goal of maintaining the child's leisure and social participation. Which is the best activity for the occupational therapist to recommend the family pursue with this child?

Answer Choices:

A. Electronic sports (e.g., Wii bowling).
B. Adapted little league baseball.
C. Wheelchair basketball.
D. Recreational swimming. ✓

Correct Answer: D.

Rationale:

Recreational swimming is a social and leisure activity that the child can participate in with family members and friends. It can also be helpful in maintaining the child's functional level as long as possible. Even when the child's Duchenne's progresses, swimming will often remain an activity that can be successfully pursued. The eye-hand coordination to play electronic sports games will likely be too difficult for the child with Duchenne's. Baseball and basketball also have mobility and coordination requirements that would be difficult for this child. In addition, at an elementary school age, wheelchair use due to Duchenne's is not usual.

Type of Reasoning: Inferential

In this question, one must make a link between the diagnosis, the age of the child, and the appropriate interventions. Here, swimming is appropriate because it encourages the maintenance of function for as long as possible. Questions such as these require one to draw conclusions based on evidence presented, which is an inferential skill. If answered incorrectly, review muscular dystrophy. An understanding of the progressive nature of this disorder is needed to select the correct answer.

B70 C8

An occupational therapist conducts an on-site accessibility assessment with a building contractor who is remodeling an apartment building. The therapist recommends modifications for doorways which do not meet minimum accessibility width standards. The contractor states the building's owner wants to exceed minimum standards without incurring unreasonable costs. Which is the most preferred doorway measurement for the occupational therapist to recommend the contractor use for the remodeling?

Answer Choices:

A. 36 inches.
B. 32 inches.
C. 34 inches.
D. 38 inches.

Correct Answer: A.

Rationale:

36 inches is the preferred doorway measurement for wheelchair accessibility that exceeds the minimum accessibility standard of 32 inches. This allows for adequate hand clearance and is sufficiently wide enough for non-standard width chairs. 34 inches may not be sufficient for wider wheelchairs. Although the 36-inch width exceeds minimum accessibility standards, it is a door frame width that is commonly used in commercial and residential construction; therefore, modification can be done in a cost-efficient manner. A 38-inch door frame width would require costly customized construction that is difficult to justify and is likely not necessary.

Type of Reasoning: Deductive
One must recall the accessibility guidelines for doorway clearances according to universal design standards. This is factual knowledge, which is a deductive reasoning skill. A doorway width of 36″ would best meet these standards and the therapist should recommend this guideline to the contractor. If answered incorrectly, review universal design standards for wheelchair accessibility, especially doorway measurements.

B71 C1

An occupational therapist works in a school system with a child with developmental delays. One of the goals of treatment is to develop pre-writing skills. The child exhibits the ability to grasp a pencil proximally with crude approximation of the thumb, index and middle fingers and the ring and little fingers slightly flexed. The therapist develops an intervention plan. Which grasp should be the focus for the implementation of intervention?

Answer Choices:
A. Digital pronate grasp.
B. Static tripod posture grasp.
C. Dynamic tripod grasp.
D. Palmar supinate grasp.

Correct Answer: C.

Rationale:
The grasp pattern described in the case is static tripod posture grasp. The next grasp pattern to be mastered after this grasp is the dynamic tripod grasp. The other grasp patterns are precursors to the static tripod grasp.

Type of Reasoning: Inferential
This question requires one to infer the intervention goal that will develop appropriate grasp for this child. This requires inferential reasoning skill, where one must draw conclusions about the described grasp pattern. In this situation, dynamic tripod grasp is the next pattern to be mastered after static tripod grasp. If answered incorrectly, review grasp patterns of the hand in children, especially dynamic tripod.

B72 C8

An older adult diagnosed three years ago with dementia, Alzheimer type has been admitted to the hospital for regulation of medication. The occupational therapist determines that the patient demonstrates diminished memory skills since the previous evaluation, but is still able to live independently at home with support and supervision. During the discharge planning meeting, which activity should the therapist recommend family members perform for the patient?

Answer Choices:
A. Weeding the garden.
B. Sorting and folding laundry.
C. Preparing cold sandwiches.
D. Cooking hot meals.

Correct Answer: D.

Rationale:
Cooking hot meals provides the main opportunity for the patient who is increasingly forgetful to be unsafe. Leaving the stove on due to memory loss can be a fire hazard. The patient can continue the other activities without compromising personal safety. In addition, weeding and sorting and folding laundry are structured and repetitive activities which can facilitate the patient's active engagement.

Type of Reasoning: Inductive
Knowledge of Alzheimer's disease and clinical judgment are the most important skills needed for answering this question, which requires inductive reasoning skill. In this case, because cooking independently presents the greatest risk for safety, the therapist should recommend that the patient refrain from this IADL upon return to home. If answered incorrectly, review safety in IADL for patients with Alzheimer's disease.

B73 C1

During an occupational therapy screening session, the therapist observes that a child bangs objects on a table-top but is unable to give up a toy upon request. The occupational therapist documents these behaviors. Which developmental level would be most accurate for the therapist to report the child's observed behaviors indicates?

Answer Choices:
A. 3–4 months. ✓
B. 7–8 months.
C. 9–10 months.
D. 11–12 months.

Correct Answer: A.

Rationale:
At 3–4 months, children are able to bang toys on a tabletop but they do not have a voluntary release. At 7–8 months children begin to be able to give up objects with an assisted release, and at 9–10 months there is more efficient release. One-year-old children have a voluntary release.

Type of Reasoning: Deductive
One must recall the developmental guidelines for children in banging toys and lack of a voluntary release. This is factual knowledge, which is a deductive reasoning skill. The functional activity described is a skill at 3–4 months developmentally. If answered incorrectly, review developmental milestones of infants in gross motor and fine motor skills.

B74 C8

Occupational therapy services are provided to the clients of a psychogeriatric unit in a skilled nursing facility. An occupational therapist presents an inservice on restraint reduction to the unit's direct care staff. Which of the following would the therapist identify as a permissible use of a restraint?

Answer Choices:
A. A bed guardrail to prevent a confused resident from wandering in the evening.
B. Prescribed medication to control a resident's agitated behavior.
C. A lap board to enhance a resident's self-directed functional behavior. ✓
D. A wheelchair with a lap belt to prevent a person with ataxic gait from falling.

Correct Answer: C.

Rationale:
A restraint is defined as anything that prevents access to the environment or to one's self. A restraint such as a lap board can enhance functional performance and is permissible with a resident's informed consent. The correct answer choice states that the individual can self-direct. This indicates that the person has the ability to give the required informed consent and that he/she can direct the staff on its removal and its desired use. The other purposes of restraints are not permissible and alternatives such as the provision of meaningful activities, adaptive aids and/or environmental modifications must be actively pursued as preventative measures.

Type of Reasoning: Deductive

This question requires recall of guidelines and principles, which is factual knowledge. Deductive reasoning skills are utilized whenever one must recall facts to solve novel problems. In this situation, the use of a lap board is the only choice that does not constitute a restraint as it does not prevent access to the environment or one's self. Review guidelines for use of restraints if answered incorrectly.

B75 C5

A client attends a work hardening program. The client arrives on time for the scheduled session but complains of significant substernal pain, extreme discomfort in the epigastric area, indigestion and nausea. Which is the best action for the occupational therapist to take in response to the client's expressed complaints?

Answer Choices:

A. Initiate the session and provide breaks and activity modifications as needed.
B. Cancel the session and immediately call emergency medical services (EMS).
C. Cancel the session and tell the client to call to reschedule when feeling better.
D. Cancel the session and call the client's physician to discuss the client's complaints.

Correct Answer: B.

Rationale:

The client is complaining of symptoms that can be the presenting signs for a myocardial infarction. This is a medical emergency and must be handled as such. The therapist must cancel the session and call for EMS to address the situation. The therapist should not delay this action by cancelling the session and having the client reschedule or waiting to speak with the primary care physician. The occupational therapist can (and should) act independently in this medical emergency.

Type of Reasoning: Evaluative

One must weigh the possible courses of action and then make a value judgment about the best course to take. This requires evaluative reasoning skill, which often utilizes guiding principles of action in order to arrive at a correct conclusion. In this case, because the patient's symptoms are indicative of a myocardial infarction, the therapist should cancel the session and call emergency medical services. Review symptoms of myocardial infarction if answered incorrectly.

B76 C2

Several residents of a skilled nursing facility report that they are bored with their individual daily range of motion exercise programs. The occupational therapist collaborates with the physical therapist to design a group format to facilitate participation in range of motion exercises. Which would be most beneficial for the therapist to recommend incorporating into the proposed group?

Answer Choices:

A. The use of several exercise videos with diverse exercise styles and music.
B. The pairing of residents to perform gentle range of motion on each other.
C. The use of exercises performed in rhythm to a marching band video.
D. The provision of coffee and cake after the group.

Correct Answer: A.

Rationale:
Adding variety to the exercise program can stimulate interest and increase socialization. The individuals can select videos that are of personal interest. Clients should not do hands-on treatment with each other. Moreover, passive range of motion is contraindicated for many diagnoses. A marching band video may be at a tempo that is too vigorous for some residents. Providing coffee and cake does not address the need to increase interest in performing daily ROM exercises.

Type of Reasoning: Inductive
One must utilize clinical knowledge and judgment to determine the exercise approach that best addresses the residents' lack of interest in participating in individual ROM exercise programs. In this case, providing a group that includes the use of several exercise videos with diverse styles and music is best. If answered incorrectly, review principles for using therapeutic activities. The integration of this knowledge is needed to determine the correct answer.

B77 C1

The parents of an 18-month-old bring their child to a free community developmental screening. The child can attend to shapes and use them appropriately. However, the parents are worried because the child cannot match shapes or manipulate different shaped objects into a shape sorter. Which is the best response for the occupational therapist to make in response to the parents' expressed concern?

Answer Choices:
A. Advise the parents that the child is showing a typical, age-appropriate skill.
B. Complete an occupational therapy evaluation of the child's cognitive skills.
C. Refer the child to the early intervention program for developmental delay.
D. Provide the parents with activity recommendations to develop shape recognition.

Correct Answer: A.

Rationale:
The child is showing an age-appropriate skill. According to established developmental milestones, the ability to recognize shapes and manipulate different shaped objects into a shape sorter does not typically develop until the age 21–24 months. The ability to attend to the shape of things and use them appropriately is typical of children aged 18–21 months. There is no additional information provided in the scenario to indicate a developmental delay that would warrant further evaluation of cognitive skills or intervention for developmental delay. There is no need to provide activities to reinforce shape recognition since the child is functioning at a developmentally appropriate level and these skills can be expected to develop typically as the child ages.

Type of Reasoning: Deductive
One must recall the developmental guidelines for 18-month-old children. This is factual knowledge, which is a deductive reasoning skill. Because the child is not expected to recognize shapes and manipulate different shaped objects into a shape sorter at 18 months, the child is demonstrating age-appropriate skills. If answered incorrectly, review the major milestones of cognitive development.

B78 C6

A young adult recently diagnosed with undifferentiated schizophrenia is referred to an occupational therapy day treatment program. Which should the occupational therapist do first with the client?

Answer Choices:
A. Determine short-term and long-term goals for program participation.
B. Model desired behaviors during occupational therapy groups.
C. Have the client complete an occupational interest checklist.
D. Encourage the client to maintain a daily log of medication intake.

Correct Answer: C.

Rationale:
Upon referral, the first step in the OT process is screening. Determining the person's occupational interests can help identify areas requiring further evaluation. One cannot establish short-term and long-term goals with the client until an evaluation is completed. It is unknown if the client has deficits in medication management. Modeling behavior is a component of the intervention process.

Type of Reasoning: Inductive
One must draw conclusions about a best approach based on the diagnosis of the client in order to arrive at a correct conclusion. This requires inferential reasoning skill. In this case, the therapist should have the person complete an occupational interest inventory. If answered incorrectly, review client-centered approaches in psychosocial practice, especially during the screening process.

B79 **C8**

An occupational therapist working in a skilled nursing facility observes a resident with cognitive disabilities don slippers by putting them on the wrong feet. The resident plans to go visit a friend on another floor and does not seem aware that the slippers are on the wrong feet. Which is the best action for the therapist to take in response to this situation?

Answer Choices:
A. Say nothing for this error may embarrass the resident.
B. Say nothing but follow the resident to the friend's room to ensure a safe arrival.
C. Ask the resident to look at the slippers to see if the error is noticed.
D. Approach the resident and advise the resident to reverse the slippers. ✓ safety concern

Correct Answer: D.

Rationale:
The slippers must be immediately reversed to ensure safety and prevent a fall. Poor or inappropriate use of footwear is a primary cause of falls. Letting the resident walk with slippers on the wrong feet is an unacceptable risk. Since the resident has cognitive deficits, he/she may not be able to notice the error and self-correct. A direct intervention done in a supportive manner is needed to ensure safety.

Type of Reasoning: Evaluative
This question requires professional judgment in a challenging situation, which is an evaluative reasoning skill. Because the resident is at risk for a fall wearing the slippers on the wrong feet, the therapist should advise the resident to reverse the slippers. In judgment situations such as these, where safety is a concern, test takers should often consider the safest, most prudent response as the best one. Review safe mobility guidelines if answered incorrectly.

B80 **C4**

An individual with Parkinson's disease exhibits difficulty moving from sitting in a chair to standing. Which technique is best for the therapist to recommend the person use to help successfully complete this functional mobility activity?

Answer Choices:
A. Rise from the chair while sitting with buttocks against the back of the chair.
B. Extend both legs so that both feet are in front of the chair while rising.
C. Sit at the edge of the chair and rock back and forth before rising. ✓
D. Rise while weight-bearing on one foot and pushing up with both arms.

Correct Answer: C.

Rationale:
One of the most common problems that persons with Parkinson's disease have is difficulty with the initiation of movement. Rocking back and forth prior to moving from sit-to-stand provides the person with vestibular and proprioceptive input that can help facilitate movement. Rising from the chair while sitting with buttocks against the back of the chair increases the difficulty of the activity, so it is not appropriate. Rising with extended legs or while weight-bearing on one foot are incorrect as they employ inappropriate body mechanics, and may be unsafe.

Type of Reasoning: Inductive
This question requires one to determine the best technique to recommend for a functional mobility activity. This requires inductive reasoning skill, where clinical judgment is paramount in arriving at a correct conclusion. For this situation, the therapist should instruct the person to sit at the edge of the chair and rock back and forth before rising. If answered incorrectly, review techniques to improve the functional mobility of persons with Parkinson's disease.

B81 C8

An occupational therapist provides an accessibility consultation to a business that has hired a new employee who uses a wheelchair for mobility. The only entrance to the business has four steps, each seven inches high. Which ramp length is best for the therapist to recommend the business have constructed?

Answer Choices:
A. 14 feet.
B. 28 feet.
C. 35 feet.
D. 46 feet

Correct Answer: B.

Rationale:
Accessibility guidelines state that the ramp should be constructed with one foot of ramp length for each inch of rise. The total rise for these steps is 28 inches; therefore the ramp should be 28 feet long. The other options do not meet these guidelines.

Type of Reasoning: Deductive
This question requires recall of guidelines, which is factual knowledge. Deductive reasoning skills are utilized whenever one must recall facts to find ideal solutions. In this situation, accessibility guidelines indicate that for every one inch of rise, there should be one foot of ramp; therefore the ramp should be 28 feet long. Review accessibility guidelines, especially ramp construction, if answered incorrectly.

B82 C8

A middle school-aged child with right upper extremity amelia attends occupational therapy to learn how to dress independently. Which of the following is most beneficial for the occupational therapist to focus on during intervention?

Answer Choices:
A. Donning and doffing a variety of shirt types of personal preference.
B. Donning and doffing only shirts that can be donned overhead.
C. Donning and doffing shirts that button in the front.
D. Donning and doffing shirts with Velcro tabs sewn on to replace buttons.

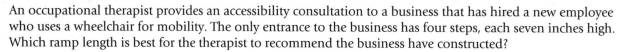

Correct Answer: A.

Rationale:
A child with amelia, or absence of one arm, can easily learn to use a diversity of dressing techniques for a variety of shirt types. This is the best way to engage a pre-adolescent in treatment for it allows the pre-adolescent to make personal decisions about clothing. This choice reflects incorporation of the child's developmental levels, motivation level, and therapeutic use of self to work with the child's interests. The child can don and doff different types of shirts with no need to limit choices. Velcro tabs are appropriate for someone with decreased fine motor skills and/or strength, but are not indicated in this situation.

Type of Reasoning: Inductive
This requires one to understand the nature of amelia, and based on this knowledge; choose the most appropriate dressing activity. This requires inductive reasoning skill, where clinical judgment is paramount in arriving at a correct conclusion. In this case, working on a variety of shirt types of personal preference is the best recommendation for this patient. If answered incorrectly, review information on amelia and principles of activity adaptation. The integration of this knowledge is required to determine the correct answer.

B83 C7

An occupational therapist plans intervention for an individual with cognitive perceptual deficits. In deciding whether to use a dynamic interactional approach or a deficit-specific approach which is most important for the occupational therapist to consider?

Answer Choices:
A. The client's auditory processing skills.
B. The availability of familial support.
C. The client's social interaction skills.
D. The client's problem-solving skills.

Correct Answer: A.

Rationale:
The dynamic interactional approach utilizes awareness questioning to help the individual detect errors, estimate task difficulty and predict outcomes. Therefore, the therapist must consider the client's level of auditory processing skills to determine if adaptations or modifications are needed when implementing this approach. If an individual has severe auditory processing deficits, it may indicate a need to use a deficit-specific approach, for cognitive perceptual remediation. Family support, social interaction skills and problem-solving skills can all influence intervention, but they are not determining factors in selecting which theoretical approach to use in this case.

Type of Reasoning: Inferential
One must link the dynamic interactional approach to the functional skill in order to determine which skill is most important to consider. This requires inferential reasoning, where one must consider the primary features of the dynamic interactional approach and then determine the skill that is primarily utilized. In this case, auditory processing is the most utilized skill. If answered incorrectly, review the dynamic interactional approach.

B84 C1

A child with developmental delay has mastered the ability to cut simple figure shapes with scissors. Which is scissor activity is best for the occupational therapist to next introduce to the child?

Answer Choices:
A. Cutting simple geometric figures.
B. Cutting complex figure shapes. ✓
C. Cutting multiple circles.
D. Cutting additional simple figure shapes.

Correct Answer: B.

Rationale:
The ability to use scissors to cut complex figure shapes is the next developmental task after the acquisition of the ability to cut simple figure shapes. In typically developing children, these abilities develop between the ages of four and six. The abilities to cut circles and cut geometric shapes are earlier developmental scissors skill tasks (typically emerging between the ages of three and four). In this scenario, it states that the child has mastered the specified task. Since it is typical to use a developmental frame of reference with children with developmental delays, the therapist would introduce activities that employ the next developmental skill.

Type of Reasoning: Deductive
One must recall the developmental guidelines for children in cutting figure shapes with a scissors. This is factual knowledge, which is a deductive reasoning skill. One must recall the next developmental ability in this situation, which is to cut out complex figure shapes. If answered incorrectly, review developmental milestones of scissor skills in children.

B85 C9

A high school student is referred to occupational therapy for ADL training. The student has not received occupational therapy services for the past seven years. The student has non-spastic cerebral palsy resulting in right side hemiparesis and decreased muscle tone. The student plans to attend college and live on-campus. During a transition planning meeting, the student's teacher reports the student has had several accidents during a meal preparation class (i.e., incurring cuts when using a knife and burning hands when taking items out of the oven). As part of the transition plan, the occupational therapist will teach the student adaptive techniques used in a kitchen setting to compensate for right side weakness. Which of the following adaptations should the therapist recommend to improve the student's independence in preparing meals safely?

Answer Choices:
A. Prepare foods that do not require cutting.
B. Use a microwave oven to cook food.
C. Use a weighted knife to cut food.
D. Use oven mitts that extend to the elbows. ✓

Correct Answer: D.

Rationale:
Non-spastic cerebral palsy will exhibit decreased or fluctuating muscle tone and can include hemiparesis which indicates the arm and leg on one side of the body is weakened. Adaptations to an activity or the environment can prevent injuries in the kitchen and support independence during meal preparation. Using oven mitts that cover the forearms is a practical adaptation that will prevent burns when handling hot baking dishes in both the oven and microwave. The adaptation will allow the student a choice in using an oven or the microwave during meal preparation. Cutting food items regularly occurs when preparing meals. Rather than limiting meal preparation options, cutting food can be easily modified by using a cutting board with prongs to help secure the food item, using a rocker knife for one-handed cutting or using a finger guard to prevent cutting injuries. Weighted utensils may be recommended to reduce tremors which have not been identified as a problem.

Type of Reasoning: Inductive

This question requires one to apply knowledge of adaptive techniques for safe meal preparation in order to arrive at a correct conclusion. This necessitates clinical judgment, which is an inductive reasoning skill. For this scenario, the therapist should recommend using oven mitts that extend to the elbow to prevent burns when handling hot items. If answered incorrectly, review adaptive strategies used during meal preparation tasks.

B86 C2

An individual recently discharged from an acute psychiatric unit interviews for a position in a transitional employment program (TEP). The person answers the interviewing therapist's questions in a direct yet subdued manner and rarely looks at the therapist. Which is most accurate for the therapist to document in the summary of the interview?

Answer Choices:

A. The individual should have medications evaluated before starting the TEP.
B. The individual demonstrated limited eye contact.
C. The individual exhibited poor social interaction skills.
D. The individual appeared depressed.

Correct Answer: B.

Rationale:

The only factual answer is that the individual demonstrated limited eye contact as evidenced by rarely looking at the therapist. The other answers are based upon conjecture as to the meaning or precipitant to this decreased eye contact. Individuals from many cultures are not comfortable with direct eye contact. One cannot assume that this behavior is due to depression, poor social interaction skills or the need for medication. The subdued answers can be due to cultural and/or personality factors.

Type of Reasoning: Analytical

This question requires the test taker to determine the functional deficit of the patient, which is an analytical reasoning skill. Questions of this nature often call upon the test taker to determine a diagnosis based on a functional description of deficits. Based on this information, the description indicates that the person exhibits limited eye contact. Review documentation guidelines if answered incorrectly.

B87 C5

An adult is hospitalized and diagnosed with mild chronic obstructive pulmonary disease (COPD). During the discharge planning session, the person identifies a desire to exercise regularly. Which of the following should the occupational therapist recommend the client pursue?

Answer Choices:

A. The hospital wellness program's yoga group.
B. Low-impact aerobics at a local gym.
C. Weight-lifting under the direction of a personal trainer.
D. Jogging in a local park with friends.

Correct Answer: A.

Rationale:

The yoga and stretching program put the least amount of pressure on the pulmonary and cardiovascular systems. Also, the program is monitored by hospital personnel. All of the other activities can stress the cardiovascular and pulmonary systems too much. Also, they are not monitored by health care professionals familiar with COPD.

Type of Reasoning: Inferential
One must consider the diagnosis and needs of the client in order to choose the best exercise program for the patient. For patients with COPD, a monitored exercise program with the least amount of pressure on the pulmonary and cardiovascular systems is best. Questions that ask for a best course of action or what will best consider a patient's needs often necessitate inferential reasoning skill. If answered incorrectly, review information on exercise guidelines for patients with COPD.

B88 C2

An individual who is acutely psychotic has been brought to the hospital by a legal guardian. The individual neither responds to questions nor attends to visual stimuli in the room. Who should the therapist collaborate with to determine the individual's short-term goals?

Answer Choices:
A. The guardian.
B. The individual.
C. The psychiatrist.
D. The case manager.

Correct Answer: A.

Rationale:
An individual decides goals in conjunction with the therapist except when the person is unable to take care of self, is a danger to self or others, or is unable to participate in the process. Since the person cannot respond, it would be in the individual's best interest to have the guardian take the place of the individual. The case manager and psychiatrist are important members of the team with whom the therapist will collaborate, but they cannot set goals for the individual. Goal-setting must take into account the individual's perspective and they will not have this personal awareness. The guardian would be the person most informed about the individual's life situation, roles, values, needs and desires; all critical to the formulation of relevant goals.

Type of Reasoning: Evaluative
One must determine a best course of action, given the information provided and the value assigned by the test taker for each of the possible courses of action. In this situation, because the patient cannot participate in goal setting, the guardian and therapist should be involved in goal-setting until the individual can participate. Evaluative reasoning questions often require one to assign value to a course of action or situations in order to determine an ideal solution.

B89 C2

In an outpatient rehabilitation clinic, an occupational therapist is treating a high-school student with spina bifida resulting in full motor paralysis and sensory deficits below L1 spinal cord level. The client is a competitive swimmer and is able to transfer independently from the wheelchair to the pool without an assistive device. The client's goal is to learn how to mount and ride a horse. Which is best for the therapist to do initially to help the client attain this goal?

Answer Choices:

A. Implement a home-based transfer training program for the client's family to learn how to assist with mounting a horse.
B. Develop an exercise program for the client to do at home on a daily basis to increase upper extremity strength.
C. Encourage the client to extend scheduled swimming sessions and practice mounting large inflatable tubes in the pool.
D. Consult with a stable owner to discuss alternative methods of mounting a horse.

Correct Answer: D.

Rationale:

Consulting with a stable owner would be the best option initially to determine other ways to mount a horse. Based upon this information, the therapist can plan an appropriate intervention. Implementing a home-based transfer training program for the family may be relevant after determining the possible ways the client can safely mount a horse. Since the client is a competitive swimmer and can transfer independently to the floor, upper extremity strength is not a problem. The activity demands of mounting large inflatable tubes in a pool are not the same as the activity demands of mounting a horse. The ability to mount tubes in a pool would not generalize to mounting a horse.

Type of Reasoning: Inductive

For this item, one must determine the best course of action for an individual with spina bifida. The test taker must have knowledge of the diagnosis and be able to effectively use activity analysis skills to come to a correct conclusion. For this situation, it would be best for the therapist to consult with a stable owner to discuss alternative methods of mounting a horse. If answered incorrectly, review information on spina bifida and activity analysis guidelines.

B90 C1

An occupational therapist provides intervention to develop independent feeding skills in an 18-month-old child with significant developmental delays. The child has mastered the ability to hold a spoon and bang it on the tray of the high chair. The child can also hold and suck on a cracker. Which activity is best for the therapist to provide next during intervention?

Answer Choices:

A. Finger-feeding soft foods.
B. Scooping food and bringing it to the mouth.
C. Taking cereal from a spoon held by the therapist.
D. Bringing a filled spoon to the mouth.

Correct Answer: A.

Rationale:

The next developmental milestone after holding and banging a spoon is finger-feeding soft foods. Due to the child's developmental delay, an occupational therapist would work on the acquisition of feeding skills according to normal developmental milestones. The typical developmental sequence of feeding is: taking cereal from a spoon (5–7 months), self-feeding by sucking a cracker (6–9 months), holding and banging a spoon (6–9 months), finger-feeding soft foods (9–13 months), bringing a filled spoon to mouth (12–14 months), scooping food and bringing it to the mouth (15–18 months). See Table 5-5 in Chapter 5 for more details on the developmental sequence of self-feeding. In working with a child with developmental disabilities, it is the child's developmental age, not his/her chronological age which guides intervention.

Type of Reasoning: Deductive
One must recall the developmental guidelines for feeding infants with developmental delays. This is factual knowledge, which is a deductive reasoning skill. First, the test taker must determine what developmental age the child is performing feeding and then determine the next developmental milestone for that skill. In this case, the child is developmentally at 9 months and finger-feeding soft foods is the next milestone for feeding. If answered incorrectly, review developmental milestones of infant feeding.

B91 C9

The residents of a halfway house plan a community leisure activity for a Saturday. Two residents state that they cannot participate in Saturday activities due to religious observances. The other residents express strong interest in the activity. Which is the occupational therapist's best response to this situation?

Answer Choices:
A. Schedule an in-house Saturday leisure activity for the two observant residents.
B. Explore with the group an alternative schedule for a community leisure activity. ✓
C. Schedule an in-house Saturday leisure activity for all residents.
D. Recommend the two observant members seek approval from their religious leadership to attend the Saturday activity.

Correct Answer: B.

Rationale:
All residents should be provided with the opportunity to engage in the community leisure activity. Facilitating the group's exploration of alternative scheduling can result in all residents' needs being met. Engaging in an on-site activity is not congruent with the residents' statement that they could not participate in activities on Saturday. It is inappropriate to advise group members to seek the approval of their religious leadership to engage in an activity that is inconsistent with their religious beliefs. Finding an alternative schedule for a community activity that all residents can participate in does not prevent the other residents from engaging in community activities of interest on a Saturday.

Type of Reasoning: Evaluative
One must weigh the possible courses of action and then make a value judgment about the best course to take. This requires evaluative reasoning skill, which often utilizes guiding principles of action in order to arrive at a correct conclusion. In this case, because not all residents can attend the leisure activity due to religious observances, the most appropriate recommendation is for the group to explore an alternative schedule for the activity.

Multiple Choice Scenario Item B.II.

Questions B92 to B96 are based on the following information.

An individual is transferred from an acute care hospital to a sub-acute rehabilitation unit in a long-term care facility. The patient incurred a left cerebral vascular accident (CVA) in the middle cerebral artery (MCA) one week ago. The individual is referred to occupational therapy. The referral states that the patient has right hemiplegia and a subluxed right shoulder.

B92 C4

The occupational therapist meets with the nursing staff that will be providing primary care to the patient at the patient's bedside. The occupational therapist recommends that the direct care staff position the patient in left sidelying. Which is the best bed position for the therapist to recommend for placement of the patient's right arm?

Answer Choices:

A. In 90° of humeral abduction and internally rotated.
B. Protracted with arm forward on a pillow and the elbow extended or slightly flexed.
C. On the person's side, adducted and internally rotated.
D. In 90° of abduction of the humerus with neutral rotation.

Correct Answer: B.

Rationale:

The best position of the upper extremities for sleeping or bed rest is to place the affected arm on a pillow in a position which ensures that the shoulder is approximated and that the extremity is well supported. Excess abduction can cause the joint capsule to loosen and reduce the stability of the humeral head in the glenoid fossa. It is important to avoid traction of the affected arm to ensure adequate positioning of the humerus with the scapula and to prevent subluxation. Correct positioning means putting the involved arm in slight abduction. 90° of abduction is excessive.

Type of Reasoning: Inferential

One must infer or draw conclusions about the optimal positioning of the affected upper extremity in side-lying. One must understand the reasons for the positioning of the extremity in order to prevent further problems from developing, which requires inferential reasoning skill. In this situation, positioning the extremity on a pillow in slight abduction is best.

B93 C4

The occupational therapist also advises the direct care staff on proper positioning of the patient's right arm while the patient is seated in a wheelchair. Which is the most appropriate recommendation for the therapist to make for positioning of the patient's right arm?

Answer Choices:

A. Rest the person's arm on a wheelchair lap board.
B. Rest the arm in the person's lap with the hands folded.
C. Wear a resting hand splint to avoid joint contractures.
D. Have the person wear a shoulder sling throughout the day.

Correct Answer: A.

Rationale:

Proper positioning is important in addressing shoulder subluxations. Positioning must avoid shoulder traction, scapular downward rotation and weight on the shoulder. Lap boards are ideal for positioning in a wheelchair. They promote proper shoulder positioning and protect the arm from hanging over the side of the wheelchair and getting caught in the wheel during mobility. Wearing a shoulder sling for prolonged periods is contraindicated as long-term use can result in soft-tissue contractures, edema and the development of pain syndromes. Shoulder slings can be used to support a flaccid shoulder for short and controlled periods of time. A resting hand splint is beneficial for wrist and hand positioning, but does not address the shoulder subluxation.

Exam B

Type of Reasoning: Inductive
This question requires one to determine the best approach for treating subluxation of the shoulder. This requires inductive reasoning skill, where clinical judgment is paramount in arriving at a correct conclusion. For this situation, positioning the arm to rest on a lapboard is best. If answered incorrectly, review treatment guidelines and positioning recommendations for patients with shoulder subluxation.

B94 **C7**

While completing the screening, the occupational therapist observes that the patient uses only the left side to participate in activities. The therapist suspects that the patient has unilateral neglect and difficulties with body scheme. Which should the therapist have the patient do during the OT evaluation to determine if these deficits are present?

Answer Choices:
A. Point to various body parts named by the therapist.
B. Complete an upper extremity dressing evaluation. ✓
C. Complete the draw-a-person test.
D. Complete a body puzzle.

Correct Answer: B.

Rationale:
The best way to evaluate for unilateral neglect and difficulties with body scheme is to have the person physically complete a dressing evaluation. Pointing to named body parts, draw-a-person and body puzzles address somatognosis, one element of body scheme.

Type of Reasoning: Analytical
This question requires one to analyze the various evaluation techniques and then determine which one most effectively assesses unilateral neglect and body scheme dysfunction together. An upper extremity dressing evaluation is the only choice that evaluates both. Analytical reasoning skills are utilized for this question, as one must take the pieces of information provided, determine their meaning and match this to an appropriate solution.

B95 **C7**

During the initial ADL evaluation, the therapist notes that the patient consistently spills food due to an inability to adjust movements while cutting food and moving the food from the plate to the mouth. Which deficit does this behavior most likely indicate?

Answer Choices:
A. Ideational apraxia.
B. Asomatognosia.
C. Motor apraxia. ✓
D. Tactile agnosia.

Correct Answer: C.

Rationale:
Motor apraxia (also known as ideomotor apraxia) is the loss of access to kinesthetic memory so that purposeful movement cannot be achieved due to ineffective motor planning; although sensation, movement, and coordination are intact. Ideational apraxia is a breakdown in the knowledge of what is to be done or how to perform an action or use an object. Asomatognosia is a body scheme disorder that results in diminished awareness of body structure and a failure to recognize body parts as one's own. Tactile agnosia, also known as astereognosis is the inability to recognize objects, forms, shapes and sizes by touch alone.

Type of Reasoning: Analytical
This question requires the test taker to determine the functional deficit of the patient, which is an analytical reasoning skill. Questions of this nature often call upon the test taker to determine a diagnosis based on a functional description of deficits. Based on this information, the symptoms of the patient indicate the deficit of motor apraxia, which should be reviewed if answered incorrectly.

B96 C4

Upon evaluation, the therapist determines that the patient has right homonymous hemianopsia. The therapist provides recommendations to modify the patient's room to enhance independence. Which are the most appropriate recommendations for the therapist to make for the placement of the patient's telephone and radio?

Answer Choices:
A. Telephone on the left side and the radio on the left side.
B. Telephone on the right side and the radio on the right side.
C. Telephone on the right side and the radio on the left side.
D. Telephone on the left side and the radio on the right side. ✓

Correct Answer: D.

Rationale:
The telephone must be placed within the person's intact visual field (which, in this case, is left) so that the person can readily access it in case of emergency. However, the radio can be placed outside of the person's visual field (right, in this case), to encourage the person to scan the environment. If the person initially has trouble locating the radio, it will not pose any danger to him/her. The occupational therapist can use the radio as a tool to increase scanning skills during intervention sessions.

Type of Reasoning: Inductive
Clinical knowledge and judgment are the most important skills needed for answering this question, which requires inductive reasoning skill. Knowledge of the diagnosis and most appropriate clinical outcomes is essential to choose the best solution. In this case, the therapist should recommend that the telephone is placed on the left and the radio on the right side. This best addresses the person's safety as well as improving function in scanning the environment.

B97 C8

In an outpatient rehabilitation clinic, an occupational therapist is developing a fall prevention group for at risk elderly clients with Parkinson's disease. The clients live alone and have had at least three falls within the past six months. When presenting strategies to prevent falls, which is the most common risk factor for falls in the elderly that the therapist should review with the clients?

Answer Choices:
A. Ascending and descending stairs. ✓
B. Dressing while seated in a chair.
C. Walking with a walker with wheels.
D. Transferring out of the shower with grab bars.

Correct Answer: A

Rationale:
Most falls occur during normal activities of daily living, including bending, getting up and down from a seated surface, turning, walking and ascending and descending stairs. Using assistive devices in the correct manner reduces fall risk and completing activities of daily living while seated is a safe modification to the activity of dressing.

Type of Reasoning: Inferential
For this item, the test taker must determine the most common risk factors for falls in the elderly. This necessitates inferential reasoning skill, where one determines what is likely to be true in a therapeutic situation. For this scenario, ascending and descending stairs are the most common risk factor for falls in the elderly. Review fall prevention guidelines if answered incorrectly.

B98 C9

An occupational therapist working in a school system must incorporate the Individuals with Disabilities Education Act (IDEA) in the program. In which of the following locations should the therapist provide intervention?

Answer Choices:
A. Regular classroom while general education classes are not in session.
B. Special education classroom while other children with disabilities are present.
C. Regular classroom while general education classes are in session. ✓
D. Private occupational therapy room designed for children with disabilities.

Correct Answer: C.

Rationale:
The guidelines from IDEA emphasize that a child's needs be served in an inclusive manner that enables the child to have full access to the general education curriculum, focusing on participation in a general education classroom. The other options are too restrictive and do not facilitate inclusion in general education.

Type of Reasoning: Deductive
One must recall IDEA guidelines in order to arrive at a correct conclusion. This requires deductive reasoning skill, where knowledge of protocols and guidelines are paramount in choosing the correct answer. In this situation, therapy intervention in a regular classroom while general education classes are in session is the only location that provides inclusive treatment. If answered incorrectly, review IDEA guidelines and inclusive services in the classroom.

B99 C8

An occupational therapist conducts an in-service at an outpatient wheelchair clinic for individuals with central nervous system dysfunction. According to the principles of wheelchair prescription, which of the following statements is accurate for the therapist to make during the presentation?

Answer Choices:
A. Firm seats are needed to provide stability. ✓
B. Soft seats are needed to prevent decubiti.
C. Back heights should be extended to facilitate weight shifting. ✗
D. Seat angles should be 45° to prevent falling forward. ✗

Correct Answer: A.

Rationale:
Firm seats provide stability and a solid base for seating systems that can be used to prevent decubiti, contractures and deformities, and to increase sitting tolerance, proper positioning and functional abilities. Soft seats are contraindicated as they do not provide sufficient pressure relief. Soft seats can "collapse" under pressure and can increase the risk of decubiti. Extended back heights increase the difficulty of weight shifting because the person cannot hook his/her arm around the push handle. The recommended seat angle ranges from 80°–110°.

Type of Reasoning: Deductive

This question requires recall of guidelines and principles, which is factual knowledge. Deductive reasoning skills are utilized whenever one must recall facts to solve everyday problems. In this situation, the therapist is accurate in stating that firm seats are needed to provide stability. Review wheelchair prescription guidelines if answered incorrectly.

B100 C9

An occupational therapist working in an outpatient clinic observes the clinic's administrative assistant leaving patient records open on the clinic's reception counter. The assistant has left the clinic to go for lunch. Which action is best for the therapist to take in response to this observation?

Answer Choices:
A. Remind the administrative assistant of the need to keep patient records private when the assistant returns from lunch.
B. Immediately contact the administrative assistant's direct supervisor to report this observation.
C. Pick up the records and place them in a location out of public view.
D. Discuss the issue with the clinic's director during their next scheduled supervision session.

Correct Answer: C.

Rationale:
The therapist must act to protect patient privacy. The HIPAA Privacy Rule requires that all providers protect patient confidentiality in all forms (i.e., oral, written and electronic). Charts and any documentation with patients' names or other identifiers must be stored out of public view and in secure locations. Reminding the administrative assistant of documentation privacy requirements when the assistant returns, contacting the administrative assistant's direct supervisor and discussing the issue with the clinic's director do not address the immediate need for the therapist to take action that makes sure no patient record is visible to anyone in the reception area.

Type of Reasoning: Evaluative

This question requires the test taker to weigh the merits of the courses of action presented and determine the approach that will most effectively resolve the issue. This requires evaluative reasoning skill. For this situation, the therapist should pick up the records and place them in a location out of public view to protect patient privacy. If answered incorrectly, review HIPAA guidelines and the protection of patient privacy.

B101 C2

An occupational therapist works in a program for survivors of domestic violence. Which of the following would the therapist do when using a client-centered approach?

Answer Choices:
A. Offer specific concrete behavioral suggestions for dealing with confrontations.
B. Respond to the participants' self-deprecating comments with positive feedback on personal characteristics. ✗
C. Reinforce only the participants' neutral comments about themselves and personal skills. ✗
D. Reflectively paraphrase the participants' statements to help clarify their feelings.

Exam B

Correct Answer: D.

Rationale:
The main principle of client-centered therapy is that it is directed by the person. An intervention goal when working with survivors of domestic violence is to increase their awareness of feelings. Since the expression of feelings can be difficult for survivors of domestic violence, the best client-centered approach is to accept the person unconditionally and reflect back what he/she is saying in a nonjudgmental manner. Offering concrete suggestions is too directive and is not a component of client-centered therapy. The therapist should use techniques to encourage the participants' to generate their own personal strategies for behavioral change. In the client-centered approach, the therapist should withhold judgment on self-deprecating comments. Survivors of domestic violence often have decreased self-efficacy and typically will deflect positive feedback. To foster self-esteem, the therapist can be most effective by providing opportunities for the person to discover positive attributes and feelings independent of the viewpoints of others.

Type of Reasoning: Inferential
This question requires one to determine a best course of action based on the information provided, which is an inferential reasoning skill. For this situation, paraphrasing the participants' statements to help clarify feelings is best. If answered incorrectly, review information on the client-centered practices and the characteristics of survivors of domestic violence. The correct answer requires the integration of this information.

B102 C8

A patient is recovering from a right CVA resulting in severe left hemiplegia and visuospatial deficits. The person's left lower extremity has pitting edema. Which wheelchair would be best for the occupational therapist to recommend for this patient?

Answer Choices:
A. A powered wheelchair with a joystick control and dual elevating leg rests.
B. A lightweight active duty wheelchair with dual elevating leg rests.
C. A one-arm drive chair with an elevating leg rest on the left.
D. A hemiplegic chair with an elevating leg rest on the left.

Correct Answer: D.

Rationale:
A hemiplegic chair has a low seat height ($17\frac{1}{2}$ inches as compared to the standard seat height of $19\frac{1}{2}$ inches) and is the best choice for this patient. The patient can propel it using both the unaffected hand and leg. An elevating leg rest for the left side is needed to address the edema in the patient's left lower extremity. There is no need for an elevating leg rest for the right lower extremity. A one-arm drive wheelchair has both drive mechanisms located on one wheel. A person can propel this type of wheelchair by using one hand. A one-arm drive wheelchair is contraindicated for patients with cognitive or perceptual deficits (as in this case) as they can be confusing to learn to propel accurately. The electric wheelchair with joystick would also be difficult for a person with visuospatial deficits. In addition, an electric wheelchair is significantly more expensive, less transportable, requires increased maintenance and would be difficult to justify for reimbursement.

Type of Reasoning: Analytical
A number of important symptoms are described in this exam item and the test taker must analyze all of the symptoms (not just some) in order to make the best choice in wheelchair prescription. When balancing the edema issues, hemiplegia and visuospatial deficits, one must conclude that a hemi chair with elevating leg rest provides the safest, most effective means of mobility and addresses all the deficits mentioned. If answered incorrectly, review wheelchair prescription guidelines.

B103 C8

An older adult with a diagnosis of osteoarthritis in both knees is referred to inpatient occupational therapy. During screening, the patient expresses a desire to return home to live alone independently. Which should the occupational therapist do first in response to the patient's stated goal?

Answer Choices:

A. Recommend adaptations to the patient's home environment to increase safety.
B. Evaluate the patient's BADL and IADL using a standardized measure.
C. Teach the patient energy conservation techniques to use during IADL tasks.
D. Train the patient in a home resistive exercise program to build strength and ROM.

Correct Answer: B.

Rationale:

The patient has just been screened for occupational therapy services so the next step in the occupational therapy process is to evaluate the person's functional abilities. Osteoarthritis is isolated to specific joints and is not systemic in nature. By evaluating the patient's BADL and IADL, the occupational therapist can determine the activity demands of the BADL and IADL the patient performs while keeping in mind the specific joints that are affected. Once this information is obtained, then the occupational therapist can make informed recommendations based upon his/her observations and clinical reasoning to decrease excessive loading and repetitive use of these joints. Simple adaptations, such as moving items higher (onto counters, etc.) can be recommended and energy conservation techniques can be taught based upon the evaluation results. Resistive exercise programs are contraindicated for persons with osteoarthritis.

Type of Reasoning: Inferential

One must determine the best approach for evaluation of this patient, given his/her stated desires and diagnosis. This requires inferential reasoning skill, where one must infer or draw conclusions about the approach that will result in the best functional outcome. In this case, evaluation of the patient's daily activities using a standardized measure is the best approach to learn about his/her ability to safely return home, managing the symptoms of osteoarthritis. Review evaluation guidelines and home management assessments if answered incorrectly. Integration of this knowledge with an understanding of the impact osteoarthritis has on BADL and IADL is required to determine a correct answer.

B104 C3

An older teenager with a congenital right below-elbow amputation had never wanted a prosthesis before. Now the teen wants a prosthesis "to look good at the prom and more 'normal' when doing things with my friends." Which action would be most beneficial for the occupational therapist to take to meet the client's expressed needs?

Answer Choices:

A. Recommend a prosthesis with a cosmetic passive hand.
B. Recommend a prosthesis with a voluntary opening hook.
C. Recommend a prosthesis with a myoelectrically controlled hand.
D. Recommend counseling to explore the client's sudden preoccupation with body image.

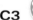

Correct Answer: C.

Rationale:
The best choice is a prosthesis that meets the teen's expressed need for a cosmetically appealing device which can also be used to perform functional age-appropriate bilateral fine motor activities, such as text messaging, or playing video games. Although a prosthesis can be used for purely cosmetic reasons, it would be best to provide the teen with a device that he/she could use to increase functional performance when doing activities with friends. A passive cosmetic hand can be used for grasping large objects like a beach ball or to hold an object on a table but has no moving parts for grasp and release, so it would not be the most functional choice. Although a voluntary opening hook would enable the teen to perform functional activities, recommending this would not respect the teen's expressed desire for a cosmetically appealing device. Recommending counseling based on an interpretation of the teen's request as a preoccupation with body image is judgmental. This action also violates the person's rights of autonomy.

Type of Reasoning: Inductive
This question requires the test taker to determine through clinical judgment which course of action will best address the client's request and provide optimal functioning. This requires inductive reasoning skill, where clinical judgment plus prediction of how a course of action will result in future benefit is accentuated. In this case, a prosthesis with a myoelectrically controlled hand is the best choice to facilitate function and fulfill the client's wishes. Review upper extremity prosthetic options if answered incorrectly.

B105 C3

An adult is referred to occupational therapy for ADL training. The patient incurred a fracture of the right proximal humerus and is using a shoulder immobilizer for the first two weeks to aid healing and help control pain. The patient is right hand dominant. Which activity will be the most difficult for the patient?

Answer Choices:
A. Putting on a pullover top.
B. Completing online banking.
C. Taking off a winter coat.
D. Brushing their teeth.

Correct Answer: A.

Rationale:
Treatment of a proximal fracture of the humerus includes non-operative treatment using a sling or shoulder immobilizer with no shoulder mobility for the first two weeks followed by exercises to slowly increase the range of motion or surgery. Since there is a period of immobilization patients need to learn how to complete ADL using modified techniques. While the person could use a one-handed technique to don a pullover top, this would put too much strain on the upper extremity and may cause increased pain. A safer alternative to dressing the upper body is to wear tops with front opening closures (i.e., zippers, buttons or snaps). Because coats have front openings, taking off a winter coat would not pose greatest difficulty. The keyboarding required to complete online banking can be adapted by having the person use the non-injured upper extremity. The patient can learn a one-handed technique to brush their teeth.

Type of Reasoning: Inferential
This question requires one to infer what is likely to be true of a therapeutic situation based on knowledge of the diagnosis and functional limitations. Questions of this nature require inferential reasoning skill. For this case, based on knowledge of the limitations with recent humeral fractures, donning a pullover top would present the most difficulty for this patient. Review self-care techniques for patients with decreased mobility if answered incorrectly.

B106 C6

An occupational therapist is treating an individual with Parkinson's disease in an outpatient setting. The therapist observes that the person attends regularly but has little energy and does not seem to be performing the prescribed home program. Which is the best action for the therapist to take in response to these observations?

Answer Choices:
A. Advise the physician to complete a referral for a psychiatric evaluation. ✗
B. Tell the person that the completion of the home program is vital to recovery. ✗
C. Interview the person and complete a standardized depression scale. ✓
D. Defer intervention until the person's depression is treated.

Correct Answer: C.

Rationale:
A standardized depression scale provides objective data and an interview can obtain the person's subjective experience and viewpoints. Together this information can be used to determine the reasons for the person's observable behaviors, namely lethargy and decreased motivation to practice what is being learned in therapy. A referral for a psychiatric evaluation would be premature at this point as the cause of the person's behavior is not known. The person's lack of energy and noncompliance can be due to other factors that are not psychiatric in nature. For example, the individual could be providing care for a spouse and not have time for a home program and/or for adequate sleep. Telling a person the importance of a home program does not directly deal with the issue of lack of follow through. In addition, there is nothing in the scenario to indicate that the person is not aware of the importance of compliance. Since it is not known if the person's behaviors are due to depression, it would not be appropriate to defer treatment. If the person is depressed, the treatment for depression can be provided concurrently with the treatment for the person's physical limitations.

Type of Reasoning: Inferential
One must infer or draw conclusions about a likely course of action, given the information presented. This is an inferential reasoning skill, where knowledge of a therapeutic approach, such as identifying what the symptoms indicate in this situation, is essential to choosing a correct solution. In this case, the therapist should perform a standardized depression scale and interview the person. Review symptoms of depression if answered incorrectly.

B107 C9

An occupational therapist working for a home care agency provides an inservice to new employees on Medicare reimbursement guidelines for durable medical equipment (DME). Which item would the therapist describe as reimbursable by Medicare?

Answer Choices:
A. A raised toilet seat for a patient after a hip replacement.
B. A reacher for a person with arthritis in both hips.
C. A walker for a person who cannot ambulate in the home without one. ✓
D. Grab bars in the bathroom for a person who cannot bathe or toilet without them.

Correct Answer: C.

Rationale:
The walker is covered by Medicare. The others are not. The criteria for durable medical equipment to be reimbursable by Medicare are that the item must be necessary and reasonable to treat an illness or incidence of decreased functioning. The item must have a medical purpose, be used repeatedly and not useful in the absence of an illness.

Type of Reasoning: Deductive

This question requires one to recall Medicare reimbursement guidelines, which is factual knowledge. Deductive reasoning skills are utilized whenever one must recall concrete principles and guidelines to draw conclusions. The only item listed that is considered a medical necessity by Medicare is a walker when issued for a person who cannot ambulate in the home without one. Review Medicare guidelines for reimbursement of DME if answered incorrectly.

B108 C4

An individual has had a brain tumor removed from the cerebellum. The occupational therapist conducts a screening to determine the need for further evaluation. During the screening the therapist observes deficits that indicate the need for further evaluation. Which would be most relevant for the therapist to evaluate based on this screening?

Answer Choices:
A. Proprioception and coordination. ✓
B. Tactile and sensory integration.
C. Vision and visual-perception.
D. Audition and communication.

Correct Answer: A.

Rationale:

The cerebellum receives input from the proprioceptive pathways and modulates the smooth coordination of voluntary movements. Therefore, a tumor in this area would affect proprioception and coordination. These deficits would be evident upon screening. Further evaluation would be needed to determine the extent of the brain tumor's effect on these areas. Tactile and sensory integration skills would be most affected by damage to the parietal lobe. Vision and visual-perceptual skills would be most affected by damage to the occipital lobe. Audition and communication abilities would be most affected by damage to the temporal lobe.

Type of Reasoning: Inferential

One must have knowledge of the functional anatomy of the brain to arrive at a correct conclusion since tumors in a specific lobe would compromise its function. This is an inferential reasoning skill where knowledge of clinical guidelines and judgment based on facts are utilized to reach conclusions. In this situation, the screening will most likely indicate a need for further evaluation of proprioception and coordination skills since these are functions of the cerebellum. If answered incorrectly, review the functional anatomy of the brain. Understanding the effects of a tumor on typical neurological functioning is key to selecting the correct answer.

B109 C3

A client participates in occupational therapy for intervention following a rotator cuff injury. The therapist provides progressive resistive exercises. When grading these exercises, which of the following is best for the therapist to increase?

Answer Choices:
A. The amount of resistance provided with a stronger level of therapy band. ✓
B. The range of motion involved in completing the exercises. ✗
C. The proximal load on the muscles the client uses during the exercises. distal load
D. The repetitions of external rotation exercises with less distal weight. endurance

Correct Answer: A.

Rationale:
Resistive exercises serve to increase strength of muscles from fair plus to normal through adequate ROM. Increasing the resistance level of therapy band is the best method provided to progressively grade the resistive exercises. This approach can increase the person's strength. Increasing the ROM of an exercise helps to increase the available ROM of the muscle, but not strength. Progressively increasing strength, the focus of resistive exercise, would be helped by increasing the distal load on the muscles, not necessarily by increasing the proximal load on muscles. Increased repetitions with decreased distal weight can increase endurance but not specifically strength.

Type of Reasoning: Inductive
One must utilize clinical knowledge and judgment to determine the exercise approach that progressively grades resistance. In this case, a stronger level of therapy band is the ideal way to foster greater resistance out of the choices provided. If answered incorrectly, review progressive resistive exercise guidelines, including exercise programming for a patient post rotator cuff injury.

B110 C1

A toddler attends an early intervention program as a result of developmental delay. Over the past two weeks, the toddler has successfully completed the activities the occupational therapist has provided in order to develop a palmar grasp. Which action should the therapist take next in response to the child's progress?

Answer Choices:
A. Continue providing the child with the activities to refine palmar grasp.
B. Review the initial evaluation to determine new goals.
C. Provide activities to develop a radial palmar grasp.
D. Provide activities to develop an ulnar palmar grasp.

Correct Answer: C.

Rationale:
The child has exhibited mastery of a palmar grasp. The next developmental level of grasp after a palmar grasp is a radial palmar grasp. Ulnar palmar grasp is the developmental precursor to palmar grasp. If the initial evaluation determined there was a need to work on the development of grasp, intervention can proceed to the next level without re-evaluation or the establishment of new goals.

Type of Reasoning: Deductive
One must recall the developmental milestones of grasp patterns for children. This is factual knowledge, which is a deductive reasoning skill. In this case, after the development of a palmar grasp, the next level is the development of a radial palmar grasp. If answered incorrectly, review development of grasp patterns in children.

B111 C1

A child with congenital anomalies has severe developmental delay. The child demonstrates motor and cognitive skills at the nine-month level. Which is the best adaptation for the occupational therapist to use during intervention to develop the child's visual and auditory awareness?

Answer Choices:
A. A hand-held rattle of the child's favorite cartoon character.
B. A wrist bracelet with blinking lights that makes noise when moved.
C. A button switch that activates a CD player when the switch is pressed.
D. A communication device that offers selections of "yes" and "no."

Correct Answer: C.

Rationale:
The button switch encourages the child to develop the developmentally appropriate skill of cause and effect. Visual stimulation is provided when the child focuses on the device to activate it. Activating the CD player provides auditory feedback. The rattle is an activity that is developmentally appropriate for a child at the three- to six-month level. The wrist bracelet is an activity that is developmentally appropriate for the child at the three- to six-month level. The communication device is an activity that is developmentally appropriate at the level of 12 to 18 months.

Type of Reasoning: Inferential
One must infer or draw conclusions about each of the four possible choices. The key to answering this question correctly is matching an activity to the child's developmental age and current needs. In this situation, a button switch that activates a CD player helps to develop cause and effect for this child who functions at a nine-month level. If answered incorrectly, review developmental milestones and appropriate activities for the nine-month level and other developmental levels.

B112 C4

An adult incurred an injury to the anterior spinal artery at the T12 level. The occupational therapist completes a sensory evaluation with this client. Which sensation is most likely for the therapist to document that the individual has retained?

Answer Choices:
A. Proprioception.
B. Pain.
C. Light touch.
D. Temperature.

Correct Answer: A.

Rationale:
Proprioception is maintained with the condition of anterior spinal cord syndrome, which is caused by damage to the anterior spinal artery or anterior spinal cord. Dorsal (posterior) columns transmit proprioceptive information. The others are aspects of sensation that are impaired or absent in anterior spinal cord syndrome.

Type of Reasoning: Inferential
This question provides the diagnosis and the test taker must determine what is and is not affected by this injury. This is an inferential reasoning skill. For this case, an anterior spinal artery injury would preserve proprioception, as it transmitted through the dorsal columns in the spine. If answered incorrectly, review symptoms of anterior spinal artery damage and other spinal tracts.

B113 C9

An occupational therapy administrator implements a quality improvement program at a large private hand therapy clinic. The administrator determines that the clinic's occupational therapy assistants (OTAs) are not completing their assigned initial screenings in a timely manner. This has resulted in scheduling delays for complete functional evaluations. Which initial action is most effective for the administrator to take in response to this situation?

Answer Choices:

A. Counsel the OTAs on the need to adhere to screening schedules.
B. Examine the organizational structure of the screening process.
C. Assign the occupational therapists to complete all screenings.
D. Redesign the screening to simplify the process.

Correct Answer: B.

Rationale:

A fundamental principle of quality improvement (QI) is to view problems and limitations as opportunities to explore organizational improvement needs. Blame for identified problems is not attributed to any person within the organization. Counseling the OTAs and reassigning screening to the occupational therapists may not effectively address the underlying reason for the delays in screening. Before redesigning the screening process, the administrator must first examine the organizational structure of the screening process to be able to identify the needed organizational change.

Type of Reasoning: Inductive

This question requires one to determine the most appropriate initial action for addressing delays in completing initial screenings. This requires inductive reasoning skill, where clinical judgment is paramount in arriving at a correct conclusion. For this situation, the administrator should examine the organizational structure of the screening process. If answered incorrectly, review QI guidelines.

B114 C9

An occupational therapist designs a qualitative research study to examine the efficacy of an after-school play-based program for the development of social interaction skills. Which method of data collection is best for the therapist to use?

Answer Choices:

A. The therapist's observations of the participating children in the classroom and during recess.
B. The completion of a social skills Likert-scale questionnaire by the participants' teachers.
C. The completion of a social skills Likert-scale questionnaire by the participants' parents.
D. The administration of a social skills evaluation pre- and post-intervention.

Correct Answer: A.

Rationale:

Qualitative research is a form of descriptive research that studies people individually or collectively in their natural social and cultural contexts. It involves direct observation in naturalistic settings, such as observing children in their classroom and during recess. The completion of Likert-scale questionnaires and the administration of an evaluation are research methods that are used to collect quantitative data; therefore, they would not be used in a qualitative study.

Type of Reasoning: Deductive

One must recall the guidelines for qualitative research methods in order to arrive at a correct conclusion. This requires deductive reasoning skill, where factual knowledge is essential to choosing the correct solution. The only qualitative method listed in this case is the therapist observation of the children. Review qualitative research methods if answered incorrectly.

B115 **C3**

A person fell and sustained bilateral Colles' fractures. The client wore bilateral short-arm casts for six weeks. After cast removal, the client began OT sessions to increase endurance and strength prior to returning to work. The client tends to work hard when performing resistive exercises with both wrists. The therapist monitors the client for overexertion. Which behavior indicates overexertion?

Answer Choices:
A. Decreased respiration rate during resistive wrist flexion.
B. Increased ability to achieve full ROM of the wrist.
C. Complaints of pain in the wrist extensors.
D. Consistent strength in wrist extension activities.

Correct Answer: C.

Rationale:
Complaints of pain can be a sign of overexertion. The others are signs of adequate performance, not overexertion.

Type of Reasoning: Inferential
The test taker must reason which observation would likely indicate overexertion. Inferential reasoning skill is used as one must draw conclusions about the statements provided based upon clinical knowledge of therapeutic exercise. For this situation, complaints of pain often indicate overexertion. Review exercises approaches for Colles' fracture and signs of overexertion if answered incorrectly.

B116 **C9**

The administrator of a home care agency tells the occupational therapist to submit all intervention plans to the client's third party payers, prior to the implementation of treatment. Which is the most accurate term for the therapist to use when documenting these actions?

Answer Choices:
A. Concurrent review.
B. Peer review.
C. Utilization review.
D. Prospective review.

Correct Answer: D.

Rationale:
The evaluation and approval of proposed intervention plans by third party payers is called prospective review. Concurrent review is the evaluation of ongoing intervention programs. Peer review is a system in which the quality of work by a group of health professionals is reviewed by their peers. Utilization review is a plan to review the use of resources within a facility to determine medical necessity and cost efficiency.

Type of Reasoning: Deductive
This question requires recall of guidelines and principles, which is factual knowledge and a deductive reasoning skill. In this situation, the therapist submitting all intervention plans to a third party payer prior to implementation of treatment is an example of a prospective review. Review characteristics of prospective payment systems and methods of program evaluation and continuous quality improvement if answered incorrectly.

B117 C3

An individual is recovering from deep partial thickness burns on the upper extremities, chest and lower neck. The occupational therapist provides equipment to prevent positions that can result in contractures. Which are the most important positions for the therapist to prevent?

Answer Choices:
A. Positions of comfort. ✓
B. Anti-deformity positions.
C. Positions resulting in edema.
D. Positions of pain.

Correct Answer: A.

Rationale:
The position of comfort is often assumed by individuals recovering from burns. This position occurs when the person assumes the protective postures of adduction and flexion of the upper extremities, flexion of the hips and knees and plantar flexion of the ankles. This position does decrease discomfort but it is non-functional and can result in contractures. The anti-deformity position is the desired position. It is the opposite of the position of comfort. While preventing edema is important in burn rehabilitation, the question is about the prevention of contractures. Positions of pain and discomfort are unavoidable for persons recovering from deep partial thickness burns. These burns involve the epidermis and deep portion of the dermis, hair follicles and sweat glands, and are often very painful.

Type of Reasoning: Inductive
Clinical knowledge and judgment are the most important skills needed for answering this question, which requires inductive reasoning skill. Knowledge of the diagnosis and most appropriate positioning given the severity of the burns is essential to choosing the ideal solution. In this case, the patient should avoid positions of comfort. If answered incorrectly, review positioning guidelines for patients with full thickness burns.

B118 C2

A cooking group meets for $1\frac{1}{2}$ hours each week at a partial hospitalization program. During the group, members do not smoke, they wait for everyone to be served before eating and they clean up after the meal. When reporting these observations, which of the following is the most accurate statement for the therapist to make?

Answer Choices:
A. The group protocol is clear.
B. Group norms are being followed. – accepted behaviors
C. Group sanctions are effective.
D. A diversity of group roles is evident.

Correct Answer: B.

Rationale:
Group norms are the expected and accepted behaviors in a group. These norms establish an atmosphere of mutual respect, safety and support. Sanctions are implemented only in a group if members' behaviors fall outside ✗ of the group's norms and are considered deviant. The scenario does not provide sufficient information to determine members' group roles. A group protocol outlines the group's membership criteria, goals and activities.

Type of Reasoning: Analytical
This question provides a description of a functional activity and the test taker must determine the likely definition of such an activity. This is an analytical reasoning skill, as questions of this nature often ask one to analyze descriptors of functional skills to determine the overall skill involved. In this situation, the activity demonstrates that group norms are being followed.

B119　C5

An older adult recovering from a myocardial infarction is referred to occupational therapy for a home care evaluation. The referral states that the client has high blood pressure and medication-related orthostatic hypotension. Which precaution is most important for the occupational therapist to observe with this client?

Answer Choices:
A. Adherence to dietary restrictions during meal preparation activities.
B. Avoidance of activities that require movement against gravity.
C. Delay of the OT evaluation until the client's medications are stabilized.
D. Avoidance of activities that require sudden postural changes. ✓

Correct Answer: D.

Rationale:
Orthostatic hypotension or postural hypotension is an excessive drop in blood pressure that occurs upon assuming an upright position. All functional activities have components that are against gravity so these cannot be avoided during treatment. Adherence to dietary restrictions during meal preparation activities is important, but the question is about an evaluation session not an intervention session. The side effect of orthostatic hypotension may not be remediated and the patient's need for OT evaluation cannot wait.

Type of Reasoning: Evaluative
This question requires one to weigh the merits of each of the possible courses of action, which is an evaluative reasoning skill. After weighing the patient's symptoms and current status, the test taker should determine that avoidance of activities that require sudden postural changes is most important. If answered incorrectly, review activity precautions and treatment guidelines for orthostatic hypotension.

B120　C8

An occupational therapist measures a person for a wheelchair. The widest point across the person's hips and thighs is 16 inches and the greatest length from the person's posterior portion of the buttocks to the popliteal fossa is 18 inches. Which wheelchair seat dimensions should the therapist recommend?

Answer Choices:
A. 18 inches wide by 20 inches deep.
B. 18 inches wide by 18 inches deep.
C. 16 inches wide by 18 inches deep.
D. 18 inches wide by 16 inches deep. ✓

Correct Answer: D.

Rationale:
To determine the width of a wheelchair seat, two inches are added to the measurement of the widest point across the hips and thighs. This allows for clearance on the sides to prevent rubbing and to allow the individual to wear heavier material clothing without it being cumbersome. To determine the depth of a wheelchair seat, two inches are subtracted from the measurement of the length from the posterior portion of the buttocks to the popliteal fossa. This prevents rubbing and potential decubiti formation in the posterior knee region, while also allowing maximum swing length. In the case, the person's measurements were 16 inches wide by 18 inches long; therefore, the resulting seat measurement is 18 inches wide by 16 inches deep.

Type of Reasoning: Deductive
One must recall the guidelines for wheelchair prescription. This is factual knowledge, which is a deductive reasoning skill. In this situation, because the individual's measurements were 16 inches wide by 18 inches long, the seat dimensions should be 18 inches wide by 16 inches deep. If answered incorrectly, review wheelchair prescription guidelines for adults.

B121 C5

An occupational therapist provides bed mobility training for an individual recovering from a left CVA. The therapist notes that the person's right calf is swollen and warm. The person complains that it is painful. Which action should the therapist take initially?

Answer Choices:
A. Elevate the leg and provide retrograde massage.
B. Advise the person to tell the physician about the symptoms during the physician's next bedside visit.
C. Continue with the training and document the symptoms in the medical record.
D. Contact the charge nurse immediately to report symptoms.

Correct Answer: D.

Rationale:
The signs and symptoms in this scenario are indicative of deep vein thrombosis (DVT). DVT, an inflammation of a vein in association with the formation of a thrombus is often a complication of CVAs or the result of prolonged bed rest. DVT is a medical emergency that must be handled immediately by medical staff. While it would be appropriate to elevate the legs, massage is contraindicated. The other answers are inappropriate because they delay the acquisition of needed medical care.

Type of Reasoning: Evaluative
This question requires a value judgment in an urgent situation, which is an evaluative reasoning skill. In this situation, the symptoms indicate a DVT, which is a medical emergency. Essential to arrive at a correct conclusion in situations such as these, is determining when symptoms indicate an emergency and recognizing appropriate measures to remedy the situation. Review symptoms of DVT, especially appropriate courses of action if answered incorrectly.

B122 C8

An individual with bilateral proximal weakness identifies a goal of independence in self-feeding. Which equipment is most beneficial for the occupational therapist to recommend for goal attainment?

Answer Choices:
A. Extended long-handled utensils.
B. Built-up handled utensils.
C. An electric feeder.
D. Mobile arm supports.

Correct Answer: D.

Rationale:
Mobile arm supports can effectively compensate for upper extremity weakness. Extended long-handled utensils are indicated for individuals with decreased ROM. Built-up handled utensils are indicated for individuals with decreased grasp. An electric feeder is indicated for individuals with no functional use of the upper extremities.

Type of Reasoning: Inductive
This question requires one to determine the most appropriate equipment for an individual based on the person's limitations. This requires inductive reasoning skill, where clinical judgment is paramount in arriving at a correct conclusion. For this situation, mobile arm supports are most appropriate in order to enhance self-feeding. If answered incorrectly, review indications for use of mobile arm supports.

B123 **C6**

A homemaker and parent is hospitalized for depression and prescribed Parnate to treat depressive symptoms. The patient's hobbies are gardening and jogging. Upon discussing the functional effects of medications with the patient, which is the most important precaution for the occupational therapist to review?

Answer Choices:
A. Photosensitivity.
B. Dietary restrictions.
C. Orthostatic hypotension.
D. Amenorrhea.

Correct Answer: B.

Rationale:
Parnate is a monoamine oxidase inhibitor (MAOI). It has serious side effects when a person eats foods that contain the amino acid tyramine. Tyramine increases blood pressure and may lead to stroke or other cardio-vascular reactions. Photosensitivity, orthostatic hypotension and amenorrhea can be side effects of psychiatric medications but they are not typically a major concern of MAOIs. These side effects are more of a concern with anti-psychotic medications.

Type of Reasoning: Deductive
One must recall the precautions for psychotropic medications in order to arrive at a correct conclusion. This requires deductive reasoning skill, where factual knowledge is essential to choosing the correct solution. Adherence to dietary restrictions is required when taking an MAOI, such as Parnate. Review precautions for MAOIs if answered incorrectly.

B124 **C9**

An occupational therapist establishes a program for a new acute psychiatric unit at a community hospital. The therapist designs the physical layout of the occupational therapy department to include storage for arts and crafts materials. Which of the following should the therapist recommend to store arts and crafts materials?

Answer Choices:
A. A ventilated locked metal cabinet accessible only to staff. ✓
B. Open shelving accessible to patients.
C. Shelving next to a sink for easy clean up.
D. A locked closet outside of the intervention area to ensure safety.

Correct Answer: A.

Rationale:
Arts and crafts materials may include flammable, hazardous materials such as paint, stain and thinners. These must be kept in ventilated metal cabinets in accordance with fire safety guidelines. Since these supplies are also toxic and potentially dangerous, access to them must be controlled by staff; therefore, a locked storage unit is required. The other options do not meet fire safety needs.

Type of Reasoning: Inferential
One must have knowledge of safety guidelines given the clinical setting in order to arrive at a correct conclusion. This is an inferential reasoning skill where knowledge of clinical guidelines and judgment based on facts are utilized to reach conclusions. In this case, the therapist should recommend a ventilated locked metal cabinet accessible only to staff. If answered incorrectly, review safety guidelines for storage of equipment in acute psychiatric settings.

Exam B

B125 C3

A person with arthrogryposis undergoes serial casting with weekly cast changes of the right wrist. Upon cast removal during the fourth week, the therapist notes a small open area $^1/_4$ cm by $^1/_4$ cm and a red rash over the ulnar styloid. Which is the therapist's best response to these observations?

Answer Choices:

A. Pad the area and apply another cast.
B. Refer the individual to the wound care team.
C. Fabricate a static splint that does not impede on the ulnar styloid.
D. Contact the physician and describe the observations.

Correct Answer: D.

Rationale:
The physician needs to be informed of the therapist's observations. The physician can then make a decision whether to recast, dress the open area, refer to the wound care team, fabricate a new splint or employ other action.

Type of Reasoning: Evaluative
This question requires one to determine a best course of action after weighing the four possible choices. This requires evaluation of the strength and merits of the four choices, which necessitates evaluative reasoning skill. In this situation, the therapist should refer the patient to the physician for a medical evaluation of the seriousness of the wound.

B126 C8

A school-based occupational therapist consults with a teacher regarding a non-speaking student who uses a wheelchair and an augmentative communication device. The teacher reports that the student has been making many errors on the communication device but that no difficulties had been observed when the student used the device in the past. Which is the most effective initial action for the therapist to take in response to the teacher's report?

Answer Choices:

A. Advise the teacher to contact the student's parents and recommend that they bring the child to a physician for an examination.
B. Reassess the student's motor and communication abilities to determine needed modifications.
C. Evaluate the position of the student in the wheelchair and the device on the wheelchair.
D. Reposition the communication device on the wheelchair to facilitate access and increase accuracy.

Correct Answer: C.

Rationale:
Even minor changes in a person's positioning can impact on his/her access to an assistive device; therefore, the therapist's initial action must be to evaluate the position of the student and the device. Based upon the results of this assessment, the therapist may provide recommendations for positioning the student and/or for placement of the device. Referring the student's parents to contact a physician for a physical examination, reassessing the student's motor and communication abilities and repositioning the communication device are not initial steps indicated at this time.

Type of Reasoning: Inferential
One must determine the most likely cause of the communication difficulty, given the diagnosis and limitations of the student. This requires inferential reasoning skill, where one must draw conclusions based on the information presented. In this situation, the therapist should evaluate the position of the student in the wheelchair and the device on the wheelchair, as improper positioning can affect the use of an augmentative communication device. If answered incorrectly, review positioning of augmentative devices on wheelchairs.

B127 **C6**

An occupational therapist plans individual and group activities for a child with oppositional defiant disorder. Which is most important for the therapist to address during group activities?

Answer Choices:
A. The child's willingness to take on a variety of group roles.
B. The child's ability to attend to and complete a task. ✓
C. The child's distorted body image.
D. The child's self-regulation of energy and activity levels.

Correct Answer: B.

Rationale:
Children with oppositional defiant disorder tend to have difficulties with impulse control, attention span and short-term memory and exhibit argumentative and resentful behaviors. These deficits often affect the ability to complete tasks and can hinder adaptive role functioning. A child does not have to be willing to take on a variety of roles to benefit from group activities. Some find security and stability in the same type role. This stability can be healthy as long as the role contributes to productive behavior. Distorted body image is more indicative of anorexia nervosa, bulimia nervosa or body dysmorphia. Difficulties with energy and activity levels relate more to hyperactivity disorder than to oppositional defiant disorder.

Type of Reasoning: Inductive
This question requires one to recall the typical features of a client with oppositional defiant disorder and then to determine what would be an important skill to address in therapy. This necessitates inductive reasoning skill, where the test taker must couple knowledge of the diagnosis with clinical judgment to arrive at a correct conclusion. In this case, it is most important for the therapist to address the child's ability to attend to and complete a task. If answered incorrectly, review symptoms of oppositional defiant disorder and therapeutic approaches.

B128 **C2**

A single parent with rheumatoid arthritis and two school-aged children reports difficulty completing a home exercise program. The parent states that multiple familial, work and home management responsibilities fill the day and additional activities cannot fit into the day. Which is the best action for the occupational therapist to take in response to these realities?

Answer Choices:
A. Explain and reinforce the importance of active range of motion exercises for remediation of dysfunction.
B. Provide intervention to develop time management skills and enable temporal adaptation.
C. Incorporate the parent's engagement in a diversity of role activities into the home program. ✓
D. Increase the frequency of OT sessions to compensate for lack of follow-through with the home program.

Correct Answer: C.

Rationale:
The performance of role activities requires the individual to actively range joints which is the purpose of an exercise program. Incorporating AROM into one's daily routine can be more easily implemented than adding a specific exercise regimen. Some people find pure rote exercise uninteresting. In addition, since activity and the pursuit of occupational roles is the foundation of OT, this choice provides the most theoretically consistent action. Reminding the individual of the importance of AROM, providing time management intervention and/or increasing the frequency of the OT sessions ignore the reality of a single parent's busy life. The person has reported nothing to indicate a lack of understanding of the importance of AROM, poor time management skills or temporal dysfunction. Increasing the frequency of OT sessions would just add further demands to the parent's already busy schedule and is not indicated.

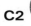

Type of Reasoning: Evaluative

This question requires a value judgment, which is an evaluative reasoning skill. In this situation, the patient has indicated that he/she has little time to complete a home exercise program. Therefore the test taker should look for a solution that addresses the patient's concerns, but also still provides opportunities for functional activity. The only solution that addresses both concerns is to incorporate the patient's engagement in a diversity of role activities into the home program. Review principles of client-centered practice and approaches to home program development if answered incorrectly.

B129 C4

An individual with a spinal cord injury (SCI) at the level of T-1 is practicing a stand pivot transfer in the OT department of a rehabilitation center. The patient complains of dizziness and nausea. Which action is most important for the occupational therapist to take first?

Answer Choices:

A. Call for help according to facility procedures.
B. Return the patient to the wheelchair for a five minute rest break.
C. Return the person to the wheelchair and immediately recline it.
D. Return the patient to the wheelchair and transport the patient back to rest in bed.

Correct Answer: C.

Rationale:

Individuals with SCIs are at risk for orthostatic hypotension. Complaints of dizziness and nausea are indications of orthostatic hypotension and require an immediate response. Reclining the individual in his/her wheelchair will return blood pressure to a normal range. The other choices do not address the need for immediate remediation of this crisis.

Type of Reasoning: Evaluative

This question requires professional judgment based on knowledge of the symptoms and safety guidelines, which is an evaluative reasoning skill. Because the patient's symptoms indicate orthostatic hypotension, the therapist should return the person to the wheelchair and immediately recline it to relieve symptoms. Review care guidelines for orthostatic hypotension, especially in SCI if answered incorrectly.

B130 C6

An individual attends a community day treatment program to assist in recovery from major depression. The client has fair eye contact and responds verbally to interactions initiated by others. The person's cognition is intact. Which group level is best for the occupational therapist to recommend this client attend?

Answer Choices:

A. Project.
B. Parallel.
C. Cooperative.
D. Mature.

Correct Answer: A.

Rationale:

A project group utilizes short term activities that require the participation of two or more people. Tasks are shared and the focus is on interaction rather than task completion. This level is appropriate for someone who is socially responsive to others with intact cognition. A parallel group does not require any interaction for task completion. This group is too low-level for this individual because it would not provide the opportunity to use and build existing social skills. Cooperative and mature groups require members to be self-expressive and meet socio-emotional roles. These groups are too high-level for the individual at this point.

Type of Reasoning: Inductive
One must utilize clinical knowledge and judgment to determine the group level that most appropriately facilitates interaction with this individual. This requires inductive reasoning skill. In this case, a project group is most appropriate to facilitate sharing and interaction. If answered incorrectly, review types of groups, especially project level groups.

B131 C4

An adolescent with spina bifida at the C-8 level wants to access the new computerized play system that was received as a birthday gift. Which is the best adaptation for the occupational therapist to recommend the adolescent use to access this system?

Answer Choices:
A. A chin switch. C3-4
B. A tenodesis splint. C6
C. A dorsal wrist splint with a universal cuff. C5
D. A joystick control. ✓

Correct Answer: D.

Rationale:
At the level of C-8, the teenager can independently use a joystick control. A chin switch would be indicated for a C3/C4 level lesion; a tenodesis splint is indicated for a C-6 level lesion; and a dorsal splint with a universal cuff is indicated for a C-5 level lesion.

Type of Reasoning: Inductive
This question requires one to determine the most appropriate recommendation for an adolescent with cervical spina bifida. This requires inductive reasoning skill, where clinical judgment and knowledge of the diagnosis, including functional abilities, are paramount in arriving at a correct conclusion. For this situation, the occupational therapist should recommend a joystick control. If answered incorrectly, review functional abilities of persons with spina bifida, especially C-8 level.

B132 C8

A college is converting an historical building into wheelchair accessible dormitory space. To allow for a 360° turning radius, which dimensions are best for the occupational therapist to recommend as the minimum space between the students' desk and bed?

Answer Choices:
A. 4 feet by 4 feet.
B. 5 feet by 5 feet. ✓
C. 6 feet by 6 feet.
D. 7 feet by 7 feet.

Correct Answer: B.

Rationale:
A 360° turning radius requires a minimum clearance of at least 5 feet by 5 feet. 4 feet by 4 feet is too small. 6 feet by 6 feet and 7 feet by 7 feet are more than the minimum standard. While exceeding minimal standards is desirable, it is not always attainable and the question is asking for the minimum.

Type of Reasoning: Deductive
This question requires recall of guidelines and principles, which is factual knowledge. Deductive reasoning skills are utilized whenever one must recall facts to solve therapeutic issues. In this situation, accessibility guidelines indicate a minimum space clearance of 5 feet by 5 feet. Review building accessibility guidelines for wheelchair use if answered incorrectly.

B133 C9

An occupational therapist working for a home care agency is vacationing and sees a colleague at an all-day concert. Upon return from the vacation, the therapist notices that this colleague had billed for a full-day of home visits on the day of the concert. Which action is best for the therapist to take first in response to this situation?

Answer Choices:
A. Inform the home care supervisor.
B. Contact the state regulatory board.
C. Contact the National Board for Certification of Occupational Therapy.
D. Ask the colleague to clarify the situation.

Correct Answer: A.

Rationale:
The therapist must inform the home care supervisor who can then investigate the employee's behavior according to the agency's guidelines. This investigation may result in the supervisor contacting the state regulatory board or NBCOT. Speaking to a colleague to clarify a situation prior to reporting it to a supervisor can often be an appropriate initial step. However, in this case, the person has committed potential fraud. This situation is very serious and must be brought immediately to the attention of a supervisor.

Type of Reasoning: Evaluative
This question requires a value judgment in an ethical situation, which is an evaluative reasoning skill. In this situation, because the therapist has witnessed unethical (and potentially illegal) behavior, the therapist should inform the home care supervisor. Ethical situations such as these often rely upon the OT Code of Ethics to provide guiding principles of action. This ethical situation violates Principle 6, the code of veracity, which means to be truthful and accurate in documenting services.

B134 C2

A caregiver support group meets weekly at a senior center. A new member attends the group for the third time and listens intently. The person nods in agreement when others speak, but does not participate verbally. Which action is most effective for the occupational therapist to take to facilitate the individual's engagement in the group?

Answer Choices:
A. Reiterate the group's norm that active participation is expected from all group members.
B. Ask the individual several questions to encourage verbal participation.
C. Invite the individual to join in the discussion, if the person would like.
D. Refer the individual to the center's social worker for individual, non-group counseling.

Correct Answer: C.

Rationale:
Inviting the individual to join the discussion acknowledges his/her membership and supports attention and active listening but it does not pressure the person to speak before ready. It can take time for an individual to feel comfortable sharing personal thoughts with a group of people who may have been just acquaintances (or even strangers) prior to this group membership. It is inappropriate to pressure for verbal participation before a person is ready. Individual counseling can be helpful, but it is no substitute for the therapeutic benefits of a group. In addition, group members can benefit from a group discussion without verbally participating. These benefits can include many of Yalom's curative factors including universality, instillation of hope and the gaining of specific information.

Type of Reasoning: Inductive
One must utilize clinical knowledge and judgment to determine the best approach for this group situation. This requires inductive reasoning skill. In this case, because the new member has not initiated conversation, it is best to invite the member to join in the discussion if desired. If answered incorrectly, review group dynamics and methods of facilitating discussion.

B135 C2

An occupational therapist accepts a job in an after-school program. The program provides services for adolescents at risk for mental health problems due to their history of being victims of abuse. The therapist decides that an activity group to elicit the adolescents' thoughts and feelings in a safe atmosphere would be instrumental to their recovery. Which group would be most relevant for the therapist to design?

Answer Choices:
A. A task-oriented group.
B. An instrumental group.
C. A topical group.
D. A thematic group.

Correct Answer: A.

Rationale:
The purpose of a task-oriented group is to increase members' awareness of feelings, thoughts, needs, values and behaviors through the process of choosing, planning and implementing a group activity. Activities are selected for their expressive characteristics so that participants can project their feelings and study their behaviors. A topical group is a verbal group that focuses on the discussion of activities members are engaged in (concurrent) or will be engaged in (anticipatory) outside of the group. The purpose is to improve activity performance through problem-solving. An instrumental group is designed for individuals with chronic disabilities who are functioning at their highest level with no anticipation for improvement. The aim of this group is to provide a supportive, safe, structured environment that maintains function, prevents regression and promotes quality of life. A thematic group assists members in acquiring the knowledge, skills and/or attitudes to perform a specific set of skills independently.

Type of Reasoning: Analytical
This question provides a description of a group and the test taker must determine the type of group that would achieve the goals of the program. This is an analytical reasoning skill, as questions of this nature often ask one to analyze descriptors of functional activities or situations to determine the type of activity involved. In this situation the group description is that of a task-oriented group, which should be reviewed if answered incorrectly.

B136 **C1**

An elementary school student with hypotonic cerebral palsy receives school-based occupational therapy to improve fine motor skills. The child holds a thick marker with a static tripod grasp and holds a No. 2 pencil with a gross grasp. The occupational therapist revises the intervention plan based on the child's attained skills. Which grasp would be best for the therapist to address next in the revised occupational therapy intervention plan?

Answer Choices:
A. Dynamic tripod with the thick marker. ✗
B. Static tripod with a pencil. ✓
C. Lateral pinch with a thick marker. ✗
D. Dynamic tripod with a pencil.

Correct Answer: B.

Rationale:
Developmentally, the best way to progressively grade the grasp is to work on static tripod with a thinner object before going to work on dynamic tripod. A lateral pinch is not an effective grasp for holding a thick marker.

Type of Reasoning: Inductive
This question requires one to determine the most appropriate modification to the intervention plan to reflect progress to the next developmental stage of grasp. This requires inductive reasoning skill, where clinical judgment is paramount in arriving at a correct conclusion. In this situation, a short-term goal of improving static tripod grasp with a pencil is the best modification to the intervention plan based on current ability. If answered incorrectly, review developmental patterns of hand grasp for writing.

B137 **C6**

A young adult with a 10-year history of serious and persistent mental illness is being discharged home in two days. The client collaborates with the care coordination team to plan discharge with the client's primary family members. The team consists of a psychiatrist, a registered nurse, a social worker and an occupational therapist. The team conducts a pre-discharge family meeting to provide family members with information to assist them in supporting the client's recovery. Which is the most relevant information for the occupational therapist to provide to the client's primary family members at this meeting?

Answer Choices:
A. Family role activity suggestions and potential adaptations. ✓
B. The therapeutic effects and potential side effects of medications.
C. Advocacy strategies and consumer/family resources.
D. Family dynamics information and family support groups.

Correct Answer: A.

Rationale:
The occupational therapist is the only one on the identified care coordination team who is qualified to provide information about role activities and potential activity adaptations. The ability of a client to engage in meaningful activities in the home and resume relevant role activities can facilitate positive family functioning and support recovery. The other choices are all relevant but other members of the team can provide this information.

Type of Reasoning: Inferential

One must determine the most appropriate information to provide for the family of a person with serious and persistent mental illness prior to discharge home. This requires inferential reasoning skill, where one draws conclusions based on information presented. In this situation, the most appropriate information to provide is family role activity suggestions and potential adaptations. If answered incorrectly, review discharge planning guidelines and the functional impact of serious and persistent mental illness. The integration of this knowledge is required for a correct answer.

B138 C4

A Sensory Profile completed by a caregiver indicates that an elementary school-aged child has modulation impairments and sensation seeking patterns. The occupational therapist observes the child frequently wandering, bumping into objects in the room and fidgeting. Which is the best intervention approach for the therapist to use to address this child's deficits?

Answer Choices:

A. Strategies to increase random sensory input and encourage high physical activity at home.
B. An obstacle course which requires diverse movements for varied proprioceptive and tactile input.
C. Sensory experiences that focus on body awareness and grading control during play activities.
D. A sensory diet which includes controlled sensory input integrated into the child's daily routine.

Correct Answer: D.

Rationale:

The use of skilled clinical observation is important when evaluating and planning intervention for children with sensory processing deficits. Because they create sensation for themselves, their behavior tells us what sensory input they need. Children who rock and fidget require vestibular input to help them attend and learn. Children with proprioceptive problems often rely on visual and/or verbal cues to know how to move their bodies and they often appear clumsy, bumping into objects in their environments. It is important to provide caregivers with a written sensory diet to implement on a daily basis in the child's home and school environments to facilitate carryover.

Type of Reasoning: Inductive

This question requires one to draw upon knowledge of effective therapy processes in order to determine the best approach for this child. This requires inductive reasoning skill. In this situation, the therapist should provide a sensory diet which includes controlled sensory input to integrate into the child's daily routine at home and school. If answered incorrectly, review sensory integration and sensory modulation guidelines.

B139 C8

An occupational therapist provides home care services to a neonate with significant developmental delays. Two hours before the next scheduled home visit, the child's parent informs the therapist that one of three older children has developed chicken pox. While the other children do not show signs of chicken pox, the parent expresses concern that they are contagious. Which is the therapist's best response to this situation?

Answer Choices:

A. Cancel the scheduled session and reschedule after two weeks have passed.
B. Complete the scheduled session using airborne precautions.
C. Complete the scheduled session using standard precautions.
D. Complete the scheduled session using droplet precautions.

Correct Answer: B.

Rationale:
There is no need to cancel the scheduled session. Standard precautions are used in all clinical situations. Chickenpox is a disease transmitted by airborne droplet nuclei that remain suspended in the air; therefore, airborne precautions are warranted. Wearing respiratory protection (i.e., a mask) provides sufficient protection. Droplet precautions are used with individuals known or suspected to be infected with serious illness microorganisms transmitted by large particle droplets that can be generated by the person during talking, sneezing, coughing (e.g., rubella, mumps, pertussis, influenza).

Type of Reasoning: Evaluative
One must weigh the possible courses of action and then make a value judgment about the best course to take. This requires evaluative reasoning skill, which often utilizes guiding principles of action in order to arrive at a correct conclusion. In this case, because there is the presence of an airborne virus, the therapist should complete the session using airborne precautions. Review precautions for airborne viruses if answered incorrectly.

B140 C8

An individual with borderline personality disorder incurred a back injury while working as a stock person for a large warehouse. The individual attends a work hardening program. The occupational therapist evaluates the individual and determines that the client's level of productivity is just below the warehouse minimum standards. The individual complains of pain when lifting the heaviest of boxes. The client frequently becomes angry and verbally abusive in response to directions or feedback. Which is the most important initial focus of the work hardening program for this individual?

Answer Choices:
A. An increase in productivity to meet minimum standards.
B. An increase in productivity to exceed minimum standards.
C. The development of affective work behavior skills.
D. The development of strength and ergonomic lifting abilities.

Correct Answer: C.

Rationale:
Affective work behavior skills include social responsiveness, attitude toward the job and relationships with supervisors and coworkers. The individual is exhibiting significant deficits in these areas by becoming agitated and verbally abusive. These behaviors put the client at risk for not being able to maintain employment upon return to work. Increasing work productivity and developing ergonomic lifting abilities and strength can be addressed during the course of the work hardening program. The individual's inappropriate work behavior skills must be immediately addressed for the individual to be able to benefit from this program.

Type of Reasoning: Inductive
This question requires one to determine the best approach for improving function for a client in a work hardening setting. This requires inductive reasoning skill, where clinical judgment is paramount in arriving at a correct conclusion. In this situation, given the individual's behaviors, the therapist should focus on the development of affective work behavior skills. If answered incorrectly, review treatment guidelines for work hardening settings, especially work behavior skills.

B141 C9

An older client with a diagnosis of late onset dementia of the Alzheimer type lives with family members. On the last three occasions, the client attended OT sessions with bruises and cuts on both legs. When asked about this, the client replies that a family member caused these injuries. Which is the first action the occupational therapist should take?

Answer Choices:
A. Confirm the client's statements with the family.
B. Immediately report potential abuse according to the facility policy. ✓
C. Call the police to report elder abuse.
D. Administer a cognitive evaluation before taking further action.

Correct Answer: B.

Rationale:
This situation may indicate elder abuse. The therapist must report the findings according to established facility protocols. It is not within the realm of an entry-level therapist's area of expertise to investigate, judge or confirm child, adult and/or elder abuse. The role of the therapist is to report suspected abuse to professionals who are qualified to investigate the incident. Even though the person claimed to have been abused, the therapist should not directly call the police. A professional skilled in the investigation of potential abuse must investigate and decide the most appropriate course of action, which may or may not include a police report. The evaluation of cognitive skills can determine the elder's cognitive level; however, this choice does not address the issue of potential abuse.

Type of Reasoning: Evaluative
This question requires one to determine a best course of action, given the information provided by the person. The test taker must understand that the elder's disclosure of potential abuse needs to be reported for investigation by appropriate agencies. The person's diagnosis of dementia, Alzheimer's type does not mitigate this requirement. Questions that require one to weigh the merits of each choice often require evaluative reasoning skills. If answered incorrectly, review guidelines on reporting suspected elder abuse.

B142 C4

A client with a lower brain stem injury is referred to occupational therapy. During the evaluation, which reflex would the person most likely demonstrate?

Answer Choices:
A. Tonic lumbar.
B. Body-on-body righting.
C. Tonic labyrinthine. ✓
D. Labyrinthine righting.

Correct Answer: C.

Rationale:
The lower brain stem mediates the tonic labyrinthine reflex. The other answer choices are all righting reactions that are mediated in the upper brain stem.

Type of Reasoning: Deductive
One must review each of the reflexes presented and recall which one is mediated at the lower brain stem level. This requires factual recall of knowledge, which is a deductive reasoning skill. In this case, the tonic labyrinthine reflex is mediated at the lower brain stem level, whereas all the others are mediated by the upper brain stem. Review brain stem reflexes if answered incorrectly.

B143 C2

Ten members of a community reintegration group are not working well together and show decreased levels of trust. The occupational therapist's goal is to enhance the level of cohesiveness in the group. To begin the next group session, which is the best action for the therapist to take?

Answer Choices:

A. Read inspirational phrases to increase motivation.
B. Verbally review the goals and purposes of the group.
C. Have each person contribute a line about childhood memories to group poem.
D. Ask each person to talk about silly mistakes to provide some levity.

Correct Answer: B.

Rationale:
The best choice is to verbally review the goals and purpose of the group. This helps to direct the focus of the members onto the reason(s) that they are participating in the group. This reinforcement of a shared purpose can help develop cohesion. The therapist can then provide activities that build on this commonality. Inspirational phrases can help instill a positive attitude but they do not address the need to develop group cohesion. Using individual member's input to compile a group poem can be an activity that could increase cohesiveness. However, some group members may have had less than wonderful childhood experiences and may be reticent to share a childhood memory with persons that with whom they are not close. Consequently, this activity may be more detrimental than helpful. One way to decrease cohesiveness is to require self-disclosure in a group with decreased levels of trust. As a result, the topic of silly mistakes is also not a good group discussion focus for it is not likely to facilitate trust, openness and willingness to share.

Type of Reasoning: Inferential
One must determine which course of action will result in improved group cohesiveness. This requires inferential reasoning where one must draw conclusions about each course of action as achieving the ultimate purpose of group cohesion. In this case, verbally reviewing the goals and purposes of the group will best enhance group cohesion. If answered incorrectly, review characteristics of cohesive groups and group facilitation techniques.

B144 C7

An individual with developmental disabilities scores a Level 3 on the Allen Cognitive Level Test. Which activities should the occupational therapist include in the intervention plan to help meet the client's functional needs?

Answer Choices:

A. Community mobility activities such as taking a bus.
B. Home management activities such as preparing a food shopping list.
C. Self-care activities such as brushing teeth.
D. Leisure activities such as completing a 50-piece puzzle.

Correct Answer: C.

Rationale:
An individual who scores a Level 3 on the Allen's Cognitive Level Test can perform basic repetitive tasks. Level 3 is the beginning of using the hands to manipulate objects, but task completion requires proprioceptive cues (e.g., physical prompts to perform the hand to mouth movement needed to brush teeth). The other activities require cognitive skills that are not present at Level 3, according to Allen's model.

Type of Reasoning: Inductive
One must utilize clinical knowledge and judgment to determine the most appropriate activities for this patient. This requires inductive reasoning skill. In this case, because the patient is functioning at Level 3, the therapist should choose self-care activities, such as brushing teeth in the intervention plan. If answered incorrectly, review Allen's cognitive disabilities model and intervention approaches for patients functioning at Level 3.

B145 C1

An occupational therapist observes that an 18-month-old child is not able to creep more than a few steps. When the child looks up, both hips and knees flex and the child ends up W sitting with both arms extended and propped forward. When documenting this observation, which is most accurate for the occupational therapist to report the child is demonstrating?

Answer Choices:

A. Typical development of locomotion skills.
B. The influence of the symmetrical tonic neck reflex (STNR) resulting in delayed gross motor skills.
C. An obligatory asymmetrical tonic neck reflex (ATNR) resulting in delayed gross motor skills.
D. An intact tonic labyrinthine reflex which facilitates balance responses.

Correct Answer: B.

Rationale:

A persistent STNR would cause extension of upper extremities. The described motor behavior is not normal. An ATNR would cause the child to collapse to one side. Tonic labyrinthine reflex would cause a total body extended posture.

Type of Reasoning: Analytical

This question requires the test taker to determine the functional deficit of the child, which is an analytical reasoning skill. Questions of this nature often call upon the test taker to determine a diagnosis based on a functional description of deficits. Based on this information, the demonstration of W sitting with arms extended indicate influence of the STNR reflex resulting in delayed gross motor skills. Review STNR reflex pattern if answered incorrectly.

B146 C8

An occupational therapist provides caregiver training to the spouse of an individual with cerebellar cortical degeneration. The focus of the session is on community mobility using a wheelchair. The individual is dependent upon the spouse's assistance for mobility. Which of the following is most effective for the therapist to recommend the spouse do when descending a steep grade?

Answer Choices:

A. Go down backwards with all wheelchair wheels maintaining contact with the ground surface.
B. Tilt the wheelchair backward to its gravitational balance point and then go down forward.
C. Tilt the wheelchair backward to its gravitational balance point and then go down backward.
D. Push forward as on flat surfaces but lean body back for extra drag.

Correct Answer: A.

Rationale:

Proceeding down a steep grade backwards with all wheelchair wheels maintaining contact with the ground enables the spouse to use body weight to slow the chair's momentum. If the spouse tires, he/she can readily stop and use his/her body weight to hold the chair in place while putting the wheelchair brakes on. Pushing the chair in a forward position can be dangerous on a steep grade, for if the spouse loses his/her grip and/or tires, it could be very difficult to regain control of the situation. Maintaining the chair in a backward tilt position while going backwards is an unnecessary use of energy and can greatly contribute to the caregiver's physical fatigue.

Type of Reasoning: Inductive
Clinical knowledge and judgment are the most important skills needed for answering this question, which requires inductive reasoning skill. Knowledge of safety guidelines in mobility utilizing a wheelchair is essential to arriving at a correct conclusion. In this case, the therapist should recommend descending a steep grade backwards with all wheelchair wheels in contact with the ground. Review community wheelchair mobility guidelines if answered incorrectly.

B147 C3

An adult has been referred to occupational therapy. The individual demonstrates decreased ROM in the dominant hand secondary to a nerve injury. Active thumb ROM for the IP and MP is within normal limits. Active ROM of the IPs of all four fingers is 0°–60°. The individual wants to be able to hold a knife, spoon and fork. Which utensils are best for the therapist to recommend to this person?

Answer Choices:
A. Utensils with cylindrical foam handles, 1½″ in diameter. ✓
B. Standard utensils with no adaptations. ✗
C. Utensils with custom-built handles made of low temperature thermoplastic splinting material. ✗
D. Utensils held in a universal cuff. —no grasp

Correct Answer: A.

Rationale:
The foam handle accommodates to the 60° ROM of the IPs of the fingers to hold the utensils. Without an adapted handle, the person can use only pad-to-pad grasp, which is unstable. A custom handle is most commonly used for someone with spasticity or with more difficulty holding the utensil than mentioned in the scenario. A universal cuff is used by someone who has no functional grasp.

Type of Reasoning: Analytical
This question provides detailed information about a client's ROM in an affected hand and the test taker must determine how this information relates to functional grasp for holding utensils. This requires analytical reasoning, where the precise meaning of data must be analyzed in order to make a determination for functioning. In this situation, a cylindrical foam handle would be the best recommendation.

B148 C5

The population of an urban homeless shelter includes individuals with histories of chronic alcohol abuse who are at risk for developing peripheral neuropathy. The occupational therapist consulting at this shelter monitors the residents' status to ensure early detection of this problem. Which is the most important observed status change for the therapist to report?

Answer Choices:
A. Progressive deterioration in visual acuity. ✗
B. Progressive deterioration of sensorimotor functions of the lower extremities ✓
C. Rapid onset of intention tremors. ✗
D. Rapid loss of sensorimotor functions of the facial and neck muscles. ✗

Correct Answer: B.

Rationale:
Peripheral neuropathy is a syndrome of sensory, motor, reflex and vasomotor symptoms, with symptoms exhibited according to the distribution of the affected nerve. Its etiology includes diabetes, Lyme disease, multiple sclerosis, alcoholism, metabolic or infectious diseases. It has a slow and progressive onset and course. It does not result in a rapid loss of function, deterioration of visual acuity or the onset of intention tremors. Treatment of the underlying systemic disorder (e.g., diabetes) can slow progression. In general, recovery takes extended time.

Type of Reasoning: Inferential
One must link knowledge of peripheral neuropathy to the symptoms presented in order to arrive at a correct conclusion. This requires inferential reasoning skill, where one must draw conclusions based on evidence presented. In this case the most relevant status change for the therapist to assess is the progressive deterioration of sensorimotor functions in the lower extremities. Review symptoms of peripheral neuropathy if answered incorrectly.

B149 **C4**

A middle school student with learning disabilities exhibits no behavioral problems in the classroom. However, whenever the class is in a line waiting to switch classrooms, the student becomes agitated and often pushes classmates. The occupational therapy consultant advises the teacher that this behavior may be indicative of an underlying problem. Which of the following is most accurate for the therapist to identify as a potential disorder warranting further evaluation?

Answer Choices:
A. Gravitational insecurity.
B. A conduct disorder.
C. Antisocial tendencies.
D. Tactile defensiveness.

Correct Answer: D.

Rationale:
The tactile stimuli due to closeness of peers in a line can become overwhelming to an individual with tactile defensiveness. The behavior described in the scenario is not reflective of behavior indicative of the other disorders listed.

Type of Reasoning: Analytical
This question provides symptoms and the test taker must determine the likely cause for them. This is an analytical reasoning skill, as questions of this nature often ask one to analyze a group of symptoms in order to determine a diagnosis. In this situation the symptoms indicate tactile defensiveness, which should be reviewed if answered incorrectly.

Multiple Choice Scenario Item B. III.

Questions B150 to B152 are based on the following information.

An individual recovering from flexor tendon repair surgery is two days post operation. The surgeon refers the client to occupational therapy with a prescription to use the Kleinert protocol to guide intervention.

B150 **C3**

The occupational therapist plans the client's early mobilization program. Which is the most appropriate exercise routine for the occupational therapist to use within the limits of a dorsal block splint?

Answer Choices:
A. Active flexion/passive extension.
B. Active flexion/active extension.
C. Active extension/passive flexion. ✓
D. Passive flexion/passive extension.

Correct Answer: C.

Rationale:
The Kleinert protocol in the early phase (0–4 weeks post-surgery) has the person performing active extension and passive flexion within the limits of a dorsal block splint. The Duran protocol, which also can be used post-surgery for flexor tendon repairs, uses passive flexion and passive extension within the limits of a dorsal block splint. Active flexion is contraindicated for post flexor tendon repair surgery because the tendon repair can rupture when actively flexed.

Type of Reasoning: Deductive
This question requires recall of guidelines and principles, which is factual knowledge. Deductive reasoning skills are utilized whenever one must recall facts to solve clinical problems. In this situation, the therapist should provide active extension and passive flexion within the limits of the dorsal blocking splint. Review exercise guidelines post flexor tendon repair, especially the Kleinert protocol if answered incorrectly.

B151 **C3**

The occupational therapist meets with the client to ensure compliance with the prescribed splinting protocol. Which is the most important outcome of this session?

Answer Choices:
A. The client's adherence to a written splint wearing schedule.
B. The client's ability to independently don and doff the splint.
C. The client's understanding of the purpose(s) and procedure(s) of the splint protocol. ✓
D. The completion of functional training in the use of the splint.

Correct Answer: C.

Rationale:
If a client understands the purposes and procedures of the splint protocol he/she will become a collaborative partner in the intervention programs. The other choices are important components of a splinting intervention program and may be required by accrediting bodies (e.g., documentation of functional training and the individual's ability to don/doff a splint). However, the success of these interventions and the attainment of client compliance rely on the client's understanding of the splint protocol's purpose(s) and procedure(s).

Type of Reasoning: Inductive
This question requires one to determine the most important factor to ensure compliance with a splinting protocol. This requires inductive reasoning skill, where clinical judgment is paramount in arriving at a correct conclusion. For this situation, ensuring the client understands the purpose(s) and procedure(s) of the splint protocol are most important. If answered incorrectly, review guidelines for improving compliance with splinting protocols.

B152 C3

The client is now seven weeks postoperation. Which are the most appropriate intervention activities for the occupational therapist to use with this client?

Answer Choices:

A. Home management activities such as doing laundry.
B. Light activities of daily living such as grooming.
C. Strengthening exercises using high resistance theraband.
D. Passive exercises using a dynamic splint.

Correct Answer: B.

Rationale:
According to the Kleinert protocol, light ADL are introduced 6–8 weeks post operation. Strengthening activities and heavier work activities (such as laundry) are introduced 8–12 weeks post operation. The use of a dynamic splint is indicated immediately and up to 4 weeks post operation.

Type of Reasoning: Deductive
This question requires recall of guidelines and principles, which is factual knowledge. Deductive reasoning skills are utilized whenever one must recall facts to solve novel problems. In this situation, the Kleinert protocol indicates that a patient seven weeks postoperation can engage in light ADL. Review the Kleinert protocol if answered incorrectly.

B153 C1

During an intervention session in a school, the occupational therapist observes a young child turn the pages of a book. The therapist identifies this behavior as an example of an in-hand manipulation task. Which task should the occupational therapist document the child is capable of performing?

Answer Choices:

A. Shift.
B. Simple rotation.
C. Translation.
D. Translation without stabilization.

Correct Answer: A.

Rationale:
Turning the pages of a book involves a linear movement of each page on the finger surface. This allows for repositioning of the page relative to the pads of the fingers while the thumb remains opposed. Simple rotation is not correct as this involves a turning/rolling of an object held at the finger pads with the fingers acting as a unit and the thumb in opposition (e.g., unscrewing a bottle cap). Translation is incorrect as this involves linear movement of an object from the palm to the fingers or fingers to the palm. The activity of turning pages does not use the palm with stabilization or without stabilization.

Type of Reasoning: Analytical
This question provides a description of a functional activity and the test taker must determine the likely definition of such an activity. This is an analytical reasoning skill, as questions of this nature often ask one to analyze descriptors of functional skills to determine the overall skill involved. In this situation, the activity is that of the in-hand manipulation task of shift, which should be reviewed if answered incorrectly.

B154 **C8**

A rehabilitation hospital is interested in starting a driver rehabilitation program. Which must the occupational therapist hired to develop this program do first?

Answer Choices:
A. Determine the cost of commercially available driving rehabilitation programs.
B. Develop admission criteria for program participants.
C. Develop a marketing plan to obtain referrals.
D. Learn the state's driving laws and requirements. ✓

Correct Answer: D.

Rationale:
State laws and regulations regarding the mandatory reporting of driving ability post illness or injury are essential for a therapist developing a driver rehabilitation program. The therapist would need to know state laws and regulations prior to setting admission criteria or a marketing plan. While cost is an important aspect of program development it is not the greatest priority. Knowledge and adherence to state laws are essential to avoid potential program liability.

Type of Reasoning: Inductive
Clinical knowledge and judgment are the most important skills needed for answering this question, which requires inductive reasoning skill. In this case, the therapist must first learn the state's driving laws and requirements in order to proceed with development of a driver rehabilitation program. Review program development guidelines, especially driver rehabilitation guidelines if answered incorrectly.

B155 **C3**

An individual recovering from hepatitis, type C has decreased upper and lower extremity muscle strength and hypertension. Six months ago the client had an angioplasty and is very fearful of having a heart attack. Which should the occupational therapist instruct the client to perform to increase muscle strength?

Answer Choices:
A. Isotonic exercises. ✓
B. Isometric exercises.
C. Contract-relax exercise.
D. Muscle contractions and holds.

Correct Answer: A.

Rationale:
Isotonics are the only exercises listed that are not contraindicated for a person with hypertension or heart disease. The other choices describe isometric exercises or activities which include isometric elements and are contraindicated in this case.

Type of Reasoning: Inferential
One must determine the most appropriate exercise for an individual, given knowledge of the presenting diagnoses. This requires inferential reasoning skill, where one must infer or draw conclusions about a best course of action. In this situation, the therapist should recommend isotonic exercises, as this is the only exercise listed that is not contraindicated for individuals with hypertension or heart disease. Review exercise guidelines for individuals with hypertension and heart disease if answered incorrectly.

B156 **C9**

During a home care intervention planning meeting, the team discusses a client with a right CVA. The physical therapist states the individual's ambulatory status is now within functional limits. Physical therapy services will be discontinued because the person is no longer homebound. The occupational therapist reports that the individual is frequently confused during home management task performance and becomes extremely anxious when community activities are discussed. Which recommendation should the therapist make?

Answer Choices:

A. Refer the individual to a psychiatrist for a mental status evaluation.

B. Continue OT services as the person should continue to be considered homebound.✓

C. Discontinue OT services as they are non-reimbursable since the person is no longer considered homebound.

D. Contact the physician to discuss the need for OT services on an outpatient basis and for psychosocial counseling.

Correct Answer: B.

Rationale:

The individual can be considered homebound for cognitive and psychosocial deficits. Discontinuing services can place the individual at risk because the person will not receive evaluation or intervention for his/her demonstrated cognitive and psychosocial deficits. There is no need for a consultation with a physician at this point. OT practitioners can continue to provide services in this scenario without physician input.

Type of Reasoning: Inductive

Clinical knowledge and judgment are the most important skills needed for answering this question, which requires inductive reasoning skill. Knowledge of the diagnosis and best courses of action is essential to choose the best solution. In this case, because the person is considered homebound for cognitive and psychosocial deficits, the team's best approach is to continue OT services. Review home health care treatment guidelines and criteria for homebound status if answered incorrectly.

B157 **C6**

An older adult with Parkinson's disease has a secondary diagnosis of depression. During home-based occupational therapy service provision, the client exhibits increased confusion and disorientation. Which action is best for the home-care occupational therapist to advise the client's primary caregiver to take in response to the client's change in status?

Answer Choices:

A. Obtain an evaluation from a neurologist to determine if dementia has begun. ✗

B. Seek support from a caregiver's respite program. ✗

C. Discuss placement alternatives with the social worker. ✗

D. Contact the client's psychiatrist for a medication evaluation. ✓

Correct Answer: D.

Rationale:

Depression can result in confusion and disorientation; therefore, the first action should be to consult with a psychiatrist to determine the need for anti-depressants. Depression is a reversible cause of dementia and should be ruled out prior to seeing a neurologist. See Table 10-1 in Chapter 10 for a listing of reversible causes of dementia. It is premature to advise the spouse to seek respite or alternative placements because it is not known if these cognitive deficits are permanent.

Type of Reasoning: Evaluative
This question requires professional judgment based on guiding principles, which is an evaluative reasoning skill. Because the individual is exhibiting confusion and disorientation, the therapist should contact the elder's psychiatrist for a medication evaluation. This way the therapist can determine the next most appropriate course of action based on an evaluation from the psychiatrist. Review symptoms of depression in the elderly if answered incorrectly.

B158 C5

An adult with amyotrophic lateral sclerosis frequently coughs and chokes when eating finely chopped foods and drinking thin liquids. The speech pathologist and occupational therapist collaborate and recommend a videofluoroscopy procedure. Which behavioral information would be most relevant for the occupational therapist to include on the referral?

Answer Choices:
A. The client demonstrates minimal limitations in cognitive level.
B. The client is able to consume chopped foods and apple juice with no difficulty.
C. The client demonstrates only oral stage problems during eating.
D. The client cannot tolerate therapy focused on improving feeding and swallowing skills.

Correct Answer: A.

Rationale:
The client with minimal cognitive limitations can be a candidate for the procedure. If a person can progress to swallowing thin liquids, a videofluoroscopy is usually not necessary. The client that shows only oral stage problems also does not need a videofluoroscope to rule out swallowing difficulties, which is the goal of the videofluoroscopy procedure. The client who tolerates therapies has a better chance of improvement and could benefit from the procedure. If the client with a swallowing disorder cannot tolerate therapy, an alternative intervention, such as a gastronomy tube, would be indicated.

Type of Reasoning: Inductive
This question requires one to determine, through clinical judgment, the indications for when to recommend videofluoroscopy. This requires inductive reasoning skill, where one must match the client's current status to the candidacy guidelines for the procedure. In this situation, a client is a candidate if there are minimal cognitive limitations. Review indications for videofluoroscopy if answered incorrectly.

B159 C5

An adult recently diagnosed with scleroderma receives occupational therapy services to deal with the functional changes caused by this disease. Which recommendation is best for the occupational therapist to make to this individual?

Answer Choices:
A. Dress in lightweight clothing for thermal comfort.
B. Dress in layers for neutral warmth.
C. Use pull-on clothing to ease donning and doffing.
D. Use Velcro/or a button hook to ease fastening.

Correct Answer: B.

Rationale:
Scleroderma is a systemic disease of unknown etiology. Symptoms are grouped into the CREST syndrome which includes calcinosis, Raynaud's phenomenon, esophageal dysfunction, sclerodactyly of fingers and toes and telangiectasis or red spots covering the hands, feet, forearms, face and hips. The systemic sclerosis of internal organs can be life threatening. A common early (and ongoing) symptom of scleroderma is poor circulation, as in Raynaud's phenomenon which is characterized by episodic vasospasm in the small peripheral arteries and arterioles. This phenomenon usually affects the hands, and at times the feet. It is often precipitated by exposure to cold. Dressing in layers can compensate for this problem. Lightweight clothing would not address the person's need for warmth. The use of pull on clothing, Velcro fasteners and/or a button hook may be indicated if the disease progresses to the point that the individual develops contractures. However, these are not indicated for a person recently diagnosed with the disorder.

Type of Reasoning: Inductive
One must utilize clinical knowledge and judgment to determine the best recommendation for the patient with scleroderma. Knowledge of scleroderma and guidelines to minimize effects of the disease are critical in order to arrive at a correct conclusion. In this case, the best recommendation is for the patient to dress in layers for neutral warmth. If answered incorrectly, review characteristics of scleroderma.

B160 C3

An individual is status post carpal tunnel release. When the occupational therapist conducts a sensory test for sharp/dull (pain), the person reports dull as sharp on the palmar surface of the thumb and index finger. All other responses were correct. Which is accurate for the therapist to document about the individual's sensation?

Answer Choices:
A. Impaired for pain along C5 and C6 dermatomes.
B. Hypersensitive along the ulnar nerve distribution of the palmar surface of the hand.
C. Hypersensitive along the median nerve distribution of the thumb and index fingers. ✓
D. Absent for pain along the median nerve distribution.

Correct Answer: C.

Rationale:
The individual is so sensitive that when touched with a dull stimulus he/she reports it as "sharp." Therefore, the sensation is not absent, but rather hypersensitive at the median nerve distribution. Impairment at C5 and C6 would also involve the loss of sensation in the upper arm and forearm. Ulnar nerve distribution involves the ring and little fingers.

Type of Reasoning: Analytical
This question provides symptoms and the test taker must determine the likely cause for them. This is an analytical reasoning skill, as questions of this nature often ask one to analyze a group of symptoms in order to determine a diagnosis. In this situation the symptoms indicate hypersensitivity in the median nerve distribution of the thumb and index finger. Review symptoms of median nerve disorders if answered incorrectly.

B161 **C8**

The family of a two year-old in a spica cast asks the occupational therapist to modify the child's car seat. The child cannot fit safely in the car seat due to the cast. Which action is best for the therapist to take in response to this request?

Answer Choices:
A. Pad the area between the car seat and the child's back with a pillow to accommodate for the lack of hip flexion.
B. Recommend the family purchase a car seat designed for a child with a spica cast. ✓
C. Cut down the sides of the car seat to allow the cast to hang out of the sides of the car seat.
D. Tell the family to use the current car seat and tighten up the straps to hold in the child.

Correct Answer: B.

Rationale:
The child needs a car seat adapted for a child in a spica cast that has been crash tested. A variety of specialized car seats are available. Therapists and other pediatric care providers can become trained in fitting specialized car seats. Padding the area between the child and the car seat and cutting the car seat would compromise its integrity and is unsafe. The current car seat is not safe and cannot be made safer by tightening the strap.

Type of Reasoning: Inductive
The test taker must determine the safest course of action in this scenario, which requires clinical judgment, an inductive reasoning skill. Being able to predict what may happen as a result of such actions, the test taker should conclude that purchasing a car seat made for a child with a spica cast is the best and safest choice. If answered incorrectly, review pediatric adaptive car seats.

B162 **C4**

A Level II fieldwork student's first assigned case is an individual with right hemiplegia. The supervising therapist reminds the student that primitive reflexes can emerge when someone incurs a CVA. The therapist demonstrates this point by rotating the client's head to the right and stating that the observed response demonstrates a subtle asymmetrical tonic neck reflex (ATNR). The therapist asks the student to describe the client's reaction that resulted in the therapist's interpretation. Which is most accurate for the student to state the client is exhibiting based on this observation?

Answer Choices:
A. Increased flexor tone of the right upper extremity.
B. Increased extensor tone of the left upper extremity.
C. Increased extensor tone of the right upper extremity. ✓
D. Increased extensor tone in both upper extremities.

Correct Answer: C.

Rationale:
Rotating the head to one side facilitates the ATNR. When observing ATNR, one will see flexion of the skull side of the body, and extension of the "face" side. Therefore, when assessing an adult patient with right hemiplegia and rotating the head to the right, one would note an increase in extension tone in the right upper extremity.

Type of Reasoning: Deductive
This question requires recall of guidelines and principles, which is factual knowledge. Deductive reasoning skills are utilized whenever one must recall clinical guidelines. In this situation, the student should report the observation of increased extensor tone in the right upper extremity. Review ATNR reflex in adults with CVA if answered incorrectly.

B163 C5

An individual with a spinal cord injury at C-7 reports noticeable redness on the ischial tuberosity during self-examination with a mirror. Which action is most effective for the occupational therapist to recommend in response to client's observations?

Answer Choices:
A. Integrate weight shifting into daily activities. ✓
B. Use a tilt-in-space wheelchair.
C. Use an angled foam cushion.
D. Self-direct caregivers to assist with weight shifting at least once every 30 minutes.

Correct Answer: A.

Rationale:
During rehabilitation, a person with a spinal cord injury must be instructed on the need to relieve pressure on a consistent basis. A person with a spinal cord injury at the level of C-7 can perform depression transfers so the ability to perform weight shifting for pressure relief is intact. The person is reporting the early signs of skin breakdown so it is vital that the person integrates weight shifting into daily activities. This is a very effective way to prevent decubitus ulcers. Since the person is able to weight shift independently, a tilt-in-space wheelchair and self-directing caregivers to assist with weight shifting are two modifications that are at too low a level for this scenario. An angled foam cushion would position the person in a manner that would increase weight on the ischial tuberosity. This would be contraindicated.

Type of Reasoning: Inductive
One must utilize clinical knowledge and judgment to determine the recommendation that best addresses the individual's issue. This requires inductive reasoning skill. In this case, the therapist should recommend weight shifting into daily activities to prevent pressure sores. If answered incorrectly, review pressure relief activities for individuals with cervical spinal cord injury and the functional abilities of the different levels of SCI. Integration of this knowledge is required for a correct answer.

B164 C6

A graduate student with an anxiety disorder reports feeling confused about the future. During the OT evaluation, the client relates decreased feelings of competence for a chosen field of study and overall poor personal causation. Which is the best initial action for the therapist to take in response to the client's stated concerns?

Answer Choices:
A. Administer a vocational interest inventory.
B. Provide activities related to the client's chosen field of study.
C. Refer the client to the state office of vocational and educational services.
D. Establish short-term goals with high potential for attainment. ✓

Correct Answer: D.

Rationale:
Decreased personal causation and feelings of incompetence are common symptoms of anxiety disorders. The establishment of short-term goals with high potential for attainment can provide the individual with the success experiences needed to develop a sense of competence and improve personal causation. Once these skills are developed, the need for further vocational exploration and/or services can be determined.

Type of Reasoning: Inferential
One must determine the most appropriate initial action for this patient, given the symptoms described. This requires inferential reasoning, where one must draw conclusions based on the evidence presented. In this situation, the occupational therapist should establish short-term goals with high potential for achievement. If answered incorrectly, review intervention planning guidelines for patients with anxiety disorders.

B165 C7

An occupational therapist completes a cognitive screening for a person with chronic schizophrenia, undifferentiated type. The therapist uses Allen's cognitive disabilities model to guide the evaluation process. During the screening, the person is able to imitate the whipstitch but cannot imitate the single cordovan stitch. Based upon these results, the occupational therapist determines that further evaluation is indicated. Which ability is most relevant for the therapist to assess?

Answer Choices:
A. Performance of multi-step tasks using overt trial and error problem-solving.
B. Performance of multi-step tasks using analytical reasoning.
C. Performance of simple tasks independently using visual cues.
D. Performance of simple tasks with long-term repetitive training.

Correct Answer: C.

Rationale:
According to the Allen Cognitive Level (ACL) test, a person who is able to imitate a whipstitch but not able to imitate a cordovan stitch is at a cognitive level of 4. According to Allen's cognitive disabilities model, a person at Level 4 is able to complete simple tasks independently. However, the person relies heavily on visual clues. Since the screening indicated that the person is likely at this level, further evaluation is needed to provide more specifics about the person's abilities and limitations. According to Allen's cognitive disabilities model, a person at Level 3 can perform simple tasks with long-term repetitive training. Since this level is lower than the level identified in the screening, the OT would not begin evaluation here. According to Allen's cognitive disabilities model, a person who can use overt trial and error problem-solving is at Level 5, while the use of analytical reasoning is indicative of Level 6. These levels are higher than the level screened, so evaluation would also begin here.

Type of Reasoning: Analytical
This question requires the test taker to determine the functional deficit of the patient, which is an analytical reasoning skill. Questions of this nature often call upon the test taker to determine a diagnosis based on a functional description of deficits. Based on this information, the person should be further evaluated for the ability to perform simple tasks independently using visual cues. Review ACL testing, especially cognitive level of 4 if answered incorrectly.

B166 C4

An occupational therapist works with a child with pervasive developmental disabilities in order to improve self-care skills. In teaching the child to brush teeth, the therapist places the toothbrush in the child's hand and guides it to the mouth. To help the child learn to complete the activity the therapist uses the somatosensory system. Which of the following is most effective for the therapist to use next during intervention with this child?

Answer Choices:
A. Tell the child to brush up and down.
B. Provide hand-over-hand assistance to brush the child's teeth.
C. Touch the child's hand to prompt hand-to-mouth movements.
D. Instruct the child to follow a pictorial sequence card depicting tooth-brushing.

Correct Answer: B.

Rationale:
In providing hand-over-hand assistance, the occupational therapist is using tactile, proprioceptive and movement stimuli to cue the child. The somatosensory system is inclusive of these sensory systems. Providing auditory, tactile or visual input does not provide sufficient input for the child to learn the task.

Type of Reasoning: Inferential
One must have knowledge of somatosensory interventions in children with pervasive developmental disabilities in order to choose the best intervention approach. This is an inferential reasoning skill where one must infer or draw conclusions about a best course of action. For this case, the occupational therapist should next provide hand-over-hand assistant to brush the child's teeth. If answered incorrectly, review sensory system terminology and interventions using a somatosensory approach.

B167 C9

A pre-school aged child with recurring headaches and decreased gross and fine motor skills is hospitalized on an acute care unit for a diagnostic work-up. Just prior to the occupational therapy evaluation, the parents are told that their child has cancer. The parents are upset when they bring their child to the evaluation session. Which are the best actions for the therapist to take in response to this situation?

Answer Choices:
A. Recommend the parents speak to their spiritual advisor or the social worker and proceed with the OT session.
B. Cancel the OT session and recommend the parents speak to their spiritual advisor or the social worker.
C. Spend the OT session providing support to the parents and addressing the parents' acceptance of the diagnosis.
D. Recommend the parents speak to their spiritual advisor or the social worker and reschedule the OT session for later in the week.

Correct Answer: A.

Rationale:
The best actions are recommending the parents speak to a source of help and comfort and then proceed with the session. The therapist can provide this recommendation in a supportive and empathetic manner and then complete the scheduled evaluation. The child needs an occupational therapy evaluation as part of the diagnostic work-up. The therapist can help the family adjust to and accept the diagnosis via therapeutic activities during the OT session. However, the provision of counseling is most appropriately provided by pastoral care and/or social work practitioners. Moreover, in a medical model setting, these services would not be reimbursable if administered by an occupational therapist. Cancelling or rescheduling the session is not necessary and in a hospital setting it is highly unlikely that immediate re-appointments would be available.

Type of Reasoning: Evaluative
One must weigh the possible courses of action and then make a value judgment about the best course to take. This requires evaluative reasoning skill, which often utilizes guiding principles of action in order to arrive at a correct conclusion. For this case, because the parents are obviously upset, the therapist should refer the family to their spiritual advisor or the social worker.

B168 C8

After six months of rehabilitation for a T-2 spinal cord injury, a patient is being discharged. The occupational therapist conducts a home visit to evaluate accessibility. The individual lives with two roommates in an apartment in a private home. The doorway measurements currently range from 30–32 inches throughout the apartment. The patient's landlord is amenable to making changes in the apartment but has no financial resources. Which recommendation is best for the therapist to make for independent accessibility in the apartment?

Answer Choices:
A. Install offset hinges on all doors.
B. Remove doorframes of doorways less than 32 inches and install wider frames.
C. Remove all doors except for the apartment entrance door.
D. Remove all doorframes and install 36 inch wide doorframes.

Correct Answer: A.

Rationale:
Offset hinges can increase a doorway's width by 2 inches which would result in all doorways meeting or exceeding minimum accessibility standards. It is not necessary to widen the doorways any further. In addition, physically removing doorframes and then installing wider ones is costly. This extra expense is not warranted. While the removal of all doors can increase accessibility it also eliminates privacy which may not be desirable when living with two other individuals.

Type of Reasoning: Inductive
Clinical knowledge and judgment are the most important skills needed for answering this question, which requires inductive reasoning skill. Reasoning the most realistic and cost effective solution to the problem at hand is important in choosing the best solution. In this case, the best solution is to install offset hinges on all doors. Review home adaptations for persons who use wheelchairs if answered incorrectly.

B169 C3

An individual recovering from myasthenia gravis has fair minus (F–) muscle strength in both upper extremities. The occupational therapist develops an intervention plan to include the goal of increasing muscle strength. According to the biomechanical approach, which should the therapist work on with the patient during intervention?

Answer Choices:
A. Complete active ROM with gravity decreased.
B. Complete active ROM against gravity.
C. Incomplete active ROM against gravity.
D. Complete active ROM against gravity and slight resistance.

Correct Answer: B.

Rationale:
The next muscle grade after a minus Fair (F–) is fair (F) which indicates the ability of the body part to move through its complete ROM against gravity. An F– muscle grade indicates a body part can move through its incomplete ROM (more than 50%) against gravity. An F+ muscle grade indicates a body part can move through its complete ROM against gravity and slight resistance. The ability to move a body part through complete ROM with gravity decreased is indicative of a poor (P) muscle grade.

Type of Reasoning: Deductive
This question requires recall of guidelines and principles, which is factual knowledge. Deductive reasoning skills are utilized whenever one must recall facts to solve problems. In this situation, one should recall the definition of the next grade above F– in order to arrive at a correct conclusion. Review muscle grades obtained from manual muscle testing if answered incorrectly.

B170 C6

A high school student with a diagnosis of borderline personality disorder and a history of self-abusive behaviors attends a transitional school-to-work program co-lead by an occupational therapist and an occupational therapy assistant (OTA). During the vocational skills group, the student expresses feelings of hopelessness about the future and questions the point of participating in the program. The student asks to leave the group due to being too tired to concentrate as a result of sleepless nights. The occupational therapist asks the OTA to assume leadership of the group while the therapist addresses the student's concerns. Which action is best for the therapist to take in response to the student's statements?

Answer Choices:
A. Pull the student aside from the group and ask if the student is feeling self-destructive.
B. Allow the student to leave the group after reminding the student to relay concerns to the guidance counselor.
C. Support the validity of the student's feelings and encourage the student to remain in the group.
D. Remind the student that in a work setting the norm is to work even if fatigued.

Correct Answer: A.

Rationale:
All statements of hopelessness and a lack of future vision must be taken seriously, as they can indicate a suicide risk. This is especially important in this case since there is a history of self-destructive behavior. Pulling the student aside from the group allows for the maintenance of confidentiality. The student's reports of sleep disturbances, concentration difficulties and feelings of hopelessness can reflect an increase in depression. If the student is allowed to leave the group, there is a risk that self-destructive behavior (or even suicide) may occur. Validating the student's feelings and reinforcing workplace norms do not deal safely with a potential immediate crisis.

Type of Reasoning: Evaluative
This question requires professional judgment based on guiding principles, which is an evaluative reasoning skill. Because the client is stating feelings of hopelessness and lack of future vision, the therapist should ask the client if he/she is feeling self-destructive. This way the therapist can determine the most appropriate course of action based on this information. Review symptoms of suicidal ideations if answered incorrectly.

Exam C

Examination C

Simulation Test Item C.I.

Opening Scene:

An older adult with moderate rheumatoid arthritis of the hips, knees, shoulders and hands is admitted to a subacute rehabilitation facility after a hospital stay. The patient was hospitalized after a fall at home from a syncopal episode. The patient is deconditioned and fatigues easily. The patient complains of moderate pain in the shoulders and hands. The occupational therapist receives a physician order for evaluation and intervention.

Section A

The occupational therapist is preparing to evaluate the patient to determine functional abilities and premorbid status. Which of the following approaches should the therapist include during the evaluation? Choose all that apply.

1. C2 Interview the patient to learn about past performance in the patient's prior living situation.

Feedback: The patient describes living alone in a 2nd-story apartment, preparing meals daily and cleaning the apartment and completing laundry tasks weekly.

Outcome and Rationale: Interviewing a patient to determine performance in a prior living situation will yield valuable information about the patient's level of independence and performance expectations upon return home. This is a positive outcome so points would be awarded for this selection.

2. C8 Administer a leisure interest inventory.

Feedback: The patient states a primary focus of getting back home and is not worried about leisure pursuits right now.

Outcome and Rationale: While leisure interests are important to many individuals and can be relevant to consider during rehabilitation, functional performance in motor skills and activities of daily living (ADL) are the primary focus of a subacute rehabilitation facility. Older adults in these settings are often covered under Medicare, which will not reimburse for leisure skills and interests. This choice does not cause harm nor does it move the person forward in the intervention process; therefore, it would be considered a neutral selection. Points would neither be awarded nor deducted for its selection.

3. C3 Conduct manual muscle testing of both upper extremities.

Feedback: The patient cries out in pain as the therapist begins testing the shoulders and asks the therapist to stop.

Outcome and Rationale: Manual muscle testing is contraindicated with individuals who have rheumatoid arthritis (RA) due to its potential to invoke pain and damage delicate joint tissues that are destroyed as part of the disease. Selecting this action would cause harm; consequently, its selection would result in the deduction of points.

4. C3 Perform an active range-of-motion (ROM) evaluation to tolerance.

Feedback: The patient moves the shoulders in flexion and abduction to ½ the normal range. All other joints move slowly but through normal ranges with pain in the shoulders and hands.

Outcome and Rationale: Active ROM evaluation can provide valuable information about the patient's ability to tolerate motion, potential for pain and ultimately to engage in everyday tasks using his/her available range to complete ADL. This is a positive outcome so points would be awarded for this selection.

5. C3 Administer a subjective pain inventory.

Feedback: The patient indicates that the pain is throbbing in both hands and shoulders at a level 6 with activity and a level 3 at rest on the analog scale.

Outcome and Rationale: A subjective pain inventory can provide valuable information about the patient's subjective pain perceptions, including what exacerbates and remedies the pain, current measures utilized to decrease the pain and location of such pain. Therapists can then use this information to assist the patient in the safe completion of ADL and instrumental activities of daily living (IADL). This is a positive outcome so points would be awarded for this selection.

6. C3 Determine the patient's ability to ambulate to the bathroom without an assistive device.

Feedback: The patient becomes unsteady after a few steps and stumbles, requiring intervention from the therapist to prevent a fall.

Outcome and Rationale: The therapist needs to finish the evaluation before asking a patient to ambulate without a device. Though the information provided does not indicate a level of performance in mobility, one should infer that a person with moderate RA in the hips and knees will not tolerate ambulation without some type of support to ensure safe mobility. Failing to provide this assistance exhibits poor judgment and harm to the patient was the result. Consequently, this selection would result in the deduction of points.

7. C8 Provide a long-handled bath sponge to the patient.

Feedback: The patient thanks the therapist for the device and wants to know how to use it.

Outcome and Rationale: A bath sponge may be needed and helpful, but this should be issued after the evaluation. It is not a harmful action, but it would be more beneficial to wait and determine after a complete ADL evaluation that this is needed and provide appropriate training in its use. Although this was a premature action, no harm was done. Consequently, it would be considered a neutral selection and points would neither be awarded nor deducted for its selection.

8. C9 Collaborate with the facility's social worker to determine the patient's previous use of home-based services.

Feedback: The social worker states the patient used no home-based services previously.

Outcome and Rationale: While collaborating with other team members is typically a positive action, it is the occupational therapist's responsibility to interview the patient to receive first-hand information about the patient's prior use of home-based services, if any. In this situation, the collaboration does not yield enough information to have a complete understanding of the patient's use of services. Although this was not an effective action, no harm was done. Consequently, it would be considered a neutral selection and points would neither be awarded nor deducted for its selection.

Section B

Evaluation results reveal that the patient lived alone in a 2nd-story apartment with an elevator. The patient reports preparing daily meals and weekly apartment cleaning and laundering of clothes prior to hospitalization. The patient describes experiencing joint pain and fatigue during these IADL tasks. The patient currently has normal active ROM with the exception of both shoulders, which are limited to ½ normal ROM. The shoulders are red and warm to the touch. Strength is fair in both shoulders and hands. All other UE joints demonstrate good strength. Which activities and/or modalities should the occupational therapist choose to implement during intervention? Choose all that apply.

1. C3 Hot packs on bilateral shoulders and hands for relief of pain.

Feedback: The patient complains that the heat is making the pain worse and asks the therapist to remove them.

Outcome and Rationale: Heat is contraindicated in patients with RA where signs of acute inflammation are present in the affected joints. The results above indicate that the patient's shoulders display redness (erythema) and increased temperature, which a therapist should conclude are indicative of an acute inflammatory process. Consequently, this selection would result in the deduction of points.

2. C3 Meal preparation activities with supplies located in high and low cupboards to simulate the home environment.

Feedback: The patient attempts the task but cannot reach up or down sufficiently.

Outcome and Rationale: Meal preparation is a good IADL to focus on. The issue in this circumstance is asking the patient to retrieve items from high and low areas when the patient has limited shoulder ROM and pain in the hips and knees. The ideal situation would be to adapt the activity to make supply retrieval successful. The given choice will likely not result in harm, but is not ideal to request it, as the occupational therapist should anticipate this will be difficult for the patient. This choice would be considered a neutral selection and points would neither be awarded nor deducted for its selection.

3. C3 Energy conservation training during cleaning tasks.

Feedback: The patient learns to pace during the activities and describes feeling less fatigued performing the tasks.

Outcome and Rationale: Energy conservation is clearly an indicated activity and is tied to what the patient needs to complete at home. Because the patient was admitted for rehabilitation due to deconditioning and the patient's diagnosis is chronic in nature, energy conservation is a good choice to help him/her be successful at home. This is a positive outcome so points would be awarded for this selection.

4. C3 Simulated completion of laundry tasks with education on proper body positioning.

Feedback: The patient learns how to complete laundry tasks while protecting the joints from increased pain and potential injury.

Outcome and Rationale: Laundry is an important activity that the patient needs to learn how to do safely, especially as it relates to protecting the joints. Simulating the task while providing education on joint protection will help reduce pain and increase independence. This is a positive outcome so points would be awarded for this selection.

5. C3 Theraband exercises to build upper body strength.

Feedback: The patient complains of pain in the shoulders and hands while trying to complete the task and stops.

Outcome and Rationale: High resistance activities are clearly contraindicated in people with moderate RA due to the potential to invoke pain and cause tissue damage. Strengthening should be limited to functional activities that are low in resistance to protect the affected joints. Since this action causes harm, its selection would result in the deduction of points.

6. C8 Feeding tasks using built-up utensils.

Feedback: The patient states an ability to feed without the built-up utensils and does not like how different they look.

Outcome and Rationale: The information provided in the case scenario does not indicate a need to focus on feeding or to build up utensils. While it may be valid for some people, in this case it was not needed, but at the same time not harmful to the patient. Therefore, this action would be considered a neutral selection and points would neither be awarded nor deducted for its selection.

7. C8 Practice in the retrieval of ADL items using a standard reacher.

Feedback: The patient likes the idea of a reacher, but states that the trigger mechanism hurts the fingers.

Outcome and Rationale: A reacher can be very helpful for patients with RA. The key is to provide an easy squeeze reacher that encourages a mass grasp pattern to close the device, not a trigger handle. Trigger handles can provide too much resistance on small finger joints. In this case it is not harmful, but not ideal to provide. Therefore, it would be considered a neutral selection and points would neither be awarded nor deducted for its selection.

8. C3 Instruction in gentle upper extremity stretching activities to be completed outside of therapy time.

Feedback: The patient states that the stretching helps decrease joint stiffness.

Outcome and Rationale: Gentle stretching is indicated in people with rheumatoid arthritis to prevent stiffness and loss of range of motion. The low to no resistance activity is safe and effective in maintaining joint integrity and can also alleviate morning stiffness and pain. This is a positive outcome so points would be awarded for this selection.

Section C

The patient has progressed in treatment and the rehabilitation team is planning for discharge. The patient can now complete basic and instrumental ADL with modified independence and use of a cane for mobility. The team wants to ensure that the patient is able to safely and independently live alone. The occupational therapist takes the patient to the patient's 2nd-story apartment for an evaluation. What abilities should the therapist assess during this home evaluation? Choose all that apply.

1. C8 Ability to ascend stairs up to the patient's 2nd-story apartment.

Feedback: The patient states the apartment building has an elevator and does not climb the stairs.

Outcome and Rationale: The ability to climb stairs is not a pivotal task for this patient, especially given the diagnosis of RA. Therefore, ascending stairs is not the most important focus. However, it is not harmful either. Therefore, this action would be considered a neutral selection and points would neither be awarded nor deducted for its selection.

2. C8 Independence in opening food packaging.

Feedback: The patient states that he/she buys easy-open packages and has family members open difficult packages when visiting.

Outcome and Rationale: Opening food packaging is a needed task, but is not an important focus for a home evaluation. There is no indication that this is a functional difficulty that would require evaluation in the patient's home. This choice does not cause harm nor does it move the person forward in the intervention process; therefore, it would be considered a neutral selection and points would neither be awarded nor deducted for its selection.

3. C8 Transfer performance to the couch, chairs, bed and toilet.

Feedback: The patient states that standing up from low surfaces is difficult and would like help in making this task easier.

Outcome and Rationale: Transfers are a pivotal part of a home evaluation in order to determine if the patient can safely move on and off various surfaces without falling or getting stuck. This is a positive outcome so points would be awarded for this selection.

4. C8 Ability to open and close the apartment door and manage locks.

Feedback: The patient takes extra time to complete the task due to difficulty operating the door knob and locking mechanisms.

Outcome and Rationale: Safety is paramount during all home evaluations. The patient must be able to leave the apartment quickly and with ease in case of emergency and secure it to be safe. Based upon the observed difficulties, the therapist can recommend adaptive devices and/or strategies to make these operations easier. This is a positive outcome so points would be awarded for this selection.

5. C8 Ability to descend stairs from the apartment to the first floor.

Feedback: The patient states that this will be helpful in case the elevator is out of order.

Outcome and Rationale: The ability to descend stairs is an important task, not only in case the elevator is not operational, but more so in an emergency, such as a fire. This is vital for safety so points would be awarded for this selection.

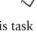

6. C8 Ability to safely stand on a step stool to retrieve high items in kitchen cupboards.

Feedback: The patient is very unsteady, reports discomfort with using a step stool and refuses to complete the task.

Outcome and Rationale: Though the patient may have previously used a step stool, the occupational therapist should know that the patient's diagnosis and presenting symptoms makes using a step stool neither practical nor safe. Rather than evaluating the ability to complete an unsafe activity, the therapist should assist the patient in relocating out-of-reach items to avoid the use of the step stool. This selection could result in a dangerous situation; consequently, it would result in the deduction of points.

7. C3 Independence in tub transfer, including sitting down in the tub.

Feedback: The patient struggles and complains of pain in the hips and knees when attempting to lower body into the tub.

Outcome and Rationale: Tub transfers are important. However, given the diagnosis of RA, it is unrealistic and unsafe to ask the patient to transfer down into the tub. Instead the occupational therapist should encourage the use of a tub bench for safe bathing. Since this action caused pain to the patient and is potentially dangerous, its selection would result in the deduction of points.

8. C8 Ability to walk to laundry room while transporting light laundry items.

Feedback: The patient ambulates with a cane while carrying the items. The therapist recommends a rolling transport cart.

Outcome and Rationale: Laundry is a task that was focused on in the clinic and an activity that the patient previously performed; therefore, its performance in the home certainly needs to be assessed during a home evaluation. The occupational therapist should suggest alternatives to carrying items in order to protect the joints. This is an action that will increase the patient's independence and safety. This is a good outcome and points would be awarded for this selection.

9. C3 Ability to pick up items on the floor while crouching.

Feedback: The patient attempts to crouch, complains of pain in the hips and knees and refuses to complete the task.

Outcome and Rationale: Patients do drop items on the floor from time to time. However, crouching is contraindicated with RA due to the pain and stress on the hips and knees. Instead, the patient should use a reacher to retrieve items or use an alternate bending technique to pick up items that does not provide excess stress on the joints. Since this action is contraindicated and caused pain to the patient, its selection would result in the deduction of points.

Simulation Test Item C.II.

Opening Scene:

A pediatrician refers a child who is 3 years 10 months old to an occupational therapy private practice for evaluation and intervention for developmental delay. The physician's note accompanying the referral states that the child was born full term with no complications and that two siblings aged 6 and 9 have no medical problems or developmental delays. The physician note state the parents specifically requested a referral to a private practitioner because they did not want their child to be "labeled" as delayed by the local school system. However, the parents are concerned that their youngest child "does not do things the same way" as their older children did when they were younger.

Section A

When the parents and child come to the initial session, the therapist observes the child walking and running around the room and walking up and down the stairs. The child asks to play with toys. The therapist observes the child successfully picking up coins but the child has difficulty placing the coins in the slot of a toy cash register. The child has difficulty turning the pages in a coloring book and grasps a crayon with a digital pronate grasp. Which additional action(s) should the therapist take during the initial session to evaluate the child's capabilities? Choose all that apply.

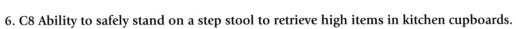

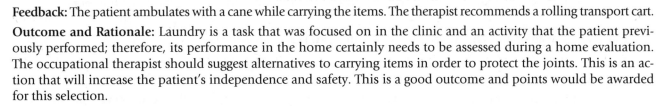

1. C1 Evaluate the child's baseline gross motor skills using a standardized scale.

Feedback: The child easily completes all gross motor activities presented during this assessment.

Outcome and Rationale: The child was observed to walk and run around the room and walk up and down the stairs. These behaviors indicate that the child's gross motor skills are developing typically and do not indicate a need for a gross motor assessment. See Table 5-3 for the developmental sequence of walking and Table 5-4 for the developmental sequence of stair climbing. Although the completion of this assessment did not provide new information about this child, the validation of the child's attainment of gross motor developmental milestones can be comforting to the parents. Therefore, this option would be considered neutral and no points would be awarded or deducted for its selection.

2. C2 Question parents about potential events that could have caused the child's delay.

Feedback: The parents become upset with the therapist.

Outcome and Rationale: The purpose of an initial session is to build rapport with the child and parents and complete an evaluation of the child's abilities and limitations. It is not necessary or appropriate to inquire about potential precipitants to a child's developmental delay during an initial evaluation session. This line of inquiry can be perceived as prejudicial, accusatory and/or an invasion of privacy by the parents. If the attainment of etiological information is important to the development of an intervention plan, the therapist should obtain this information from the referring physician. Since this action is negative, its selection would result in the deduction of points.

3. C1 Evaluate the child's reach, grasp, release and in-hand manipulation skills.

Feedback: The child exhibits developmentally appropriate reach and release skills. The child has difficulty with palm to finger translation, simple rotation and shift of objects.

Outcome and Rationale: The therapist's observations of the child's play indicated the need to evaluate the child's fine motor skills. The ability to pick up coins is indicative of intact finger-to-palm translation which is typically developed at 12 to15 months of age. Difficulty placing the coins in the slot of a toy cash register indicates a deficit in the ability to use palm-to finger translation, a skill which typically develops at age 2 to $2\frac{1}{2}$ years. Difficulty in turning the pages in a book indicates a deficit in shift, a skill which typically develops at age 3 to $3\frac{1}{2}$ years. The ability to grasp a crayon using a digital pronate grasp is a skill that is typically developed at the age 2 to 3 years. The evaluation of the child's fine motor skills provided relevant information about the child's developmental level and functional capabilities which the therapist can use to develop an intervention plan. This is a good outcome and the selection of this positive action would result in the awarding of points.

4. C2 Refer the child to the local school system's prekindergarten program.

Feedback: The parents state that they prefer to work with a private practitioner.

Outcome and Rationale: The focus of this section is about evaluation. A referral is not a method of evaluation. The selection of this action represents a lack of understanding of the occupational therapy (OT) process. Most important, the physician had noted that the parents had specifically requested a referral to a private practitioner. It is the parents' choice and right to obtain treatment in the private sector and not through the school system. Referring the child to the school system is an action that is counter to the parents, expressed wishes. As a result, this action is negative and its selection would result in the deduction of points.

5. C2 Discuss the scope of school-based occupational therapy services with the parents.

Feedback: The parents state that they understand but still do not want to "go that route."

Outcome and Rationale: The child may or may not be a candidate for school-based occupational therapy services. However, educating the parents about school-based occupational therapy can provide information on the scope of services that may be of value to their child, if needed in the future. This information can contribute to an open discussion about the parents' perception that their child will be 'labeled' if he/she receives school-based occupational therapy. However, it is not an evaluation method, which is the focus of this section. While this action did not advance the child in the OT process, it did not cause harm. As a result, this action is neutral and no points would be awarded or deducted for its selection.

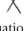

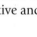

6. C1 Administer the Miller Assessment for Preschoolers (MAP™).

Feedback: The child demonstrates non-verbal delays in fine motor skills and no delays in gross motor, cognitive, verbal or non-verbal skills.

Outcome and Rationale: The Miller Assessment for Preschoolers (MAP™) is a standardized task performance measure that assesses cognitive, sensory, motor and verbal and non-verbal abilities. Combined abilities, which include a complex tasks index, are also measured. The specific items used during the evaluation's administration are determined by the age of the child being evaluated. The MAP™ is standardized for children age 2 years 9 months to age 5 years 8 months. The child's performance on the standardized items is compared to established norms. Supplemental non-standardized observations may also be included in the evaluation process. The MAP™ is a developmental measure that can provide baseline information about the child's functional abilities which can be used for intervention planning. As a result, this action is positive and its selection would result in the awarding of points.

7. C1 Administer the Bruininks-Oseretsky Test of Motor Proficiency™ (BOT-2).

Feedback: The child is unable to complete the evaluation activities.

Outcome and Rationale: The BOTMP is used to assess gross motor and fine motor speed, agility, strength and coordination for children aged 4 to 21 years. While this assessment is a good one, it is not standardized for this child's age group. As a result, the information obtained from this evaluation would not be valid. The selection of this action reflects a lack of knowledge about this standardized assessment and would result in the deduction of points.

8. C1 Administer the Pediatric Evaluation of Disability Inventory (PEDI).

Feedback: The child's social function is within normal limits. Mild delays in self-care and fine motor skills (e.g., difficulty with clothing fastening) are evident.

Outcome and Rationale: The PEDI is a standardized behavior checklist and rating scale that assesses capabilities and detects functional deficits to determine a child's developmental level. It provides a baseline of social, self-care and mobility skills for children aged 6 months to 7 years. The score forms include the areas of functional skills, caregiver assistance and activity modifications. The information can be obtained by interview of parents in combination with therapist observation. The administration of the PEDI provides information that can help the therapist develop a relevant intervention plan. As a result, this action is positive and its selection would result in the awarding of points.

9. C8 Ask the parents to describe the child's performance in ADL.

Feedback: The parents state that their child is independent in ADL performance except for fastening clothing and using a spoon and fork to feed self.

Outcome and Rationale: The parents' report about their child's capabilities can provide the therapist with relevant information upon which to base a family-centered intervention plan. This is a positive outcome and the selection of this action would result in the awarding of points.

Section B

The occupational therapist collaborates with the parents to develop an intervention plan focused on improving the child's fine motor skills to complete functional tasks including fastening clothing and using a spoon and fork to feed self. The parents report that their child often becomes frustrated when attempting these tasks. During the evaluation, it was determined that the child has developmentally appropriate reach and release skills, but grasp is delayed. The child has difficulty with palm-to-finger translation, simple rotation and shift of objects. The child can open and close scissors in a controlled fashion and snips at the edges of construction paper. The child was observed during the evaluation session to enjoy coloring and playing in the clinic's child-size kitchen. Which activities are best for the occupational therapist to have the child engage in during intervention? Choose all that apply.

1. C1 Practice spearing and eating small pieces of fruit with a child-size fork.

Feedback: The child becomes frustrated with the difficulty of holding the fork.

Outcome and Rationale: Although the parents identified the use of a spoon and fork to self-feed as a desired outcome of occupational therapy, they also reported that their child often becomes frustrated with his/her difficulty with this task. In addition, the evaluation determined that the child has delays in grasp and in-hand manipulation skills. Therefore, OT intervention should first address the development of these skills by using activities that include the grasping and manipulating of objects, without the expectation of self-feeding. After the development of these skills, the use of utensils to self-feed can be introduced. Interventions to develop the use of eating utensils should begin with the use of a spoon prior to a fork, since the unskilled use of a fork can cause injury to the child. The inclusion of an intervention activity that uses a fork prior to the development of essential requisite skills reflects a poor understanding of the child's developmental level and functional capabilities. As a result, this action is negative and points would be deducted for its selection.

2. C1 Engage in play kitchen activities to "cook," "stir," "serve," and "eat" a meal.

Feedback: The child effectively grasps and manipulates various objects during the activities.

Outcome and Rationale: The active movements and variety of tools used in this activity can enhance the child's refinement of functional grasp and his/her development of in-hand manipulation skills. In addition, this play activity is developmentally appropriate and can be fun, which can facilitate the child's active engagement in intervention. These outcomes are positive; therefore, the selection of this action would result in the awarding of points.

3. C1 Pick up coins and drop into an open box.

Feedback: The child easily completes this activity.

Outcome and Rationale: In this case scenario, it was noted that the child successfully picked up coins, which indicates intact finger-to-palm translation. However, the child had difficulty placing the coins in a slot. The focus of intervention should be on developing needed skills. It would be more effective to provide an intervention activity that enables the child to develop skills in palm-to-finger translation by requiring the child to move coins within the hand to place the coins in a slot rather than in an open box. While this activity does not directly address the child's deficits it can provide the child with a sense of mastery, which is important in this case since the parents reported that their child often becomes frustrated when attempting these tasks. Therefore, this option is neutral. No points would be awarded or deducted for its selection.

4. C1 Practice unbuttoning 2-inch buttons using dress-up clothes during a pretend play situation.

Feedback: The child initially unbuttons with difficulty. After several sessions of therapy, the child progresses to unbuttoning with ease.

Outcome and Rationale: The stated focus of this section was on the development of fine motor skills to complete functional tasks including the fastening of clothing. Since the first step in the developmental sequence of fastening clothing is to unbutton large buttons, practicing the unbuttoning of 2-inch buttons is an effective intervention activity. After the child masters the ability to unbutton large buttons with ease, intervention should progress to buttoning large buttons and then to unbuttoning smaller buttons, followed by buttoning smaller buttons. Developing fastening skills by using dress-up clothes during a pretend play situation can be particularly effective since symbolic play is typical of children aged 2 to 4 years. In addition, this activity can facilitate carryover to dressing at home. Since this action is developmentally appropriate and addresses an identified intervention focus, it is positive. As a result, the selection of this action would result in the awarding of points.

5. C1 Play 'hand hide and seek' to hide small objects in the palm of one hand and then place them in the opposite hand.

Feedback: The child initially has difficulty with this activity. After two weeks of therapy, the child completes this activity with ease.

Outcome and Rationale: The activity enhances both finger-to-palm translation and palm-to-finger translation, essential components of fine motor coordination and dexterity for ADL. This action is developmentally appropriate and addresses an identified intervention focus; therefore, it is positive. As a result, the selection of this action would result in the awarding of points.

6. C1 Cut out circles using a child scissors and place them on a shape board. X

Feedback: The child struggles with turning the scissors to cut a circle.

Outcome and Rationale: The child was reported as being able to open and close scissors in a controlled fashion and snip at the edges of construction paper. These skills are typical of a 2- to 3-year-old child. Prior to being able to cut circles, the child needs to develop the ability to coordinate the lateral direction of the scissors, cut a straight forward line and cut simple geometric shapes. These skills all typically develop between 3 to 4 years of age. The ability to cut circles comes after the acquisition of these skills, typically at 3½ to 4½ years old. When working with a child with a developmental delay, it is typical to use a developmental frame of reference. Therefore, the therapist should introduce activities that employ the child's current skills while developing the ability to perform the skill that is next in the typical developmental sequence. Since cutting circles skips over several key steps in the development of scissor skills, the selection of this option reflects a poor understanding of the developmental sequence of scissoring. In addition, the introduction of an activity that is beyond a child's capability will be frustrating to the child. As a result, this action is negative and its selection would result in the deduction of points.

7. C1 Cut paper strips using a child scissors and use them to construct a paper chain. ✓

Feedback: The child successfully cuts in a lateral direction to make paper strips.

Outcome and Rationale: The child was reported as being able to open and close scissors in a controlled fashion and snip at the edges of construction paper. The next skill in scissoring is the ability to coordinate the lateral direction of the scissors and cut a straightforward line. When working with a child with a developmental delay, it is typical to use a developmental frame of reference. Therefore, the therapist should introduce activities that employ the child's current skills, while developing the ability to perform the skill that is next in the typical developmental sequence. The cutting of paper strips can help the child work on using the scissors to cut laterally and then in a straight line. In addition, the child's in-hand manipulation skills can be developed and refined by the folding of the paper strips into circles to construct a paper chain. Since this option is developmentally appropriate, it is positive. Its selection would result in the awarding of points.

8. C1 Practice coloring large shapes with a crayon held in a digital pronate grasp. O

Feedback: The child scribbles with a crayon on each shape.

Outcome and Rationale: The child was observed to grasp the crayon with a digital pronate grasp. This is a skill that is typically developed at the age of 2 to 3 years. When working with a child with a developmental delay, it is typical to use a developmental frame of reference. Therefore, the therapist should introduce activities that develop the child's ability to perform the skill that is next in the typical developmental sequence. In this case, that would be the development of the ability to grasp using a static tripod posture. While this activity did not advance the child in the OT process, it did not cause harm. As a result, this action is neutral and no points would be awarded or deducted for its selection.

Section C

After three weeks of twice weekly occupational therapy sessions, the child can unbutton 2-inch buttons, use scissors to cut paper laterally and in a straight line and effectively grasp various tools during play activities. The child exhibits good finger-to-palm and palm-to-finger translation and the ability to shift objects. The child colors shapes using a static tripod posture. The therapist modifies the child's intervention plan to reflect this progress. Which activities should the therapist include in the modified plan to further achieve the goal of improving the child's fine motor skills to complete functional tasks? Choose all that apply.

1. C1 Practice buttoning 2-inch buttons using dress-up clothes during a pretend play situation. ✓

Feedback: The child initially buttons with difficulty. After several sessions of therapy, the child progresses to buttoning with ease.

Outcome and Rationale: The child has developed the ability to unbutton 2-inch buttons, therefore, the intervention should progress to buttoning 2-inch buttons and then to unbuttoning smaller buttons. After the child masters this skill, intervention should focus on buttoning smaller buttons. Developing fastening skills by using dress-up clothes during a pretend play situation can be particularly effective since symbolic play is typical of children aged 2 to 4 years. In addition, this activity can facilitate carryover to dressing at home. Since this action is developmentally appropriate and addresses an identified intervention focus, it is positive. As a result, the selection of this action would result in the awarding of points.

2. C1 Provide the parents with a home program that includes practice in unbuttoning front 2-inch buttons.

Feedback: The child independently unbuttons the buttons.

Outcome and Rationale: The child has developed the skill to unbutton 2-inch buttons. Providing the parent with a home program to support this skill development can help the child acquire a sense of mastery. However, this action does not move the child forward in the intervention process. As a result, it is neutral and points would not be awarded or deducted for its selection.

3. C1 Practice snapping snaps on a dressing clown.

Feedback: The child cannot snap the snaps.

Outcome and Rationale: According to the typical developmental sequence of dressing skills, the ability to snap occurs after the ability to button. The child has developed the ability to unbutton 2-inch buttons and needs to develop the ability to button 2-inch buttons and unbutton and button smaller buttons prior to learning to snap. The selection of this option reflects a poor understanding of the developmental sequence of fastening skills. In addition, the introduction of an activity that is beyond a child's capability will be frustrating to the child. As a result, this action is negative and its selection would result in the deduction of points.

4. C1 Instruct the parents to have the child zip zippers that are placed on track during the child's daily dressing routine.

Feedback: The child independently zips zippers.

Outcome and Rationale: The child has developed the skill to unbutton large buttons. One of the next developmental tasks after mastery of this skill is the zipping of zippers that have been placed on track. Providing the parent with a dressing activity that can be incorporated into the family's daily routine can support the child's skill development in fastening. This can also help the child acquire a sense of mastery. These are positive outcomes; therefore, the selection of this action would be awarded points.

5. C1 Have the child use a child fork and spoon to "feed" self and stuffed animal "guests" during a pretend party.

Feedback: The child feeds "guests" and self with a child fork and spoon.

Outcome and Rationale: The child has demonstrated effective grasp during OT sessions, so it is appropriate to work on having the child use these skills to develop the ability to use a spoon and fork. Using a play activity to develop functional skills is a primary form of intervention in pediatric OT practice. Having the child pretend to feed self and stuffed animal "guests" during a party can be a very effective method for developing the ability to use a spoon and fork. These skills can then be used during the child's "real-life" feeding situations. Pretending stuffed animals are guests at a party is a form of symbolic play, which is developmentally the typical play of children aged 2 to 4 years. Since this action is developmentally appropriate and facilitates the child's acquisition of desired feeding skills, it is positive. As a result, the selection of this action would result in the awarding of points.

6. C8 Provide the child with adaptive grips for crayons.

Feedback: The child colors with the adapted crayons.

Outcome and Rationale: Adaptive grips are a compensatory approach which is used when intervention is not expected to result in functional improvements. For example, adaptive grips are appropriate when a child's grasp is limited due to poor fine motor control, weakness and/or abnormal tone. In this case, the child is still showing progress in the development of fine motor skills. The child can hold a crayon using a static tripod posture so it is better to continue working on the improvement of grasp prior to providing a compensatory approach. The selection of this option reflects a lack of understanding of the appropriate approaches to use with a child with developmental delay who is capable of progress. Therefore, it is a negative action and its selection would result in the deduction of points.

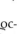

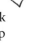

7. C1 Instruct the parents to have the child play simple games that require the moving of pieces across a game board with their older children.

Feedback: The child effectively moves the game pieces across the board.

Outcome and Rationale: The picking up and moving of pieces to play a board game with siblings will enable the child to use a variety of grasp skills in a fun manner. Depending on the size and the shape of the game pieces, the child may use a pincer grasp which typically develops at 10 months old, a fine pincer grasp which typically develops at 12 months old or a radial digital grasp which typically develops at 8 months old. Based on the information provided, the child possesses these skills; therefore, this action does not move the child forward in the intervention process. However, providing the parent with a home program to support intact skills can help the child acquire a sense of mastery. As a result, this action is neutral and points would not be awarded or deducted for its selection.

8. C1 Have the child cut out simple geometric shapes using a child scissors and place them on a shape board.

Feedback: The child successfully cuts the shapes and places them on the shape board.

Outcome and Rationale: The child was reported as being able to use scissors to cut paper laterally and in a straight line. The next skill in scissoring is the ability to cut out simple geometric shapes. When working with a child with a developmental delay, it is typical to use a developmental frame of reference. Therefore, the therapist should introduce activities that employ the child's current skills, while developing the ability to perform the skill that is next in the typical developmental sequence. Since this option is developmentally appropriate, it is positive. Its selection would result in the awarding of points.

Simulation Test Item C.III.

Opening Scene:

An occupational therapist working on a locked inpatient psychiatric unit receives a referral for occupational therapy for a young adult who was just admitted. The physician reports that the client is exhibiting symptoms of bipolar disorder, manic episode, with anxiety. The client graduated from college 8 months ago. The client was fired from a job as a bank teller 3 weeks ago. The client resides with a younger sibling in their parents' single family home.

Section A

Within 24 hours of admission, the occupational therapist meets with the client to complete an evaluation. What evaluation approaches should the occupational therapist use? Choose all evaluation approaches that apply to this client and situation.

1. C9 Ask the client to clarify information obtained from the client's parents regarding behaviors they have observed since the client lost the teller job.

Feedback: The client is surprised to learn that the therapist obtained personal information without permission.

Outcome and Rationale: Information from the family can be helpful but HIPPA regulations require that the client sign authorization for the therapist to talk with anyone outside the interdisciplinary team. The selection of this action reflects poor judgment and unfamiliarity with HIPPA regulations and would result in the deduction of points.

2. C6 Verbally administer the Role Checklist.

Feedback: The client indicates that the roles of friend and hobbyist (woodworker) are highly valued and presently pursued, but the valued role of worker is difficult to maintain.

Outcome and Rationale: The Role Checklist provides information about the client's ability to engage in meaningful roles. It is an appropriate measure to use to evaluate the client's occupational interests. The information obtained will be helpful toward designing a relevant intervention plan for this client. Consequently, this selection would result in the awarding of points.

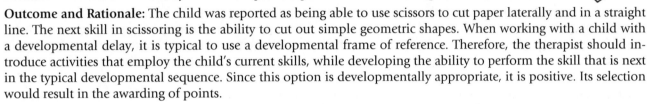

3. C6 Assess the client's reality orientation.

Feedback: The client states the day of the week, the date and the weather correctly.

Outcome and Rationale: The assessment of reality orientation is a component of the mental status examination (MSE) which would have been completed upon admission. The results of the MSE would be recorded in the client's chart and reviewed during the screening process. It would not be relevant to reassess the client's mental status because the client's diagnosis does not indicate psychotic features. Manic symptoms are unlikely to shift the client's orientation to person, place, time and situation. While the reassessment of the client's mental status is not indicated in this case, this action does not cause harm. Therefore, it would be considered neutral and no points would be awarded or deducted for its selection.

4. C6 Assess cognition by having the client purchase coffee in the hospital's main cafeteria.

Feedback: The client cannot leave the unit for this activity.

Outcome and Rationale: The client was admitted within the last 24 hours to a locked inpatient psychiatric unit. It would be unsafe to take the client off the unit given the likelihood of impulsive behavior, distractibility and secondary diagnosis of anxiety. The selection of this evaluation reflects a poor understanding of the client's current functional level and the safety procedures that are characteristic of a locked inpatient unit. Consequently, points would be deducted for this choice.

5. C6 Interview the client using the Canadian Occupational Performance Measure (COPM).

Feedback: The client reports no difficulty with self-care but acknowledges financial instability and difficulty completing work tasks. The client wants to work and live independently.

Outcome and Rationale: Learning what the client sees as strengths and limitations is useful in developing an intervention plan. The client was recently fired from a job. The client wants to resume working to earn money as a way to achieve the goal of living independently. The COPM uncovers the client's priorities and can help the therapist structure activities that develop the client's work potential. Since unemployment is often a secondary effect of mental illness, this is a relevant focus. Obtaining information about the client's priorities is a good outcome; therefore, points would be awarded for this selection.

6. C6 Observe the client during a morning community meeting.

Feedback: The therapist observes that the client is talkative and interrupts other speakers.

Outcome and Rationale: Community meetings are typically part of an inpatient psychiatric unit program, with leadership shared among interdisciplinary staff. Observation of the client during this non-structured activity is one way to gather information, but it is a method that is not unique to occupational therapy. The occupational therapist would gather little new information about how the client engages in purposeful activity or occupational roles with this action. Consequently, no progress would be made toward completing a functional evaluation. However, this is an innocuous action and it would be considered neutral. No points would be awarded or deducted for its selection.

Section B

At the end of the evaluation session, the occupational therapist collaborates with the client to develop an intervention plan based on information obtained from the referral and initial evaluation. They determine that the development of skills to live independently and engage in the valued roles of worker, hobbyist (i.e., woodworker) and friend will be the focus of intervention. Which approaches and activities are most effective for the occupational therapist to use in designing and implementing the intervention plan? Choose all that apply.

1. C6 Speak in short sentences using clear, calm and direct speech.

Feedback: The client responds to the therapist's guidance and instructions.

Outcome and Rationale: Verbal communications are an important aspect of the therapeutic use of self. Clear, calm and direct speech can be used to develop rapport. It can also provide a context for symptom management by helping the client attend during intervention. This can be helpful for a person distracted by symptoms of mania. While this action does not provide a direct approach for the design or implementation of the intervention plan to meet the identified goals, it is supportive and it does not cause harm. Therefore, this action would be considered a neutral selection and no points would be added or deducted.

2. C6 Include the client in a money management group focused on budgeting future earnings from work.

Feedback: The client attends the unit's money management group.

Outcome and Rationale: While the management of future earnings would be a relevant long-term goal for this client, it is too complex for the client to work on attaining during an acute manic episode. To be admitted to an inpatient unit, the client would have symptoms that seriously hindered functional performance. During inpatient hospitalization, the therapist's role is to help the client manage symptoms to set the stage for the client's future ability to engage in postdischarge treatment. An outpatient setting would be the appropriate place to work on the development of financial management skills. Choosing this option would demonstrate poor understanding of inpatient acute care, symptoms of mania and the time needed for medication management to be effective. Points would be deducted for this selection.

3. C2 Provide the client with step-by-step instructions to complete a structured woodworking activity.

Feedback: The client builds a model airplane.

Outcome and Rationale: The choice of a structured woodworking activity is well supported by the client's interest in woodworking. The provision of a structured activity and step-by-step instructions are essential for successful task performance when a person has manic symptoms. Typically, mania results in poor attention, decreased concentration, lack of planning and poor organization. The therapist's provision of a breakdown of task steps can enable the client's successful performance of a valued activity. The therapist will then have the opportunity to help the client reflect on how the activity was structured for success. This process can increase the client's understanding of effective behavior management and is supportive of the client's recovery. This selection directly addresses the functional limitations imposed by mania and effectively enables goal attainment; therefore, it would be awarded points.

4. C6 Include the client in a cooperative social skills group focused on social etiquette to reduce pressured speech.

Feedback: The client frequently interrupts group members to give personal examples of proper social etiquette.

Outcome and Rationale: Mania is characterized by pressured speech, flight of ideas, distractibility and grandiosity, all symptoms that would be increased when a person's illness exacerbates to the point of requiring hospitalization. In addition to the presenting symptoms of mania, the therapist can also expect the client to have behaviors associated with these symptoms, such as poor concentration and limited self-awareness, which would make participation in a group discussion very difficult. The client's symptoms and accompanying behaviors are not appropriate for inclusion in a cooperative social skills group. A group at a project or parallel level would be appropriate for this client. Including the client in a group that is above the client's functional level is counter-therapeutic. The client's manic behaviors would disrupt the group and the resulting reactions of group members would present a challenging group dynamic for the therapist to manage. This action would not be helpful to the client or group members. Its selection reflects poor knowledge of the symptoms of acute mania, the developmental levels of groups and group norms. Consequently, it would result in the deduction of points.

5. C6 Have the client unpack and organize personal belongings.

Feedback: The client pulls everything out of the suitcase.

Outcome and Rationale: To require hospitalization and admission to an inpatient unit, the client would have to be very symptomatic. Based on the client's diagnosis and presenting symptoms, it would be expected that the client would have difficulty concentrating, planning and organizing. This organizational activity could be helpful once symptoms have been managed pharmacologically, but more than 24 hours would be needed for this to occur. The selection of this action reflects an incomplete understanding of bipolar disorder, manic episode and poor activity analysis skills. However, it does not cause harm or disrupt the care of any other clients on the inpatient unit; therefore, it would be considered a neutral response. No points would be awarded or deducted for this selection.

6. C2 Guide the client in completing a goal-planning sheet that lists long- and short-term goals with steps to achieve them.

✓

Feedback: The client fills the sheet with many goals and their steps and asks for another sheet of paper.

Outcome and Rationale: Stating goals, and more importantly, reasonable steps to achieve them, is a useful approach in an acute hospital with a short length of stay. Putting thoughts on paper is an approach that can lessen anxiety and help the client stop racing thoughts. Additionally, this activity can help the therapist learn more about the client's desired outcomes for intervention. It can also help the therapist determine what may be interfering with the client's goal attainment if the client's stated steps are not relevant or realistic. The therapist can then guide the client to establish and structure realistic task-related steps to achieve desired goals. Even though many goals will likely not be attainable during this hospitalization due to the client's mania and the short length of stay on an inpatient unit, this activity will provide the therapist with information about what is important to the client. This knowledge can help the therapist engage the client in treatment activities during the inpatient hospitalization and assist in making relevant discharge plan recommendations. Consequently, this would be a useful intervention and its selection would be awarded points.

Section C

The occupational therapist determines that the client's grandiosity, racing thoughts and anxiety resulted in the client setting unrealistic goals and plans. The therapist provides intervention to develop the client's symptom management skills by using recognition of functional status and engagement in mood-congruent activities to achieve goals. How should the occupational therapist engage the client in the revised intervention program? Choose all of the goal-directed activity approaches and activity demands that are best for this client and this situation.

1. C6 In a scrapbooking group, encourage the client to make a page using shared decorative paper, stickers and pens to create a unique design.

X

Feedback: The client has difficulty choosing page layout, materials and supplies.

Outcome and Rationale: The client in a manic phase of bipolar disorder would approach this task in a disorganized manner. The client would have difficulty negotiating for shared materials and supplies, making the task difficult for other group members. The resulting psychosocial reactions would present a challenging group dynamic for the therapist to manage using therapeutic use of self. This action would not be helpful to the client or group members. The consequences of this action should have been anticipated; therefore, its selection would result in the deduction of points.

2. C2 In a cooking group, suggest that the client cut shapes to construct a gingerbread house, providing templates and directions.

✓

Feedback: The client initiates and readily follows step-by-step directions.

Outcome and Rationale: Choosing an activity with task steps and required skills similar to an activity known to be interesting (i.e., woodworking) to the client is a good choice. Because bipolar disorder interferes with executive functions of the brain, structuring the activity with directions and patterns would lessen information processing demands and lend itself to greater potential for success. Additionally, this activity can be individualized so the client can work on the task alone in a parallel group or in an assembly line fashion in a project group. This action would allow for the activity to be meaningful, graded for task demands and social interaction and organized to minimize stress. This would facilitate goal attainment and symptom management. Consequently, points would be awarded for this action.

3. C2 Assign the client the unit chore of tidying magazines and shelving books in the day room.

O

Feedback: The client assembles the magazines haphazardly and randomly shelves books.

Outcome and Rationale: Unit chores can simulate home management activities, but in this action, they are not structured as a therapeutic intervention. Instead, there is little structure other than the outcome needed to keep the unit in order. Assigning tasks without skilled intervention is not a therapeutic approach, so this would not be effective.

However, there is no harm done to the client by this action. As a result this action would result in a neutral outcome. No points would be awarded or deducted for this selection.

4. C2 Ask the client to describe what was challenging in the client's recent job as a bank teller.

Feedback: The client describes negative attributes of the bank supervisor, co-workers and the teller station environment.

Outcome and Rationale: This action uses self-report to gather information which can be informative, but it is not an intervention approach. The therapist's provision of simulated, structured work tasks would be an effective intervention that would provide the client with an effective way to evaluate work performance and develop needed skills. While obtaining the client's description of past work experiences is not a therapeutic intervention, it is not a detrimental action. Consequently, the selection of this option would not be awarded or deducted points.

5. C2 Have the client help decorate the unit for an upcoming holiday using supplies from a storage box of last year's decorations.

Feedback: The client rummages through the box, excitedly pulling out random decorations.

Outcome and Rationale: The therapist has provided an activity on the unit, but it has not been structured to facilitate goal attainment for this client. Instead, it fosters the client's manic behaviors by its lack of structure, unclear definition of roles for client participation and laissez-faire leadership approach. The aim of inpatient hospitalization is to facilitate symptom management, so this is not a good action. Points would be deducted for the therapist's lack of planning, poor activity analysis and absent structuring of activity demands to address individual goals in a therapeutic activity.

6. C2 Give the client three magazines and verbal instructions of sequential steps to make a picture collage of work and leisure interests.

Feedback: The client completes the collage of work and leisure interests.

Outcome and Rationale: This activity structure enables the client with mania to successfully engage in and complete an activity. It can be completed in a parallel group which is at the appropriate group level for this client. The process of completing the collage can be used to explore the client's current mood and its effect on function. For example, was the client's selection of pictures haphazard and random or focused and deliberate? This structured task also provides an opportunity to evaluate the client's task skills such as decision making, attention, concentration, organization and ability to follow directions. These are fundamental skills for work. The therapist and client can discuss the client's task performance and its relationship to the skills needed to successfully perform work tasks that are inherent in employment. The completion of a collage also provides a concrete visual that can be used by the therapist and client to examine the client's interests in more depth. In a facility with a short length of stay, this structured activity is appropriate. Processing the client's performance in this activity with the client is a positive first step to orient the client to a self-management approach for a chronic illness. This is a strong therapeutic action and points would be awarded for its selection.

Section D

The occupational therapist contributes to discharge planning for the client. In considering recommendations to make to the interdisciplinary team, the therapist integrates the client's goals, evaluation results and performance in occupational therapy intervention over the 4-day length of stay. What should the occupational therapist do to prepare the client for discharge? Choose all of the actions that are effective for this client and this situation.

1. C8 Refer the client to the state office of vocational services for an evaluation of job skills and job placement.

Feedback: The client makes an appointment for the week after discharge.

Outcome and Rationale: Four days is an insufficient time for medications and behavioral therapy approaches to have made the substantial impact on client's functional level that would be needed for the client to be able to engage in a vocational assessment for job placement. Consequently, it is premature to recommend work evaluation and job placement because it is probable that the client could not succeed in any type of job without more sustained symptom management and behavioral change. Although the client could make an appointment, beginning to search for work when symptoms are not well controlled would cause stress and facilitate symptom exacerbation. Because this action shows poor understanding of psychopharmacology and the realistic limitations of short-term inpatient acute psychiatric care on a client's functional level, points would be deducted for this selection.

2. C2 Using guidelines established with the client, work with the client and family to structure household chores congruent with realistic expectations.

Feedback: The client and family come to a predischarge meeting to explore the client's role in household management.

Outcome and Rationale: The ultimate aim of occupational therapy for persons with chronic mental illnesses is helping them learn how to manage daily life so that symptoms are not exacerbated by activity demands or psychosocial stressors. During hospitalization, the therapist and client evaluate the client's performance in a variety of situations, identify early warning signs while engaging in activity and collaborate on ways the client might change the activity, how it is done and under what conditions. Working with the client during hospitalization to begin the process of self-management and transferring that information to the family prior to discharge would be an asset to the client. This action is consistent with occupational therapy practice guidelines and indicates the ability to make sound discharge recommendations. Consequently, its selection would be awarded points.

3. C9 Provide feedback to the client's former bank supervisor on optimal ways to structure the bank teller job for the client.

Feedback: The client is angry that the therapist called the bank supervisor.

Outcome and Rationale: The client is understandably angry and the therapist's action in this situation is grounds for disciplinary action. HIPPA guidelines make it unethical for the therapist to make contact with anyone outside the hospital without specific written consent of the client. The client was fired from the bank teller job, so working with the client's previous supervisor is not helpful and has implications for the client's future employment. This action shows poor procedural reasoning and unethical conduct, so points would be deducted for this choice.

4. C6 Provide the client with a list of foods not allowed on the low monoamine diet (LMA) diet and encourage the client to contribute to meal preparation.

Feedback: The client reviews what foods are not allowed on the LMA diet.

Outcome and Rationale: It is important for the therapist to know the foods that cause high blood pressure for clients who are on monoamine oxidase inhibitors. These medications are used for people with major depressive disorder, not for those with bipolar disorder. Encouraging the client to participate in meal planning is a useful recommendation, but the orientation to the low monoamine (LMA) diet may be confusing to the client However, this specialized diet orientation is not harmful to the client. Consequently, this action is neutral and no points would be awarded or deducted for its selection.

5. C9 Refer the client to occupational therapy services that are part of the hospital's outpatient day program.

Feedback: The client agrees to come to the day program 3 days a week and attend occupational therapy.

Outcome and Rationale: The short length of stay for acute hospitalization is intended to begin medication and symptom management, reduce severe symptoms, and evaluate the client for discharge placement. Outpatient occupational therapy intervention would follow from inpatient services and extend the client's transition to community living, whether in another facility or home. Engaging the client in therapeutic activities as an outpatient provides the occupational therapist with further opportunities to evaluate symptoms and needs, continue collaborating with the client on self-management strategies and provide feedback on performance to the interdisciplinary team. Because this action demonstrates sound clinical judgment, points would be awarded for its selection.

6. C8 Collaborate with the client to identify community activities that the client can participate in when willing and able.

Feedback: The client agrees to look for volunteer work and sign up for an adult education class in wood carving.

Outcome and Rationale: The client is expected to begin a transition from hospitalization to increasingly more independent function. This action would offer a long-term view of building tolerance for work and community involvement. During transition to discharge, the client's evaluation of community activities is central to self-management. This action lends itself to helping the client link function and volition. Because this action describes the role of occupational therapy in fostering self-management, it is a good choice for this client. Points would be awarded for selection of this action.

Multiple Choice Test Items C1–170

C1 C8

An occupational therapist conducts a home evaluation for an individual who uses a wheelchair for functional mobility. The only entrance to the home has five steps, a total of 35 inches in height. Which ramp length should the therapist recommend the family have constructed to enable accessibility to the home?

Answer Choices:
A. 17.5 feet long.
B. 35 feet long.
C. 48 feet long.
D. 70.5 feet long.

Correct Answer: B.

Rationale:
Accessibility guidelines state that the ramp should be constructed with 1 foot of ramp length for each inch of rise. The others do not meet these guidelines.

Type of Reasoning: Deductive
This question requires recall of guidelines, which is factual knowledge. Deductive reasoning skills are utilized whenever one must recall facts to find ideal solutions. In this situation, accessibility guidelines indicate that for every 1 inch of rise, there should be 1 foot of ramp. Review community accessibility guidelines if answered incorrectly.

C2 C3

An occupational therapist works with a survivor of a house fire. The client has burns on both hands that limit thumb mobility. The client identifies a personal goal of being able to pick up and hold cans to enable independent shopping and meal preparation activities. Which movement of the thumb should the goal statement include as the desired functional outcome?

Answer Choices:
A. Carpometacarpal (CMC) palmar abduction.
B. CMC extension.
C. Metacarpophalangeal (MCP) flexion.
D. Interphalangeal (IP) flexion.

Correct Answer: A.

Rationale:
CMC palmar abduction is the major movement required of the thumb to pick up cans. CMC extension places the thumb in a hitchhiking position, which makes picking up a can very difficult. MCP and IP flexion alone will not expand the web space to pick up a can.

Type of Reasoning: Analytical
This question provides a description of a functional activity and the test taker must determine the major movement that is required in performing this functional activity. This is an analytical reasoning skill, as questions of this nature often ask one to analyze functional skills to determine the overall skill involved. In this situation the functional activity is performed using CMC palmar abduction and should be the focus of the long-term goal. Review movement patterns of the thumb if answered incorrectly.

C3 C7

A person diagnosed with dementia, Alzheimer type is evaluated by an occupational therapist. Although the client demonstrates diminished memory skills, the therapist determines that the patient is still able to live at home with supportive structure. The therapist collaborates with the client to identify activities to include in a structured routine that enables the client's continued occupational performance. Which activity is best for the occupational therapist to recommend to the client?

Answer Choices:
A. Cooking dinner.
B. Doing laundry.
C. Walking with a neighbor.
D. Watching television.

Correct Answer: C.

Rationale:
Walking with a neighbor can meet the person's needs for social participation and physical exercise. This is an activity that can be safely pursued even with memory deficits. Cooking is unsafe for a person with memory deficits. Leaving the stove on due to memory loss can be a fire hazard. Doing laundry requires memory of multiple steps that would make this task difficult. While watching television is safe for a person with a cognitive deficit, it is passive activity that does not support the use of intact abilities.

Type of Reasoning: Inductive
One must utilize clinical judgment in order to determine the best activity to recommend for a client with Alzheimer's disease. This requires knowledge of the diagnosis and best activities to promote social participation and physical exercise, which necessitates inductive reasoning skill. For this situation, the occupational therapist should recommend walking with a neighbor. If answered incorrectly, review therapeutic activity guidelines for persons with Alzheimer's disease, especially activities that promote socialization and physical exercise.

C4 C6

During an intervention session, a client complains of dry mouth due to prescribed medications. What is the most effective strategy for the occupational therapist to suggest to the client to manage this side effect?

Answer Choices:

A. Suck on ice.
B. Suck on hard candies.
C. Drink iced tea.
D. Sip water.

Correct Answer: D.

Rationale:

Sipping water is the best choice to relieve dry mouth. Sucking ice and/or hard candies presents a possible choking risk. Hard candies might present a dietary risk for some clients. Iced tea contains caffeine, which can increase dehydration. Large amounts of caffeinated beverages can cause serious reactions when taken with certain medications such as monoamine oxidase inhibitors (MAOIs).

Type of Reasoning: Evaluative

This question requires one to evaluate the merits of the four possible choices and determine which will most effectively remedy the clients' symptoms. This requires evaluative reasoning skill. For this situation, sips of water is the best and the safest remedy for dry mouth. If answered incorrectly, review information on side effects of psychotropic medications and compensatory techniques.

C5 C8

An adult diagnosed with multiple sclerosis (MS) over 10 years ago experiences an exacerbation of symptoms. The individual's principle complaint is decreased strength and endurance. The person can ambulate short distances with a cane in the home and uses a wheelchair outside of the home. The client asks for suggestions to enable independent home maintenance. Which is the best positioning recommendation for the occupational therapist to suggest the person use during meal preparation?

Answer Choices:

A. Sitting in the wheelchair with a tray table.
B. Sitting at the kitchen table.
C. Leaning against the counter while standing.
D. Leaning against a tall stool while standing.

Correct Answer: B.

Rationale:

Multiple sclerosis (MS) is characterized by fluctuations in abilities. The best choice for an activity that will be performed frequently is to perform the activity in an adequately supported position. The avoidance of fatigue is important in the management of MS. Doing meal preparation while sitting at the kitchen table achieves these aims and uses the person's natural context. There is no need indicated in this scenario for the use of a wheelchair and a tray. The client can do meal preparation activities with readily available supports. Standing might require using too much energy and does not provide good support or stability for performing the fine motor aspects of meal preparation. Leaning against the counter or a stool requires more energy, and does not provide good support or stability for performing the fine motor aspects of meal preparation, and may not be safe.

Type of Reasoning: Inductive

This question requires clinical judgment to determine which position would be optimal for a client with MS given the current status and symptoms presented. For this client, sitting at the kitchen table is best as it provides the appropriate stability and reinforces the natural context during meal preparation. If answered incorrectly, review meal preparation strategies for clients with MS.

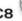

C6 C4

An occupational therapist provides occupational therapy services in a patient's room. The patient has left hemiplegia and is able to recognize the therapist after the therapist talks with the patient for a while. The patient is unable to recognize the faces of family members when they enter the room to visit. The family members become upset by this behavior. Which deficit should the therapist explain to the family members as the most likely reason for the patient's behavior?

Answer Choices:
A. Ideational apraxia.
B. Anosognosia.
C. Visual agnosia. ✓
D. Asomatognosia.

Correct Answer: C.

Rationale:
All of the choices are indicative of perceptual dysfunction. This patient is most likely experiencing visual agnosia, which is an inability to recognize familiar objects despite normal function of the eyes and optic tracts. Once the family members talk with the patient, he/she will likely be able to recognize them by their voices. Ideational apraxia is the inability to perform a purposeful motor act, either automatically or upon command. Anosognosia is the frank denial, neglect or lack of awareness of the presence or severity of one's paralysis. Asomatognosia is an impairment in body scheme.

Type of Reasoning: Analytical
In this question, one must recall the meaning of the four choices provided and apply them to the patient's symptoms described above. This requires analytical reasoning, which often requires one to determine the meaning of symptoms or deficits. For this situation, the symptoms are indicative of visual agnosia, which should be reviewed if answered incorrectly.

C7 C3

A restaurant employee incurred a fracture to the left humerus. After cast removal, the patient received occupational therapy and now demonstrates $\frac{3}{5}$ strength of the left triceps and full ROM of the left elbow. To increase elbow function in order to perform work-related tasks, which activity is most effective for the occupational therapist to next include during intervention?

Answer Choices:
A. Storing plates and glasses on shelves at chest height. ✓
B. Wiping off a table while standing.
C. Carrying a tray of dishes from the table to the sink.
D. Wiping off a counter at chest height.

Correct Answer: A.

Rationale:
Storing plates at chest height is a resistive activity against gravity, one of the best ways to increase strength in a muscle to attain full elbow ROM. Wiping the table at stomach level is an isotonic activity, gravity assisted. Carrying a tray of dishes is an isometric activity. Wiping a counter at chest height is isotonic with the effects of gravity decreased.

Type of Reasoning: Inductive
One must utilize clinical knowledge and judgment to determine the functional activity that would provide resistive activity of the triceps. In this case, storing plates and glasses on shelves at chest height is the ideal way to implement a resistive activity for the triceps. If answered incorrectly, review resistive and strengthening exercises.

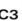

C8 C2

A home care occupational therapist seeks to enhance an elder's compliance with the occupational therapy intervention program. After discussing the goals of the program with the person, which intervention is most effective for the therapist to use?

Answer Choices:
A. Provide the individual with limited opportunities for practice of skills to decrease boredom.
B. Use multiple, variable instructions to ensure retention of new learning.
C. Integrate previously learned strategies into new activities to facilitate generalization. ✓
D. Teach family members positive techniques to reinforce activity performance in the home.

Correct Answer: C.

Rationale:
Discussion of personal goals with the individual and the utilization of familiar activities and learning strategies will increase compliance with treatment since the person has played an active part in designing his/her individualized goals and treatment program. Investment in treatment is an important factor in motivation and compliance. Providing the individual with limited practice of new skills can decrease compliance because he/she will have a smaller number of successful experiences. This can increase feelings of hopelessness. The use of new or complex learning strategies can also be frustrating and decrease the likelihood of success during the treatment session. Discussing the person's goals with his/her family members and providing them with methods of positive reinforcement can be helpful but this can only be done with the individual's permission. Additionally, this does not directly address the individual who is the person that the therapist needs to engage.

Type of Reasoning: Inferential
One must determine the most appropriate method for enhancing compliance with a treatment program, given the information provided. This requires inferential reasoning skill, where one must infer or draw conclusions about a best course of action. In this situation, the therapist should discuss the goals of the program with the person and utilize previously learned strategies for retention of new material. If answered incorrectly, review and reflect on approaches to increase compliance with therapy programs.

C9 C3

In measuring the ROM of a client's elbow, the occupational therapist records a flexion measurement of 145°. Which is most accurate for the therapist to document based on this measurement?

Answer Choices:
A. Hypomobility.
B. Dysfunctional elbow ROM.
C. Hypermobility.
D. Normal elbow ROM. ✓

Correct Answer: D.

Rationale:
Normal elbow ROM is zero degrees to 135°–150°. Individual variation in the end range of elbow flexion is normal due to differences in muscle mass of the biceps and the forearm as they meet at the end range. Having 145° of flexion is normal. ROM outside of these parameters would be atypical. Hypermobility would be evident if the person extended the elbow beyond zero and hypomobility would be indicated if the person could not flex within the normal range.

Type of Reasoning: Analytical
This question provides a functional description and the test taker must determine the likely indicator of the description. This is an analytical reasoning skill, as questions of this nature often ask one to analyze a group of symptoms or functional indicators in order to determine a diagnosis or outcome. In this situation the description indicates typical ROM of the elbow, which should be reviewed if answered incorrectly.

C10 C8

An individual is 5'11" and is of average weight for this height. Following a recent traumatic brain injury (TBI), the person has flaccid hemiparesis and demonstrates poor righting and equilibrium responses in standing. Which wheelchair is best for the occupational therapist to recommend for this client?

Answer Choices:
A. A power wheelchair.
B. A light weight, standard size wheelchair. ✓
C. A reclining, hemi-height wheelchair.
D. A one-arm drive, standard size wheelchair. TBI

Correct Answer: B.

Rationale:
A standard size and lightweight wheelchair is the best one for this individual. It is light and therefore easy to push. It is the best size, given the person's height. The client is too tall for a hemi-height wheelchair whose seat is lower to the ground to allow for propulsion with one's lower extremities. Power wheelchairs are used for persons with significant functional deficits that preclude the ability to propel a manual wheelchair, for example, an individual with quadriparesis/quadriplegia. One-arm-drive wheelchairs are difficult to learn to use effectively. This difficulty may be exacerbated by the residual deficits of the client's recent TBI.

Type of Reasoning: Inductive
One must utilize clinical knowledge and judgment to determine the wheelchair that is most appropriate for the described individual. This requires inductive reasoning skill. In this case, a light weight, standard size wheelchair is most appropriate. If answered incorrectly, review wheelchair prescription guidelines, especially for the deficits described in this scenario.

C11 C5

An individual with a C3 spinal cord injury is participating in a community mobility group at a shopping mall. The client expresses the desire to return to the rehabilitation center due to a pounding headache. The occupational therapist notices the client is sweating profusely. Which is the best initial action for the therapist to take in response to this observation and request?

Answer Choices:
A. Check the client's urinary catheter and collecting bag. ✓
B. Call the rehabilitation center's transportation department to relay the client's request.
C. Escort the client to outside of the mall to cool off in the fresh air.
D. Immediately activate the recline feature of the patient's tilt-in-space wheelchair.

Correct Answer: A.

Rationale:
Profuse sweating and headaches are signs of autonomic dysreflexia. This is an extreme rise in blood pressure caused by a noxious stimulus, which must be treated immediately by removing the stimulus. A blocked catheter and overfilled urine bag are common precipitants to this complication and could result in a medical emergency in persons with a spinal cord injury. Other common stimuli include sitting on sharp objects, a tight abdominal binder, pressure stockings that have rolled down or excess pressure on the buttocks. The patient should be placed in an upright position to help manage the rise in blood pressure.

Type of Reasoning: Evaluative
One must weigh the possible courses of action and then make a value judgment about the best course to take. This requires evaluative reasoning skill, where an understanding of what the symptoms indicate is pivotal to arriving at a correct conclusion. For this case, the symptoms indicate autonomic dysreflexia and the therapist's first action should be to check the catheter line to remove the noxious stimulus causing the dangerous rise in blood pressure. If answered incorrectly, review symptoms of autonomic dysreflexia.

C12 C4

An occupational therapist works with an individual recovering from traumatic brain injury who demonstrates behaviors consistent with Level VII of the Rancho Level of Cognitive Functioning Scale. The client is a resident in a transitional living program. Which is the most important focus for the therapist to include in the client's intervention plan?

Answer Choices:
A. The provision of a high degree of environmental structure to decrease confusion and ensure safety.
B. The development of strategies to accurately and safely complete IADL with minimal assistance.
C. The development of adaptive techniques to accurately and safely complete BADL with moderate assistance.
D. The provision of maximum assistance to accurately and safely complete IADL.

Correct Answer: B.

Rationale:
A person at Level VII of the Rancho Level of Cognitive Functioning Scale is able to appropriately complete highly familiar tasks such as BADL with minimal assistance. At this level, the person can learn to use strategies to accurately and safely complete IADL with minimal assistance.

Type of Reasoning: Inductive
While this question does require one to recall the Rancho Level of Cognitive Functioning Scale and the guidelines for treatment provided within these levels, one must utilize inductive reasoning skill to determine the most important focus for intervention within the individual's current abilities and limitations. This necessitates clinical judgment, which is an inductive reasoning skill. For this case, the therapist should focus on the development of strategies to accurately and safely complete IADL with minimal assistance. Refer to the Rancho Level of Cognitive Functioning Scale if answered incorrectly.

C13 C8

An occupational therapist who is a driver rehabilitation specialist provides on-the-road evaluation for an individual recovering from a right cerebrovascular accident (CVA). The individual is right dominant and has regained sensorimotor functions in the affected extremity. Which is most important for the therapist to assess during the on-the-road evaluation?

Answer Choices:
A. Tactical aspects of driving.
B. Operational aspects of driving.
C. Ergonomic aspects of driving.
D. Social aspects of driving.

Correct Answer: A.

Rationale:
The tactical aspects of driving involve the ability to respond to changes in road conditions and traffic/driving risks. Therefore, intact cognitive skills are necessary. Since a CVA can result in residual cognitive deficits, the therapist must assess these abilities in an on-the-road evaluation. Clinical assessments may not provide the real-life challenges to cognitive abilities that typically occur while driving. Operational aspects of driving involve the ability to steer, brake and turn. Since the person in this scenario has intact dominant upper and lower extremities and functional return on his/her affected side, there is no reason to assess his/her physical driving abilities or the ergonomic aspects of driving. The social aspects of driving are not an evaluation focus in driver rehabilitation.

Type of Reasoning: Inferential
One must infer or draw conclusions about a likely course of action, given the information presented. This is an inferential reasoning skill, where knowledge of a therapeutic approach, such as the on-the-road driver evaluation in this situation, is essential to choosing a correct solution. In this case, it is most important for the therapist to assess tactical aspects of driving. Review the driver rehabilitation assessment guidelines if answered incorrectly.

C14 C3

An occupational therapist evaluates a person who complains of persistent wrist pain after painting a house three weeks ago. The patient demonstrates signs and symptoms consistent with de Quervain's tenosynovitis. Which assessment measure should the therapist use to confirm the diagnosis?

Answer Choices:
A. Finkelstein's test.
B. Phalen's test.
C. Froment's sign.
D. Craig's test.

Correct Answer: A.

Rationale:
Finkelstein's test is specific for reproducing the pain associated with de Quervain's tenosynovitis of the abductor pollicis longus and extensor pollicis brevis. Froment's sign is used to identify ulnar nerve dysfunction. Phalen's test identifies median nerve compression in the carpal tunnel. Craig's test is used by physical therapists to identify an abnormal femoral antetorsion angle.

Type of Reasoning: Deductive
This question requires factual recall of knowledge of provocative tests for de Quervain's tenosynovitis. In this case, the appropriate test is Finkelstein's test, which reproduces the pain of the abductor pollicis longus (APL) and extensor pollicis brevis (EPB) tendons associated with de Quervain's. Refer to provocative testing of the hand or wrist and de Quervain's tenosynovitis if answered incorrectly.

C15 C7

During an occupational therapy group, a person receiving electroconvulsive therapy (ECT) treatments complains about short-term memory loss. Which should the therapist do in response to the client's stated concerns?

Answer Choices:

A. Provide cues during activities to compensate for memory loss.
B. Immediately contact the psychiatrist to inform him/her of this symptom development.
C. Tell the person to inform the psychiatrist of this symptom development.
D. Reassure the person that short-term memory loss is a typical response to ECT.

Correct Answer: A.

Rationale:
Short-term memory loss is typical after ECT; therefore, there is no need to inform the psychiatrist. However, reassuring the person that this loss is typical does not address the problem at hand. Providing cues can effectively help the individual deal with this memory loss and allow effective engagement in meaningful activities.

Type of Reasoning: Inductive
This question requires one to determine the best approach for assisting a person who is dealing with short-term memory loss after ECT. This requires inductive reasoning skill, where clinical judgment is paramount in arriving at a correct conclusion. For this situation, the therapist should provide cues during activities to compensate for the loss. If answered incorrectly, review effects of ECT treatment on cognitive functioning.

C16 C1

An ambulatory elder adult with hemiparesis and presbycusis is moving in with an adult child's family. The family hires an occupational therapist to provide information to help them maintain the elder's functional ability in the home. Which should the occupational therapist recommend?

Answer Choices:

A. Remove knobs from the stove when the elder is home alone.
B. Speak directly, clearly and slowly to the elder.
C. Add bright color strips to the edge of each stair tread.
D. Provide lists of the sequence of routine tasks.

Correct Answer: B.

Rationale:
Presbycusis is an age-related sensorineural loss that results in decreased hearing. Speaking directly, clearly and slowly can help ensure that the elder hears what the family is saying. This will enable the elder to participate fully in family interactions. There is nothing in the situation to indicate the need for any of the other suggestions, as no cognitive or visual deficits are noted.

Type of Reasoning: Inferential
One must have knowledge of presbycusis and presenting symptoms in order to determine the best recommendation for this situation. This is an inferential reasoning skill where knowledge of clinical guidelines and judgment based on facts are utilized to reach conclusions. In this situation, the OT should recommend speaking directly, clearly and slowly to the elder. If answered incorrectly, review presbycusis and intervention approaches.

Exam C

C17 C8

An occupational therapist provides caregiver education to the spouse of a client with Alzheimer's disease and a secondary diagnosis of left CVA. The client is dependent upon a wheelchair for mobility and has been deemed cognitively incompetent. The spouse reports that the client becomes restless at meal times, consistently undoes the lap belt, and tries to get up from the wheelchair. The spouse reports that the need to constantly say "sit down" is personally exhausting and often increases the client's agitation. Frequently, neither one eats dinner. Which is the most effective recommendation for the therapist to make to the spouse?

Answer Choices:

A. Allow the spouse to get up when restless and provide dinner to the client at a later time.
B. Use a wheelchair lap tray to serve several smaller meals to the client at intervals throughout the day.
C. Hire a home care attendant to assist the client at meal times and provide some respite to the spouse.
D. Use a wheelchair lap tray to serve the client large meals at breakfast, lunch and dinner.

Correct Answer: B.

Rationale:

The client must be considered at risk for falling if he/she is allowed to get up because a person deemed dependent upon a wheelchair for mobility has significant motor deficits. A lap tray is a permissible and reasonable restraint if it is necessary to maintain a person's safety, if it allows for increased function and if less restrictive restraints have been attempted. A family member can approve the use of this device if a person is not cognitively intact. These criteria apply to this case. A lap belt has been applied but it has not been successful. A lap tray with food on it can provide physical and sensory cues necessary to keep the client seated for a time that is sufficient for eating a small meal. It is advisable to provide small meals at frequent intervals rather than three large meals when a person has significant cognitive impairments. Hiring a home care attendant can relieve the spouse's caregiver stress, but it does not address the client's risk of falling when attempting to get up from the wheelchair. It is unlikely that this behavior would cease for a home care attendant.

Type of Reasoning: Inductive

Clinical knowledge and judgment are the most important skills needed for answering this question, which requires inductive reasoning skill. Knowledge of the diagnosis and most appropriate recommendations is essential to choosing the best solution. In this case, recommending use of a lap tray to serve several smaller meals throughout the day is most appropriate. If answered incorrectly, review treatment guidelines for persons with Alzheimer's disease and principles of fall prevention and restraint reduction.

C18 C8

During a topical work preparation group for individuals recovering from mental illness, a member expresses concern about answering questions related to personal psychiatric history during a job interview. Which action is best for the occupational therapist to take in response to these expressed concerns?

Answer Choices:

A. Refer the client to a vocational rehabilitation counselor.
B. Encourage the other members of the group to share their interview experiences.
C. Lead a group discussion on the legal rights afforded in the interview process.
D. Support the client in not disclosing past psychiatric history.

Correct Answer: C.

Rationale:
A primary purpose of a topical group is to develop knowledge about a particular area of performance. Since members of the group may not be aware of all of their legal rights in an interview, it is most important for the occupational therapist to lead a discussion about this issue. Americans with Disabilities Act (ADA) protections concerning the disclosure of medical histories are invaluable for all members to know. This knowledge can help the individual make an informed decision about disclosure. For example, if the person can perform the essential functions of a job, there is no compelling reason to disclose a past medical history. There is no need to refer the individual to a vocational rehabilitation counselor as this area is within the OT's domain of practice. While encouraging members to share experiences and supporting a client's decision are both relevant, it is more important for the occupational therapist to share information about ADA.

Type of Reasoning: Evaluative
This question requires a value judgment, which is an evaluative reasoning skill. Having an understanding of the ADA, the test taker should conclude that the best response in this situation is to discuss the legal rights afforded in the interview process with the group members. Review ADA regulations related to job interviewing if answered incorrectly.

C19 C3

A carpenter incurred a short below-elbow amputation. The client plans to return to work. Which components would be most important for the occupational therapist to recommend for the client's prosthesis?

Answer Choices:
A. A fixed-elbow socket and a lightweight Teflon-coated terminal device.
B. A cable-driven elbow socket and a heavy-duty serrated grid terminal device.
C. A fixed-elbow socket and a heavy-duty serrated grip terminal device.
D. A cable-driven elbow socket and lightweight Teflon-coated terminal device.

Correct Answer: C.

Rationale:
An individual with a short below-elbow amputation will require a fixed-elbow socket to provide stability because natural forearm rotation is not possible. A carpenter will need a heavy-duty serrated grid terminal device to hold tools and nails.

Type of Reasoning: Inferential
One must link the individual's diagnosis to the prostheses presented in order to determine which prosthesis would best meet the individual's needs. This requires inferential reasoning, where one must draw conclusions about the likely needs of an individual based on an understanding of the carpenter's occupation. In this case a fixed-elbow socket and heavy-duty serrated grip terminal device would best meet the carpenter's needs. Review prosthetic options and features for below-elbow amputations if answered incorrectly.

C20 **C6**

An individual with schizophrenia continues to experience hallucinations. Which action should the occupational therapist take when the individual begins to actively hallucinate during an occupational therapist project group?

Answer Choices:
A. Redirect the individual's attention back to the project. ✓
B. Provide tactile reassurance to the individual.
C. Verbally reassure the individual that the hallucination is not real.
D. Use humor to divert the individual's attention away from the hallucination.

Correct Answer: A.

Rationale:
The best action to take when a person is experiencing a hallucination is to redirect attention back to the project in which the person has been engaged using a calm, matter-of-fact tone. This can help the person focus on reality. It can also be helpful to reinforce any misinterpretations of environmental noises and events, since hallucinations often result from faulty interpretations of external stimuli. Explaining that a hallucination is not real and/or trying to minimize the stress caused by a hallucinatory experience would not be effective, since by definition hallucinations are real sensory experiences to the person. Entering into a dialogue about these experiences could lead to arguing about their reality, which would be counterproductive. Uninvited touch can be inappropriate in some cultures and can be threatening during hallucinations. The other choices are ineffective ways to reinforce reality for the client who is hallucinating.

Type of Reasoning: Inductive
One must determine a best course of action through clinical judgment, based on the information provided, which is an inductive reasoning skill. For this situation, the question inquires about the best way to help a patient who is actively hallucinating. The best response would be to redirect the individual back to the activity at hand. If answered incorrectly, review information on schizophrenia and management of hallucinations.

C21 **C8**

A fifth-grade student is having difficulty self-feeding and frequently spills beverages. The student has non-spastic cerebral palsy resulting in fluctuating muscle tone and poor motor control. Which is best for the occupational therapist to recommend the student use to improve independence in self-feeding and minimize spillage?

Answer Choices:
A. A sippy cup ✗
B. Both hands to hold the cup ✗
C. A cup with a handle. ✗
D. A straw. ✓

Correct Answer: D

Rationale:
Using a straw to drink from a cup is an easy and age-appropriate adaptation to prevent spills. A sippy cup is developmentally inappropriate for a fifth-grader and should only be used if there is no age-appropriate alternative. Fluctuating muscle tone will result in the muscles relaxing and contracting involuntarily and make purposeful movements difficult to control. Using both hands to hold a cup or using a cup with a handle may not prevent spills secondary to the child's fluctuating muscle tone.

Type of Reasoning: Inductive
For this question, the test taker must utilize clinical judgment to determine the best feeding recommendation for a child with cerebral palsy. This requires knowledge of the diagnosis and adaptive methods in order to arrive at a correct conclusion. In this situation, it is best to recommend that the child use a straw, which will reduce the likelihood of spilling liquids when drinking. Review feeding strategies for children with cerebral palsy if answered incorrectly.

C22 C6

An entry-level occupational therapist implements a therapeutic feeding program in a skilled nursing facility. During a therapeutic feeding session, a 97-year-old resident with dementia, non-Alzheimer's type, becomes upset and cries for his/her mother. Which should the therapist say in response to the resident's statements?

Answer Choices:
A. "Remember that you are now in a nursing home and your mother is not here."
B. "You must miss your mother, tell me about her."
C. "Remember your mother passed away years ago."
D. "I will tell the nurse that you want your mother contacted."

Correct Answer: B.

Rationale:
This response validates the person's feelings and provides him/her with the opportunity to reminisce about a pleasant memory. Even a few minutes of reminiscing can provide solace to the individual, which can help calm him/her. This can then enable the resident to reengage in the feeding activity. Individuals with dementia generally respond well to validation therapy and reminiscence activities. Asking the individual to recall that his/her mother is deceased and/or not available is inappropriate for they are asking the resident to remember something that is no longer part of his/her reality. Telling the person that that there is a potential for his/her mother to be contacted is offering an action that cannot be completed in reality. In addition, it does not address the individual's valid feelings which need to be addressed at the moment.

Type of Reasoning: Evaluative
This question requires professional judgment based on guiding principles, which is an evaluative reasoning skill. Most important in this situation is to validate the person's feelings. This way the therapist can provide an opportunity to reminisce without asking the person to recall something that is not part of his/her reality. Review validation strategies for persons with dementia if answered incorrectly.

C23 C4

A client has a 3-year history of multiple sclerosis. One of the client's disabling symptoms is a persistent and severe diplopia, which leaves the client frequently nauseated and unable to complete desired activities. Which adaptive strategy is most effective for the occupational therapist to recommend the client use during BADL and IADL?

Answer Choices:
A. Wear magnifying glasses.
B. Wear prism glasses.
C. Wear shaded glasses.
D. Wear an eye patch on one eye.

Correct Answer: D.

Rationale:
Double vision (diplopia) can be managed by patching one eye. Patients are typically on an eye-patching schedule that alternates the eye that is patched. Loss of depth perception can be expected with eye patching but is not as disabling as diplopia. The other options do not correct diplopia.

Type of Reasoning: Inferential
The test taker must infer or draw conclusions about how the four possible treatment options will be the best remedy for diplopia. This requires knowledge of the condition of diplopia and how eye patching is the most effective choice for remedying the condition, which is an inferential reasoning skill. For this case, the therapist should recommend that the client wear an eye patch. Review information about treatment of diplopia if answered incorrectly.

Multiple Choice Scenario Item C.I.

Questions C24 to C28 are based on the following information.

A young adult recently diagnosed with depression and anorexia nervosa is a consumer of services at a psychosocial clubhouse. The client attends individual OT sessions once a week and several evening and weekend groups. When completing an activities schedule and questionnaire, the client identifies the clubhouse groups and part-time work as an editorial assistant as the only activities completed each week. In high school the client was captain of the swim team, played tennis and worked in an after-school activities program for young children.

C24 C6

The client attends a goal-setting group for persons with depression. Which is the most helpful approach for the occupational therapist leading this group to take with the group members?

Answer Choices:
A. Encourage the members to discuss long-range planning.
B. Say as little as possible to allow the members to do most of the talking.
C. Remain cheerful and upbeat to alleviate the members' depression.
D. Facilitate reality-testing of the members' negative thinking.

Correct Answer: D.

Rationale:
People with depression often interpret events and the behaviors of themselves and others with unfounded or exaggerated negativity. Developing the members' ability to test and correct negative thinking is an important precursor to developing the ability to set goals. Long-range planning is limited when an individual is initially adjusting to a new diagnosis. In addition, persons with depression often have difficulty with this ability. Persons with depression may also have difficulty independently initiating conversation. Cheerful, upbeat behavior may be offensive as it can highlight the members' depressed mood and appear to minimize the group members' affective state. This can bring the therapist's empathy into question.

Type of Reasoning: Inferential
One must determine the most helpful intervention approach for individuals with major depression. This requires inferential reasoning skill, where one must draw conclusions based on the information presented. In this situation, the therapist should facilitate reality testing of negative thinking. If answered incorrectly, review group treatment guidelines for individuals with major depression.

C25 C2

During an individual session with the occupational therapist, the client states, "I don't know what I want to work on. I don't really know what my goals are." Which is the most appropriate action for the occupational therapist to take?

Answer Choices:

A. Defer the development of an intervention plan until the individual has determined personal goals.
B. Establish a short-term goal related to improving the individual's goal-setting skills.
C. Initiate a discussion with the individual about what is personally important.
D. Contact the individual's psychiatrist to request a medication evaluation.

Correct Answer: C.

Rationale:

It is best for the therapist to engage the person in the goal-setting process by exploring personal values and priorities. This answer choice is client-centered, employs therapeutic use of self, and incorporates patient's rights. It is also helpful for the establishment of rapport with the individual. Deferring the development of an intervention plan does not provide the client with the opportunity to participate in this planning process nor does it provide the opportunity to facilitate the ability to articulate personal preferences. Setting up a short-term goal to improve goal-setting skills without the input of the individual is vague and would not contribute to a client-directed intervention plan. This is a violation of the ethical principle of autonomy. There is nothing in the scenario to indicate the need for a medication evaluation.

Type of Reasoning: Evaluative

One must determine which of the four possible courses of action will best establish a therapeutic rapport and incorporate the patient's rights. This requires evaluative reasoning, where the test taker must determine which course of action is most valuable and effective. In this situation, the therapist should initiate discussion about what the client finds important. If answered incorrectly, review information on client-centered treatment planning.

C26 C8

The client expresses interest in the pursuit of additional activities outside of the clubhouse and work. Which is the most appropriate avocational resource for the therapist to recommend that the client explore?

Answer Choices:

A. A local fitness center for exercise classes.
B. The town swimming pool for open swimming sessions.
C. The area soup kitchen for volunteer opportunities.
D. A local community center for volunteer opportunities.

Correct Answer: D.

Rationale:

This suggestion can support the client's altruistic interests while providing a diversity of potential activity pursuits. Exercise and swimming can be contraindicated for persons with anorexia nervosa because they often engage in these activities in an excessive (sometimes self-abusive) manner that is counterproductive to healthy leisure. Volunteering in a soup kitchen is altruistic but persons recovering from eating disorders often find food-related activities difficult

Exam C

Type of Reasoning: Inductive

One must utilize clinical knowledge and judgment to determine the most appropriate avocational resource for this patient. In this case, given an understanding of the nature of anorexia, the therapist should consider the local community center for volunteer opportunities. If answered incorrectly, review the diagnostic criteria and behavioral manifestations of eating disorders and depression and intervention guidelines for avocational activities. The integration of this knowledge is required to correctly answer this question.

C27 C8

During the clubhouse vocational support group, the client reports difficulty keeping track of the job tasks that need to be completed each day. Which is the most appropriate recommendation for the occupational therapist to make to the client?

Answer Choices:

A. Write down directions for each task that needs to be completed.
B. Keep a daily log of completed tasks.
C. Develop and use a checklist of tasks to be completed each day. ✓
D. Ask the work supervisor to provide verbal cues through the workday.

Correct Answer: C.

Rationale:

Developing a daily 'to do' checklist provides a clear visual cue of what needs to be accomplished. The client can check off each job task as he/she completes it and immediately see what job tasks must still be accomplished. This can provide the needed organizational structure to complete all job tasks each day. There is nothing in the scenario to indicate that the person does not know how to perform his/her job tasks; therefore, there is no need for the person to write down directions for each task. Keeping a log of each completed job task will help the person to know what has been accomplished, but it provides no organizational cue regarding what remains to be done. There is nothing in the scenario to indicate that the person cannot independently perform his/her daily work tasks; therefore, there is no need for the supervisor's cueing.

Type of Reasoning: Inductive

This question requires one to determine the best approach for assisting a client in keeping track of job tasks. This requires inductive reasoning skill, where clinical judgment is paramount to arriving at a correct conclusion. For this case, the therapist's most appropriate recommendation is to develop and use a checklist of tasks to be completed each day. If answered incorrectly, one should review vocational training guidelines, especially organizational behaviors and compensatory strategies.

C28 C2

The clubhouse members attain a level of cohesion which enables them to perform at a cooperative level. Two members of a community integration group disagree with the others on the details of a group project. How should the occupational therapist leading this group respond to this conflict?

Answer Choices:

A. Clarify all viewpoints and facilitate the members in decision making.
B. Listen to all viewpoints and suggest that members vote to determine the project details.
C. Mediate only when the members have reached a deadlocked situation. ✗
D. Encourage the members to explore alternative methods to resolve the conflict. ✓

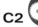

Correct Answer: D.

Rationale:
In a cooperative group, the therapist acts as an advisor. Group members are mutually responsible for giving feedback and meeting group needs. The therapist's interventions should facilitate group problem solving rather than direct the course of actions or decisions. Waiting until a group is deadlocked would not be beneficial to group cohesion.

Type of Reasoning: Evaluative
One must weigh the merits of the courses of action in order to arrive at a correct conclusion. This requires evaluative reasoning skill, where judgment based on values and principles is paramount to choosing the best solution. In this situation, where two members disagree in a cooperative level group, the therapist should encourage the members to explore alternative methods to resolve the conflict. Review cooperative group guidelines if answered incorrectly.

C29 C9

An occupational therapist wants to develop an after-school program for obese adolescents who have diabetes or who are at risk for developing diabetes. Which program development action should the therapist take first?

Answer Choices:
A. Obtain statistical data about adolescent obesity to support the need for the program to the school administrators.
B. Survey the adolescents about their occupational performance to determine program focus.
C. Survey OT practitioners about services they provide to obese adolescents to determine program focus.
D. Review the professional literature to obtain ideas for activities to include in the program.

Correct Answer: B.

Rationale:
The development of new services would require a needs assessment to determine the necessity and focus of services. The information obtained from surveying potential participants is an excellent way to ensure that the program developed will meet a real unmet need. While statistics can support the rationale for a program, specific information about the target population is more relevant. In addition, prior to marketing a program, one should first determine its focus. Practitioner viewpoints and professional literature do not substantiate an unmet need that would require a program to be developed.

Type of Reasoning: Inferential
This question requires one to utilize knowledge of program development guidelines in order to determine the first approach for development of a program. This requires one to reason which action will have the most effective outcome, which is an inferential reasoning skill. For this situation, the occupational therapist should survey the adolescents about their occupational performance in order to determine the adolescents' needs. This will ensure that the program's focus is relevant to the targeted population. If answered incorrectly, review program development guidelines.

C30 C5

An older adult is referred to occupational therapy for intervention to develop independence in the performance of activities of daily living. During a dressing session, the occupational therapist notices a persistent area of redness over the sacrum that is still evident after the patient has been upright for 30 minutes. The client reports the area is itchy. Based on this observation, which of the following is most accurate for the therapist to document as needing attention in a revised intervention plan?

Answer Choices:
A. A stage I pressure ulcer. ✓
B. A stage II pressure ulcer.
C. A stage III pressure ulcer.
D. A stage IV pressure ulcer.

Correct Answer: A.

Rationale:
A stage I pressure ulcer is characterized by a defined area of persistent redness. Skin is intact with visible, non-blanchable redness over a localized area, typically over a bony prominence (the sacrum in this example). Additional changes include alterations in skin temperature (warmth or coolness), tissue consistency (firm or soft) and sensation (pain, itching). A stage II ulcer involves the dermis with partial thickness loss which presents as a shallow open ulcer that can be shiny or dry. A stage II ulcer can also present as a blister that is intact or open/ruptured. The wound bed is a red pink color without slough or bruising. Stages I and II are considered partial thickness ulcers. A stage III pressure ulcer involves full thickness tissue loss with subcutaneous fat possibly visible. The depth of tissue loss is not obscured if slough (i.e., dead matter/necrotic tissue) is present. Bone, tendon or muscle are not exposed or directly palpable. Stage IV involves full thickness tissue loss with bone, tendon or muscle visible or directly palpable. Osteomyelitis is possible if stage IV ulcers extend into muscle, fascia, tendon and/or the joint capsule. While nursing staff in medical model settings typically assume the responsibility for skin and risk assessments, OT practitioners can (and should) contribute to this process. OT intervention plans should be written to address concerns related to the maintenance of skin integrity. Prevention is the most effective intervention. Effective techniques include the use of wheelchair cushions, flotation pads and pressure-relief bed aids to distribute pressure over a larger skin surface and the training of the individual and/or caregivers in positioning and weight-shifting techniques and schedules and in proper skin care.

Type of Reasoning: Analytical
This question provides a description of a condition and the test taker must determine what the symptoms indicate. This is an analytical reasoning skill. For this case, the symptoms described indicate a stage I pressure ulcer. Review pressure ulcer stages, especially stage I, if answered incorrectly.

C31 C2

An occupational therapist conducts a caregiver education workshop on positioning techniques for family caregivers. At the conclusion of the class, the caregivers will be expected to utilize the skills taught. Which is the most effective method for the therapist to use when teaching these techniques?

Answer Choices:
A. Therapist demonstration of general techniques followed by individualized discussion with each caregiver.
B. An oral multimedia presentation including PowerPoint slides and handouts of positioning techniques for diverse disorders.
C. Therapist demonstration of techniques followed by a lab with caregivers practicing positioning on each other. ✓
D. A question and answer session to address the specific individual positioning concerns of the caregivers.

Correct Answer: C.

Rationale:
A variety of teaching methods including demonstration, practice and discussion has the best chance of reinforcing learning in a diverse group. Using only oral teaching methods will not likely enable the participants to develop the needed positioning skills. Psychomotor skills are best learned by practice, not lecture or question and answer. Feedback should include both knowledge of performance and knowledge of results.

Type of Reasoning: Inferential

One must infer to draw a conclusion about the best approach for educating a group of individuals. Because the group may have differing needs and abilities in learning information, one must provide a variety of approaches to delivering the information. Inferential reasoning requires one to use knowledge of therapeutic approaches to determine which approach will result in the most effective outcome. For this case, demonstration of the techniques by the therapist and the caregivers practicing the techniques on each other is most effective. Review principles of teaching and caregiver education if answered incorrectly.

C32 C3

A patient is recovering from a right total hip replacement (posterolateral incision, cementless fixation). Which is the best type of bed-to-wheelchair transfer for the occupational therapist to teach the patient to use?

Answer Choices:

A. Stand-pivot transfer to the surgical side.
B. Stand-pivot transfer to the non-surgical side.
C. Lateral slide transfer using a transfer board.
D. Squat-pivot transfer to the surgical side.

Correct Answer: B.

Rationale:

During initial healing, it is important to protect the hip from dislocation or subluxation of the prosthesis. With a posterolateral incision, excessive hip flexion, internal rotation and adduction past neutral are contraindicated. This is minimized by transferring to the non-surgical side. Full ROM of the operated hip is also contraindicated.

Type of Reasoning: Deductive

This question requires one to recall posterolateral hip precautions and the guidelines for bed-to-wheelchair transfers of patients with total hip replacements in order to arrive at a correct conclusion. The recall of factual guidelines and information necessitates deductive reasoning skill. For this case, the therapist should perform a stand-pivot transfer to the non-surgical side. Review guidelines for transferring patients with hip replacements if answered incorrectly.

C33 C9

An occupational therapy assistant (OTA) employed in a work-hardening program in a rehabilitation facility demonstrates limited skills when evaluating clients' body mechanics. The OTA demonstrates excellent skills in other areas of evaluation and intervention. In the OTA's initial performance appraisal, which is best for the supervising occupational therapist to suggest to the OTA?

Answer Choices:

A. The development of a plan of action to acquire service competence in the evaluation of body mechanics.
B. Assignment to another area of OT service delivery until service competence in the evaluation of body mechanics is established.
C. The completion of evaluations of clients' body mechanics under routine supervision of an occupational therapist experienced in the evaluation of body mechanics.
D. The completion of a continuing education course in body mechanics to increase knowledge about this area of practice.

Correct Answer: A.

Rationale:
In order to complete an evaluation, an OTA must demonstrate service competence in each area of evaluation and for each evaluation tool. Therefore, the best option is for the OTA to work out a plan to develop service competence in the assessment of body mechanics. There is no need to assign the OTA to another area of OT service delivery as long as the services the OTA is providing are under the supervision of an occupational therapist. An OTA without established service competence cannot evaluate under routine supervision since this level of supervision involves limited direct contact between the supervisor and supervisee. A continuing education course can help increase knowledge, but it does not ensure competence in the actual performance of an evaluation.

Type of Reasoning: Evaluative
This question requires one to weigh the merits of each of the possible courses of action in order to determine a best solution. This requires evaluative reasoning skill, where the value of principles and guidelines are used to choose a best solution. For this case, developing a plan of action with an experienced occupational therapist to improve skills in evaluating body mechanics is the best choice. If answered incorrectly, review standards for OTA supervision and service competence.

C34 C6

An occupational therapist leads an outpatient wellness program. An individual with obsessive-compulsive disorder asks for suggestions to manage symptoms that are interfering with life satisfaction. Which is the most beneficial recommendation for the therapist to make to the individual?

Answer Choices:
A. Approach activities in a nonchalant manner without high expectations.
B. Engage in concrete activities that can be broken down into simple steps.
C. Redirect thoughts and energies into meaningful activities.
D. Set limits on the number of activities done in a day.

Correct Answer: C.

Rationale:
The focus of OT in a wellness program is to help individuals attain and maintain life satisfaction through the engagement in meaningful activities. Individuals with obsessive-compulsive disorder have recurring and persistent thoughts (obsessions) and the need to engage in repetitious or ritualistic behaviors (compulsions) that interfere with functional activities; therefore, redirecting thoughts and energy into meaningful activities can be an effective behavior management strategy. Approaching activities in a nonchalant manner without high expectations and limiting the number of activities performed during a day would not address the person's need to refocus thoughts and behaviors away from his/her obsessions and compulsions. Engaging in activities that can be broken down into simple steps is helpful for persons with cognitive deficits. Individuals with obsessive-compulsive disorders typically do not have cognitive deficits.

Type of Reasoning: Inductive
This question requires one to determine the most appropriate recommendation for a person with obsessive-compulsive disorder. This requires inductive reasoning skill, where clinical judgment is paramount to arriving at a correct conclusion. For this situation, the therapist should suggest redirecting thoughts and energies into meaningful occupations. If answered incorrectly, review treatment guidelines for persons with obsessive-compulsive disorder.

C35 C8

A high school senior with Friedreich's ataxia is working on developing keyboarding skills in a school-to-work transition program. While assessing the student's capabilities for computer keyboarding, the occupational therapist observes signs of dysmetria. Which is the most appropriate adaptation for the occupational therapist to recommend to increase the effectiveness of the student's keyboarding skills?

Answer Choices:
A. An eye-gaze input system.
B. A key guard overlay.
C. A voice-activated input system.
D. A reduced size keyboard.

Correct Answer: B.

Rationale:
Dysmetria is the overshooting (hypermetria) or the undershooting (hypometria) of a target. It would be observed during a keyboarding activity as frequent misses of the desired key, either hitting keys above, below or next to the targeted key. A key guard overlay provides raised separations between each key. This enables the individual to place his/her finger into the desired key space and prevents the person's finger from "jumping" to keys above, below or next to the targeted key. An individual with Friedreich's ataxia has poor coordination of all muscles, including ocular muscles rendering an eye-gaze input system ineffective. Dysarthria is also characteristic of Friedreich's ataxia, which limits the efficacy of a voice-activated system. A reduced size keyboard has smaller keys and controls. It is indicated for a person with decreased ROM and good fine motor skills.

Type of Reasoning: Inferential
One must have knowledge of Friedreich's ataxia and typical deficits in order to choose the best adaptation for keyboarding skills. This is an inferential reasoning skill where one must infer or draw conclusions based on information presented. If answered incorrectly, review characteristics of Friedreich's ataxia and keyboarding adaptations for persons with mobility impairments. The integration of this knowledge is required to determine a correct answer.

C36 C4

An occupational therapist works with a patient who incurred a right CVA. The patient has homonymous hemianopsia. Which is the most effective compensatory strategy for the therapist to use initially with this patient?

Answer Choices:
A. Teach the patient to turn the head to the affected left side.
B. Provide printed notes on the left side telling the patient to look to the left.
C. Place the patient's plate and eating utensils on the left side of the bed tray.
D. Rearrange the patient's room so while the patient is in bed the left side is facing the doorway.

Correct Answer: A.

Rationale:
Homonymous hemianopsia results in the loss of ½ of the visual field in each eye (nasal half of one eye and temporal half of other eye) which corresponds to the side of the sensorimotor deficit incurred by the CVA. A patient with a right CVA will have left homonymous hemianopsia. Left homonymous hemianopsia results in an inability to receive information from the left side. Initially, the patient needs to be made aware of his/her deficit and instructed to compensate by turning the head to the affected left side. Providing printed notes on the left side and placing the patient's eating utensils on the left side will not be effective as these items will not be within the person's intact visual field. Initially, items should be placed on the person's right (unaffected side) so that the patient can successfully complete tasks and interact with the environment. As the person develops awareness of the deficit, additional compensatory strategies include moving items to the midline and then to the affected left side and teaching the person to scan from the right to midline to the left.

Type of Reasoning: Analytical
For this question, the test taker must consider the best initial strategy for a patient with homonymous hemianopsia in order to arrive at a correct conclusion. This requires analytical reasoning skill, where deficits are analyzed in order to determine a most effective approach to addressing the deficits. For this case, teaching the patient to turn his/her head is what needs to occur first when compensating for the functional effects of homonymous hemianopsia. Review intervention approaches for homonymous hemianopsia if answered incorrectly.

C37 C3

An individual recently had a left transfemoral amputation as a result of the complications of diabetes. The client is 2 years' status-post a right transtibial amputation as a result of the same precipitant. The client is referred to OT for preprosthetic interventions. The referral notes that the complications of neuromas and phantom limb pain are present in the left residual limb. Which intervention is best for the occupational therapist to implement during the first session?

Answer Choices:
A. Upper extremity strengthening with emphasis on the biceps.
B. Percussion to the left lower extremity's residual limb.
C. Upper extremity strengthening with emphasis on the triceps.
D. Lower extremity dressing with emphasis on donning and doffing prostheses.

Correct Answer: C.

Rationale:
Strengthening the upper extremities, especially the triceps, will facilitate independence in transfers. Neuromas are nerve endings that are adhered to scar tissue. Since neuromas can be very painful, percussion to the left residual limb and donning/doffing of the left prosthesis is contraindicated at this time. Given that the right amputation is 2 years' status-post, it is likely that the client has achieved independence in donning and doffing the right prosthesis.

Type of Reasoning: Inferential
One must link the patient's diagnosis and current symptoms to the interventions presented in order to determine which intervention would be best to address current deficits. This requires inferential reasoning, where one must infer or draw conclusions based on facts and evidence. In this case, upper extremity strengthening, especially the triceps, is most important in order to facilitate independence in transfers. Review intervention approaches for clients with lower extremity amputations if answered incorrectly.

C38 C8

A person blinded in an accident begins an occupational therapy program for persons with vision loss. The occupational therapist collaborates with the individual to develop an intervention plan. Which should be included in the plan as an initial focus of intervention?

Answer Choices:

A. Developing the client's computer skills.
B. Adapting meal preparation techniques.
C. Exploring vocational interests.
D. Organizing the client's morning routine.

Correct Answer: D.

Rationale:

Organizing the morning routine is most appropriate as an initial goal to help the individual effectively and independently complete his/her personal activities of daily living. This can help the person feel confident, and serve as a basis for organizing the rest of the person's home and work routine. The development of meal preparation skills would initially focus on non-cooked foods and meals. Typically, one of the most frightening areas for the newly blinded person is the use of the stove because of the risk of burns and danger of fire, so developing skills to cook hot meals would be a long-term goal. The development of computer skills and vocational interests would be better choices for long-term intervention, if the client identifies these as a personal goal.

Type of Reasoning: Inferential

One must infer or draw conclusions about the best initial focus for OT with a person who has experienced recent visual loss. The key to arriving at a correct conclusion is determining which approach fosters confidence and provides a starting point for future community reentry activity. Organization of the morning routine is the most appropriate approach for achieving this goal. If answered incorrectly, review therapeutic approaches for patients with recent visual loss.

C39 C9

An adult with a right CVA begins occupational therapy to improve grooming and dressing skills. The client refuses to work with a female therapist and insists on working with a male therapist. The OT supervisor reviews the department's case load and finds that the department's sole male therapist has limited experience working with individuals with CVA. Which action is best for the supervisor to take next in response to this situation?

Answer Choices:

A. Encourage the individual to work with the female therapist currently assigned and assure the client of the therapist's skill and competence.
B. Contract with a per diem male therapist to work with the client and provide the needed interventions.
C. Assign the male therapist to work with the individual and provide supervision for the therapist.
D. Modify the intervention goals to include activities that are more comfortable for the individual when working with a female therapist.

Correct Answer: C.

Rationale:
This is the choice that respects the person's autonomy. The client's preference for working only with a male therapist can be due to a cultural, religious and/or personal reason(s), all of which should be honored. Therefore, this is a request that should be granted. While the male therapist has little direct experience working with persons with CVA, the evaluation and intervention of personal ADL is an area of entry-level OT practice that does not typically require specialized training. However, it would be helpful to provide the therapist with supervision regarding the application of these fundamental skills to persons with CVA. The supervisor is responsible to help the therapist develop the skills needed for best practice. Encouraging the client to do something that is uncomfortable violates the person's rights. Modifying the goals is not appropriate as goal modification must be based on an assessment of the client's abilities. In addition, the established goals are relevant and should be addressed.

Type of Reasoning: Evaluative
This question requires one to evaluate all of the potential courses of action and determine which one best considers the patient's needs and provides effective care. Questions that require one to weigh the merits of potential courses of action require evaluative reasoning skills. In this situation, the first action for the supervisor would be to have the male therapist work with the individual and provide supervision for the therapist.

C40 C1

An occupational therapist provides intervention for a 4-year-old with developmental delays characterized by the persistence of primitive postural reflexes. The child demonstrates age-appropriate cognitive skills. Which is the best play activity for the therapist to incorporate into the child's intervention?

Answer Choices:
A. Spinning on a swing.
B. Putting a puzzle together.
C. Lying on the floor and playing a game of marbles.
D. Pretending to be an explorer crawling through caves.

Correct Answer: D.

Rationale:
Pretending to crawl through caves can help facilitate the integration of primitive postural reflexes. It is also imaginative, which is appropriate play for a 4-year-old. Spinning on a swing is a fast vestibular activity indicated for treatment of sensory integration dysfunction. This activity could increase abnormal reflex activity in this child. Putting a puzzle together and playing marbles require fine motor skills and dexterity and would be too advanced for a child with the persistence of primitive postural reflexes.

Type of Reasoning: Inductive
One must utilize clinical knowledge and judgment to determine the therapeutic approach that would be best for the child. In this case, pretending to be an explorer crawling through caves is best given the child's age and limitations. If answered incorrectly, review the developmental levels of play and the impact of primitive postural reflexes on motor function. The integration of this knowledge is required to determine the correct answer.

C41 C5

An occupational therapist has scheduled a discharge planning session with an individual recovering from hip replacement surgery. In preparation for this session, the therapist reviews the nursing reports and learns that the person has mycobacterium tuberculosis (TB) which is currently in the dormant phase. Which type of precautions should the therapist use when entering the patient's room?

Answer Choices:
A. Standard.
B. Airborne.
C. Droplet.
D. Contact.

Correct Answer: A.

Rationale:
Standard precautions are observed in all clinical situations. The additional use of airborne precautions is required when working with persons known or suspected to be infected with a serious illness transmitted by airborne nuclei that remain suspended in the air and can be dispersed widely by air currents within a room. When in the active phase, mycobacterium TB, measles, and chickenpox are transmitted in this manner. Airborne precautions include the use of a respiratory isolation room and the wearing of respiratory protection (i.e., a mask) when entering the room. Airborne precautions are not needed when TB is dormant as is the case in this scenario. Droplet precautions are used for persons known or suspected to be infected with serious illness microorganisms transmitted by large particle droplets that can be generated by the individual during talking, sneezing and coughing (e.g., rubella, mumps, pertussis, influenza). Contact precautions are used for persons known or suspected to be infected or colonized with a serious illness transmitted by direct contact (hand or skin-to-skin contact) or contact with items in the patient's environment.

Type of Reasoning: Deductive
One must recall the guidelines for standard and transmission-based precautions. This is factual knowledge, which is a deductive reasoning skill. Because mycobacterium TB is dormant, one should recall that this is no longer an airborne illness and only standard precautions need to be observed. If answered incorrectly, review standard precautions and transmission-based precautions, especially guidelines for working with individuals with active vs. dormant TB.

C42 C6

An individual hospitalized for the first time due to a brief psychotic episode attends an occupational therapy group. During task performance, the occupational therapist notices that the person is restless with hand tremors and shaking legs. Which of the following should the therapist document that the person seems to be exhibiting?

Answer Choices:
A. Akinesia.
B. Pseudo-parkinsonism.
C. Akathisia.
D. Tardive dyskinesia.

Correct Answer: C.

Rationale:
Akathisia is a side effect of antipsychotic medications that is exhibited by restlessness, hand tremors and shaky legs. Akinesia is also a potential side effect, but this is evident by a lack of movement. Akinesia is also a negative symptom of schizophrenia. Pseudo-parkinsonism is also a side effect that appears as behaviors similar to the symptoms of advanced Parkinson's disease; that is, rigidity, pill-rolling tremors, masked face and a shuffling gait. Tardive dyskinesia is an irreversible neurological condition caused by prolonged use of neuroleptic medications. It would not be evident in someone being treated initially with neuroleptic medications.

Type of Reasoning: Analytical

This question provides symptoms and the test taker must determine the cause for such symptoms. This is an analytical reasoning skill, as questions of this nature often ask one to analyze a group of symptoms in order to determine a diagnosis. In this situation the symptoms indicate akathisia, which should be reviewed if answered incorrectly.

C43 C4

An occupational therapist works on feeding with a toddler who has a hyperactive gag reflex. What should the therapist do to decrease the gag reflex?

Answer Choices:

A. Have the child suck through straws of progressively longer lengths.
B. Walk a tongue depressor from the front of the tongue to its back.
C. Quickly ice the child's throat laterally.
D. Have the child blow bubbles.

Correct Answer: B.

Rationale:

Walking a tongue depressor from the front of the tongue to the back can desensitize a hyperactive gag reflex. The other interventions do not address a hyperactive gag reflex. Sipping on a straw can increase the sucking reflex. Quick icing is a traditional Rood technique that theoretically stimulates a muscle group. This technique has no evidence to support its use and should not be used in current practice. Stimulating the neck muscles would not influence a gag reflex.

Type of Reasoning: Inductive

This question requires one to determine the best approach for decreasing a hyperactive gag reflex. This requires inductive reasoning skill, where clinical judgment is paramount to arriving at a correct conclusion. For this situation, the therapist should walk a tongue depressor from the front to the back of the tongue. If answered incorrectly, review treatment guidelines for a hyperactive gag reflex.

C44 C8

A client in the descending phase of Guillain-Barré syndrome has bilateral shoulder strength of 2/5. The client fatigues easily. Which equipment should the occupational therapist recommend to enhance the person's performance of activities of daily living?

Answer Choices:

A. An overhead suspension sling.
B. Long-handled utensils and tools.
C. Angled/curved-handled utensils and tools.
D. An environmental control unit.

Correct Answer: A.

Rationale:
The overhead suspension sling is best suited for individuals presenting with proximal weakness with muscle grades in the 1/5 to 3/5 range. Long-handled and curved utensils and tools are useful for individuals with range of motion limitations. Environmental control units are used for individuals who have significant motor deficits, proximally and distally, and who cannot independently perform tasks such as controlling the switches on electronic equipment.

Type of Reasoning: Inferential
One must infer or draw conclusions about a likely course of action, given the information presented. This is an inferential reasoning skill, where knowledge of a therapeutic approach, such as providing equipment to enhance functioning in this situation, is essential to choosing a correct solution. In this case, the therapist should choose an overhead suspension sling. If answered incorrectly, review the diagnostic criteria and functional impact of Guillain-Barré syndrome and adaptive equipment for persons with proximal weakness. Integration of this knowledge is required to answer this item correctly.

C45 C9

An occupational therapist working in an outpatient pediatric clinic has been seeing a child for sensory processing deficits. After 12 treatment sessions a denial letter for services has been received. The letter states that the diagnosis and the treatment do not meet the requirements of the policy. The parents who are aware of the denial want the therapist to change the child's diagnosis code in order to receive reimbursement. What is the best way for the therapist to respond?

Answer Choices:
A. Discharge the child from OT and provide a home sensory program for follow-up by the parents.
B. Encourage the parents to seek an alternate insurance carrier to receive improved coverage for services.
C. Explain to the parents that the current diagnosis cannot be changed in order to receive reimbursement.
D. Encourage the parents to set up a payment plan with the clinic's accounting department.

Correct Answer: C.

Rationale:
It is against the AOTA Code of Ethics of veracity to change a diagnosis in order to receive payment from an insurance company. If there was an error in the diagnosis when the bill was submitted for payment to the insurance company or if the occupational therapist actually assigned an incorrect diagnosis code by mistake, then the diagnosis could be corrected and resubmitted with a letter of explanation. However, in this scenario, there is nothing to indicate the code was incorrect. Therefore the code cannot be changed. Discharging the child deprives the child of needed skilled treatment. It is not the therapist's place to suggest changes in insurance carriers and it also does not solve the current situation. While setting up a payment plan may be needed, it does not address the parent's request to change the code.

Type of Reasoning: Evaluative
This question requires one to weigh the merits of the course of actions presented and determine which action effectively addresses the issue at hand. This requires judgment based on guiding principles, which is an evaluative reasoning skill. For this situation, the therapist should explain to the parents that the current diagnosis cannot be changed in order to receive reimbursement as it violates ethical principles. If answered incorrectly, review the AOTA Code of Ethics, especially veracity.

C46 **C8**

An intervention plan for a person with a complete lesion of the spinal cord at the C6 level has been developed by the client and occupational therapist. Which activity should be included in this plan as a goal for the client to develop the ability to independently perform?

Answer Choices:
A. Typing with a mouth stick. ✗
B. Transferring using depression transfers. ✗
C. Donning pants while in bed.
D. Feeding using a suspension sling or mobile arm support. ✗

Correct Answer: C.

Rationale:
A person with a C6 spinal cord injury (SCI) can independently don underwear and pants while lying in bed. Minimal assistance is needed to don socks and shoes. Therefore, intervention would focus on developing the ability to don pants while lying in bed. A person with a C6 SCI uses a sliding board to transfer; depression transfers are possible at the C7 level. The client with a complete SCI at the C6 level does not need a mouth stick to type or a suspension sling/mobile arm support to feed. Therefore, intervention is not needed to develop these abilities.

Type of Reasoning: Deductive
This question requires factual recall of functional abilities according to spinal level lesions. Specifically, one must recall the expected outcomes of a patient with C6 complete injury. Therefore, dressing the lower extremities is most aligned with C6 functioning. Review functional outcomes of cervical level injuries if answered incorrectly.

C47 **C8**

An occupational therapist completes an ergonomic examination of a computer programmer and the programmer's workstation. Which is the best recommendation for the therapist to make to ensure the programmer uses ideal wrist and elbow positioning?

Answer Choices:
A. Elevate the keyboard to increase wrist flexion.
B. Use a keyboard rest to maintain a neutral wrist position. ✓
C. Lower the keyboard to increase wrist extension.
D. Add armrests to support elbows in 90° of flexion.

Correct Answer: B.

Rationale:
Work involving increased wrist deviation from a neutral posture in either flexion/extension or radial/ulnar deviation has been associated with increased reports of carpal tunnel syndrome and other wrist and hand problems. Therefore, using a keyboard rest to maintain a neutral wrist position is the best recommendation for the therapist to make to ensure the programmer uses ideal wrist and elbow positioning.

Type of Reasoning: Deductive
This question requires one to recall the proper ergonomic guidelines for workstation function. This is factual information, which is a deductive reasoning skill. In this scenario, it is important to prevent wrist and elbow dysfunction by facilitating neutral wrist positioning when using a keyboard. Review ergonomic workstation evaluation guidelines if answered incorrectly.

C48 C3

A therapist in a rehabilitation hospital receives a physician's order to evaluate a patient who has metastatic bone cancer with pathologic fracture of the ribs. The physician requests information about the patient's ability to tolerate resistive activities of the upper extremities. Which action is best for the occupational therapist to take in response to this request?

Answer Choices:
A. Complete a manual muscle test with less than full resistance.
B. Provide isometric strengthening exercises for the upper extremities.
C. Evaluate tolerance during functional ADL tasks.
D. Initiate theraband stretches and report tolerance to physician.

Correct Answer: C.

Rationale:
A patient with metastatic bone cancer with pathological fractures is at high risk for fractures from higher resistance activities. In this situation, manual muscle testing should be deferred and information about tolerating resistive activities can be gained through lower resistance ADL activities, such as bathing, dressing and feeding. The therapist should not conduct muscle testing, even with less than full resistance. Resistive exercises, whether isometric or isotonic, are also not ideal in this situation for two reasons: it can cause a fracture to occur and a patient with rib fractures should not engage in high-resistive-upper body exercises due to pain.

Type of Reasoning: Inferential
This situation requires one to determine a best course of action, given the diagnosis and current status. Despite the physician requesting information about tolerance for resistive activities, one should infer that given the diagnosis, manual muscle testing is contraindicated due to the high risk for fractures. However, this does not preclude performing any resistive activities. This type of decision making requires inferential reasoning skill, where one must draw a conclusion about the consequences of each of the four possible courses of action. If answered incorrectly, review assessment guidelines for people with metastatic bone cancer.

C49 C1

An older adult with persistent balance difficulty and a history of recent falls (two in the last 3 months) receives home care occupational therapy services. During the initial session, which client factors are most important for the occupational therapist to consider?

Answer Choices:
A. Spinal musculoskeletal changes secondary to degenerative joint disease.
B. Cardiovascular endurance and level of dyspnea during IADL.
C. Mental functions of attention and orientation during functional mobility.
D. Sensory functions and sensory organization of balance.

Correct Answer: D.

Rationale:
A critical component of balance control is sensory input from somatosensory, visual, and vestibular receptors and overall sensory organization of inputs. With age, these systems undergo changes that can compromise the person's balance and safety. Therefore, these are the most important client factors for the occupational therapist to consider during intervention. There is no information in the scenario to indicate that the person has a cognitive deficit, degenerative joint disease or a cardiopulmonary disorder.

Type of Reasoning: Inductive
This case scenario requires the test taker to combine knowledge of the somatosensory system and possible reasons for falls in order to arrive at the correct conclusion. A key facet of this question is in the terms "initial session" and "most important." These words should cause the test taker to focus on what should come first in a sequence of intervention events and what is most important for the patient. This requires the use of clinical judgment, which is an inductive reasoning skill. For this case, sensory functions and sensory organization of balance are most important. Review intervention approaches for balance deficits in older adults if answered incorrectly.

C50 **C9**

A rehabilitation facility is completing a utilization review. The occupational therapist on the utilization review committee contributes to the process by submitting a detailed report about the reasons for, costs of and outcomes of a specific aspect of occupational therapy service delivery. Which information is most relevant for the occupational therapist to include in this utilization review report?

Answer Choices:
A. The therapeutic use of the OT department's activity of daily living apartment. ✓
B. The splinting and adaptive equipment prescribed to clients prior to discharge.
C. The use of personal care aides to provide morning self-care assistance to clients.
D. The craft and art materials used during leisure exploration groups.

Correct Answer: A.

Rationale:
Utilization review involves the analysis of the use of the resources within a facility. It examines the medical necessity and cost efficiency of these resources. An ADL apartment would be considered a facility resource. Splints, adaptive equipment, crafts and art materials are supplies, not facility resources. Personal care aides are personnel resources, not facility resources.

Type of Reasoning: Inferential
One must have knowledge of utilization review guidelines in order to arrive at a correct conclusion. This is an inferential reasoning skill where knowledge of guidelines and judgment based on facts are utilized to reach conclusions. In this situation the utilization review would include therapeutic use of the OT department's ADL equipment. If answered incorrectly, review utilization guidelines.

C51 **C2**

An occupational therapist works at a psychosocial clubhouse. The therapist is leading a closed group on stress management that has been together for several months. One of the members shares some concerns about personal safety at home. Which is the therapist's best response to the member's expressed concerns?

Answer Choices:
A. Tell the individual you will privately talk about the concerns after the group.
B. Immediately send the individual to see the clubhouse's social worker.
C. Assure the individual that the concerns reflect normal anxieties.
D. Invite the individual to share more details about the concerns. ✓

Correct Answer: D.

Rationale:
It can be very difficult for an individual to share concerns about personal safety. This person clearly felt safe in this group and sufficiently comfortable with the therapist and members to be able to voice these concerns. Therefore, the therapist should seize the opportunity to obtain more information about the nature of the person's concerns. Delaying the attainment of this information until after the group is not necessary and can have the risk that the person will change his/her mind. Even the minute delay caused by having the person go see the social worker can be long enough for the person to decide that he/she does not want to disclose any further information. In addition, the person may not have a rapport or therapeutic relationship with the social worker and may not be comfortable sharing personal information. Assuring the person that these anxieties are normal minimizes his/her feelings and can be dangerous if the individual is truly unsafe at home.

Type of Reasoning: Evaluative
This question requires professional judgment based on guiding principles, which is an evaluative reasoning skill. The best response in this situation is to invite the individual to share more details about the concern for personal safety. This way the therapist can determine the most appropriate course of action based on further information.

C52 C2

An adolescent with Duchenne muscular dystrophy refuses to use mobile arm supports (MAS) because "they look so big and stupid." Which action should the occupational therapist take first in response to the client's statement?

Answer Choices:
A. Collaborate with a rehabilitation engineer to design a more compact device.
B. Explore other options with the client to perform activities that do not use the MAS. ✓
C. Provide several logical reasons for using the MAS to enhance functional performance.
D. Discharge the client and follow up with after 1 month to reassess interest in the MAS.

Correct Answer: B.

Rationale:
The most appropriate first action is exploring ways the client can do activities without requiring the use of the mobile arm supports. This response is an example of therapeutic use of self and a client-centered approach. Developing a different design for a mobile arm support is a long-term option that may not be feasible. Providing logical reasons for using the mobile arm supports is not the best initial response as it ignores the client's feelings of frustration and is not a client-centered approach. There is no need to discharge the client from treatment. The issue needs to be addressed now, not in 1 month.

Type of Reasoning: Inductive
This question requires one to determine the best approach for addressing the patient's concerns about using mobile arm supports. This requires inductive reasoning skill, where clinical judgment is paramount to arriving at a correct conclusion. For this situation, the therapist should explore other options for activity performance that do not use the arm supports.

C53 C4

Two weeks after beginning kindergarten, a 5-year-old with myelomeningocele develops sudden onset of headaches, vomiting, irritability and 'sunken' appearance of eyes without signs of a fever. When the occupational therapist reports the child's presenting symptoms to the child's physician, which condition should the therapist identify as a concern?

Answer Choices:

A. Stomach flu.
B. Tethered cord.
C. School anxiety.
D. Shunt malfunction.

Correct Answer: D.

Rationale:

These identified symptoms, along with seizures, are all symptoms of shunt malfunction. Shunt malfunction is a medical emergency. Stomach flu might be a possible reason for several of these symptoms, but given the clustering of the symptoms, the child should be checked for shunt malfunction. The signs of tethered cord include difficulties with bowel and bladder, gait disturbances, and/or foot deformities. A child may have a tendency to complain of stomachaches and other complaints to avoid school, if anxious. However, school anxiety would not include physical evidence of illness such as sunken eyes.

Type of Reasoning: Analytical

This question provides a group of symptoms and the test taker must determine the likely cause and inform the physician since the probable cause of the symptoms is a potential medical emergency. This requires analytical reasoning, where one must determine the precise meaning of the information presented. For this case, shunt malfunction is the most likely cause and should be reported. If answered incorrectly, review shunts for myelomeningocele and symptoms of malfunction.

C54 C1

A child with autism receives home care occupational therapy intervention services. The parent identifies a primary goal of developing the child's independent toileting skills. The child is completely dependent and the parent reports not attempting toilet training for several years. The therapist collaborates with the parent to establish the first intervention goal for the child. Which behavior should this goal address?

Answer Choices:

A. The child's ability to sit on the toilet with supervision.
B. The child's ability to verbally tell someone of the need to go to the bathroom.
C. The child's ability to indicate when the diaper is wet or soiled.
D. The child's ability to non-verbally indicate the need to go to the bathroom.

Correct Answer: C.

Rationale:

The first toileting skill that must be developed is the child's recognition of being wet or soiled. This typically occurs at 12 months. Subsequent toileting skills such as sitting on the toilet with supervision and indicating the need to go to the bathroom can develop after this initial recognition of being wet or soiled.

Type of Reasoning: Inferential

One must have knowledge of the typical developmental sequence of toilet skills and toilet training guidelines in order to arrive at a correct conclusion. This is an inferential reasoning skill where knowledge of guidelines and judgment based on facts are utilized to reach conclusions. In this situation, the first intervention goal would be to have the child indicate when his diaper is wet or soiled. If answered incorrectly, review the typical developmental sequence of toilet skills and toilet training guidelines for children.

C55 C7

An occupational therapist is providing intervention for an individual recovering from a CVA who has residual body neglect. The therapist is using a deficit-specific approach to intervention. Which type of activities is best for the therapist to use with this client?

Answer Choices:

A. Unilateral using the affected upper extremity.
B. Unilateral using the non-affected upper extremity.
C. Tasks that require right/left discrimination.
D. Bilateral using both upper extremities.

Correct Answer: D.

Rationale:

A basic principle of intervention for body neglect, according to a deficit-specific approach, is to provide bilateral activities. During these activities, the therapist can guide the affected extremity through the activity, if needed. Providing unilateral activities does not work on the identified deficits. The provision of tasks that require discrimination of right/left is indicated for spatial relations dysfunction.

Type of Reasoning: Deductive

One must recall the guidelines for use of a deficit-specific approach for body neglect. This is factual knowledge, which is a deductive reasoning skill. In this situation, the most appropriate activities for the therapist to use under this approach are bilateral with use of both upper extremities. If answered incorrectly, review deficit-specific approach to treatment with CVA.

C56 C5

A person is diagnosed with chronic obstructive pulmonary disease (COPD). The occupational therapist instructs the individual on breathing exercises to use to control respiration rate during activities. The therapist tells the person to inhale as if smelling roses. How should the therapist tell the person to exhale?

Answer Choices:

A. As if blowing out 20 lit candles on a birthday cake.
B. As if blowing forcibly to relight a dying campfire.
C. As if flickering a lit candle.
D. In quick short, multiple breaths.

Correct Answer: C.

Rationale:

When one exhales to flicker a lit candle, one uses pursed lip breathing. Pursed lip breathing is a method of controlled breathing which requires the individual to purse his/her lips while exhaling. This slows the exhalation process and improves the carbon dioxide exchange. This decreases one's rate of breathing and prevents airway collapse. The other descriptions do not result in pursed lip breathing.

Type of Reasoning: Inductive
This question requires one to determine the best approach for performing exercises for COPD. This requires inductive reasoning skill, where clinical judgment is paramount to arriving at a correct conclusion. For this situation, the person should exhale as if flickering a lit candle. If answered incorrectly, review pursed lip breathing strategies for persons with cardiopulmonary disorders.

C57 C9

An assisted-living facility has received a grant to purchase capital items that can be used to increase the independence of its residents. Which is best for the occupational therapy consultant to recommend for the use of these grant funds?

Answer Choices:
A. The purchase of adaptive equipment that residents can borrow when needed.
B. The purchase of a computer-based driver rehabilitation program.✓
C. The hiring of more personal care attendants.
D. The construction of an ADL training apartment. *live in own apartments*

Correct Answer: B.

Rationale:
A capital expense is an item that is above a fixed amount, typically $1000.00. A computer-based driver rehabilitation program is a capital expense which would be appropriate for this setting. Since the residents of assisted-living facilities tend to be elderly, the need to evaluate driving abilities and provide appropriate interventions to ensure safe driving is an important focus. Adaptive equipment and staff are considered direct expenses, for they are related to service provision. An ADL apartment does meet the criteria of a capital expense, but it would not be needed in an assisted-living facility because the residents live in their own apartments. Interventions to increase independence are most beneficial when conducted in a person's own living space.

Type of Reasoning: Inferential
One must infer or draw conclusions about a likely course of action, given the information presented. This is an inferential reasoning skill, where knowledge of a therapeutic approach, such as the purchase of capital equipment, is essential to choosing a correct solution. In this case, the therapist should choose to purchase a computer-based driver rehabilitation program. Review criteria for capital expenses if answered incorrectly.

C58 C8

An occupational therapist working in a spinal cord injury unit evaluates a client for bowel and bladder training. The client and therapist set a goal of independence in all aspects of bowel and bladder care, including skin inspection. Which of the following is the highest or most severe level of complete spinal cord injury the client can have to be able to achieve this goal?

Answer Choices:
A. C7–8.✓
B. C4–5.
C. C5.
D. C6.

Correct Answer: A.

Rationale:
These skills correspond to the C7–8 level. Individuals with SCIs at the other levels do not have the fine motor control to perform the skills independently.

Type of Reasoning: Deductive
This question requires factual recall of functional abilities according to spinal level lesions. Specifically, one must recall the expected outcomes of a patient with a complete C7–8 injury. Therefore, a client with this level of injury could be expected to be independent in bowel and bladder care and skin inspection. Review functional outcomes of cervical-level injuries if answered incorrectly, especially bowel and bladder care.

C59 C6

A person is recovering from a major cardiac infarct. During the initial occupational therapy session, the patient loudly and vigorously expresses plans to immediately resume a daily rigorous exercise routine. The occupational therapist reports the individual's plan to the cardiac rehabilitation team and explains that the individual appears to be in which of the following disability adjustment stages?

Answer Choices:
A. Shock.
B. Denial.
C. Acting out.
D. Acceptance.

Correct Answer: B.

Rationale:
During the psychosocial adjustment to disability/illness, denial is characterized by unrealistic expectations of recovery and a minimization of one's difficulties. Shock is characterized by emotional numbness, depersonalization and reduced speech and mobility. Acceptance is reflected in the acknowledgement of the situation and the development of a new self-concept reflective of one's assets and potentialities. Acting out is a term used to describe behavior that challenges societal norms.

Type of Reasoning: Analytical
This question provides a description of a behavior and the test taker must draw conclusions about what the behavior indicates. This is an analytical reasoning skill, as questions of this nature often ask one to analyze descriptors and symptoms in order to determine a diagnosis or draw a conclusion. In this situation the behavior indicates denial. If answered incorrectly, review disability adjustment.

C60 C1

A 6-year-old begins prosthetic training with a right below-elbow myoelectric prosthesis. To learn to operate the terminal device, the occupational therapist implements intervention using age-appropriate play activities. Which activity is best for the therapist to first include during intervention?

Answer Choices:
A. Assembling building blocks.
B. Squeezing a squeeze toy.
C. Playing board games.
D. Stacking 1-inch blocks.

Correct Answer: A.

Rationale:
In prosthetic training, the person first learns to open and close the terminal device. Assembling building blocks provides the opportunity to develop this skill and it is the most appropriate activity for the child of this age. A squeeze toy is appropriate for a child up to 2 years of age. The pieces of board games are small and will require an advanced level of skill in operating the terminal device. Stacking blocks is appropriate for a preschool child.

Type of Reasoning: Inferential
One must determine the best activity for a child with a below-elbow myoelectric prosthesis. The key is to choose the activity that is age appropriate and focuses on opening and closing the terminal device. In this situation, assembling building blocks provides opportunities to practice opening and closing the device and is age appropriate for a 6-year-old. If answered incorrectly, review the developmental levels of play and principles of prosthetic training. The integration of this knowledge is required to determine the correct answer.

C61 C2

An occupational therapist meets with a patient with fibromyalgia who has had difficulty meeting intervention goals. The patient complains of being hurt and frustrated in attempts to resolve pain and fatigue issues. Which is the most effective technique for the therapist to use to help the patient increase insight into this situation?

Answer Choices:
A. Offer a variety of options for pain management.
B. Reflect the patient's verbal expressions back to the patient.
C. Refer the patient to a specialized pain management center.
D. Repeat the patient's exact words back to the patient.

Correct Answer: B.

Rationale:
Reflection involves expressing the feeling behind the patient's words and is an effective technique to facilitate self-reflection and develop insight. Repeating the exact words or parroting is not effective because this means merely stating the words without a focus on the emotions behind the words. Offering options for pain treatment and a referral to a pain management center can be helpful for managing the patient's pain but these options do not address the question's stated focus on increasing the client's insight.

Type of Reasoning: Inductive
Clinical knowledge and judgment are the most important skills needed for answering this question, which requires inductive reasoning skill. Knowledge of interpersonal skills and how to respond to a patient who expresses frustration is key to arriving at a correct conclusion. In this case, reflection is the most effective technique for this patient to express the feelings behind the patient's words.

C62 C9

An occupational therapist designs a research project to study the efficacy of training nursing assistants in feeding techniques for individuals residing in a skilled nursing facility who have dementia. Before implementing the study, from whom must the occupational therapist first obtain consent?

Answer Choices:
A. The facility's institutional review board.
B. The residents who will be the study's sample.
C. The designated representatives of residents who will be the study's sample.
D. The nursing assistants who will participate in the training.

Correct Answer: A.

Rationale:
Researchers must obtain institutional review board (IRB) approval for all human subject research. This ensures that research participants are not placed at risk. Once IRB approval is obtained, informed consent from the study's participants must be obtained. Since the residents have dementia resulting in cognitive deficits, their ability to give informed consent is compromised. Therefore, consent must be obtained from their designated representatives.

Type of Reasoning: Deductive
This question requires recall of guidelines and principles, which is factual knowledge. Deductive reasoning skills are utilized whenever one must recall facts and protocols to solve problems. In this situation, the initial action in implementing a study is to obtain consent from the facility's IRB. Review the research process, especially guidelines for human subject research and IRB consent if answered incorrectly.

C63 C9

An occupational therapist leads a community integration group for individuals with mild intellectual disabilities who reside in a group home. During a travel training session, a member of the group slips while going up the stairs of a bus. The client quickly gets up, pays the fare, sits down and jokingly states, "Good thing I bounce well." Which action should the occupational therapist take after assessing that the person is not injured?

Answer Choices:
A. Cancel the planned activity and return to the group home to file an occurrence report.
B. Ask the bus driver to radio for an ambulance to obtain a medical assessment to validate that the client was not injured.
C. Continue with the planned activity and file an occurrence report upon return to the group home. ✓
D. Continue with the activity and ask the client to report any development of symptoms related to the fall.

Correct Answer: C.

Rationale:
Upon determination that the client has not been injured there is no need to cancel the planned activity. It is standard policy to file a report about any incidents that involve clients but occurrence reports about minor events do not have to be done immediately. There is no information in the scenario provided to indicate a need to call an ambulance. Asking the client to report any symptoms related to the fall is appropriate, but it is not the most important action for the occupational therapist to take. Proper documentation is a professional and legal requirement that must be met.

Type of Reasoning: Evaluative
This question requires a value judgment in a situation regarding safety, which is an evaluative reasoning skill. In this situation, the most prudent procedure should be followed given the individual's status, which is to continue with the planned activity and file an occurrence report upon return to the group home. Review guidelines for reporting occurrences if answered incorrectly.

C64 C8

An older adult is referred to occupational therapy with a diagnosis of osteoarthritis in both knees and elbows. The occupational therapist interviews the patient and learns that the patient desires to return home to live alone independently in a bi-level home. Which should the therapist do next?

Answer Choices:

A. Provide suggestions for adaptations to the patient's bathroom to increase safety.
B. Train the patient in energy conservation techniques to use during IADL tasks.
C. Evaluate the patient's performance of daily activities in a simulated setting.
D. Provide the patient with a home exercise program to build strength and ROM.

Correct Answer: C.

Rationale:

The person has just been referred to occupational therapy and the patient interview has indicated a need for further evaluation. By observing the person perform daily activities within a simulated setting, the occupational therapist can assess the demands of the activities the patient performs and the patient's capabilities. Because osteoarthritis is isolated to specific joints and not systemic in nature, the therapist can assess how the specific affected joints impact occupational performance. Once this information is obtained, the therapist can use clinical reasoning to make recommendations to improve occupational performance.

Type of Reasoning: Inferential

One must determine the best approach for evaluation of this patient, given the stated desires and diagnosis. This requires inferential reasoning skill, where one must infer or draw conclusions about the approach that will result in the best functional outcome. In this case, evaluation of the patient's daily activities in a simulated setting is the best approach to learn about the patient's ability to safely return home and manage the symptoms of osteoarthritis.

C65 C4

An occupational therapist uses a motor learning intervention approach to develop prehension patterns with a child recovering from a brain tumor. The therapist places small toys on a table and asks the child to pick up the toys and put them into a storage box that is also on the table. The therapist uses random practice during this activity. Which types and arrangement of toys are most effective for the therapist to provide according to the motor learning approach?

Answer Choices:

A. Toys that are exactly the same shape, size and weight in a mixed arrangement on the table.
B. Toys that are exactly the same shape, size and weight placed in a straight line on the table.
C. Toys of different shapes, sizes and weights in a mixed arrangement on the table.
D. Age-appropriate toys arranged in a developmental sequence according to the child's developmental age.

Correct Answer: C.

Rationale:

According to a motor learning approach, random practice involves the performance of several motor tasks in random order to encourage the reformulation of the solution to the presented motor problem. Each time the child picks up a small toy of a different shape, size and/or weight his/her grasp pattern must be different. This activity is consistent with random practice. Having the child pick up toys that are of the same shape, size and weight involves repeated performance of the same motor skill. This activity reflects blocked practice according to the motor learning approach. The motor learning approach does not utilize a developmental sequence.

Type of Reasoning: Inductive

This question requires one to determine the best approach for arrangement of toys for prehension according to motor learning approach and utilization of random practice. This requires inductive reasoning skill, where clinical judgment is paramount to arriving at a correct conclusion. For this situation, the toys of different shapes, sizes and weights should be placed in a mixed arrangement on the table. If answered incorrectly, review motor learning approach, especially the principle of random practice.

C66 C2

An occupational therapist reviews the positioning protocol for a premature infant with severe spastic cerebral palsy with the infant's parents. The protocol is in a written format. During the review, the therapist notices that the parents do not seem able to follow along with the protocol's text. Which action is best for the therapist to take initially in response to this observation?

Answer Choices:

A. Ask the parents if they have any concerns about positioning their infant.
B. Ask the parents if they can read and understand English.
C. Include pictures of proper positioning in the protocol.
D. Demonstrate proper positioning techniques.

Correct Answer: A.

Rationale:

This is an open-ended question that enables the parents to express any concerns that they may have about positioning their infant. These concerns may be comprehension related and/or task related. Caring for a child with severe physical disabilities can be overwhelming and the parents' perceived difficulties in following the written protocol may be due to emotional stress, not limitations in literacy. The parents may welcome the opportunity to express their concerns. The other choices are close-ended and do not facilitate an open dialogue. If the parents have difficulty understanding English or if they could benefit from pictures and/or demonstrated positions, they can express this in response to the therapist's open invitation to express concerns.

Type of Reasoning: Evaluative

This question requires professional judgment based on guiding principles, which is an evaluative reasoning skill. Because the therapist cannot completely determine the source of the parent's difficulty, the therapist should ask if there are any concerns about positioning the infant. This way the therapist can invite the parent to share any concerns in an open-ended fashion without delineating the specific challenge.

C67 C8

An occupational therapist conducts a group for long-term inmates in a forensic facility. Which of the following would be best for the therapist to focus on during the group?

Answer Choices:

A. Vocational planning strategies.
B. Remedial educational activities.
C. Money management skills.
D. Leisure management techniques.

Correct Answer: D.

Rationale:
Persons in a forensic setting have a significant amount of time that is not filled by productive or meaningful activity. A group focused on the development of leisure management skills would be an appropriate focus for a group of individuals living long-term in an environment with limited leisure opportunities. Moreover, since these inmates are there for extended time periods, the development of skills to effectively manage leisure time would benefit them on an ongoing basis. Vocational planning would be most effective for persons who are nearing their release. It would be not the most relevant group focus for persons with a lot of time remaining on their sentences. Remedial educational activities would be the focus of services provided by an educational professional, not by an occupational therapist. Role-playing is a technique that might be employed in any group rather than a primary focus of a group.

Type of Reasoning: Inferential
One must consider the information provided and infer what is likely to be a correct conclusion, which is an inferential reasoning skill. For this situation, leisure management techniques are most likely to be addressed in a group within a forensic facility. If answered incorrectly, review information on the characteristics of forensic settings and the focus of OT interventions in these settings.

C68 C3

An individual is referred to a work-hardening program for evaluation. The referral states that the person had attended another work program for 6 months but had been discharged due to lack of compliance with treatment recommendations. The physician wants the occupational therapist to determine if the person is applying maximal effort or if the person is magnifying symptoms. When measuring the grip strength of each hand to compare to established norms, which evaluation protocol will be most effective for the therapist to use?

Answer Choices:
A. One trial on the dynamometer on all five positions.
B. Three trials on the dynamometer at level #2.
C. Five trials of lateral pinch.
D. Three trials of lateral pinch.

Correct Answer: A.

Rationale:
If the person is applying maximal effort when the dynamometer is tested on all five positions a bell curve should be noted. All of the other evaluation procedures could enable the person to not apply maximum effort and readings would be below the norms.

Type of Reasoning: Inductive
This question requires one to determine the most appropriate evaluation approach for determining a person's functional ability. This requires inductive reasoning skill, where clinical judgment is paramount to arriving at a correct conclusion. For this situation, the therapist should choose one trial on the dynamometer on all five positions for each hand. If answered incorrectly, review evaluation guidelines in work rehabilitation settings.

C69 C9

A parent receiving occupational therapy in a hand clinic asks the occupational therapist to adjust his/her child's hand splint. The parent reports that the splint leaves red marks after being removed for 20 minutes. The child received the splint from a school therapist. Which is the best action for the therapist to take in response to this request?

Answer Choices:

A. Modify the splint using a heat gun.
B. Suggest that the parent have the child refrain from wearing the splint.
C. Have the pediatric therapist in the department modify the splint.
D. Call the child's therapist and have the parent express the concern.

Correct Answer: D.

Rationale:

The best choice is to have the parent directly speak to the child's therapist. The report that the splint leaves red marks 20 minutes after removal is a concern that must be handled in a timely manner. In the other choices, the therapist is providing treatment without a referral which is not in accordance with established practice standards. Moreover, this would result in the therapist acting without having any knowledge of the diagnosis or plan of care which would be unethical. The child received a splint for a reason and not wearing it could be detrimental to the child. However, the child's therapist must be advised of the situation so that he/she can plan a correct course of action.

Type of Reasoning: Evaluative

This question requires one to make a value judgment about a best course of action, which requires evaluative reasoning skill. Because the therapist is treating the parent and not the child, it is not the therapist's place to adjust the child's splint and the therapist should have the patient contact the child's therapist for follow-up.

C70 C5

A person is 5 days' post coronary artery bypass graft (CABG). The patient expresses anxiety about performing any type of activity and reports chest pain during ambulation. The cardiologist has approved activities at a metabolic equivalent (MET) level of 2–3. Which activity is best for the occupational therapist to use when initiating intervention with this person?

Answer Choices:

A. Grooming while standing at the sink.
B. Grooming in sitting.
C. Sponge bathing while sitting.
D. Performing light housework.

Correct Answer: A.

Rationale:

Grooming while standing at the sink is at a MET level of 2–3. Grooming in sitting and sponge bathing while sitting are at a 1–2 MET level. Light housework is at the 3–4 MET level.

Type of Reasoning: Deductive

One must recall MET level guidelines for cardiac rehabilitation. This is factual knowledge, which is a deductive reasoning skill. In this situation, the only activity that falls within the range of the 2–3 MET level is grooming while standing at the sink. If answered incorrectly, review MET level guidelines, especially 2–3 level.

C71 C1

A child with mild cerebral palsy (CP) receives occupational therapy intervention in a preschool setting. Which intervention approach should the therapist employ to facilitate development of typical grasp patterns?

Answer Choices:
A. Place soft foam tubing around objects to be grasped.
B. Analyze the present components of the child's grasp.
C. Analyze the missing components of the child's grasp.
D. Grade the sizes and shapes of objects to be grasped.

Correct Answer: D.

Rationale:
Gradation of the size and shape of items to be grasped enables the therapist to begin with items that are within the child's grasp capabilities and then add different items as the child's grasp abilities progress. There is no need to add soft foam tubing at this time. Soft tubing may be used as a compensation approach if the child does not develop typical grasp patterns. Analyzing the components of grasp is part of the evaluation and reevaluation process, not intervention.

Type of Reasoning: Inductive
This question requires one to determine the most appropriate intervention for a child with mild CP. This requires inductive reasoning skill, where clinical judgment is paramount to arriving at a correct conclusion. For this situation, grading the size and shapes of objects to be grasped is most appropriate. If answered incorrectly, review development of grasp patterns for children.

C72 C7

An occupational therapist receives a referral to evaluate an individual's executive functioning following a mild cerebral vascular accident. Which are the most relevant foci for this evaluation?

Answer Choices:
A. The person's initiation and planning.
B. The person's attention and memory.
C. The person's job interests and efficacy.
D. The person's spatial relations and praxis.

Correct Answer: A.

Rationale:
Executive functions are higher-level cognitive abilities that are needed to perform unstructured multistep activities and role tasks. The four main components of executive functioning are volition, planning, purposeful action and effective performance. Attention and memory are considered primary cognitive capacities that are prerequisite to higher-level cognitive abilities. The other choices do not relate to cognitive functioning.

Type of Reasoning: Inferential
One must infer or draw conclusions about a likely course of action, given the information presented. This is an inferential reasoning skill, where knowledge of a therapeutic approach, such as executive functioning in this situation, is essential to choosing a correct solution. In this case, the therapist would most likely assess the person's initiation and planning. Review executive functions if answered incorrectly.

C73 C2

During a parallel task group, one of the members appears agitated and fidgety. The member gets up and looks out the window for a few minutes and then sits back down and quietly returns to the task. This behavior continues throughout the group. Which is the occupational therapist's best response when the group member stands again?

Answer Choices:

A. Tell the group member to remain seated or leave the group.
B. Ask the other members if the group member is bothering them.
C. Say nothing to the group member and proceed with the group.
D. Inform the group member that the observed behaviors indicate a lack of readiness for this group.

Correct Answer: C.

Rationale:
Many individuals, due to the symptoms of their illness and/or medication, have difficulty remaining still. They can, however, benefit from attending a group. A parallel group does not require any interaction for task completion. Therefore, if the group member's behavior is not disturbing or disruptive to the group he/she should be allowed to benefit from this form of treatment.

Type of Reasoning: Evaluative
This question requires professional judgment based on guiding principles, which is an evaluative reasoning skill. Because the person is not disturbing the other group members with his/her behavior, the therapist should say nothing to the person. Questions such as these can be challenging. However, essential to arriving at a correct conclusion is determining if the behavior is expected or typical of the person, given his/her diagnosis. In this situation, it is typical behavior; therefore, no action needs to be taken.

C74 C6

An occupational therapist works in an adult home with a resident who has just been discharged from the hospital. The resident wants to resume participation in the gardening group, physical exercise group, and current events group. The resident takes anti-psychotic medications to manage symptoms. Which potential medication side effect should the resident be aware of, and take precautions for, prior to participating in group?

Answer Choices:

A. Akathisia.
B. Photosensitivity.
C. Akinesia.
D. Tardive dyskinesia.

Correct Answer: B.

Rationale:
Anti-psychotic medication can result in all of the side effects or conditions listed. However, photosensitivity would be of the greatest concern for this individual given the stated interest in resuming participation in the gardening group. Individuals who take psychotropic medications can incur severe sunburns if they do not take the precautions of wearing sunscreen, hats and/or long-sleeved shirts. There are no precautions to prevent akathisia or akinesia other than medication adjustments by a physician. Tardive dyskinesia is not a medication side effect. It is an irreversible neurological condition caused by prolonged use of neuroleptic medications.

Type of Reasoning: Deductive
One must recall the side effects of psychotropic medications in order to arrive at a correct conclusion. This requires deductive reasoning skill, where factual knowledge is essential to choosing the correct solution. Photosensitivity is a common side effect of anti-psychotic medications. Review side effects of psychotropic medications if answered incorrectly.

C75 C4

An occupational therapist working in early intervention meets with the parents of an infant who cries a lot and has difficulty being soothed. The parents are concerned that they are unable to comfort their child. Which is the most effective strategy for the therapist to recommend to the parents?

Answer Choices:

A. Loosely wrap the infant in a blanket.
B. Provide frequent and rapid changes in movement.
C. Do nothing, as the infant's behavior is typical.
D. Tightly wrap the infant in a blanket.

Correct Answer: D.

Rationale:

Tightly wrapping an infant in a blanket can provide controlled and consistent firm pressure that is non-aversive and soothing. The crying behavior, whether typical or indicative of a difficulty, will likely respond to this strategy. Loosely wrapping the infant provides inconsistent and variable input that can increase discomfort. Frequent and rapid changes in movement are contraindicated because they can increase tone and stimulate arousal. Whether the child's behavior is considered typical or not is irrelevant; the parents are concerned and can benefit from suggestions.

Type of Reasoning: Inductive

This question requires one to determine the best approach for an infant with difficulty being soothed. This requires inductive reasoning skill, where clinical judgment is essential to arriving at a correct conclusion. For this situation, the therapist should recommend tightly wrapping the infant in a blanket. If answered incorrectly, review treatment guidelines for infants with difficulties in being soothed.

C76 C1

An occupational therapist observes that a child can open a combination lock, open a lock with a key and turn a pencil over to erase. In documenting the child's in-hand manipulation, which is most accurate for the occupational therapist to report the child can correctly perform?

Answer Choices:

A. Finger-to-palm translation.
B. Rotation.
C. Palm-to-finger translation.
D. Shift.

Correct Answer: B.

Rationale:

The activities described involve turning or rolling. Finger-to-palm translation and palm-to-finger translation are incorrect, as no palm is involved in the performance of the described activities. Shift is incorrect for the activities do not just use a linear movement.

Type of Reasoning: Analytical

This question provides descriptions of functional activity and the test taker must determine the likely definition of such skills. This is an analytical reasoning skill, as questions of this nature often ask one to analyze descriptors of functional skills to determine the overall skill involved. In this situation the activities are descriptive of rotation. Review rotation skills in children if answered incorrectly.

C77 C8

An individual with mild cognitive deficits takes medications for multiple medical conditions. The occupational therapist works with the individual to develop the ability to safely self-administer medications. Which equipment and/or strategy should the therapist train the client to use?

Answer Choices:
A. Easy-open caps on the medication bottles.
B. A chart listing medication dosages and administration times on the refrigerator.
C. A daily pill holder with time-labeled slots for each dosage. ✓
D. Family caregiver supervision of medication administration

Correct Answer: C.

Rationale:
The use of a pill holder with slots for each dose of medication labeled with its administration time can provide the needed structure for safe self-administration of medications. A chart on a refrigerator is not as useful for the individual cannot take the chart with him/her during daily activities. Easy-open caps do not provide any organizational structure for the identified cognitive deficits. Family caregiver supervision could be needed if the person was not able to benefit from organizational strategies. The individual needs to be provided with the opportunity to develop abilities to self-administer medications to maintain autonomy. In addition, one cannot assume that there is a family caregiver available who would be able to provide the appropriate support.

Type of Reasoning: Inferential
One must determine the most appropriate recommendation for an individual with cognitive deficits. This requires inferential reasoning skill, where one must infer or draw conclusions about a best course of action. In this situation, the therapist should recommend a daily pill holder with time-labeled slots to aid in appropriate administration of medication. Review adaptive strategies for medication management if answered incorrectly.

C78 C9

An occupational therapist has been counseled twice by the director of the OT department for overcharging patients for services rendered. The behavior continues despite repeated verbal and written reprimands from the director. Which action is best for the director to take next?

Answer Choices:
A. Report the therapist's behavior to the NBCOT. ✗
B. Formulate a plan of action to modify the therapist's behaviors ✗
C. Terminate the employee according to facility procedures.
D. Follow facility procedures for reporting employee misconduct. ✓

Correct Answer: D.

Rationale:
Overcharging patients is fraud and must be stopped. The therapist has already been reprimanded for this inappropriate action and has not altered the behavior. The director must follow facility guidelines for reporting employee misconduct. The facility's director of human resources (HR) will investigate the situation and determine if it is best to place the employee on probation or terminate the employee. Probation typically includes a well-documented corrective plan of action to assure that opportunities are given to employees to modify inappropriate behaviors and that employees fully understand the consequences of their behaviors. If an employee does not correct identified behaviors of concern while he/she is on probation, the facility will have just cause for termination of the employee. Since this scenario involves fraud and the therapist has been reprimanded twice by the OT director, the HR director may determine that just cause has already been established and terminate the employee. This would most likely occur if the OT director provided adequate documentation about all communications concerning the employee's continuing misconduct and non-response to supervision. The facility must directly address the therapist's fraudulent behavior and reporting this therapist to NBCOT will not do this.

Type of Reasoning: Evaluative

One must weigh the possible courses of action and then make a value judgment about the best course of action. This requires evaluative reasoning skill, which often utilizes guiding principles of action in order to arrive at a correct conclusion. For this case, the director should follow human resources procedures for reporting employee misconduct. If answered incorrectly, review guidelines for management of OT personnel and the OT Code of Ethics.

C79 C2

An adolescent incurred a C4 spinal cord injury. During the initial session, the patient refuses to speak to the occupational therapist. The therapist supportively acknowledges the client's response. Which action should the therapist take next?

Answer Choices:

A. Set up a chin-operated, bedside extensor carpi ulnaris (ECU) to enable access to the environment.✓
B. Provide passive range of motion to prevent contractures.
C. Explain what OT can offer the adolescent to adjust to decreased abilities.
D. Ask the adolescent to tell nursing staff when personally ready for OT.

Correct Answer: A.

Rationale:

The individual immediately needs a method to access the environment. Being able to call staff, operate a TV and/or radio, answer the phone, turn on/off lights, and other basic ECU functions are important tasks for the adolescent to self-control. It is not necessary to explain what OT can offer. Some of the benefits of OT will likely become self-evident as the adolescent learns to use the ECU. This explanation can be expanded on as the adolescent begins to engage in intervention. Providing passive range of motion (PROM) ignores the patient's feelings. PROM can be provided by direct-care staff. The individual may not be ready for quite a while to collaborate with the occupational therapist due to the need to adjust to disability. While this is occurring, the therapist can still provide meaningful supportive interventions and work on developing a therapeutic relationship.

Type of Reasoning: Inductive

One must utilize clinical knowledge and judgment to determine the best action that addresses the adolescent's needs in the absence of his/her input. In this case, a chin-operated, bedside ECU is the best course of action out of the choices provided as it provides access to the environment. If answered incorrectly, review treatment guidelines, especially equipment needs for persons with a C4 injury.

C80 C5

Several patients in a cardiovascular unit are referred to occupational therapy for rehabilitation in areas of occupation. Which diagnosis would be an inclusive criterion for participation in the home management activity group conducted in the department's simulated apartment?

Answer Choices:
A. Hypotension.✓
B. Unstable angina.
C. Venous thrombosis.
D. Uncontrolled atrial arrhythmia.

Correct Answer: A.

Rationale:
Persons with hypotension can be included in a rehabilitation group that includes instrumental activities of daily living. Engagement in these activities would be contraindicated for patients with the other conditions. Unstable angina is a coronary insufficiency with risk for myocardial infarction or sudden death. The person's pain is difficult to control and it is present with low-level activity or rest. Venous thrombosis and uncontrolled atrial arrhythmia must be monitored closely and persons with these diagnoses would be better candidates for OT services that are provided bedside.

Type of Reasoning: Deductive
This question requires the test taker to recall symptoms of cardiac dysfunction and guidelines for cardiac rehabilitation. Deductive reasoning skills are utilized, as one must recall factual information about indications and contraindications for cardiac rehabilitation programs associated with certain diagnoses. In this situation, only patients with hypotension are allowed to engage in instrumental activities of daily living. If answered incorrectly, review cardiac rehabilitation guidelines, especially for patients with the identified symptoms.

An elder expresses concerns about the ability to perform daily tasks. The occupational therapist assesses that the individual has somatosensory deficits consistent with the normal aging process. The therapist recommends adaptive equipment to assist with task performance. Which adaptive equipment should the therapist recommend the person use during meal preparation and feeding?

Answer Choices:
A. Utensils with narrow, smooth grips.✗
B. Utensils with wide, textured grips.
C. A rocker knife.✗
D. Dycem pads.

Correct Answer: B.

Rationale:
Wide, textured grips will provide augmented sensory feedback to the individual and will be easier to grip than narrow, smooth handles. Somatosensory changes associated with aging include decreased tactile sensation, decreased proprioception and increased pain thresholds. A rocker knife and dycem pads would not address these deficits. A rocker knife is suitable for one-handed cutting and dycem pads are used to provide stability to an object.

Type of Reasoning: Inferential
One must have knowledge of somatosensory deficits and the aging process in order to arrive at a correct conclusion. This is an inferential reasoning skill where knowledge of deficits and judgment based on facts are utilized to reach conclusions. If answered incorrectly, review somatosensory deficits in older adults and adaptive equipment.

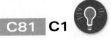

C82 C9

An occupational therapist implements intervention with five patients using a group format. The therapist charges each patient's insurance provider for individual treatments. Which of the following does this action represent?

Answer Choices:
A. An example of impairment.
B. A violation of procedural justice.
C. An established, accepted practice.
D. A correct action, if group interventions are individualized.

Correct Answer: B.

Rationale:
Procedural justice is the principle in the AOTA Code of Ethics which requires all OT personnel to comply with the laws and regulations guiding the profession and practice of occupational therapy. This includes being truthful in charging for services and meeting legal requirements for documentation. Impairment refers to being under the influence of alcohol, drugs or any substance that compromises judgment and abilities. It also includes personal issues, such as severe emotional distress, which impede the practitioner's abilities to fully engage in the OT process with clients. It is inappropriate and illegal to submit charges for individual treatments if treatment was actually performed in a group.

Type of Reasoning: Evaluative
This question requires a value judgment in an ethical situation, which is an evaluative reasoning skill. Following the OT Code of Ethics, all therapists should observe procedural justice, which is to comply with all laws and rules, including being truthful in billing for services. Therefore, the billing is a potential violation of procedural justice. Review the OT Code of Ethics if answered incorrectly, especially justice guidelines.

C83 C6

An occupational therapist implements an activity program at a hospital that provides long-term care to elderly persons with severe and persistent mental illnesses (SPMI). The occupational therapist uses a sensorimotor approach to guide the program design. Which activity is best for the therapist to incorporate into a group?

Answer Choices:
A. Ballroom dancing using pictures of feet on the floor as visual cues for dance steps.
B. Exercising along with a video routine.
C. A sing-along using songbooks and recorded music.
D. Keeping balloons afloat while music plays.

Correct Answer: D.

Rationale:
According to the sensorimotor approach, activities should not require the individuals to think about the steps needed to complete the activity. Activities should be spontaneous, "non-cortical," and fun. Keeping balloons afloat to music meets the criteria. The other activities require the individuals to think and follow some type of set, predetermined format.

Type of Reasoning: Inductive
One must utilize clinical knowledge and judgment to determine the exercise approach that best meets the criteria of a sensorimotor approach. This requires inductive reasoning skill. In this case, keeping balloons afloat while music plays is most appropriate out of the choices provided. If answered incorrectly, review sensorimotor approach for patients with SPMI.

C84 C5

An occupational therapist implements intervention for individuals on an inpatient cardiopulmonary rehabilitation unit. The therapist assesses a patient's heart rate during intervention sessions by palpating a peripheral pulse. Which of the following most accurately describes the timing the therapist should use to complete this assessment?

Answer Choices:

A. 30 seconds prior to, during and at cessation of the activity.
B. 1–2 minutes prior to, during and at cessation of the activity and 5 minutes' postactivity.
C. 1–2 minutes prior to, during and at cessation of the activity.
D. 30 seconds prior to, during and at cessation of the activity and 5 minutes' postactivity.

Correct Answer: B.

Rationale:
On an inpatient cardiopulmonary rehabilitation unit, the therapist must monitor a patient's heart rate before, during and immediately after an activity and a few minutes (e.g., 5 minutes) postactivity. Heart rate should be assessed using palpation of peripheral pulses. The most common monitoring site is the radial artery. Individuals with normal heart rhythms require only 30 seconds of palpation. Individuals receiving treatment in an inpatient cardiopulmonary rehabilitation unit will likely have irregular heart rhythms which require 1–2 minutes of palpation.

Type of Reasoning: Deductive
This question requires recall of guidelines and principles, which is factual knowledge. In this situation, the guideline for inpatient cardiac monitoring is to monitor a patient's heart rate before, during and immediately after an activity, plus a few minutes postactivity. Review cardiac monitoring guidelines for inpatient rehabilitation if answered incorrectly.

C85 C2

A person with recently diagnosed multiple sclerosis begins an outpatient program. During the initial intervention session, the client expresses difficulty concentrating on daily tasks due to chronic fatigue. Which should the occupational therapist do in response to the client's stated concerns?

Answer Choices:

A. Reassure the client that these are typical symptoms of this diagnosis.
B. Reassure the client that medications will ease these symptoms.
C. Inquire about the client's fatigue level during different tasks.
D. Evaluate the client's endurance and cognition.

Correct Answer: C.

Rationale:
The therapist must obtain further information about the individual's fatigue levels and activity patterns. This information is essential to plan intervention for energy conservation and fatigue management. In addition, this action supports the validity of the client's concern and can be helpful in providing the foundation for a therapeutic relationship. Reassurance does not acknowledge the reality of the client's concern and does not deal with the stated problem. In addition, medications may not ease the client's symptoms. The client has just begun the program so the client's abilities would have been evaluated during the admission process. There is no information provided in this exam item to indicate a need to reevaluate the client's status at this time.

Type of Reasoning: Inferential

One must have knowledge of multiple sclerosis and typical symptoms of the disease in order to choose the best response in this situation. This is an inferential reasoning skill where one must infer or draw conclusions about the information provided. For this situation, the therapist should inquire about the patient's fatigue level during various tasks. If answered incorrectly, review symptoms of multiple sclerosis.

C86 C4

An elementary school student with autism is referred to occupational therapy. One of the student's goals is to self-initiate goal-directed play to decrease the frequency of self-stimulating behaviors of hand waving and rocking. The student's verbal communication is impaired but the student compensates by using picture cards to let others know what is wanted or needed. Which of the following approaches to initiate self-play in the home environment is best for the occupational therapist to suggest to the student's parents?

Answer Choices:

A. Allow the child time to choose a play activity from several options and do not provide guidance to ensure self-directed decision making.

B. Provide limited choices using picture cards and only give verbal praise when the child participates in the chosen play activity.

C. Include the child in after-school programs to socialize with other children and provide role modeling opportunities for typical play behaviors.

D. Provide limited play choices using picture cards, encourage choosing and give verbal praise when the child chooses an activity.

Correct Answer: D

Rationale:

Autism presents as impaired development of social interactions and communication and a limited repertoire of activities of interest. Symptoms can include repetitive movements or self-stimulating behaviors. Persons with autism often do not speak. They may have a limited vocabulary and will typically not ask for help or request things. Children with autism prefer to play alone and they have a hard time sharing experiences with others. The goal of therapy is to encourage engagement in purposeful activity, self-direction, imitation and social interaction. Using the child's form of communication of picture cards, the parents can provide a choice between a limited number of play activities at home to encourage the self-directed activity of choosing a play activity. Providing verbal praise immediately after a decision is made will reinforce a positive behavior and support continued decision making over time. As the child makes decisions more readily, verbal praise can be reduced. When decision making is difficult, providing several options to choose from can be over-stimulating and cause stress. Causing stress typically increases repetitive or self-stimulating behaviors. Including the child in after-school programs can be an option when the child is able to participate in purposeful activities and benefit from learning through imitation. At this point, an after-school program will likely be too stressful, which may result in social isolation or lost opportunity for self-directed decision making. In addition, this scenario specifically asked for an intervention strategy for the parents to use in the home environment, not within the school environment.

Type of Reasoning: Inductive

This question requires the test taker to determine a best course of action, utilizing clinical judgment to reach a reasonable conclusion. This requires inductive reasoning skill. For this scenario, the therapist should provide limited play choices using picture cards, encourage choosing and give verbal praise when the child chooses an activity, as this approach uses the child's current form of communication and encourages self-directed activity. If answered incorrectly, review intervention activities for children with autism.

C87 C6

An older adult who incurred a hip fracture resides with a family caregiver. The person is referred to home-based occupational therapy services. During the initial home visit, the occupational therapist observes that the individual demonstrates impaired short-term memory, disorientation to time and situation and difficulty engaging in activities. The family caregiver expresses many concerns about the client's decreased functional capacity and reports feeling stressed. Which recommendation is best for the therapist to make first to the family caregiver?

Answer Choices:

A. Explore residential placement to ensure the client's safety.
B. Contact the local Alzheimer's Association to attain caregiver support.
C. Contact the local adult day treatment center to explore respite programs.
D. Contact the client's physician to request a complete medical evaluation.

Correct Answer: D.

Rationale:

The client's symptoms may be due to depression, dementia, or pseudo-dementia Pseudo-dementia is the development of dementia-like symptoms due to a reversible cause. Reversible causes of dementia can include poly-medication, viral or bacterial infections, urinary tract infections, gall bladder disease and metabolic problems such as thyroid disorders or poorly controlled diabetes. A complete medical evaluation is needed to determine the cause(s) of the client's behavior, prior to making any treatment or referral recommendations.

Type of Reasoning: Evaluative

This question requires professional judgment based on guiding principles, which is an evaluative reasoning skill. The client's symptoms warrant a medical evaluation; therefore, the therapist should contact the physician for evaluation in this situation. Questions such as these can be challenging as value judgments are often not concrete and require thoughtful reflection and professional knowledge.

C88 C8

An individual with a complete C5 spinal cord injury prepares for discharge. The client plans to return to work as an editor of children's books. Which adaptive equipment is best for the occupational therapist to recommend the client use to access desktop publishing programs?

Answer Choices:

A. A wrist splint in the functional position with a slot to hold a typing stick.
B. A balanced forearm orthosis with a slot to hold a typing stick.
C. A wrist-driven flexor hinge splint with a slot to hold a typing stick.
D. A universal cuff to hold a typing stick.

Correct Answer: A.

Rationale:

A wrist splint in the functional position will provide the support needed due to absence of wrist extensors and wrist flexors. A person with a C5 spinal cord injury can perform keyboarding tasks with a typing stick inserted into a splint. A balanced forearm orthosis (BFO) is used to compensate for upper extremity muscle weakness. BFOs are also called deltoid aids or suspension slings. BFOs and similar equipment solely support the upper extremity and do not provide any options for holding items as a substitute for hand function. A person at C5 does not have active wrist movements, so a wrist-driven flexor hinge splint would be ineffective. While persons with a C5 SCI can use a universal cuff to hold items (e.g., a toothbrush) during activity performance, this type of adaptive equipment does not support the wrist. Because an editor needs to do substantial computer work, the use of a splint which supports the wrist is the best recommendation.

Type of Reasoning: Inferential
One must have knowledge of C5 spinal injury and effective adaptive devices for this level of injury in order to choose the best device to enhance participation in computer skills. This is an inferential reasoning skill where knowledge of the diagnosis coupled with knowledge of the functional ability to use devices with residual upper extremity musculature is key to choosing the correct solution. If answered incorrectly, review C5 injury, intact musculature and available adaptive devices for computer work.

C89 C4

An adolescent incurred a spinal cord injury at the C5 level. During a family caregiver education session, the occupational therapist instructs family members in the provision of passive range of motion (PROM) to the patient's wrist and fingers. Which method of PROM should the therapist teach the family members to perform?

Answer Choices:
A. Extend the fingers with the wrist extended.
B. Flex the fingers with the wrist flexed.
C. Flex and extend the fingers with the wrist in a neutral position.
D. Flex the fingers with the wrist fully extended and extend the fingers with the wrist fully flexed.

Correct Answer: D.

Rationale:
A major goal of OT for a person with a SCI at C5 or C6 is to enhance the development of a tenodesis grasp. Family caregivers can perform PROM to enhance achievement of this goal. Ranging the finger flexors with the wrist extended and the finger extensors with the wrist flexed will result in shortening of the flexor tendons without compromising joint ROM. This shortening will enhance the tenodesis grasp. The other ROM patterns do not do this.

Type of Reasoning: Deductive
One must recall the guidelines for ranging in a tenodesis pattern. This is factual knowledge, which is a deductive reasoning skill. The proper ranging in this pattern is to flex the finger with the wrist fully extended and extend the fingers with the wrist fully flexed. Review tenodesis pattern and PROM if answered incorrectly.

C90 C2

A 4-year-old child with a complete myelomeningocele at the T12 level is referred for outpatient occupational and physical therapy. In setting goals with the family, the occupational therapist suggests increasing independence in dressing skills and the physical therapist recommends improving ambulation. The family wants to work on ambulation but refuse interventions to develop dressing skills. Which action is best for the occupational therapist to take first to address the family's stated preference?

Answer Choices:
A. Concur with the family that the child does not need to receive occupational therapy services.
B. Refer the family to counseling to assist them in accepting the child's functional limitations.
C. Work with the family to determine a different focus for occupational therapy intervention.
D. Reinforce the importance of independence in dressing for the child to the family.

Exam C

Correct Answer: C.

Rationale:
This addresses the child's and family's rights and allows the therapist to apply therapeutic use of self. The family refuses intervention to work on the child's dressing skills and the therapist should respect their decision. The therapist can use this opportunity to collaborate with the family to help them determine a focus for occupational therapy services that meets their child's needs. A 4-year-old with a complete myelomeningocele at the T12 level will have needs in other areas of occupation besides dressing (e.g., play). There is no information provided in the item scenario to indicate that the family needs a counseling referral. Reinforcing the importance of dressing does not respect the family's stated preference.

Type of Reasoning: Evaluative
This question requires one to primarily consider the parent's needs in order to arrive at a correct conclusion. This necessitates weighing the benefits of the four possible choices, which utilizes evaluative reasoning skills. For this situation, working with the family to determine a different focus for occupational therapy best considers the parent's preferences and respects their right to refuse certain intervention approaches.

C91 **C3**

An occupational therapist evaluates an individual with a partial tear of the supraspinatus muscle. The therapist documents the results of muscle testing. Which is most accurate for the therapist to state when reporting these results?

Answer Choices:
A. Strength is fair and the person reports pain.
B. Strength is fair and the person reports no pain.
C. Strength is good and the person reports pain.
D. Strength is good and the person reports no pain.

Correct Answer: A.

Rationale:
A partial tear results in weakness because of the tendon tear. It is painful because it is only partially torn. A complete tendon rupture results in muscle weakness but it is painless. Tendonitis would result in pain but the muscle would remain strong. Good muscle strength that is pain-free is within functional limits.

Type of Reasoning: Inferential
One must link the individual's diagnosis to the muscle signs presented in order to determine which presenting signs are most representative of a partial supraspinatus tear. This requires inferential reasoning, where one must draw conclusions about the likely presentation of a diagnosis. In this case the presentation would include fair strength and pain reported. Review clinical presentation of supraspinatus tears if answered incorrectly.

C92 **C9**

An occupational therapist accepts a position at an adult day care and respite program for elders with a variety of physical and cognitive disabilities. The therapist only has clinical experience in school-based practice. Which is the most effective way for the therapist to prepare for the professional responsibilities this new position will entail?

Answer Choices:
A. Attend caregiver support group meetings.
B. Review current literature on evidence-based elder care. ✓
C. Review area demographic information on elders with disabilities.
D. Confer with the program's administrative director.

Correct Answer: B.

Rationale:
The therapist must update his/her knowledge base about current evidence-based practices in the care of the elderly with an emphasis on physical and cognitive disabilities. A review of the professional literature can provide relevant information about effective evaluation and intervention approaches for the setting's population. Attending a caregiver group will provide information about caregiver needs but this is not the most important area for the therapist to acquire knowledge about for this new position. Information about demographics is too broad. The program's administrative director can provide relevant information about the setting's policies, but he/she would not be able to provide information on the practice of occupational therapy.

Type of Reasoning: Inductive
This question requires one to determine the most effective approach for preparing for an entry-level job role. This requires inductive reasoning skill, where clinical judgment is paramount to arriving at a correct conclusion. For this situation, the therapist should prepare by reviewing current OT literature on evidence-based elder care. Review importance of evidence-based practice if answered incorrectly.

C93 C1

An occupational therapist provides home-based services to a child with developmental delays. The child picks up and puts away toys when reminded by the parents and mimics the parents when they dry dishes and fold clothes. The family has identified a goal of including the child in home management activities. Which activity should the therapist introduce next during intervention?

Answer Choices:
A. Wiping tabletops.
B. Sorting laundry.
C. Making a bed.
D. Taking out trash.

Correct Answer: A.

Rationale:
Picking up and putting away toys when reminded and copying the parents when they do domestic chores are home management task skills that are typical of 2-year-old children. When working with a child with a developmental delay, the therapist would use a developmental frame of reference. According to the typical developmental sequence of home management tasks, wiping spills is an ability of 3-year-old children. Therefore, the next activity the therapist should work on with the child is wiping tabletops since this is consistent with normal development. The other options are too high a level at this point for this child. Sorting laundry is typically a 4-year-old skill, making a bed and taking out trash are typically 5-year-old skills.

Type of Reasoning: Deductive
One must recall the developmental sequence of home management tasks and the developmental frame of reference in order to arrive at a correct conclusion. This is factual recall of information, which necessitates deductive reasoning skill. For this situation, the therapist should introduce wiping tabletops as the next developmental activity. If answered incorrectly, refer to Chapter 5 and developmental sequence of home management tasks, as well as the developmental frame of reference. The integration of the knowledge is pivotal to answering the question correctly.

C94 C3

A client is being discharged after recovery from hip replacement surgery to live at home alone. Which is the most important equipment for the therapist to review with the client prior to discharge?

Answer Choices:
A. A rolling walker.
B. A long-handled reacher.
C. A bedside commode.
D. An emergency call system.

Correct Answer: B.

Rationale:
The client will need to observe hip precautions for several weeks. These precautions include not flexing the hip beyond 90°, which can make retrieving items very difficult. A long-handled reacher can facilitate safety and independence in numerous tasks throughout the home. A rolling walker, bedside commode, and emergency call system can be helpful to many individuals with a variety of diagnoses. However, they are not necessary for an individual recovering from hip replacement surgery with no secondary diagnosis; therefore, they are not indicated in this case.

Type of Reasoning: Inferential
One must have knowledge of hip replacement and functional activities in the home setting in order to choose the most important equipment to recommend. This is an inferential reasoning skill where knowledge of the diagnosis coupled with the benefits of each of the described equipment is pivotal to choosing the correct solution. If answered incorrectly, review the benefits of a long-handled reacher and other adaptive aides for clients with posthip replacement precautions.

C95 C9

During an accreditation self-study, the OT department personnel review all charts. An occupational therapist notices that a colleague fills out the review forms without reading the charts. Which action is best for the therapist to take in response to this observation?

Answer Choices:
A. Talk to the colleague directly.
B. Report the incident to the director of medical records.
C. Report the colleague to the accrediting agency.
D. Report the observation to the OT supervisor.

Correct Answer: D.

Rationale:
Reporting the observation to the supervisor is the best choice since the therapist directly observed a colleague committing an act that directly violates the AOTA Code of Ethics. Any overt violation of the Code of Ethics should be reported to the direct supervisor of the practitioner. The supervisor is the person who is responsible for dealing with the situation. The therapist does not need to personally talk directly to the colleague. It is not necessary to report the incident to the accrediting agency.

Type of Reasoning: Evaluative
This question requires a value judgment in an ethical situation, which is an evaluative reasoning skill. In this situation, the colleague has violated the Code of Ethics of veracity, which is to be truthful in duties. Therefore, the therapist should report the colleague's actions to the supervisor. If answered incorrectly, review the AOTA Code of Ethics, especially veracity.

Exam C

C96 C4

An individual recovering from a head trauma exhibits a motor pattern indicative of being influenced by the symmetrical tonic neck reflex (STNR). Which is most likely for the occupational therapist to observe the client having difficulty with during functional mobility?

Answer Choices:
A. Moving both arms to midline when supine.
B. Moving from lying supine to sitting.
C. Flexing the head from the supine position.
D. Extending the head from the prone position.

Correct Answer: B.

Rationale:
Moving from lying to sitting is initiated by flexion of the neck. The presence of a STNR will cause this flexion to result in increased hip extension, making it difficult to assume a sitting position. The presence of the asymmetrical tonic neck reflex can decrease the ability to bring both arms to midline when supine. Flexing the head from a supine position would be more difficult in the presence of the tonic labyrinthine supine reflex because this reflex increases extensor tone. Extending the head from a prone position would be more difficult in the presence of the tonic labyrinthine prone reflex because this reflex increases flexor tone.

Type of Reasoning: Inferential
One must have knowledge of STNR and influence of the reflex on functional activity. This is an inferential reasoning skill where knowledge of clinical guidelines and judgment based on facts are utilized to reach conclusions. In this case the presence of a STNR can affect moving from supine to sitting. If answered incorrectly, review STNR reflex and its influence on functional activities.

C97 C8

An occupational therapist provides caregiver education to the family of an individual who is dependent in all self-care. During instruction on proper wheelchair positioning, where should the therapist advise the family to place the wheelchair seatbelt?

Answer Choices:
A. At waist level.
B. Midway between waist and trunk.
C. At the widest point of the individual's midsection.
D. At hip level. ✓

Correct Answer: D.

Rationale:
Wheelchair seat belts are to extend across the hips and into the lap at a 45° angle.

Type of Reasoning: Deductive
One must recall the proper positioning of a wheelchair seat belt in order to arrive at a correct conclusion. This requires deductive reasoning skill, where factual knowledge is essential to choosing the correct solution. Standard practice is for the seat belt to be placed at the hip level at a 45° angle. Review use of seat belts in wheelchairs and proper positioning if answered incorrectly.

C98 C9

An experienced occupational therapist assumes a new position as the director of a department of 10 therapists, 4 OTAs, 3 aides and a secretary. The department is in a state of chaos with therapists complaining about case loads and poor support from the administration. Which action is most important for the new director to take first in response to this situation?

Answer Choices:

A. Request that the director of human resources complete performance appraisals on all department employees.
B. Determine the basis of the complaints to design targeted conflict-resolution strategies.
C. Organize the distribution of patients among all the therapists.
D. Offer positive feedback to all staff on performance and attitude as merited.

Correct Answer: B.

Rationale:

The new OT director should focus on determining the basis of the complaints so that he/she can identify the interpersonal, departmental and organizational conflicts that can interfere with the delivery of services to patients. Based on the findings, the OT director should implement conflict-resolution strategies that are targeted towards the identified problems. This can include reorganizing the department, redistributing work and/or providing positive feedback. However, an evaluation of the situation is needed first to determine if these approaches or others are warranted. For example, an employee may be very effective in getting all notes done, but spends too much time using the Dictaphone so that others cannot get their notes done. Offering positive feedback to this employee for completing work can actually be detrimental to the current situation. A request that the human resources director complete performance appraisals on all department employees would not be helpful toward resolving conflict in a department that is not cohesive.

Type of Reasoning: Evaluative

One must determine the best course of action by weighing the merits of each course of action. This requires evaluative reasoning, which primarily utilizes value judgments and principles to guide one's actions. In this situation, the director should implement conflict-resolution strategies after determining the difficulties.

C99 C3

An individual with a traumatic above-elbow (transhumeral) amputation has received a body-powered prosthesis. To train the person in the operation of the terminal device (TD), which of the following should the occupational therapist do initially during intervention?

Answer Choices:

A. Teach the person how to control the elbow joint.
B. Combine training of TD use with training for elbow joint movement.
C. Lock the elbow in full extension and teach only TD control.
D. Lock the elbow in 90° of flexion and teach only TD control.

Correct Answer: D.

Rationale:

Locking the elbow joint into flexion places the TD in a functional position for the completion of activities with the TD. Locking the elbow in extension would not place the TD in a position suitable for the completion of most functional activities. The question specifically asks about training for TD operation, not control of the elbow joint. Control of the elbow joint would occur independent of TD control training, because the elbow joint must be locked for TD use in an above-elbow (transhumeral) prosthesis.

Exam C

Type of Reasoning: Inductive
One must utilize clinical knowledge and judgment to determine the training approach for an individual with an above-elbow amputation (AEA). This requires inductive reasoning skill. In this case, the therapist should lock the elbow in 90° of flexion and teach only TD control. If answered incorrectly, review training guidelines for individuals with AEA and body-powered prostheses.

C100 C5

The manager of a large occupational therapy department is planning to expand the current inpatient cardio-pulmonary rehabilitation program to include outpatient services. Which information is most relevant for the manager to include in the proposal to the hospital's administrative board?

Answer Choices:
A. Data on the inpatient rehabilitation program's outcomes. ✓
B. Testimonials from patients regarding their satisfaction with the inpatient program.
C. Statistics on physician referrals to the inpatient unit and the average length of stay.
D. Literature on cardiopulmonary rehabilitation across the continuum of care.

Correct Answer: A.

Rationale:
The provision of data on the inpatient rehabilitation program's outcomes will indicate that patients are discharged when they are able to carry out activities at a 3.5 MET level. Since many instrumental activities of daily living, work and leisure activities are at MET levels greater than 3.5, there will be a documented need for a continuation of cardiopulmonary rehabilitation services on an outpatient basis. A needs assessment that provides information indicative of an unmet program need is the first component of a program proposal. Testimonials, statistics and literature do not substantiate an unmet need that would require a program to be developed.

Type of Reasoning: Inferential
One must determine the most relevant information to provide to the hospital's administrative board that would best reflect the viability of a new outpatient rehabilitation program. In this situation, providing inpatient rehabilitation program outcomes is most relevant and beneficial for the board. Questions such as these can be challenging because one must infer or draw conclusions based upon available information and make judgments about its benefit.

C101 C3

An adult with arthritis of both hands has ulnar drift of myofascial pain syndrome (MPS) during finger extension and flexion and at rest. The patient also has a lengthening of the central slips of the extensor digitorum communis tendons of the right index and middle fingers. Which of the following should the occupational therapist report the person is exhibiting?

Answer Choices:
A. Swan-neck deformities.
B. Trigger-finger deformities.
C. MP palmar subluxation-dislocations.
D. Boutonniere deformities.

Correct Answer: D.

Rationale:

A boutonniere deformity is caused by a lengthening or rupture of the extensor digitorum communis tendons and is expressed by distal interphalangeal (DIP) hyperextension and proximal interphalangeal (PIP) flexion. A swan-neck deformity can result from the rupture of the lateral slips of the extensor digitorum communis or flexor digitorum superficialis tendon and results in DIP flexion and PIP hyperextension. A trigger-finger deformity results from a thickening of the flexor digitorum superficialis tendon at the flexor tunnel, also called a tendon sheath. The affected joint tends to stay open upon attempt to close or fist the hand. Synovitis of the MP joints can cause damage to the MP ligaments with palmar dislocation in conjunction with, or independent of, ulnar drift.

Type of Reasoning: Analytical

This question requires the test taker to determine the diagnosis from a set of symptoms, which is an analytical reasoning skill. In this situation, the symptoms indicate a boutonniere deformity. If answered incorrectly, review characteristics of boutonniere deformity.

C102 C9

An occupational therapist completes a risk management report for the reaccreditation of a rehabilitation facility. In this report, which information is most important for the therapist to include?

Answer Choices:

A. Procedures for informed consent.
B. Revenue resulting from reimbursement claims.
C. Medical necessity of resources used.
D. The appropriateness of services provided.

Correct Answer: A.

Rationale:

Risk management is a process that identifies, evaluates and takes corrective action against risk. A vital component of preventing risk and doing no harm is the acquisition of informed consent. Therefore, an occupational therapy report on risk management should include the procedures for obtaining informed consent. A description of the revenue resulting from reimbursement claims would be a component of a fiscal report and/or a statistical utilization review. A description of the appropriateness of services provided is a component of peer review and retrospective review.

Type of Reasoning: Deductive

One must recall the guidelines of a risk management report in order to arrive at a correct conclusion. This requires deductive reasoning skill, where factual knowledge is essential to choosing the correct solution. In this situation, the therapist should include procedures for informed consent, which is important in preventing harm to others. Review risk management reports if answered incorrectly.

C103 C2

An occupational therapist documents an individual's performance during a stress management group. According to established documentation standards, which statement is best for the therapist to include in the daily progress note?

Answer Choices:

A. The client completed the checklist of stressors in an appropriate amount of time.
B. The client was able to identify three current life stressors.
C. The client appeared upset and tense throughout the session.
D. The client stated walking is a relaxing and enjoyable activity.

Correct Answer: B.

Rationale:
Documentation must be specific, measurable and behavioral. In this scenario, it must provide information that is objective and related to the individual's performance in group. Timely completion of an assessment does not include sufficient information about the client's performance. More specific information would need to be provided to meet documentation standards (e.g., client became upset when discussing the stress of single parenthood while having an exacerbation of multiple sclerosis). The identification of an enjoyable and relaxing activity can be relevant information to include in documentation but this statement does not directly address the person's performance in group. In addition, more specific information would need to be provided to meet documentation standards (e.g., client states he/she goes for long walks when stressed). The report of a client appearing 'upset' is subjective and does not meet documentation standards.

Type of Reasoning: Inferential
One must determine the best statement to include in a progress note regarding a client in a stress management group. Established standards for documentation require notes to be specific, measurable and behavioral. Therefore, the therapist would most appropriately document the client's ability to identify three current life stressors. If answered incorrectly, documentation guidelines should be reviewed.

C104 C4

A school system hires an occupational therapist to implement an after-school sensorimotor integration (SI) program. The occupational therapist plans a staff in-service to explain the indications, contraindications and precautions for the use of a sensory integrative approach. Which precaution is most important for the therapist to review?

Answer Choices:
A. Self-abusive behavior.
B. Seizures.
C. Somatodyspraxia.
D. Hyperresponsiveness to sensory stimuli.

Correct Answer: B.

Rationale:
Individuals with seizures often have difficulty tolerating sensory input, especially brushing and vestibular input. These types of SI approaches can trigger seizures. Many children that can benefit from a SI approach also have a secondary diagnosis of seizure disorders; therefore, it is important that response(s) to SI interventions be carefully monitored. Since sensory integrative approaches can be inhibitory, they can be indicated for children with self-abusive behaviors or hyperresponsiveness to sensory stimuli. Somatodyspraxia is a disorder in motor planning due to poor tactile perception and proprioception and it is an indication for SI intervention.

Type of Reasoning: Inductive
Clinical knowledge and judgment are the most important skills needed for answering this question, which requires inductive reasoning skill. Knowledge of the treatment technique and diagnoses contraindicated for the technique is essential to choosing the best solution. In this case, seizures is the most important precaution. Review precautions and contraindications for SI intervention if answered incorrectly.

C105 C6

An individual diagnosed with schizophrenia, undifferentiated type, is referred to a partial hospitalization program. During the initial evaluation interview, the occupational therapist observes that the client answers each question by consistently returning to the focus of the first question. Each time the therapist introduces a new topic to discuss in the interview, the client ignores this topic and returns to the original topical focus. When documenting the client's behavior, which of the following is most accurate for the therapist to report the client is demonstrating?

Answer Choices:
A. Thought blocking.
B. Perseveration.
C. Obsessive thinking.
D. Poverty of speech.

Correct Answer: B.

Rationale:
Perseveration is a persistent focus on a previous topic or behavior after a new topic or behavior is introduced. Thought blocking is the interruption of a thought process before it's carried to completion. Obsessive thinking involves the persistence of an illogical thought. Poverty of speech is speech that is limited in amount and content.

Type of Reasoning: Analytical
This question provides symptoms and the test taker must determine the likely cause for them. This is an analytical reasoning skill, as questions of this nature often ask one to analyze a group of symptoms in order to determine a diagnosis. In this situation the symptoms indicate perseveration, which should be reviewed if answered incorrectly.

C106 C3

A teenager with congenital bilateral above-elbow amputations is referred to OT to increase independence in ADL. The adolescent wants to be independent in donning and doffing shirts. Which action is best for the therapist to take first?

Answer Choices:
A. Refer the patient to a prosthetist.
B. Evaluate abdominal strength.
C. Evaluate the use of adapted equipment in dressing.
D. Evaluate trunk and lower extremity ROM.

Correct Answer: D.

Rationale:
Upon receipt of a referral, the therapist must complete an evaluation. Thus, the first step in this case is to evaluate trunk and lower extremity ROM to determine if the patient can use the lower extremities to dress, as many persons with amelia do. Hip ROM is essential to be able to don shirts with the feet. After ruling out adapted techniques, the next step would be to attempt adapted equipment. Most people who are missing both upper extremities do not use prostheses for dressing especially since the body jacket to the prosthetic arms prevents trunk flexion. Evaluation of abdominal strength might be helpful but it is not the first action to take.

Exam C

Type of Reasoning: Inferential
One must infer or draw conclusions about the first action a therapist is likely to take given a patient's diagnosis and goals. Having an understanding of amelia and typical dressing strategies is pivotal to arrive at a correct conclusion. In this case, the therapist should first evaluate trunk and lower extremity ROM. If answered incorrectly, review the characteristics of amelia and adaptive dressing strategies. The integration of this information is required to determine the correct answer.

C107 C6

A patient with a diagnosis of borderline personality disorder attends a stress management group on an inpatient psychiatric unit. During the group, the patient's roommate states that there is a pocket knife in the patient's backpack. The patient says the roommate is exaggerating and that the item is only a keychain. Which should the occupational therapist do in response to these statements?

Answer Choices:
A. Immediately inform the charge nurse. ✓
B. Immediately check the patient's backpack.
C. Check the patient's backpack after the group session.
D. Meet with the patient's individual therapist after the group session.

Correct Answer: A.

Rationale:
The possibility that there is any item on an inpatient psychiatric unit that could be used by a person to harm him/herself presents a danger to all; therefore, the charge nurse must be immediately notified. Searching the backpack may or may not produce the item and it is not the occupational therapist's role to conduct a room or person search.

Type of Reasoning: Evaluative
One must weigh the possible courses of action and then make a value judgment about the best course to take. This requires evaluative reasoning skill, which often utilizes guiding principles of action in order to arrive at a correct conclusion. For this case, because the object could harm the patient or others, the therapist should immediately contact the charge nurse. Review safety protocols for inpatient psychiatric facilities if answered incorrectly.

C108 C4

The parents of a school-aged child with Rett syndrome ask the occupational therapist for activities to do at home to help their child regain lost skills. Which of the following should the therapist include in the home program for the parents to do with their child?

Answer Choices:
A. Encourage the child to use pressure distribution techniques.
B. Use four-step sequencing cards to increase attention.
C. Give positive feedback for active ROM performance.
D. Perform passive ROM to prevent contractures. ✓

Correct Answer: D.

Rationale:
Rett syndrome is a genetic progressive disorder in which motor, cognitive, social and language skills deteriorate. If the child is school-aged, it is highly likely that the child has experienced significant functional decline. Regardless of the child's current functional level, children with this progressive condition cannot regain lost skills. Therefore, the home program must focus on maintaining function and preventing complications. Passive ROM is an activity that the parents can do to prevent contractures, which are a complication of this progressive condition. The child will not be able to respond to encouragement to use pressure distribution techniques. Since pressure relief is important to prevent the complication of skin breakdown, a more appropriate approach is to make sure that the parents are aware of correct positioning and the need to change positions frequently. The child in this scenario will not be able to attend to sequencing cards to increase attention or independently perform ROM.

Type of Reasoning: Inferential
One must link the child's diagnosis to the activities presented in order to determine which activity would be the most likely recommendation. This requires inferential reasoning, where one uses knowledge of a diagnosis to choose a best course of action. In this case passive ROM is the most likely recommendation. Review symptoms of Rett syndrome if answered incorrectly.

C109 C7

A child with short attention span and processing difficulties is referred to occupational therapy. Based on the results of a screening, the therapist decides to focus the evaluation on sensory processing performance skills. Which should the therapist evaluate?

Answer Choices:
A. Form-constancy.
B. Right-left discrimination.
C. Proprioception.
D. Spatial relations.

Correct Answer: C.

Rationale:
Proprioception is a component of sensory processing performance skills. Form-constancy, right-left discrimination and spatial relations are all part of perceptual processing.

Type of Reasoning: Deductive
This question requires recall of guidelines and principles, which is factual knowledge. Deductive reasoning skills are utilized whenever one must recall facts to solve novel problems. In this situation, one must recall the OT Practice Framework guidelines, which indicate that the performance skill of proprioception is part of sensory processing. Review the OT Practice Framework, especially sensory processing if answered incorrectly.

C110 C8

Following an exacerbation of postpolio syndrome, a client is referred to occupational therapy for a wheelchair evaluation to enable independent mobility. The client wears bilateral hip-knee-ankle-foot orthoses (HKAFOs) to provide support during independent transfers and brief standing periods throughout the workday. The client's insurance is Medicare. Which is the best seat-width measurement for the occupational therapist to recommend for the client's wheelchair prescription?

Answer Choices:

A. Two inches wider than the widest point across the individual's hips or thighs.
B. Four inches wider than the widest point across the individual's hips or thighs while wearing orthoses.
C. A standard adult seat width to ensure Medicare reimbursement.
D. Two inches wider than the point across the individual's hips or thighs while wearing orthoses.

Correct Answer: D.

Rationale:

Two inches wider than the individual's widest measurement with the orthoses on will allow for ease of movement in and out of the chair. If the width of the orthoses is not included in the seat measurement the chair will be too tight. A standard-width adult chair would not meet this individual's needs. Four inches added to the measurement while wearing orthoses would significantly increase the width of the chair. This can complicate mobility in hallways, office spaces and through doorways. Medicare does reimburse for wheelchairs that are prescribed based upon an individual's measurements.

Type of Reasoning: Inferential

One must have knowledge of HKAFOs and wheelchair prescription guidelines in order to arrive at a correct conclusion. This is an inferential reasoning skill where knowledge of clinical guidelines and judgment based on facts are utilized to reach conclusions. In this situation, the therapist should recommend a seat width two inches wider than the point across the person's hips or thighs while wearing the orthoses. If answered incorrectly, review wheelchair prescription guidelines and use of HKAFOs.

C111 C9

The parents of a child referred to occupational therapy ask the occupational therapist to treat their child who does not have insurance and bill for services in the name of their older who does have insurance. Which is the therapist's best response to this situation?

Answer Choices:

A. Deny the request.
B. Report the parents to the insurance company.
C. Refer the parents to the department supervisor.
D. Ask the family to get a referral from a physician.

Correct Answer: A.

Rationale:

This is an unethical request. The therapist must deny this type of request. It is feasible for one child to have met the limits of the insurance and no longer be eligible for benefits, or to have a preexisting condition such as cerebral palsy and not be insured by the carrier. There is no need to report the parents since no violation of the law has been committed. It can be a good idea to discuss the issue with the supervisor, but this does not preclude the reality that the occupational therapist must deny this request.

Type of Reasoning: Evaluative

This question requires a value judgment in an ethical situation, which is an evaluative reasoning skill. Following the OT Code of Ethics, all therapists should observe veracity, which is to be truthful in the delivery of services. Therefore, the correct response of the therapist is to deny the request. Review the OT Code of Ethics if answered incorrectly.

C112 **C2**

A 2-month-old infant with bilateral hip dislocation is being discharged home from an acute pediatric facility. The occupational therapist has developed a home program for the parents of this firstborn child. Which is most important for the occupational therapist to determine before instructing the parents in the details of this home program?

Answer Choices:
A. The child's insurance reimbursement plan.
B. The parents' level of formal education.
C. The family's home environment.
D. The parents' degree of anxiety.

Correct Answer: D.

Rationale:
Prior to providing the parents with details about the home program, the occupational therapist should determine the parents' level of anxiety since excess anxiety could impact their comprehension and retention of the instructions given. This is an appropriate use of interactive reasoning and can help build rapport with the parents. This can contribute to increased compliance with the prescribed home program. While the other factors may also be considered, they do not represent immediate priorities for hospital-based instruction.

Type of Reasoning: Inductive
This question requires one to utilize clinical judgment in order to determine the most important item to assess before instructing the parents in a home exercise program. This requires inductive reasoning skill. In this case, it is most important to determine the parents' degree of anxiety and attention. Review home program development guidelines in pediatric settings if answered incorrectly.

Multiple Choice Scenario Item C.II.

Questions C113 to C116 are based on the following information.

An occupational therapist working in a private clinic receives a referral for a client who incurred a nerve laceration while working as a cable installer and repair person. Upon evaluation, the therapist determines that the client exhibits maximum motor and sensory losses consistent with a radial nerve laceration below the supinator.

C113 **C3**

The occupational therapist documents the results of the evaluation. Which deformity should the therapist note that the client is exhibiting?

Answer Choices:
A. "Claw" hand.
B. Wrist drop.
C. "Ape" hand.
D. "Saturday night" palsy.

Correct Answer: B.

Rationale:
The presenting signs of a radial nerve laceration are weakness or paralysis of the extensors of the wrist, MCPs, and thumb with a characteristic wrist drop. "Ape" hand, which presents as a flattening of the thenar eminence, is indicative of a median nerve palsy. A "claw" hand is indicative of ulnar nerve palsy. "Saturday night palsy" is a term used to denote a radial nerve palsy that results from a position that compresses the radial nerve.

Type of Reasoning: Inferential
One must link the diagnosis provided to the symptoms presented in order to determine which definition most accurately represents a radial nerve laceration. This requires inferential reasoning, where one must infer or draw conclusions about a diagnosis. In this case symptoms of radial nerve laceration include weakness of the wrist, MCP and thumb extensors. Review symptoms of radial nerve lacerations if answered incorrectly

C114 C3

The occupational therapist constructs a splint to facilitate healing and promote function. Which is the most effective splint for the therapist to fabricate for this individual?

Answer Choices:
A. A dynamic extension splint. ✓
B. A figure-of-eight splint. ⎫ same
C. A dynamic flexion splint. ⎭
D. A splint to support the functional position.

Correct Answer: A.

Rationale:
A radial nerve injury below the supinator is classified as a low-level radial nerve injury. Presenting signs include incomplete extension of the fingers' and thumb's MP joints. The IP joints are extended by the interossei, but the MP joints rest in about 30° flexion. A dynamic splint that provides wrist, MP' and thumb extension is indicated for radial nerve palsy to prevent over-stretching of the extensor tendons during the healing phase. This splint also positions the hand for functional use. A figure-of-eight splint or a dynamic flexion splint is indicated for a combined median ulnar nerve injury. The functional position of wrist extension, MCP's flexion, IP's flexion and thumb abducted is not effective in radial nerve palsy intervention.

Type of Reasoning: Analytical
This question provides a description of an injury and the test taker must determine the most appropriate splint to address the injury. This is an analytical reasoning skill, as questions of this nature often ask one to analyze information in order to determine a proper course of action. In this situation the ideal splint to fabricate is a dynamic extensor splint. Review splinting for low radial nerve injury if answered incorrectly.

C115 C8

Through active participation in individual occupational therapy sessions, the client regains functional motor skills. To facilitate return to work, the occupational therapist refers the client to a local work-hardening program. This program does not have the exact equipment that the client uses in the job setting. Which action is best for the therapist at the work-hardening program to take in response to this situation?

Answer Choices:
A. Refer the client to another work-hardening program that has the equipment.
B. Order and install the equipment necessary to duplicate the work setting.
C. Perform some necessary aspects of rehabilitation in the client's work setting.
D. Duplicate the job task components as closely as possible. ✓

Correct Answer: D.

Rationale:
Work-hardening programs can use real or simulated tasks that duplicate as closely as possible the components of each client's job tasks. It is not realistic for all programs to have every possible piece of equipment related to clients' job tasks. Consequently, therapists become skilled at activity analysis and adept at simulating job tasks with the equipment that they have available. A therapist who is experienced in work-hardening can provide effective intervention without equipment that exactly matches the client's work. Therefore, there is no reason to refer the client to another facility. A reason to refer a client to another facility is the therapy staff's lack of experience and inability to provide effective intervention. It may be helpful to perform some aspects of rehabilitation during a site visit, but the logistics of this can be difficult and the therapist's ability to provide intensive therapy in a work environment would likely be limited. Therefore, the best answer is to duplicate the job tasks in the clinic.

Type of Reasoning: Evaluative
This question requires the test taker to weigh the merits of each of the possible courses of action. This necessitates evaluative reasoning skill, where value judgments are paramount to arriving at a correct conclusion. In this situation, the most appropriate action is for the therapist to duplicate the job task components as closely as possible. Questions of this nature can be challenging, as value judgments often do not have clear-cut answers. Review therapeutic approaches to job simulation in work-hardening settings if answered incorrectly.

C116 C3

The client successfully completes the work-hardening program. However, the client has residual moderate impairment in temperature perception. During the discharge planning session, the therapist discusses how this impairment may impact areas of occupation and suggests activity modifications to facilitate the client's occupational performance. What is the most appropriate recommendation for the therapist to make to the client?

Answer Choices:
A. Request reassignment to work activities that do not involve exposure to extreme temperatures.
B. Mark all potentially hot objects at home and at work with bright stickers.
C. Wear work gloves for activities involving extremes or variations in temperature.
D. Wear a protective splint during the work day and at home during home maintenance tasks.

Correct Answer: C.

Rationale:
The client should wear work gloves because of the danger of incurring a burn because of diminished temperature sensation. The work gloves can also protect the client's hands during extreme cold situations. As a cable installer and repair person, the essential functions of the client's job will frequently require him/her to work outdoors in all types of weather conditions. Reassigning the client is not needed since he/she developed the skills needed to adequately perform all essential work tasks in the work-hardening program. During the performance of work tasks, the client can easily compensate for sensory deficits by wearing work gloves. Since there is no co-morbidity of a cognitive deficit, the client can be expected to be able to remember to don gloves to protect the hands when he/she judges a situation that may involve extremes or variations in temperature. A splint would provide inadequate protection because it would not fully cover all surfaces of the hand.

Type of Reasoning: Inductive
The test taker must determine which recommendation most effectively addresses the client's current status and limitations. Because temperature perception is impaired, wearing work gloves when involved in activities that may involve extremes or variations in temperature is best to protect the client from injury. If answered incorrectly review recommendations for temperature impairments and guidelines for adaptations of work tasks.

C117 C3

An occupational therapist conducts a sensory evaluation for an individual with cubital tunnel syndrome. Which of the following is the most likely location for this person's sensory symptoms?

Answer Choices:
A. The ulnar aspect of the forearm and hand.✓
B. Along the radial nerve distribution of the hand.
C. The medial aspect of the forearm and hand.
D. Along the ulnar nerve distribution of the hand.

Correct Answer: A.

Rationale:
Cubital tunnel syndrome is an ulnar nerve compression at the elbow. Its presenting symptoms are numbness and tingling along the ulnar aspect of the forearm and hand, pain at the elbow with extreme elbow flexion, weakness of power grip and a positive Tinel's sign at the elbow.

Type of Reasoning: Inferential
One must have knowledge of cubital tunnel syndrome and presenting symptoms in order to arrive at a correct conclusion. This is an inferential reasoning skill where one must draw conclusions about a diagnosis. For this situation, the numbness and tingling would typically be reported along the ulnar aspect of the forearm and hand. If answered incorrectly, review symptoms of cubital tunnel syndrome.

C118 C9

An occupational therapist designs a quantitative research study to examine the treatment efficacy of a pain-management program. Which method of data collection is best for the therapist to use?

Answer Choices:
A. A survey with open-ended questions.
B. A survey with Likert-style questions.✓
C. A discussion with focus groups.
D. Individualized interviews with program participants.

Correct Answer: B.

Rationale:
Likert-style questions ask for data along a numerical scale, which would provide quantitative data. The other choices do not provide quantitative data.

Type of Reasoning: Deductive
One must recall the guidelines for quantitative research and methods. This is factual knowledge, which is a deductive reasoning skill. In this case, the only method that is quantitative in nature is a survey with Likert-style questions. If answered incorrectly, review quantitative research methods, especially Likert surveys.

C119 C9

A patient with fibromyalgia is receiving occupational therapy to reduce pain and promote flexibility during ADL tasks. The patient expresses the intent to discontinue treatment based on information obtained during an online search which questioned the value of therapy for fibromyalgia. Which of the following actions should the occupational therapist take first in response to the patient's statements?

Answer Choices:

A. Confront the inaccuracy of these statements and provide current evidence-based research about the benefits of therapy for persons with fibromyalgia.
B. Reassure the patient that the physician has ordered therapy; therefore, it will be beneficial.
C. Respect the patient's wishes and discontinue occupational therapy, offering to provide therapy in the future if symptoms exacerbate.
D. Inform the patient that online information can be inaccurate and provide literature about the benefits of therapy for fibromyalgia.

Correct Answer: D.

Rationale:

It is common for patients to seek out more information about their condition. The Internet can be informative and resourceful. It can also be inaccurate, incomplete and misleading. Occupational therapists are responsible for making sure patients have accurate information about their conditions in order to make informed decisions. In this case, the therapist should inform the patient of the inaccurate information and provide accurate information about exercise related to his/her condition. It is not as beneficial to directly confront the inaccuracies of this information with the latest research. This stance can be overwhelming and lead to the person feeling belittled. Reminding the patient of the physician's orders does not respect the patient's feelings or address his/her concerns. Discontinuing treatment overlooks the need to provide accurate information first to ensure the patient is making an informed decision.

Type of Reasoning: Evaluative

This situation requires one to consider the AOTA Code of Ethics guidelines of beneficence, nonmaleficence (do no harm) and autonomy (the right to refuse). This necessitates evaluative reasoning skill, where the test taker must determine a proper course of action that respects the rights of the patient while doing no harm. In this situation, the therapist should inform the patient of the inaccurate information and provide accurate information about the benefits of exercise. If answered incorrectly, review the AOTA Code of Ethics, especially beneficence, nonmaleficence and autonomy.

C120 C8

A parent admitted to a psychosocial day treatment program has a diagnosis of major depressive disorder. Results of the occupational therapy screening process indicate that the person is having difficulty performing home management tasks and caring for two young children. The occupational therapist has determined the need to gather further data regarding past and current performance. The therapist decides that the recently hired, entry-level occupational therapy assistant (OTA) will contribute to the evaluation process. Which evaluation is best for the therapist to assign to the OTA to complete?

Answer Choices:

A. A cognitive evaluation.
B. An ADL evaluation.
C. A mental status examination.
D. An occupational history interview.

Correct Answer: B.

Rationale:
OTAs are trained and qualified to perform ADL evaluations during their entry-level education. The ability to complete a cognitive evaluation, mental status examination and an occupational history interview require the establishment of the OTA's service competence prior to the assignment of these evaluation tasks. The establishment of service competency requires the acquisition of experience and continuing training. The OTA in this scenario has been recently hired and is an entry-level practitioner; therefore, service competency for these additional evaluations would not have yet been established.

Type of Reasoning: Deductive
This question requires recall of guidelines and principles, which is factual knowledge. Deductive reasoning skills are utilized whenever one must recall facts to solve clinical problems. In this situation, the OTA can contribute to the evaluation process by performing an ADL evaluation. Review supervisory guidelines for OTAs, especially the evaluation process if answered incorrectly.

C121 C2

An occupational therapist works in a school setting with adolescents with Asperger's syndrome. The need for a social skills training group is identified. One activity that the therapist plans to use in the group is roleplaying. Which is the most effective way for the therapist to determine relevant scenarios for the role-play activities?

Answer Choices:
A. Survey the teachers on social difficulties displayed in class.
B. Survey parents on social difficulties they have observed in the adolescents.
C. Review literature on adolescent social skill development.
D. Ask the group members about their social concerns.

Correct Answer: D.

Rationale:
Directly asking members about their concerns will enable the therapist to identify areas of common concern that can serve as the basis of relevant role-play scenarios. This will foster Yalom's curative factor of universality. The ability to express one's concerns and needs is especially important to adolescents since their main developmental task is to separate from parents and develop their own self-identity. Surveying others provides information on their perceptions of the adolescents' needs. This may or may not be an accurate reflection of members' needs. Reviewing developmental literature can be helpful in understanding adolescent concerns but it cannot be used to plan role-play scenarios for a specific group of adolescents with unique needs.

Type of Reasoning: Inductive
This question requires one to determine the best approach for determining group members' needs. This requires inductive reasoning skill, where clinical judgment is paramount to arriving at a correct conclusion. For this situation, the therapist should ask the group members about their social concerns. If answered incorrectly, review group intervention techniques including role playing and the functional impact of Asperger's syndrome. The integration of this knowledge is required to answer the question correctly.

C122 C3

An individual with complex regional pain syndrome (CRPS), Type I, presents with severe pain and pitting edema in the right hand. The individual has a secondary diagnosis of degenerative joint disease (DJD). Which should the occupational therapist initially recommend to the person to address these concerns?

Answer Choices:

A. Passive range of motion of wrist and fingers.
B. Retrograde massage from distal to proximal.
C. Elevation of the affected hand above the heart.
D. Retrograde massage from proximal to distal.

Correct Answer: C.

Rationale:

Elevation of the affected hand above the heart will promote venous and lymphatic drainage and decrease the hydrostatic pressure in the blood vessels. Retrograde massage is performed in a centripetal direction. It is not the initial treatment when severe pain is present. Passive range of motion is not advisable for persons with DJD.

Type of Reasoning: Inductive

This question requires one to determine the best recommendation for addressing the patient's symptoms. This requires inductive reasoning skill, where clinical judgment is paramount to arriving at a correct conclusion. For this situation, the OT should initially recommend elevation of the affected hand above the heart. If answered incorrectly, review treatment guidelines for patients with CRPS Type I and pitting edema.

C123 C6

A home care hospice occupational therapist works with a client with end-stage non-Hodgkin's lymphoma. The client is very knowledgeable about this illness and has been active in all aspects of its treatment. The client has requested activity ideas to fill the hours while family members are at work and at school. Which activity is best for the occupational therapist to suggest to this client?

Answer Choices:

A. Complete a series of progressive resistive exercises to maintain upper extremity strength and endurance.
B. Make personalized memory scrapbooks for each family member.
C. Research alternative and complementary medicine approaches on the Internet.
D. Prepare an entree and dessert for the family's evening meal.

Correct Answer: B.

Rationale:

One of the main goals of hospice care is to encourage positive life review and support the sharing of the legacy that each person leaves. Creating personal memory scrapbooks can accomplish this goal and help provide a method for the family to remember and share treasured memories while the person is still living. Progressive resistance exercises are contraindicated for someone who is terminally ill and at the end-stage of the illness. These exercises can increase exhaustion. Researching alternative and complementary health care can be beneficial for a person with a deadly illness, but it does not address the need of the person in hospice for closure with significant others. In addition, the efficacy of these approaches for end-stage illness has not been demonstrated. It would be counter-therapeutic to promote an activity that could give false hope. Preparing items for an evening meal can maintain relevant role function, but this activity does not address the end-of-life issues or needs which are the focus of hospice care.

Type of Reasoning: Inferential

One must infer or draw conclusions about a likely course of action, given the information presented. This is an inferential reasoning skill, where knowledge of a therapeutic approach, such as activities for persons with terminal illness, is essential in choosing a correct solution. In this case, the therapist should suggest making memory scrapbooks for the family. Review the intervention approaches for persons in hospice care if answered incorrectly.

C124 C9

An occupational therapist provides consultation services to a nursing home and is developing a restraint reduction program. The therapist is also a faculty member in an occupational therapy professional education program. The therapist uses this consultation experience to explain to the students the role of occupational therapy. Which of the following is most accurate for the therapist to state this consultation experience represents?

Answer Choices:

A. Direct service.
B. Primary prevention.
C. Secondary prevention.
D. Needs assessment.

Correct Answer: C.

Rationale:

Secondary prevention involves the early detection of problems in a population that have diagnoses that place them at risk for the development of complicating or secondary conditions. Residents of a nursing home have preexisting medical conditions and disabilities. A restraint reduction program's aim is to prevent the development of secondary conditions, such as deconditioning. Direct service requires the implementation of intervention with clients by the therapist. A consultant for program development is not responsible for the implementation of intervention. Primary prevention targets individuals with no preexisting conditions. Needs assessment is done to determine programming needs and would have been conducted to identify the need for the restraint reduction program.

Type of Reasoning: Analytical

This question requires the test taker to determine the type of skilled service provided according to a description, which is an analytical reasoning skill. Questions of this nature often call upon the test taker to analyze an activity based on a functional description in order to draw a correct conclusion. Based on this information, the activity is that of secondary prevention, which should be reviewed if answered incorrectly.

C125 C8

An elder resident of a skilled nursing facility becomes tearful during an occupational therapy session. The resident has a diagnosis of advanced osteoarthritis and relates that pain is causing discomfort during sexual activities. The resident expresses fear about "losing" a valued intimate relationship and asks the occupational therapist for advice. Which is the most beneficial action for the therapist to take in response to the resident's expressed concerns?

Answer Choices:

A. Refer the resident to social work for individual counseling.
B. Explore the resident's goals for sexual expression.
C. Refer the resident and the resident's significant other to social work for couples counseling.
D. Advise nursing of the resident's statements to ensure that sexual behavior is monitored.

Correct Answer: B.

Rationale:

Sexuality and sexual expression are within the practice domain of occupational therapy. It is important for the therapist to create an atmosphere that enables the person to express his/her concerns. Once the individual's goals for sexual expression are established, strategies to attain these goals can be explored. These strategies can include the use of activity analysis, gradation, modification and simplification, non-medical methods to manage pain and stiffness (e.g., warm baths), positioning alternatives, adaptive equipment, energy conservation methods and/or referral(s) to other professionals. It is inappropriate for staff to monitor consensual sexual expression of any individual, regardless of age or facility.

Type of Reasoning: Inductive

Clinical knowledge and judgment are the most important skills needed for answering this question, which requires inductive reasoning skill. Knowledge of occupational therapy's domains of practice is essential for arriving at a correct conclusion. In this case, the therapist should explore the resident's goals for sexual expression and strategies to achieve goals. Review OT guidelines for sexual expression if answered incorrectly.

C126 C5

An adolescent with a complete myelomeningocele at the T9 level is diagnosed with diabetes. The occupational therapist meets with the adolescent and a nurse practitioner to review the impact of this new diagnosis on the teen's health and daily routines. Which is most important for the therapist to emphasize during this discussion?

Answer Choices:

A. Skin inspection performed by a parent.
B. Upper extremity strengthening.
C. Self-directed pressure relief.
D. Self-initiated pressure relief.

Correct Answer: D.

Rationale:

The person with complete myelomeningocele at the T9 level has absent sensation in the lower extremities and buttocks. Therefore, frequent pressure relief is essential to prevent skin breakdown. While it is likely that the teen has previously been taught pressure relief techniques, the new diagnosis of diabetes makes a review of the importance of consistent and routine pressure relief a priority. Skin care and inspection is an important element to include in programs for people with diabetes, especially for those with absent sensation. However, it would be unlikely that an adolescent would want to have an adult inspect the skin. Upper extremity strengthening can be helpful to provide pressure relief; however, a T9 lesion does not affect the upper extremities so the adolescent's strength is likely within functional limitations. Consequently, the teen is capable of self-initiating pressure relief and does not have to self-direct the performance of this routine activity.

Type of Reasoning: Inferential

One must understand the nature of both myelomeningocele and diabetes in order to arrive at a correct conclusion. Inferential reasoning skills are utilized as the test taker must infer the nature of both of these diagnoses and then determine the most important home education guidelines based on this knowledge. In this case, self-initiated pressure relief is most important to prevent skin breakdown. If answered incorrectly, review symptoms of myelomeningocele and diabetes, especially the importance of pressure relief.

Exam C

C127 C9

An adult with hereditary ataxia receives home care occupational therapy services. Recently, the client has become more withdrawn and the client's spouse has become more verbal about caregiver strain. During an intervention session, the occupational therapist works with the client on attaining the goal of dressing independently. The therapist notices and comments on several large bruises on the middle section of the client's back. The client tearfully states that a bad fall that morning had caused these and that the progression of the ataxia is becoming too difficult to handle. Which action is best for the therapist to take in response to the observed bruises and the client's statements?

Answer Choices:

A. Provide reassurance and support of the client's legitimate feelings of loss.
B. Conduct an evaluation of the home to remove items that can contribute to falls.
C. Report the incident to the local domestic violence hotline.
D. Supportively question the client about the incident.

Correct Answer: D.

Rationale:

While persons with ataxia often do fall resulting in bruises, it would require a very unusual fall to incur bruises in the middle of the back. The possibility that the injuries were the result of an incident of domestic violence must be seriously considered given the location of the injury and the increasing evidence of caregiver strain. The client may respond to the therapist's supportive questioning and share concerns. Due to the serious nature of domestic violence, the therapist must provide the client with this opportunity to disclose. Providing reassurance and conducting a home evaluation may be relevant to the case, but they do not assess the immediate need to determine if the individual is a victim of domestic violence. Contacting the domestic violence hotline when a client has not disclosed this as a problem is premature since a shelter can only work with persons who self-disclose. This action could increase the client's fear of disclosure and escalate the situation.

Type of Reasoning: Evaluative

This question requires a value judgment in an ethical situation, which is an evaluative reasoning skill. In this situation, there is evidence of injury, which could be caused by abuse rather than a fall. Ethical situations such as these often rely upon guiding principles of action to choose best courses of action. Because the potential for abuse exists, the therapist's most appropriate course of action is to supportively question the client about the incident. Review guidelines for addressing and following up on suspected abuse if answered incorrectly.

C128 C3

After a work-related injury to the left index finger, an assembly line worker is fit with a buddy strap incorporating the index and middle fingers. In describing the primary purpose of the strap to the client, which of the following explanations is most accurate for the therapist to state?

Answer Choices:

A. "The strap provides passive ROM to the index finger."
B. "The strap reduces edema in the index finger."
C. "The strap immobilizes the index finger."
D. "The strap provides active ROM to the index finger."

Correct Answer: A.

Rationale:

The buddy strap helps to provide passive ROM to the injured finger. The buddy strap can also help to improve a deformity that has been caused by immobilization due to injury, weakness or casting. A buddy strap on the finger can sometimes result in increased edema due to restricted circulation. Elevation of the finger, retrograde massage and contrast baths are techniques that help to reduce edema. The strap immobilizes the finger IP joints and thereby limits active ROM.

Type of Reasoning: Inferential

One must infer or draw conclusions about the possible effects of a buddy strap involving the middle or index finger. The benefit is typically passive ROM to the injured finger. In order to arrive at a correct conclusion, one must understand the indications for issuing a buddy strap, which should be reviewed if answered incorrectly.

C129 C7

An occupational therapist completes the discharge plan for an individual with a right cerebral vascular accident (CVA) who has completed a 3-week inpatient rehabilitation program. The person is right-hand dominant. The patient exhibits residual cognitive perceptual deficits but seems unaware of these problems. Which discharge recommendation is best for the therapist to discuss with the patient and the patient's family?

Answer Choices:

A. An extension of length of stay.
B. A full-time home health aide.
C. Assistance with personal care.
D. Supervision for cooking.

Correct Answer: D.

Rationale:

A right CVA results in left-sided deficits, decreased judgment and diminished insight. The latter two deficits can pose a safety risk during cooking activities. Therefore, supervision is recommended. Since the person is right-hand dominant, the ability to perform many personal tasks will likely remain intact. In addition, it is highly likely that the individual has received intervention to increase the functional abilities of his/her left upper extremity (UE) and/or to develop unilateral functional skills during his/her 3-week rehabilitation program. Therefore, a full-time home health aide, personal care assistance and an extension of length of stay are not warranted.

Type of Reasoning: Inductive

One must utilize clinical knowledge and judgment to determine the recommendation that best considers the person's limitations. This requires inductive reasoning skill. In this case, recommending supervision for cooking is best out of the choices provided. If answered incorrectly, review intervention planning guidelines and IADL activity adaptations for persons with cognitive deficits and discharge options for persons with disabilities.

C130 C2

An occupational therapist steps in, at the last minute, to assist another therapist with a problem-solving skills group. Which is the most helpful action for the occupational therapist to take?

Answer Choices:

A. Split the group in two and have each therapist work with his/her own group.
B. Participate as a member of the group and supply the desired responses.
C. Support the leader with comments and questions that keep the group on focus.
D. Act as an observer and take notes for documentation.

Correct Answer: C.

Rationale:

The role of assisting a group leader is to facilitate participation of the members and the achievement of the goals of the group. Splitting members into two groups would result in the assisting therapist having no knowledge of the group's history, process or goals. In addition, the existing leader would receive no input from a co-leader. The benefit of receiving feedback from a co-leader is likely the precipitant for the group leader asking the therapist to participate. Participating as a member, an observer and/or a recorder also do not provide any co-leadership benefits.

Type of Reasoning: Inductive

Clinical knowledge and judgment are the most important skills needed for answering this question, which requires inductive reasoning skill. Knowledge of the group processes and effective co-leadership are essential to choosing the best solution. In this case, the therapist should support the leader with comments and questions that keep the group on focus. If answered incorrectly, review effective group co-leadership strategies.

C131 C3

An individual has relocated to a new area and begins treatment at an outpatient occupational therapy clinic for follow-up after rotator cuff surgery. It is 6 weeks' postoperation. Which is the most effective intervention for the occupational therapist to implement at this time?

Answer Choices:

A. An isometric strengthening program.
B. Passive range of motion.
C. Active assistive ROM.
D. An isotonic strengthening program.

Correct Answer: A.

Rationale:

Strengthening should begin with isometrics at 6 weeks and then progress to isotonics. PROM progressing to active assisted/active range of motion (AA/AROM) is the intervention for 0–6 weeks' postoperation.

Type of Reasoning: Deductive

This question requires recall of guidelines, which is factual knowledge. Deductive reasoning skills are utilized whenever one must recall facts to solve novel problems. In this situation, a patient who is 6 weeks' postoperation for rotator cuff repair can begin an isometric strengthening program. Review treatment guidelines for postsurgical rotator cuff repair if answered incorrectly.

C132 C1

A school-based occupational therapist receives a referral for evaluation from a third-grade teacher. The teacher reports difficulty with a student who has illegible handwriting, poor attending behaviors, questionable visual skills, and problems with pencil management. After speaking with the teacher, reviewing classroom work samples and reading the student's history, which action should the therapist take next?

Answer Choices:

A. Provide pencil grips and specialized paper as a trial to determine interventions.
B. Directly observe the student during a naturally occurring writing time.
C. Administer a standardized visual perceptual and visual motor assessment.
D. Administer a standardized handwriting assessment.

Correct Answer: B.

Rationale:

Skilled observation during a writing activity is an essential part of the evaluation process. Noting the student's performance in the classroom should precede standardized testing of performance skills. The observation and teacher interview should then direct the therapist to the most appropriate standardized measures if needed. Assessment needs to be completed prior to implementing interventions.

Type of Reasoning: Inductive

This question requires one to determine a best course of action, given the information provided. This requires inductive reasoning skill, where one must use clinical judgment to determine the best approach for evaluating this child. In this situation, the therapist should directly observe the student during a naturally occurring writing time. If answered incorrectly, review observational guidelines for the evaluation of functional skills and the developmental skills required for effective classroom participation. The integration of this knowledge is required for the determination of a correct answer.

C133 C4

An elementary school student is referred to occupational therapy to improve fine motor skills. The student is having difficulty drawing simple shapes (i.e., circle, square, and triangle) and cutting a straight line with scissors. Which of the following activities is best to help develop the arches of the hand and increase hand strength to improve the student's ability to grasp a writing utensil or scissors?

Answer Choices:

A. Spell vocabulary words using three-dimensional letter shapes.
B. Identify simple shapes with vision occluded.
C. Complete a puzzle lying prone on the floor.
D. Chair push-ups before tabletop activities.

Correct Answer: D.

Rationale:

Weight-bearing activities, such as chair push-ups, help develop the arches of the hand and strengthen intrinsic muscles of the hand to improve fine motor activities. Using three-dimensional letter shapes to spell vocabulary words does not provide resistance to increase muscle strength. Identifying simple shapes with vision occluded is stereognosis and does not address developing hand arches and muscle strength. Lying on the floor to complete a puzzle will provide weight bearing through the shoulder and increase shoulder stability, but it does not develop the arches of the hand or increase hand strength.

Type of Reasoning: Inductive

For this item, the test taker must utilize clinical judgment to determine a best course of action for developing the arches of the hand and increasing hand strength. This requires inductive reasoning skill, where clinical judgment is paramount to arriving at a correct conclusion. For this situation, the therapist should have the child perform chair push-ups before tabletop activities. If answered incorrectly, review hand development, guidelines for increasing strength, and principles of activity analysis. The integration of this knowledge is required to determine the therapeutic activity which would be most effective to improve the child's hand strength and develop the arches of the hand.

C134 C6

An individual with peripheral neuropathies due to diabetes is scheduled for a bilateral lower extremity (transfemoral) amputation. During an OT session to develop upper extremity strength to assist with postamputation transfers, the patient happily chats about plans to go shopping for new clothing to wear to a grandchild's wedding. After the session, which defense mechanism should the occupational therapist document that the person seems to be exhibiting?

Answer Choices:

A. Suppression.
B. Regression.
C. Displacement.
D. Projection.

Correct Answer: A.

Rationale:

Suppression is a defense mechanism that allows an individual to divert uncomfortable feelings (in this case, fear of an undesirable event) into socially acceptable feelings (in this case, anticipation of a desirable event) in order to avoid thinking about a disturbing issue. Regression is the returning to an earlier stage of development to avoid tension or conflict (e.g., an individual becomes needy or child-like during a period of stress). Displacement is the redirection of an emotion or reaction from one object to a similar but less threatening one (e.g., a child who is angry with his/her parents yells at a younger sibling). Projection is the attribution of unacknowledged characteristics or thoughts to others (e.g., someone who feels guilty interprets the statements of others as blaming him/her).

Type of Reasoning: Analytical

This question provides symptoms and the test taker must determine the likely cause for them. This is an analytical reasoning skill, as questions of this nature often ask one to analyze a group of symptoms in order to determine a diagnosis. In this situation the symptoms indicate the defense mechanism of suppression, which should be reviewed if answered incorrectly.

C135 C7

An occupational therapist works with an individual recovering from a traumatic brain injury in a rehabilitation hospital. The therapist uses a transfer of training approach to help the patient develop and carry out a daily schedule of activities upon the patient's return home. What is the most effective activity for the therapist to use during an intervention session with this client?

Answer Choices:

A. Preparation of a simple meal.
B. Organization of a list of daily activities.
C. Composition of a shopping list.
D. Completion of an interest checklist.

Correct Answer: B.

Rationale:

A transfer of training approach is a remedial/restorative approach that focuses on restoration of components to increase skill. It is deficit specific and utilizes tabletop and computer activities as treatment modalities. According to this approach, the activity of organizing a list of daily activities will help with the ability to formulate a schedule in one's home environment. Preparing a meal, composing a shopping list and completing an interest checklist are each discrete activities that would develop skills related to the performance of these activities, but they do not address the skills needed to schedule the multiple activities of a typical day.

Type of Reasoning: Inductive

This question requires the test taker to determine the most effective activity for a client with traumatic brain injury using a transfer of training approach. This is an inductive reasoning skill, as questions of this nature often ask one to utilize clinical judgment to determine therapeutic courses of action. For this case, the therapist should emphasize organization of a list of daily activities in treatment. Review transfer of training approach if answered incorrectly.

C136 C6

A person experiencing an acute manic episode is completing the admission process to an inpatient psychiatric unit. The intake coordinator has to unexpectedly complete an emergency admission. The admissions coordinator asks the occupational therapist to spend some one-to-one time with this individual until the coordinator can return to complete the intake process. Which is the best way for the occupational therapist to use this time with the client?

Answer Choices:

A. Discuss the precipitants to the hospitalization with the person.
B. Ask the person to make positive statements about him/herself.
C. Have the person do a craft activity requiring attention to detail.
D. Take a walk around the unit to orient the person.

Correct Answer: D.

Rationale:

Walking with the person can allow for some energy release which is important for a person with mania. It is a non-threatening activity that can facilitate interaction. Providing the person with an orientation may decrease the stress of admission and foster rapport. Upon admission, the person may be uncomfortable discussing precipitants to hospitalization and may have difficulty making positive statements about him/herself. Activities requiring concentration and attention can also be difficult with acute mania.

Type of Reasoning: Evaluative

This question requires one to determine the best response in an unexpected situation. This requires evaluative reasoning skill, where one must reach conclusions using value judgments. In this situation, the therapist should take a walk with the person around the unit to orient the person.

C137 C4

An adult with right hemisphere damage from a CVA is referred to occupational therapy. Which deficits will the patient most likely demonstrate upon evaluation?

Answer Choices:

A. Negative, self-deprecating comments and depression.
B. Slow responses and cautious behavior.
C. Hesitancy and fearfulness.
D. Poor judgment and difficulties with safety issues.

Correct Answer: D.

Rationale:

A patient with a right CVA will demonstrate impulsive behaviors that demonstrate poor judgment and disregard for safety. Negative, self-deprecating comments and depression can be evident when a person incurs a disability but these behaviors are not necessarily indicative of a right CVA. Slow responses, hesitancy and fearfulness and cautious behavior are indicative of a left CVA. The person's behaviors can appear slow because of the hesitancy caused by perceptual or motor planning problems.

Type of Reasoning: Inferential

This question requires one to draw conclusions based on the information presented, which is an inferential reasoning skill. Questions that ask about what to expect from a diagnosis are essentially asking one to infer information, even though one cannot be 100% sure. For this situation, the most likely symptom of this patient would be poor judgment and decreased safety. If answered incorrectly, review the typical presentations of right and left CVA.

C138 C9

A school-based occupational therapist is providing contracted per diem coverage for an occupational therapist on a disability leave. Upon reviewing the caseload, the therapist notes that 10 students have had evaluations completed during the past month. Five of these students' individualized education plans (IEPs) have also been completed by the team and approved by their families. Which is the best initial action for the therapist to take as a contract practitioner?

Answer Choices:

A. Consult with the team and family to complete the IEPs for the remaining children.
B. Conduct independent evaluations of each child.
C. Implement the IEPs that have been established and approved.
D. Report to the supervisor of the contract agency that the school has failed to comply with IEP guidelines.

Correct Answer: A.

Rationale:

The Individuals with Disabilities Act (IDEA) mandates that an IEP be written within 30 days of evaluation. This must be done as a team effort with the professionals providing their recommendations to the team and the child's family. Family consent is an essential part of the IEP process and is required by IDEA. There is nothing in the scenario to indicate a need for an additional evaluation or the reporting of the school. While it is important to implement IEPs, the first priority is to ensure that all students have an IEP within 30 days of evaluation. In addition, many aspects of the IEP can be implemented by teachers and other school personnel (e.g., resource room aides, behavioral specialists, speech-language pathologists).

Type of Reasoning: Inferential
One must infer or draw conclusions about a likely course of action, given the information presented. This is an inferential reasoning skill, where knowledge of IDEA guidelines is essential to choosing a correct solution. In this case, the therapist should consult with the team and family to complete the remaining IEPs. Review IDEA guidelines for completion of IEPs if answered incorrectly.

C139 C8

An individual with cyclothymic disorder has successfully completed a transitional employment program (TEP) and is competitively employed in a busy real estate office as an administrative assistant. The person reports feeling overwhelmed by the number of part-time real estate agents who drop off work late in the afternoon to be completed within 1–2 days. The individual contacts the TEP occupational therapist for suggestions on dealing with this work stress. Which action is most effective for the therapist to recommend the person take in response to this situation?

Answer Choices:
A. Make an appointment for a vocational skills reevaluation to determine an intervention plan to develop needed skills.
B. Make an appointment with the psychiatrist for a medication evaluation to manage anxiety.
C. Meet with the work site's direct supervisor at the end of each day to prioritize the next day's workload.
D. Organize the next day's workload at the end of each day according to the deadlines set by each agent.

Correct Answer: C.

Rationale:
Input from one's direct supervisor on the prioritization of the next day's work can be very helpful for someone who has multiple individuals giving daily work with expectations for quick completion of this work. Speaking to the supervisor will ensure that the total needs of the agency, not just the needs of individual agents, are met. Organizing the next day's work according to each agent's stated priority can result in multiple expectations for work being completed at the same time. This would be difficult to fulfill and would not decrease stress. Supervisory input for the prioritization of tasks can also help deal effectively with the potential interpersonal problems that can occur when all work is not completed for all of the agents. There is no indicated need in this scenario for a vocational reevaluation or a medication evaluation. The problem described is typical of busy offices with multiple part-time workers and can be resolved through workplace supervisory procedures.

Type of Reasoning: Inductive
One must utilize clinical knowledge and judgment to determine the most appropriate recommendation for this individual. This requires inductive reasoning skill. In this case, the OT should recommend that the individual speak to the supervisor at the end of each work day to prioritize the next day's workload. If answered incorrectly, review TEP guidelines and reasonable accommodation recommendations.

C140 C4

A middle school-aged child with a sensory processing disorder participates in weekly occupational therapy sessions in a pediatric private practice. Initial evaluation had identified the presence of symptoms consistent with a sensory-based motor disorder. The child has shown no improvement in coordination, equilibrium and motor planning for the past 2 months. The parent reports that the child continues to exhibit difficulties with play, learning and social participation. Which action is best for the therapist to take in response to these observations and parental report?

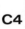

Answer Choices:

A. Provide the parent with a home program and discharge the child from therapy.
B. Refer the child to a pediatric social worker to explore potential resistance to therapy.
C. Increase the frequency of therapy to two sessions per week to increase the child's engagement.
D. Reevaluate the child to determine deficit areas that are contributing to dysfunction.

Correct Answer: D.

Rationale:

The child is not making gains in occupational therapy with the current approach to address coordination, equilibrium and motor planning and the parent is reporting ongoing dysfunction. Therefore, the occupational therapist should reevaluate the child to obtain information that can help determine an intervention plan that would more effectively meet the child's needs. Intervention focused on other performance skills and client factors may be effective and should be implemented before discharging the child. The therapist should not continue to treat the child in areas that show no progress. The child has not made gains. Increasing the frequency of occupational therapy without a revised intervention plan will not facilitate functional improvements. The identified deficits are within the domain of practice of an occupational therapist, so a referral to a social worker is not necessary. There is no information provided in the scenario to indicate that the child is resistant to therapy.

Type of Reasoning: Inferential

One must infer or draw conclusions about a best course of action, given the information provided. In this situation, reevaluation of the child is ideal in order to determine a new focus of OT intervention as the current plan is not resulting in functional gains. If answered incorrectly, review treatment planning guidelines for children with sensory processing disorders.

C141 C7

An individual is newly admitted to an acute inpatient psychiatric hospital. The occupational therapist observes that the patient is able to follow the unit routines and construct a simple craft project by following written directions with diagrams. However, the patient is not able to complete the project if the directions are missing. According to Allen's Cognitive Disability frame of reference, which level is most accurate for the therapist to document as descriptive of the individual's functional level?

Answer Choices:

A. Level two.
B. Level four.
C. Level three.
D. Level five.

Correct Answer: B.

Rationale:

Individuals at Level 4 require visual cues to complete tasks. Individuals functioning at Level 2 and Level 3, according to Allen's cognitive disabilities model, cannot follow written directions to complete a task. Individuals functioning at Level 5 can complete a simple craft project without written directions.

Type of Reasoning: Deductive

One must recall the Allen Cognitive Levels and appropriate descriptions under each level. This is factual knowledge, which is a deductive reasoning skill. For this situation, the description of patient functioning is most representative of Level 4. If answered incorrectly, review Allen Cognitive Levels.

C142 C5

A resident in a long-term care facility is able to tolerate pureed fruit, finely ground meats and mashed potatoes. The resident chokes on cereals, most raw fruits and rice. During the videofluoroscopy procedure, which foods are best for the occupational therapist to sequentially give to the client?

Answer Choices:
A. Diced and minced foods, followed by cereals and then thin liquids.
B. Diced and minced foods, followed by cereals and then thickened liquids.
C. Cereals, followed by thickened liquids and then thin liquids.
D. Pureed and strained foods followed by diced foods and then cereals.

Correct Answer: B.

Rationale:
The therapist carries out the videofluoroscopy procedure by offering foods that do not present problems at the lowest levels and progresses as possible. In this scenario, the patient shows the ability to manage Stage II foods which are mashed and pureed, so the therapist begins with foods in Stage III, such as ground, diced and minced foods and then progresses to liquids. The first step in introducing liquids is thickened liquids. All types of foods are not tested. The best place to start is with Stage III foods, not with liquids. The patient can already tolerate Stage II foods, so they would not be tested.

Type of Reasoning: Inductive
This question requires one to determine which foods to present according to the patient's current abilities and limitations. This necessitates inductive reasoning skill, where clinical judgment is paramount to arriving at a correct conclusion. In this case, starting at a level that does not present problems and then progressing from this point is ideal.

C143 C1

An individual with bilateral lower extremity amputations and cataracts is newly admitted to a skilled nursing facility. The individual retains some residual vision. During the initial evaluation, which is the most effective placement for the occupational therapist to use when presenting materials to the person?

Answer Choices:
A. To the side of the person, with no direct lighting.
B. Directly in front of the person, at eye level.
C. Directly in front of the person, at tabletop level.
D. To the side of the person, with a strong light shining.

Correct Answer: A.

Rationale:
An individual with cataracts loses central vision first; therefore, presenting evaluation materials directly in front of the person will be ineffective. Peripheral vision gradually decreases with cataracts, so presenting materials to the side will enable the person to use his/her residual vision. Individuals with cataracts have increased difficulty with glare, so indirect lighting is indicated.

Type of Reasoning: Inferential
One must have knowledge of cataracts and visual limitations in order to choose the best manner of presenting evaluation materials. This is an inferential reasoning skill where knowledge of the visual disorder and presenting deficits is pivotal to choosing the correct solution. For this situation, the therapist should present materials to the side of the person, with no direct lighting. If answered incorrectly, review the clinical presentation of cataracts and engagement in functional activities.

C144 C2

An OTA provides community mobility training for a resident in a group home for individuals with developmental disabilities. A resident successfully completes the intervention activity the OTA had designed with the occupational therapy supervisor. The OTA needs to plan the next day's intervention session but the supervising occupational therapist is on a 2-week vacation. Which is the best action for the OTA to take in response to this situation?

Answer Choices:

A. Grade the activity that the client successfully completed to its next level of difficulty.
B. Use the same activity that the resident successfully completed during the next session.
C. Delay the next treatment session until the supervisor returns from vacation and is able to provide guidance.
D. Ask the director of the residential program to assign another supervisor for the duration of the current supervisor's vacation.

Correct Answer: A.

Rationale:

OTAs are trained in activity gradation and the implementation of OT intervention; therefore, the OTA can independently plan the next treatment activity. Using the same activity would not enable the resident to progress toward goal attainment. There is no need to delay the treatment session or obtain another supervisor. In this scenario, the OTA had designed the intervention activity with the occupational therapy supervisor. This intervention planning would have involved collaboration between the two professionals and provided the OTA with a solid basis for designing the next level of activity needed to meet the established goals.

Type of Reasoning: Evaluative

One must weigh the possible courses of action and then make a value judgment about the best course to take. This requires evaluative reasoning skill, which often utilizes guiding principles of action in order to arrive at a correct conclusion. For this case, because the supervising therapist is on vacation, the OTA should grade the activity that the client completed to its next level of difficulty. Assistants are able to grade activities and implement interventions which have been developed in collaboration with the occupational therapist. Review supervisory guidelines for OTAs if answered incorrectly.

C145 C8

An individual is recovering from lumbar surgery. The patient must remain flat in bed during the initial recovery stages. The patient expresses an interest in reading from a personal collection of classic comics. Which adaptation is best for the occupational therapist to recommend the client use for reading?

Answer Choices:

A. Prism glasses.
B. A page magnifier.
C. Audiotapes of books of interest.
D. Large-print books of interest.

Correct Answer: A.

Rationale:

Prism glasses are eyeglasses that bend light by 90°. This angle enables a person who is lying on his/her back to read anything that is resting on his/her lap. This recommendation enables the individual to read his/her collection of classic comics independently, as the client wanted. The use of audiotaped books does not meet the client's expressed interest in reading comics. Large-print books and a page magnifier do not address the issue that the client must remain flat on his/her back.

Type of Reasoning: Inductive
Clinical knowledge and judgment are the most important skills needed for answering this question, which requires inductive reasoning skill. Knowledge of the diagnosis and most appropriate equipment to address the patient's limitations are essential to arriving at a correct conclusion. In this case, prism glasses is the most appropriate recommendation as it is the only device that addresses the individual's needs while maintaining the lumbar restrictions. If answered incorrectly, review information on use of prism glasses.

Multiple Choice Scenario Item C.III.

Questions C146 to C149 are based on the following information.

An individual who is scheduled for a right hip total arthroplasty (THA) is referred to occupational therapy. A posterolateral surgical approach will be used. The client has expressive aphasia resulting from a cerebral vascular accident incurred 4 years ago. Medicare is the client's only health care benefit. The client states that private payment for any health care services or equipment is not possible at this time.

C146 **C8**

What should the occupational therapist focus on during preoperative occupational therapy interventions?

Answer Choices:
A. The performance of upper and lower extremity strengthening exercises.
B. The performance of IADL tasks in a sitting rather than standing position.
C. The practice of non–weight-bearing crutch walking
D. The use of modified techniques to perform transfers and BADL.

Correct Answer: D.

Rationale:
Intervention should cover the use of modified techniques to ensure that the person maintains correct positioning during transfers and during BADL (e.g., bathing, dressing and toileting). These essential ADL will be done daily during the postoperative rehabilitation phase. The modified techniques for the performance of ADL typically include the use of equipment (e.g., long-handled sponge/shoehorn, sock aide, three-in one-commode). During the planning of these interventions, the therapist will need to consider the reality that the client's only health care benefit is Medicare and that the client reports no financial resources for the purchase of equipment. There is nothing in the question scenario to indicate that the person has decreased upper extremity strength and this answer choice does not apply to any functional outcome. Performing tasks in sitting is more stressful on the hip joint than doing them in standing and are contraindicated. Restrictions for weightbearing will depend on several factors (e.g., the integrity of the bone) that may not be determined until after the person's surgery. Interventions for postsurgery gait training are most appropriately conducted by the physical therapist.

Type of Reasoning: Inferential
One must draw conclusions about the likely preoperative training for a patient requiring a total hip replacement. Most important in this situation is to prepare the patient for postoperative rehabilitation. Therefore training in the use of equipment and skills needed for transfers and BADL is most important preoperatively. If answered incorrectly, review total hip replacement precautions.

C147 C8

Following surgery, which is the most appropriate bed-positioning intervention for the occupational therapist to recommend?

Answer Choices:

A. Side-lying with the lower extremities adducted.
B. Use of an abductor pillow between the lower extremities.
C. Use of a hospital bed to elevate the lower extremities to 90°.
D. Change of position from supine to prone every 2 hours.

Correct Answer: B.

Rationale:

An abductor pillow will prevent adduction of the operated hip, which is an important postsurgery precaution. Using a hospital bed to elevate the lower extremities to flex the hips to 90° is contraindicated because a major hip precaution is not to flex beyond 90°. Changing position from supine to prone requires rolling, which can result in internal rotation of the hip. External rotation should be avoided if an anterolateral approach is used. This is contraindicated for it can result in dislocation.

Type of Reasoning: Deductive

One must recall the postsurgery guidelines for total hip replacement. This is factual knowledge, which is a deductive reasoning skill. In this situation, the only appropriate guideline listed is to use an abductor pillow between the legs. If answered incorrectly, review posterolateral surgical approach total hip precautions, especially bed positioning.

C148 C8

The client is being discharged home. Which equipment should the occupational therapist recommend to ensure safety and independence in toileting?

Answer Choices:

A. A raised toilet seat.
B. Grab bars.
C. A three-in-one commode.
D. Non-skid mats.

Correct Answer: C.

Rationale:

The client will need to observe hip precautions for several weeks. These precautions include not flexing the hip beyond 90°. A three-in-one commode will provide the additional height needed by the individual to maintain hip precautions. It is also the only item identified that is reimbursable by Medicare. Medicare does not cover any equipment that can be useful to individuals without a disability. Self-help items such as grab bars, raised toilet seats and non-skid mats are not considered medically necessary and are not reimbursable since other people can use them.

Type of Reasoning: Inductive

One must utilize clinical knowledge and judgment to determine the equipment that will be reimbursed by Medicare and provide safety and independence. In this case, a three-in-one commode is the only equipment reimbursed by Medicare and provides needed safety and independence. If answered incorrectly, review Medicare guidelines for reimbursement of durable medical equipment.

C149 C7

How can the occupational therapist most reliably determine that hip precautions will be effectively implemented postdischarge?

Answer Choices:

A. Have the patient demonstrate the techniques that have been taught.
B. Ask the family to observe the patient once home.
C. Ask the patient to point to pictures of the hip precautions being used during activities.
D. Have the patient demonstrate positions that should be avoided.

Correct Answer: A.

Rationale:

Expressive aphasia interferes with the person's ability to verbally express him/herself. Therefore, the most effective method for assessing the individual's understanding of teaching is via demonstration. The therapist must observe the person performing the precautions during activities to ensure that the person has generalized the precautions to actually implement them during functional activities. Asking the family to observe the client may be helpful to assess carryover; however, this source can be unreliable. Family members are not trained in assessment or activity analysis and they may not accurately report details of activity performance. Pointing to pictures provides limited information. The person may recognize precautions but not use them during the performance of an activity. Therefore, the therapist will not know for sure that the individual can perform the activity appropriately. Having the individual demonstrate positions that should be avoided is contraindicated and could cause harm.

Type of Reasoning: Inductive

One must utilize clinical knowledge and judgment to determine the educational approach that best determines effectiveness and competence. This requires inductive reasoning skill. In this case, having the client demonstrate the skills that have been taught is most reliable. If answered incorrectly, review educational training guidelines for persons with CVA and aphasia.

C150 C4

A patient who incurred a right CVA asks for a bottle of water to drink. The occupational therapist gives the patient a bottle of water but the patient is unable to open it. The therapist provides instruction on opening the bottle but the patient remains unable to complete the task. After the intervention session, the therapist observes the patient independently open the bottle and drink from it. Which deficit is most relevant for the occupational therapist to further evaluate?

Answer Choices:

A. Anosognosia.
B. Ideomotor apraxia.
C. Unilateral neglect.
D. Asomatognosia.

Correct Answer: B.

Rationale:

With ideomotor apraxia, a patient cannot perform a task upon direction but can do the task when on his/her own. Anosognosia is a more severe form of neglect that is demonstrated by a lack of awareness and denial of the severity of one's paralysis. Unilateral neglect is demonstrated by a failure to respond to or report unilateral stimulus presented to the body side contralateral to the lesion. Asomatognosia is a body scheme disorder that results in diminished awareness of body structure and a failure to recognize body parts as one's own.

Type of Reasoning: Analytical
One must have a firm understanding of the difference between the cognitive-perceptual deficits of apraxia, neglect and agnosia in order to arrive at the correct conclusion. Doing so requires one to assess the differences between these deficits and determine the likely reason for this deficit, which is an analytical reasoning skill. Review the definitions of these terms and other perceptual deficits associated with CVA if answered incorrectly.

C151 C4

A preschool-aged child is hypersensitive to touch. The therapist decides to use the SI frame of reference to help the child develop the ability to adequately modulate sensory stimuli. Which technique is best for the therapist to use initially with this child?

Answer Choices:
A. Fast brushing to the child's arms in a direction opposite of hair growth.
B. Lightly moving touch to the child's abdomen and the extremities.
C. Firm pressure where the child can see the source of the stimuli.
D. Quick icing where the child cannot see the source of the stimuli.

Correct Answer: C.

Rationale:
Firm pressure and deep touch where the child can see the source of the stimuli is an effective approach for a child who is hypersensitive to touch. This technique tends to be more tolerable than light touch stimuli which tend to be aversive, especially when applied to the face, abdomen and palmar surfaces of the extremities and/or in a direction opposite of hair growth. Tactile stimuli should be applied in the direction of hair growth as this is less aversive to persons who are hypersensitive to touch. Quick icing is a technique that was used in the Rood approach in an effort to stimulate the muscles. It is an approach with no established evidence and is not used in a SI frame of reference

Type of Reasoning: Inferential
One must infer or draw conclusions about a best course of action, given the patient's diagnosis and presenting symptoms. For this child, firm pressure is the best initial technique as it is the most tolerated proprioceptive technique by a child with hypersensitivity to touch. Review proprioceptive techniques for hypersensitivity if answered incorrectly.

C152 C3

An occupational therapist provides a wellness and prevention education series to a community senior center. The topic of the week is joint protection. Which joint protection principle should the therapist include in the presentation?

Answer Choices:
A. Stand diagonally to the side of containers to be opened or closed to maximize torque.
B. Work through the pain experienced during activities by performing stretching exercises.
C. Preserve joint ROM and muscle strength by using the minimal effort required to perform an activity.
D. Start an activity only if it can be immediately stopped when it requires capacities beyond existing capabilities.

Correct Answer: D.

Rationale:
Starting an activity only if it can be immediately stopped when it requires capacities beyond existing capabilities is an important joint protection principle. The other choices are counter to joint protection principles. These principles include that one should stand directly in front of items to be opened or closed; pain should be a warning sign indicating that an activity should be modified or stopped; ROM and muscle strength can be maintained by using maximal ROM and maximal strength during activities.

Type of Reasoning: Deductive
One must recall joint protection principles in order to arrive at a correct conclusion. This requires deductive reasoning skill, where factual knowledge is key to choosing the correct solution. For this scenario, the only principle that is in keeping with proper joint protection is to start an activity only if it can be immediately stopped when it requires capacities beyond existing capabilities. Review joint protection principles if answered incorrectly.

C153 C8

A client with Charcot-Marie-Tooth disease participates in a reevaluation session at a wheelchair clinic. The client reports difficulty keeping both feet on the wheelchair's footrests. Which is the most effective action for the occupational therapist to take to address the client's stated concerns?

Answer Choices:
A. Implement an exercise routine to strengthen lower extremities.
B. Elevate the footrests.
C. Provide heel loops on the footrests.
D. Provide ankle straps on the footrests.

Correct Answer: D.

Rationale:
Ankle straps are used to prevent feet from slipping off the footrests. Charcot-Marie-Tooth disease is a neuropathic muscular atrophy characterized by progressive weakness of the distal muscles of the arms and feet. It does not respond to strengthening exercises. Elevating footrests are indicated for edema control, lower extremity (LE) extension contractures and long leg casts. They do not prevent the lower extremity from slipping off the rest. In fact, the increased pull of gravity would likely exacerbate the problem. In addition, elevated footrests greatly extend the length of a wheelchair, making it very cumbersome to maneuver in the environment. Heel loops on footrests prevent the feet only from slipping posteriorly, which would not be an adequate solution in this case.

Type of Reasoning: Inductive
One must utilize clinical knowledge and judgment to determine the most appropriate recommendation for this patient. In this case, ankle straps on the footrests is most appropriate to prevent feet from slipping off the footrests. If answered incorrectly, review footrest equipment for wheelchairs, especially ankle straps.

C154 C2

An occupational therapist consults at a day treatment program for individuals with dementia. Which groups are best for the therapist to recommend the program include?

Answer Choices:
A. Reality orientation groups.
B. Cognitive-behavioral groups.
C. Parallel groups.
D. Instrumental groups.

Correct Answer: D.

Rationale:
According to Mosey's taxonomy of groups, instrumental groups help individuals function at their highest possible level for as long as possible. They provide supportive structured environments and appropriate activities that prevent regression, maintain function and meet mental health needs. Activities can include reminiscence, arts and crafts, music, exercise, dance and any other activity that is interesting and enjoyable to the members. Reality orientation groups are contraindicated for persons with dementia who cannot remember basic facts like dates, people or places. Groups that focus on the use of memory can be very frustrating and counter-therapeutic for persons with dementia. Cognitive-behavioral groups require intact cognition and are at too high a level for persons with dementia. Parallel groups can be indicated for individuals with dementia but a schedule should not be comprised primarily of parallel groups for they are limiting in their potential for social interactions.

Type of Reasoning: Inferential
One must link the symptoms of the provided diagnosis to the type of groups presented in order to determine which group is most appropriate for individuals with dementia. This requires inferential reasoning, where one must draw conclusions about the features and benefits of each of the groups. In this case an instrumental group is most appropriate. Review Mosey's taxonomy of groups, especially instrumental groups if answered incorrectly.

C155 C3

An occupational therapist working in a hand clinic conducts an evaluation. During the evaluation, the therapist uses the Froment's sign. When documenting the outcome of this evaluation procedure, which is most accurate for the therapist to state was assessed?

Answer Choices:
A. Sensation of median nerve.
B. Motor function of the median nerve.
C. Sensation of the ulnar nerve.
D. Motor function of the ulnar nerve.

Correct Answer: D.

Rationale:
The Froment's sign assesses the motor function of the adductor pollicis which is innervated by the ulnar nerve. It involves an attempt to pinch an object firmly with the thumb. With an ulnar nerve injury, this attempt results in flexion of the distal joint of the thumb.

Type of Reasoning: Deductive
This question requires recall of guidelines and principles, which is factual knowledge. Deductive reasoning skills are utilized whenever one must recall facts to solve clinical problems. In this situation, evaluation using the Froment's sign is conducted to assess the motor function of the ulnar nerve. Review ulnar nerve palsy, especially Froment's sign if answered incorrectly.

C156 C8

An occupational therapist works with a child who has developmental delay and unintelligible speech to develop the child's functional communication skills using a communication board. The child has attained 100% accuracy in pointing to "yes" and "no" on the communication board in response to questions. The occupational therapist determines that the child should be provided with the opportunity to expand communication skills. Which action should the therapist take to help attain this goal?

Answer Choices:

A. Add two more choices such as "play" and "snack" to the communication board.
B. Reverse the positions of "yes" and "no" on the communication board to assure competence.
C. Add the options of "play," "thirsty," "hungry" and "TV" to the communication board.
D. Evaluate the child's ability to use a joystick to access a computer.

Correct Answer: A.

Rationale:

The best choice for a child with developmental delay is to maintain the consistency of the original selections and add one or two new options at a time. The best choices are to pick concrete items that the child prefers and enjoys and would therefore be interested in communicating. Reversing the position of the items will test the child's memory and ability to generalize, but would not improve his/her communication skills. With a developmental delay, it is important to be consistent to train and retain desired behaviors. The board should include the original options, not include only new options. Four would be too many new options to add at this time. Evaluating the child's ability to use a joystick does not address his/her communication skills. Using a joystick requires the ability to understand directionality, access four directions and understand cause and effect.

Type of Reasoning: Inductive

One must determine the next step in communication after determining competency in pointing to "yes" and "no." This requires inductive reasoning, where the test taker must utilize clinical judgment to determine the next course of action. For this scenario, adding two more choices to the board is the best next step. If answered incorrectly, review the characteristics of children with developmental delays and the use of augmentative communication devices for persons with communication difficulties. The integration of this knowledge is required for the determination of a correct answer.

C157 C9

An occupational therapist is working in a skilled nursing facility. The therapist is documenting current patient progress for the past 14 days and realizes that a required 7-day progress report to the client's insurance carrier had not been documented. Which should the therapist do in response to this omission?

Answer Choices:

A. Document the patient's status as of 14 days and backdate the note 1 week.
B. Write a note describing the patient's progress after 7 days of treatment and sign with the current date.
C. Call the insurance company to explain the documentation was lost due to a computer failure.
D. Describe the patient's progress after 7 days of treatment and backdate the note 1 week.

Correct Answer: B.

Rationale:

It is important to accurately document therapy progress in a timely manner. It is possible for a therapist to inadvertently miss a documentation deadline. If this occurs, the therapist should follow the AOTA Code of Ethics for veracity and document the patient's progress for the first 7 days and date it with the current date. Notes should never be backdated.

Type of Reasoning: Evaluative
This question requires one to determine a best course of action in an ethical situation. This requires evaluative reasoning skill, where one must evaluate the merits of the potential courses of action and choose the one course of action that best provides resolution, while still adhering to the Code of Ethics. For this situation, the therapist should write a note that describes the patient's progress after 7 days of treatment, dating the note with the current date. If answered incorrectly, review the AOTA Code of Ethics, especially veracity.

C158 C4

An occupational therapist working in a school system conducts a series of educational workshops for parents of children with attention deficit disorders and sensory processing disorders. The series focuses on principles of sensory integration (SI). Which of the following is most beneficial for the therapist to recommend the parents provide in the home environment?

Answer Choices:
A. A wide range of sensory stimuli including auditory, visual and tactile to increase awareness and responsivity.
B. Minimal auditory, visual and tactile sensory stimuli to decrease distractibility and responsivity.
C. A balance between structure and freedom so the child can direct his/her own actions.
D. Clear directions and structured limits to organize behavior and promote adaptive responses.

Correct Answer: C.

Rationale:
A key principle of SI theory is to structure the environment to match the child's capabilities. This 'just right' environment enables the child to direct his/her own activity participation which can then facilitate skill development. Sensory processing disorders may present along a continuum of under-responsivity (hyposensitivity) to over-responsivity (hypersensitivity) of multisensory processing and sensory seeking. Environments and activities must be tailored to the specific child. The design of an environment to increase awareness or to decrease distractibility is more consistent with a compensatory remediation approach. Providing structure and limits is more consistent with a behavioral approach.

Type of Reasoning: Inferential
One must have knowledge of attention deficit disorder and SI guidelines in order to arrive at a correct conclusion. This is an inferential reasoning skill where knowledge of clinical guidelines and judgment based on facts are utilized to reach conclusions. If answered incorrectly, review SI treatment guidelines for children with attention deficit and sensory processing disorders.

C159 C8

An individual with left hemiplegia who is right-hand dominant receives training to resume independent driving. Which adaptation is best for the occupational therapist to recommend the client use?

Answer Choices:
A. 'Palming' the steering wheel.
B. Hand controls for brake and gas pedals.
C. A spinner knob on the steering wheel.
D. Left-sided accelerator pedal.

Correct Answer: C.

Rationale:
A person who is right-hand dominant with left hemiplegia can drive one-handed using a spinner knob on the steering wheel. 'Palming' the steering wheel is not recommended for one-handed drivers, for it is easier to lose control of the vehicle. It is difficult to maintain smooth handling and turns are made much more slowly, which can be dangerous in traffic situations. There is no functional need to change a car's existing pedal arrangement.

Type of Reasoning: Inductive
Clinical knowledge and judgment are the most important skills needed for answering this question, which requires inductive reasoning skill. Knowledge of the functional limitations and most appropriate equipment for driving is essential to choosing the best solution. In this case, a spinner knob on the steering wheel is the best recommendation. Review vehicle adaptations for one-handed drivers.

C160 C3

A child with moderate arthrogryposis complains of profuse sweating when wearing bilateral night resting splints. Which of the following should the occupational therapist suggest to the child?

Answer Choices:
A. Wear only one splint each night, rotating from left to right.
B. Wear volar cock-up splints instead.
C. Wear a cotton stockinet liner under the splints.
D. Wear a splint with several 1-centimeter perforations in the splinting material.

Correct Answer: C.

Rationale:
A stockinet liner helps to absorb sweat. It is also helpful to wash and thoroughly dry the hands prior to donning splints. Wearing only one splint each night does not address sweating and cuts wearing time in half, making splints less effective. Volar cock-up splints do not address the position of the MPs and IPs and might result in increased MP and IP flexion contractures. Perforations might decrease the strength and integrity of the splinting material.

Type of Reasoning: Inferential
One must link the child's problem to the solutions presented in order to determine which solution would best address the child's complaint. This requires inferential reasoning, where one must determine which approach would most effectively remedy the problem. In this case using a stockinet liner under the splints would best address the sweating when wearing splints. If answered incorrectly, review splinting adaptations and addressing sweating while wearing splints.

C161 C9

A hospital-based occupational therapist is committed to promoting the profession to hospital staff and the general public. Which is the most effective action for the therapist to take to accomplish this goal?

Answer Choices:
A. Write an article about recent accomplishments of new OT staff members in the hospital's employee newsletter.
B. Include photos of patients participating in the new driver rehabilitation clinic in the hospital's annual report.
C. Display information sheets about major areas of OT practice on the hospital's cafeteria bulletin board.
D. Write a monthly column in a local newspaper about OT approaches for a diversity of clinical conditions.

Correct Answer: C.

Rationale:
A hospital cafeteria services both hospital staff and the general public so this would be the communication venue that would be readily accessible to both audiences. Displaying information sheets about major areas of OT practice on this bulletin board is an effective method for promoting OT. The other answer choices do include activities which can help promote OT but they do not target both hospital staff and the general public.

Type of Reasoning: Inferential
This question requires one to infer or draw a reasonable conclusion for a most effective course of action when promoting OT to staff and the public. Questions that ask about future benefits for a present course of action often require inferential reasoning skills. For this scenario, the occupational therapist should display information sheets about the major areas of practice on the hospital's cafeteria bulletin board to have the most benefit. If answered incorrectly, review guidelines for the promotion of OT.

C162 C3

An older adult with RA is provided with a functional hand splint to help prevent deformity. The occupational therapist also advises the individual about actions that can be taken to help prevent deformity. Which of the following is most important for the therapist to advise the individual to do?

Answer Choices:
A. Avoid fatigue.
B. Maintain active range of motion.
C. Increase muscle strength.
D. Do passive range of motion exercises.

Correct Answer: B.

Rationale:
The maintenance of active range of motion is a primary anti-deformity technique. Passive range of motion and resistive exercise to increase strength are contraindicated for individuals with RA. Avoiding fatigue is helpful from an energy conservation perspective but it does not prevent joint deformity.

Type of Reasoning: Inferential
One must link the individual's diagnosis to the recommendations presented in order to determine which recommendation is best to prevent deformity. This requires inferential reasoning, where one must draw conclusions about the likely course of action for a diagnosis. In this case the most appropriate recommendation is to maintain active range of motion. Review deformity prevention activities for persons with RA if answered incorrectly.

C163 C3

A carpenter complains of tingling of the left thumb, index and middle finger; weakened grasp; and night pain secondary to carpal tunnel syndrome. The left thenar eminence appears smaller and more flattened compared to the right thenar eminence. The occupational therapist collaborates with the client to develop an intervention plan. Which recommendation is best to include in this plan?

Answer Choices:
A. Wrapping wrists with elastic bandages to provide support.
B. Modification of techniques used to hold a hammer.
C. Application of hot packs upon waking to decrease pain.
D. Performance of wrist flexion and extension exercises with progressively increasing repetitions.

Correct Answer: B.

Rationale:
The symptoms provided are indicative of carpal tunnel syndrome (CTS). CTS includes sensory and motor deficits associated with median nerve compression, which can lead to permanent loss of motor and sensory functions. An important aspect in the treatment of CTS is modification of repetitive motions, especially those involved in everyday activities such as work. Elastic wraps are not supportive enough. Soft or semi-rigid splints are helpful to allow minimal wrist movement while providing sufficient stability for day use. Sometimes positional night splints may be helpful. The administration of physical agent modalities (PAMS) such as hot packs should be done under the supervision of an OT or physical therapist (PT) practitioner. In occupational therapy, PAMS are used to prepare the person for functional performance of meaningful occupations. Repetitive motions should be limited as they can exacerbate symptoms.

Type of Reasoning: Analytical
One must determine the best recommendation for a carpenter with carpal tunnel syndrome, based on an understanding of the client's occupation and diagnosis. This requires inductive reasoning skill. For this situation, the best recommendation for the intervention plan is to provide modification of techniques used to hold a hammer. Review activity adaptations for carpal tunnel syndrome if answered incorrectly.

C164 C5

A client with chronic schizophrenia attends a transitional employment program. The individual has a secondary diagnosis of Class I heart disease. The occupational therapist meets with the client and the client's work supervisor to discuss the work activities the client can safely complete. Which of the following most accurately describes the client's capacity for work?

Answer Choices:
A. Work with minimum limitations.
B. Work with no limitations.
C. Work with reasonable accommodation of frequent rest breaks.
D. Work with reasonable accommodation of no heavy lifting.

Correct Answer: B.

Rationale:
Class I heart disease requires no limitations on activities; therefore, no reasonable accommodations are needed.

Type of Reasoning: Deductive
One must recall the guidelines for activity and potential restrictions with Class I heart disease. This is factual knowledge, which is a deductive reasoning skill. For this case, the patient with Class I heart disease would have no limitations. If answered incorrectly, review Class I heart disease activity guidelines.

C165 C8

A resident of a skilled nursing facility (SNF) is severely dehydrated after a viral illness. The resident is agitated and confused. The doctor has prescribed intravenous (IV) fluid infusions, but the nursing staff is concerned that the individual will pull out the infusion line. They request that the occupational therapist provide a restraint for this resident. Which is the best action for the therapist to take in response to this request?

Answer Choices:
A. Provide soft, fleeced mittens for the person's hands.
B. Report the request to the administrator as a violation of restraint-free standards.
C. Decline the referral and explain that restraints are no longer allowed to be used in SNFs.
D. Provide a lap board as this is the least restrictive restraint.

Correct Answer: A.

Rationale:

Wearing mittens will help prevent the individual from pulling out the IV lines. Providing ones that are soft and fleeced can provide tactile input that is not noxious. While federal guidelines (i.e., Omnibus Budget Reconciliation Act (OBRA)) emphasize restraint reduction and the provision of a restraint-free environment, they also recognize the potential need to provide restraints in certain circumstances. A restraint is permissible and acceptable if it is medically necessary and temporary for lifesaving treatment. These criteria apply in this case; therefore, the therapist should not decline the request. The wearing of mittens can sufficiently deter the person from pulling out the IV line. If the person begins to rub the IV line with his/her hands even while wearing the mittens, the therapist may need to recommend the use of bilateral soft elbow splints that fix the elbows at 20°–30° of flexion. The splints would prevent the person from accessing the IV line. However, this is a more restrictive solution so it would only be allowed after the failure of less restrictive methods. A lap tray would not limit the person's upper extremity mobility and thus would not be effective.

Type of Reasoning: Inductive

Clinical knowledge and judgment are the most important skills needed for answering this question, which requires inductive reasoning skill. Knowledge of the federal guidelines for use of restraints and most appropriate courses of action are essential to choosing the best solution. In this case, the therapist should provide soft, fleeced mittens for the person's hands. Review restraint utilization guidelines in SNFs if answered incorrectly.

C166 C3

An occupational therapist works with a person who incurred full thickness burns to both arms. Which intervention approach would be most effective for the therapist to provide to control hypertrophic scar formation?

Answer Choices:

A. Axillary splints applied in the airplane position.
B. Compression garments.
C. Wound grafting.
D. Elevation of the areas just above heart level.

Correct Answer: B.

Rationale:

Custom-made compression garments provide equal pressure over the entire area to prevent scarring. They must be worn 23 hours a day for approximately 12 months, or until the scar and wound maturation is complete. Airplane splints are used to prevent tightening of the axilla area which would result in the inability to horizontally abduct the arm. Wound grafting is used as biological dressing to provide wound covering and pain relief. Elevation of the areas just above heart level is a technique to reduce upper extremity edema.

Type of Reasoning: Inferential

One must determine the most effective approach to control hypertrophic scar formation in order to arrive at a correct conclusion. This requires one to determine what course of action will result in the best therapeutic outcome, which is an inferential reasoning skill. For this case, compression garments are most effective. Review intervention approaches for burns if answered incorrectly.

C167 C8

A teenager with Duchenne muscular dystrophy can no longer snap blue jeans or zip zippers. Which recommendation is best for the occupational therapist to make to this client?

Answer Choices:

A. Replace snaps and zippers with Velcro.
B. Replace snaps and zippers with large buttons.
C. Use a zipper pull to zip jeans and leave the snaps unsnapped.
D. Purchase and wear elastic waist pants.

Correct Answer: A.

Rationale:

Muscular dystrophy is a progressive condition. The therapist must be able to assist the person in adjusting to its progressive nature and provide options that maintain independence as long as possible. Velcro can be more easily managed than snaps or zippers. It can also be easily sewn into the jeans and pants that the adolescent already owns. Buttoning large buttons and using a zipper pull are not the best solutions due to the progressive loss of dexterity, coordination and strength that occurs with Duchenne muscular dystrophy. Elastic waist pants facilitate the process of donning pants but they do not address the identified difficulty of fastening jeans. This recommendation would not allow the adolescent to continue wearing jeans and pants in his current wardrobe. In addition, the style of elastic waist pants may not be acceptable to a teenaged boy. Recall that Duchenne muscular dystrophy is sex-linked and only affects males.

Type of Reasoning: Inductive

This question requires clinical judgment to determine which action would best address the teenager's needs and foster independence in dressing. Questions that require one to determine which course of action will result in the best outcome often require inductive reasoning skills. If answered incorrectly, review information on clothing adaptations and/or the sequelae of Duchenne muscular dystrophy. A correct answer requires one to analyze the activity adaptations provided to find the one activity that best matches the teen's capabilities.

C168 C5

An occupational therapist evaluates the feeding abilities of a patient who had a CVA 2 weeks ago. The therapist observes that the patient's dentures seem to slip when attempting to chew food. Which is the best action for the therapist to take in response to this situation?

Answer Choices:

A. Complete a referral to a dentist.
B. Continue the evaluation using only soft foods.
C. Develop an intervention plan to teach the individual compensation methods.
D. Request that nursing staff reapply denture adhesive prior to all feeding activities.

Correct Answer: A.

Rationale:

Dentures slip or move due to improper fit. Poorly fitting dentures must be evaluated and corrected by a dentist. It is inappropriate to continue the evaluation or plan intervention prior to ensuring that the individual's dentures are properly fitted. Reapplying denture adhesive does not address the underlying problem and can lead to additional problems if the individual chews with ill-fitting dentures (e.g., temporomandibular joint [TMJ] pain).

Type of Reasoning: Inferential

One must infer or draw conclusions about a likely course of action, given the information presented. This is an inferential reasoning skill, where knowledge of a therapeutic course of action is essential to choosing a correct solution. In this case, the therapist should refer the person to a dentist. Review referral guidelines for oral motor disorders in adults if answered incorrectly.

C169 C6

An occupational therapist conducts the preadmission screening for a supported housing program with several levels of care. The therapist receives a referral for an individual with chronic schizophrenia, disorganized type, with residual symptoms of circumstantiality, flat affect, and decreased attention. Which screening tool is best for the therapist to use with this client?

Answer Choices:
A. A semi-structured interview.
B. An ADL checklist.
C. A structured cooking task.
D. A weekly activity schedule.

Correct Answer: C.

Rationale:
A structured cooking task can be used to screen for a diversity of cognitive skills (e.g., ability to follow directions and problem solve, awareness of safety) and home management abilities (e.g., use of kitchen equipment, level of cleanliness) that can help determine the need for further evaluation to assist with selecting the level of supported housing that is most appropriate for the individual. A semi-structured interview can be helpful in determining the person's interests and goals but it is not an effective screening for functional skill level. In addition, the person exhibits circumstantiality, which may make it difficult for him/her to provide useful answers to the interview questions. An ADL checklist can assess knowledge of an activity/skill but it does not assess performance; therefore, its usefulness is limited. A weekly activity schedule can provide information about an individual's time use and ability to complete a structured task, but it is a paper and pen task that has limited applicability to screening for housing placement recommendations.

Type of Reasoning: Inferential
One must determine the most appropriate screening tool, given the diagnosis provided and current deficits. This requires inferential reasoning skill, where one must draw conclusions based on the information presented. In this situation, a structured cooking task is most appropriate. If answereds incorrectly, review screening guidelines for persons with schizophrenia.

C170 C8

A local pharmacy hires an occupational therapist to consult on the redesign of the pharmacy's customer service area. Which height should the therapist recommend the pharmacy counter be no higher than?

Answer Choices:
A. 29 inches.
B. 31 inches.
C. 33 inches.
D. 35 inches.

Correct Answer: B.

Rationale:
The recommended maximal height for countertops is 31 inches, according to the American National Standards Institute (ANSI) guidelines for buildings and facilities. The other choices do not meet these criteria.

Type of Reasoning: Deductive
This question requires recall of guidelines and principles, which is factual knowledge. Deductive reasoning skills are utilized whenever one must recall facts to solve novel problems. In this situation, following ANSI guidelines, the counter should be no higher than 31 inches. Review ANSI standards for buildings and facilities if answered incorrectly.

Index

Note: *f* denotes figure; *n*, note; and *t*, table.

B

C

D

E

Q

R